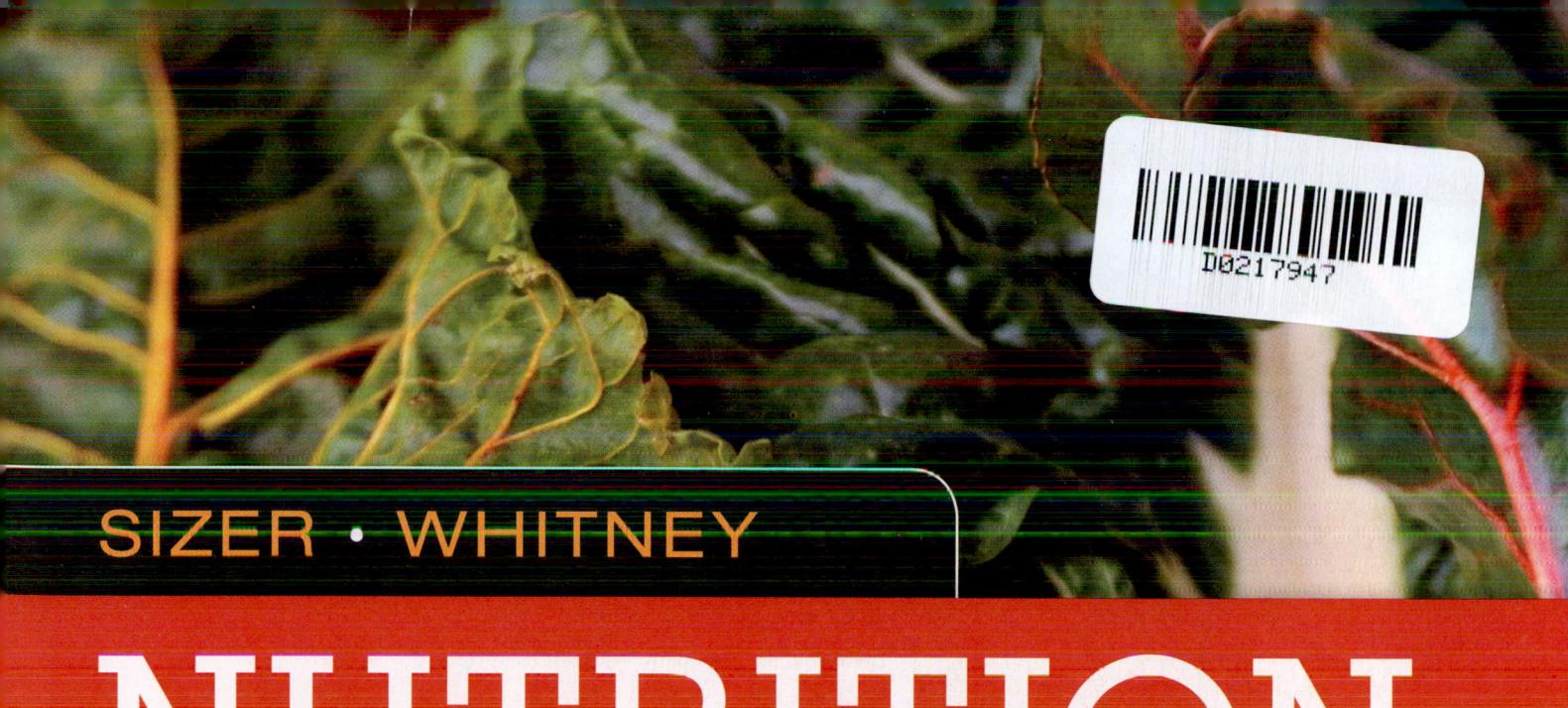

SIZER • WHITNEY

NUTRITION
Concepts and Controversies

FOURTEENTH EDITION

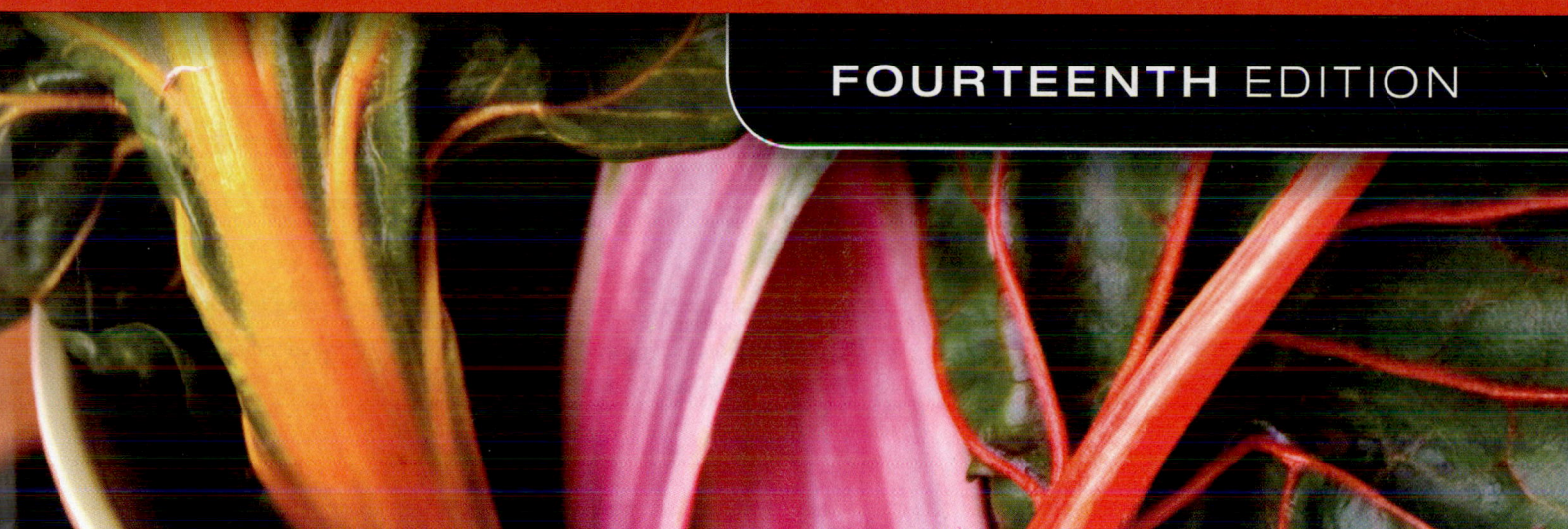

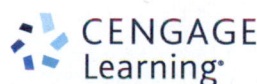

CENGAGE
Learning®

Australia • Brazil • Mexico • Singapore • United Kingdom • United States

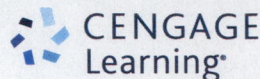

**Nutrition: Concepts & Controversies,
Fourteenth Edition**
Frances Sienkiewicz Sizer and Ellie Whitney

Product Manager: Krista Mastroianni

Content Developer: Miriam Myers

Product Assistant: Victor Luu

Marketing Manager: Tom Ziolkowski

Content Project Manager: Carol Samet

Art Director: Michael Cook

Manufacturing Planner: Karen Hunt

Production Service: Heidi Allgair,
    Cenveo® Publisher Services

Photo Researcher: Lumina Datamatics

Text Researcher: Lumina Datamatics

Text Designer: Tani Hasegawa, Michael Cook

Cover Designer: Michael Cook

Cover Image: Dave Le/Moment/Getty Images

Compositor: Cenveo® Publisher Services

For product information and technology assistance, contact us at
Cengage Learning Customer & Sales Support, 1-800-354-9706.

For permission to use material from this text or product,
submit all requests online at **www.cengage.com/permissions.**
Further permissions questions can be e-mailed to
permissionrequest@cengage.com.

Library of Congress Control Number: 2015936118

ISBN: 978-1-305-62799-4

Loose-leaf Edition:
ISBN: 978-1-305-63938-6

Cengage Learning
20 Channel Center Street
Boston MA 02210
USA

Cengage Learning is a leading provider of customized learning solutions
with employees residing in nearly 40 different countries and sales in more
than 125 countries around the world. Find your local representative at
www.cengage.com.

Cengage Learning products are represented in Canada by Nelson
Education, Ltd.

To learn more about Cengage Learning Solutions, visit **www.cengage.com.**

Purchase any of our products at your local college store or at our preferred
online store **www.cengagebrain.com.**

Printed in the United States of America
Print Number: 01   Print Year: 2016

About the Authors

Frances Sienkiewicz Sizer

M.S., R.D.N., F.A.N.D., attended Florida State University where, in 1980, she received her B.S., and in 1982 her M.S., in nutrition. She is certified as a charter Fellow of the Academy of Nutrition and Dietetics. She is a founding member and vice president of Nutrition and Health Associates, an information and resource center in Tallahassee, Florida, that maintains an ongoing bibliographic database tracking research in more than 1,000 topic areas of nutrition. Her textbooks include *Life Choices: Health Concepts and Strategies*; *Making Life Choices*; *The Fitness Triad: Motivation, Training, and Nutrition*; and others. She also authored *Nutrition Interactive*, an instructional college-level nutrition CD-ROM that pioneered the animation of nutrition concepts in college classrooms. She consults with an advisory board of professors from around the nation, and attends workshops on innovations in nutrition education. She has lectured at universities and at national and regional conferences and supports local hunger and homelessness relief organizations in her community.

To my family, near and far, and especially to Joan Spencer Webb.

—*Fran*

Eleanor Noss Whitney

Ph.D., received her B.A. in biology from Radcliffe College in 1960 and her Ph.D. in biology from Washington University, St. Louis, in 1970. Formerly on the faculty at Florida State University and a dietitian registered with the Academy of Nutrition and Dietetics, she now devotes full time to research, writing, and consulting in nutrition, health, and environmental issues. Her earlier publications include articles in *Science*, *Genetics*, and other journals. Her textbooks include *Understanding Nutrition*, *Understanding Normal and Clinical Nutrition*, *Nutrition and Diet Therapy*, and *Essential Life Choices* for college students and *Making Life Choices* for high school students. Her most intense interests presently include energy conservation, solar energy uses, alternatively fueled vehicles, and ecosystem restoration. She is an activist who volunteers full-time for the Citizens Climate Lobby.

To Max, Zoey, Emily, Rebecca, Kalijah, and Duchess with love.

—*Ellie*

Brief Contents

Contents

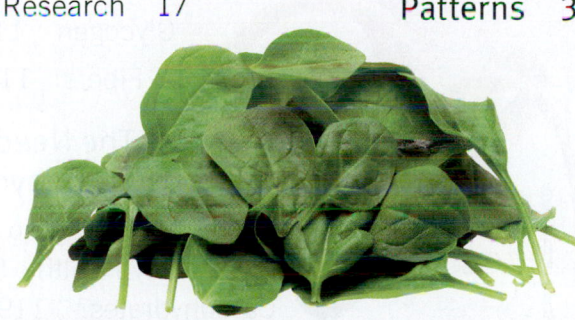
Norman Chan/Shutterstock.com

v

iStockphoto.com/Floortje

CHAPTER 5

The Lipids: Fats, Oils, Phospholipids, and Sterols 160

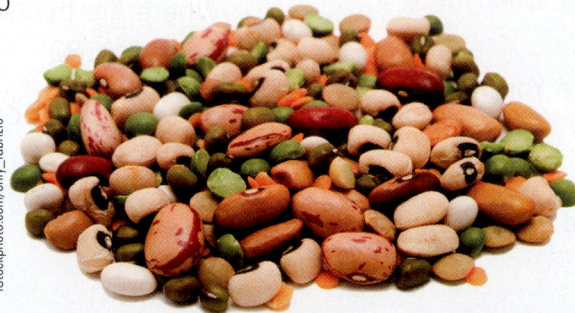

iStockphoto.com/only_fabrizio

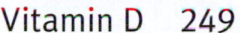
Evgeny Karandaev/Shutterstock.com

CHAPTER 9

Energy Balance and Healthy Body Weight 343

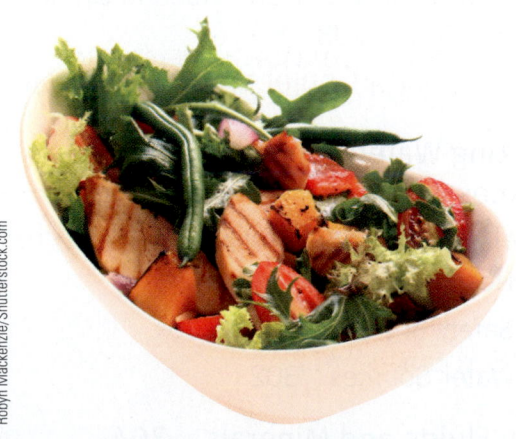

Robyn Mackenzie/Shutterstock.com

Nativarnia/Shutterstock.com

CHAPTER 11

Diet and Health 428

CHAPTER 12

Food Safety and Food Technology 470

Viktar Malyshchyts/Shutterstock.com

iStockphoto.com/marmo81

CHAPTER 15

Hunger and the Future of Food   599

Appendixes

Preface

A billboard in Louisiana reads, "Come as you are. Leave different," meaning that once you've seen, smelled, tasted, and listened to Louisiana, you'll never be the same. This book extends the same invitation to its readers: come to nutrition science as you are, with all of the knowledge and enthusiasm you possess, with all of your unanswered questions and misconceptions, and with the habits and preferences that now dictate what you eat.

But leave different. Take with you from this study a more complete understanding of nutrition science. Take a greater ability to discern between nutrition truth and fiction, to ask sophisticated questions, and to find the answers. Finally, take with you a better sense of how to feed yourself in ways that not only please you and soothe your spirit but nourish your body as well.

For over 35 years, *Nutrition: Concepts and Controversies* has been a cornerstone of nutrition classes across North America, serving the needs of students and professors. In keeping with our tradition, in this, our 14th edition, we continue exploring the ever-changing frontier of nutrition science, confronting its mysteries through its scientific roots. We maintain our sense of personal connection with instructors and learners alike, writing for them in the clear, informal style that has become our trademark.

Pedagogical Features

Throughout these chapters, features tickle the reader's interest and inform. For both verbal and visual learners, our logical presentation and our lively figures keep interest high and understanding at a peak. The photos that adorn many of our pages add pleasure to reading.

Many tried-and-true features return in this edition: Each chapter begins with What Do You Think? questions to pique interest. What Did You Decide? at the chapter's end asks readers to draw conclusions. A list of Learning Objectives (LO) offers a preview of the chapter's major goals, and the LO reappear under section headings to make clear the main take-away messages. Do the Math margin features challenge readers to solve nutrition problems, with examples provided. My Turn features invite the reader to hear stories from students in nutrition classes around the nation offer solutions to real-life situations. Think Fitness reminders alert readers to links among nutrition, fitness, and health. Food Feature sections act as bridges between theory and practice; they are practical applications of the chapter concepts. The consumer sections,

Workmans Photos/
Shutterstock.com

entitled A Consumer's Guide To . . ., lead readers through an often bewildering marketplace with scientific clarity, preparing them to move ahead with sound marketplace decisions. Each Consumer's Guide ends with review questions to improve recall of the main points.

By popular demand, we have retained our Snapshots of vitamins and minerals, which now reflect the 2015 Daily Values. These concentrated capsules of information depict food sources of vitamins and minerals, present DRI values, and offer the chief functions of each nutrient along with deficiency and toxicity symptoms.

New or major terms are defined in the margins of chapter pages or in nearby tables, and they also appear in the Glossary at the end of the book. The reader who wishes to locate any term can quickly do so by consulting the Index, which lists the page numbers of definitions in boldface type.

Two useful features close each chapter. First, our popular Concepts in Action diet and exercise tracking activities integrate chapter concepts with the Diet & Wellness Plus program. The second is the indispensible Self Check that provides study questions, with answers in Appendix G to provide immediate feedback to the learner.

Controversies

The Controversies of this book's title invite you to explore beyond the safe boundaries of established nutrition knowledge. These optional readings, which appear at the end of each chapter, delve into current scientific topics and emerging controversies. These fast-changing topics are relevant to nutrition science today.

Chapter Contents

Chapter 1 begins the text with a personal challenge to students. It asks the question so many people ask of nutrition educators—"Why should people care about nutrition?" We answer with a lesson in the ways in which nutritious foods affect diseases and present a continuum of diseases from purely genetic in origin to those almost totally preventable by nutrition. After presenting some beginning facts about the genes, nutrients, bioactive food components, and nature of foods, the chapter goes on to present the *Healthy People* goals for the nation. It concludes with a discussion of scientific research and quackery.

Chapter 2 brings together the concepts of nutrient standards, such as the Dietary Reference Intakes, and diet planning using the Dietary Guidelines for

Americans 2015–2020. Chapter 3 presents a thorough, but brief, introduction to the workings of the human body from the genes to the organs, with major emphasis on the digestive system and its microbiota. Chapters 4–6 are devoted to the energy-yielding nutrients—carbohydrates, lipids, and protein. Controversy 4 has renewed its focus on theories and fables surrounding the health effects of added sugars in the diet. Controversy 5, new to this edition, considers the scientific debate surrounding lipid guidelines.

Chapters 7 and 8 present the vitamins, minerals, and water. Chapter 9 relates energy balance to body composition, obesity, and underweight and provides guidance on lifelong weight maintenance. Chapter 10 presents the relationships among physical activity, athletic performance, and nutrition, with some guidance about products marketed to athletes. Chapter 11 applies the essence of the first 10 chapters to disease prevention.

Chapter 12 delivers urgently important concepts of food safety. It also addresses the usefulness and safety of food additives, including artificial sweeteners and artificial fats, and explains the widely varying effects of processing on nutrients in foods. Chapters 13 and 14 emphasize the importance of nutrition through the life span, with issues surrounding childhood obesity in Controversy 13. Chapter 14 includes nutrition advice for feeding preschoolers, schoolchildren, teens, and the elderly.

Chapter 15 devotes attention to hunger and malnutrition, both in the United States and throughout the world. It also touches on the vast network of problems that threaten the future food supply, and explores sustainable diets as part of the solution.

Our Message to You

Our purpose in writing this text, as always, is to enhance our readers' understanding of nutrition science. We also hope the information on this book's pages will reach beyond the classroom into our readers' lives. Take the information you find inside this book home with you. Use it in your life: nourish yourself, educate your loved ones, and nurture others to be healthy. Stay up with the news, too—for despite all the conflicting messages, inflated claims, and even quackery that abound in the marketplace, true nutrition knowledge progresses with a genuine scientific spirit, and important new truths are constantly unfolding.

New to This Edition

Every section of each chapter of this text reflects the changes in nutrition science occurring since the last edition. The changes range from subtle shifts of emphasis to entirely new sections that demand our attention. Appendix F supplies current references; older references may be viewed in previous editions, available from the publisher.

Chapter 1
- New introductory section on water.
- Defines *NHANES*.
- Defines *registered dietitian nutritionist (RDN)*.

- Condensed and enhanced Tables C1–2 and C1–3.
- Condensed Tables C1–5 and C1–6.

Chapter 2
- Integration of the Dietary Guidelines for Americans 2015–2020.
- New table of shortfall and overconsumed nutrients.
- Defines *empty calories*.
- Introduces the American Diabetes Association's *Choose Your Foods* lists.
- New figure of dining-out trends.
- Updated labeling discussion and new figure to illustrate proposed changes to the Nutrition Facts Panel.
- Newly approved Daily Values used in inside back cover, figures, and discussions.
- New front of package labeling information and figure.
- New phytochemical Point/Counterpoint table.

Chapter 3
- Clarified Figure 3–4.
- New section to introduce microbiota of the intestinal tract.
- New table of definitions of common digestive disorders.
- New Point/Counterpoint table summarizing issues of alcohol and health.

Chapter 4
- Expanded coverage of the health effects of fermentable fibers and their products.
- New coverage and table of the glycemic index.
- New nutrition guidelines for diabetes.
- New section on relationship between obesity and diabetes.
- Updated table of diabetes diagnostic criteria.
- New figure illustrating sugar alcohols on a label.
- New table of added sugar intake through the life span.
- New coverage of added sugars and blood pressure.
- New Point/Counterpoint table on the health effects of added sugars.

Chapter 5
- Expanded coverage of dietary fat and satiety.
- Updated lipid intake recommendations.
- New emphasis on fat sources in Mediterranean eating patterns.
- Updated presentation of fast food choices.
- New figure explaining the Supplement Facts panel of a fish oil supplement.
- New Do the Math feature on percentages of fat in ground meats.
- New practical tips for consuming fish and seafood in Food Feature.
- New Controversy on scientific debate surrounding lipid guidelines, concluding with new eating patterns approach.
- New Point, Counterpoint table on lipid guidelines debate.

Chapter 6
- Expanded section on gluten-free diets, celiac disease, and gluten sensitivity.

- New discussion of protein labeling.
- New figure highlighting protein labeling.
- New Point/Counterpoint table on vegetarian and meat-containing diets.

Chapter 7
- Introduces the role of obesity in vitamin D deficiency.
- New table highlighting current research on the role of vitamin D in disease.
- New Daily Values for vitamins reflected in the Snapshots.
- New explanation of food fortification with B vitamins.
- New Point/Counterpoint table on arguments for and against dietary supplements.

Chapter 8
- New sports-drink labeling figure in Consumer's Guide.
- New Daily Values for minerals throughout the Snapshots.
- Revised and updated graph on sodium intakes of U.S. adults.
- Revised and updated graph on calcium sources in the U.S. diet.
- New presentation of lifetime plan for healthy bones.
- New Point/Counterpoint table on arguments for and against calcium supplements.

Chapter 9
- New table on underweight, overweight, and obesity in U.S. adults.
- New table presents American College of Cardiology/American Heart Association Task Force Guidelines.
- New coverage of intermittent fasting for weight control.
- Updated table of eating patterns for weight loss to reflect recent research and reviews.
- New figure and text coverage of calorie labels on restaurant menus.
- New section on potential benefits and risks, including nutrient deficiency risks, of obesity surgery.
- Added Contrave and Saxenda information.
- New discussion of the idea of binge eating as addiction.

Chapter 10
- New table on benefits of fitness.
- New discussion of exercise factors as molecular links between physical activity and health.
- Condensed and reorganized fitness sections.
- New major section on the body's three energy systems that support physical activity.
- Explains the "train low, compete high" theory.
- Expanded coverage of protein intakes for athletes.
- New table of protein-rich snacks for athletes.
- New coverage of vitamin D for athletes.
- Added DMAA and DMBA as unsafe supplements for athletes.

Chapter 11
- Enhanced the table of selected nutrients' roles in immune function.

- Newly revised tables of recommendations and strategies to reduce the risk of CVD and recommendations and strategies to reduce the risk of cancer.
- Emphasizes the role of obesity as a major risk factor for other chronic diseases throughout the chapter.
- New information related to the 2013 American College of Cardiology/American Heart Association guidelines for assessment of CVD risk and lifestyle modifications for reducing the risk of heart disease.
- New emphasis on risks and benefits of alternative therapies.
- New figure summarizing the relationship between risks and benefits.

Chapter 12
- Updated hand washing figure to reflect new guidelines.
- New table on how to wash produce.
- New figure depicting imported food in the U.S. diet.
- Updated figure on organic food labels.
- New table on natural toxins.
- New discussion of arsenic in apple juice and rice.
- New discussion of artificial sweeteners and GI flora.

Chapter 13
- New discussion of choline during pregnancy.
- New table of complications associated with smoking during pregnancy.
- New discussion of the importance of zinc in complementary foods for breastfed infants.
- Restructured and simplified table of nutrient supplements for infants.
- Reorganized Controversy 13.
- New table of physical complications of obesity during childhood.
- New figure demonstrating how to read a growth chart.
- New figure of sleep, screen time, and obesity in children.

Chapter 14
- Updated energy intake needs for children.
- New table of healthy snack ideas from each food group.
- Updated USDA Eating Pattern calorie intakes for children.
- New figure of physical symptoms of lead toxicity in children.
- New discussion on vitamin D and PMS.
- Increased coverage of dietary protein and muscle protein synthesis in the elderly.
- Caffeine information from the *Scientific Report of the 2015 Dietary Guidelines Advisory Committee*.

Chapter 15
- Title change reflects current trends in sustainability research.
- New table of U.S. food security terms.
- New figure of expenditures for U.S. food programs.
- Reorganized world hunger and malnutrition section.
- New figure on mid-upper arm circumference.
- Defines *wasting*, *stunting*, and *marasmic kwashiorkor*.

Appendixes:

Appendix D: Presents the 2014 Food Lists for Diabetes and Weight Management.

Appendix E: Presents Eating Patterns recommended by the 2015–2020 Dietary Guidelines for Americans: Healthy U.S.-Style, Healthy Vegetarian, and Healthy Mediterranean-Style, and support materials for the Mediterrranean diet.

Appendix H: Offers tables and figures to support physical activity.

Appendix I: New appendix of selected nutrient chemical structures.

Ancillary Materials

Students and instructors alike will appreciate the innovative teaching and learning materials that accompany this text.

MindTap: A new approach to highly personalized online learning. Beyond an eBook, homework solution, digital supplement, or premium website, MindTap is a digital learning platform that works alongside your campus LMS to deliver course curriculum across the range of electronic devices in your life. MindTap is built on an "app" model allowing enhanced digital collaboration and delivery of engaging content across a spectrum of Cengage and non-Cengage resources.

Instructor Companion Site: Everything you need for your course in one place! This collection of book-specific lecture and class tools is available online via www.cengage.com/login. Access and download PowerPoint presentations, images, instructor's manual, videos, and more.

Test Bank with Cognero: Cengage Learning Testing Powered by Cognero is a flexible online system that allows you to:

- Author, edit, and manage test bank content from multiple Cengage Learning solutions.

- Create multiple test versions in an instant.

- Deliver tests from your LMS, your classroom, or wherever you want.

Diet & Wellness Plus: Diet & Wellness Plus helps you understand how nutrition relates to your personal health goals. Track your diet and activity, generate reports, and analyze the nutritional value of the food you eat. Diet & Wellness Plus includes over 75,000 foods as well as custom food and recipe features. The new Behavior Change Planner helps you identify risks in your life and guides you through the key steps to make positive changes.

Global Nutrition Watch: Bring currency to the classroom with Global Nutrition Watch from Cengage Learning. This user-friendly website provides convenient access to thousands of trusted sources, including academic journals, newspapers, videos, and podcasts, for you to use for research projects or classroom discussion. Global Nutrition Watch is updated daily to offer the most current news about topics related to nutrition.

Acknowledgments

Our thanks to our partners Linda Kelly DeBruyne and Sharon Rolfes for decades of support. Thank you, Spencer Webb, RD, CSCS, for your guidance in Chapter 10 (and for getting us into shape, too). Thank you, K. Autumn Ehsaei, R.D.N., for generating our orderly endnote lists. And to Kathy Guilday, the Queen of Minutiae, many heartfelt thanks for your meticulous work and cheerful nature.

We are also grateful to the nutrition professionals who updated sections of this edition.

- Linda DeBruyne, M.S., R.D.N. (Chapter 11 and Chapter 13). Linda received her master's degree in nutrition from Florida State University and is a founding member of Nutrition and Health Associates. She also coauthors the college nutrition texts *Nutrition and Diet Therapy* and *Nutrition for Health and Health Care*.

- Crystal Clark Douglas, Ph.D., R.D.N./L.D.N. (Controversy 13 and Chapter 14). Crystal holds a doctoral degree in nutrition sciences from the University of Alabama at Birmingham and is the coauthor of multiple peer-reviewed publications. After teaching nutrition at Florida State University, she has maintained her professional skills working as a clinical dietitian and continuing to write on topics in nutrition.

- Shannon Dooies Gower-Winter, M.S., R.D.N./L.D.N. (Controversy 2, Chapter 7, and Chapter 8). Shannon graduated from Florida State University with her master's degree in nutrition. She has taught nutrition at Florida State University and lectured on topics related to childhood nutrition throughout the state. She currently conducts research in the area of nutritional neuroscience, where her work focuses on various roles of zinc in the brain. Her research has been presented at regional and national scientific conferences, and she has coauthored multiple articles in peer-reviewed journals.

Our special thanks to our publishing team—Miriam Myers, Heidi Allgair, and Carol Samet—for their hard work and dedication to excellence. Thank you to our marketing manager, Tom Ziolkowski, for ensuring that our text finds the hands of its readers.

We would also like to thank Chimborazo Publishing, Inc. for their work on the student and instructor ancillaries for the 14th edition, which includes the test bank, instructor's manual, and PowerLecture.

Reviewers of Recent Editions

As always, we are grateful for the instructors who took the time to comment on this revision. Your suggestions were invaluable in strengthening the book and suggesting new lines of thought. We hope you will continue to provide your comments and suggestions.

Alex Kojo Anderson, *University of Georgia, Athens*
Sharon Antonelli, *San Jose City College*
L. Rao Ayyagari, *Lindenwood University*

James W. Bailey, *University of Tennessee*
Ana Barreras, *Central New Mexico Community College*
Karen Basinger, *Montgomery College*
Leah Carter, *Bakersfield College*
Melissa Chabot, *SUNY at Buffalo*
Janet Colson, *Middle Tennessee State University*
Priscilla Connors, *University of North Texas*
Karen Davidowitz Corbin, *The Translational Research Institute for Metabolism and Diabetes*
Monica L. Easterling, *Wayne County Community College District*
Katie Faulk, *Pacific Oregon University*
Shannon Gower-Winter, *Florida State University*
Jena Nelson Hall, *Butte Community College*
Charlene G. Harkins, *University of Minnesota, Duluth*
Sharon Anne Himmelstein, *Central New Mexico Community College*
Rachel Johnson, *University of Vermont*
Judy Kaufman, *Monroe Community College*
David Lightsey, *Bakersfield College*
Craig Meservey, *New Hampshire Technical Institute*

Liza Marie Mohanty, *Olive-Harvey College*
Eimear M. Mullen, *Northern Kentucky University*
Suzanne Linn Nelson, *University of Colorado at Boulder*
Steven Nizielski, *Grand Valley State University*
Carmen Nochera, *Grand Valley State University*
David J. Pavlat, *Central College*
Begoña Cirera Perez, *Chabot College*
Cydne Perry, *Shepherd University*
Liz Quintana, *West Virginia University*
Janice M. Rueda, *Wayne State University*
Donal Scheidel, *University of South Dakota*
Carole A. Sloan, *Henry Ford Community College*
Leslie S. Spencer, *Rowan University*
Ilene Sutter, *California State University, Northridge*
Sue Ellen Warren, *El Camino College*
Barbara P. Zabitz, *Wayne County Community College District*
Joseph Zielinski, *SUNY at Brockport*
Nancy Zwick, *Northern Kentucky University*

1

Food Choices and Human Health

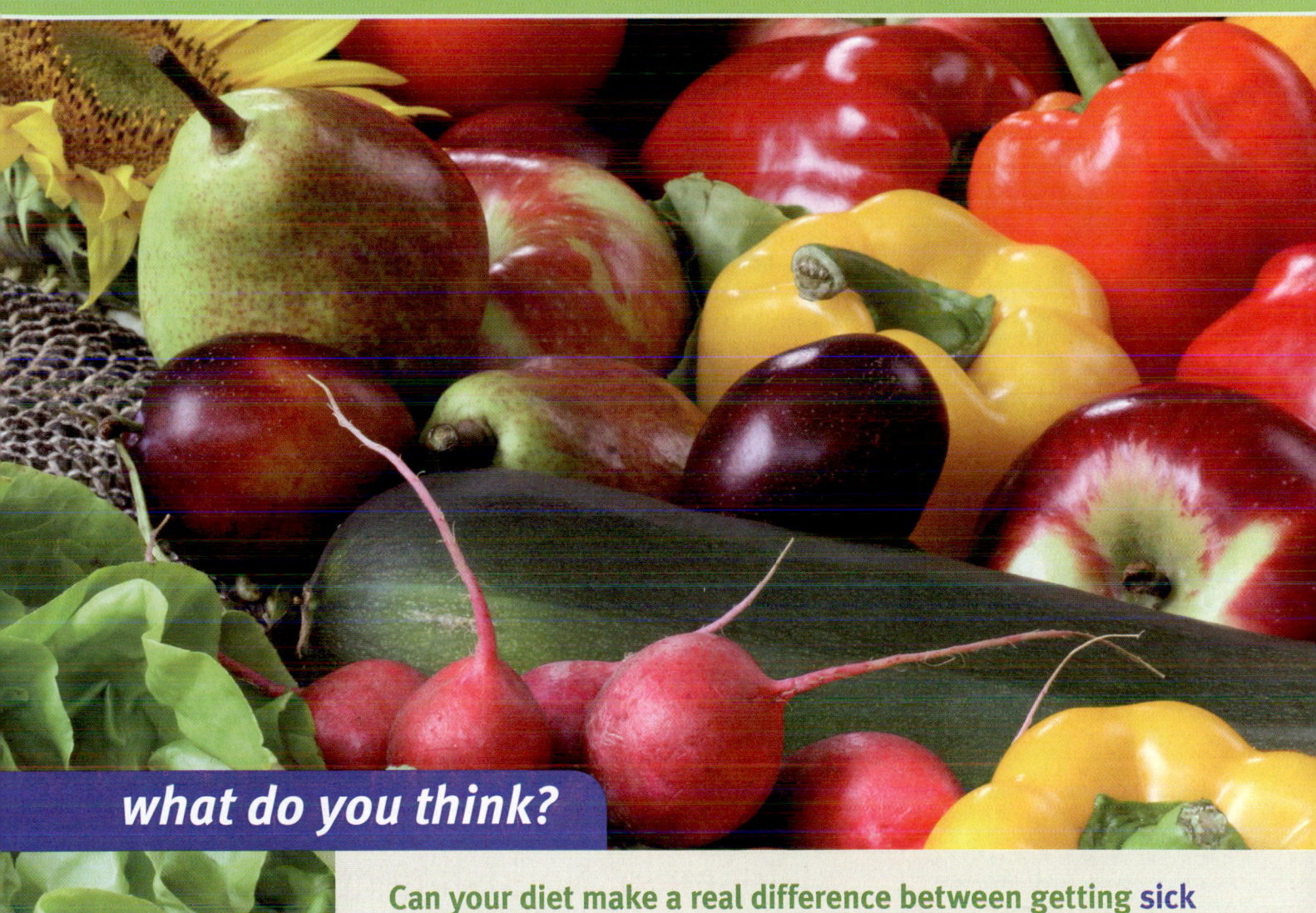

what do you think?

Can your diet make a real difference between getting **sick** or staying **healthy**?

Are **supplements** more powerful than food for ensuring good nutrition?

What makes your favorite foods your **favorites**?

Are **news and media nutrition reports** informative or confusing?

Learning Objectives

After reading this chapter, you should be able to accomplish the following:

LO 1.1 Discuss the impact of food choices on a person's health.

LO 1.2 List seven major categories of nutrition and weight-related objectives included in the publication *Healthy People 2020*.

LO 1.3 Specify the six classes of nutrients.

LO 1.4 Recognize the challenges and solutions to choosing a health-promoting diet.

LO 1.5 Describe the science of nutrition.

LO 1.6 Explain the significance of behavior change in improving a person's diet.

LO 1.7 Discuss the importance of nutrient density in creating an effective diet plan.

LO 1.8 Evaluate the authenticity of nutrition information sources.

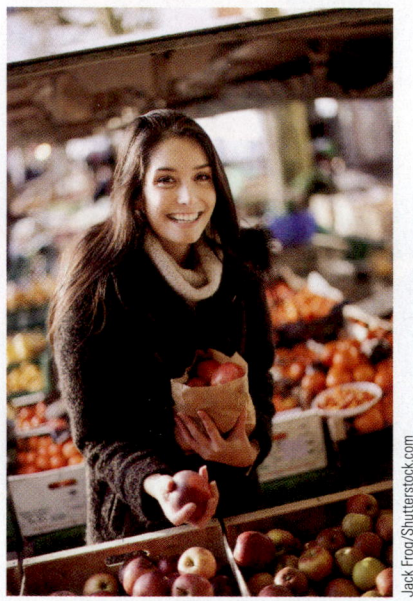

When you choose foods with nutrition in mind, you can enhance your own well-being.

Jack Frog/Shutterstock.com

food medically, any substance that the body can take in and assimilate that will enable it to stay alive and to grow; the carrier of nourishment; socially, a more limited number of such substances defined as acceptable by each culture.

nutrition the study of the nutrients in foods and in the body; sometimes also the study of human behaviors related to food.

diet the foods (including beverages) a person usually eats and drinks.

nutrients components of food that are indispensable to the body's functioning. They provide energy, serve as building material, help maintain or repair body parts, and support growth. The nutrients include water, carbohydrate, fat, protein, vitamins, and minerals.

I f you care about your body, and if you have strong feelings about **food**, then you have much to gain from learning about **nutrition**—the science of how food nourishes the body. Nutrition is a fascinating, much talked-about subject. Each day, newspapers, Internet websites, radio, and television present stories of new findings on nutrition and heart health or nutrition and cancer prevention, and at the same time, advertisements and commercials bombard us with multicolored pictures of tempting foods—pizza, burgers, cakes, and chips. If you are like most people, when you eat you sometimes wonder, "Is this food good for me?" or you berate yourself, "I probably shouldn't be eating this."

When you study nutrition, you learn which foods serve you best, and you can work out ways of choosing foods, planning meals, and designing your **diet** wisely. Knowing the facts can enhance your health and your enjoyment of eating while relieving your feelings of guilt or worry that you aren't eating well.

This chapter addresses these "why," "what," and "how" questions about nutrition:

- *Why* care about nutrition? Why be concerned about the **nutrients** in your foods? Why not just take supplements?

- *What* are the nutrients in foods, and what roles do they play in the body? What are the differences between vitamins and minerals?

- *What* constitutes a nutritious diet? How can you choose foods wisely, for nutrition's sake? What factors motivate your choices?

- *How* do we know what we know about nutrition? How does nutrition science work, and how can a person keep up with changing information?

Controversy 1 concludes the chapter by offering ways to distinguish between trustworthy sources of nutrition information and those that are less reliable.

A Lifetime of Nourishment

LO 1.1 Discuss the impact of food choices on a person's health.

If you live for 65 years or longer, you will have consumed more than 70,000 meals, and your remarkable body will have disposed of 50 tons of food. The foods you choose most often have cumulative effects on your body.[1]* As you age, you will see and feel those effects—if you know what to look for.

Your body renews its structures continuously, and each day, it builds a little muscle, bone, skin, and blood, replacing old tissues with new. It may also add a little fat if

---

*Reference notes are found in Appendix F.

you consume excess food energy (calories) or subtract a little if you consume less than you require. Some of the food you eat today becomes part of "you" tomorrow.

The best food for you, then, is the kind that supports the growth and maintenance of strong muscles, sound bones, healthy skin, and sufficient blood to cleanse and nourish all parts of your body. This means you need food that provides not only the right amount of energy but also sufficient nutrients—that is, enough water, carbohydrates, fats, protein, vitamins, and minerals. If the foods you eat provide too little or too much of any nutrient today, your health may suffer just a little today. If the foods you eat provide too little or too much of one or more nutrients every day for years, then in later life you may suffer severe disease effects.

A well-chosen diet supplies enough energy and enough of each nutrient to prevent **malnutrition**. Malnutrition includes deficiencies, imbalances, and excesses of nutrients, alone or in combination, any of which can take a toll on health over time.

KEY POINTS

- The nutrients in food support growth, maintenance, and repair of the body.
- Deficiencies, excesses, and imbalances of energy and nutrients bring on the diseases of malnutrition.

The Diet and Health Connection

Your choice of diet profoundly affects your health, both today and in the future. Only two common lifestyle habits are more influential: smoking and using other forms of tobacco and drinking alcohol in excess. Of the leading causes of death listed in Table 1–1, four—heart disease, cancers, strokes, and diabetes—are directly related to nutrition, and another—accidents—is related to drinking alcohol.

Many older people suffer from debilitating conditions that could have been largely prevented had they known and applied the nutrition principles known today. The **chronic diseases**—heart disease, diabetes, some kinds of cancer, dental disease, and adult bone loss—all have a connection to poor diet. These diseases cannot be prevented by a good diet alone; they are to some extent determined by a person's genetic constitution, activities, and lifestyle. Within the range set by your genetic

Table 1–1

Leading Causes of Death in the United States

	Percentage of Total Deaths
1. **Heart disease**	23.7
2. **Cancers**	22.9
3. Chronic lung diseases	5.7
4. **Strokes**	5.1
5. Accidents	4.9
6. Alzheimer's disease	3.4
7. **Diabetes mellitus**	2.9
8. Pneumonia and influenza	2.1
9. Kidney disease	1.8
10. Suicide	1.5

Note: The diseases highlighted in bold have relationships with diet.

Source: J. Xu and coauthors, Mortality in the United States, 2012, NCHS Data Brief 168, October 2014.

malnutrition any condition caused by excess or deficient food energy or nutrient intake or by an imbalance of nutrients. Nutrient or energy deficiencies are forms of undernutrition; nutrient or energy excesses are forms of overnutrition.

chronic diseases degenerative conditions or illnesses that progress slowly, are long in duration, and lack an immediate cure; chronic diseases limit functioning, productivity, and the quality and length of life. Examples include heart disease, cancer, and diabetes.

Figure 1–1

Nutrition and Disease

Not all diseases are equally influenced by diet. Some are almost purely genetic, like the anemia of sickle-cell disease. Some may be inherited (or the tendency to develop them may be inherited in the genes) but may be influenced by diet, like some forms of diabetes. Some are purely dietary, like the vitamin and mineral deficiency diseases.

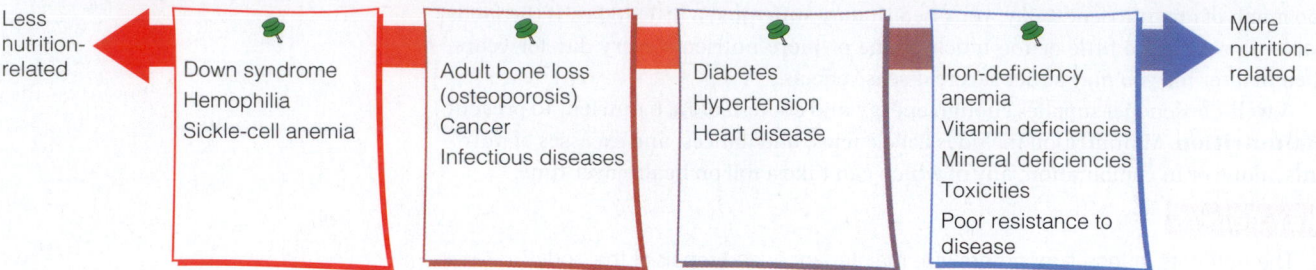

Less nutrition-related

Down syndrome
Hemophilia
Sickle-cell anemia

Adult bone loss (osteoporosis)
Cancer
Infectious diseases

Diabetes
Hypertension
Heart disease

Iron-deficiency anemia
Vitamin deficiencies
Mineral deficiencies
Toxicities
Poor resistance to disease

More nutrition-related

inheritance, however, the likelihood of developing these diseases is strongly influenced by your daily choices.

KEY POINT

- Nutrition profoundly affects health.

Genetics, Nutrition, and Individuality

Consider the role of genetics. Genetics and nutrition affect different diseases to varying degrees (see Figure 1–1). The **anemia** caused by sickle-cell disease, for example, is purely hereditary and thus appears at the left of Figure 1–1 as a genetic condition largely unrelated to nutrition. Nothing a person eats affects the person's chances of contracting this anemia, although nutrition therapy may help ease its course. At the other end of the spectrum, iron-deficiency anemia most often results from undernutrition. Diseases and conditions of poor health appear all along this continuum, from almost entirely genetically based to purely nutritional in origin; the more nutrition-related a disease or health condition is, the more successfully sound nutrition can prevent it.

Furthermore, some diseases, such as heart disease and cancer, are not one disease but many. Two people may both have heart disease but not the same form; one person's cancer may be nutrition-related, but another's may not be. Individual people differ genetically from each other in thousands of subtle ways, so no simple statement can be made about the extent to which diet can help any one person avoid such diseases or slow their progress.

The identification of the human **genome** establishes the entire sequence of the **genes** in human **DNA**. This work has, in essence, revealed the body's instructions for making all of the working parts of a human being. The human genome is 99.9% the same in all people; all of the normal variations such as differences in hair color, as well as variations that result in diseases such as sickle-cell anemia, lie in the 0.1% of the genome that varies. Nutrition scientists are working quickly to apply this new wealth of knowledge to benefit human health. Later chapters expand on the emerging story of nutrition and the genes.

KEY POINTS

- Diet influences long-term health within the range set by genetic inheritance.
- Nutrition has little influence on some diseases but strongly affects others.

Other Lifestyle Choices

Besides food choices, other lifestyle choices affect people's health. Tobacco use and alcohol and other substance abuse can destroy health. Physical activity, sleep, emotional stress, and other environmental factors can also modify the severity of some diseases.

anemia a blood condition in which red blood cells, the body's oxygen carriers, are inadequate or impaired and so cannot meet the oxygen demands of the body.

genome (GEE-nome) the full complement of genetic information in the chromosomes of a cell. In human beings, the genome consists of about 35,000 genes and supporting materials. The study of genomes is *genomics*. Also defined in the Controversy section of Chapter 11.

genes units of a cell's inheritance; sections of the larger genetic molecule DNA (deoxyribonucleic acid). Each gene directs the making of one or more of the body's proteins.

DNA an abbreviation for deoxyribonucleic (dee-OX-ee-RYE-bow-nu-CLAY-ick) acid, the thread-like molecule that encodes genetic information in its structure; DNA strands coil up densely to form the chromosomes (Chapter 3 provides more details).

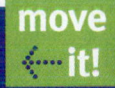
Why should people bother to be physically active? A person's daily food choices can powerfully affect health, but the combination of nutrition and physical activity is more powerful still. People who combine regular physical activity with a nutritious diet can expect to receive at least some of these benefits:

- Reduced risks of cardiovascular diseases, diabetes, certain cancers, hypertension, and other diseases.
- Increased endurance, strength, and flexibility.
- More cheerful outlook and less likelihood of depression.
- Improved mental functioning.

- Feeling of vigor.
- Feeling of belonging—the companionship of sports.
- Stronger self-image.
- Reduced body fat and increased lean tissue.
- A more youthful appearance, healthy skin, and improved muscle tone.
- Greater bone density and lessened risk of adult bone loss in later life.
- Increased independence in the elderly.
- Sound, beneficial sleep.
- Faster wound healing.
- Reduced menstrual symptoms.
- Improved resistance to infection.

If even half of these benefits were yours for the asking, wouldn't you step up to claim them? In truth, they are yours to claim, at the price of including physical activity in your day. Chapter 10 explores the topics of fitness and physical activity.

start now! ···⟩ Ready to make a change? Go to Diet & Wellness Plus online and track your physical activities—all of them—for three days. (The Concepts in Action activity at the end of this chapter will use this information.) After you have recorded your activities, see how much time you spent exercising at a moderate to vigorous level. Could you increase your level and amount of activity?

Physical activity is so closely linked with nutrition in supporting health that most chapters of this book offer a feature called Think Fitness, such as the one above.

KEY POINT

- Life choices, such as being physically active or using tobacco or alcohol, can improve or damage health.

Healthy People: Nutrition Objectives for the Nation

LO 1.2 List seven major categories of nutrition and weight-related objectives included in the publication *Healthy People 2020*.

In its publication *Healthy People*, the U.S. Department of Health and Human Services sets specific 10-year objectives to guide national health promotion efforts.[2] The vision of *Healthy People 2020* is a society in which all people live long, healthy lives. Table 1–2 (p. 6) provides a quick scan of the nutrition and weight-related objectives set for this decade. The inclusion of nutrition and food-safety objectives shows that public health officials consider these areas to be top national priorities.

In 2015, the nation's health report was mixed: the number of adults meeting physical activity and muscle strengthening guidelines increased from 18 percent to over 20 percent of the population, but most people's diets still lacked enough vegetables, and obesity rates were creeping higher among people aged two years and older.[3] To fully meet the current *Healthy People* goals, our nation must take steps to change its habits.

The next section shifts our focus to the nutrients at the core of nutrition science. As your course of study progresses, the individual nutrients will become like old friends, revealing more and more about themselves as you move through the chapters.

KEY POINT

- Each decade, the U.S. Department of Health and Human Services sets health and nutrition objectives for the nation.

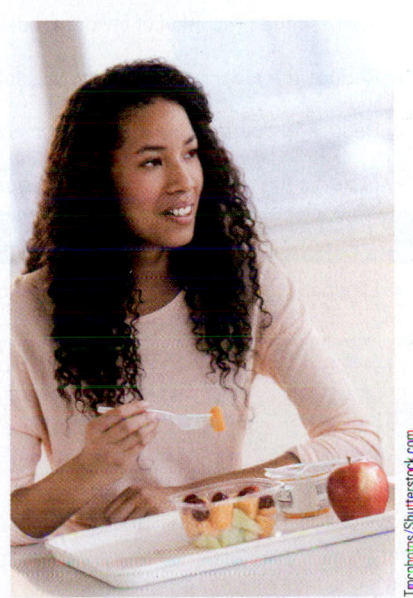

The aim of Healthy People 2020 *is to help people live long, healthy lives.*

Table 1–2

Healthy People 2020, Selected Nutrition and Body Weight Objectives

Many other Objectives for the Nation are available at www.healthypeople.gov.

Chronic Diseases

- Reduce the proportion of adults with osteoporosis.
- Reduce the death rates from cancer, diabetes, heart disease, and stroke.
- Reduce the annual number of new cases of diabetes.

Food Safety

- Reduce outbreaks of certain infections transmitted through food.
- Reduce severe allergic reactions to food among adults with diagnosed food allergy.

Maternal, Infant, and Child Health

- Reduce the number of low birthweight infants and preterm births.
- Increase the proportion of infants who are breastfed.
- Reduce the occurrence of fetal alcohol syndrome (FAS).
- Reduce iron deficiency among children, adolescents, women of childbearing age, and pregnant women.
- Reduce blood lead levels in children.
- Increase the number of schools offering breakfast.

Food and Nutrient Consumption

- Increase vegetables, fruits, and whole grains in the diets of those aged 2 years and older, and reduce solid fats and added sugars.

Eating Disorders

- Reduce the proportion of adolescents who engage in disordered eating behaviors in an attempt to control their weight.

Physical Activity and Weight Control

- Increase the proportion of children, adolescents, and adults who are at a healthy weight.
- Reduce the proportions of children, adolescents, and adults who are obese.
- Reduce the proportion of people who engage in no leisure-time physical activity.
- Increase the proportion of schools that require daily physical education for all students.

Food Security

- Eliminate very low food security among children in U.S. households.

Source: www.healthypeople.gov.

The Human Body and Its Food

LO 1.3 Specify the six classes of nutrients.

energy the capacity to do work. The energy in food is chemical energy; it can be converted to mechanical, electrical, thermal, or other forms of energy in the body. Food energy is measured in calories, defined on page 8.

As your body moves and works each day, it must use **energy**. The energy that fuels the body's work comes indirectly from the sun by way of plants. Plants capture and store the sun's energy in their tissues as they grow. When you eat plant-derived foods such as fruits, grains, or vegetables, you obtain and use the solar energy they

Table 1–3

Elements in the Six Classes of Nutrients

The nutrients that contain carbon are organic.

	Carbon	Oxygen	Hydrogen	Nitrogen	Minerals
Carbohydrate	✓	✓	✓		
Fat	✓	✓	✓		
Protein	✓	✓	✓	✓	b
Vitamins	✓	✓	✓	✓a	b
Minerals					✓
Water		✓	✓		

a All of the B vitamins contain nitrogen; amine means nitrogen.
b Protein and some vitamins contain the mineral sulfur; vitamin B_{12} contains the mineral cobalt.

have stored. Plant-eating animals obtain their energy in the same way, so when you eat animal tissues, you are eating compounds containing energy that came originally from the sun.

The body requires six kinds of nutrients—families of molecules indispensable to its functioning—and foods deliver these. Table 1–3 lists the six classes of nutrients. Four of these six are **organic**; that is, the nutrients contain the element carbon derived from living things.

Meet the Nutrients

The human body and foods are made of the same materials, arranged in different ways (see Figure 1–2). When considering quantities of foods and nutrients, scientists often measure them in **grams**, units of weight.

Figure 1–2

Components of Food and the Human Body

Foods and the human body are made of the same materials.

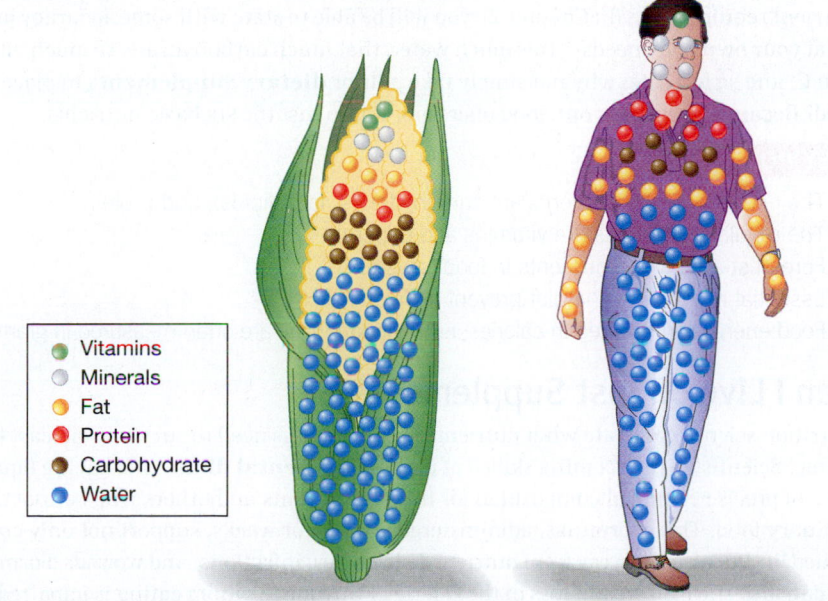

- ● Vitamins
- ○ Minerals
- ● Fat
- ● Protein
- ● Carbohydrate
- ● Water

organic carbon containing. Four of the six classes of nutrients are organic: carbohydrate, fat, protein, and vitamins. Organic compounds include only those made by living things and do not include compounds such as carbon dioxide, diamonds, and a few carbon salts.

grams units of weight. A gram (g) is the weight of a cubic centimeter (cc) or milliliter (ml) of water under defined conditions of temperature and pressure. About 28 grams equal an ounce.

Table 1–4
Calorie Values of Energy-Yielding Nutrients

The energy a person consumes in a day's meals comes from these three energy-yielding nutrients; alcohol, if consumed, also contributes energy.

Energy Nutrient	Energy
Carbohydrate	4 cal/g
Fat (lipid)	9 cal/g
Protein	4 cal/g

Note: Alcohol contributes 7 cal/g that the human body can use for energy. Alcohol is not classed as a nutrient, however, because it interferes with growth, maintenance, and repair of body tissues.

The Energy-Yielding Nutrients   Of the four organic nutrients, three are **energy-yielding nutrients**, meaning that the body can use the energy they contain. The carbohydrates and fats (fats are also called lipids) are especially important energy-yielding nutrients. As for protein, it does double duty: it can yield energy, but it also provides materials that form structures and working parts of body tissues. (Alcohol yields energy, too—see the note to Table 1–4).

Vitamins and Minerals   The fourth and fifth classes of nutrients are the vitamins and the minerals, sometimes referred to as *micronutrients* because they are present in tiny amounts. These provide no energy to the body. A few minerals serve as parts of body structures (calcium and phosphorus, for example, are major constituents of bone), but all vitamins and minerals act as regulators. As regulators, the vitamins and minerals assist in all body processes: digesting food; moving muscles; disposing of wastes; growing new tissues; healing wounds; obtaining energy from carbohydrate, fat, and protein; and participating in every other process necessary to maintain life. Later chapters are devoted to these six classes of nutrients.

Water   Although last on the list, water is foremost in quantity among the six classes of nutrients. The body constantly loses water, mainly through sweat, breath, and urine, and that water must constantly be replaced. Without sufficient water, the body's cells cannot function.

The Concept of Essential Nutrients   When you eat food, then, you are providing your body with energy and nutrients. Furthermore, some of the nutrients are **essential nutrients**, meaning that if you do not ingest them, you will develop deficiencies; the body cannot make these nutrients for itself. Essential nutrients are found in all six classes of nutrients. Water is an essential nutrient; so is a form of carbohydrate; so are some lipids, some parts of protein, all of the vitamins, and the minerals important in human nutrition.

Calorie Values   Food scientists measure food energy in kilocalories, units of heat. This book uses the common word ***calories*** to mean the same thing. It behooves the person who wishes to control food energy intake and body fatness to learn the calorie values of the energy nutrients, listed in Table 1–4. The most energy-rich of the nutrients is fat, which contains 9 calories in each gram. Carbohydrate and protein each contain only 4 calories in a gram. Weight, measure, and other conversion factors needed for the study of nutrition are found in Appendix C at the back of the book.

Scientists have worked out ways to measure the energy and nutrient contents of foods. They have also calculated the amounts of energy and nutrients various types of people need—by gender, age, life stage, and activity. Thus, after studying human nutrient requirements (in Chapter 2), you will be able to state with some accuracy just what your own body needs—this much water, that much carbohydrate, so much vitamin C, and so forth. So why not simply take pills or **dietary supplements** in place of food? Because, as it turns out, food offers more than just the six basic nutrients.

energy-yielding nutrients   the nutrients the body can use for energy—carbohydrate, fat, and protein. These also may supply building blocks for body structures. Also called *macronutrients*.

essential nutrients   the nutrients the body cannot make for itself (or cannot make fast enough) from other raw materials; nutrients that must be obtained from food to prevent deficiencies.

calories   units of energy. In nutrition science, the unit used to measure the energy in foods is a kilocalorie (also called *kcalorie* or *Calorie*): it is the amount of heat energy necessary to raise the temperature of a kilogram (a liter) of water 1 degree Celsius. This book follows the common practice of using the lowercase term *calorie* (abbreviated *cal*) to mean the same thing.

KEY POINTS

- The energy-yielding nutrients are carbohydrates, fats (lipids), and protein.
- The regulator nutrients are vitamins and minerals.
- Foremost among the nutrients in food is water.
- Essential nutrients in the diet prevent deficiencies.
- Food energy is measured in calories; nutrient quantities are often measured in grams.

Can I Live on Just Supplements?

Nutrition science can state what nutrients human beings need to survive—at least for a time. Scientists are becoming skilled at making **elemental diets**—life-saving liquid diets of precise chemical composition for hospital patients and others who cannot eat ordinary food. These formulas, administered for days or weeks, support not only continued life but also recovery from nutrient deficiencies, infections, and wounds. Formulas can also stave off weight loss in the elderly or anyone in whom eating is impaired.

Formula diets are essential to help sick people to survive, but they do not enable people to thrive over long periods. Even in hospitals, elemental diet formulas do not support optimal growth and health and may even lead to medical complications. Although serious problems are rare and can be detected and corrected, they show that the composition of these diets is not yet perfect for all people in all settings.

Lately, marketers have taken these liquid supplement formulas out of the medical setting and have advertised them heavily to healthy people of all ages as "meal replacers" or "insurance" against malnutrition. The truth is that real food is superior to such supplements. Most healthy people who eat a nutritious diet need no dietary supplements at all.

Food Is Best Even if a person's basic nutrient needs are perfectly understood and met, concoctions of nutrients still lack something that foods provide. Hospitalized clients who are fed nutrient mixtures through a vein often improve dramatically when they can finally eat food. Something in real food is important to health—but what is it? What does food offer that cannot be provided through a needle or a tube? Science has some partial explanations, some physical and some psychological.

In the digestive tract, the stomach and intestine are dynamic, living organs, changing constantly in response to the foods they receive—even to just the sight, aroma, and taste of food. When a person is fed through a vein, the digestive organs, like unused muscles, weaken and grow smaller. Medical wisdom now dictates that a person should be fed through a vein for as short a time as possible and that real food taken by mouth should be reintroduced as early as possible. The digestive organs also release hormones in response to food, and these send messages to the brain that bring the eater a feeling of satisfaction: "There, that was good. Now I'm full." Eating offers both physical and emotional comfort.

Complex Interactions Foods are chemically complex. In addition to their nutrients, foods contain **phytochemicals**, compounds that confer color, taste, and other characteristics to foods. Some may be **bioactive** food components that interact with metabolic processes in the body and may affect disease risks. Even an ordinary baked potato contains hundreds of different compounds. Nutrients and other food components interact with each other in the body and operate best in harmony with one another. In view of all this, it is not surprising that food gives us more than just nutrients. If it were otherwise, *that* would be surprising.

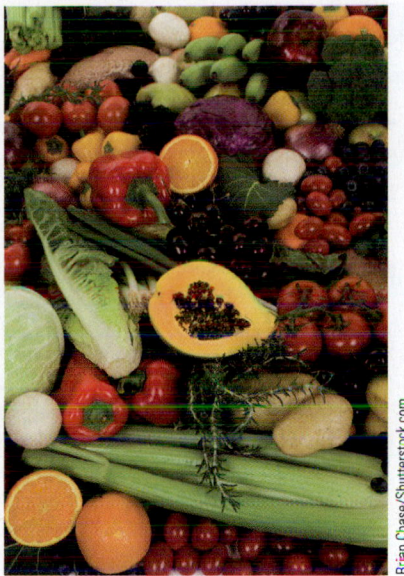

Some foods offer phytochemicals in addition to the six classes of nutrients.

Brian Chase/Shutterstock.com

KEY POINTS

- Nutritious food is superior to supplements for maintaining optimal health.
- Most healthy people who eat a nutritious diet do not need supplements at all.

The Challenge of Choosing Foods

LO 1.4 Recognize the challenges and solutions to a health-promoting diet.

Well-planned meals convey pleasure and are nutritious, too, fitting your tastes, personality, family and cultural traditions, lifestyle, and budget. Given the astounding numbers and varieties available, a consumer can easily lose track of what individual foods contain and how to put them together into a health-promoting diet. A few definitions and basic guidelines can help.

The Abundance of Foods to Choose From

A list of the foods available 100 years ago would be relatively short. It would consist mostly of **whole foods**—foods that have been around for a long time, such as vegetables, fruits, meats, milk, and grains (see Table 1–5 for a glossary of food types, p. 10). These foods have been called basic, unprocessed, natural, or farm foods. By whatever name, choosing a sufficient variety of these foods each day is an easy way to obtain a nutritious diet. On a given day, however, well over 80 percent of our population

dietary supplements pills, liquids, or powders that contain purified nutrients or other ingredients (see Controversy in Chapter 7).

elemental diets diets composed of purified ingredients of known chemical composition; intended to supply all essential nutrients to people who cannot eat foods.

phytochemicals compounds in plant-derived foods (*phyto*, pronounced FYE-toe, means "plant").

bioactive having chemical or physical properties that affect the functions of the body tissues. See also the Controversy in Chapter 2.

Table 1–5

Glossary of Food Types

- **enriched foods** and **fortified foods** foods to which nutrients have been added. If the starting material is a whole, basic food such as milk or whole grain, the result may be highly nutritious. If the starting material is a concentrated form of sugar or fat, the result is likely to be less nutritious.
- **fast foods** restaurant foods that are available within minutes after customers order them—traditionally, hamburgers, French fries, and milkshakes; more recently, salads and other vegetable dishes as well. These foods may or may not meet people's nutrient needs, depending on the selections made and on the energy allowances and nutrient needs of the eaters.
- **functional foods** whole or modified foods that contain bioactive food components believed to provide health benefits, such as reduced disease risks, beyond the benefits that their nutrients confer. However, all nutritious foods can support health in some ways; Controversy 2 provides details.
- **medical foods** foods specially manufactured for use by people with medical disorders and administered on the advice of a physician.
- **natural foods** a term that has no legal definition but is often used to imply wholesomeness.

- **organic foods** understood to mean foods grown without synthetic pesticides or fertilizers. In chemistry, however, all foods are made mostly of organic (carbon-containing) compounds.
- **processed foods** foods subjected to any process, such as milling, alteration of texture, addition of additives, cooking, or others. Depending on the starting material and the process, a processed food may or may not be nutritious.
- **staple foods** foods used frequently or daily—for example, rice (in East and Southeast Asia) or potatoes (in Ireland). If well chosen, these foods are nutritious.
- **ultra-processed foods** a term used to describe products of manufacturing made from industrial ingredients and additives, such as sugars, refined starches, fats, imitation flavors and colors, or industrial remnants, such as meat fats and scraps, with little or no whole food added. They are often high in fat, sugar, salt, and calories, and heavily advertised.
- **whole foods** milk and milk products; meats and similar foods such as fish and poultry; vegetables, including dried beans and peas; fruits; and grains. These foods are generally considered to form the basis of a nutritious diet. Also called *basic foods*.

consumes too few servings of fruit and vegetables each day.[4] And when people do choose to eat a vegetable, the one they most often choose is potatoes, usually prepared as French fries. Such choices, repeated over time, make development of chronic diseases more likely.

The number of foods supplied by the food industry today is astounding. Tens of thousands of foods now line the market shelves—many are processed mixtures of the basic ones, and some are constructed entirely from highly processed ingredients. Ironically, this abundance often makes it more difficult, rather than easier, to plan a nutritious diet.

The food-related terms defined in Table 1–5 reveal that all types of food—including **fast foods**, **processed foods**, and **ultra-processed foods**—offer various constituents to the eater. You may also hear about **functional foods**, a marketing term coined to identify those foods containing substances, natural or added, that might

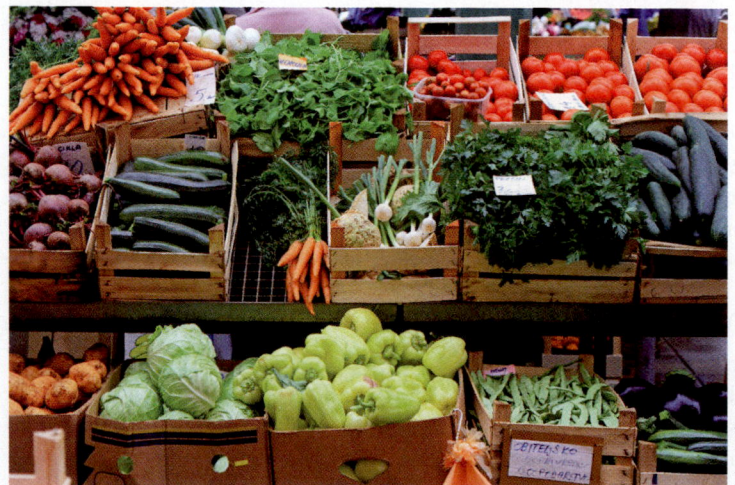

All foods once looked like this . . .

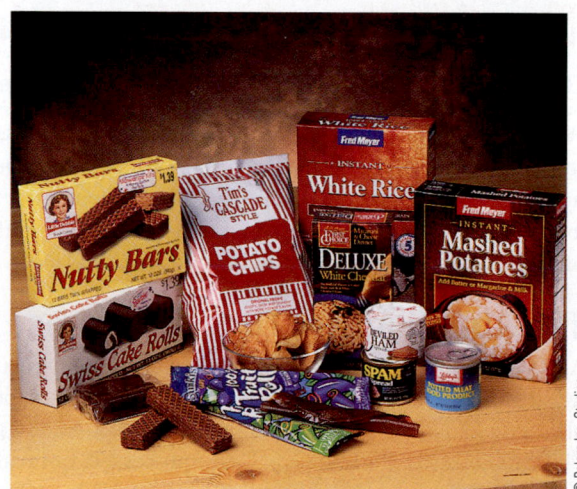

. . . but now many foods look like this.

lend protection against chronic diseases. The trouble with trying to single out the most health-promoting foods is that almost every naturally occurring food—even chocolate—is functional in some way with regard to human health.[5]

The extent to which foods support good health depends on the calories, nutrients, and phytochemicals they contain. In short, to select well among foods, you need to know more than their names; you need to know the foods' inner qualities. Even more important, you need to know how to combine foods into nutritious diets. Foods are not nutritious by themselves; each is of value only insofar as it contributes to a nutritious diet. A key to wise diet planning is to make sure that the foods you eat daily, your **staple foods**, are especially nutritious.

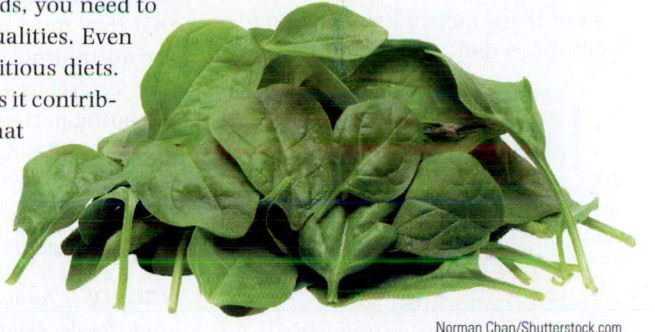
Norman Chan/Shutterstock.com

KEY POINT

- Foods that form the basis of a nutritious diet are whole foods, such as ordinary milk and milk products; meats, fish, and poultry; vegetables and dried peas and beans; fruits; and grains.

How, Exactly, Can I Recognize a Nutritious Diet?

A nutritious diet is really an **eating pattern**, a habitual way of choosing foods, with five characteristics. First is **adequacy**: the foods provide enough of each essential nutrient, fiber, and energy. Second is **balance**: the choices do not overemphasize one nutrient or food type at the expense of another. Third is **calorie control**: the foods provide the amount of energy you need to maintain appropriate weight—not more, not less. Fourth is **moderation**: the foods do not provide excess fat, salt, sugar, or other unwanted constituents. Fifth is **variety**: the foods chosen differ from one day to the next. In addition, to maintain a steady supply of nutrients, meals should occur with regular timing throughout the day. To recap, then, a nutritious diet is an eating pattern that follows the A, B, C, M, V principles: Adequacy, Balance, Calorie control, Moderation, and Variety.

Adequacy   Any nutrient could be used to demonstrate the importance of dietary adequacy. Iron provides a familiar example. It is an essential nutrient: you lose some every day, so you have to keep replacing it, and you can get it into your body only by eating foods that contain it.* If you eat too few of the iron-containing foods, you can develop iron-deficiency anemia. With anemia, you may feel weak, tired, cold, sad, and unenthusiastic; you may have frequent headaches; and you can do very little muscular work without disabling fatigue. Some foods are rich in iron; others are notoriously poor. If you add iron-rich foods to your diet, you soon feel more energetic. Meat, fish, poultry, and **legumes** are in the iron-rich category, and an easy way to obtain the needed iron is to include these foods in your diet regularly.

Balance   To appreciate the importance of dietary balance, consider a second essential nutrient, calcium. A diet lacking calcium causes poor bone development during the growing years and increases a person's susceptibility to disabling bone loss in adult life. Most foods that are rich in iron are poor in calcium. Calcium's richest food sources are milk and milk products, which happen to be extraordinarily poor iron sources. Clearly, to obtain enough of both iron and calcium, people have to balance their food choices among the types of foods that provide both nutrients. Balancing the whole diet to provide enough of every one of the 40-odd nutrients the body needs for health requires considerable juggling, however. As you will see in Chapter 2, food group plans ease this task by clustering rich sources of nutrients into food groups that will help you to achieve both dietary adequacy and balance within an eating pattern that meets your needs.

Calorie Control   Energy intakes should not exceed or fall short of energy needs. Named *calorie control*, this characteristic ensures that energy intakes from food balance energy expenditures required for body functions and physical activity.

---

*A person can also take supplements of iron, but as later discussions demonstrate, eating iron-rich foods is preferable.

eating pattern the combination of foods and beverages that constitute an individual's complete dietary intake over time; a person's usual diet.

adequacy the dietary characteristic of providing all of the essential nutrients, fiber, and energy in amounts sufficient to maintain health and body weight.

balance the dietary characteristic of providing foods of a number of types in proportion to each other, such that foods rich in some nutrients do not crowd out of the diet foods that are rich in other nutrients.

calorie control the dietary characteristic of controlling energy intake; a feature of a sound diet plan.

moderation the dietary characteristic of providing constituents within set limits, not to excess.

variety the dietary characteristic of providing a wide selection of foods—the opposite of monotony.

legumes (leg-GOOMS, LEG-yooms) beans, peas, and lentils, valued as inexpensive sources of protein, vitamins, minerals, and fiber that contribute little fat to the diet. Also defined in Chapter 6.

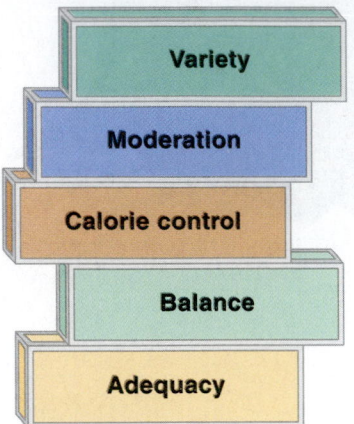

Eating such a diet helps to control body fat content and weight. The many strategies that promote this goal appear in Chapter 9.

Moderation   Intakes of certain food constituents such as saturated fats, added sugars, and salt should be limited for health's sake. Some people take this to mean that they must never indulge in a delicious beefsteak or hot-fudge sundae, but they are misinformed: moderation, not total abstinence, is the key.[6] A steady diet of steak and ice cream might be harmful, but once a week as part of an otherwise healthful eating pattern, these foods may have little impact; as once-a-month treats, these foods would have practically no effect at all. Moderation also means that limits are necessary, even for desirable food constituents. For example, a certain amount of fiber in foods contributes to the health of the digestive system, but too much fiber leads to nutrient losses.

Variety   As for variety, nutrition scientists agree that people should not eat the same foods, even highly nutritious ones, day after day, for a number of reasons. First, a varied diet is more likely to be adequate in nutrients. Second, some less-well-known nutrients and phytochemicals could be important to health, and some foods may be better sources of these than others. Third, a monotonous diet may deliver large amounts of toxins or contaminants. Such undesirable compounds in one food are diluted by all the other foods eaten with it and are diluted still further if the food is not eaten again for several days. Finally, variety adds interest—trying new foods can be a source of pleasure.

Variety applies to nutritious foods consumed within the context of all of the other dietary principles just discussed. Relying solely on the principle of variety to dictate food choices could easily result in a low-nutrient, high-calorie eating pattern with a variety of nutrient-poor snack foods and sweets. If you establish the habit of using all of the principles just described, you will find that choosing a healthful diet becomes as automatic as brushing your teeth or falling asleep. Establishing the A, B, C, M, V habit (summed up in Figure 1–3) may take some effort, but the payoff in terms of improved health is overwhelming. Table 1–6 takes an honest look at some common excuses for *not* eating well.

KEY POINT

- A well-planned diet is adequate, balanced, moderate in energy, and moderate in unwanted constituents and offers a variety of nutritious foods.

Why People Choose Foods

Eating is an intentional act. Each day, people choose from the available foods, prepare the foods, and decide where to eat, which customs to follow, and with whom to dine. Many factors influence food-related choices.

Table 1–6
What's Today's Excuse for Not Eating Well?

If you find yourself saying, "I know I should eat well, but I'm too busy" (or too fond of fast food, or have too little money, or a dozen other excuses), take note:

- *No time to cook.* Everyone is busy. Convenience packages of fresh or frozen vegetables, jars of pasta sauce, and prepared meats and salads make nutritious meals in little time.
- *Not a high priority.* Priorities change drastically and instantly when illness strikes—better to spend a little effort now nourishing your body's defenses than to spend enormous resources later fighting illnesses.
- *Crave fast food and sweets.* Occasional fast-food meals and sweets in moderation are acceptable in a nutritious diet.
- *Too little money.* Eating right often costs no more than eating poorly. Chips, colas, snack cakes, and premium ice cream cost as much or more per serving as nutritious foods.[a]
- *Take vitamins instead.* Vitamin pills or even advertised "nutritional drinks" cannot make up for consistently poor food choices.

[a]For a discussion of this topic, see A. Carlson and E. Frazão, *Are healthy foods really more expensive? It depends on how you measure the price*, Economic Research Service EIB-96, *May 2012*, available at www.ers.usda.gov/publications/eib-economic-information-bulletin/eib96.aspx.

Cultural and Social Meanings Attached to Food

Like wearing traditional clothing or speaking a native language, enjoying traditional **cuisines** and **foodways** can be a celebration of your own or a friend's heritage. Sharing **ethnic foods** can be symbolic: people offering foods are expressing a willingness to share cherished values with others. People accepting those foods are symbolically accepting not only the person doing the offering but also the person's culture. Developing **cultural competence** is particularly important for professionals who help others to achieve a nutritious diet.[7]

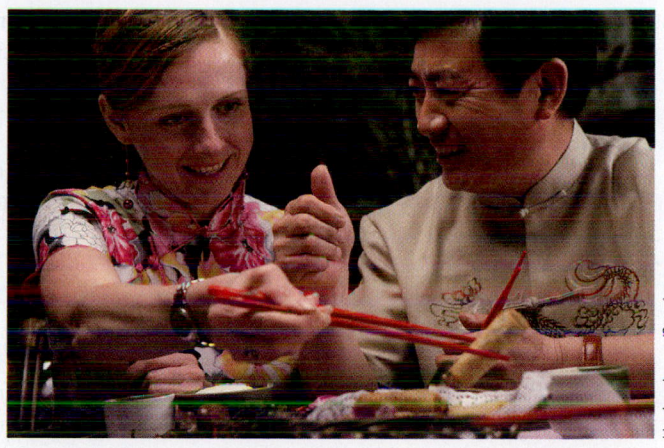

Sharing traditional food is a way of sharing culture.

Cultural traditions regarding food are not inflexible; they keep evolving as people move about, learn about new foods, and teach each other. Today, some people are ceasing to be **omnivorous** and are becoming **vegetarians**. Vegetarians often choose this lifestyle because they honor the lives of animals or because they have discovered the health and other advantages associated with eating patterns rich in beans, whole grains, fruits, nuts, and vegetables. The Chapter 6 Controversy explores the strengths and weaknesses of both the vegetarian's and the meat eater's diets.

Factors That Drive Food Choices

Taste prevails as the number-one factor driving people's food choices, with price following closely behind.[8] Consumers also value convenience so highly that they are willing to spend almost half of their food budget on meals prepared outside the home. They frequently eat out, bring home ready-to-eat meals, or have food delivered. In their own kitchens, they want to prepare a meal in 15 to 20 minutes, using only a few ingredients. Such convenience has a cost in terms of nutrition, however: eating away from home reduces intakes of fruit, vegetables, milk, and whole grains. It also increases intakes of calories, saturated fat, sodium, and added sugars.[9] Convenience doesn't have to mean that nutrition is out the window, however. This chapter's Food Feature (p. 21) explores the trade-offs of time, money, and nutrition that many busy people face today.

Many other factors—psychological, physical, social, and philosophical—also influence how people choose which foods to eat. Some factors include:

- *Advertising.* The media have persuaded you to consume these foods.
- *Availability.* They are present in the environment and accessible to you.
- *Cost.* They are within your financial means.
- *Emotional comfort.* They can make you feel better for a while.
- *Habit.* They are familiar; you always eat them.
- *Personal preference and genetic inheritance.* You like the way these foods taste.
- *Positive or negative associations.*[10] *Positive:* They are eaten by people you admire, or they indicate status, or they remind you of fun. *Negative:* They were forced on you, or you became ill while eating them.
- *Region of the country.* They are foods favored in your area.
- *Social norms.* Your companions are eating them, or they are offered and you feel you can't refuse them.[11]
- *Values or beliefs.* They fit your religious tradition, square with your political views, or honor the environmental ethic.
- *Weight.* You think they will help to control body weight.
- *Nutrition and health benefits.* You think they are good for you.

College students often choose to eat at fast-food and other restaurants to socialize, to get out, to save time, or to date; they are not always conscious of their body's need for nutritious food.

cuisines styles of cooking.

foodways the sum of a culture's habits, customs, beliefs, and preferences concerning food.

ethnic foods foods associated with particular cultural subgroups within a population.

cultural competence having an awareness and acceptance of one's own and others' cultures and abilities, leading to effective interactions with all kinds of people.

omnivorous people who eat foods of both plant and animal origin, including animal flesh.

vegetarians people who exclude from their diets animal flesh and possibly other animal products such as milk, cheese, and eggs.

Nutrition understanding depends upon a firm base of scientific knowledge. The next section describes the nature of such knowledge and addresses one of the "how" questions posed earlier in this chapter: How do we know what we know about nutrition?

The Science of Nutrition

LO 1.5 Describe the science of nutrition.

Nutrition is a science—a field of knowledge composed of organized facts. Unlike sciences such as astronomy and physics, nutrition is a relatively young science. Most nutrition research has been conducted since 1900. The first vitamin was identified in 1897, and the first protein structure was not fully described until the mid-1940s. Because nutrition science is an active, changing, growing body of knowledge, scientific findings often seem to contradict one another or are subject to conflicting interpretations. Bewildered consumers complain in frustration, "Those scientists don't know anything. If they don't know what's true, how am I supposed to know?"

Yet many facts in nutrition are known with great certainty. To understand why apparent contradictions sometimes arise in nutrition science, we need to look first at what scientists do.

The Scientific Approach

In truth, it is a scientist's business not to know. Scientists obtain facts by systematically asking honest, objective questions—that's their job. Following the scientific method (outlined in Figure 1–4), they attempt to answer scientific questions. They design and conduct various experiments to test for possible answers (see Figure 1–5, and Table 1–7 on p. 16). When they have ruled out some possibilities and found evidence for others, they submit their findings not to the news media but to boards of reviewers composed of other scientists who try to pick the findings apart. Finally, the work is published in scientific journals where still more scientists can read it. Then the news reporters read it and write about it, and the public can read about it, too.

KEY POINTS

- Nutrition is a young and fast-growing science.
- Scientists ask questions and then design research experiments to test possible answers.
- Researchers follow the scientific method and apply it to various research study designs.

Scientific Challenge

An important truth in science is that one experiment does not "prove" or "disprove" anything. Even after publication, other scientists try

Figure 1–4

The Scientific Method

Research scientists follow the scientific method. Note that most research projects result in new questions, not final answers. Thus, research continues in a somewhat cyclical manner.

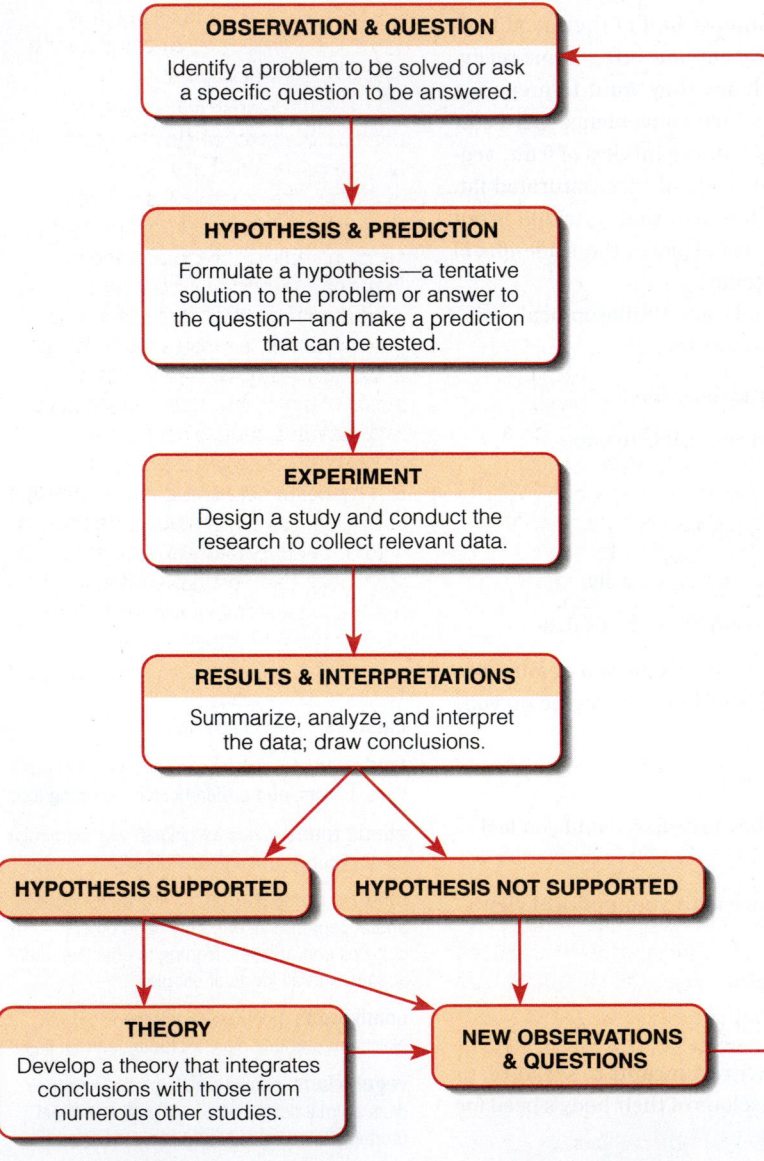

OBSERVATION & QUESTION
Identify a problem to be solved or ask a specific question to be answered.

HYPOTHESIS & PREDICTION
Formulate a hypothesis—a tentative solution to the problem or answer to the question—and make a prediction that can be tested.

EXPERIMENT
Design a study and conduct the research to collect relevant data.

RESULTS & INTERPRETATIONS
Summarize, analyze, and interpret the data; draw conclusions.

HYPOTHESIS SUPPORTED

HYPOTHESIS NOT SUPPORTED

THEORY
Develop a theory that integrates conclusions with those from numerous other studies.

NEW OBSERVATIONS & QUESTIONS

Figure 1–5
Examples of Research Design

Case Study

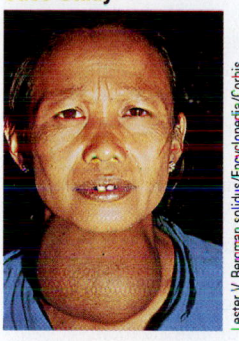

"This person eats too little of nutrient X and has illness Y."

Epidemiological Study

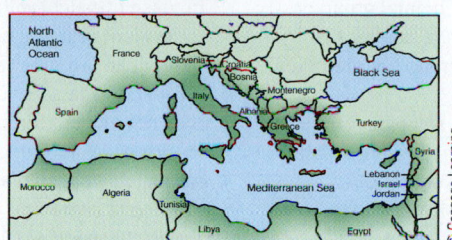

"This country's food supply contains more nutrient X, and these people suffer less illness Y."

Intervention Study

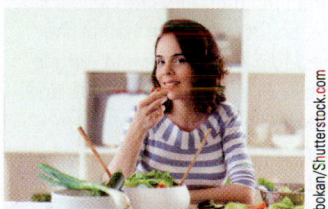

"Let's add foods containing nutrient X to some people's food supply and compare their rates of illness Y with the rates of others who don't receive the nutrient."

Laboratory Study

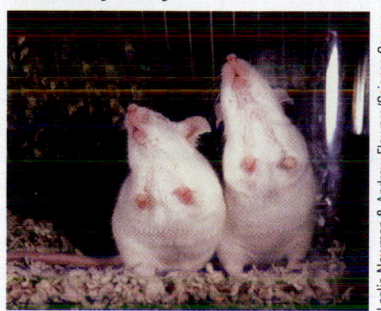

"Now let's prove that a nutrient X deficiency causes illness Y by inducing a deficiency in these rats."

The type of study chosen for research depends upon what sort of information the researchers require. Studies of individuals (**case studies**) yield observations that may lead to possible avenues of research. A study of a man who ate gumdrops and became a famous dancer might suggest that an experiment be done to see if gumdrops contain dance-enhancing power.

Studies of whole populations (**epidemiological studies**) provide another sort of information. Such a study can reveal a **correlation**. For example, an epidemiological study might find no worldwide correlation of gumdrop eating with fancy footwork but, unexpectedly, might reveal a correlation with tooth decay.

Studies in which researchers actively intervene to alter people's eating habits (**intervention studies**) go a step further. In such a study, one set of subjects (the **experimental group**) receives a treatment, and another set (the **control group**) goes untreated or receives a **placebo** or sham treatment. If the study is a **blind experiment**, the subjects do not know who among the members receives the treatment and who receives the sham. If the two groups experience different effects, then the treatment's effect can be pinpointed. For example, an intervention study might show that withholding gumdrops, together with other candies and confections, reduced the incidence of tooth decay in an experimental population compared to that in a control population.

Finally, **laboratory studies** can pinpoint the mechanisms by which nutrition acts. What is it about gumdrops that contributes to tooth decay: their size, shape, temperature, color, ingredients? Feeding various forms of gumdrops to rats might yield the information that sugar, in a gummy carrier, promotes tooth decay. In the laboratory, using animals or plants or cells, scientists can inoculate with diseases, induce deficiencies, and experiment with variations on treatments to obtain in-depth knowledge of the process under study. Intervention studies and laboratory experiments are among the most powerful tools in nutrition research because they show the effects of treatments.

---

to duplicate the work of the first researchers to support or refute the original finding.

Only when a finding has stood up to rigorous, repeated testing in several kinds of experiments performed by several different researchers is it finally considered confirmed. Even then, strictly speaking, science consists not of facts that are set in stone but of *theories* that can always be challenged and revised. Some findings, though, like the theory that the earth revolves about the sun, are so well supported by observations and experimental findings that they are generally accepted as facts. What we "know" in nutrition is confirmed in the same way—through years of replicating study findings. This slow path of repeated studies stands in sharp contrast to the media's desire for today's latest news.[12]

To repeat: the only source of valid nutrition information is slow, painstaking, authentic scientific research. We believe a nutrition fact to be true because it has

Table 1-7

Research Design Terms

- **blind experiment** an experiment in which the subjects do not know whether they are members of the experimental group or the control group. In a *double-blind experiment*, neither the subjects nor the researchers know to which group the members belong until the end of the experiment.
- **case studies** studies of individuals. In clinical settings, researchers can observe treatments and their apparent effects. To prove that a treatment has produced an effect requires simultaneous observation of an untreated similar subject (a *case control*).
- **control group** a group of individuals who are similar in all possible respects to the group being treated in an experiment but who receive a sham treatment instead of the real one. Also called *control subjects*. See also *experimental group* and *intervention studies*.
- **controlled clinical trial** a research study design that often reveals effects of a treatment on human beings. Health outcomes are observed in a group of people who receive the treatment and are then compared with outcomes in a control group of similar people who received a placebo (an inert or sham treatment). Ideally, neither subjects nor researchers know who receives the treatment and who gets the placebo (a double-blind study).

- **correlation** the simultaneous change of two factors, such as the increase of weight with increasing height (a *direct* or *positive* correlation) or the decrease of cancer incidence with increasing fiber intake (an *inverse* or *negative* correlation). A correlation between two factors suggests that one may cause the other but does not rule out the possibility that both may be caused by chance or by a third factor.
- **epidemiological studies** studies of populations; often used in nutrition to search for correlations between dietary habits and disease incidence; a first step in seeking nutrition-related causes of diseases.
- **experimental group** the people or animals participating in an experiment who receive the treatment under investigation. Also called *experimental subjects*. See also *control group* and *intervention studies*.
- **intervention studies** studies of populations in which observation is accompanied by experimental manipulation of some population members—for example, a study in which half of the subjects (the *experimental subjects*) follow diet advice to reduce fat intakes, while the other half (the *control subjects*) do not, and both groups' heart health is monitored.
- **laboratory studies** studies that are performed under tightly controlled conditions and are designed to pinpoint causes and effects. Such studies often use animals as subjects.
- **placebo** a sham treatment often used in scientific studies; an inert, harmless medication. The *placebo effect* is the healing effect that the act of treatment, rather than the treatment itself, often has.

been supported, time and again, in experiments designed to rule out all other possibilities. For example, we know that eyesight depends partly on vitamin A because:

- In case studies, individuals with blindness report having consumed a steady diet devoid of vitamin A; and

- In epidemiological studies, populations with diets lacking in vitamin A are observed to suffer high rates of blindness; and

- In intervention studies (**controlled clinical trials**), vitamin A–rich foods provided to groups of vitamin A–deficient people reduce their blindness rates dramatically; and

- In laboratory studies, animals deprived of vitamin A and only that vitamin begin to go blind; when it is restored soon enough in the diet, their eyesight returns; and

- Further laboratory studies elucidated the molecular mechanisms for vitamin A activity in eye tissues; and

- Replication of these studies provides the same results.

    Now we can say with certainty, "Eyesight depends upon sufficient vitamin A."

KEY POINTS

- Single studies must be replicated before their findings can be considered valid.
- A theory is strengthened when results from follow-up studies with a variety of research designs support it.

Can I Trust the Media to Deliver Nutrition News?

The news media are hungry for new findings, and reporters often latch onto hypotheses from scientific laboratories before they have been fully tested. Also, a reporter who lacks a strong understanding of science may misunderstand or misreport complex scientific principles.[13] To tell the truth, sometimes scientists get excited about their findings, too, and leak them to the press before they have been through a rigorous review by the scientists' peers. As a result, the public is often exposed to late-breaking nutrition news stories before the findings are fully confirmed. Then, when the hypothesis being tested fails to hold up to a later challenge, consumers feel betrayed by what is simply the normal course of science at work.

The real scientists are trend watchers. They evaluate the methods used in each study, assess each study in light of the evidence gleaned from other studies, and modify little by little their picture of what may be true. As evidence accumulates, the scientists become more and more confident about their ability to make recommendations that apply to people's health and lives. The Consumer's Guide section (p. 19) offers some tips for evaluating news stories about nutrition.

Sometimes media sensationalism overrates the importance of even true, replicated findings. For example, the media eagerly report that oat products lower blood cholesterol, a lipid indicative of heart disease risk. Although the reports are true, they often fail to mention that eating a nutritious diet that is low in certain fats is still the major step toward lowering blood cholesterol. They also may skip over important questions: How much oatmeal must a person eat to produce the desired effect? Do little oat bran pills or powders meet the need? Do oat bran cookies? If so, how many cookies? For oatmeal, it takes a bowl and a half daily to affect blood lipids. A few pills or cookies do not provide nearly so much and certainly cannot undo all the damage from a high-fat meal.

Today, the cholesterol-lowering effect of oats is well established. The whole process of discovery, challenge, and vindication took almost 10 years of research. Some other lines of research have taken much longer. In science, a single finding almost never makes a crucial difference to our knowledge, but like each individual frame in a movie, it contributes a little to the big picture. Many such frames are needed to tell the whole story.

KEY POINT

- News media often sensationalize single-study findings and so may not be trustworthy sources.

National Nutrition Research

As you study nutrition, you are likely to hear of findings based on ongoing nationwide nutrition and health research projects.[14] A national food and nutrient intake survey, called *What We Eat in America*, reveals what we know about the population's food and supplement intakes. It is conducted as part of a larger research effort, the **National Health and Nutrition Examination Surveys (NHANES)**, that also

My Turn

watch it!

Lose Weight While You Sleep!

See a student talking about how he learned the truth about nutrition claims made in advertising.

Visit www.cengagebrain.com to access MindTap, a complete digital course that includes this video and other resources.

Gabriel

© Cengage Learning

National Health and Nutrition Examination Surveys (NHANES) a program of studies designed to assess the health and nutritional status of adults and children in the United States by way of interviews and physical examinations.

conducts physical examinations and measurements and laboratory tests. Boiled down to its essence, NHANES involves:

- Asking people what they have eaten and
- Recording measures of their health status.

Past NHANES results have provided important data for developing growth charts for children, guiding food fortification efforts, developing national guidelines for reducing chronic diseases, and many other beneficial programs. Some agencies involved with these efforts are listed in Table 1–8.

KEY POINT

- National nutrition research projects, such as NHANES, provide data on U.S. food consumption and nutrient status.

Table 1–8

Nutrition Research and Policy Agencies

These agencies are actively engaged in nutrition policy development, research, and monitoring:

- Centers for Disease Control and Prevention (CDC)
- U.S. Department of Agriculture (USDA)
- U.S. Department of Health and Human Services (DHHS)
- U.S. Food and Drug Administration (FDA)

Changing Behaviors

LO 1.6 Explain the significance of behavior change in improving a person's diet.

Nutrition knowledge is of little value if it only helps people to make A's on tests. The value comes when people use it to improve their diets. To act on knowledge, people must change their behaviors, and while this may sound simple enough, behavior change often takes substantial effort.

The Process of Change

Psychologists often describe the six stages of behavior change, offered in Table 1–9. Knowing where you stand in relation to these stages may help you move along the path toward achieving your goals. When offering diet help to others, keep in mind that their stages of change can influence their reaction to your message.

Table 1–9

The Stages of Behavior Change

Stage	Characteristics	Actions
Precontemplation	Not considering a change; have no intention of changing; see no problems with current behavior.	Collect information about health effects of current behavior and potential benefits of change.
Contemplation	Admit that change may be needed; weigh pros and cons of changing and not changing.	Commit to making a change and set a date to start.
Preparation	Preparing to change a specific behavior, taking initial steps, and setting some goals.	Write an action plan, spelling out specific parts of the change. Set small-step goals; tell others about the plan.
Action	Committing time and energy to making a change; following a plan set for a specific behavior change.	Perform the new behavior. Manage emotional and physical reactions to the change.
Maintenance	Striving to integrate the new behavior into daily life and striving to make it permanent.	Persevere through lapses. Teach others and help them achieve their own goals. (This stage can last for years.)
Adoption/Moving On	The former behavior is gone, and the new behavior is routine.	After months or a year of maintenance without lapses, move on to other goals.

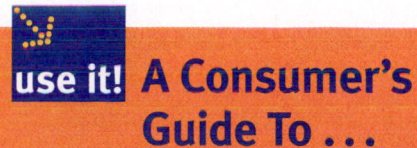
Reading Nutrition News

At a coffee shop, Nick, a health-conscious consumer, sets his cup down on the Lifestyle section of the newspaper. He glances at the headline—"Eating Fat OK for Heart Health!"—and jumps to a wrong conclusion: "Do you mean to say that I could have been eating burgers and butter all this time? I can't keep up! As soon as I change my diet, the scientists change their story." Nick's frustration is understandable. Like many others, he feels betrayed when, after working for years to make diet changes for his health's sake, headlines seem to turn dietary advice upside down. He shouldn't blame science, however.

Tricks and Traps

The trouble started when Nick was "hooked" by a catchy headline. Media headlines often seem to reverse current scientific thought because new "breakthrough" studies are exciting; they grab readers' attention and make them want to buy a newspaper, book, or magazine. (By the way, you can read the true story behind changing lipid intake guidelines in Controversy 5.) Even if Nick had read the entire newspaper article, he could have still been led astray by phrases like "Now we know" or "The truth is." Journalists use such phrases to imply finality, the last word.[1]* In contrast, scientists use tentative language, such as "may" or "might," because they know that the conclusions from one study will be challenged, refined, and even refuted by others that follow.

Markers of Authentic Reporting

To approach nutrition news with a trained eye, look for these signs of a scientific approach:

- When an article describes a scientific study, that study should have been published in a peer-reviewed journal, such as the *American Journal of Clinical Nutrition*. An unpublished study may or may not be valid; the reader has no way of knowing because the study lacks scrutiny by other experts.

- The news item should describe the researchers' methods; in truth, few popular reports provide these details. It matters whether the study participants numbered 8 or 80,000 or whether researchers personally observed participants' behaviors or relied on self-reports given over the telephone, for example.

- The report should define the study subjects—were they single cells, animals, or human beings? If they were human beings, the more you have in common with them (age and gender, for example), the more applicable the findings may be for you.

- Valid reports also present new findings in the context of previous research. Some reporters in popular media regularly follow developments in a research area and thus acquire the background knowledge needed to report meaningfully. They strive for adequacy, balance, and completeness, and they cover such things as cost of a treatment, potential harms and benefits, strength of evidence, and who might stand to gain from potential sales relating to the finding.**

- For a helpful *scientific* overview of current topics in nutrition, look for review articles written by experts. They regularly appear in scholarly journals such as *Nutrition Reviews*. A relative of the review article, the meta-analysis, uses the power of a computer to combine and reanalyze the results of many previously published studies on a single topic. The results of a

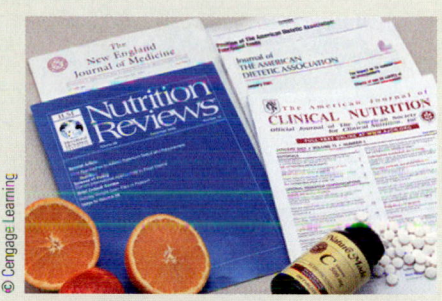

For the whole story on a nutrition topic, read articles from peer-reviewed journals such as these. A review journal examines all available evidence on major topics. Other journals report details of the methods, results, and conclusions of single studies.

meta-analysis study often do not apply to individuals, however.[2]

The most credible source of scientific nutrition information is the scientific journal. The Controversy section following this chapter addresses other sources of nutrition information and misinformation.

Moving Ahead

Develop a critical eye, and let scientific principles guide you as you read nutrition news. When a headline touts a shocking new "answer" to a nutrition question, approach it with caution. It may indeed be a carefully researched report that respects the gradual nature of scientific discovery and refinement, but more often it is a sensational news flash intended to grab your attention and your media dollars.

Review Questions[†]

1. To keep up with nutrition science, the consumer should _____.

   a. seek out the health and fitness sections of newspapers and magazines and read them with a trained eye

(continued)

*Reference notes are found in Appendix F.

**An organization that promotes valid health-care reporting is HealthNewsReview.org, available at www.healthnewsreview.org/.

[†]Answers to Consumer's Guide review questions are found in Appendix G.

b. read studies published in a peer-reviewed journal, such as the *American Journal of Clinical Nutrition*

c. look for review articles published in peer-reviewed journals, such as *Nutrition Reviews*

d. all of the above

2. To answer nutrition questions _____.

a. watch for articles that include phrases such as "Now we know" or "The answer is" that put nutrition issues to rest

b. look to science for answers, with the expectation that scientists will continually revise their understandings

c. realize that problems in nutrition are probably too complex for consumers to understand

d. a and c

3. Scholarly review journals such as *Nutrition Reviews* _____.

a. are behind the times when it comes to nutrition news

b. discuss all available research findings on a topic in nutrition

c. are filled with medical jargon

d. are intended for use by practitioners only, not students

Taking Stock and Setting Goals

To make a change, you must first become aware of a problem. Some problems, such as *never* consuming a vegetable, are easy to spot. More subtle dietary problems, such as failing to meet your need for calcium, may be hidden but can have serious repercussions for health. Tracking food intakes over several days' time and then comparing intakes to standards (see Chapter 2) can reveal all sorts of interesting tidbits about strengths and weaknesses of your eating pattern.

Once a weakness is identified, setting small, achievable goals to correct it becomes the next step to making improvements. The most successful goals are set for specific behaviors, not overall outcomes. For example, if losing 10 pounds is the desired outcome, goals should be set in terms of food intakes and physical activity to help achieve weight loss. After goals are set and changes are under way, a means of tracking progress increases the likelihood of success.

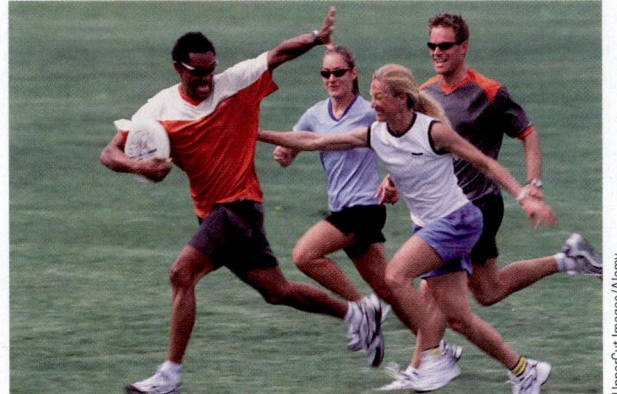

Many people need to change their daily routines to include physical activity.

UpperCut Images/Alamy

Start Now

You may, as you progress through this text, want to change some of your own habits. To help you, little reminders entitled "Start Now" close each chapter's Think Fitness section (on p. 5 in this chapter) with an invitation to visit this book's website, where you can take inventory of your current behaviors, set goals, track progress, and practice new behaviors until they become as comfortable and familiar as the old ones were.

KEY POINTS

- Behavior change follows a predictable pattern.
- Setting goals and monitoring progress facilitate behavior change.

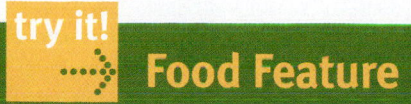
How Can I Get Enough Nutrients Without Consuming Too Many Calories?

LO 1.7 Discuss the importance of nutrient density in creating an effective diet plan.

In the United States, only a tiny percentage of adults manage to choose an eating pattern that achieves both adequacy and calorie control. The foods that can help in doing so are foods richly endowed with nutrients relative to their energy contents; that is, they are foods with high **nutrient density**. Figure 1–6 is a simple depiction of this concept. Consider calcium sources, for example. Ice cream and fat-free milk both supply calcium, but a cup of rich ice cream contributes more than 350 calories, whereas a cup of fat-free milk has only 85—and almost double the calcium. Most people cannot, for their health's sake, afford to choose foods without regard to their energy contents. Those who do very often exceed calorie allowances while leaving nutrient needs unmet.

Among foods that often rank high in nutrient density are the vegetables, particularly the nonstarchy vegetables such as dark leafy greens (cooked and raw), red bell peppers, broccoli, carrots, mushrooms, and tomatoes.[15] These inexpensive foods take time to prepare, but time invested in this way pays off in nutritional health. Twenty minutes spent peeling and slicing vegetables for a salad is a better investment in nutrition than 20 minutes spent fixing a fancy, high-fat, high-sugar dessert. Besides, the dessert ingredients often cost more money and strain the calorie budget, too.

Time, however, is a concern to many people. Today's working families, college students, and active people of all ages may have little time to devote to food preparation. Busy cooks should seek out convenience foods that are

nutrient-dense, such as bags of ready-to-serve salads, ready-to-cook fresh vegetables, refrigerated prepared low-fat meats and poultry, canned beans, and frozen vegetables. A tip for lower-cost convenience is to double the amount of whole vegetables for a recipe; wash, peel, and chop them; and then refrigerate or freeze the extra to use on another day.*

*For freezing instructions, see www.fsis.usda.gov/wps/portal/fsis/topics/food-safety-education/get-answers/food-safety-fact-sheets/safe-food-handling/freezing-and-food-safety. For other tips on low-cost, convenient, and healthy eating, see www.choosemyplate.gov/budget/index.html.

Dried fruit and dry-roasted nuts require only that they be kept on hand and make a tasty, nutritious topper for salads and other foods. To round out the meal, fat-free milk or yogurt is both nutritious and convenient. Other convenience selections, such as most pot pies, many frozen pizzas, ramen noodles, and "pocket" style sandwiches, are less nutritious overall because they contain too few vegetables and too many calories, making them low in nutrient density. The Food Features of later chapters offer many more tips

Figure 1–6

A Way to Judge Which Foods Are Most Nutritious

These two breakfasts provide about 500 calories each, but they differ greatly in the nutrients they provide per calorie. Note that the sausage in the larger breakfast is lower-calorie turkey sausage, not the high-calorie pork variety. Making small changes like this at each meal can add up to large calorie savings, making room in the diet for more servings of nutritious foods and even some treats.

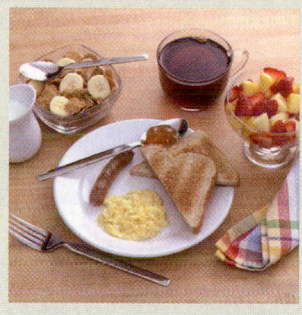

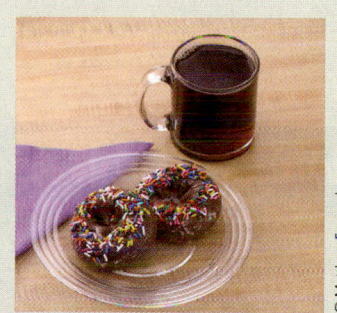

© Matthew Farruggio

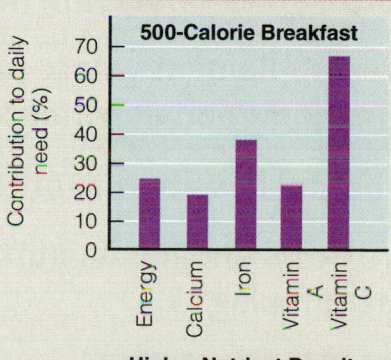

Higher Nutrient Density

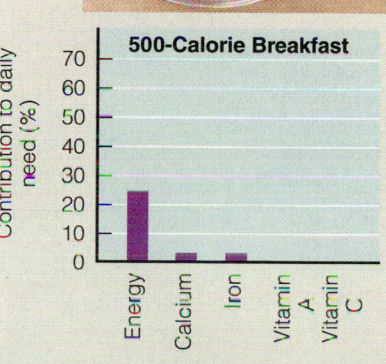

Lower Nutrient Density

nutrient density a measure of nutrients provided per calorie of food. A *nutrient-dense food* provides vitamins, minerals, and other beneficial substances with relatively few calories.

for choosing convenient and nutritious foods.

All of this discussion leads to a principle that is central to achieving nutritional health: No particular foods must be included or excluded in the diet. Instead, your eating pattern—the way you combine foods into meals and the way you arrange meals to follow one another over days and weeks—determines how well you are nourishing yourself.[16] Nutrition is a science, not an art, but it can be used artfully to create a pleasing, nourishing diet. The remainder of this book is dedicated to helping you make informed choices and combine them artfully to meet all the body's needs.

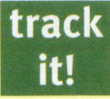

track it! DIET & WELLNESS **PLUS+** Concepts in Action

Track Your Diet

After each Food Feature section in this text, exercises like this one provide an ongoing diet analysis activity that asks you to apply what you've learned in the chapter to your own diet. To do so, access the Diet & Wellness Plus (D&W+) program that accompanies this book. Then do the following:

1. From the Home page of the D&W+ program (after entering your personal data), select the Reports tab from the red navigation bar, and then select DRI Report. Click Save as PDF button. You will now have a list of the appropriate DRI values for calories, carbohydrates, and fat for your Profile.

2. For the next three days, with pencil and paper, keep track of everything you eat and drink. Be honest and careful in your record keeping. Measure or estimate amounts of foods and beverages you consume, as well as margarine or butter, salt, cream sauces, gravies, pasta sauce, ketchup, relish, jams, jellies, and other add-ons. Even a slice of tomato and a lettuce leaf on a sandwich count toward the day's intake. Distribute your data among meals for each day: breakfast, lunch, dinner, and snacks.

3. Keep track of your physical activity for all three of those days. Record all the minutes spent walking or biking to class, working out, vacuuming rugs, washing cars, playing sports, dancing with friends, or any other nonsedentary behavior. Hold onto these data: you'll need them in chapters to come.

4. From the Home page of D&W+, select the Track Diet tab, select a date, and enter each food item you recorded for day one into the Search area. Select a new date and repeat for day two and day three. When finished, for each date, select the Reports tab and go to Intake vs. Goals. Choose all meals and read the report. What information on the report most surprised you?

5. From the Reports tab, go to Energy Balance. Using day two (from the three-day diet intake), choose all meals and generate a report. Was your calorie intake more or less than the recommended calories (kcal) for your Profile? Was it higher or lower than you expected? You will analyze your energy balance in more detail later, in Chapter 9.

what did you decide?

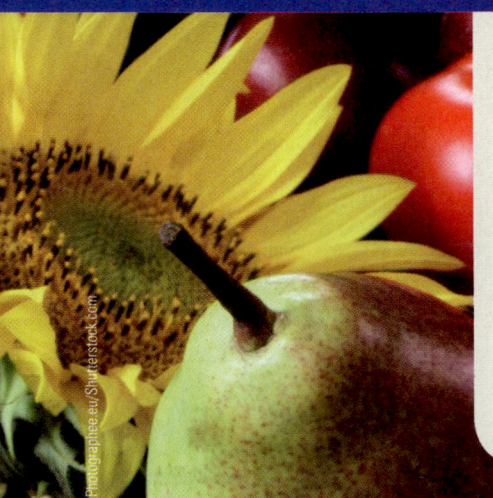

Can your diet make a real difference between getting sick or staying healthy?

Are supplements more powerful than food for ensuring good nutrition?

What makes your favorite foods your favorites?

Are news and media nutrition reports informative or confusing?

Self Check

1. (LO 1.1) Both heart disease and cancer are due to genetic causes, and diet cannot influence whether they occur.
   T   F

2. (LO 1.1) Some conditions, such as _____, are almost entirely nutrition related.
   a. cancer
   b. Down syndrome
   c. iron-deficiency anemia
   d. sickle-cell anemia

3. (LO 1.2) The nutrition objectives for the nation, as part of *Healthy People 2020*,
   a. envision a society in which all people live long, healthy lives.
   b. track and identify cancers as a major killer of people in the United States.
   c. set U.S. nutrition- and weight-related goals, one decade at a time.
   d. a and c.

4. (LO 1.2) According to a national 2010 health report,
   a. most people's diets lacked enough fruits, vegetables, and whole grains.
   b. most people were sufficiently physically active.
   c. the number of overweight people was declining.
   d. the nation had fully met the previous *Healthy People* objectives.

5. (LO 1.3) Energy-yielding nutrients include all of the following except _____.
   a. vitamins   c. fat
   b. carbohydrates   d. protein

6. (LO 1.3) Organic nutrients include all of the following except _____.
   a. minerals   c. carbohydrates
   b. fat   d. protein

7. (LO 1.3) Both carbohydrates and protein have 4 calories per gram.
   T   F

8. (LO 1.4) One of the characteristics of a nutritious diet is that the diet provides no constituent in excess. This principle of diet planning is called _____.
   a. adequacy   c. moderation
   b. balance   d. variety

9. (LO 1.4) Which of the following is an example of a processed food?
   a. carrots   c. nuts
   b. bread   d. watermelon

10. (LO 1.4) People most often choose foods for the nutrients they provide.
    T   F

11. (LO 1.5) Studies of populations in which observation is accompanied by experimental manipulation of some population members are referred to as _____.
    a. case studies
    b. intervention studies
    c. laboratory studies
    d. epidemiological studies

12. (LO 1.5) An important national food and nutrient intake survey, called *What We Eat in America*, is part of
    a. NHANES.
    b. FDA.
    c. USDA.
    d. none of the above.

13. (LO 1.6) Behavior change is a process that takes place in stages.
    T   F

14. (LO 1.6) A person who is setting goals in preparation for a behavior change is in a stage called *Precontemplation*.
    T   F

15. (LO 1.7) A slice of peach pie supplies 357 calories with 48 units of vitamin A; one large peach provides 42 calories and 53 units of vitamin A. This is an example of _____.
    a. calorie control
    b. nutrient density
    c. variety
    d. essential nutrients

16. (LO 1.7) A person who wishes to meet nutrient needs while not overconsuming calories is wise to master
    a. the concept of nutrient density.
    b. the concept of carbohydrate reduction.
    c. the concept of nutrients per dollar.
    d. French cooking.

17. (LO 1.8) "Red flags" that can help to identify nutrition quackery include
    a. enticingly quick and simple answers to complex problems.
    b. efforts to cast suspicion on the regular food supply.
    c. solid support and praise from users.
    d. all of the above.

18. (LO 1.8) In this nation, stringent controls make it difficult to obtain a bogus nutrition credential.
    T   F

Answers to these Self Check questions are in Appendix G.

Sorting the Imposters from the Real Nutrition Experts

LO 1.8 Evaluate the authenticity of nutrition information sources.

From the time of snake oil salesmen in horse-drawn wagons to today's Internet sales schemes, nutrition **quackery** has been a problem that often escapes government regulation and enforcement. To avoid being sitting ducks for quacks, consumers themselves must distinguish between authentic, useful nutrition products or services and a vast array of faulty advice and outright scams.

Each year, consumers spend a deluge of dollars on nutrition-related services and products from both legitimate and fraudulent businesses. Each year, nutrition and other health **fraud** diverts tens of *billions* of consumer dollars from legitimate health care.

More Than Money at Stake

When scam products are garden tools or stain removers, hoodwinked consumers may lose a few dollars and some pride. When the products are ineffective, untested, or even hazardous "dietary supplements" or "medical devices," consumers stand to lose the very

thing they are seeking: good health. When a sick person wastes time with quack treatments, serious problems can advance while proper treatment is delayed. And ill-advised "dietary supplements" have inflicted dire outcomes, even liver failure, on previously well people who took them in hopes of *improving* their health.

Information Sources

When asked, most people name television as their primary source of nutrition knowledge, with magazine articles a close second, and the Internet gaining quickly from behind.[1]* Sometimes these sources provide sound, scientific, trustworthy information. More often, though, **infomercials**, **advertorials**, and **urban legends** (defined in Table C1–1) pretend to inform but in fact aim primarily to sell products by making fantastic promises for health or weight loss with minimal effort and at bargain prices.

Reference notes are found in Appendix F.

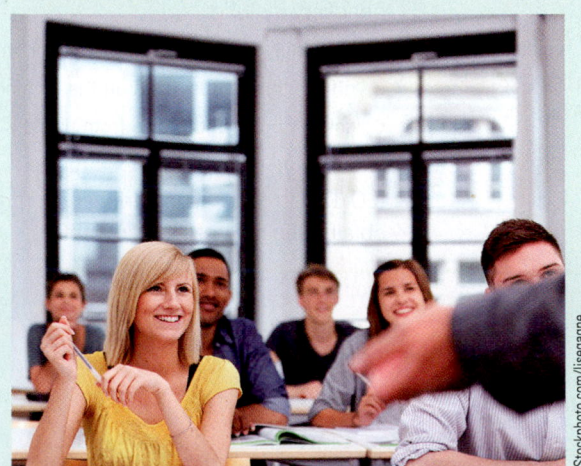

Who speaks on nutrition?

Table C1–1
Quackery and Internet Terms

- **advertorials** lengthy advertisements in newspapers and magazines that read like feature articles but are written for the purpose of touting the virtues of products and may or may not be accurate.
- **anecdotal evidence** information based on interesting and entertaining, but not scientific, personal accounts of events.
- **fraud** or **quackery** the promotion, for financial gain, of devices, treatments, services, plans, or products (including diets and supplements) claimed to improve health, well-being, or appearance without proof of safety or effectiveness. (The word *quackery* comes from the term *quacksalver*, meaning a person who quacks loudly about a miracle product—a lotion or a salve.)
- **infomercials** feature-length television commercials that follow the format of regular programs but are intended to convince viewers to buy products and not to educate or entertain them. The statements made may or may not be accurate.
- **Internet (the Net)** a worldwide network of millions of computers linked together to share information.
- **urban legends** stories, usually false, that may travel rapidly throughout the world via the Internet, gaining strength of conviction solely on the basis of repetition.
- **websites** Internet resources composed of text and graphic files, each with a unique URL (Uniform Resource Locator) that names the site (for example, www.usda.gov).
- **World Wide Web** (the Web, commonly abbreviated **www**) a graphical subset of the Internet.

How can people learn to distinguish valid nutrition information from misinformation? Some quackery is easy to identify—like the claims of the salesman in Figure C1–1—whereas other types are more subtle. Between the extremes of accurate scientific data and intentional quackery lies an abundance of nutrition misinformation.[†]

[†] Quackery-related definitions are available from the National Council Against Health Fraud, www.ncahf.org/pp/definitions.html. Consumers with questions or suspicions about fraud can contact the FDA on the Internet at www.FDA.gov or by telephone at (888) INFO-FDA.

An instructor at a gym, a physician, a health-food store clerk, an author of books, or an advocate for a "cleansing diet" product or weight-loss gadget may sincerely believe that the recommended nutrition regimen is beneficial. But what qualifies these people to give nutrition advice? Would following their advice be helpful or harmful? To sift the meaningful nutrition information from the rubble, you must learn to identify both.

Chapter 1 explained that valid nutrition information arises from scientific research and does not rely on **anecdotal evidence** or testimonials.

Scientists who use animals in their research do not apply their findings directly to human beings. And science is first published in peer-reviewed journals. Table C1–2 lists some sources of this authentic nutrition information.

Nutrition on the Net

If you have a question, the **World Wide Web** on the **Internet** has an answer. The "Net" offers convenient access to high-quality knowledge banks, such as in scientific journals, but it also delivers an abundance of incomplete, misleading,

Figure C1–1

Earmarks of Nutrition Quackery

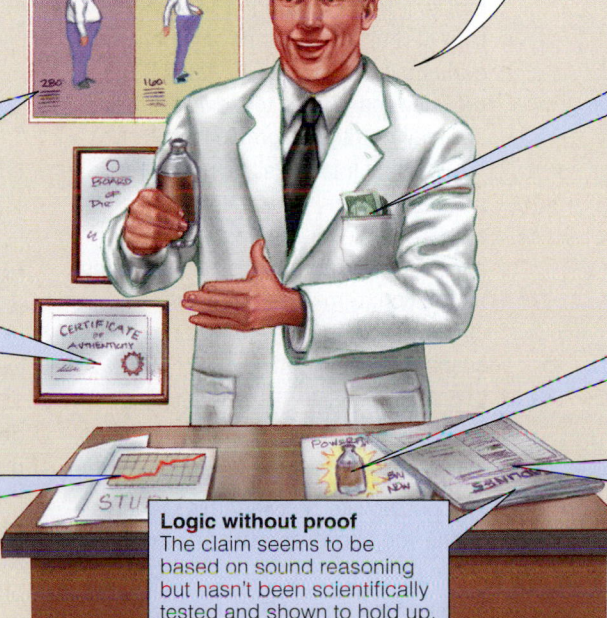

Too good to be true
Enticingly quick and simple answers to complex problems. Says what most people want to hear. Sounds magical.

Suspicions about food supply
Urges distrust of the current methods of medicine or suspicion of the regular food supply. Provides "alternatives" for sale under the guise of freedom of choice. May use the term "natural" to imply safety.

Testimonials
Support and praise by people who "felt healed," "felt younger," "lost weight," and the like as a result of using the product or treatment.

Fake credentials
Uses title "doctor," "university," or the like but has created or bought the title—it is not legitimate.

Unpublished studies
Cites scientific studies but not studies published in reliable journals.

A **SCIENTIFIC BREAKTHROUGH**! FEEL **STRONGER**, LOSE WEIGHT. **IMPROVE** YOUR MEMORY ALL WITH THE HELP OF **VITE-O-MITE**! OH SURE, YOU MAY HAVE HEARD THAT **VITE-O-MITE** IS NOT ALL THAT WE SAY IT IS, BUT THAT'S WHAT THE FDA WANTS YOU TO THINK! **OUR DOCTORS** AND SCIENTISTS SAY IT'S THE ULTIMATE VITAMIN SUPPLEMENT. SAY "NO!" TO THE WEAKENED VITAMINS IN TODAY'S FOODS. **VITE-O-MITE** INCLUDES **POTENT SECRET INGREDIENTS** THAT YOU CANNOT GET WITH ANY OTHER PRODUCT! ORDER RIGHT NOW AND WE'LL SEND YOU ANOTHER FOR FREE!

Persecution claims
Claims of persecution by the medical establishment or a fake government conspiracy or claims that physicians "want to keep you ill so that you will continue to pay for office visits."

Authority not cited
Studies cited sound valid but are not referenced, so that it is impossible to check and see if they were conducted scientifically.

Motive: personal gain
Those making the claim stand to make a profit if it is believed.

Advertisement
Claims are made by an advertiser who is paid to promote sales of the product or procedure. (Look for the word "Advertisement" in tiny print somewhere on the page.)

Latest innovation/Time-tested
Fake scientific jargon is meant to inspire awe. Claims of being "ancient remedies" are meant to inspire trust.

Logic without proof
The claim seems to be based on sound reasoning but hasn't been scientifically tested and shown to hold up.

Table C1–2

Credible Sources of Nutrition Information

Professional health organizations, government health agencies, volunteer health agencies, and consumer groups provide consumers with reliable nutrition information. Some credible sources include:

- Government agencies
  Department of Agriculture (USDA)
  www.usda.gov
  Department of Health and Human Services (DHHS)
  www.hhs.gov
  Food and Drug Administration (FDA)
  www.fda.gov
  World Health Organization, United Nations (WHO)
  www.who.int/en
- Journals
  American Journal of Clinical Nutrition
  www.ajcn.org
  Journal of the Academy of Nutrition and Dietetics
  http://www.andjrnl.org
  New England Journal of Medicine
  www.nejm.org
  Nutrition Reviews
  www.ilsi.org
- Reputable consumer and professional groups
  Academy of Nutrition and Dietetics
  www.eatright.org
  American Council on Science and Health
  www.acsh.org
  American Medical Association
  www.ama-assn.org
  Feeding America
  http://feedingamerica.org
  International Food Information Council Foundation
  www.foodinsight.org
- Volunteer health agencies
  American Cancer Society
  www.cancer.org
  American Diabetes Association
  www.diabetes.org
  American Heart Association
  www.heart.org

Table C1–3

Is This Site Reliable?

To judge whether an Internet site offers reliable nutrition information, answer the following questions.

- **Who is responsible for the site?** Clues can be found in the three-letter "tag" that follows the dot in the site's name. For example, "gov" and "edu" indicate government and university sites, usually reliable sources of information.
- **Do the names and credentials of information providers appear? Is an editorial board identified?** Many legitimate sources provide e-mail addresses or other ways to obtain more information about the site and the information providers behind it.
- **Are links with other reliable information sites provided?** Reputable organizations almost always provide links with other similar sites because they want you to know of other experts in their area of knowledge. Caution is needed when you evaluate a site by its links, however. Anyone, even a quack, can link a webpage to a reputable site without the organization's permission. Doing so may give the quack's site the appearance of legitimacy, just the effect the quack is hoping for.
- **Is the site updated regularly?** Nutrition information changes rapidly, and sites should be updated often.
- **Is the site selling a product or service?** Commercial sites may provide accurate information, but they also may not, and their profit motive increases the risk of bias.
- **Does the site charge a fee to gain access to it?** Many academic and government sites offer the best information, usually for free. Some legitimate sites do charge fees, but before paying up, check the free sites. Chances are good you'll find what you are looking for without paying.

or inaccurate information. Simply put: anyone can publish anything on the Internet. For example, popular self-governed Internet "encyclopedia" **websites** allow anyone to post information or change others' postings on all topics. Information on the sites may be correct, but it may not be—readers must evaluate it for themselves. Table C1–3 provides some clues to judging the reliability of nutrition information websites.

Personal Internet sites, known as "weblogs" or "blogs," contain the author's personal opinions and are not often reviewed by experts before posting. In addition, e-mail messages often circulate hoaxes and scare stories. Be suspicious when:

- Someone other than the sender or some authority you know wrote the contents.
- A phrase like "Forward this to everyone you know" appears anywhere in the piece.
- The piece states, "This is not a hoax"; chances are it is.

- The information seems shocking or something that you've never heard from legitimate sources.
- The language is overly emphatic or sprinkled with capitalized words or exclamation marks.
- No references are offered or, if present, are of questionable validity when examined.
- Websites such as www.quackwatch.org or www.urbanlegends.com have debunked the message.

In contrast, one of the most trustworthy Internet sites for scientific investigation is the National Library of Medicine's PubMed website, which provides free access to over 10 million abstracts (short descriptions) of research papers published in scientific journals around the world.[2] Many abstracts provide links to full articles posted on other sites. The site is easy to use and offers instructions for beginners. Figure C1–2 introduces this resource.

PubMed (www.ncbi.nlm.nih.gov/pubmed): Internet Resource for Scientific Nutrition References

The U.S. National Library of Medicine's PubMed website offers tutorials to help teach the beginner to use the search system effectively. Often, simply visiting the site, typing a query in the search box, and clicking *Search* will yield satisfactory results.

For example, to find research concerning calcium and bone health, typing in "calcium bone" nets almost 3,000 results. To refine the search, try setting limits on dates, types of articles, languages, and other criteria to obtain a more manageable number of abstracts to peruse.

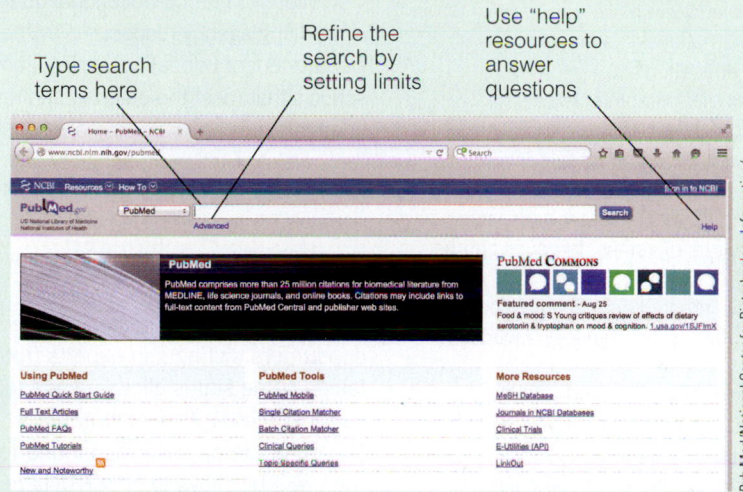

Type search terms here   Refine the search by setting limits   Use "help" resources to answer questions

PubMed/National Center for Biotechnology Information/ U.S. National Library of Medicine/NIH

Who Are the True Nutrition Experts?

Most people turn to their physicians for dietary advice, but physicians vary in their knowledge of nutrition. Physicians have extensive training in human biochemistry and physiology, the bedrocks of nutrition science, but typical medical schools in the United States do not require students to take a comprehensive nutrition course, such as the class taken by students reading this text.[3] Less than half of medical schools require even 25 hours of nutrition instruction. By comparison, your current nutrition class provides an average of 45 hours of instruction.

The exceptional physician has a specialty area in clinical nutrition and is highly qualified to advise on nutrition. Membership in the Academy of Nutrition and Dietetics or the Society for Clinical Nutrition, whose journals are cited many times throughout this text, can be a clue to a physician's nutrition knowledge.

Fortunately, the credential that indicates a qualified nutrition expert is easy to spot—you can confidently call on a **registered dietitian nutritionist (RDN)**. Additionally, some states require that **nutritionists** and **dietitians** obtain a **license to practice**. Meeting state-established criteria in addition to **registration** with the **Academy of Nutrition and Dietetics** certifies that an expert is the genuine article. Table C1–4 defines nutrition specialists along with other relevant terms.

RDNs are easy to find in most communities because they perform a multitude of duties in a variety of settings (see Table C1–5).[4] They work in foodservice operations, pharmaceutical companies, sports nutrition programs, corporate wellness programs, the food industry, home health agencies, long-term care institutions, private practice, community and public health settings, cooperative extension offices,[§] research centers, universities, hospitals, health

[§]*Cooperative extension agencies are associated with land grant colleges and universities and may be found in the telephone book's government listings or on the Internet.*

maintenance organizations (HMO), and other facilities. In hospitals, they may offer **medical nutrition therapy** as part of patient care, or they may run the foodservice operation, or they may specialize as **certified diabetes educators (CDE)** to help people with diabetes manage the disease. **Public health nutritionists** play key roles in government agencies as expert consultants and advocates or in direct service delivery.[5] The roles are so diverse that many pages would be required to cover them thoroughly.

In some facilities, a **dietetic technician** assists registered dietitian nutritionists in both administrative and clinical responsibilities. A dietetic technician has been educated and trained to work under the guidance of a registered dietitian nutritionist; upon passing a national examination, the technician earns the title **dietetic technician, registered (DTR)**.

Detecting Fake Credentials

In contrast to RDNs and other credentialed nutrition professionals, thousands of people possess fake nutrition degrees and claim to be nutrition counselors, nutritionists, or "dietists." These and other such titles may sound meaningful, but most of these people lack the established credentials of the Academy of Nutrition and Dietetics–sanctioned dietitian. If you look closely, you can see signs that their expertise is fake.

Educational Background

Take, for example, a nutrition expert's educational background. The minimum standards of education for a dietitian specify a bachelor of science (BS) degree in food science and human nutrition (or related fields) from an **accredited** college or university. Such a degree generally requires four to five years of study.

In contrast, a fake nutrition expert may display a degree from a six-week course of study; such a degree is simply not the same. In some cases, schools posing as legitimate institutions are actually **diploma mills**—fraudulent businesses that sell certificates of competency to anyone who pays the

- **Academy of Nutrition and Dietetics (AND)** the professional organization of dietitians in the United States (formerly the American Dietetic Association). The Canadian equivalent is the Dietitians of Canada (DC), which operates similarly.
- **accredited** approved; in the case of medical centers or universities, certified by an agency recognized by the U.S. Department of Education.
- **certified diabetes educator (CDE)** a health-care professional who specializes in educating people with diabetes to help them manage their disease through medical means and lifestyle changes. Work experience, extensive training, and passing an examination are required to achieve CDE status.
- **dietetic technician** a person who has completed a two-year academic degree from an accredited college or university and an approved dietetic technician program. A **dietetic technician, registered (DTR)** has also passed a national examination and maintains registration through continuing professional education.
- **dietitian** a person trained in nutrition, food science, and diet planning. See also *registered dietitian nutritionist*.
- **diploma mill** an organization that awards meaningless degrees without requiring students to meet educational standards. Diploma mills are not the same as diploma forgers (providing fake diplomas and certificates bearing the names of real, respected institutions). While virtually indistinguishable from authentic diplomas, forgeries can be unveiled by checking directly with the institution.
- **license to practice** permission under state or federal law, granted on meeting specified criteria, to use a certain title (such as *dietitian*) and to offer certain services. Licensed dietitians may use the initials LD after their names.
- **medical nutrition therapy** nutrition services used in the treatment of injury, illness, or other conditions; includes assessment of nutrition status and dietary intake and corrective applications of diet, counseling, and other nutrition services.
- **nutritionist** someone who studies nutrition. Some nutritionists are RDNs, whereas others are self-described experts whose training is questionable and who are not qualified to give advice. In states with responsible legislation, the term applies only to people who have master of science (MS) or doctor of philosophy (PhD) degrees from properly accredited institutions.
- **public health nutritionist** a dietitian or other person with an advanced degree in nutrition who specializes in public health nutrition.
- **registered dietitian nutritionist (RDN)** food and nutrition experts who have earned at least a bachelor's degree from an accredited college or university with a program approved by the Academy of Nutrition and Dietetics (or the Dietitians of Canada). The dietitian must also serve in an approved internship or coordinated program, pass the registration examination, and maintain professional competency through continuing education.[a] Many states also require licensing of practicing dietitians. Also called *registered dietitian (RD)*.
- **registration** listing with a professional organization that requires specific course work, experience, and passing of an examination.

[a] *The five content areas of the registration examination for dietitians are food and nutrition; clinical and community nutrition; education and research; food and nutrition systems; and management. New emphasis is placed on genetics, cultural competency, complementary care, and reimbursement.*

fees, from under a thousand dollars for a bachelor's degree to several thousand for a doctorate. To obtain these "degrees," a candidate need not read any books or pass any examinations, and the only written work is a signature on a check. Here are a few red flags to identify these scams:

- A degree is awarded in a very short time—sometimes just a few days.

- A degree can be based entirely on work or life experience.

- An institution provides only an e-mail address, with vague information on physical location.

- It provides sample styles of certificates and diplomas for choosing.

- It offers a choice of graduation dates to appear on a diploma.

Selling degrees is big business; networks of many bogus institutions are often owned by a single entity. In 2011, more than 2,600 such diploma and accreditation mills were identified, and 2,000 more were under investigation.

Accreditation and Licensure

Lack of proper accreditation is the identifying sign of a fake educational institution. To guard educational quality, an accrediting agency recognized by the U.S. Department of Education certifies those schools that meet the criteria defining a complete and accurate schooling, but in the case of nutrition, quack accrediting agencies cloud the picture. Fake nutrition degrees are available from schools "accredited" by more than 30 phony accrediting agencies.**

State laws do not necessarily help consumers distinguish experts from fakes; some states allow anyone to use the title *dietitian* or *nutritionist*. But other states have responded to the need by allowing only RDNs or people with certain graduate degrees and state licenses to call themselves dietitians. Licensing provides a way to identify people who have met minimum standards of education and experience.

A Failed Attempt to Fail

To dramatize the ease with which anyone can obtain a fake nutrition degree, one writer paid $82 to enroll in

** *To find out whether an online school is accredited, write the Distance Education and Training Council, Accrediting Commission, 1601 Eighteenth Street, NW, Washington, D.C. 20009; call 202-234-5100; or visit their website (www.detc.org).*

To find out whether a school is properly accredited for a dietetics degree, visit the U.S. Department of Education's Database of Accredited Postsecondary Institutions and Programs at http://ope.ed.gov/accreditation/Search.aspx. You can also write the Academy of Nutrition and Dietetics, Division of Education and Research, 120 South Riverside Plaza, Suite 2000, Chicago, Illinois 60606–6995: call 800-877-1600; or visit their website (www.eatright.org/caade).

The American Council on Education publishes Accredited Institutions of Postsecondary Education Programs, a directory of accredited institutions, professionally accredited programs, and candidates for accreditation that is available at many libraries. For additional information, write the American Council on Education, One Dupont Circle NW, Suite 800, Washington, D.C. 20036; call 202-939-9382; or visit their website (www.acenet.edu).

Table C1–5

Professional Responsibilities of Registered Dietitian Nutritionists

Registered dietitian nutritionists perform varied and important roles in the workforce. This table lists just a few responsibilities of just a few specialties.

Specialty	Sample Responsibilities
Public Health Nutrition	▪ Influence nutrition policy, regulations, and legislation. ▪ Plan, coordinate, administer, and evaluate food assistance programs. ▪ Consult with agencies; plan and manage budgets.
Hospital Health Care/Clinical Care	▪ Design and implement disease prevention services. ▪ Order therapeutic diets independently. ▪ Coordinate patient care with other health-care professionals. ▪ Assess client nutrient status and requirements. ▪ Provide client care and diet plan counseling.
Foodservice Management	▪ Plan and direct an institution's foodservice system, from kitchen to delivery. ▪ Plan and manage budgets; develop products; market services.
Laboratory Research	▪ Design, execute, and interpret food and nutrition research. ▪ Write and publish research articles in peer-reviewed journals and lay publications. ▪ Provide science-based guidance to nutrition practitioners. ▪ Write and manage grants.
Education	▪ Write curricula to deliver to students nutrition knowledge that is appropriate for their goals and that meets criteria of accrediting agencies and professional groups. ▪ Teach and evaluate student progress; research, write, and publish.
Health and Wellness	▪ Design and implement research-based programs for individuals or populations to improve nutrition, health, and physical fitness.

Sources: B. Boyce, CMS final rule on therapeutic diet orders means new opportunities for RDNs, Journal of the Academy of Nutrition and Dietetics 114 (2014): 1326–1328. S. H. Laramee and M. Tate, Dietetics Workforce Demand Study Task Force Supplement: An introduction, Journal of the Academy of Nutrition and Dietetics, 112 (2012): S7–S9.

a nutrition diploma mill that billed itself as a correspondence school. She made every attempt to fail, intentionally giving all wrong answers to the examination questions. Even so, she received a "nutritionist" certificate at the end of the course, together with a letter from the "school" officials explaining that they were sure she must have misread the test.

Would You Trust a Nutritionist Who Eats Dog Food?

In a similar stunt, Mr. Eddie Diekman was named a "professional member" of an association of nutrition "experts." For his efforts, Eddie received a diploma suitable for framing and displaying. Eddie is a cocker spaniel. His owner, Connie B. Diekman, then president of

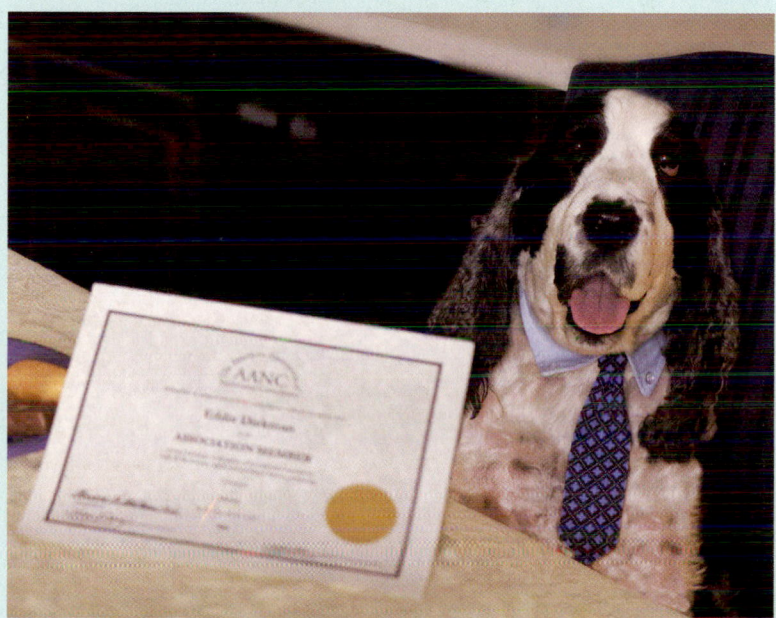

© Courtesy of eatright.org

Eddie displays his professional credentials.

the American Dietetic Association, paid Eddie's tuition to prove that he could be awarded the title "nutritionist" merely by sending in his name.

Staying Ahead of the Scammers

In summary, to stay one step ahead of the nutrition quacks, check a provider's qualifications. First, look for the degrees and credentials listed after the person's name (such as MD, RDN, MS, PhD, or LD). Next find out what you can about the reputations of the institutions that awarded the degrees. Then call your state's health-licensing agency and ask if dietitians are licensed in your state. If they are, find out whether the person giving you dietary advice has a license—and if not, find someone better qualified. Your health is your most precious asset, and protecting it is well worth the time and effort it takes to do so.

Critical Thinking

1. This class will give you the skills to learn how to separate legitimate nutrition claims from those that are questionable. To help practice the skills needed to separate fact from fiction, describe how you would respond to the following situation:

   A friend has started taking ginseng, a supplement that claims to help her lose weight. You are thinking of trying ginseng, but you want to learn more about the herb and its effects before deciding. What research would you do, and what questions would you ask your friend to determine if ginseng is a legitimate weight loss product?

2. Recognizing a nutrition authority that you can consult for reliable nutrition information can be difficult because it is so easy to acquire question-able nutrition credentials. Read the education and experience of the "nutrition experts" described below and put them in order, beginning with the person with the strongest and most trustworthy nutrition expertise and ending with the person with the weakest and least trustworthy nutrition expertise.

   1. A dietetic technician, registered (DTR) working in a clinic

   2. A highly successful athlete/coach who has a small business as a nutrition counselor and sells a line of nutrition supplements

   3. An individual who has completed 30 hours of nutrition training through the American Association of Nutrition Counseling

   4. A registered dietitian nutritionist (RDN) associated with a hospital

2 Nutrition Tools—Standards and Guidelines

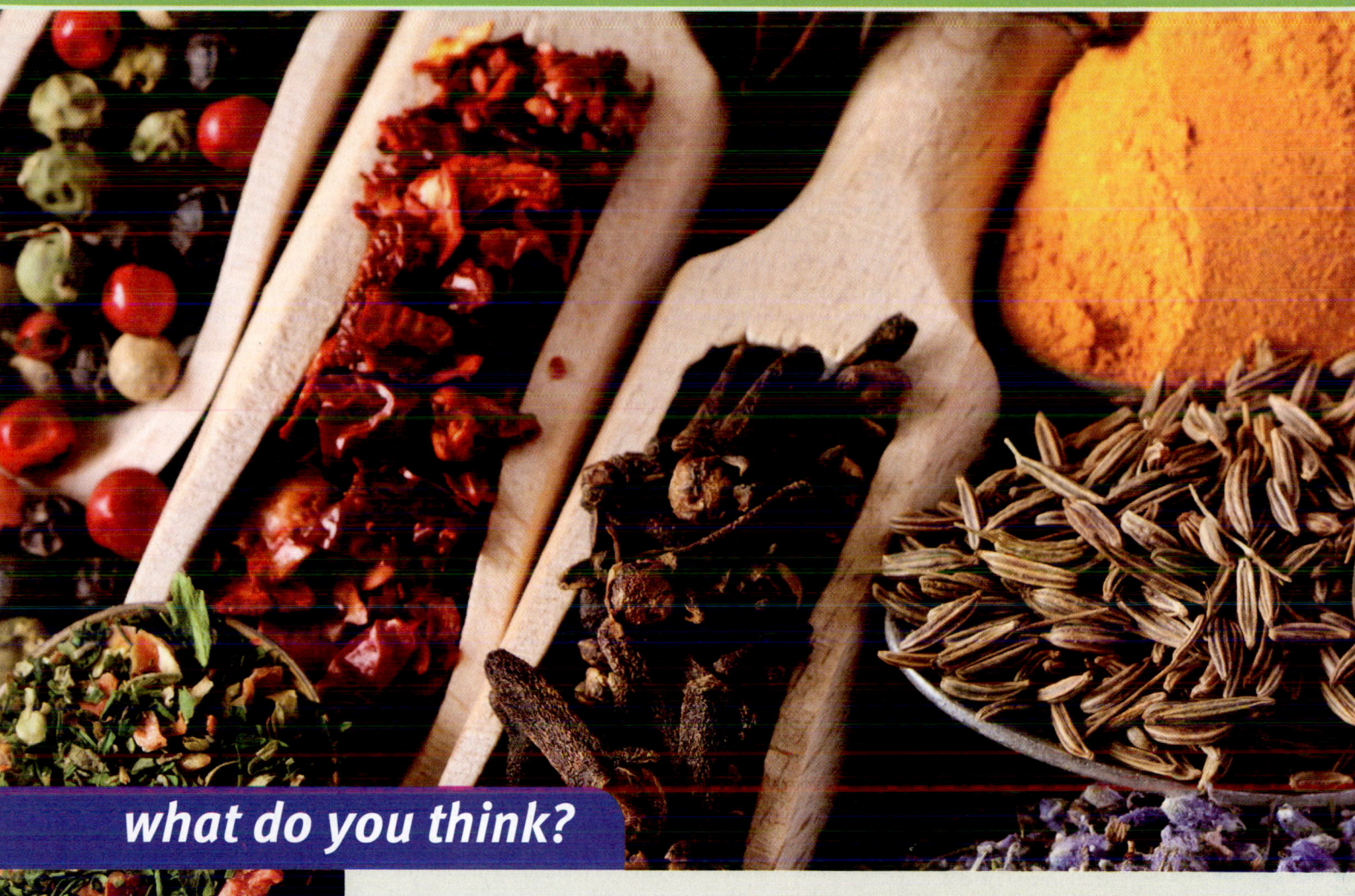

what do you think?

How can you tell **how much of each nutrient** you need to consume daily?

Are **government dietary recommendations** too simplistic to be of help?

Are the health claims on food labels **accurate and reliable**?

Can certain **"superfoods"** boost your health with more than just nutrients?

Learning Objectives

After completing this chapter, you should be able to accomplish the following:

LO 2.1 State the significance of Dietary Reference Intakes (DRI) and Daily Values as nutrient standards.

LO 2.2 Specify how the Dietary Guidelines for Americans work as part of an overall U.S. dietary guidance system.

LO 2.3 Explain the use of the USDA Eating Patterns to plan a nutritious diet.

LO 2.4 Given the required number of calories, discuss a healthful diet plan by applying the USDA Eating Patterns.

LO 2.5 Discuss the information included on food labels.

LO 2.6 Estimate the benefits of a nutrient-dense meal plan through comparison with a meal plan that does not take nutrient density into account.

LO 2.7 Summarize the potential health effects of phytochemicals from both food sources and supplements.

E ating well is easy in theory—just choose foods that supply appropriate amounts of the essential nutrients, fiber, phytochemicals, and energy without excess intakes of fat, sugar, and salt, and be sure to get enough physical activity to help balance the foods you eat. In practice, eating well proves harder to do. Many people are overweight, or are undernourished, or suffer from nutrient excesses or deficiencies that impair their health—that is, they are malnourished. You may not think that this statement applies to you, but you may already have less than optimal nutrient intakes without knowing it. Accumulated over years, the effects of your habits can seriously impair the quality of your life.

Putting it positively, you can enjoy the best possible vim, vigor, and vitality throughout your life if you learn now to nourish yourself optimally. To learn how, you first need some general guidelines and the answers to several basic questions. How much of each nutrient and how many calories should you consume? Which types of foods supply which nutrients? How much of each type of food do you have to eat to get enough? And how can you eat all these foods without gaining excess weight? This chapter begins by identifying some ideals for nutrient and energy intakes and ends by showing how to achieve them.

Nutrient Recommendations

LO 2.1 State the significance of Dietary Reference Intakes (DRI) and Daily Values as nutrient standards.

Nutrient recommendations are sets of standards against which people's nutrient and energy intakes can be measured. Nutrition experts use the recommendations to assess intakes and to offer advice on amounts to consume. Individuals may use them to decide how much of a nutrient they need and how much is too much.

Dietary Reference Intakes

The standards in use in the United States and Canada are the **Dietary Reference Intakes (DRI)**. A committee of nutrition experts from the two countries develops, publishes, and updates the DRI.* The DRI committee has set values for all of the vitamins and minerals, as well as for carbohydrates, fiber, lipids, protein, water, and energy.

Another set of nutrient standards is practical for making comparisons among packaged foods. These are the **Daily Values**, familiar to anyone who has read a food

Dietary Reference Intakes (DRI) a set of five lists of values for measuring the nutrient intakes of healthy people in the United States and Canada. The lists are Estimated Average Requirements (EAR), Recommended Dietary Allowances (RDA), Adequate Intakes (AI), Tolerable Upper Intake Levels (UL), and Acceptable Macronutrient Distribution Ranges (AMDR).

Daily Values nutrient standards used on food labels and on grocery store and restaurant signs. Based on nutrient recommendations for a general 2,000-calorie diet, they allow consumers to compare foods with regard to nutrients and calorie contents.

---

*This is a committee of the Food and Nutrition Board of the National Academy of Sciences' Institute of Medicine, working in association with Health Canada.

label. Nutrient standards—the DRI and Daily Values—are used and referred to so often that they are printed on the inside front and back cover pages of this book: DRI lists—inside front cover, pages A, B, and C; Daily Values—inside back cover, page Y.

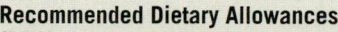
StockPhotosArt/Shutterstock.com

KEY POINTS

- The Dietary Reference Intakes are U.S. and Canadian nutrient intake standards.
- The Daily Values are U.S. standards used on food labels.

The DRI Lists and Purposes

For each nutrient, the DRI establish a number of values, each serving a different purpose. The values that most people find useful are those that set goals for nutrient intakes (RDA, AI, and AMDR, described next) and those that describe nutrient safety (UL, addressed later). In total, the DRI include five sets of values:

1. **Recommended Dietary Allowances (RDA)**—adequacy
2. **Adequate Intakes (AI)**—adequacy
3. **Tolerable Upper Intake Levels (UL)**—safety
4. **Estimated Average Requirements (EAR)**—research and policy
5. **Acceptable Macronutrient Distribution Ranges (AMDR)**—healthful ranges for energy-yielding nutrients

RDA and AI—Recommended Nutrient Intakes

A great advantage of the DRI values lies in their applicability to the diets of individuals.[†] People may adopt the RDA and AI as their own nutrient intake goals. The AI values are not the scientific equivalent of the RDA, however.

The RDA form the indisputable bedrock of the DRI recommended intakes because they derive from solid experimental evidence and reliable observations—they are expected to meet the needs of almost all healthy people. AI values, in contrast, are based as far as possible on the available scientific evidence but also on some educated guesswork. Whenever the DRI committee members find insufficient evidence to generate an RDA, they establish an AI value instead. This book refers to the RDA and AI values collectively as the DRI recommended intakes.

EAR—Nutrition Research and Policy

The EAR, also set by the DRI committee, establish the average nutrient requirements for given life stages and gender groups that researchers and nutrition policy makers use in their work. Public health officials may also use them to assess the prevalence of inadequate intakes in populations and make recommendations.[2] The EAR values form the scientific basis upon which the RDA values are set (a later section explains how).

UL—Safety

Beyond a certain point, it is unwise to consume large amounts of any nutrient, so the DRI committee sets the UL to identify potentially toxic levels of nutrient intake. Usual intakes of a nutrient below its UL have a low risk of causing illness; with chronic intakes above the UL, risks rise. The UL are indispensable to consumers who take supplements or consume foods and beverages to which vitamins or minerals have been added—a group that includes almost everyone. Public health officials also rely on UL values to set safe upper limits for nutrients added to our food and water supplies.

Nutrient needs fall within a range, and a danger zone exists both below and above that range. Figure 2–1 illustrates this point. People's tolerances for high doses of nutrients vary, so caution is in order when nutrient intakes approach the UL values (listed on the inside front cover, p. C).

Some nutrients lack UL values. The absence of a UL for a nutrient does not imply that it is safe to consume it in any amount, however. It means only that insufficient data exist to establish a value.

[†] Reference notes are found in Appendix F.

Recommended Dietary Allowances (RDA) nutrient intake goals for individuals; the average daily nutrient intake level that meets the needs of nearly all (97 to 98 percent) healthy people in a particular life stage and gender group.

Adequate Intakes (AI) nutrient intake goals for individuals; the recommended average daily nutrient intake level based on intakes of healthy people in a particular life stage and gender group and assumed to be adequate. Set when scientific data are insufficient to allow establishment of an RDA value.

Tolerable Upper Intake Levels (UL) the highest average daily nutrient intake level that is likely to pose no risk of toxicity to almost all healthy individuals of a particular life stage and gender group.

Estimated Average Requirements (EAR) the average daily nutrient intake estimated to meet the requirement of half of the healthy individuals in a particular life stage and gender group; is used in nutrition research and policy making and is the basis upon which RDA values are set.

Acceptable Macronutrient Distribution Ranges (AMDR) values for carbohydrate, fat, and protein expressed as percentages of total daily caloric intake; ranges of intakes set for the energy-yielding nutrients that are sufficient to provide adequate total energy and nutrients while minimizing the risk of chronic diseases.

Figure 2–1

The Naïve View versus the Accurate View of Optimal Nutrient Intakes

Consuming too much of a nutrient endangers health, just as consuming too little does. The DRI recommended intake values fall within a safety range, with the UL marking tolerable upper levels.

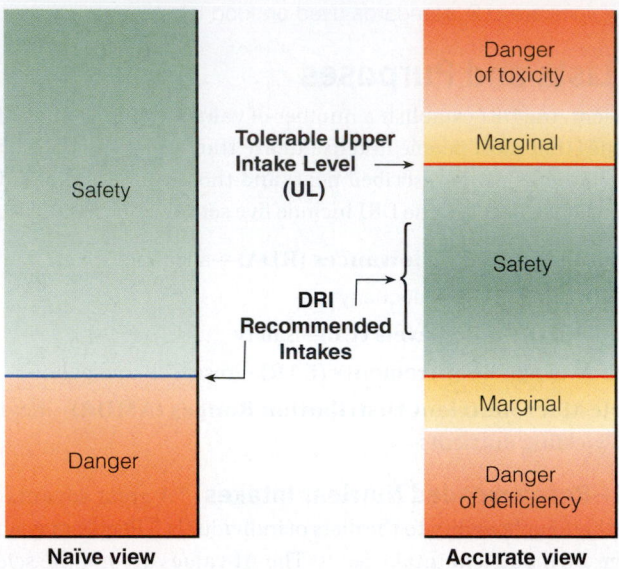

Naïve view   **Accurate view**

AMDR—Calorie Percentage Ranges The DRI committee also sets healthy ranges of intake for carbohydrate, fat, and protein known as Acceptable Macronutrient Distribution Ranges. Each of these three energy-yielding nutrients contributes to the day's total calorie intake, and their contributions can be expressed as a percentage of the total. According to the committee, a diet that provides adequate energy in the following proportions can provide adequate nutrients while minimizing the risk of chronic diseases:

- 45 to 65 percent of calories from carbohydrate.
- 20 to 35 percent of calories from fat.
- 10 to 35 percent of calories from protein.

The chapters on the energy-yielding nutrients revisit these ranges.

To judge a day's meals against the AMDR requires knowing the calories and grams of energy nutrients in the foods, and then performing the calculations shown in the margin, a daunting prospect to most consumers. Policy-makers who develop food-based guidelines (described later) take into account the principles of the DRI standards, making it easier for consumers to meet their goals.[3]

KEY POINTS

- The DRI set nutrient intake goals for individuals, standards for researchers and public policy makers, and tolerable upper limits.
- RDA, AI, EAR, and UL are all DRI standards, along with AMDR ranges for energy-yielding nutrients.

Understanding the DRI Recommended Intakes

Nutrient recommendations have been much misunderstood. One young woman posed this question: "Do you mean that some bureaucrat says that I need exactly the same amount of vitamin D as everyone else? Do they really think that 'one size fits all'?" In fact, the opposite is true.

Do the Math

Calculate the percentage of calories from an energy nutrient in a day's meals by using this general formula:

(A nutrient's calorie amount ÷ total calories) × 100

Calculate the percentage of calories from protein in a day's meals:

A day's meals provide 50 grams of protein and 1,754 total calories.

1. Convert the protein *grams* to protein *calories* (protein provides 4 calories per gram):

   50 g protein × 4 cal per g = ____ cal from protein

2. Using your answer above, apply the general formula:

   (protein calorie amount ÷ total calories) × 100

   (____ ÷ 1,754) × 100 = ____ percent calories from protein.

Follow the same procedure when considering carbohydrate (4 cal per g) and fat (9 cal per g).

DRI for Population Groups   The DRI committee acknowledges differences among individuals and takes them into account when setting nutrient values. It has made separate recommendations for specific groups of people—men, women, pregnant women, lactating women, infants, and children—and for specific age ranges. Children aged 4 to 8 years, for example, have their own DRI recommended intakes. Each individual can look up the recommendations for his or her own age and gender group. Within each age and gender group, the committee advises adjusting nutrient intakes in special circumstances that may increase or decrease nutrient needs, such as illness or smoking. Later chapters provide details about who may need to adjust intakes of which nutrients.

For almost all healthy people, a diet that consistently provides the RDA or AI amount for a specific nutrient is very likely to be adequate in that nutrient. On average, you should try to get 100 percent of the DRI recommended intake for every nutrient over time to ensure an adequate intake.

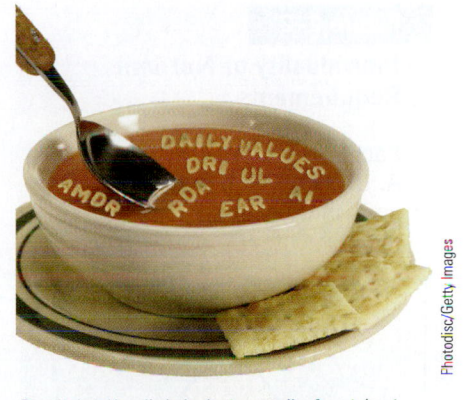

Don't let the "alphabet soup" of nutrient intake standards confuse you. Their names make sense when you learn their purposes.

Other Characteristics of the DRI Recommended Intakes   The following facts will help put the DRI recommended intakes into perspective:

- The values are based on available scientific research to the greatest extent possible and are updated to reflect current scientific knowledge.

- The values are based on the concepts of probability and risk. The DRI recommended intakes are associated with a low probability of deficiency for people of a given life stage and gender group, and they pose almost no risk of toxicity for that group.

- The values are set for optimal intakes, not minimum requirements. They include a generous safety margin and meet the needs of virtually all healthy people in a specific age and gender group.

- The values are set in reference to certain indicators of nutrient adequacy, such as blood nutrient concentrations, normal growth, or reduction of certain chronic diseases or other disorders, rather than prevention of deficiency symptoms alone.

- The values reflect daily intakes to be achieved on average, over time. They assume that intakes will vary from day to day and are set high enough to ensure that the body's nutrient stores will meet nutrient needs during periods of inadequate intakes lasting several days to several months, depending on the nutrient.

The DRI Apply to Healthy People Only   The DRI are designed for health maintenance and disease prevention in healthy people, not for the restoration of health or repletion of nutrients in those with deficiencies. Under the stress of serious illness or malnutrition, a person may require a much higher intake of certain nutrients or may not be able to handle even the DRI amount. Therapeutic diets take into account the increased nutrient needs imposed by certain medical conditions, such as recovery from surgery, burns, fractures, illnesses, malnutrition, or addictions.

KEY POINTS

- The DRI set separate recommendations for specific groups of people at different ages.
- The DRI intake recommendations (RDA and AI) are up-to-date, optimal, and safe nutrient intakes for healthy people in the United States and Canada.

How the Committee Establishes DRI Values— An RDA Example

A theoretical discussion will help to explain how the DRI committee goes about setting DRI values. Suppose we are the DRI committee members with the task of setting an RDA for nutrient X (an essential nutrient).[‡] Ideally, our first step will be to find out how much of that nutrient various healthy individuals need. To do so, we review studies of deficiency states, nutrient stores and their depletion, and the factors influencing

---

[‡]This discussion describes how an RDA value is set; to set an AI value, the committee would use some educated guesswork, as well as scientific research results, to determine an approximate amount of the nutrient most likely to support health.

Figure 2–2

Individuality of Nutrient Requirements

Each square represents a person. A, B, and C are Mr. A, Mr. B, and Mr. C. Each has a different requirement.

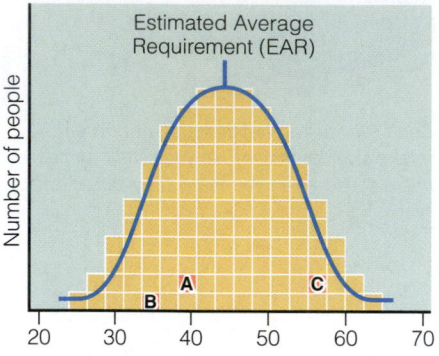

them. We then select the most valid data for use in our work. Of the DRI family of nutrient standards, the setting of an RDA value demands the most rigorous science and tolerates the least guesswork.

Determining Individual Requirements

One experiment we would review or conduct is a **balance study**. In this type of study, scientists measure the body's intake and excretion of a nutrient to find out how much intake is required to balance excretion. For each individual subject, we can determine a **requirement** to achieve balance for nutrient X. With an intake below the requirement, a person will slip into negative balance or experience declining stores that could, over time, lead to deficiency of the nutrient.

We find that different individuals, even of the same age and gender, have different requirements. Mr. A needs 40 units of the nutrient each day to maintain balance; Mr. B needs 35; Mr. C needs 57. If we look at enough individuals, we find that their requirements are distributed as shown in Figure 2–2—with most requirements near the midpoint (here, 45) and only a few at the extremes.

Accounting for the Needs of the Population
To set the value, we have to decide what intake to recommend for everybody. Should we set it at the mean (45 units in Figure 2–2)? This is the Estimated Average Requirement for nutrient X, mentioned earlier as valuable to scientists and policy makers but not appropriate as an individual's nutrient goal. The EAR value is probably close to everyone's minimum need, assuming the distribution shown in Figure 2–2. (Actually, the data for most nutrients indicate a distribution that is much less symmetrical.) But if people took us literally and consumed exactly this amount of nutrient X each day, half the population would begin to develop nutrient deficiencies and, in time, even observable symptoms of deficiency diseases. Mr. C (at 57 units) would be one of those people.

Perhaps we should set the recommendation for nutrient X at or above the extreme—say, at 70 units a day—so that everyone will be covered. (Actually, we didn't study everyone, and some individual we didn't happen to test might have an even higher requirement.) This might be a good idea in theory, but what about a person like Mr. B who requires only 35 units a day? The recommendation would be twice his requirement, and to follow it, he might spend money needlessly on foods containing nutrient X to the exclusion of foods containing other vital nutrients.

The Decision
The decision we finally make is to set the value high enough so that 97 to 98 percent of the population will be covered but not so high as to be excessive (Figure 2–3 illustrates such a value). In this example, a reasonable choice might be 63 units a day. Moving the value further toward the extreme would pick up a few additional people, but it would inflate the recommendation for most people, including Mr. A and Mr. B. The committee makes judgments of this kind when setting the DRI recommended intakes for many nutrients. Relatively few healthy people have requirements that are not covered by the DRI recommended intakes.

KEY POINT

- The DRI intake recommendations are based on scientific data and generously cover the needs of virtually all healthy people in the United States and Canada.

Setting Energy Requirements

In contrast to the recommendations for nutrients, the value set for energy, the **Estimated Energy Requirement (EER)**, is not generous; instead, it is set at a level predicted to maintain body weight for an individual of a particular age, gender, height, weight, and physical activity level consistent with good health. The energy DRI values reflect a balancing act: enough food energy is critical to support health and life, but too much energy causes unhealthy weight gain. Because even small amounts of excess energy consumed day after day cause unneeded weight gain and increase chronic disease risks, the DRI committee did not set a Tolerable Upper Intake Level for energy.

Figure 2–3

Nutrient Recommended Intake: RDA Example

Intake recommendations for most vitamins and minerals are set so that they will meet the requirements of nearly all people (boxes represent people).

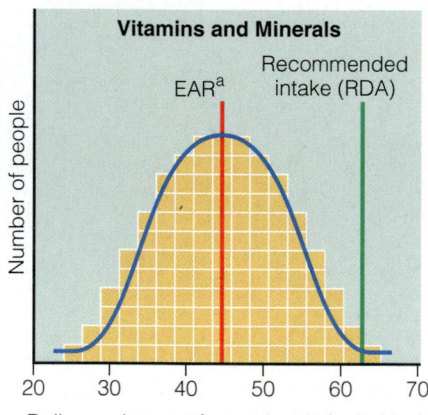

^aEstimated Average Requirement

balance study a laboratory study in which a person is fed a controlled diet and the intake and excretion of a nutrient are measured. Balance studies are valid only for nutrients like calcium (chemical elements) that do not change while they are in the body.

- Estimated Energy Requirements are predicted to maintain body weight and to discourage unhealthy weight gain.

Why Are Daily Values Used on Labels?

On learning about the Daily Values, many people ask why yet another set of nutrient standards is needed for food labels—why not use the DRI? The reason they are not used is that DRI values for a nutrient vary, sometimes widely, to address the different nutrient needs of different population groups. Food labels, in contrast, must list a single value for each nutrient that may be used by anyone who picks up a package of food and reads the label.[4]

The Daily Values reflect the highest level of nutrient need among all population groups, from children of age 4 years through aging adults; for example, the Daily Value for iron is 18 milligrams (mg), an amount that far exceeds a man's RDA of 8 mg (but that meets a young woman's high need precisely). Thus, the Daily Values are ideal for allowing general comparisons among *foods*, but they cannot serve as nutrient intake goals for individuals. The recently updated Daily Values are listed on the inside back cover, p. Y.

- The Daily Values are standards used solely on food labels to enable consumers to compare the nutrient values of foods.

Dietary Guidelines for Americans

LO 2.2   Specify how the Dietary Guidelines for Americans work as part of an overall U.S. dietary guidance system.

Many countries set dietary guidelines to answer the question, "What should I eat to stay healthy?" In this country, the U.S. Department of Agriculture publishes its *Dietary Guidelines for Americans* as part of a national nutrition guidance system. While the DRI values set nutrient intake goals, the Dietary Guidelines for Americans offer food-based strategies for achieving them. If everyone followed their advice, people's energy intakes and most of their nutrient needs would fall into place.[5§] Table 2–1 (p. 38) lists the 2015–2020 Dietary Guidelines and their key recommendations.

> **Appendix B** offers more about the 2015 Dietary Guidelines, along with World Health Organization guidelines.

The Guidelines Promote Health   People who follow the Dietary Guidelines— that is, those who do not overconsume calories, who take in enough of a variety of nutrient-dense foods and beverages, and who make physical activity a habit—often enjoy the best possible health. Only a few people in this country meet this description, however. Instead, about half of American adults suffer from one or more *preventable* chronic diseases related to poor diets and sedentary lifestyles.

How Does the U.S. Diet Compare with the Guidelines?   The Dietary Guidelines committee reviewed nationwide survey results reflecting current nutrient intakes, along with biochemical assessments and other forms of evidence. The results are clear: important needed nutrients are undersupplied by the current U.S. diet, while other, less healthful nutrients are oversupplied (see Table 2–2). Figure 2–4 (p. 39) shows that, typically, people take in far too few nutritious foods from most food groups when compared with the ideals of the Dietary Guidelines for Americans (discussed fully in the next section). They also take in too many calories and too much red and processed meat, refined grains, added sugars, sodium, and saturated fat.

Note that the Dietary Guidelines for Americans do not require that you give up your favorite foods or eat strange, unappealing foods. They advocate achieving a healthy dietary pattern through wise food and beverage choices and not by way of

§The USDA Eating Patterns may not provide the DRI recommended intake of vitamin D or potassium.

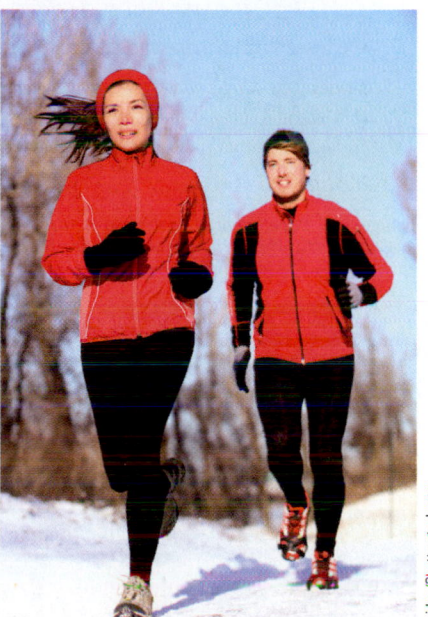

The Dietary Guidelines recommend physical activity to help balance calorie intakes to achieve and sustain a healthy body weight.

Maridav/Shutterstock.com

requirement   the amount of a nutrient that will just prevent the development of specific deficiency signs; distinguished from the DRI recommended intake value, which is a generous allowance with a margin of safety.

Estimated Energy Requirement (EER)   the average dietary energy intake predicted to maintain energy balance in a healthy adult of a certain age, gender, weight, height, and level of physical activity consistent with good health.

Table 2–1

Dietary Guidelines for Americans 2015–2020: Guidelines and Recommendations

The Dietary Guidelines and key recommendations for healthy eating patterns should be applied in their entirety to people 2 years of age and older; they are interconnected and each component can affect the others.

Dietary Guidelines	Key Recommendations
1. *Follow a healthy eating pattern across the lifespan.* All food and beverage choices matter. Choose a healthy eating pattern at an appropriate calorie level to help achieve and maintain a healthy body weight, support nutrient adequacy, and reduce the risk of chronic disease.	**Consume a healthy eating pattern that accounts for all foods and beverages within an appropriate calorie level.** *A healthy eating pattern includes:* ■ A variety of vegetables from all of the subgroups—dark green, red and orange, legumes (beans and peas), starchy, and other. ■ Fruits, especially whole fruits.
2. *Focus on variety, nutrient density, and amount.* To meet nutrient needs within calorie limits, choose a variety of nutrient-dense foods across and within all food groups in recommended amounts.	■ Grains, at least half of which are whole grains. ■ Fat-free or low-fat dairy, including milk, yogurt, cheese, and /or fortified soy beverages. ■ A variety of protein foods, including seafood, lean meats and poultry, eggs, legumes (beans and peas), and nuts, seeds, and soy products.

3. *Limit calories from added sugars and saturated fats and reduce sodium intake.* Consume an eating pattern low in added sugars, saturated fats, and sodium. Cut back on foods and beverages higher in these components to amounts that fit within healthy eating patterns.	■ Oils.
	
	A healthy eating pattern limits:
	■ Saturated fats and *trans* fats, added sugars, and sodium.
	  ■ Consume less than 10 percent of calories per day from added sugars.
	  ■ Consume less than 10 percent of calories per day from saturated fats.

4. *Shift to healthier food and beverage choices.* Choose nutrient-dense foods and beverages across and within all food groups in place of less healthy choices. Consider cultural and personal preferences to make these shifts easier to accomplish and maintain.	■ Consume less than 2,300 milligrams per day of sodium. ■ If alcohol is consumed, it should be consumed in moderation—up to one drink per day for women and up to two drinks per day for men—and only by adults of legal drinking age.
5. *Support healthy eating patterns for all.* Everyone has a role in helping to create and support healthy eating patterns in multiple settings nationwide, from home to school to work to communities.	**Meet the *Physical Activity Guidelines for Americans.***

Source: U.S. Department of Health and Human Services and U.S. Department of Agriculture, 2015–2020 Dietary Guidelines for Americans, 8th edition (2015), available at http://health.gov/dietaryguidelines/2015/guidelines/.

Table 2–2

Shortfall Nutrients and Overconsumed Nutrients

The Dietary Guidelines committee compared average U.S. nutrient intakes with DRI recommendations and identified nutrients that are chronically under- or over-consumed, indicating a need for change in U.S. eating habits. Added sugars, not listed, are also overconsumed, but no DRI standard exists for added sugars.

Shortfall nutrients: Chronically undersupplied by diets of many people ages 2 years and older:

■ Vitamin A	■ Calcium
■ Vitamin C	■ Iron (for some girls and women; see Chapter 8)
■ Vitamin D	■ Magnesium
■ Vitamin E	■ Fiber
■ Folate	■ Potassium

Overconsumed nutrients: Chronically oversupplied by the diets of many people ages 2 years and older:

■ Saturated fat	■ Sodium

Source: U.S. Department of Agriculture and U.S. Department of Health and Human Services, Scientific Report of the 2015 Dietary Guidelines Advisory Committee (2015), D-1:89, available at www.health.gov.

nutrient or dietary supplements except when medically necessary. With a little planning and a few adjustments, almost anyone's diet can contribute to health instead of disease. Part of the plan must also be to increase physical activity to help achieve and sustain a healthy body weight, and this chapter's Think Fitness box (p. 42) offers some guidelines, while Chapter 10 provides details.

Figure 2–4

How Does the Typical U.S. Diet Stack Up?

The average U.S. diet needs improvements—more whole grains, fewer refined grains, more vegetables and fruit, and more milk—to meet intake goals. In addition, most Americans greatly exceed recommendations for added sugars, saturated fats, and sodium.

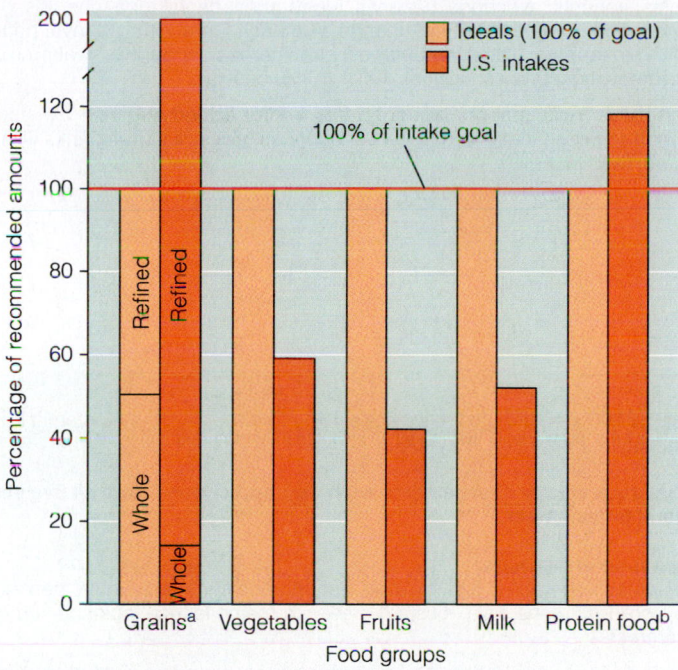

^aAt least half of the grain selections should be whole grains.
^bIntake of the seafood subgroup is only 44 percent of recommended levels.

Our Two Cents' Worth If the experts who develop the Dietary Guidelines for Americans were to ask us, our focus would fall on this recommendation: choose carefully, but enjoy your food. The joys of eating are physically beneficial to the body because they trigger health-promoting changes in the nervous, hormonal, and immune systems. When the food is nutritious as well as enjoyable, then the eater obtains all the nutrients needed to support proper body functioning, as well as for the healthy skin, glossy hair, and natural attractiveness that accompany robust health.[6] Remember to enjoy your food.

KEY POINTS

- The Dietary Guidelines for Americans address problems of undernutrition and overnutrition.
- They recommend following a healthful eating pattern and being physically active.
- Key nutrients of concern are lacking in many U.S. diets; others are oversupplied.

Diet Planning with the USDA Eating Patterns

LO 2.3 Explain the use of the USDA Eating Patterns to plan a nutritious diet.

Diet planning connects nutrition theory with the food on the table, and a few minutes invested in meal planning can pay off richly in better nutrition. To help people achieve the goals of the Dietary Guidelines for Americans, the USDA employs a **food group plan** known as the USDA Eating Patterns. Figure 2–5 (pp. 40–41)

food group plan a diet-planning tool that sorts foods into groups based on their nutrient content and then specifies that people should eat certain minimum numbers of servings of foods from each group.

Figure 2–5

USDA Food Groups and Subgroups

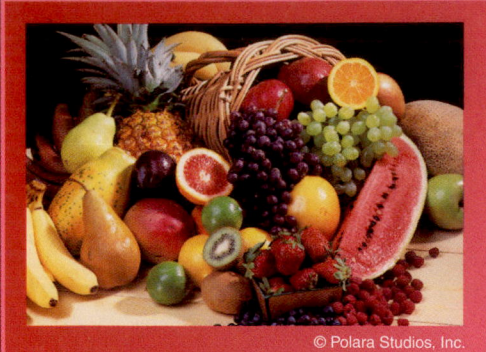

© Polara Studios, Inc.

1 c fruit =
1 c fresh, frozen, cooked, or canned fruit
½ c dried fruit
1 c 100% fruit juice

Fruits contribute folate, vitamin A, vitamin C, potassium, and fiber.

Consume a variety of fruits, and choose whole or cut-up fruits more often than fruit juice.

Apples, apricots, avocados, bananas, blueberries, cantaloupe, cherries, grapefruit, grapes, guava, honeydew, kiwi, mango, nectarines, oranges, papaya, peaches, pears, pineapples, plums, raspberries, strawberries, tangerines, watermelon; dried fruit (dates, figs, prunes, raisins); 100% fruit juices

Limit these fruits that contain solid fats and/or added sugars:
Canned or frozen fruit in syrup; juices, punches, ades, and fruit drinks with added sugars; fried plantains

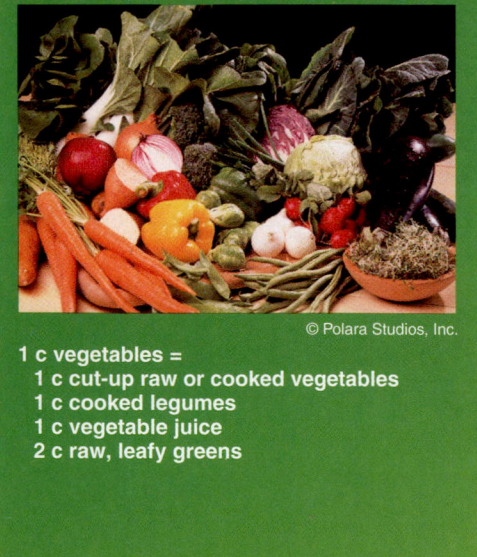

© Polara Studios, Inc.

1 c vegetables =
1 c cut-up raw or cooked vegetables
1 c cooked legumes
1 c vegetable juice
2 c raw, leafy greens

Vegetables contribute folate, vitamin A, vitamin C, vitamin K, vitamin E, magnesium, potassium, and fiber.

Consume a variety of vegetables each day, and choose from all five subgroups several times a week.

Vegetables subgroups:
Dark green vegetables: Broccoli and leafy greens such as arugula, beet greens, bok choy, collard greens, kale, mustard greens, romaine lettuce, spinach, turnip greens, watercress

Red and orange vegetables: Carrots, carrot juice, pumpkin, red bell peppers, sweet potatoes, tomatoes, tomato juice, vegetable juice, winter squash (acorn, butternut)

Legumes: Black beans, black-eyed peas, garbanzo beans (chickpeas), kidney beans, lentils, navy beans, pinto beans, soybeans and soy products such as tofu, split peas, white beans

Starchy vegetables: Cassava, corn, green peas, hominy, lima beans, potatoes

Other vegetables: Artichokes, asparagus, bamboo shoots, bean sprouts, beets, brussels sprouts, cabbages, cactus, cauliflower, celery, cucumbers, eggplant, green beans, green bell peppers, iceberg lettuce, mushrooms, okra, onions, seaweed, snow peas, zucchini

Limit these vegetables that contain solid fats and/or added sugars:
Baked beans, candied sweet potatoes, coleslaw, french fries, potato salad, refried beans, scalloped potatoes, tempura vegetables

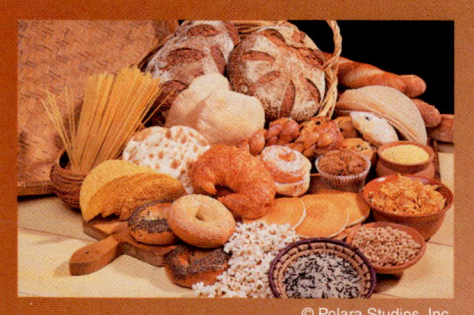

© Polara Studios, Inc.

1 oz grains =
1 slice bread
½ c cooked rice, pasta, or cereal
1 oz dry pasta or rice
1 c ready-to-eat cereal flakes
3 c popped popcorn

Grains contribute folate, niacin, riboflavin, thiamin, iron, magnesium, selenium, and fiber.

Make most (at least half) of the grain selections whole grains.

Grains subgroups:
Whole grains: amaranth, barley, brown rice, buckwheat, bulgur, cornmeal, millet, oats, quinoa, rye, wheat, and wild rice and whole-grain products such as breads, cereals, crackers, and pastas; popcorn

Enriched refined products: bagels, breads, cereals, pastas (couscous, macaroni, spaghetti), pretzels, white rice, rolls, tortillas

Limit these grains that contain solid fats and/or added sugars:
Biscuits, cakes, cookies, cornbread, crackers, croissants, doughnuts, fried rice, granola, muffins, pastries, pies, presweetened cereals, taco shells

Art © Cengage Learning 2013

Figure 2–5

USDA Food Groups and Subgroups (continued)

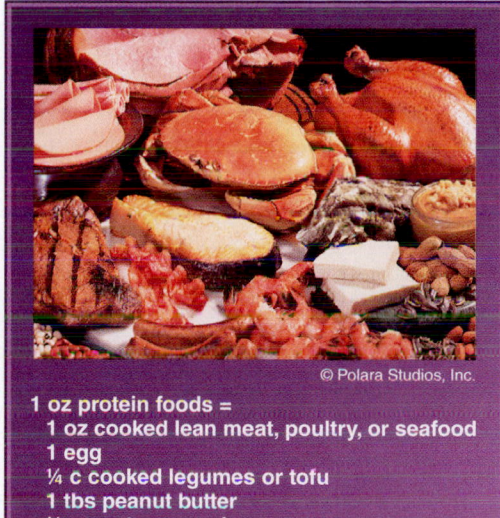

© Polara Studios, Inc.

1 oz protein foods =
- **1 oz cooked lean meat, poultry, or seafood**
- **1 egg**
- **¼ c cooked legumes or tofu**
- **1 tbs peanut butter**
- **½ oz nuts or seeds**

Protein foods contribute protein, essential fatty acids, niacin, thiamin, vitamin B_6, vitamin B_{12}, iron, magnesium, potassium, and zinc.

Choose a variety of protein foods from the three subgroups, including seafood in place of meat or poultry twice a week.

Protein foods subgroups:
Seafood: Fish (catfish, cod, flounder, haddock, halibut, herring, mackerel, pollock, salmon, sardines, sea bass, snapper, trout, tuna), shellfish (clams, crab, lobster, mussels, oysters, scallops, shrimp)

Meats, poultry, and eggs: Lean or low-fat meats (fat-trimmed beef, game, ham, lamb, pork, veal), poultry (no skin), eggs

Nuts, seeds, and soy products: Unsalted nuts (almonds, cashews, filberts, pecans, pistachios, walnuts), seeds (flaxseeds, pumpkin seeds, sesame seeds, sunflower seeds), legumes, soy products (textured vegetable protein, tofu, tempeh), peanut butter, peanuts

Limit these protein foods that contain solid fats and/or added sugars:
Bacon; baked beans; fried meat, seafood, poultry, eggs, or tofu; refried beans; ground beef; hot dogs; luncheon meats; marbled steaks; poultry with skin; sausages; spare ribs

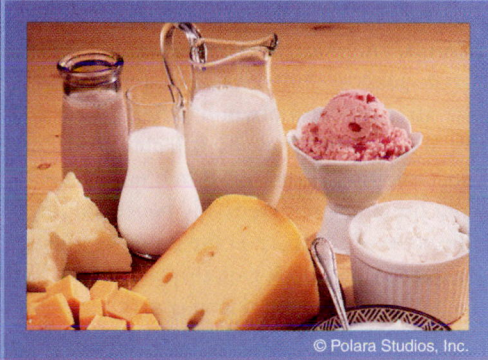

© Polara Studios, Inc.

1 c milk or milk product =
- **1 c milk, yogurt, or fortified soy milk**
- **1½ oz natural cheese**
- **2 oz processed cheese**

Milk and milk products contribute protein, riboflavin, vitamin B_{12}, calcium, potassium, and, when fortified, vitamin A and vitamin D.

Make fat-free or low-fat choices. Choose other calcium-rich foods if you don't consume milk.

Fat-free or 1% low-fat milk and fat-free or 1% low-fat milk products such as buttermilk, cheeses, cottage cheese, yogurt; fat-free fortified soy milk

Limit these milk products that contain solid fats and/or added sugars:
2% reduced-fat milk and whole milk; 2% reduced-fat and whole-milk products such as cheeses, cottage cheese, and yogurt; flavored milk with added sugars such as chocolate milk, custard, frozen yogurt, ice cream, milk shakes, pudding, sherbet; fortified soy milk

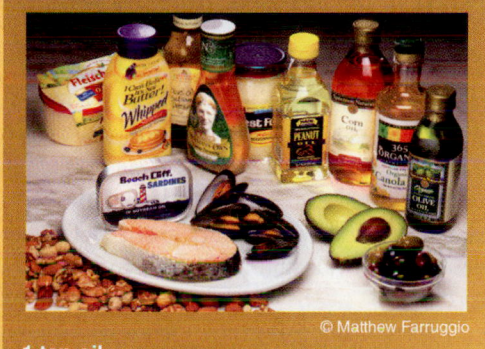

© Matthew Farruggio

1 tsp oil =
- **1 tsp vegetable oil**
- **1 tsp soft margarine**
- **1 tbs low-fat mayonnaise**
- **2 tbs light salad dressing**

Oils are not a food group, but are featured here because they contribute vitamin E and essential fatty acids.

Use oils instead of solid fats, when possible.

Liquid vegetable oils such as canola, corn, flaxseed, nut, olive, peanut, safflower, sesame, soybean, sunflower oils; mayonnaise, oil-based salad dressing, soft *trans* fat-free margarine; unsaturated oils that occur naturally in foods such as avocados, fatty fish, nuts, olives, seeds (flaxseeds, sesame seeds), shellfish

Limit these solid fats:
Butter, animal fats, stick margarine, shortening

Art © Cengage Learning 2013

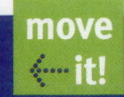
Recommendations for Daily Physical Activity

The USDA's Physical Activity Guidelines for Americans suggest that to maintain good health, adults should engage in about 2½ hours of moderate physical activity each week.[7] A brisk walk at a pace of about 100 steps per minute (1,000 steps over 10 minutes) constitutes "moderate" activity. In addition:

- Physical activity can be intermittent, 10 minutes here and there, throughout the week.

- Resistance activity (such as weight-lifting) can be a valuable part of the exercise total for the week.

For weight control and additional health benefits, more than this minimum amount of physical activity is required. Details can be found in Chapter 10.

start now! ···⟩ Ready to make a change? Set a goal of 30 minutes per day of physical activity (walking, jogging, biking, weight training, etc.), and then track your actual activity for five days. You can use the Track Activity feature of Diet & Wellness Plus.

---

displays the food groups used in this plan. By using the plan wisely and by learning about the energy-yielding nutrients, vitamins, and minerals in various foods (as you will in coming chapters), you can achieve the goals of a nutritious diet first mentioned in Chapter 1: adequacy, balance, calorie control, moderation, and variety.

If you design your diet around this plan, it is assumed that you will obtain adequate and balanced amounts of the two dozen or so essential nutrients and hundreds of potentially beneficial phytochemicals because all of these compounds are distributed among the same foods. It can also help you to limit calories and potentially harmful food constituents.

> Phytochemicals and their potential biological actions are explained in **Controversy 2**.

The Food Groups and Subgroups

Figure 2–5 defines the major food groups and their subgroups. The USDA specifies portions of various foods within each group (left column of Figure 2–5) that are nutritional equivalents and thus can be treated interchangeably in diet planning. It also lists the key nutrients provided by foods within each group, information worth noting and remembering. The foods in each group are well-known contributors of the key nutrients listed, but you can count on these foods to supply many other nutrients as well. Note also that the figure sorts foods within each group by **nutrient density**.

Vegetables Subgroups and Protein Foods Subgroups   Not every vegetable supplies every key nutrient attributed to the Vegetables group, so the vegetables are sorted into subgroups by their nutrient contents. All vegetables provide valuable fiber and the mineral potassium, but many from the "red and orange vegetables" subgroup are known for their vitamin A content; those from the "dark green vegetables" provide a wealth of folate; "starchy vegetables" provide abundant carbohydrate; and "legumes" supply substantial iron and protein.

The Protein Foods group falls into subgroups, too. All protein foods dependably supply iron and protein, but their fats vary widely. "Meats" tend to be higher in saturated fats that should be limited. "Seafood" and "nuts, seeds, and soy products" tend to be low in saturated fats while providing essential fats that the body requires.

Grains Subgroups and Other Foods   Among the grains, the foods of the "whole grains" subgroup supply fiber and a wide variety of nutrients. Refined grains lack many of these beneficial compounds but provide abundant energy. The Dietary Guidelines suggest that at least half of the grains in a day's meals be whole grains

nutrient density a measure of nutrients provided per calorie of food. A *nutrient-dense food* provides vitamins, minerals, and other beneficial substances with relatively few calories. Also defined in Chapter 1.

or that at least three servings of whole-grain foods be included in the diet each day. (Grain serving sizes in 1-ounce equivalents are listed in Figure 2–5.)

Spices, herbs, coffee, and tea provide few, if any, nutrients but can add flavor and pleasure to meals. Some, such as tea and spices, are particularly rich in potentially beneficial phytochemicals—see this chapter's Controversy section.

Variety among and within Food Groups   Varying food choices, both among the food groups and within each group, helps to ensure adequate nutrient intakes and also protects against consuming large amounts of toxins or contaminants from any one food. Achieving variety may require some effort, but knowing which foods fall into which food groups eases the task.

KEY POINTS

- The USDA Eating Patterns divide foods into food groups based on key nutrient contents.
- People who consume the specified amounts of foods from each group and subgroup achieve dietary adequacy, balance, and variety.

Choosing Nutrient-Dense Foods

To help people control calories and achieve and sustain a healthy body weight, the Dietary Guidelines instruct consumers to base their diets on the most nutrient-dense foods from each group. Unprocessed or lightly processed foods are generally best because many processes strip foods of beneficial nutrients and fiber and others add salt, sugar, or fat. As mentioned, Figure 2–5 identifies many nutrient-dense food choices in each food group and points out some foods of lower **nutrient density** to give you an idea of which are which.

> Nutrient density was explained in **Chapter 1**, page 21.

Uncooked (raw) oil is worth notice in this regard. Oil is pure, calorie-rich fat and is therefore low in nutrient density, but a small amount of raw oil from sources such as avocados, olives, nuts, and fish, or even raw vegetable oil, provides vitamin E and essential lipids that other foods lack. High temperatures used in frying destroy these nutrients, however, so the recommendation specifies *raw* oil.

Solid Fats, Added Sugars, and Alcohol Reduce Nutrient Density   **Solid fats** deliver saturated fat and *trans* fat, terms that will become familiar after reading Chapter 5. Sugars in all their forms (described in Chapter 4) deliver carbohydrate calories. Figure 2–6 (p. 44) demonstrates how solid fats and added sugars add **empty calories** to foods, reducing their nutrient density. Solid fats include:

- Naturally occurring fats, such as milk fat and meat fats.
- Added fats, such as butter, cream cheese, hard margarine, lard, sour cream, and shortening.

Added sugars include:

- All caloric sweeteners, such as brown sugar, candy, honey, jelly, molasses, soft drinks, sugar, and syrups.

The USDA suggests that intakes of solid fats and added sugars not exceed a daily suggested total, listed in Table 2–3 of the next section.

Alcoholic beverages are a top contributor of empty calories to the diets of many U.S. adults, but they provide few nutrients.[8] People who drink alcohol should monitor and moderate their intakes, not to exceed one drink a day for women and two for men. People in many circumstances should never drink alcohol (see Controversy 3).

KEY POINTS

- Following the USDA Eating Patterns requires choosing nutrient-dense foods most often.
- Solid fats, added sugars, and alcohol should be limited.

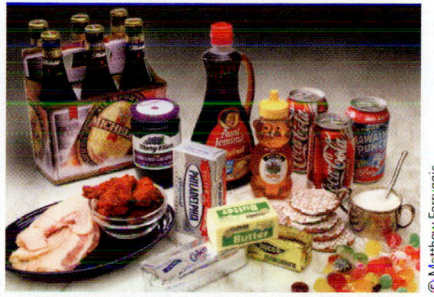

Solid fats, added sugars, and alcohol should be limited.

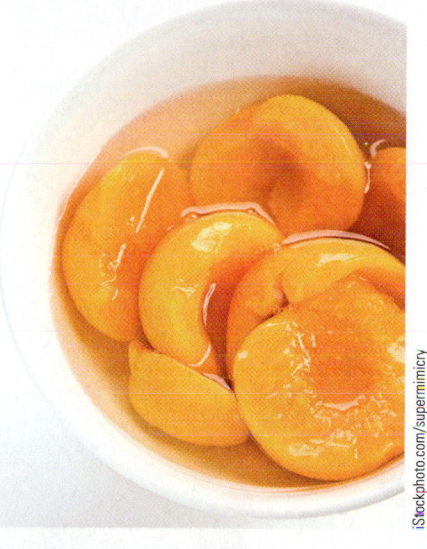

The heavy syrup in a cup of these canned peaches adds 135 empty calories of added sugar. The peaches alone provide only 60 calories.

solid fats fats that are high in saturated fat and usually not liquid at room temperature. Some common solid fats include butter, beef fat, chicken fat, pork fat, stick margarine, coconut oil, palm oil, and shortening.

empty calories calories provided by added sugars and solid fats with few or no other nutrients. Other empty calorie sources include alcohol, and highly refined starches, such as corn starch or potato starch, often found in ultra-processed foods.

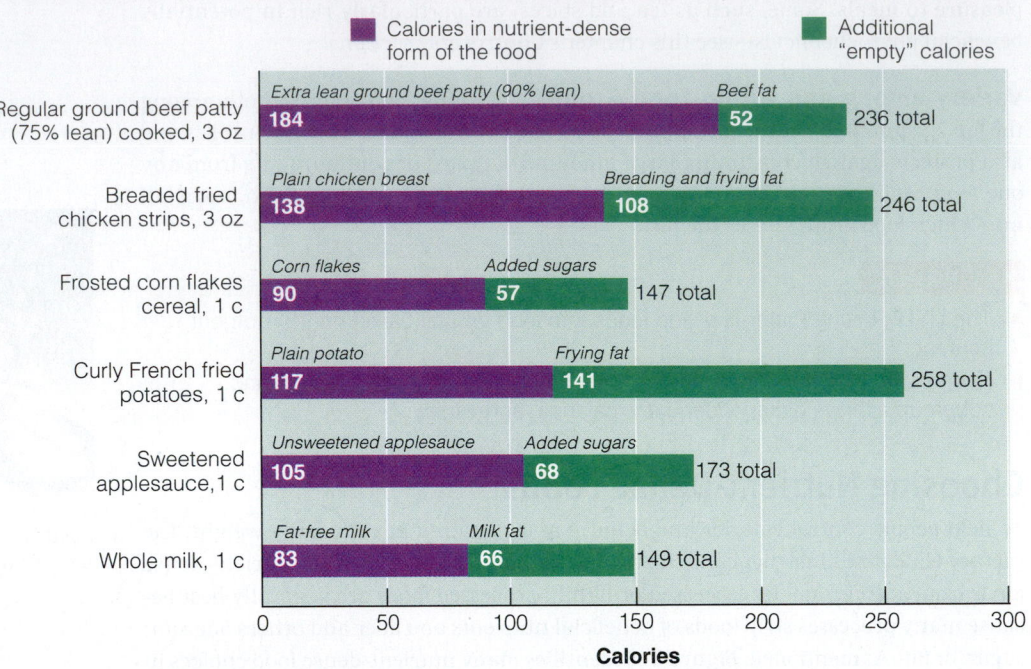

Our completed diet plan is shown in Figure 2–15 (p. 58) in the Food Feature of this chapter. We chose healthy U.S.-style foods, but many other choices are possible, so long as they adhere to the principles of the Dietary Guidelines for Americans.

Diet Planning Application

LO 2.4 Given the required number of calories, discuss a healthful diet plan by applying the USDA Eating Patterns.

The USDA Eating Patterns specify the amounts of food needed from each food group to create a healthful diet for a given number of calories. Look at the top line of Table 2–3 and find yourself among the people described there (for other calorie levels, see Table E–1 of Appendix E). Then look at the column of numbers below for amounts from each food group that meet your calorie need. Note that the more energy spent on physical activity each day, the greater the calorie need.

For vegetables and protein foods, intakes should be divided among all the subgroups over a week's time, as shown in Table 2–4. Look across the top row for your calorie level (obtained from Table 2–3)—a healthful diet includes the listed amounts of the Vegetables and Protein Foods subgroups each *week*. It is not necessary to eat foods from every subgroup each day.

With judicious selections, the diet can supply all the necessary nutrients and provide some luxury items as well. A sample diet plan demonstrates how the theory of the USDA Eating Patterns translates to food on the plate.

The diet planner begins by assigning each of the food groups to meals and snacks, as shown in Table 2–5. Then the plan can be filled out with real foods to create a menu. For example, the breakfast in Table 2–5 calls for 1 ounce of grains, 1 cup of milk, and ½ cup of fruit. Here's one possibility for this meal:

1 cup ready-to-eat cereal = 1 ounce grains

1 cup fat-free milk = 1 cup milk

1 medium banana = ½ cup fruit

Our completed diet plan is shown in Figure 2–15 (p. 58) in the Food Feature of this chapter. We chose healthy U.S.-style foods, but many other choices are possible, so long as they adhere to the principles of the Dietary Guidelines for Americans.

iStockphoto.com/Floortje

Table 2–3

USDA Healthy U.S.-Style Eating Pattern: Daily Amounts from Each Food Group[a]

Calories[a]	Sedentary Women: 51+ yr	Sedentary Women: 26–50 yr	Sedentary Women: 19–25 yr Active Women: 61+ yr Sedentary Men: 61+ yr	Active Women: 31–60 yr Sedentary Men: 41–60 yr	Active Women: 19–30 yr Sedentary Men: 21–40 yr	Active Men: 36–55 yr	Active Men: 19–35 yr
	1,600	1,800	2,000	2,200	2,400	2,800	3,000
Fruits	1½ c	1½ c	2 c	2 c	2 c	2½ c	2½ c
Vegetables[b]	2 c	2½ c	2½ c	3 c	3 c	3½ c	4 c
Grains	5 oz	6 oz	6 oz	7 oz	8 oz	10 oz	10 oz
Protein Foods[b]	5 oz	5 oz	5½ oz	6 oz	6½ oz	7 oz	7 oz
Milk	3 c	3 c	3 c	3 c	3 c	3 c	3 c
Oils	5 tsp	5 tsp	6 tsp	6 tsp	7 tsp	8 tsp	10 tsp
Solid fats[c]	8 g (1½ tsp)	11 g (2½ tsp)	18 g (4 tsp)	18 g (4 tsp)	23 g (5 tsp)	26 g (5½ tsp)	31 g (6½ tsp)
Added sugars[c]	14 g (3½ tsp)	19 g (5 tsp)	30 g (7½ tsp)	32 g (8 tsp)	39 g (10 tsp)	45 g (11½ tsp)	53 g (13½ tsp)

Note: In addition to gender, age, and activity levels, energy needs vary with height and weight (see Chapter 9 and Appendix H).

[a]*Other healthy eating patterns and additional calorie and activity levels are found in Appendix E.*

[b]*Divide these amounts among the vegetables and protein foods subgroups as specified in Table 2–4.*

[c]*In addition to fats and sugars, refined starches, more nutrient-dense foods, or alcohol can fill the calories remaining after needs are met (see Appendix E).*

Source: U.S. Department of Health and Human Services and U.S. Department of Agriculture, 2015–2020 Dietary Guidelines for Americans, *8th edition (2015), available at http://health.gov/dietaryguidelines/2015/guidelines/.*

Table 2–4

Weekly Amounts from Vegetables and Protein Foods Subgroups

Table 2–3 specifies total intakes per *day.* This table shows those amounts dispersed among five Vegetables and three Protein Foods subgroups per *week.*

Vegetables Subgroups	1,600 cal	1,800 cal	2,000 cal	2,200 cal	2,400 cal	2,800 cal	3,000 cal
Dark green	1½ c	1½ c	1½ c	2 c	2 c	2½ c	2½ c
Red and orange	4 c	5½ c	5½ c	6 c	6 c	7 c	7½ c
Legumes	1 c	1½ c	1½ c	2 c	2 c	2½ c	3 c
Starchy	4 c	5 c	5 c	6 c	6 c	7 c	8 c
Other	3½ c	4 c	4 c	5 c	5 c	5½ c	7 c
Protein Foods Subgroups							
Seafood	8 oz	8 oz	8 oz	9 oz	10 oz	10 oz	10 oz
Meat, poultry, eggs	23 oz	23 oz	26 oz	28 oz	31 oz	33 oz	33 oz
Nuts, seeds, soy products	4 oz	4 oz	5 oz	5 oz	5 oz	6 oz	6 oz

Source: U.S. Department of Agriculture and U.S. Department of Health and Human Services, Scientific Report of the 2015 Dietary Guidelines Advisory Committee *(2015):* Table D1.10, 100–101, available at www.health.gov.

This diet plan is one of many possibilities for a day's meals. Figure 2–15, Monday's Meals (p. 58), illustrates the completed diet plan.

Food Group	Recommended Amounts	Breakfast	Lunch	Snack	Dinner	Snack
Fruits	2 c	½ c		½ c	1 c	
Vegetables	2½ c		1 c		2 c	
Grains	6 oz	1 oz	2 oz	½ oz	2 oz	½ oz
Protein Foods	5½ oz		2 oz		3½ oz	
Milk	3 c	1 c		1 c		1 c
Oils	6 tsp		2 tsp		4 tsp	

Figure 2–7

USDA MyPlate

Note that vegetables and fruits occupy half the plate and that the grains portion is slightly larger than the portion of protein foods. A diet that follows the USDA Intake Food Patterns reflects these ideals.

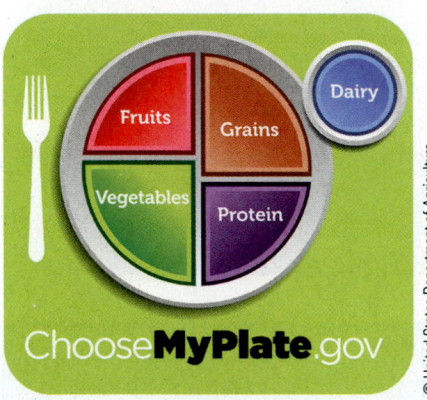

© United States Department of Agriculture

Note that our plan meets nutrient needs with about 150 calories to spare—enough for about two extra fruit servings (around 140 calories), another quarter-portion of spaghetti (115 calories), or a 12-ounce canned soft drink (150 calories). Alternatively, the diet planner endeavoring to lose weight can choose to skip such foods to create a needed calorie deficit.

KEY POINT

- The USDA Eating Patterns for various calorie levels can guide food choices in diet planning.

MyPlate Educational Tool

For consumers with Internet access, the USDA's MyPlate online suite of educational tools makes applying the USDA Eating Patterns easier.[9] Figure 2–7 displays its graphic image. Computer-savvy consumers will find an abundance of MyPlate support materials and diet assessment tools on the website (www.choosemyplate.gov). Those without computer access can achieve the same diet-planning goals by following this chapter's principles and working with pencil and paper, as illustrated later.

KEY POINT

- The concepts of the USDA Eating Patterns are demonstrated in the MyPlate online educational tools.

My Turn — watch it! **Right Size—Supersize?**

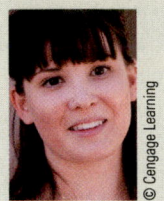

Stephanie

© Cengage Learning

Do you often overeat when you eat out? Listen to a student talk about making healthy choices in restaurants.

Visit www.cengagebrain.com to access MindTap, a complete digital course that includes this video and other resources.

Flexibility of the USDA Eating Patterns

Although they may appear rigid, the USDA Eating Patterns can actually be quite flexible once their intent is understood. For example, the user can substitute fat-free yogurt for fat-free milk because both supply the key nutrients for the Milk and Milk Products group. Legumes, an extraordinarily nutrient-rich food, provide many of the nutrients that characterize the Protein Foods group, but they also constitute a Vegetables subgroup, so legumes in a meal can count as a serving of either meat or vegetables. Consumers can adapt the plan to mixed dishes such as casseroles and to national and cultural foods as well, as Figure 2–8 illustrates.

See **Appendix E** for vegetarian and Mediterranean eating patterns, and **Controversy 6** for vegetarian diet planning.

Vegetarians can use adaptations of the USDA Eating Patterns in making sound food choices, too. The food group that includes the meats also includes nuts, seeds, and products made from soybeans. The Vegetables group includes legumes, counted as protein foods for vegetarians. In the food group that includes milk, soy drinks and soy milk (beverages made from soybeans) can fill the same nutrient needs, provided that they are fortified with calcium, riboflavin, vitamin A, vitamin D, and vitamin B_{12}. Therefore, for all sorts of careful diet planners, the USDA Eating Patterns provide a general road map for designing a healthful diet.

KEY POINT

- The USDA Eating Patterns can be used with flexibility by people with different eating styles.

Figure 2–8

A Sampling of Ethnic Food Choices

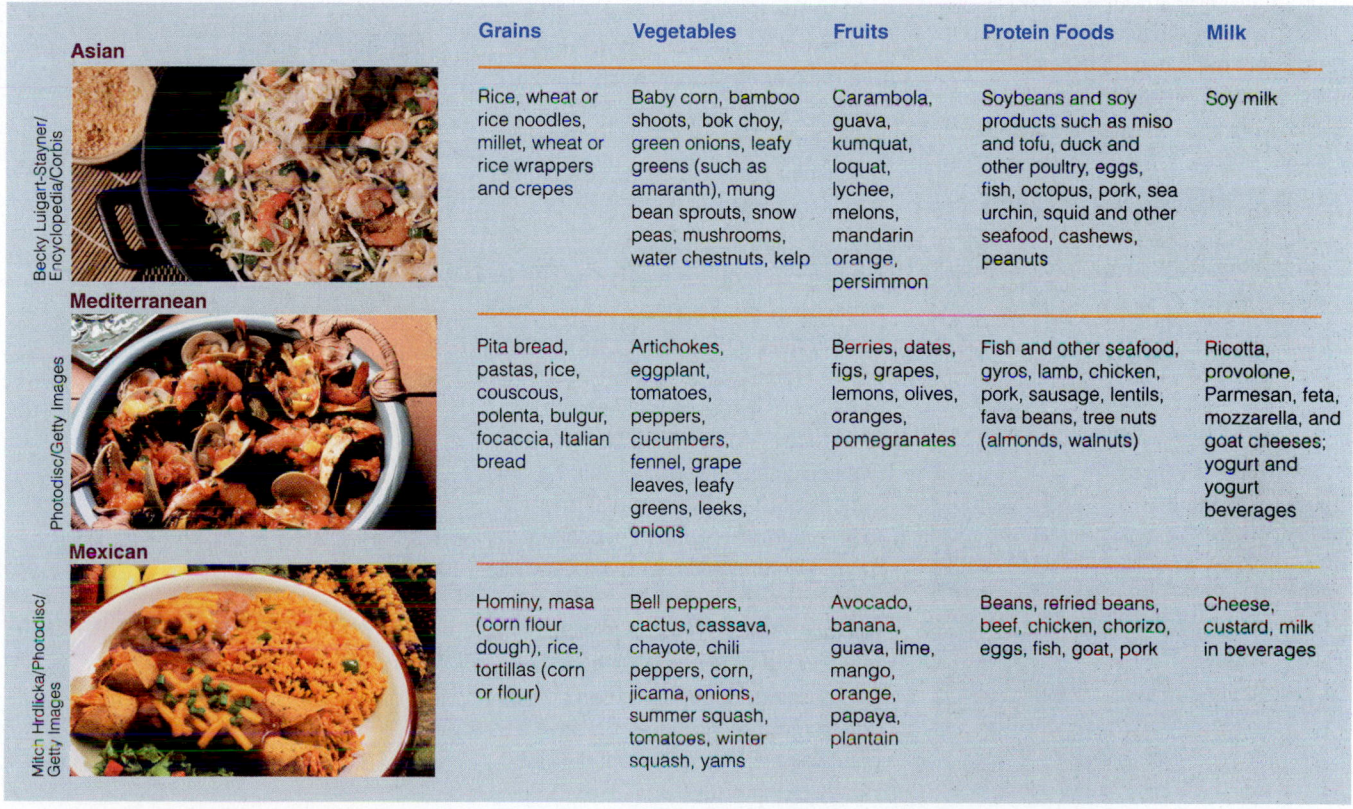

	Grains	Vegetables	Fruits	Protein Foods	Milk
Asian	Rice, wheat or rice noodles, millet, wheat or rice wrappers and crepes	Baby corn, bamboo shoots, bok choy, green onions, leafy greens (such as amaranth), mung bean sprouts, snow peas, mushrooms, water chestnuts, kelp	Carambola, guava, kumquat, loquat, lychee, melons, mandarin orange, persimmon	Soybeans and soy products such as miso and tofu, duck and other poultry, eggs, fish, octopus, pork, sea urchin, squid and other seafood, cashews, peanuts	Soy milk
Mediterranean	Pita bread, pastas, rice, couscous, polenta, bulgur, focaccia, Italian bread	Artichokes, eggplant, tomatoes, peppers, cucumbers, fennel, grape leaves, leafy greens, leeks, onions	Berries, dates, figs, grapes, lemons, olives, oranges, pomegranates	Fish and other seafood, gyros, lamb, chicken, pork, sausage, lentils, fava beans, tree nuts (almonds, walnuts)	Ricotta, provolone, Parmesan, feta, mozzarella, and goat cheeses; yogurt and yogurt beverages
Mexican	Hominy, masa (corn flour dough), rice, tortillas (corn or flour)	Bell peppers, cactus, cassava, chayote, chili peppers, corn, jicama, onions, summer squash, tomatoes, winter squash, yams	Avocado, banana, guava, lime, mango, orange, papaya, plantain	Beans, refried beans, beef, chicken, chorizo, eggs, fish, goat, pork	Cheese, custard, milk in beverages

Becky Luigart-Stayner/Encyclopedia/Corbis

Photodisc/Getty Images

Mitch Hrdlicka/Photodisc/Getty Images

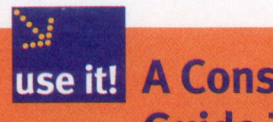
Controlling Portion Sizes at Home and Away

"May I take your order, please?" Put on the spot when eating out, a diner must quickly choose from a large, visually exciting menu. No one brings a scale to a restaurant to weigh portions, and physical cues used at home, such as measuring cups are, well, at home. Restaurant portions have no standards. When ordering "a burger," for example, the sandwich may arrive resembling a 2-ounce kids' sandwich or a ¾-pound behemoth. Even at home, portion sizes can be mystifying—how much spaghetti is enough?

How Big Is Your Bagel?

When college students are asked to bring "medium-sized" foods to class, they reliably bring bagels weighing from 2 to 5 ounces, muffins from 2 to 8 ounces, baked potatoes from 4 to 9 ounces, and so forth. Knowledge of appropriate daily amounts of food is crucial to controlling calorie intakes, but consumers need help to estimate portion sizes, whether preparing a meal at home or choosing from a restaurant menu.

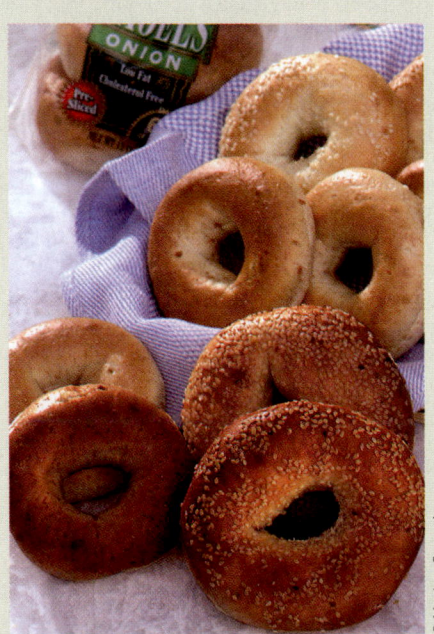

How much does your bagel weigh?

Practice with Weights and Measures

At home, practice makes perfect. To estimate the size of food portions, remember these common objects:

- 3 ounces of meat = the size of the palm of a woman's hand or a deck of cards
- 1 medium potato or piece of fruit = the size of a tennis ball
- 1½ ounces cheese = the size of a 9-volt battery
- 1 ounce lunch meat or cheese = 1 slice
- 1 cup cooked pasta = the size of a baseball
- 1 pat (1 tsp) butter or margarine = a slice from a quarter-pound stick of butter about as thick as 150 pages of this book (pressed together).
- Most ice cream scoops hold ¼ cup = a lump about the size of a golf ball. (Test the size of your scoop—fill it with water and pour the water into a measuring cup. Now you have a handy device to measure portions at home—use the scoop to serve mashed potatoes, pasta, vegetables, rice, and cereals.)

Among volumetric measures, 1 "cup" refers to an 8-ounce measuring cup (not a teacup or drinking glass) filled to level (not heaped up, or shaken, or pressed down). Tablespoons and teaspoons refer to measuring spoons (not flatware), filled to level (not rounded or heaping). Ounces signify weight, not volume. Two ounces of meat, for example, refers to one-eighth of a pound of cooked meat. One ounce (weight) of crispy rice cereal measures a full cup (volume), but take care: 1 ounce of granola cereal measures only ¼ cup. The Table of Food Composition, Appendix A, can help in determining serving sizes because it lists both weights and volumes for a wide variety of foods.

Buy New Bowls

Take a moment to consider the size of your plates, bowls, utensils, and other tableware. Tableware seems to function as a sort of visual gauge for sizing up food portions. In research, people eating from large containers often eat more per sitting than those eating from smaller ones (details in Chapter 9). Thus, if your plates look more like serving platters, try using luncheon-sized plates instead. The same holds true for bowls and spoons; if yours are overly large, invest in smaller ones.

Colossal Cuisine in Restaurants

Figure 2–9 shows that, over the past four decades, consumers have doubled the percentage of their food budgets spent on foods eaten away from home.[1]*

Figure 2–9

Dining Out Trends, United States, 1970–2012

People today are spending a greater proportion of their total food budgets on restaurant meals and other foods eaten away from home.

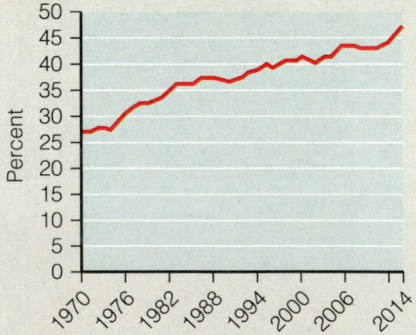

Source: Economic Research Service, U.S. Department of Agriculture, Food Expenditures, 2013, available at www.ers.usda.gov/topics/food-choices-health/food-consumption-demand/food-away-from-home.aspx.

* Reference notes are found in Appendix F.

© Matthew Farruggio

Figure 2–10

A Shift toward Colossal Cuisine

The portion sizes of many foods have increased dramatically over past decades.

Food	Typical 1970s	Today's colossal
Cola	10 oz bottle, 120 cal	40–60 oz fountain, 580 cal
French fries	about 30, 475 cal	about 50, 790 cal
Hamburger	3–4 oz meat, 330 cal	6–12 oz meat, 1,000 cal
Bagel	2–3 oz, 230 cal	5–7 oz, 550 cal
Steak	8–12 oz, 690 cal	16–22 oz, 1,260 cal
Pasta	1 c, 200 cal	2–3 c, 600 cal
Baked potato	5–7 oz, 180 cal	1 lb, 420 cal
Candy bar	1½ oz, 220 cal	3–4 oz, 580 cal
Popcorn	1½ c, 80 cal	8–16 c tub, 880 cal

Note: Calories are rounded values for the largest portions in a given range.
Source: USDA.

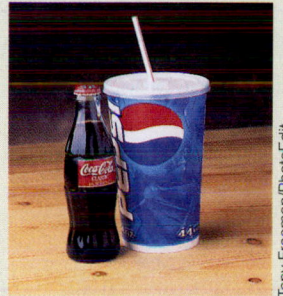
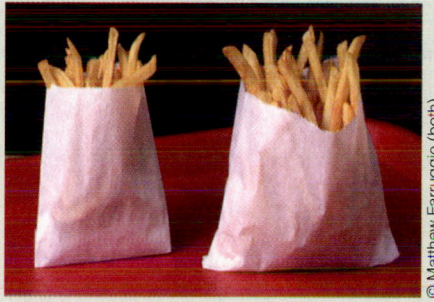
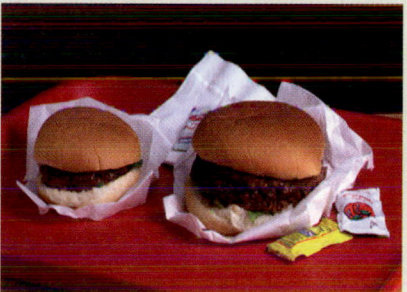

1970s   Today   1970s   Today   1970s   Today

Two other trends occurred at the same time: food portions grew larger and therefore more caloric (Figure 2–10), and people's body weights increased to new, unhealthy levels. Taken together, these trends suggest that restaurant food portions may be affecting public health.

Figure 9–9 of Chapter 9 illustrates calorie information on a restaurant menu.

A new law requires all chain restaurants with 20 or more locations, including fast-food restaurants, to post calorie information on menus and menu boards for each standard food item.[†] Without such a gauge readily at hand, consumers most

[†]*Compliance enforcement is planned to begin in December 2016.*

often underestimate the calories in restaurant foods.[2] In local non–chain restaurants where such information may be lacking, people must learn to judge portions on their own.

When portions seem excessively large or calorie-rich, use creative solutions to cut them down to size: order a half portion, ask that half of a regular portion be packaged for a later meal, order a child's portion, or split an entrée with a friend.

Moving Ahead

Portion control is a habit—and a way to defend against overeating. When cooking at home, have measuring tools at the ready. When dining out, your tools are your practiced abilities to judge portion sizes. Then, when the waiter asks, "Are you ready to order?" the savvy consumer, armed with portion size know-how, answers confidently, "Yes."

Review Questions[††]

1. American restaurant portions are stable and consistent; use them as a guide to choosing portion sizes. T F

2. Experimenting with portion sizes at home is a valuable exercise in self-education. T F

3. When consumers guess at the calorie values in restaurant food portions, they generally overestimate. T F

[††]*Answers to Consumer's Guide questions are found in Appendix G.*

Food Lists for Diabetes and Weight Management

A different kind of diet-planning tool, the Food Lists for Diabetes and Weight Management (formerly the Exchange System; see Appendix D), was developed for use by people with diabetes but can be useful to anyone wishing to control calories. The lists provide estimated grams of carbohydrate, fat, saturated fat, and protein in standardized food portions, as well as their calorie values. These are average gram values for whole groups of foods, so they often differ from the exacting values given for individual foods in Appendix A. With the calorie estimates (Table 2–6) committed to memory, people can make an informed approximation of the energy-yielding nutrients and calories in

Table 2–6

Estimating Calories with Food Lists for Diabetes and Weight Management

These calorie values are estimates for average portions of foods within various categories. Appendix D provides details about the calorie values of individual foods on these lists.

Food Lists	Calories
Starch	80
1 slice bread	
½ c cooked cereals, most grains, legumes, and starchy vegetables	
⅓ c pasta or rice	
1 oz low-fat crackers	
Sweets[a]	70
1 tbs sugar	
1 tbs syrup	
1 frozen juice bar	
Fruits	60
Milk and Milk Substitutes	
1 c fat-free, low-fat milk (0–1%)	100
⅔ c (6 oz) fat-free yogurt (plain or Greek)	100
1 c reduced-fat milk (2%)	120
1 c whole milk	160
Nonstarchy Vegetables	25
Proteins[b]	
1 oz lean	45
1 oz medium-fat	75
1 oz high-fat	100
Fats	45
1 tsp oil or solid fat	
1 tbs salad dressing	
Alcohol (½ ounce ethanol without mixers; details in Controversy 3)	100

[a]Sweets, desserts, baked goods, and beverages vary widely in calorie contents; see Appendix D for details.

[b]Plant-based proteins vary in calorie contents.

Source: Adapted from American Diabetes Association and Academy of Nutrition and Dietetics, Choose Your Foods: Food Lists for Diabetes (2014), available from www.diabetes.org (catalog no. 310X14) or www.eatright.org (order no. 5601-13).

almost any food they might encounter. To explore the usefulness of this powerful aid to diet planning, spend some time studying Appendix D.

- The Food Lists for Diabetes group foods that are similar in carbohydrate, fat, and protein to facilitate control of energy nutrient and calorie consumption.

The Last Word on Diet Planning

All of the dietary changes required to improve nutrition may seem daunting or even insurmountable at first, and taken all at once, they may be. However, small steps taken each day can add up to substantial dietary changes over time. If everyone would begin, today, to take such steps, the rewards in terms of less risk of diabetes, obesity, heart disease, and cancer along with a greater quality of life with better health would prove well worth the effort.

Checking Out Food Labels

LO 2.5   Discuss the information included on food labels.

A potato is a potato and needs no label to tell you so. But what can a package of potato chips tell you about its contents? By law, its label must list the chips' ingredients—potatoes, oil, and salt—and its **Nutrition Facts** panel must also reveal details about their nutrient composition. If the oil is high in saturated fat, the label will reveal it (more about fats in Chapter 5). In addition to required information, labels may make optional statements about the food being delicious, or good for you in some way, or a great value. Some of these comments, especially some that are regulated by the Food and Drug Administration (FDA), are reliable. Many others are marketing tools, based more on salesmanship than science.

What Food Labels Must Include

The Nutrition Education and Labeling Act of 1990 set the requirements for certain label information to ensure that food labels truthfully inform consumers about the nutrients and ingredients in the package. Every packaged food must state the following:

- The common or usual name of the product.
- The name and address of the manufacturer, packer, or distributor.
- The net contents in terms of weight, measure, or count.
- The nutrient contents of the product (Nutrition Facts panel).
- The ingredients in descending order of predominance by weight and in ordinary language.
- Essential warnings, such as alerts about ingredients that often cause allergic reactions or other problems.

Not every package need display information about every vitamin and mineral. A large package, such as a box of cereal, must provide all of the information just listed. A smaller label, such as the label on a can of tuna, provides some of the information in abbreviated form. The tiniest of labels, such as on a roll of candy rings, provides only a phone number to call for nutrient information.

The Nutrition Facts Panel   Most shoppers read food labels, and when they do, they often rely on the Nutrition Facts panel, like the one shown in Figure 2–11 on p. 52.[10] Grocers also voluntarily post placards or offer handouts in produce and other departments to provide consumers with similar nutrition information for the most popular fresh fruits, vegetables, and seafoods.

Notice in Figure 2–11 that only the top portion of a food's Nutrition Facts panel conveys information specific to the food inside the package. The bottom portion is identical on every label—it stands as a reminder of the Daily Values.

Nutrition Facts   on a food label, the panel of nutrition information required to appear on almost every packaged food. Grocers may also provide the information for fresh produce, meats, poultry, and seafood.

Figure 2–11

What's on a Food Label?

This cereal label maps out the locations of information needed to make wise purchases. The text provides details about each label section. Note that Nutrition Facts panels on real packages are printed in black and white; color is added to this demonstration and to the label on p. 53 to facilitate the discussions.

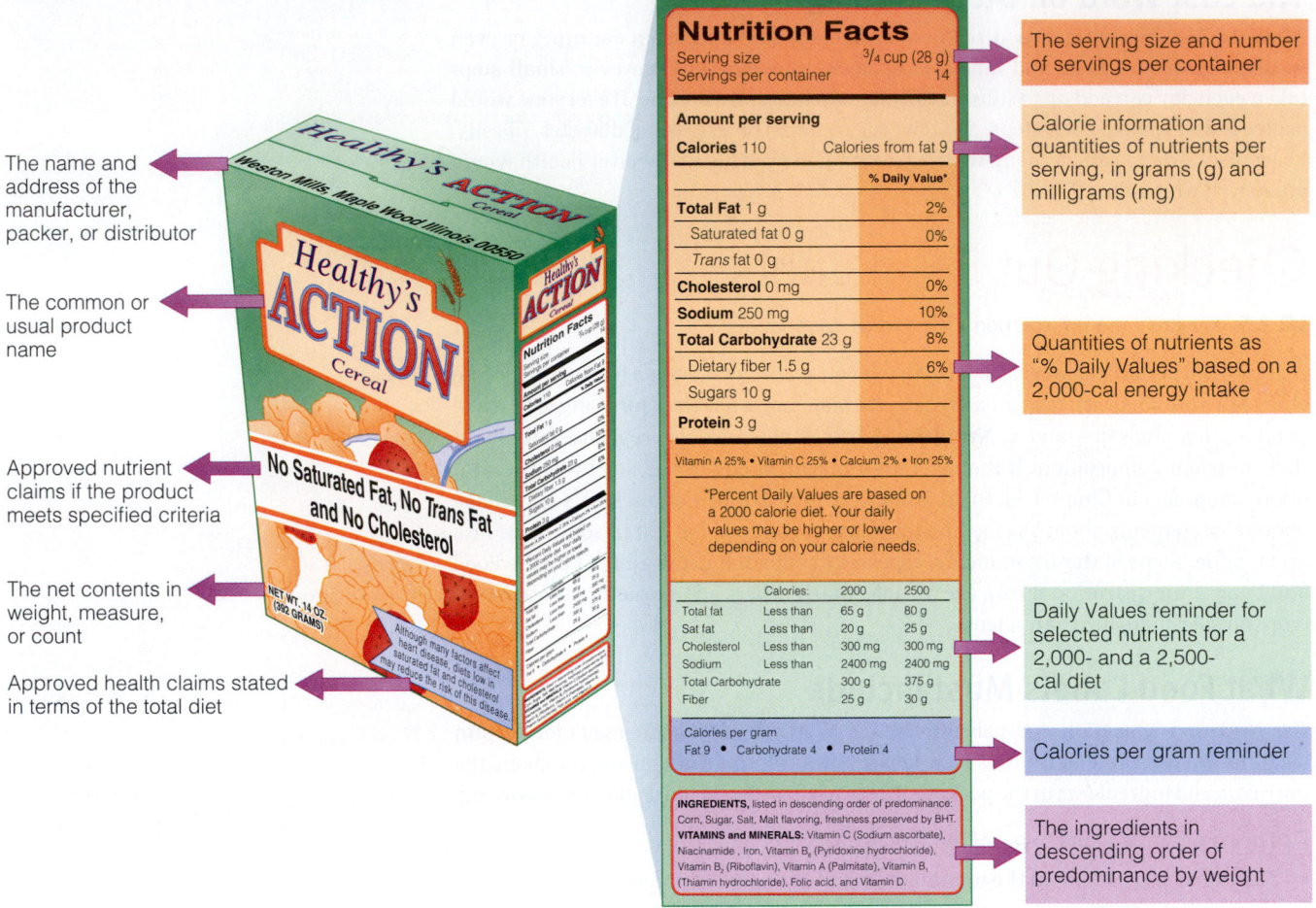

Figure 2–11 points out where the following may be found on a label (from top to bottom):

- *Serving size.* A common household and metric measure of a single serving that provides the calorie and nutrient amounts listed. A serving of chips may be 10 chips, so if you eat 50 chips, you will have consumed five times the calorie and nutrient amounts listed on the label. Keep in mind that label serving sizes are not recommendations. They simply reflect amounts that people typically consume in a serving.

- *Servings per container.* Number of servings per box, can, or package.

- *Calories/calories from fat.* Total food energy per serving and energy from fat per serving.

- *Nutrient amounts and percentages of Daily Values,* including:

  - *Total fat.* Grams of fat per serving with a breakdown showing grams of *saturated fat* and *trans fat* per serving.

  - *Cholesterol.* Milligrams of cholesterol per serving.

  - *Sodium.* Milligrams of sodium per serving.

- *Total carbohydrate.* Grams of carbohydrate per serving, including starch, fiber, and sugars, with a breakdown showing grams of dietary *fiber* and *sugars*. The sugars include those that occur naturally in the food plus any added during processing.
- *Protein.* Grams of protein per serving.

Other nutrients present in significant amounts in the food may also be listed on the label. The percentages of the Daily Values (see the inside back cover, p. Y) are given in terms of a 2,000-calorie diet.

- *Daily Values and calories-per-gram reminder.* This portion lists the Daily Values for a person needing 2,000 or 2,500 calories a day and provides a calories-per-gram reminder as a handy reference.

The FDA's New Nutrition Facts Panel A new Nutrition Facts panel is currently under construction. The new label will reflect up-to-date nutrition information and present it in an easy-to-read format.[11] Among the proposed updates, listed serving sizes will better reflect portions people typically consume. For example, most people eat an entire 19-ounce can of ready-to-eat soup for a meal, but the can's label currently claims that it holds two servings. Such serving size discrepancies will be resolved for many foods. In addition, bigger, bolder type and use of common measures, such as cups, will allow consumers to more quickly grasp the number of calories in a single serving. Figure 2–12 highlights these and other important changes to the Nutrition Facts panel that consumers may soon begin to see on food packaging.

Ingredients List An often neglected but highly valuable body of information is the list of ingredients. The product's ingredients must be listed in descending order of predominance by weight.

Knowing how to read an ingredients list puts you many steps ahead of the naïve buyer. Anyone diagnosed with a food allergy quickly learns to use these lists for spotting "off-limits" ingredients in foods. In addition, you can glean clues about the nature of the food. For example, consider the ingredients list on an orange drink powder whose first three entries are "sugar, citric acid, orange flavor." You can tell that sugar is the chief ingredient. Now consider a canned juice whose ingredients list begins with "water, orange juice concentrate, pineapple juice concentrate." This product is clearly made of reconstituted juice. Water is first on the label because it is the main constituent of juice. Sugar is nowhere to be found among the ingredients because no sugar has been added. Sugar occurs naturally in juice, though, so the label does specify sugar grams; details are in Chapter 4.

Now consider a cereal whose entire list contains just one item: "100 percent shredded wheat." No question, this is a whole-grain food with nothing added. Finally, consider a cereal whose first six ingredients are "puffed milled corn, corn syrup, sucrose, honey, dextrose, salt." If you recognize that corn syrup, sucrose, honey, and dextrose are all different versions of sugar (and you will after Chapter 4), you might guess that this product contains close to half its weight as added sugar.

More about Percentages of Daily Values The nutrient percentages of Daily Values ("% Daily Value") on labels are for a single serving of food, and they are based on the Daily Values set for a 2,000-calorie diet. For example, if a food contributes 4 milligrams of iron per serving and the Daily Value is 18 milligrams, then a serving of that food provides 22 percent of the Daily Value for iron.

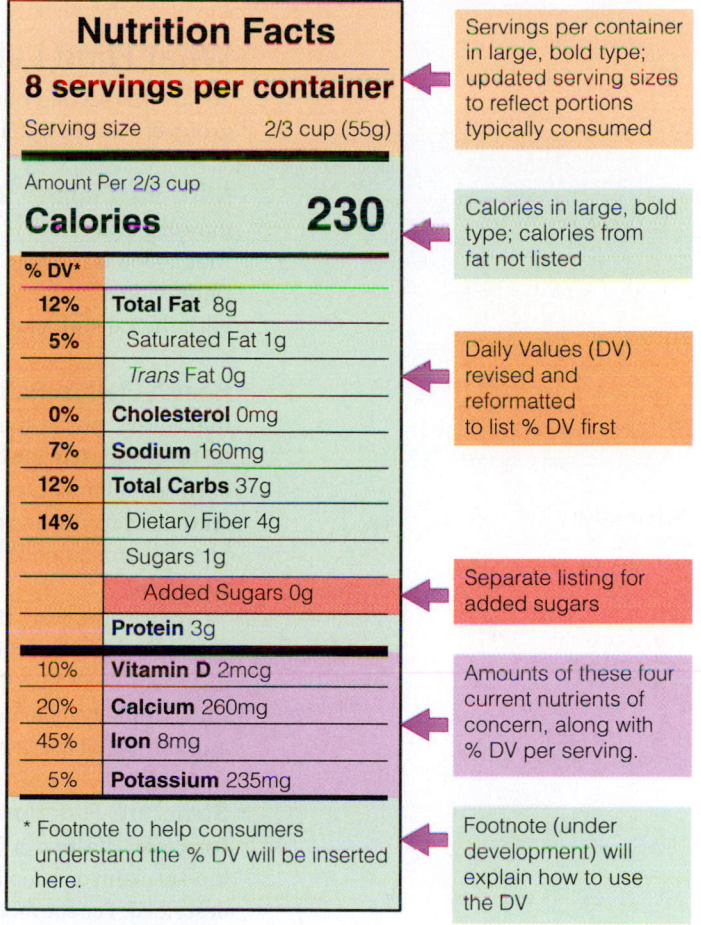

Servings per container in large, bold type; updated serving sizes to reflect portions typically consumed

Calories in large, bold type; calories from fat not listed

Daily Values (DV) revised and reformatted to list % DV first

Separate listing for added sugars

Amounts of these four current nutrients of concern, along with % DV per serving.

Footnote (under development) will explain how to use the DV

Of course, though the Daily Values are based on a 2,000-calorie diet, people's actual calorie and nutrient needs vary widely. This makes the Daily Values most useful for comparing one food with another and less useful as nutrient intake targets for individuals. Still, by examining a food's general nutrient profile, you can determine whether the food contributes "a little" or "a lot" of a nutrient and whether it contributes "more" or "less" than another food.

What Food Labels *May* Include

So far, this section has presented the accurate and reliable food label facts. Another group of reliable statements are the **nutrient claims**.

Nutrient Claims: Reliable Information
A food that meets specified criteria may display certain approved nutrient claims on its label. These claims—for example, that a food is "low" in cholesterol or a "good source" of vitamin A—are based on the Daily Values. Table 2–7 provides a list of these regulated, reliable label terms along with their definitions.

Health Claims: Reliable and Not So Reliable
In the past, the FDA held manufacturers to the highest standards of scientific evidence before allowing them to place **health claims** on food labels. A health claim describes a relationship between a food or its components and a disease or health condition. When a label stated "Diets low in sodium may reduce the risk of high blood pressure," for example, consumers could be sure that the FDA had substantial scientific support for the claim.

Today, however, the FDA also allows similar-sounding health claims that are backed by weaker evidence. These are "qualified" claims in the sense that labels bearing them must also state the strength of the scientific evidence backing them up. Unfortunately, consumers cannot distinguish between scientifically reliable claims and those that are less so.

Structure-Function Claims: Best Ignored
Even less reliable are **structure-function claims**. A label-reading consumer is much more likely to encounter this kind of claim on a food or supplement label than the more regulated health claims just described. For the food manufacturer, printing a *health claim* involves acquiring FDA permission, a time-consuming and expensive process. Instead, the manufacturer can print a similar-looking structure-function claim that requires only FDA notification and no prior approval. Figure 2–13 compares claims on food labels.

Figure 2–13
Label Claims

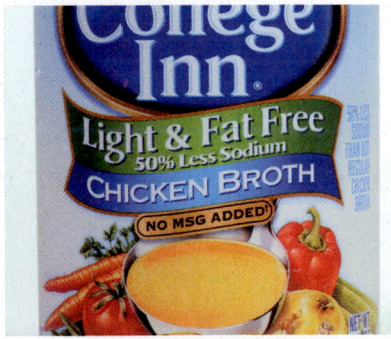

Nutrient claim

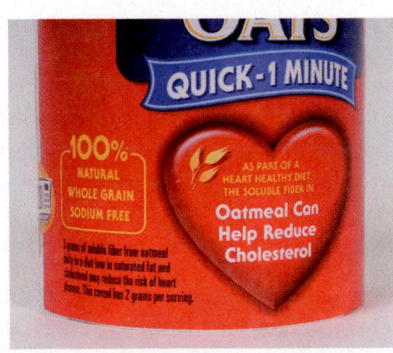

Health claim

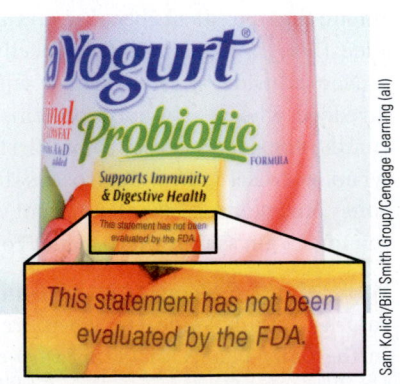

Structure-function claim

Table 2–7

Some Reliable Nutrient Claims on Food Labels

Energy Terms

- **low calorie** 40 calories or fewer per serving.
- **reduced calorie** at least 25% lower in calories than a "regular," or reference, food.
- **calorie free** fewer than 5 calories per serving.

Fat Terms (Meat and Poultry Products)

- **extra lean**[a]
  less than 5 g of total fat *and*
  less than 2 g of saturated fat and *trans* fat combined, *and*
  less than 95 mg of cholesterol per serving.
- **lean**[a]
  less than 10 g of total fat *and*
  less than 4.5 g of saturated fat and *trans* fat combined, *and*
  less than 95 mg of cholesterol per serving.

Fat Terms (All Products)

- **fat free** less than 0.5 g of fat per serving.
- **less saturated fat** 25% or less saturated fat and *trans* fat combined than the comparison food.
- **low fat** 3 g or less of total fat per serving.[a]
- **low saturated fat** 1 g or less of saturated fat and less than 0.5 g of *trans* fat per serving.
- **reduced saturated fat**
  at least 25% less saturated fat *and*
  reduced by more than 1 g of saturated fat per serving compared with a reference food.
- **saturated fat free or *trans* fat free**
  less than 0.5 g of saturated fat *and*
  less than 0.5 g of *trans* fat per serving.

Fiber Terms

- **high fiber** 5 g or more per serving. (Foods making high-fiber claims must fit the definition of low fat, or the level of total fat must appear next to the high-fiber claim.)
- **good source of fiber** 2.5 g to 4.9 g per serving.
- **more** or **added fiber** at least 2.5 g more per serving than a reference food.

Sodium Terms

- **low sodium** 140 mg or less of sodium per serving.
- **reduced sodium** at least 25% lower in sodium than the regular product.
- **sodium free** less than 5 mg per serving.
- **very low sodium** 35 mg or less of sodium per serving.

Other Terms

- **good source** 10 to 19% of the Daily Value per serving.
- **high in** 20% or more of the Daily Value for a given nutrient per serving; synonyms include "rich in" and "excellent source."
- **less, fewer, reduced** containing at least 25% less of a nutrient or calories than a reference food. This may occur naturally or as a result of altering the food. For example, pretzels, which are usually low in fat, can claim to provide less fat than potato chips, a comparable food.
- **light** this descriptor has three meanings on labels:
  1. A serving provides one-third fewer calories or half the fat of the regular product.
  2. A serving of a low-calorie, low-fat food provides half the sodium normally present.
  3. The product is light in color and texture, so long as the label makes this intent clear, as in "light brown sugar."

[a] *The word* lean *as part of the brand name (as in "Lean Supreme") indicates that the product contains fewer than 10 g of total fat per serving.*

nutrient claims FDA-approved food label statements that describe the nutrient levels in food. Examples: "fat free" or "less sodium."

health claims FDA-approved food label statements that link food constituents with disease or health-related conditions. Examples: "Soluble fiber from daily oatmeal in a diet low in saturated fat and trans fat may reduce the risk of heart disease" or "A diet low in total fat may reduce the risk of some cancers."

structure-function claims legal but largely unregulated statements permitted on labels of foods and dietary supplements, describing the effect of a substance on the structure or function of the body, but that omit references to diseases. Example: "Supports immunity and digestive health" or "Builds strong bones."

A problem is that, to a reasonable consumer, the two kinds of claims may appear identical:

- "Lowers cholesterol" (FDA-approved health claim)
- "Helps maintain normal cholesterol levels" (less-regulated structure-function claim)

Such valid-appearing but unreliable structure-function claims diminish the credibility of all health-related claims on labels. In the world of marketing, current label laws put the consumer on notice: "Let the buyer beware."

Front-of-Package Shortcuts   Some consumers find the detailed Nutrition Facts panels on food labels to be daunting. For them, easy-to-read icons of abbreviated data on the front of the package would make it quick and easy to grasp the most important nutrient information and speed comparisons among packaged foods.[12] Currently, food industry groups are working to develop a standardized set of icons for the fronts of packages, such as those shown in Figure 2–14. Their goal is to help consumers of various ages, income brackets, and literacy levels more easily compare foods and make sound choices based on nutrition.[13]

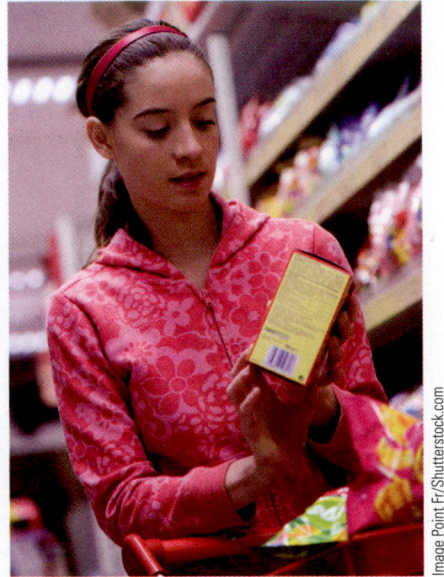

Food labels provide clues for nutrition sleuths.

KEY POINTS

- Food labels may contain reliable nutrient claims and approved health claims but may also contain structure-function claims of varying reliability.
- Front-of-package icons speed consumers' comprehension of nutrient information.

Figure 2–14
Facts Up Front

Facts Up Front is a voluntary labeling initiative, developed by food manufacturing and marketing groups.

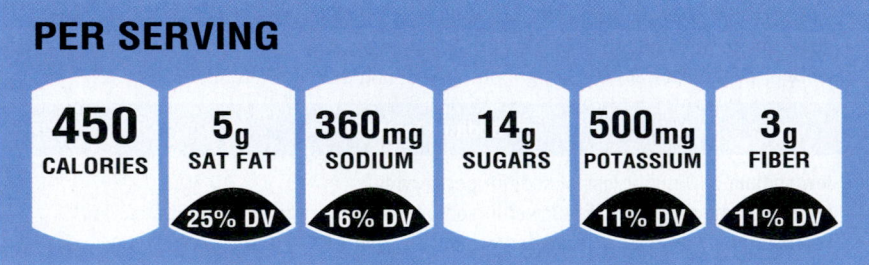

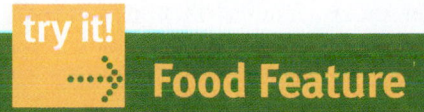
Getting a Feel for the Nutrients in Foods

LO 2.6 Estimate the benefits of a nutrient-dense meal plan through comparison with a meal plan that does not take nutrient density into account.

Figures 2–15 and 2–16 (pages 58, 59) illustrate a playful contrast between two days' meals. Monday's meals were selected according to the recommendations of this chapter and follow the sample menu of Table 2–5, shown earlier, p. 46. Tuesday's meals were chosen more for convenience and familiarity than out of concern for nutrition.

Comparing the Nutrients

How can a person compare the nutrients that these sets of meals provide? One way is to look up each food in a table of food composition, write down the food's nutrient values, and compare each one to a standard such as the DRI recommended intakes for nutrients, as we've done in Figures 2–15 and 2–16. By this measure, Monday's meals are the clear winners in terms of meeting nutrient needs within a calorie budget. Tuesday's meals oversupply calories and saturated fat while undersupplying fiber and critical vitamins and minerals.

Another useful exercise is to compare the total amounts of foods provided by a day's meals with the recommended amounts from each food group. A tally of the cups and ounces of foods consumed is provided in both Figures 2–15 and 2–16. The totals are then compared with USDA Eating Patterns in the tabular portion of the figures.

Monday's Meals in Detail

Monday's meals provide the necessary servings from each food group along with a small amount of oil needed for health, and the energy provided falls well within the 2,000-calorie allowance. A closer look at Monday's foods reveals that the whole-grain cereal at breakfast, whole-grain sandwich roll at lunch, and whole-grain crackers at snack time meet the recommendation to obtain at least half of the day's grain servings from whole grains.

For the Vegetables subgroups, dark green vegetables, orange vegetables, and legumes are represented in the dinner salad, and "other vegetables" are prominent throughout. To repeat: it isn't necessary to choose vegetables from each subgroup every day, and the person eating this day's meals will need to include vegetables from other subgroups throughout the week. In addition, Monday's eating plan has room to spare for additional servings of favorite foods or for some sweets or fats.

Tuesday's Meals in Detail

Tuesday's meals, though abundant in oils, meats, and enriched grains, completely lack fruit and whole grains and are too low in vegetables and milk to provide adequate nutrients. Tuesday's meals supply too much saturated fat and sugar, as well as excessive meats and refined grains, pushing the calorie total well above the day's allowance. A single day of such fare poses little threat to the eater, but a steady diet of Tuesday's meals presents a high probability of nutrient deficiencies and weight gain and greatly increases the risk of developing chronic diseases in later life.

Using Programs and Apps—or Not

If you have access to a computer or a "smart" cellular phone with a diet-planning application, it can be a time saver—diet analysis programs and apps perform all of these calculations at lightning speed. Working them out for yourself, using paper and a sharp pencil with a big eraser, may seem a bit old-fashioned. But there are times when using electronic gadgets may not be practical—such as when hurrying to make decisions in the cafeteria or at a fast-food counter—where real-life food decisions must be made quickly.

People who work out diet analyses for themselves on paper and those who put extra time into studying, changing, and reviewing their computer diet analysis often learn to "see" the nutrients in foods (a skill you can develop by the time you reach Chapter 10). They can quickly assess their food options and make informed choices at mealtimes, without electronic assistance. People who fail to develop such skills must wait until they can input their food data into their computer programs or apps to find out how well they did after the fact.

Figure 2–15

Monday's Meals—Nutrient-Dense Choices

Breakfast

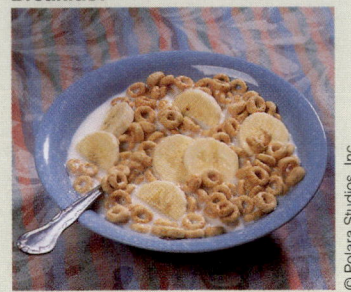

Lunch

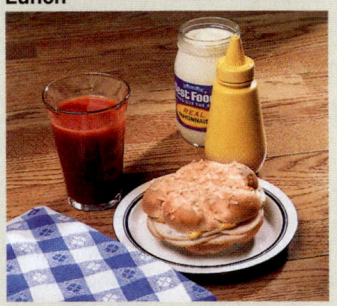

Afternoon snack

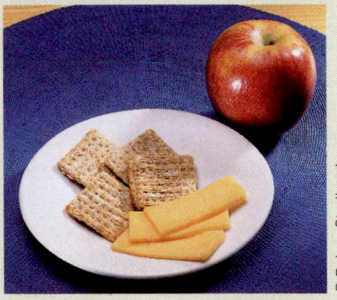

Dinner

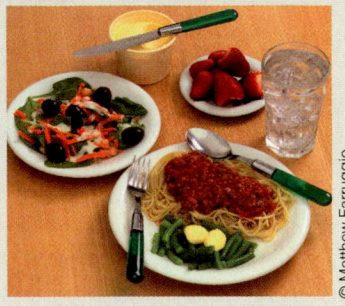

Bedtime snack

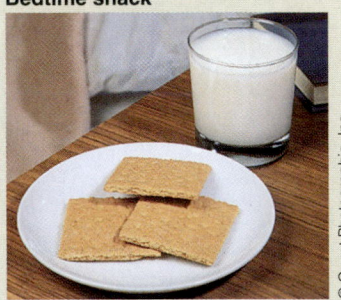

© Polara Studios, Inc.
© Matthew Farruggio
© Quest Photographic, Inc.

Foods	Food Group Amounts	Energy (cal)	Saturated Fat (g)	Fiber (g)	Vitamin C (mg)	Calcium (mg)
Before heading off to class, a student eats breakfast:						
1 c whole-grain cold cereal	1 oz grains	108	—	3	14	95
1 c fat-free milk	1 c milk	100	—	—	2	306
1 medium banana (sliced)	½ c fruit	105	—	3	10	6
Then goes home for a quick lunch:						
1 roasted turkey sandwich on 2-oz whole-grain roll with 1½ tsp low-fat mayonnaise	2 oz meat / 2 oz grains / 1½ tsp oils	343	4	2	—	89
1 c low-salt vegetable juice	1 c vegetables	50	—	1	60	27
While studying in the afternoon, the student eats a snack:						
4 whole-wheat reduced-fat crackers	½ oz grains	86	1	2	—	—
1½ oz low-fat cheddar cheese	1 c milk	74	2	—	—	176
1 medium apple	½ c fruit	72	—	3	6	8
That night, the student makes dinner:						
A salad:						
1¾ c raw spinach leaves						
¼ c shredded carrots	1 c vegetables	19	—	2	18	61
¼ c garbanzo beans	1 oz legumes	71	—	3	2	19
5 lg olives and 2 tbs oil-based salad dressing	2 tsp oils	76	1	1	—	2
A main course:						
1 c spaghetti with meat and tomato sauce	2 oz grains / 2½ oz meat	425	3	5	15	56
½ c green beans	1 c vegetables	22	—	2	6	29
2 tsp soft margarine	2 tsp oils	67	1	—	—	—
And for dessert:						
1 c strawberries	1 c fruit	49	—	3	89	24
Later that evening, the student enjoys a bedtime snack:						
3 graham crackers	½ oz grains	90	—	—	—	—
1 c fat-free milk	1 c milk	100	—	—	2	306
Totals:		**1,857**	**12**	**30**	**224**	**1,204**
DRI recommended intakes:[a]		2,000	<20[b]	25	75	1,000
Percentage of DRI recommended intakes:		93%	60%	120%	299%	120%

Intakes Compared with Recommended Amounts

Food Group	Breakfast	Lunch	Snack	Dinner	Snack	Monday's Totals	Recommended Amounts
Fruits	½ c		½ c	1 c		2 c	2 c
Vegetables		1 c		2 c		3 c	2½ c
Grains	1 oz	2 oz	½ oz	2¼ oz	½ oz	6 oz	6¼ oz
Protein foods		2 oz		3½ oz		5½ oz	5½ oz
Milk	1 c		1 c		1 c	3 c	3 c
Oils		1½ tsp		4 tsp		5½ tsp	6 tsp
Calorie allowance						1,857 cal	2,000 cal

[a]DRI values for a sedentary woman, age 19–30. Other DRI values are listed on the inside front cover, page B.

[b]The 20-g value listed is the maximum allowable saturated fat for a 2,000-cal diet. The DRI recommends consuming less than 10% of calories from saturated fat.

Figure 2–16

Tuesday's Meals—Less-Nutrient-Dense Choices

Breakfast

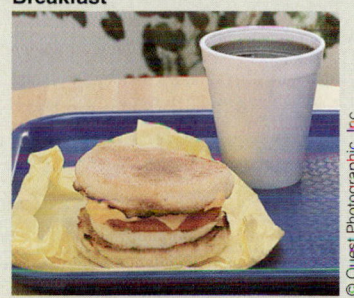

Foods	Food Group Amounts	Energy (cal)	Saturated Fat (g)	Fiber (g)	Vitamin C (mg)	Calcium (mg)
Today, the student starts the day with a fast-food breakfast:						
1 c coffee	2 oz grains	5	—	—	—	—
1 English muffin with egg, cheese, and bacon	2 oz protein foods 1 c milk	436	9	2	—	266
Between classes, the student returns home for a quick lunch:						
1 peanut butter and jelly sandwich on white bread	2 oz grains 1 oz protein foods	426	4	3	—	93
1 c whole milk	1 c milk	156	6	—	4	290
While studying, the student has:						
12 oz diet cola	—	—	—	—	—	—
Bag of chips (14 chips)[a]		105	2	—	4	—
That night for dinner, the student eats:						
A salad:						
1c lettuce						
1 tbs blue cheese dressing	1/2 c vegetables	84	2	1	2	23
A main course:						
6 oz steak	6 oz protein foods	349	6	—	—	27
1/2 baked potato	1/2 c vegetables	161	—	4	17	26
1 tbs butter		102	7	—	—	3
1 tbs sour cream[b]		31	2	—	—	17
12 oz diet cola		—	—	—	—	—
And for dessert:						
4 sandwich-type cookies	1 oz grains	158	2	1	—	—
Later on, a bedtime snack:						
2 cream-filled snack cakes	2 oz grains	250	2	2	—	20
1 c herbal tea		—	—	—	—	—
Totals:		**2,263**	**42**	**13**	**27**	**765**
DRI recommended intakes:[c]		2,000	<20[d]	25	75	1,000
Percentage of DRI recommended intakes:		113%	210%	52%	36%	77%

Lunch

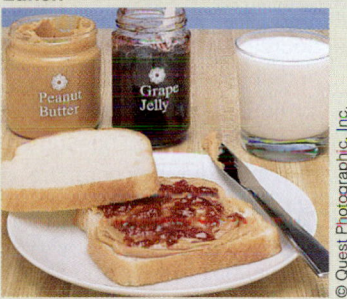

Afternoon snack

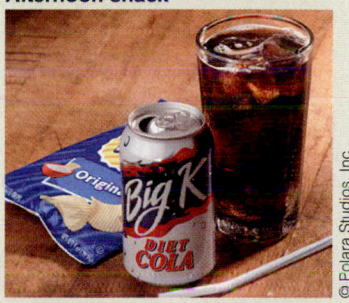

Dinner

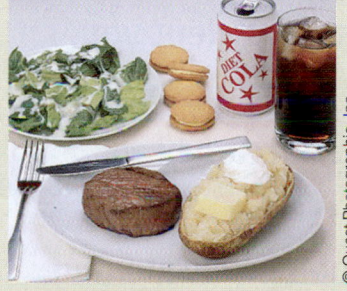

Bedtime snack

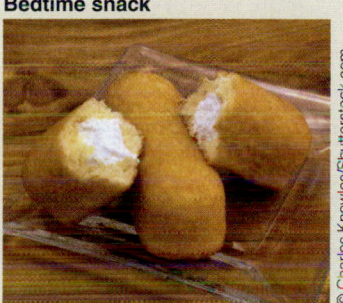

Intakes Compared with Recommended Amounts

Food Group	Breakfast	Lunch	Snack	Dinner	Snack	Tuesday's Totals	Recommended Amounts
Fruits						0 c	2 c
Vegetables			a	1 c		1 c	2 1/2 c
Grains	2 oz	2 oz		1 oz	2 oz	7 oz	6 oz
Protein foods	2 oz	1 oz		6 oz		9 oz	5 1/2 oz
Milk	1 c	1 c				2 c	3 c
Oils						7 1/2 tsp[b]	6 tsp
Calorie allowance						2,263 cal	2,000 cal

[a]The potato in 14 potato chips provides less than 1/2 c vegetables.

[b]The saturated fats of steak, butter, and sour cream are among the solid fats and do not qualify as oils.

[c]DRI values for a sedentary woman, age 19–30. Other DRI values are listed on the inside front cover, page B.

[d]The 20-g value listed is the maximum allowable saturated fat for a 2,000-cal diet. The DRI recommends consuming less than 10% of calories from saturated fat.

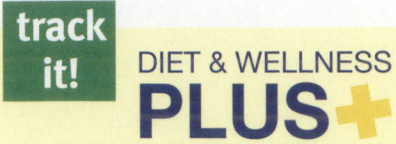

track it!

DIET & WELLNESS
PLUS+ Concepts in Action

Compare Your Intakes with USDA Guidelines

The purpose of this chapter's exercise is to give you a feel for the nutrients in food and to help you consider your sources of solid fats and added sugars. Use the Diet & Wellness Plus (D&W+) program to help you evaluate your nutritional intake and needs.

1. From the Home page of D&W+ select the Reports tab and select MyPlate Analysis. Choose day one of your three-day diet intake (from Chapter 1). Choose all meals for that day. Did your intake for that day conform to the MyPlate pattern? Did you consume too few foods from any particular food group(s)? Which, if

any, were lacking? Using Table 2–3 (p. 45) and Figure 2–5 (pp. 40–41) to guide you, suggest ways that you might realistically change your intake to better conform to the USDA Eating Patterns.

2. What about fat? Select the Reports tab; then select Macronutrient Ranges. Did your fat intake fall between 20 and 35 percent of your total energy? Did you take in enough raw oils to meet your need (see Table 2–3, p. 45)? Which ones? Change your date to include all three days of your record. How does your single day's fat intake compare with your three-day average?

3. The bottom lines of Table 2–3 specifiy an upper intake limit of calories from solid fats and added sugars. Select

the Track Diet tab and look over your day's food list. Which foods were less nutrient-dense choices?

4. A great feature of the D&W+ program is its Source Analysis Report, which allows you to list food sources of calories (kcal) or specific nutrients in order of pre-dominance. From the Reports tab, select Source Analysis, select day three, and choose all meals. Which foods provided most to your calorie intake on that day? If you consumed vegetables, how did they compare with other calorie sources? In later chapters, you'll use this report again to analyze various nutrients in your diet.

---

what did you decide?

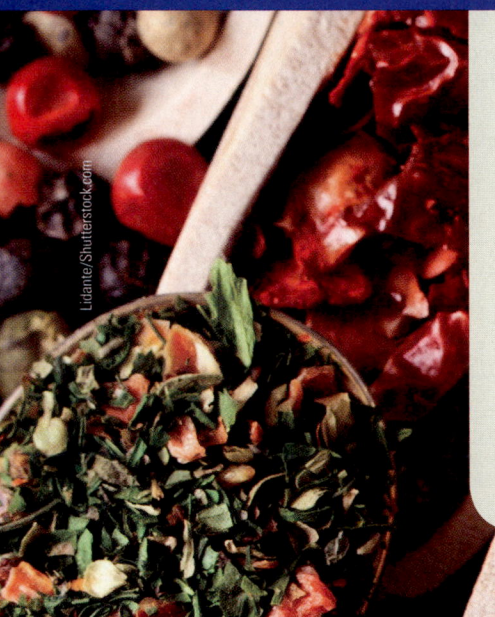

Lidiante/Shutterstock.com

How can you tell **how much of each nutrient** you **need to consume daily?**

Are **government dietary recommendations** too **simplistic to be of help?**

Are the health claims on food labels **accurate and reliable?**

Can certain **"superfoods"** boost your health with more than just nutrients?

Self Check

1. (LO 2.1) The nutrient standards in use today include all of the following *except* _____.
   a. Adequate Intakes (AI)
   b. Daily Minimum Requirements (DMR)
   c. Daily Values (DV)
   d. a and c

2. (LO 2.1) The Dietary Reference Intakes (DRI) were devised for which of the following purposes?
   a. to set nutrient goals for individuals
   b. to suggest upper limits of intakes, above which toxicity is likely
   c. to set average nutrient requirements for use in research
   d. all of the above

3. (LO 2.1) The energy intake recommendation is set at a level predicted to maintain body weight.
   T   F

4. (LO 2.1) The DRI are for all people, regardless of their medical history.
   T   F

5. (LO 2.2) Which of the following is *not* an action that could help meet the ideals of the Dietary Guidelines for Americans?
   a. increase intakes of vegetables
   b. increase intakes of nutrient-dense foods
   c. reduce intakes of artificial ingredients
   d. increase intakes of whole grains

6. (LO 2.2) The Dietary Guidelines for Americans recommend physical activity to help balance calorie intakes to achieve and sustain a healthy body weight.
   T   F

7. (LO 2.3) According to the USDA Eating Patterns, which of the following vegetables should be limited?
   a. carrots
   b. avocados
   c. baked beans
   d. potatoes

8. (LO 2.3) The USDA Eating Patterns recommend a small amount of daily oil from which of these sources?
   a. olives
   b. nuts
   c. vegetable oil
   d. all of the above

9. (LO 2.3) People who choose not to eat meat or animal products need to find an alternative to the USDA Eating Patterns when planning their diets.
   T   F

10. (LO 2.4) To plan a healthy diet that correctly assigns the needed amounts of food from each food group, the diet planner should start by consulting
    a. USDA Eating Patterns.
    b. Dietary Reference Intakes.
    c. sample menus.
    d. none of the above.

11. (LO 2.4) A properly planned diet controls calories by excluding snacks.
    T   F

12. (LO 2.5) Which of the following values is found on food labels?
    a. Recommended Dietary Allowances
    b. Dietary Reference Intakes
    c. Daily Values
    d. Estimated Average Requirements

13. (LO 2.5) By law, food labels must name the ingredients in descending order of predominance by weight and in ordinary language.
    T   F

14. (LO 2.5) To be labeled "low fat," a food must contain 3 grams of fat or less per serving.
    T   F

15. (LO 2.6) One way to evaluate any diet is to compare the total food amounts that it provides with those recommended by the USDA Eating Patterns.
    T   F

16. (LO 2.6) A carefully planned diet has which of these characteristics?
    a. It contains sufficient raw oil.
    b. It contains no solid fats or added sugars.
    c. It contains all of the Vegetables subgroups.
    d. a and c

17. (LO 2.7) Various whole foods contain so many different phytochemicals that consumers should focus on eating a wide variety of foods instead of seeking out a particular phytochemical.
    T   F

18. (LO 2.7) As natural constituents of foods, phytochemicals are safe to consume in large amounts.
    T   F

Answers to these Self Check questions are in Appendix G.

Tomatoes

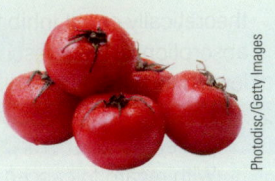

People around the world who eat the most tomatoes, about five tomato-containing meals per week, are less likely to suffer from cancers of the esophagus, prostate, or stomach than those who avoid tomatoes. Among phytochemical candidates for promoting this effect is **lycopene**, a red pigment found in guava, papaya, pink grapefruit, tomatoes (especially cooked tomato products, such as sauce), and watermelon.

Two actions of lycopene could, theoretically, inhibit cancer development. First, lycopene and its by-products are antioxidants that could inhibit the growth of cancer cells. Rats with liver cancer that were fed lycopene three times per week had greater antioxidant activity, smaller tumors, and better survival than controls.[26] A recent meta-analysis showed that when postmenopausal women consumed more lycopene, their risk for developing ovarian cancer decreased slightly, but most research to date is still inconclusive.[27] Second, in the skin, lycopene and some of its chemical relatives act as a sort of internal sunscreen, filtering high-energy wavelengths of visible light. This action may protect skin from the damaging sun rays that cause many skin cancers.[‡28]

In contrast to today's media lore, the FDA concludes that no or very little solid evidence links lycopene or tomato consumption with reduced cancer risks. Something else about tomato-eating people may be reducing their risks. Supplements of lycopene seem less harmful than those of its chemical cousins beta-carotene and **lutein**, however, which clearly raise the risk of lung cancer in smokers.[29]

Tea

Everywhere, headlines attribute almost magical benefits to tea—it's a current media darling. People in Asia who drink two cups or more of green tea each day die less often from digestive tract cancers than nondrinkers, possibly due

‡ *The other carotenoid relatives of lycopene are lutein and zeaxanthin—more about them in Chapter 7.*

to the antioxidant activity of polyphenols found in green tea.[30] Black tea, the type most U.S. consumers drink, is a major contributor of flavonoids to the diet. A recent study showed that drinking 4 cups of black tea per day reduced the risk of stroke in both men and women.[31]

Green tea consumption has the potential to reduce oxidative stress and inflammation and to reduce the levels of harmful blood lipids and blood pressure. Indeed, compiled evidence from 13 short-term controlled human studies supports the idea that green tea may improve blood pressure levels and reduce blood lipid concentrations, regardless of whether the subjects took green tea extracts or drank the tea itself.[32] Long-term controlled human studies are needed to confirm these findings, however. As for cancer, a review of 17 studies concluded that the evidence for a link between green tea and reduced cancer risk was mixed and more research is needed.[33]

In any case, high-dose supplements of green tea extract have been linked with liver toxicity and high intakes of green tea with kidney problems.[34] Concentrated flavonoids from tea may also decrease the absorption of some medications, thereby altering drug effectiveness.[35] A USDA analysis of popular name-brand green tea supplements concluded that, while some were of good quality, others lacked any trace of green tea components, and in still others, the flavonoids had decomposed, or undeclared additives were present. Supplement quality cannot be judged from label information, not even in leading brand-name pills.

Grapes and Wine

Purple grape juice and red wine contain a number of flavonoids, and among them is a small amount of **resveratrol**.[36] Resveratrol shows promise in research as a disease fighter.[37] In laboratory studies, resveratrol demonstrates the potential to reduce harmful tissue

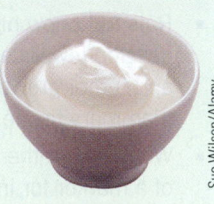

inflammation that often accompanies cancer, diabetes, obesity, and heart disease and to oppose heart disease development in many other ways.[38] In high doses, resveratrol has also demonstrated some anticancer activities, but such doses are larger than those attainable by diet, and some border on toxic doses.[39] Also to its credit are studies in which resveratrol seemed to extend the life of mice, fish, flies, worms, and yeast cells.[40] To date, not enough evidence exists to conclude that any of these effects are true in human beings.

Hints come from population studies, in which people who regularly consume red wine, grapes and their products, and other fruits and vegetables have a lower incidence of cardiovascular disease than others.[41] As tempting as it may be to conclude that grapes and red wine prevent human diseases, the controlled clinical human trials needed to confirm that people actually benefit from consuming them are still lacking.[42] (Controversy 3 compares the potential risks and benefits of drinking alcohol.)

Yogurt

Yogurt is a special case among superfoods. Being a milk product, yogurt lacks typical flavonoids or other phytochemicals from plants. Instead, it contains living *Lactobacillus* or other bacteria that ferment milk into products like yogurt or the liquid yogurt beverage **kefir**. Such microorganisms, called **probiotics**, can set up residence in the digestive tract and alter its functioning in ways that are claimed to reduce colon cancer, ulcers, and other digestive problems; to reduce allergies; or to improve immunity and resistance to infections. The types and ratios of organisms that make up the microbial colonies of the intestine are also under investigation for their roles in diseases such as diabetes and obesity.[43] *Lactobacillus* and other microbes can help correct the diarrhea that often follows antibiotic drug use.[44]

However, there is cause for concern when it comes to the safety of probiotic supplementation among certain groups of people. Read Table C2–3 to learn more. Additional research is needed to clarify potential benefits or risks from probiotics.[45]

Other foods provide **prebiotics**—that is, nondigestible carbohydrates or other constituents upon which the microbes in the digestive tract can feed.[46] A fed colony multiplies rapidly, creating by-products that are sometimes associated with certain health benefits, such as a decrease in disease-related inflammation of the colon.[47]

Table C2–3

Phytochemicals and Health: Point, Counterpoint

Arguments arise about whether large intakes of phytochemicals in superfoods or supplements might help or harm health. The arguments for loading up on certain phytochemicals are listed on the left; the opposing evidence, which calls for moderation, is offered on the right.

Points Made In Favor	Counterpoints Made Against
1. *Protection from oxidation.* In levels obtainable from foods, certain phytochemicals may protect DNA and other cellular structures from oxidative damage.	1. *Damage from oxidation.* At high levels, obtainable only from supplements, these same phytochemicals may increase oxidative damage to DNA and other structures.
2. *Disease prevention.* Diets rich in phytochemicals are shown to benefit health through their anti-inflammatory and anti-cancer properties; they also may protect against cardiovascular and neurodegenerative diseases.	2. *Disease progression.* No benefits are associated with supplements of phytochemicals. In large doses, phytochemicals also inhibit absorption of certain vitamins or minerals and thus may promote disease progression.
3. *Safe for people.* Phytochemicals are safe because they are "natural"—they arise in food. Examples: ■ *Lignans support health.* Dietary lignans may have protective effects against cancers, including breast and prostate cancers. ■ *Probiotic benefits.* Probiotics, the microorganisms of the large intestine, may have beneficial effects, including improvements in antibiotic-induced diarrhea, digestive diseases, obesity, and immunity.	3. *Unproven safety.* "Natural" does not mean "safe." All substances, even water and vitamins, are hazardous in large amounts. Examples: ■ *Lignans impede health.* High daily lignan intakes, particularly from supplements, can interfere with vitamin and mineral absorption, posing a risk of nutrient deficiencies. Digestive distress is also likely. ■ *Probiotic harms.* Probiotic supplements may be safe for most healthy people, but patients with pancreatic diseases and those with weakened immunity have contracted serious infections after consuming them.
4. *Just a few foods.* Certain "superfoods" are the richest sources of phytochemicals. These few foods should be eaten every day.	4. *A variety of foods.* Focusing on a few select "superfoods" to the exclusion of other whole foods may limit the expected health benefits. Tens of thousands of phytochemicals exist in virtually all foods from plants, but only a few have been studied, making variety the best strategy. Also, foods from plants often contain natural toxins, another reason to choose a wide variety of foods.
5. *Evidence is good enough.* Existing evidence is good enough to recommend that people take supplements of purified phytochemicals.	5. *Not enough evidence.* Evidence for the safety of isolated phytochemical supplements in human beings is lacking, and evidence for potential harm is mounting.
6. *Healthy label claims.* Product labels on phytochemical supplements claim potent health benefits, so they must be true.	6. *Unreliable label claims.* Phytochemical labels can make structure-function claims that sound good but are generally based on weak or nonexistent scientific evidence.
7. *Sufficient regulation and oversight.* Phytochemical supplements must be safe because reliable businesses—even pharmacies—sell them.	7. *Lack of oversight.* No regulatory body oversees the safety of phytochemicals sold to consumers. No studies are required to prove their safety or effectiveness before they are sold.

Data Sources: L. Haghighat and N. F. Crum-Cianflone, The potential risks of probiotics among HIV-infected persons. Bacteraemia due to Lactobacillus acidophilus and review of the literature, International Journal of STD and AIDS *(2015),* epub ahead of print, doi:10.1177/0956462415590725; M. G. Redman, E. J. Ward, and R. S. Phillips, The efficacy and safety of probiotics in people with cancer: A systematic review, Annals of Oncology: Official Journal of the European Society for Medical Oncology *25 (2014):* 1919–1929; B. Hooper and R. Frazier, Polyphenols in the diet: Friend or foe? Nutrition Bulletin *37 (2012):* 297–308; C. R. Hooijmans and coauthors, The effects of probiotic supplementation on experimental acute pancreatitis: A systematic review and meta-analysis, PLoS One *7 (2012):* e48811; A. L. Lobb, Science in liquid dietary supplement promotion: The misleading case of mangosteen juice, Hawaii Journal of Medicine and Public Health *71 (2012):* 46–48.

Phytochemical Supplements

No doubt exists that diets rich in legumes, vegetables, fruits, and other whole foods reduce the risks of heart disease and cancer, but isolating the responsible food, nutrient, or phytochemical has proved difficult. Foods deliver thousands of bioactive food components, all within a food matrix that maximizes their availability and effectiveness.[48] Broccoli, and particularly **broccoli sprouts**, may contain as many as 10,000 different phytochemicals—each with the potential to influence some action in the body. These foods are under study for their potential to defend against cancers at the DNA level, and Chapter 11 comes back to them.[49]

Even if it were known with certainty which foods protect against which diseases, most isolated supplements, even the most promising ones, fail to actually prevent diseases when they are administered in research.[50] Worse, some such supplements can interfere with and reduce the effectiveness of standard drugs given to people with serious illnesses.[51] Such food and drug inter-

actions are of critical importance, and the Controversy section of Chapter 14 is devoted to them.

Users and sellers of phytochemical supplements argue that people have been consuming foods containing phytochemicals for tens of thousands of years and because the body can handle phytochemicals in foods, it stands to reason that supplements of those phytochemicals are safe as well. Such thinking raises concerns among scientists, though. The latter point out that the body is equipped to handle the dilute phytochemicals of whole foods but not concentrated supplement doses.[52] Consider the facts about phytochemical supplements and health in Table C2–3.

The Concept of Functional Foods

Virtually all whole foods have some special value in supporting health and are therefore functional foods. Modest evidence suggests that cranberries may help to prevent some urinary tract infections, for example.[53] Manufactured functional

foods, however, often consist of ultra-processed foods that are fortified with nutrients or enhanced with particular bioactive food components (such as herbs) for which little or no supporting evidence of benefit exists.

Such novel foods raise questions:

- Is such a food really a food or a **drug**?
- Which is the better choice for the health-conscious diet planner: to eat a food with additives and hope for a benefit or to adjust the diet in ways known to support health?
- Is it a greater benefit to eat fried snack foods and candy bars sprinkled with phytochemicals than to obtain these and other beneficial substances from whole foods?
- What about smoothies packed with medicinal herbs—are these foods safe to consume regularly? Are they safe for children?

The Final Word

In light of all of the evidence for and against phytochemicals and functional foods, a moderate approach is warranted. People who eat abundant and varied fruits and vegetables each day may cut their risk for many diseases by as much as half. Replacing some meat with soy foods may reduce those risks further. Table C2–4 offers some tips for consuming the whole foods known to provide phytochemicals.

A piece of advice: don't try to single out a few superfoods or phytochemicals for their magical health effects, and ignore the hype about packaged products—no evidence exists to support their use. Instead, take a no-nonsense approach and choose a wide variety of whole grains, legumes, nuts, fruits, and vegetables in the context of an adequate, balanced, and varied diet to receive all of the health benefits these foods can offer.[54]

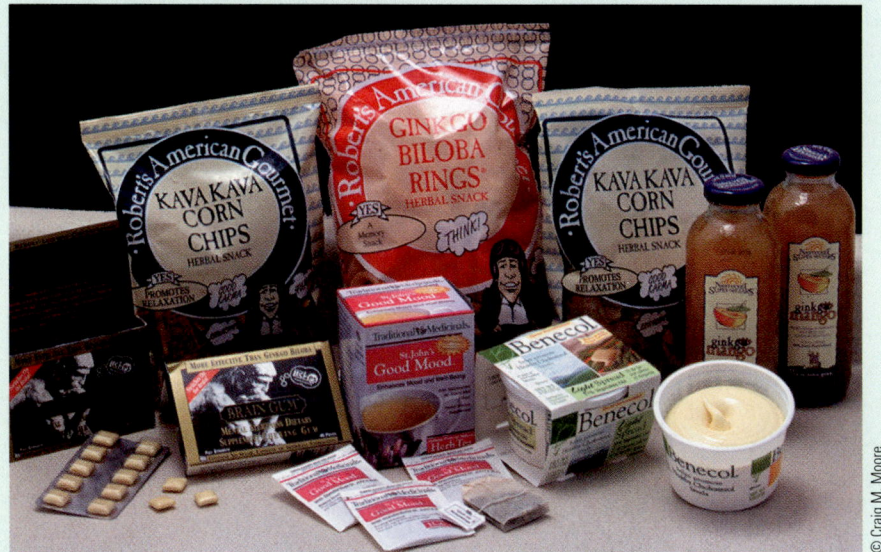

© Craig M. Moore

Functional foods currently on the market promise to "enhance mood," "promote relaxation and good karma," "support alertness," and "benefit memory," among other claims.

Table C2–4

Tips for Consuming Phytochemicals

- Eat more fruit. The average U.S. diet provides little more than ½ cup of fruit a day. Remember to choose juices and raw, dried, or cooked fruits at mealtimes, as well as for snacks. Choose dried fruit in place of candy.
- Increase vegetable portions. Double the normal portion of cooked plain, nonstarchy vegetables. Dip cut raw vegetables into yogurt-based dips for snacks.
- Use herbs and spices. Cookbooks offer ways to include parsley, basil, garlic, hot peppers, oregano, turmeric, and other phytochemical-rich seasonings.
- Replace some meat. Replace some of the meat in the diet with grains, legumes, and vegetables. Oatmeal, soy meat replacer, or grated carrots mixed with ground meat and seasonings make a luscious, nutritious meat loaf, for example.
- Add grated vegetables. Carrots in chili or meatballs, celery and squash in spaghetti sauce, and similar combinations add phytochemicals without greatly changing the taste of the food.
- Try new foods. Try a new fruit, vegetable, or whole grain each week. Walk through vegetable aisles and visit farmers' markets. Read recipes. Try tofu, fortified soy milk, or soybeans in cooking.

Critical Thinking

1. Divide into two groups. One group will argue in support of using superfoods, and one group will argue against the use of superfoods. During the debate, be sure to answer the following questions:

   - What is a superfood, and is it appropriate to classify a given food as a superfood?

   - Are there foods that you can reliably say have the characteristics of a superfood? Describe the research you have consulted to support the classification of a food as a superfood.

2. Describe a situation when the intake of a phytochemical supplement or a functional food would be appropriate. Give reasons for using a phytochemical supplement or functional food, and also give reasons against its use.

3 The Remarkable Body

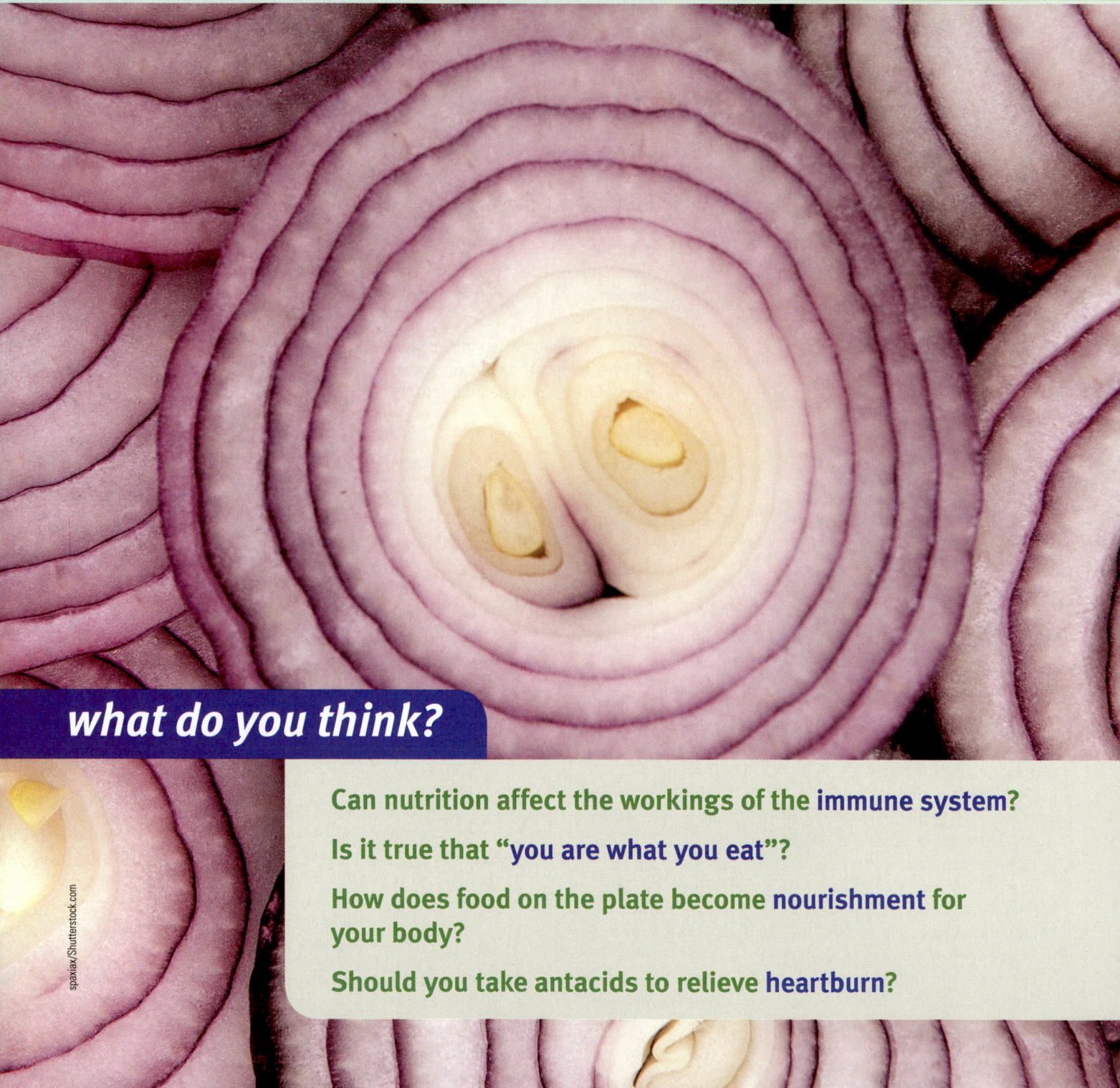

spaxiax/Shutterstock.com

what do you think?

Can nutrition affect the workings of the **immune system**?

Is it true that **"you are what you eat"**?

How does food on the plate become **nourishment** for your body?

Should you take antacids to relieve **heartburn**?

Learning Objectives

After reading this chapter, you should be able to accomplish the following:

LO 3.1 Name six basic needs of the body's cells.

LO 3.2 Summarize the exchange of materials as the body fluids circulate around the tissues.

LO 3.3 Summarize the interactions between the hormonal and nervous systems and nutrition.

LO 3.4 Specify the significance of nutrition in the proper functioning of the immune system.

LO 3.5 Summarize how the digestive system provides nutrients to the body tissues.

LO 3.6 Outline the symptoms of eight common digestive problems related to nutrition.

LO 3.7 Specify the excretory functions of the lungs, liver, kidneys, and bladder.

LO 3.8 Explain how body tissues store excess nutrients.

LO 3.9 Compare the effects of moderate and heavy alcohol consumption.

At the moment of conception, you received genes in the form of DNA from your mother and father, who, in turn, had inherited them from their parents, and so on into history. Since that moment, your genes have been working behind the scenes, directing your body's development and functioning. Many of your genes are ancient in origin and are little changed from genes of thousands of centuries ago, but here you are—living with the food, the luxuries, the smog, the contaminants, and all the other pleasures and problems of the 21st century. There is no guarantee that a diet haphazardly chosen from today's foods will meet the needs of your "ancient" body. Unlike your ancestors, who nourished themselves from the wild plants and animals surrounding them, you must learn how your body works, what it needs, and how to select foods to meet its needs.

The Body's Cells

LO 3.1 Name six basic needs of the body's cells.

The human body is composed of trillions of **cells**, and none of them knows anything about food. *You* may get hungry for fruit, milk, or bread, but each cell of your body needs nutrients—the vital components of foods. The ways in which the body's cells cooperate to obtain and use nutrients are the subjects of this chapter.

Each of the body's cells is a self-contained, living entity (see Figure 3–1, p. 72), but at the same time, it depends on the rest of the body's cells to supply its needs. Among the cells' most basic needs are energy and the oxygen with which to burn it. Cells also need water to maintain the environment in which they live. They need building blocks and control systems. They especially need the nutrients they cannot make for themselves—the essential nutrients first described in Chapter 1—which must be supplied from food. The first principle of diet planning is that the foods we choose must provide energy and the essential nutrients, including water.

As living things, cells also die off, although at varying rates. Some skin cells and red blood cells must replenish themselves every 10 to 120 days, repectively. Cells lining the digestive tract replace themselves every 3 days. Under ordinary conditions, many muscle cells reproduce themselves only once every few years. Liver cells have the ability to reproduce quickly and do so whenever repairs to the organ are needed. Certain brain cells do not reproduce at all; if damaged by injury or disease, they are lost forever.

The cells work in cooperation with each other to support the whole body. Gene activity within each cell determines the nature of that work.

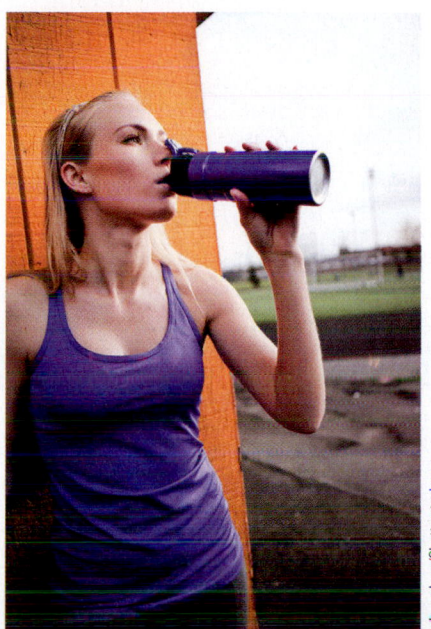

All the body's cells live in water.

cells the smallest units in which independent life can exist. All living things are single cells or organisms made of cells.

Figure 3–1
A Cell (Simplified Diagram)

This cell has been greatly enlarged; real cells are so tiny that 10,000 can fit on the head of a pin.

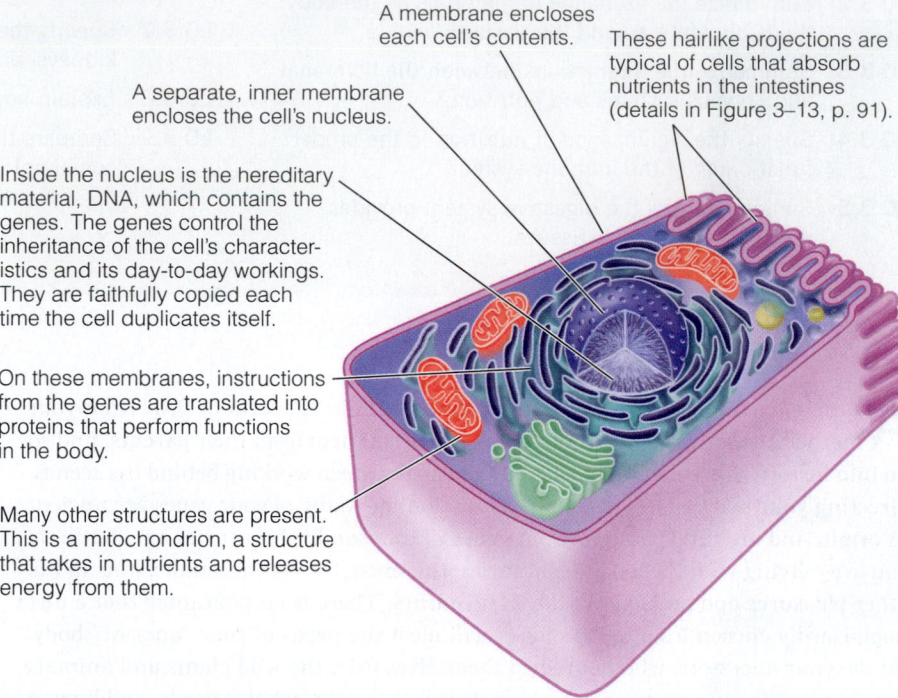

A membrane encloses each cell's contents.

These hairlike projections are typical of cells that absorb nutrients in the intestines (details in Figure 3–13, p. 91).

A separate, inner membrane encloses the cell's nucleus.

Inside the nucleus is the hereditary material, DNA, which contains the genes. The genes control the inheritance of the cell's characteristics and its day-to-day workings. They are faithfully copied each time the cell duplicates itself.

On these membranes, instructions from the genes are translated into proteins that perform functions in the body.

Many other structures are present. This is a mitochondrion, a structure that takes in nutrients and releases energy from them.

Genes Control Functions

Each gene is a blueprint that directs the production of one or more proteins, such as an **enzyme** that performs cellular work. Genes also provide the instructions for all of the structural components cells need to survive (see Figure 3–2). Each cell contains a complete set of genes, but different ones are active in different types of cells. For example, in some intestinal cells, the genes for making digestive enzymes are active, but the genes for making keratin in nails and hair are silent; in some of the body's **fat cells**, the genes for making enzymes that metabolize fat are active, but the digestive enzyme genes are silent. Certain nutrients are involved in activating and silencing genes in ways that are just starting to be revealed.

> Connections between nutrition and gene activities are emerging in the field of nutritional genomics, described in **Controversy 11.**

Genes affect the way the body handles its nutrients. Certain variations in some of the genes alter the way the body absorbs, metabolizes, or excretes nutrients from the body. Occasionally, a gene variation can cause a lifelong malady—that is, an **inborn error of metabolism**—that may require a special diet to minimize its potential to harm the body. An example is the inborn error **phenylketonuria**, in which a genetic variation compromises the body's ability to handle the amino acid phenylalanine. People with this condition must carefully limit their intakes of phenylalanine, so food manufacturers are required to print warning labels on foods, such as certain artificial sweeteners, that contain it.

Nutrients also affect the genes. For example, the concentrations of certain nutrients in the body fluids and tissues influence the genes to make more or less of certain proteins. These changes, in turn, alter body functions in ways that ultimately hold meaning for health and disease.

enzyme any of a great number of working proteins that speed up a specific chemical reaction, such as breaking the bonds of a nutrient, without undergoing change themselves. Enzymes and their actions are described in Chapter 6.

fat cells cells that specialize in the storage of fat and form the fat tissue. Fat cells also produce fat-metabolizing enzymes; they also produce hormones involved in appetite and energy balance (see Chapter 9).

inborn error of metabolism a genetic variation present from birth that may result in disease.

phenylketonuria an inborn error of metabolism that interferes with the body's handling of the amino acid phenylalanine, with potentially serious consequences for the brain and nervous system in infancy and childhood.

Figure 3–2

From DNA to Living Cells

DNA is the large molecule that encodes all genetic information in its structure; genes are units of a cell's inheritance situated along the DNA strands.

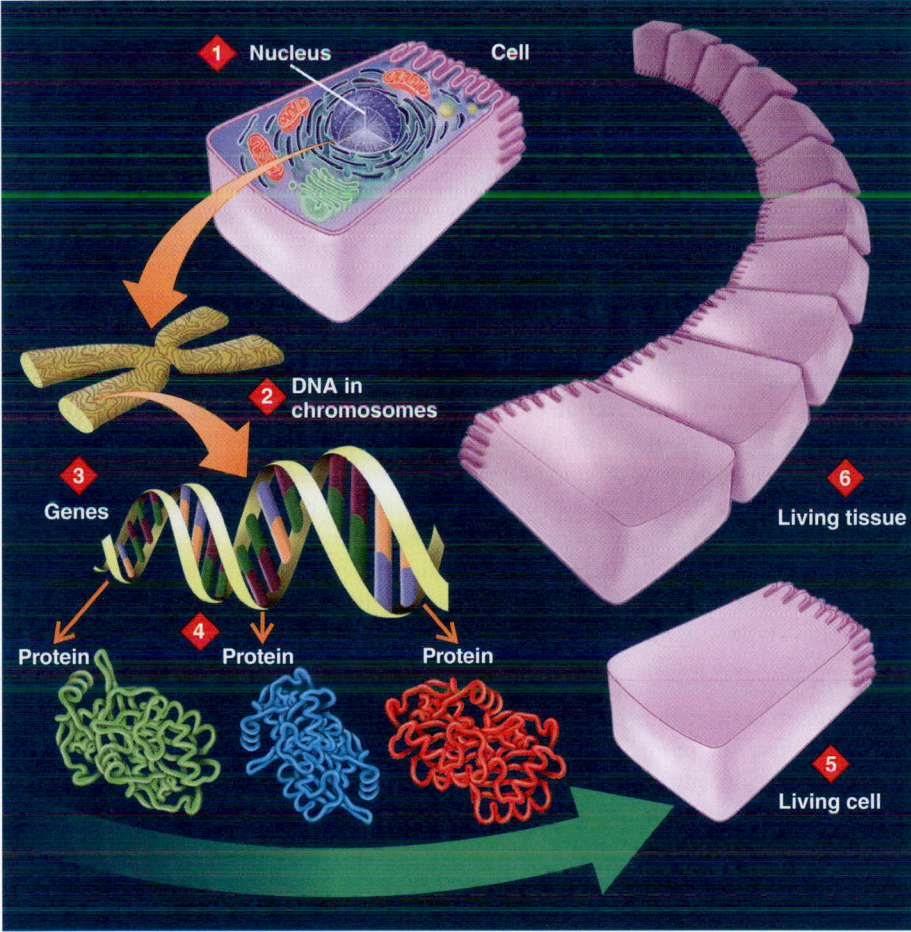

Nucleus **Cell**

1

DNA in chromosomes

2

Genes

3

Protein **Protein** **Protein**

4

Living tissue

6

Living cell

5

1 Each cell's nucleus contains DNA — the material of heredity in all living things.

2 Long strands of human DNA coil into 23 pairs of chromosomes. If the strands of DNA in all the body's cells were uncoiled and laid end to end, they would stretch to the sun and back four hundred times. Yet DNA strands are so tiny that about 5 million of them could be threaded at once through the eye of a needle.

3 Genes contain instructions for making proteins. Genes are sections along the strands of DNA that serve as templates for the building of proteins. Some genes are involved in building just one protein; others are involved in building more than one.

4 Many other steps are required to make a protein. See Figure 6–6 of Chapter 6.

5 Proteins do the work of living cells. Cells employ proteins to perform essential functions and provide structures.

6 Communities of functioning cells make up the living tissue.

Cells, Tissues, Organs, Systems

Cells are organized into **tissues** that perform specialized tasks. For example, individual muscle cells are joined together to form muscle tissue, which can contract. Tissues, in turn, are grouped together to form whole **organs**. In the organ we call the heart, for example, muscle tissues, nerve tissues, connective tissues, and others all work together to pump blood. Some body functions are performed by several related organs working together as part of a **body system**. For example, the heart, lungs, and blood vessels cooperate as parts of the cardiorespiratory system to deliver oxygen to all the body's cells. The next few sections present the body systems with special significance to nutrition.

KEY POINTS

- The body's cells need energy, oxygen, and nutrients, including water, to remain healthy and do their work.
- Genes direct the making of each cell's protein machinery, including enzymes.
- Specialized cells are grouped together to form tissues and organs; organs work together in body systems.

tissues systems of cells working together to perform specialized tasks. Examples are muscles, nerves, blood, and bone.

organs discrete structural units made of tissues that perform specific jobs. Examples are the heart, liver, and brain.

body system a group of related organs that work together to perform a function. Examples are the circulatory system, respiratory system, and nervous system.

The Body Fluids and the Cardiovascular System

LO 3.2 Summarize the exchange of materials as the body fluids circulate around the tissues.

Body fluids supply the tissues continuously with energy, oxygen, and nutrients, including water. The fluids constantly circulate to pick up fresh supplies and deliver wastes to points of disposal. Every cell continuously draws oxygen and nutrients from those fluids and releases carbon dioxide and other waste products into them.

The Body's Fluids   The body's circulating fluids are the **blood** and the **lymph**. Blood travels within the **arteries**, **veins**, and **capillaries**, as well as within the heart's chambers (see Figure 3–3). Lymph travels in separate vessels of its own.

Circulating around the cells are other fluids such as the **plasma** of the blood, which surrounds the white and red blood cells, and the fluid surrounding muscle cells (see Figure 3–4, p. 76). The fluid surrounding cells (**extracellular fluid**) is derived from the blood in the capillaries; it squeezes out through the capillary walls and flows around the outsides of cells, permitting exchange of materials.

Some of the extracellular fluid returns directly to the bloodstream by reentering the capillaries. The fluid remaining outside the capillaries forms lymph, which travels around the body by way of lymph vessels. The lymph eventually returns to the bloodstream near the heart where a large lymph vessel empties into a large vein. In this way, all cells are served by the cardiovascular system.

The fluid inside cells (**intracellular fluid**) provides a medium in which all cell reactions take place. Its pressure also helps the cells to hold their shape. The intracellular fluid is drawn from the extracellular fluid that bathes the cells on the outside.

Blood Circulation   All the blood circulates to the **lungs**, where it picks up oxygen and releases carbon dioxide wastes from the cells. Then the blood returns to the heart, where the pumping heartbeats push this freshly oxygenated blood from the lungs out to all body tissues. As the blood travels through the rest of the cardiovascular system, it delivers materials cells need and picks up their wastes.

As it passes through the digestive system, the blood delivers oxygen to the cells there and picks up most nutrients other than fats and their relatives from the **intestine** for distribution elsewhere. Lymphatic vessels pick up most fats from the intestine and then transport them to the blood (see Figure 3–5, p. 77). All blood leaving the digestive system is routed directly to the **liver**, which has the special task of chemically altering the absorbed materials to make them better suited for use by other tissues. Later, in passing through the **kidneys**, the blood is cleansed of wastes (look again at Figure 3–3). Note that the blood carries nutrients from the intestine to the liver, which releases them to the heart, which pumps them to the waiting body tissues.

Water, Nutrients, and the Blood   To ensure efficient circulation of fluid to all your cells, you need an ample fluid intake. This means consuming sufficient water to replace the water lost each day. Cardiovascular fitness is essential, too, and it requires attention to both nutrition and physical activity. Healthy red blood cells also play a role, for they carry oxygen to all the other cells, enabling them to use fuels for energy. Since red blood cells arise, live, and die within about four months, your body replaces them constantly, a manufacturing process that requires many essential nutrients from food. Consequently, the blood is very sensitive to malnutrition and often serves as an indicator of disorders caused by dietary deficiencies or imbalances of vitamins or minerals.

KEY POINTS

- Blood and lymph deliver needed materials to all the body's cells and carry waste materials away from them.
- The cardiovascular system ensures that these fluids circulate properly among all tissues.

---

blood the fluid of the cardiovascular system; composed of water, red and white blood cells, other formed particles, nutrients, oxygen, and other constituents.

lymph (LIMF) the fluid that moves from the bloodstream into tissue spaces and then travels in its own vessels, which eventually drain back into the bloodstream (see Figure 3–5, p. 77).

arteries blood vessels that carry blood containing fresh oxygen supplies from the heart to the tissues (see Figure 3–3).

veins blood vessels that carry blood, with the carbon dioxide it has collected, from the tissues back to the heart (see Figure 3–3).

capillaries minute, weblike blood vessels that connect arteries to veins and permit transfer of materials between blood and tissues (see Figures 3–3 and 3–4).

plasma the cell-free fluid part of blood and lymph.

extracellular fluid fluid residing outside the cells that transports materials to and from the cells.

intracellular fluid fluid residing inside the cells that provides the medium for cellular reactions.

lungs the body's organs of gas exchange. Blood circulating through the lungs releases its carbon dioxide and picks up fresh oxygen to carry to the tissues.

intestine the body's long, tubular organ of digestion and the site of nutrient absorption.

liver a large, lobed organ that lies just under the ribs. It filters the blood, removes and processes nutrients, manufactures materials for export to other parts of the body, and destroys toxins or stores them to keep them out of the circulatory system.

kidneys a pair of organs that filter wastes from the blood, make urine, and release it to the bladder for excretion from the body.

Figure 3-3

Blood Flow in the Cardiovascular System

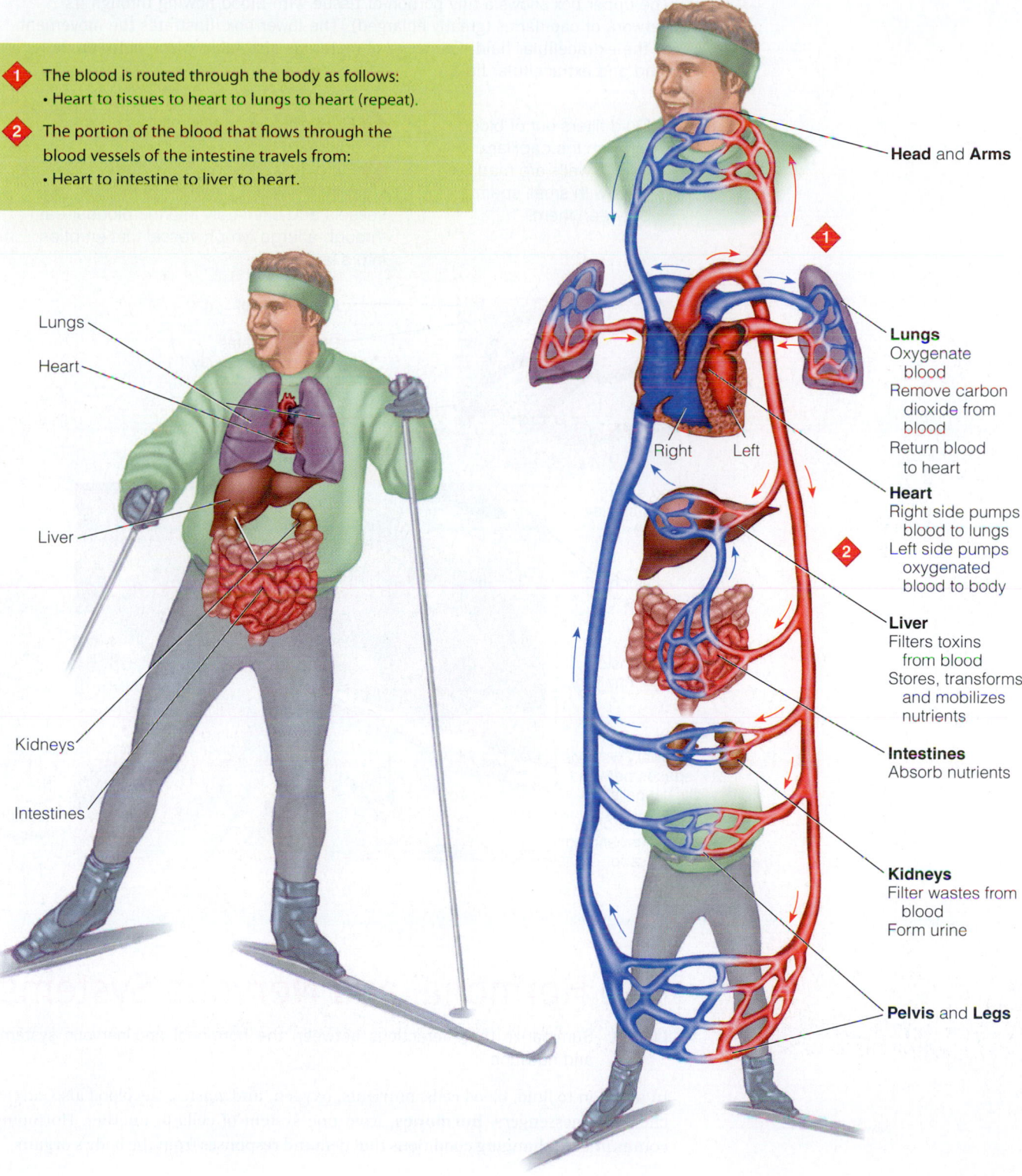

1 The blood is routed through the body as follows:
- Heart to tissues to heart to lungs to heart (repeat).

2 The portion of the blood that flows through the blood vessels of the intestine travels from:
- Heart to intestine to liver to heart.

Lungs

Heart

Liver

Kidneys

Intestines

Right   Left

Head and **Arms**

1

Lungs
Oxygenate blood
Remove carbon dioxide from blood
Return blood to heart

Heart
Right side pumps blood to lungs
Left side pumps oxygenated blood to body

2

Liver
Filters toxins from blood
Stores, transforms, and mobilizes nutrients

Intestines
Absorb nutrients

Kidneys
Filter wastes from blood
Form urine

Pelvis and **Legs**

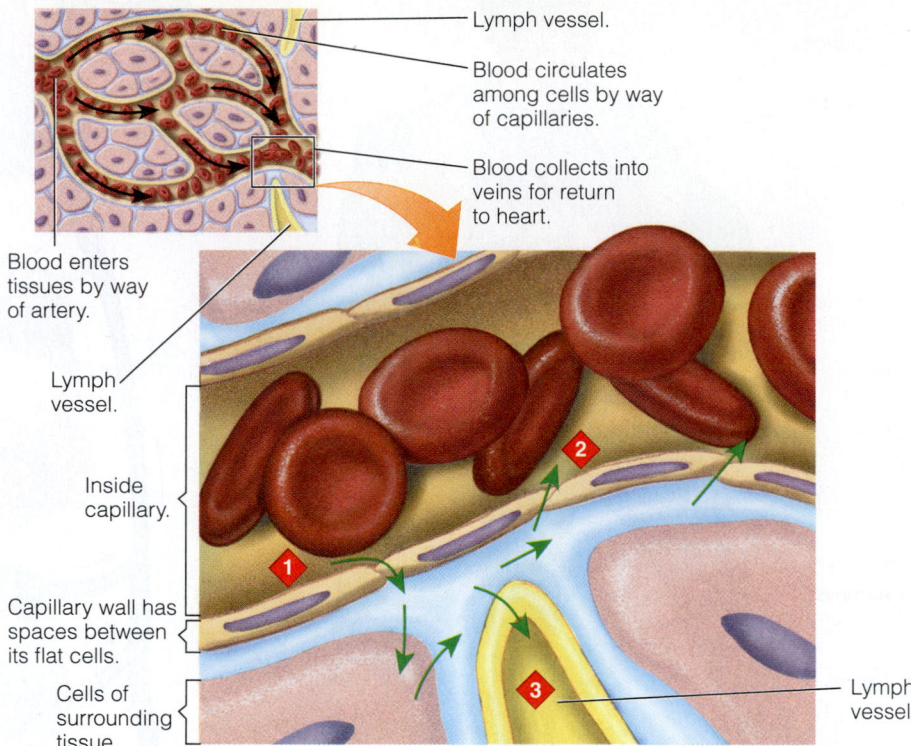

Figure 3–4

How the Body Fluids Circulate around Cells

The upper box shows a tiny portion of tissue with blood flowing through its network of capillaries (greatly enlarged). The lower box illustrates the movement of the extracellular fluid. Exchange of materials also takes place between cell fluid and extracellular fluid.

1 Fluid filters out of blood through the capillary, whose walls are made of cells with small spaces between them.

2 Fluid may enter a capillary and rejoin the bloodstream.
3 Fluid may enter a lymph vessel to join the lymphatic fluids. Lymph flows through the vessels and ultimately into the bloodstream through a large lymph vessel that empties into a large vein.

Lymph vessel.

Blood circulates among cells by way of capillaries.

Blood collects into veins for return to heart.

Blood enters tissues by way of artery.

Lymph vessel.

Inside capillary.

Capillary wall has spaces between its flat cells.

Cells of surrounding tissue.

Lymph vessel.

The Hormonal and Nervous Systems

LO 3.3 Summarize the interactions between the hormonal and nervous systems and nutrition.

In addition to fluid, blood cells, nutrients, oxygen, and wastes, the blood also carries chemical messengers, **hormones**, from one system of cells to another. Hormones communicate changing conditions that demand responses from the body's organs.

What Do Hormones Have to Do with Nutrition?

Hormones are secreted and released directly into the blood by organs known as glands. Glands and hormones abound in the body. Each gland monitors a condition and produces one or more hormones to regulate it. Each hormone acts as a messenger that stimulates various organs to take appropriate actions.

hormones chemicals that are secreted by glands into the blood in response to conditions in the body that require regulation. These chemicals serve as messengers, acting on other organs to maintain constant conditions.

Figure 3–5

Lymph Vessels and the Bloodstream—Nutrient Flow through the Body

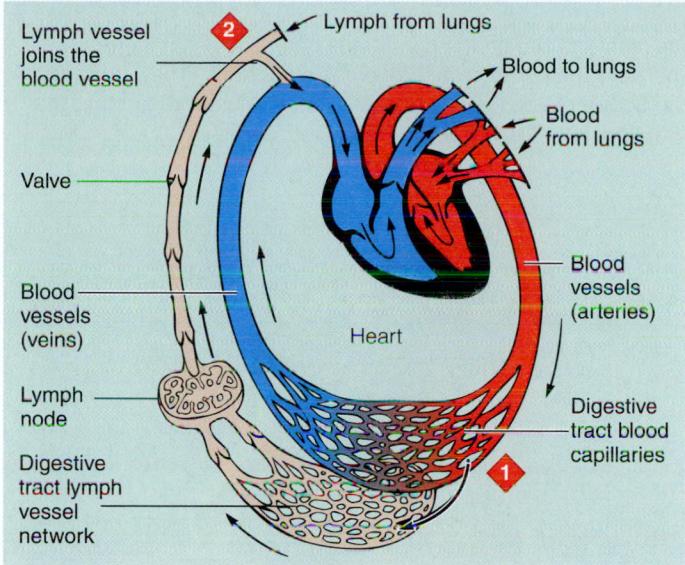

 Lymph vessel joins the blood vessel — Lymph from lungs

Blood to lungs

Blood from lungs

Valve

Blood vessels (veins)

Heart

Lymph node

Digestive tract lymph vessel network

Blood vessels (arteries)

Digestive tract blood capillaries

1. Nutrients are absorbed via two kinds of vessels in the intestines: blood capillaries and small lymph vessels. The capillaries lead to larger blood vessels that lead to the liver.

2. The lymph in the lymph vessels carries most of the absorbed dietary fat to the large vein near the heart. Some lymph vessels are depicted in Figure 3–13 (lower right, p. 91).

For example, when the **pancreas** (a gland) detects a high concentration of the blood's sugar, glucose, it releases **insulin**, a hormone. Insulin stimulates muscle and other cells to remove glucose from the blood and to store it. The liver also stores glucose. When the blood glucose level falls, the pancreas secretes another hormone, **glucagon**, to which the liver responds by releasing into the blood some of the glucose it stored earlier. Thus, a normal blood glucose level is maintained.

Nutrition affects the hormonal system. In people who become very thin, for example, an altered hormonal balance causes their bones to lose minerals and weaken. Overly thin women may also cease to menstruate, a process regulated by hormones.

The hormonal system also affects nutrition. Hormones:

- Carry messages to regulate the digestive system in response to meals or fasting.

- Inform the brain about the degree of body fatness.

- Help to regulate hunger and appetite.

- Influence appetite changes during a woman's menstrual cycle and in pregnancy.

- Regulate the body's reaction to stress, suppressing hunger and digestion.

In addition, an altered hormonal state contributes to the loss of appetite that sick people often experience. When there are questions about a person's nutrition or health, the state of that person's hormones is often part of the answer.

KEY POINT

- Glands secrete hormones that act as messengers to help regulate body processes.

How Does the Nervous System Interact with Nutrition?

The body's other major communication system is, of course, the nervous system. With the brain and spinal cord as central controllers, the nervous system receives and integrates information from sensory receptors all over the body—sight, hearing, touch, smell, taste, and others—which communicate to the brain the state of both

pancreas an organ with two main functions. One is an endocrine function—the making of hormones such as insulin, which it releases directly into the blood (*endo* means "into" the blood). The other is an exocrine function—the making of digestive enzymes, which it releases through a duct into the small intestine to assist in digestion (*exo* means "out" into a body cavity or onto the skin surface).

insulin a hormone from the pancreas that helps glucose enter cells from the blood (details in Chapter 4).

glucagon a hormone from the pancreas that stimulates the liver to release glucose into the bloodstream.

Figure 3–6

Cutaway Side View of the Brain Showing the Hypothalamus and Cortex

The hypothalamus monitors the body's conditions and sends signals to the brain's thinking portion, the cortex, which decides on actions. The pituitary gland is called the body's master gland, referring to its roles in regulating the activities of other glands and organs of the body.

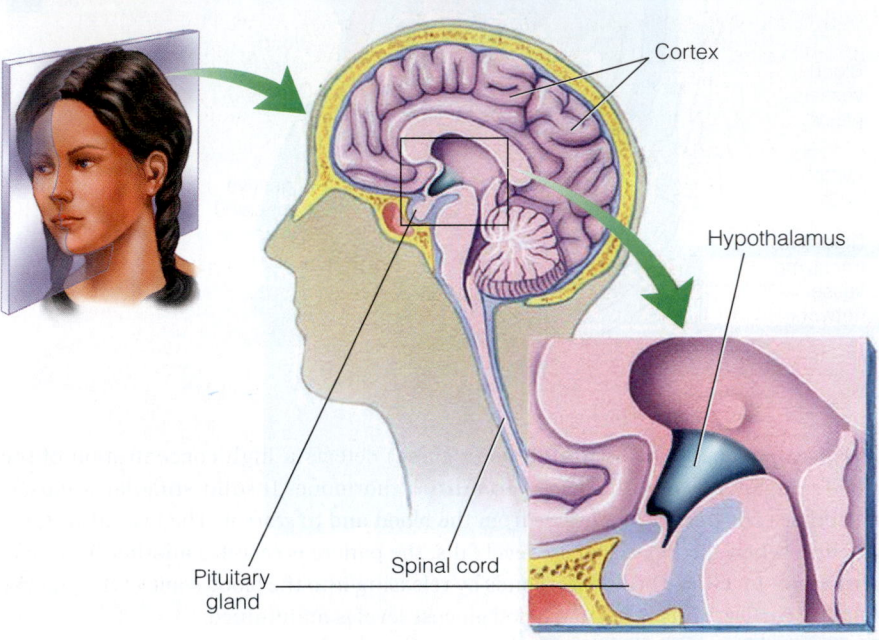

the outer and the inner worlds, including the availability of food and the need to eat. The nervous system also sends instructions to the muscles and glands, telling them what to do.

The nervous system's role in hunger regulation is coordinated by the brain. The sensations of hunger and appetite are perceived by the brain's **cortex**, the thinking, outer layer. Deep inside the brain, the **hypothalamus** (see Figure 3–6) monitors many body conditions, including the availability of nutrients and water. To signal hunger, the physiological need for food, the digestive tract sends messages to the hypothalamus by way of hormones and nerves. The signals also stimulate the stomach to intensify its contractions and secretions, causing hunger pangs (and gurgling sounds). When your brain's cortex perceives these hunger sensations, you want to eat. The conscious mind of the cortex, however, can override such signals, and a person can choose to delay eating despite hunger or to eat when hunger is absent.

In a marvelous adaptation of the human body, the hormonal and nervous systems work together to enable a person to respond to physical danger. Known as the **fight-or-flight reaction**, or the *stress response*, this adaptation is present with only minor variations in all animals, showing how universally important it is to survival. When danger is detected, nerves release **neurotransmitters**, and glands supply the compounds **epinephrine** and **norepinephrine**. Every organ of the body responds, and **metabolism** speeds up. The pupils of the eyes widen so that you can see better; the muscles tense up so that you can jump, run, or struggle with maximum strength; breathing quickens and deepens to provide more oxygen. The heart races to rush the oxygen to the muscles, and the blood pressure rises so that the fuel the muscles need for energy can be delivered efficiently. The liver pours forth glucose from its stores,

cortex the outermost layer of something. The brain's cortex is the part of the brain where conscious thought takes place.

hypothalamus (high-poh-THAL-uh-mus) a part of the brain that senses a variety of conditions in the body, such as temperature, glucose content, salt content, and others. It signals other parts of the brain or body to adjust those conditions when necessary.

fight-or-flight reaction the body's instinctive hormone- and nerve-mediated reaction to danger. Also known as the *stress response*.

neurotransmitters chemicals that are released at the end of a nerve cell when a nerve impulse arrives there. They diffuse across the gap to the next cell and alter the membrane of that second cell to either inhibit or excite it.

epinephrine (EP-ih-NEFF-rin) the major hormone that elicits the stress response.

norepinephrine (NOR-EP-ih-NEFF-rin) a compound related to epinephrine that helps to elicit the stress response.

metabolism the sum of all physical and chemical changes taking place in living cells; includes all reactions by which the body obtains and spends the energy from food.

and the fat cells release fat. The digestive system shuts down to permit all the body's systems to serve the muscles and nerves. With all action systems at peak efficiency, the body can respond with amazing speed and strength to whatever threatens it.

In ancient times, stress usually involved physical danger, and the response to it was violent physical exertion. In the modern world, stress is seldom physical, but the body reacts the same way. What stresses you today may be a checkbook out of control or a teacher who suddenly announces a pop quiz. Under these stresses, you are not supposed to fight or run, as your ancient ancestors did. You smile at the "enemy" and suppress your fear. But your heart races, you feel it pounding, and hormones still flood your bloodstream with glucose and fat.

Your number-one enemy today is not a saber-toothed tiger prowling outside your cave but a disease of modern civilization: heart disease. Years of fat and other constituents accumulating in the arteries and stresses that strain the heart often lead to heart attacks, especially when a body accustomed to chronic underexertion experiences sudden high blood pressure. Daily exercise as part of a healthy lifestyle releases pent-up stress and helps to protect the heart.

KEY POINT

- The nervous system and hormonal system regulate body processes, respond to the need for food, govern the act of eating, regulate digestion, and call for the stress response when needed.

The Immune System

LO 3.4 Specify the significance of nutrition in the proper functioning of the immune system.

Many of the body's tissues cooperate to maintain defenses against infection, and all these tissues depend on an ample supply of nutrients to function properly. The skin presents a physical barrier, and the body's cavities (lungs, mouth, digestive tract, and others) are lined with membranes that resist penetration by invading **microbes** and other unwanted substances. These linings are highly sensitive to vitamin and other nutrient deficiencies, and health-care providers inspect both the skin and the inside of the mouth to detect signs of malnutrition. (Later chapters present details of the signs of deficiencies.) If an **antigen**, or foreign invader, penetrates the body's barriers, the **immune system** rushes in to defend the body against harm.

Immune Defenses

Of the 100 trillion cells that make up the human body, one in every hundred is a white blood cell. The actions of two types of white blood cells, the phagocytes and the **lymphocytes**, known as T-cells and B-cells, are of interest:

- **Phagocytes**. These scavenger cells travel throughout the body and are the first to defend body tissues against invaders. When a phagocyte recognizes a foreign particle, such as a bacterium, the phagocyte forms a pocket in its own outer membrane, engulfing the invader. The phagocytes may then attack the invader with oxidizing chemicals in an "oxidative burst" or may otherwise digest or destroy it. Phagocytes also leave a chemical trail that helps other immune cells to find the infection and join the defense.

- **T-cells**. Killer T-cells are lymphocytes that "read" and "remember" the chemical messages put forth by phagocytes to identify invaders. The killer T-cells then seek out and destroy all foreign particles having the same identity. T-cells defend against fungi, viruses, parasites, some bacteria, and some cancer cells. They also pose a formidable obstacle to a successful organ transplant—the physician must prescribe immunosuppressive drugs following surgery to hold down the T-cells' attack against the "foreign" organ. Another group, helper T-cells, does not attack invaders directly but helps other immune cells to do so.

microbes bacteria, viruses, fungi, or other organisms invisible to the naked eye, some of which cause diseases. Also called *microorganisms*.

antigen a microbe or substance that is foreign to the body.

immune system a system of tissues and organs that defend the body against antigens, foreign materials that have penetrated the skin or body linings.

lymphocytes (LIM-foh-sites) white blood cells that participate in the immune response; B-cells and T-cells.

phagocytes (FAG-oh-sites) white blood cells that can ingest and destroy antigens. The process by which phagocytes engulf materials is called *phagocytosis*. The Greek word *phagein* means "to eat."

T-cells lymphocytes that attack antigens. *T* stands for the thymus gland of the neck, where the T-cells are stored and matured.

- **B-cells**. B-cells respond rapidly to infection by releasing invader-fighting proteins, **antibodies**, into the bloodstream. Antibodies travel to the site of the infection and stick to the surface of the foreign particles, killing or inactivating them. Like T-cells, B-cells retain a chemical memory of each invader, and if the encounter recurs, the response is swift. Immunizations work this way: a disabled or harmless form of a disease-causing organism is injected into the body so that the B-cells can learn to recognize it. Later, if the live infectious organism invades, the B-cells quickly release antibodies to destroy it.

In addition to the phagocytes and lymphocytes, the immune system includes many other categories of white blood cells and many organs and tissues. To function properly, all of these cells and organs depend on a steady flow of nutrients, delivered to the bloodstream from the digestive system.

Inflammation

When tissues become injured or irritated, they undergo **inflammation**, a condition of increased white blood cells, redness, heat, pain, swelling, and sometimes loss of function of the affected body part. Inflammation is the immune system's normal, healthy response to cell injury.

Many diseases, particularly chronic diseases of later life, such as heart disease, diabetes, and a severe type of arthritis, are associated with chronic tissue inflammation. When chronic, low-grade, unrelieved inflammation exists in chronic diseases, it often foretells an increase in both the severity of the disease and the risk of death from the disease. An important predictor of inflammation is being overweight.[1]* The links among diet, inflammatory processes, and diseases are currently topics of intense research, and later chapters revisit them.

The Digestive System

LO 3.5 Summarize how the digestive system provides nutrients to the body tissues.

When your body needs food, your brain and hormones alert your conscious mind to the sensation of hunger. Then, when you eat, your taste buds guide you in judging whether foods are acceptable.

Taste buds on the tongue contain surface structures that detect five basic chemical tastes: sweet, sour, bitter, salty, and umami (ooh-MOM-ee), the Asian name for *savory*. These basic tastes, along with aroma, texture, temperature, and other flavor elements, affect a person's experience of a food's flavor. In fact, the human ability to detect a food's aroma is thousands of times more sensitive than the sense of taste. The nose can detect just a few molecules responsible for the aroma of frying bacon, for example, even when they are diluted in several rooms full of air.

Why Do People Like Sugar, Salt, and Fat?

Sweet, salty, and fatty foods are almost universally desired, but most people have aversions to bitter and sour tastes (see Figure 3–7).[2] The enjoyment of sugars is inborn and encourages people to consume ample energy, especially in the form of foods containing carbohydrates, which provide the energy fuel for the brain.[3] The pleasure

B-cells lymphocytes that produce antibodies. *B* stands for bursa, an organ in the chicken where B-cells were first identified.

antibodies proteins, made by cells of the immune system, that are expressly designed to combine with and inactivate specific antigens.

inflammation the immune system's response to cellular injury characterized by an increase in white blood cells, redness, heat, pain, and swelling. Inflammation plays a role in many chronic diseases.

* Reference notes are found in Appendix F.

Figure 3–7

The Innate Preference for Sweet Taste

This newborn baby is (a) resting; (b) tasting distilled water; (c) tasting sugar; (d) tasting something sour; and (e) tasting something bitter

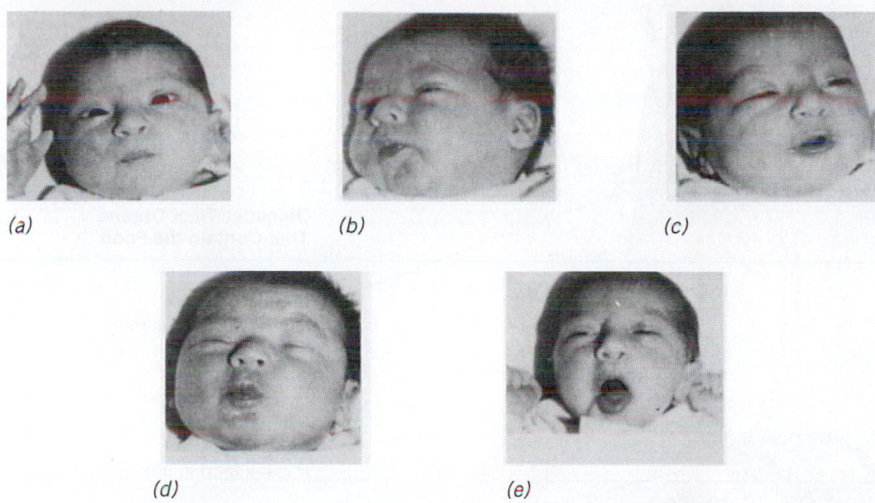

(a)   (b)   (c)

(d)   (e)

Source: Courtesy of Classic studies of J.E. Steiner, in Taste and Development: The Genesis of Sweet Preference, *ed. J.M. Weiffenbach, HHS publication no. NIH 77-1068 (Bethesda, MD: U.S. Department of Health and Human Services, 1977), pp. 173–189, with permission of the author.*

of a salty taste prompts eaters to consume sufficient amounts of two very important minerals—sodium and chloride. Likewise, foods containing fats provide concentrated energy and essential nutrients needed by all body tissues. The aversion to bitterness, universally displayed in infants, discourages consumption of potentially dangerous substances containing bitter toxins and also affects people's food preferences later on. People with greater aversion to bitter tastes are apt to avoid foods with slightly bitter flavors, such as turnips and broccoli.

The instinctive liking for sugar, salt, and fat can lead to drastic overeating of these substances. Sugar has become widely available in pure form only in the last hundred years, so it is relatively new to the human diet. Although salt and fat are much older, today all three substances are added liberally to foods by manufacturers to tempt us to eat their products.

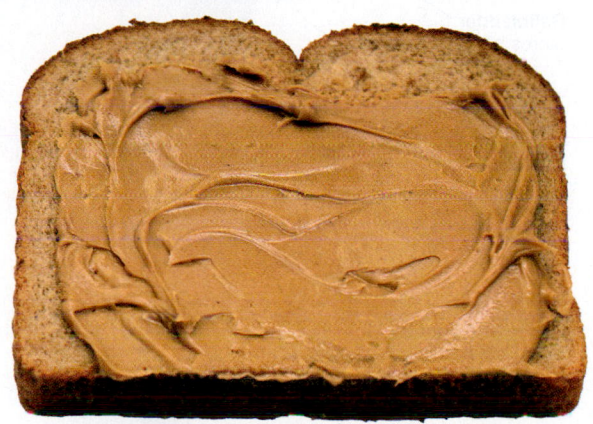

KEY POINT

- The preference for sweet, salty, and fatty tastes is inborn and can lead to overconsumption of foods that offer them.

The Digestive Tract

Once you have eaten, your brain and hormones direct the many organs of the **digestive system** to **digest** and **absorb** the complex mixture of chewed and swallowed food. A diagram showing the digestive tract and associated organs appears in Figure 3–8. The tract itself is a flexible, muscular tube extending from the mouth through the throat, esophagus, stomach, small intestine, large intestine, and rectum to the anus, for a total length of about 26 feet. The human body surrounds this digestive canal. When you swallow something, it still is not inside your body—it is only inside the inner bore of this tube. Only when a nutrient or other substance passes through the wall of the digestive tract does it actually enter the body's tissues. Many things pass into the digestive tract and out again, unabsorbed. A baby playing with

digestive system the body system composed of organs that break down complex food particles into smaller, absorbable products. The *digestive tract* and *alimentary canal* are names for the tubular organs that extend from the mouth to the anus. The whole system, including the pancreas, liver, and gallbladder, is sometimes called the *gastrointestinal*, or *GI*, system.

digest to break molecules into smaller molecules; a main function of the digestive tract with respect to food.

absorb to take in, as nutrients are taken into the intestinal cells after digestion; the main function of the digestive tract with respect to nutrients.

Figure 3–8

The Digestive System

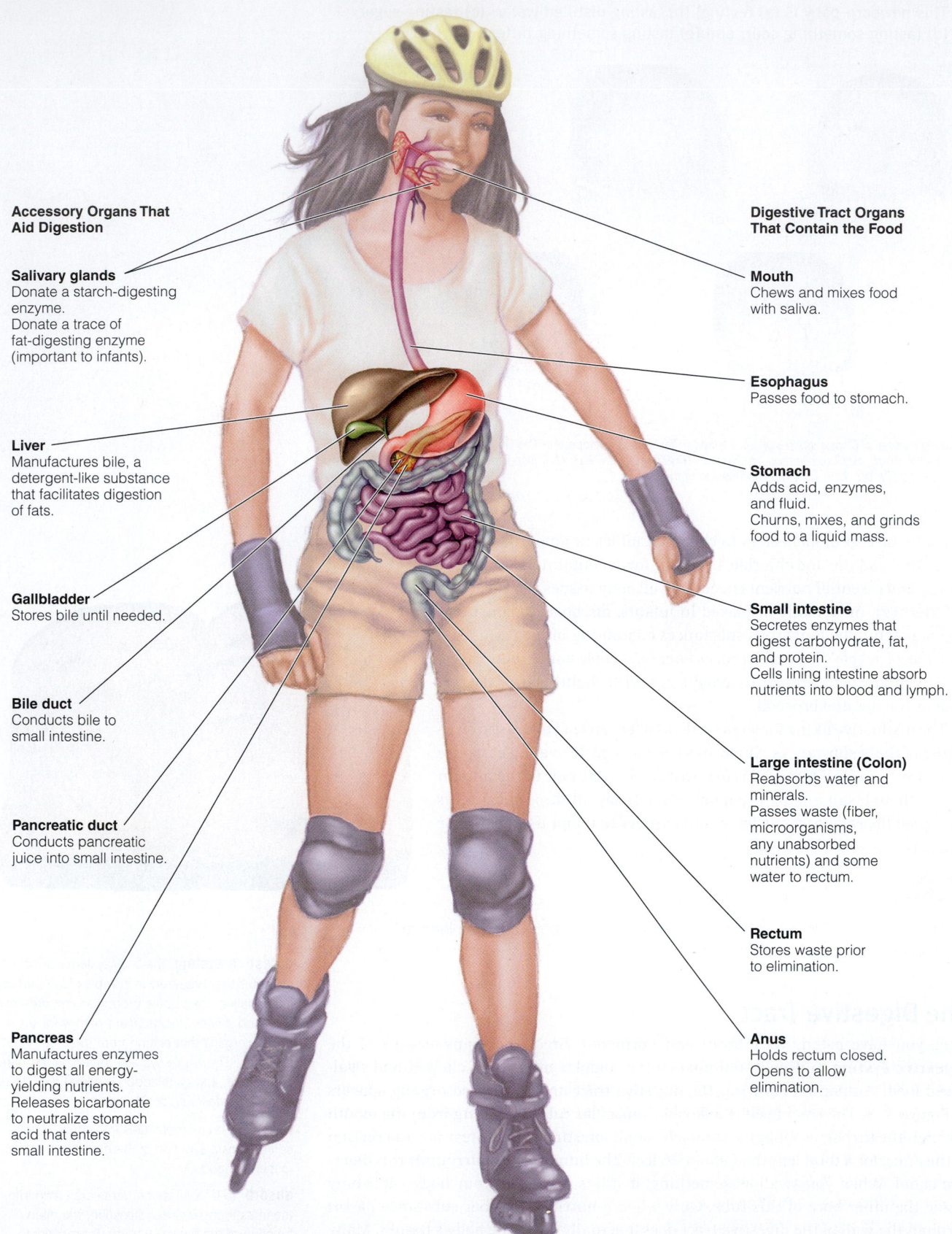

Accessory Organs That Aid Digestion

Salivary glands
Donate a starch-digesting enzyme.
Donate a trace of fat-digesting enzyme (important to infants).

Liver
Manufactures bile, a detergent-like substance that facilitates digestion of fats.

Gallbladder
Stores bile until needed.

Bile duct
Conducts bile to small intestine.

Pancreatic duct
Conducts pancreatic juice into small intestine.

Pancreas
Manufactures enzymes to digest all energy-yielding nutrients.
Releases bicarbonate to neutralize stomach acid that enters small intestine.

Digestive Tract Organs That Contain the Food

Mouth
Chews and mixes food with saliva.

Esophagus
Passes food to stomach.

Stomach
Adds acid, enzymes, and fluid.
Churns, mixes, and grinds food to a liquid mass.

Small intestine
Secretes enzymes that digest carbohydrate, fat, and protein.
Cells lining intestine absorb nutrients into blood and lymph.

Large intestine (Colon)
Reabsorbs water and minerals.
Passes waste (fiber, microorganisms, any unabsorbed nutrients) and some water to rectum.

Rectum
Stores waste prior to elimination.

Anus
Holds rectum closed.
Opens to allow elimination.

Figure 3–9

Peristaltic Wave Passing Down the Esophagus and Beyond

Peristalsis moves the digestive tract contents.

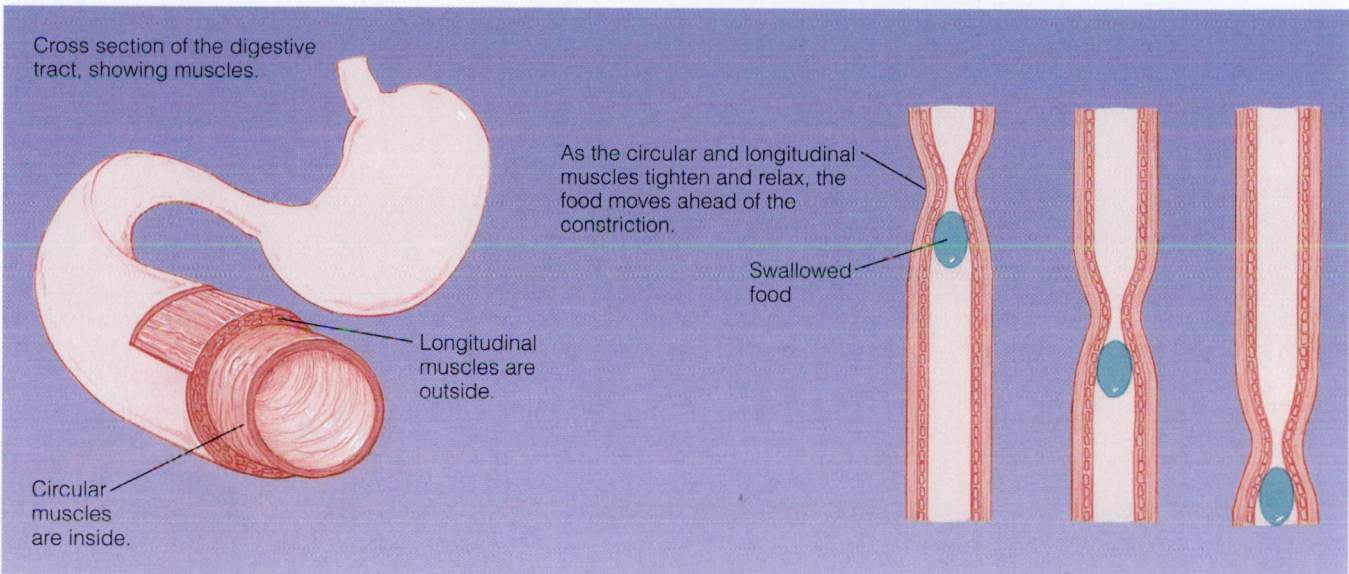

Cross section of the digestive tract, showing muscles.

As the circular and longitudinal muscles tighten and relax, the food moves ahead of the constriction.

Swallowed food

Longitudinal muscles are outside.

Circular muscles are inside.

beads may swallow one, but the bead will not really enter the body. It will emerge from the digestive tract within a day or two.

The digestive system's job is to digest food to its components and then to absorb the nutrients and some nonnutrients, leaving behind the substances, such as fiber, that are appropriate to excrete. To do this, the system works at two levels: one, mechanical; the other, chemical.

KEY POINTS

- The digestive tract is a flexible, muscular tube that digests food and absorbs its nutrients and some nonnutrients.
- Ancillary digestive organs, such as the pancreas and gallbladder, aid digestion.

The Mechanical Aspect of Digestion

The job of mechanical digestion begins in the mouth, where large, solid food pieces such as bites of meat are torn into shreds that can be swallowed without choking. Chewing also adds water in the form of saliva to soften rough or sharp foods, such as fried tortilla chips, to prevent them from tearing the esophagus. Saliva also moistens and coats each bite of food, making it slippery so that it can pass easily down the esophagus.

Nutrients trapped inside indigestible skins, such as the hulls of seeds, must be liberated by breaking these skins before they can be digested. Chewing bursts open kernels of corn, for example, which would otherwise traverse the tract and exit undigested. Once food has been mashed and moistened for comfortable swallowing, longer chewing times provide no additional advantages to digestion. In fact, for digestion's sake, a relaxed, peaceful attitude during a meal aids digestion much more than chewing for an extended time.

The stomach and intestines then take up the task of liquefying foods through various mashing and squeezing actions. The best known of these actions is **peristalsis**, a series of squeezing waves that start with the tongue's movement during a swallow and pass all the way down the esophagus (see Figure 3–9). The stomach and the intestines also push food through the tract by waves of peristalsis. Besides these actions,

peristalsis (perri-STALL-sis) the wavelike muscular squeezing of the esophagus, stomach, and small intestine that pushes their contents along.

Figure 3–10

The Muscular Stomach

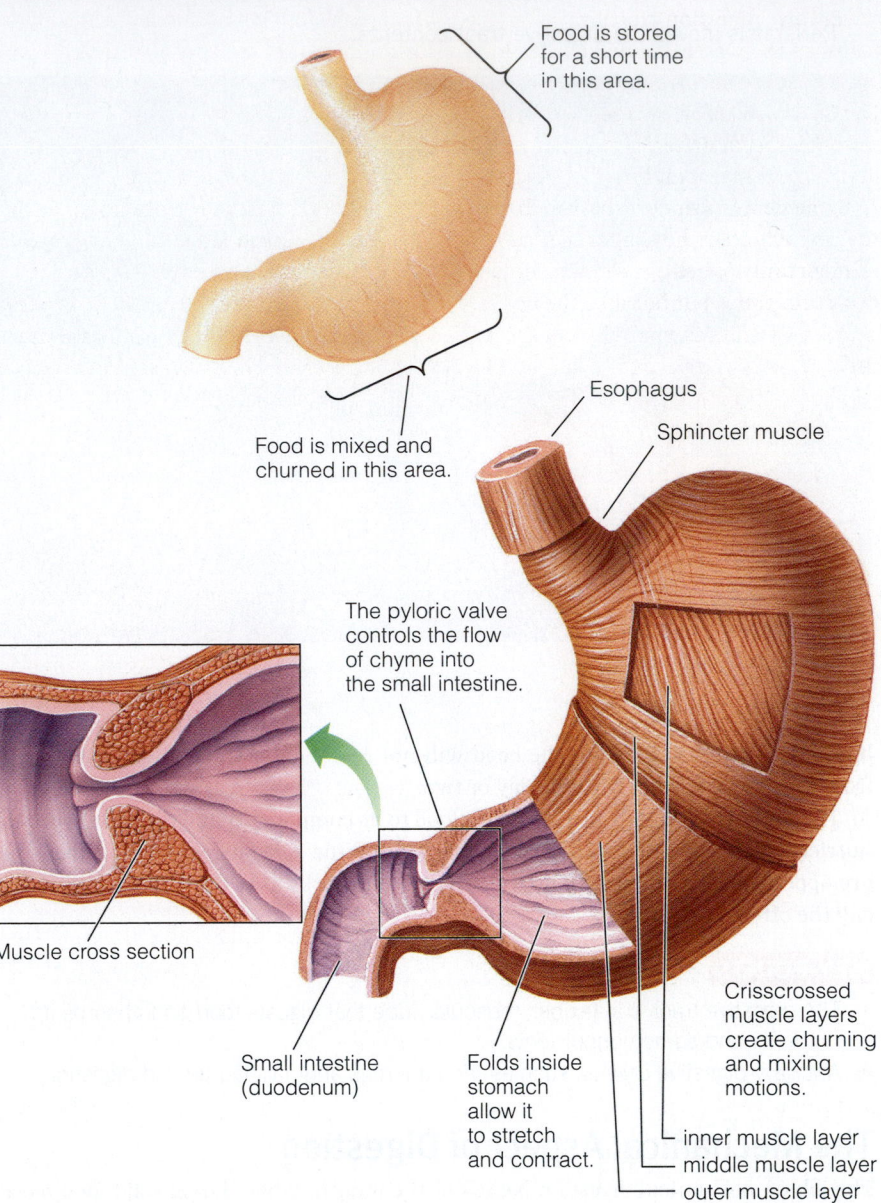

Food is stored for a short time in this area.

Food is mixed and churned in this area.

Esophagus

Sphincter muscle

The pyloric valve controls the flow of chyme into the small intestine.

Muscle cross section

Small intestine (duodenum)

Folds inside stomach allow it to stretch and contract.

Crisscrossed muscle layers create churning and mixing motions.

inner muscle layer
middle muscle layer
outer muscle layer

stomach a muscular, elastic, pouchlike organ of the digestive tract that grinds and churns swallowed food and mixes it with acid and enzymes, forming chyme.

sphincter (SFINK-ter) a circular muscle surrounding, and able to close, a body opening.

chyme (KIME) the fluid resulting from the actions of the stomach upon a meal.

pyloric (pye-LORE-ick) **valve** the circular muscle of the lower stomach that regulates the flow of partly digested food into the small intestine. Also called *pyloric sphincter*.

small intestine the 20-foot length of small-diameter intestine, below the stomach and above the large intestine, which is the major site of digestion of food and absorption of nutrients.

the **stomach** holds swallowed food for a while and mashes it into a fine paste; the stomach and intestines also add water so that the paste becomes more fluid as it moves along.

Figure 3–10 shows the muscular stomach. Notice the circular **sphincter** muscle at the base of the esophagus. It squeezes the opening at the entrance to the stomach to narrow it and prevent the stomach's contents from creeping back up the esophagus as the stomach contracts. Swallowed food remains in a lump in the stomach's upper portion, squeezed little by little to its lower portion. There the food is ground and churned thoroughly, ensuring that digestive chemicals mix with the entire thick, liquid mass, now called **chyme**. Chyme bears no resemblance to the original food. The starches have been partly split, proteins have been uncoiled and clipped, and fat has separated from the mass.

The stomach also acts as a holding tank. The muscular **pyloric valve** at the stomach's lower end (look again at Figure 3–10) controls the exit of the chyme, allowing only a little at a time to be squirted forcefully into the **small intestine**. Within a few hours after a meal, the stomach empties itself by means of these powerful squirts. The small intestine contracts rhythmically to move the contents along its length.

By the time the intestinal contents have arrived in the **large intestine** (also called the **colon**), digestion and absorption are nearly complete. The colon's task is mostly to reabsorb the water donated earlier by digestive organs and to absorb minerals, leaving a paste of fiber and other undigested materials, the **feces**, suitable for excretion. The fiber provides bulk against which the muscles of the colon can work. The rectum stores this fecal material to be excreted at intervals. From mouth to rectum, the transit of a meal is accomplished in as short a time as a single day or as long as three days.

Some people wonder whether the digestive tract works best at certain hours in the day and whether the timing of meals can affect how a person feels. Timing of meals is important to feeling well, not because the digestive tract is unable to digest food at certain times but because the body requires nutrients to be replenished every few hours. Digestion is virtually continuous, being limited only during sleep and exercise. For some people, eating late may interfere with normal sleep. As for exercise, it is best pursued a few hours after eating because digestion can inhibit physical work (see Chapter 10 for details).

KEY POINTS

- The mechanical digestive actions include chewing, mixing by the stomach, adding fluid, and moving the tract's contents by peristalsis.
- After digestion and absorption, wastes are excreted.

The Chemical Aspect of Digestion

Several organs of the digestive system secrete special digestive juices that perform the complex chemical processes of digestion. Digestive juices contain enzymes that break down nutrients into their component parts (Table 3–1 presents some enzyme terms). The digestive organs that release digestive juices are the salivary glands, the stomach, the pancreas, the liver, and the small intestine. Their secretions were listed previously in Figure 3–8 (on p. 82).

In the Mouth   Digestion begins in the mouth. An enzyme in saliva starts rapidly breaking down starch, and another enzyme initiates a little digestion of fat, especially the digestion of milk fat (important in infants). Saliva also helps maintain the health of the teeth in two ways: by washing away food particles that would otherwise foster decay and by neutralizing decay-promoting acids produced by bacteria in the mouth.

In the Stomach   In the stomach, protein digestion begins. Cells in the stomach release **gastric juice**, a mixture of water, enzymes, and **hydrochloric acid**. This strong acid mixture is needed to activate a protein-digesting enzyme and to initiate digestion of protein—protein digestion is the stomach's main function. The strength of an acid solution is expressed as its **pH**. The lower the pH number, the more acidic the solution; solutions with higher pH numbers are more basic. As Figure 3–11 (p. 86) demonstrates, saliva is only weakly acidic; the stomach's gastric juice is much more strongly acidic. Notice on the right-hand side of Figure 3–11 that the range of tolerance for the blood's normal pH is exceedingly small.

Upon learning of the powerful digestive juices and enzymes within the digestive tract, students often wonder how the tract's own cellular lining escapes being digested along with the food. The answer: specialized cells secrete a thick, viscous substance known as **mucus**, which coats and protects the digestive tract lining.

In the Intestine   In the small intestine, the digestive process gets under way in earnest. The small intestine is *the* organ of digestion and absorption, and it finishes what the mouth and stomach have started. The small intestine works with the precision of a laboratory chemist. As the thoroughly liquefied and partially digested nutrient mixture arrives there, hormonal messengers signal the gallbladder to contract

---

large intestine the portion of the intestine that completes the absorption process.

colon the large intestine.

feces waste material remaining after digestion and absorption are complete; eventually discharged from the body.

gastric juice the digestive secretion of the stomach.

hydrochloric acid a strong, corrosive acid of hydrogen and chloride atoms, produced by the stomach to assist in digestion.

pH a measure of acidity on a point scale. A solution with a pH of 1 is a strong acid; a solution with a pH of 7 is neutral; a solution with a pH of 14 is a strong base.

mucus (MYOO-cus) a slippery coating of the digestive tract lining (and other body linings) that protects the cells from exposure to digestive juices (and other destructive agents). The adjective form is *mucous* (same pronunciation). The digestive tract lining is a *mucous membrane*.

Figure 3–11

pH Values of Digestive Juices and Other Common Fluids

A substance's acidity or alkalinity is measured in pH units. Each step down the scale indicates a tenfold increase in concentration of hydrogen particles, which determine acidity. For example, a pH of 2 is 1,000 times stronger than a pH of 5.

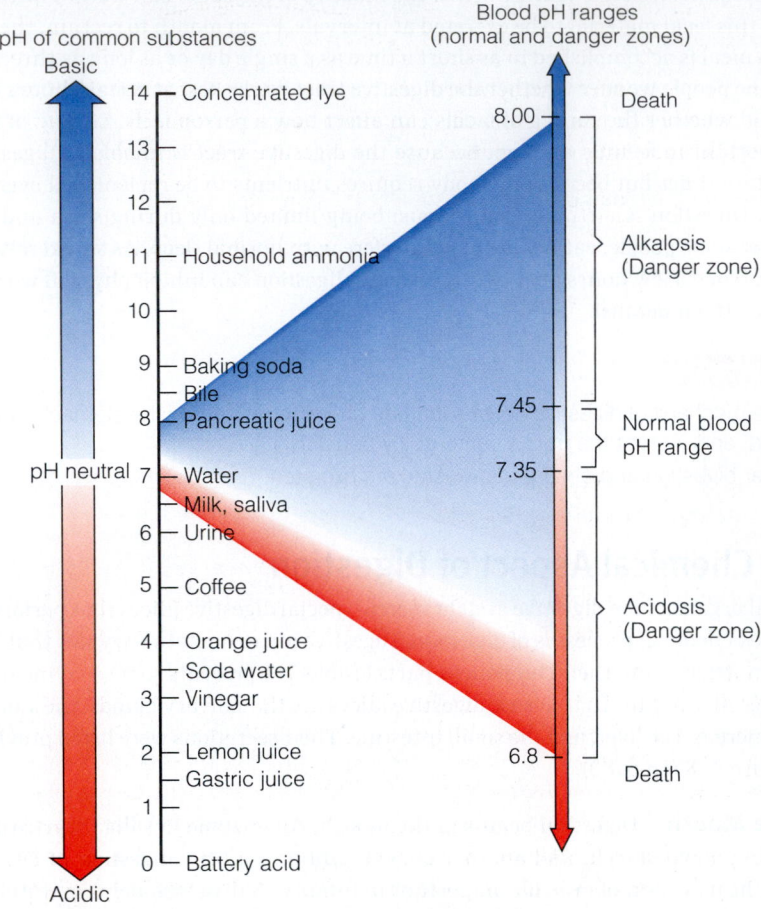

pH of common substances

Basic	
14	Concentrated lye
13	
12	
11	Household ammonia
10	
9	Baking soda
	Bile
8	Pancreatic juice
pH neutral 7	Water
	Milk, saliva
6	Urine
5	Coffee
4	Orange juice
	Soda water
3	Vinegar
2	Lemon juice
	Gastric juice
1	
0	Battery acid
Acidic	

Blood pH ranges (normal and danger zones)

8.00 — Death

Alkalosis (Danger zone)

7.45 —
Normal blood pH range
7.35 —

Acidosis (Danger zone)

6.8 — Death

and to squirt the right amount of **bile**, an **emulsifier**, into the intestine. Other hormones notify the pancreas to release **pancreatic juice**, containing the alkaline compound **bicarbonate**, in amounts precisely adjusted to neutralize the stomach acid that has reached the small intestine. All these actions alter the intestinal environment to perfectly support the work of the digestive enzymes.

Meanwhile, as the pancreatic and intestinal enzymes act on the chemical bonds that hold the large nutrients together, smaller and smaller pieces are released into the intestinal fluids. The cells of the intestinal wall also hold some digestive enzymes on their surfaces; these enzymes perform last-minute breakdown reactions required before nutrients can be absorbed. Finally, the digestive process releases pieces small enough for the cells to absorb and use. Digestion by human enzymes and absorption of carbohydrate, fat, and protein are essentially complete by the time the intestinal contents enter the colon. Water, fiber, and some minerals, however, remain in the tract.

KEY POINTS

- Chemical digestion begins in the mouth, where food is mixed with an enzyme in saliva that acts on carbohydrates.
- Digestion continues in the stomach, where stomach enzymes and acid break down protein.
- Digestion progresses in the small intestine, where the liver and gallbladder contribute bile that emulsifies fat, and the pancreas and small intestine, donate enzymes that break down food to nutrients.

bile a cholesterol-containing digestive fluid made by the liver, stored in the gallbladder, and released into the small intestine when needed. It emulsifies fats and oils to ready them for enzymatic digestion (described in Chapter 5).

emulsifier (ee-MULL-sih-fire) a compound with both water-soluble and fat-soluble portions that can attract fats and oils into water, combining them.

pancreatic juice fluid secreted by the pancreas that contains both enzymes to digest carbohydrates, fats, and proteins and sodium bicarbonate, a neutralizing agent.

bicarbonate a common alkaline chemical; a secretion of the pancreas; also the active ingredient of baking soda.

Microbes in the Digestive Tract

Certain remnants of food, largely fibers, not digested by human enzymes in the small intestine are often broken down by billions of living inhabitants in the colon, collectively called the **microbiota**. A healthy digestive tract is home to up to 100 *trillion* microbes of many species; the bacteria alone outnumber the cells of the body tenfold.[4] Bacteria in the colon are so efficient at fermenting and breaking down substances from food that they have been likened to a body organ specializing in nutrient salvage. Table 3–2 (p. 88) presents a summary of digestion, including the actions of the bacteria.

Bacterial Activities   Digestive tract bacteria harvest energy from undigested food substances and use it to sustain themselves and to proliferate. In the process, they yield smaller molecules that the body can absorb and use.[5] For example, bacteria:

- Ferment many indigestible fibers, producing short fatty acids that provide many colon cells with most of their needed energy.

- Break down any undigested protein or unabsorbed amino acids that reach the colon, producing ammonia and other compounds.[†]

- Break down and help to recycle components of bile.

- Chemically alter certain drugs and phytochemicals, changing their effects on the body.

Bacteria produce several vitamins, too, but in amounts insufficient to meet the body's needs, so these vitamins must be obtained from the diet.

Good or Bad Bacteria?   The intestinal bacteria may affect many body systems. Microbes generate compounds that communicate with such diverse tissues as muscle, adipose tissue (see Chapter 9), and even the brain in ways that alter the body's use and storage of energy.[6] They also deliver messages to the immune system, affecting health and disease. Research suggests that, when the mix of bacterial species falls out of balance, potentially harmful bacteria proliferate, producing substances that increase inflammation and that are associated with obesity, diabetes, several intestinal conditions, fatty liver disease, certain cancers, and even asthma.[7]

Food intake largely controls the mix of species in intestinal bacteria. A steady diet of meats, fats, and ultra-processed foods (defined Chapter 1) lacks the beneficial bacterial hitchhikers that ride into the digestive system in yogurt or other foods that contain live cultures. Such a diet is also stripped of the fibers upon which beneficial bacteria feed, and lacking proper food, beneficial colonies collapse. Then, lacking competition, less helpful, and even harmful, species rapidly multiply. Maintaining a healthy microbiota is simple: consume an adequate diet of mostly whole foods to provide the fiber upon which beneficial bacteria can thrive.

Enterococcus faecalis, *one of the thousands of bacterial species living in the human digestive tract.*

KEY POINTS

- A substantial population of intestinal bacteria scavenges and breaks down fibers and other undigested compounds.
- The colon absorbs and uses products of bacterial metabolism; the bacteria and their products also interact with other organs and tissues.
- Diet strongly influences the composition and metabolism of the intestinal bacteria.

Are Some Food Combinations More Easily Digested Than Others?

People sometimes wonder if the digestive tract has trouble digesting certain foods in combination—for example, fruit and meat. Proponents of fad "food-combining" diets claim that the digestive tract cannot perform certain digestive tasks at the same time, but this is a gross underestimation of the tract's capabilities. The digestive system

microbiota the mix of microbial species of a community; for example, all of the bacteria, fungi, and viruses present in the human digestive tract. The term *microbiome* refers to the collective genes of such a community.

[†]Bacterial action on lipid is insignificant.

Table 3–2
Summary of Digestion

	Mouth	Stomach	Small Intestine, Pancreas, Liver, and Gallbladder	Large Intestine (Colon)
Sugar and Starch	The salivary glands secrete saliva to moisten and lubricate food; chewing crushes and mixes it with a salivary enzyme that initiates starch digestion.	Digestion of starch continues while food remains in the upper storage area of the stomach. In the lower digesting area of the stomach, hydrochloric acid and an enzyme in the stomach's juices halt starch digestion.	The pancreas produces a starch-digesting enzyme and releases it into the small intestine. Cells in the intestinal lining possess enzymes on their surfaces that break sugars and starch fragments into simple sugars, which then are absorbed.	Undigested carbohydrates reach the large intestine and are partly broken down by intestinal bacteria.
Fiber	The teeth crush fiber and mix it with saliva to moisten it for swallowing.	No action.	Fiber binds cholesterol and some minerals.	Most fiber is excreted with the feces; some fiber is digested by bacteria in the large intestine.
Fat	Fat-rich foods are mixed with saliva. The tongue produces traces of a fat-digesting enzyme that accomplishes some breakdown, especially of milk fats. The enzyme is stable at low pH and is important to digestion in nursing infants.	Fat tends to rise from the watery stomach fluid and foods and float on top of the mixture. Only a small amount of fat is digested. Fat is last to leave the stomach.	The liver secretes bile; the gallbladder stores it and releases it into the small intestine. Bile emulsifies the fat and readies it for enzyme action. The pancreas produces fat-digesting enzymes and releases them into the small intestine to split fats into their component parts (primarily fatty acids), which then are absorbed.	Some fatty materials escape absorption and are carried out of the body with other wastes.
Protein	Chewing crushes and softens protein-rich foods and mixes them with saliva.	Stomach acid (hydrochloric acid) works to uncoil protein strands and to activate the stomach's protein-digesting enzyme. Then the enzyme breaks the protein strands into smaller fragments.	Enzymes of the small intestine and pancreas split protein fragments into smaller fragments or free amino acids. Enzymes on the cells of the intestinal lining break some protein fragments into free amino acids, which then are absorbed. Some protein fragments are also absorbed.	Resident bacteria break down small amounts of undigested protein and amino acids; any remaining residue is carried out of the body with the feces. Normally, almost all food protein is digested and absorbed.
Water	The mouth donates watery, enzyme-containing saliva.	The stomach donates acidic, watery, enzyme-containing gastric juice.	The liver donates a watery juice containing bile. The pancreas and small intestine add watery, enzyme-containing juices; pancreatic juice is also alkaline.	The large intestine reabsorbs water and some minerals.

adjusts to whatever mixture of foods is presented to it. The truth is that all foods, regardless of identity, are broken down by enzymes into the basic molecules that make them up. The next section reviews the major processes of digestion by showing how the nutrients in a mixture of foods are handled.

If "I Am What I Eat," Then How Does a Peanut Butter Sandwich Become "Me"?

The process of rendering foods into nutrients and absorbing them into the body fluids is remarkably efficient. Within about 24 to 48 hours of eating, a healthy body digests and absorbs about 90 percent of the carbohydrate, fat, and protein in a meal. Figure 3–12 illustrates a typical 24-hour transit time through the digestive system. Next, we follow a peanut butter and banana sandwich on whole-wheat sesame seed bread through the tract.

In the Mouth In each bite, food components are crushed, mashed, and mixed with saliva by the teeth and the tongue. The sesame seeds are crushed and torn open by the teeth, which break through the indigestible fiber coating so that digestive enzymes can reach the nutrients inside the seeds. The peanut butter is the "extra crunchy" type, but the teeth grind the chunks to a paste before the bite is swallowed. The carbohydrate-digesting enzyme of saliva begins to break down the starch of the bread, banana, and peanut butter to sugars. Each swallow triggers a peristaltic wave that travels the length of the esophagus and carries one chewed bite of sandwich to the stomach.

In the Stomach The stomach collects bite after swallowed bite in its upper storage area, where starch continues to be digested until the gastric juice mixes with the salivary enzymes and halts their action. Small portions of the mashed sandwich are pushed into the digesting area of the stomach, where gastric juice mixes with the mass. Acid in the gastric juice unwinds proteins from the bread, seeds, and peanut butter; then an enzyme clips the protein strands into pieces. The sandwich has now become chyme. The watery, carbohydrate- and protein-rich part of the chyme enters the small intestine first; a layer of fat follows closely behind.

In the Small Intestine Some of the sweet sugars in the banana require so little digesting that they begin to cross the linings of the small intestine immediately on contact. Nearby, the liver donates bile through a duct into the small intestine. The bile blends the fat from the peanut butter and seeds with the watery, enzyme-containing digestive fluids. The nearby pancreas squirts enzymes into the small intestine to break down the fat, protein, and starch in the chemical soup that just an hour ago was a sandwich. The cells of the small intestine itself produce enzymes to complete these processes. As the enzymes do their work, smaller and smaller chemical fragments are liberated from the chemical soup and are absorbed into the blood and lymph through the cells of the small intestine's wall. Vitamins and minerals are absorbed here, too. They all eventually enter the bloodstream to nourish the tissues.

In the Large Intestine (Colon) Only fiber fragments, fluid, and some minerals are absorbed in the large intestine. The fibers from the seeds, whole-wheat bread, peanut butter, and banana are partly digested by the bacteria living in the colon, and some of the products are absorbed. Most fiber is not digested, however, and it passes out of the colon along with some other components, excreted as feces.

Figure 3–12

Typical Digestive System Transit Times

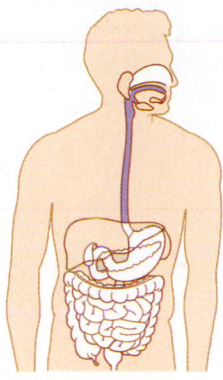
Time in mouth, less than a minute.

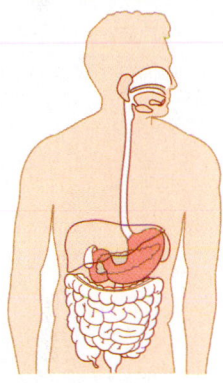
Time in stomach, about 1–2 hours.

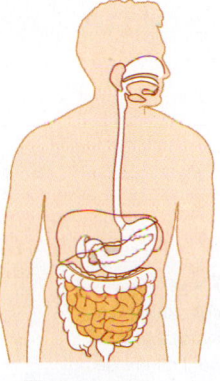
Time in small intestine, about 7–8 hours.*

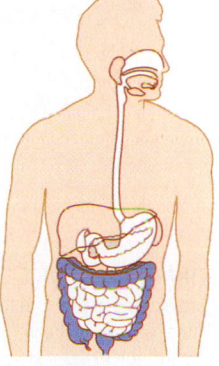
Time in colon, about 12–14 hours.*

*Based on a 24-hour transit time. Actual times vary widely.

- The mechanical and chemical actions of the digestive tract efficiently break down foods to nutrients and then large nutrients to their smaller building blocks.

Absorption and Transport of Nutrients

Once the digestive system has broken down food to its nutrient components, the rest of the body awaits their delivery. First, though, every molecule of nutrient must traverse one of the cells of the intestinal lining. These cells absorb nutrients from the mixture within the intestine and deposit the water-soluble compounds in the blood and the fat-soluble ones in the lymph. The cells are selective: they recognize that some nutrients may be in short supply in the diet. Take the mineral calcium, for example. The less calcium in the diet, the greater the percentage of calcium the intestinal cells absorb from the intestinal contents. The cells are also extraordinarily efficient: they absorb enough nutrients to nourish all the body's other cells.

The Intestine's Absorbing Surface

The cells of the intestinal tract lining are arranged in sheets that poke out into millions of finger-shaped projections (**villi**). Every cell on every villus has a brushlike covering of tiny hairlike projections (**microvilli**) that can trap the nutrient particles. Each villus (projection) has its own capillary network and a lymph vessel, so that, as nutrients move across the cells, they can immediately mingle with the body fluids. Figure 3–13 provides a close look at these details.

The small intestine's lining, villi and all, is wrinkled into thousands of folds, so its absorbing surface is enormous. If the folds, and the villi that poke out from them, were spread out flat, they would cover a third of a football field. The billions of cells of that surface weigh only 4 to 5 pounds, yet they absorb enough nutrients to nourish the other 150 or so pounds of body tissues.

Nutrient Transport in the Blood and Lymph Vessels

After the nutrients pass through the cells of the villi, the blood and lymph vessels transport the nutrients to their ultimate consumers, the body's cells. The lymph vessels initially transport most of the products of fat digestion and the fat-soluble vitamins, ultimately conveying them into a large blood vessel near the heart. The blood vessels directly transport the products of carbohydrate and protein digestion, most vitamins, and the minerals from the digestive tract to the liver. Thanks to these two transportation systems, every nutrient soon arrives at the place where it is needed.

Nourishment of the Digestive Tract

The digestive system's millions of specialized cells are themselves exquisitely sensitive to an undersupply of energy, nutrients, or dietary fiber. In cases of severe undernutrition with too little energy and nutrients, the absorptive surface of the small intestine shrinks. The surface may be reduced to a tenth of its normal area, preventing it from absorbing what few nutrients a limited food supply may provide. Without sufficient fiber to provide an undigested bulk for the tract's muscles to push against, the muscles become weak from lack of exercise. Malnutrition that impairs digestion is self-perpetuating because impaired digestion makes malnutrition worse.

The digestive system's needs are few, but important. The body has much to say to the attentive listener, stated in a language of symptoms and feelings that you would be wise to study. The next section takes a lighthearted look at what your digestive tract might be trying to tell you.

- The digestive system feeds the rest of the body and is itself sensitive to malnutrition.
- The folds and villi of the small intestine enlarge its surface area to facilitate nutrient absorption through countless cells to the blood and lymph, which deliver nutrients to all the body's cells.

villi (VILL-ee, VILL-eye) fingerlike projections of the sheets of cells lining the intestinal tract. The villi make the surface area much greater than it would otherwise be (*singular*: villus).

microvilli (MY-croh-VILL-ee, MY-croh-VILL-eye) tiny, hairlike projections on each cell of every villus that greatly expand the surface area available to trap nutrient particles and absorb them into the cells (*singular*: microvillus).

Chapter 3 The Remarkable Body

Figure 3–13

Details of the Small Intestinal Lining

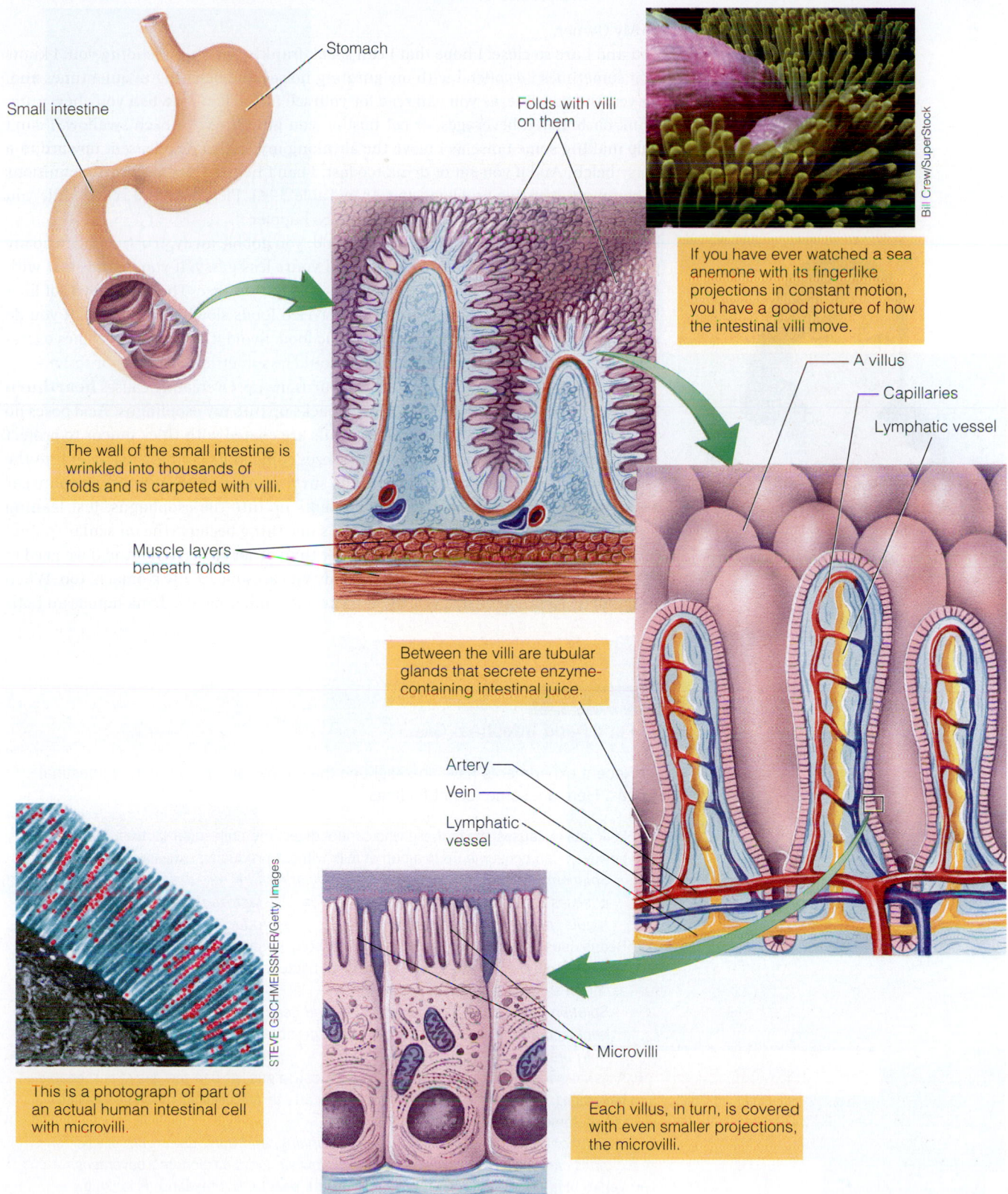

Stomach

Small intestine

Folds with villi on them

Bill Crew/SuperStock

If you have ever watched a sea anemone with its fingerlike projections in constant motion, you have a good picture of how the intestinal villi move.

A villus

Capillaries

Lymphatic vessel

The wall of the small intestine is wrinkled into thousands of folds and is carpeted with villi.

Muscle layers beneath folds

Between the villi are tubular glands that secrete enzyme-containing intestinal juice.

Artery

Vein

Lymphatic vessel

STEVE GSCHMEISSNER/Getty Images

This is a photograph of part of an actual human intestinal cell with microvilli.

Microvilli

Each villus, in turn, is covered with even smaller projections, the microvilli.

A Letter from Your Digestive Tract

LO 3.6 Outline the symptoms, prevention, and treatment of eight common digestive problems.

To My Owner,

You and I are so close; I hope that I can speak frankly without offending you. I know that sometimes I *do* offend with my gurgling noises and belching at quiet times and, oh yes, the gas. But, as you can read for yourself in Table 3–3, when you chew gum, drink carbonated beverages, or eat hastily, you gulp air with each swallow. I can't help making some noise as I move the air along my length or release it upward in a noisy belch. And if you eat or drink too fast, I can't help getting **hiccups** (definitions of common digestive problems appear in Table 3–4). Please sit and relax while you dine. You will ease my task, and we'll both be happier.

Also, when someone offers you a new food, you gobble away, trusting me to do my job. I try. It would make my life easier, and yours less gassy, if you would start with small amounts of new foods, especially those high in fiber. The breakdown of fiber by bacteria produces gas, so introduce fiber-rich foods slowly. But, please, if you do notice more gas than normal from a specific food, avoid it. If the gas becomes excessive, check with a physician. The problem could be something simple—or serious.

When you eat or drink too much, it just burns me up. Overeating causes **heartburn** because the acidic juice from my stomach backs up into my esophagus. Acid poses no problem to my healthy stomach, whose walls are coated with thick mucus to protect them. But when my too-full stomach squeezes some of its contents back up into the esophagus, the acid burns its unprotected surface. Also, those tight jeans you wear constrict my stomach, squeezing the contents up into the esophagus. Just leaning over or lying down after a meal may do the same thing because the muscular sphincter separating the two spaces is much looser than other sphincters. And if we need to lose a few pounds, let's get at it—excess body fat can squeeze my stomach, too. When heartburn is a problem, do me a favor: try to eat smaller meals; drink liquids an hour

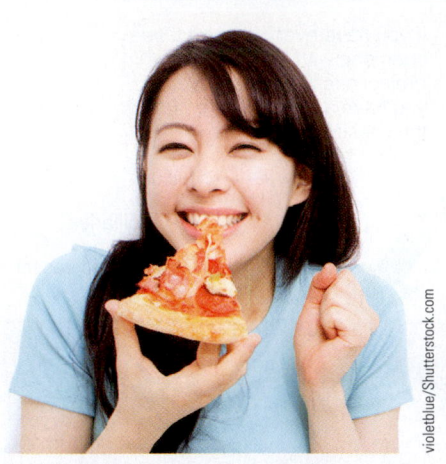

What is your digestive tract trying to tell you?

violetblue/Shutterstock.com

Table 3–3
Foods and Intestinal Gas

Recent experiments have shed light on the causes and prevention of intestinal gas. Here are some recent findings.

- Milk intake causes gas in those who cannot digest the milk sugar lactose. Most people, however, can consume up to a cup of milk without producing excessive gas.
  Solution: Drink up to 4 ounces of fluid milk at a sitting, or substitute reduced-fat cheeses or yogurt without added milk solids. Use lactose-reduced products, or treat regular products with lactose-reducing enzyme products.
- Beans cause gas because some of their carbohydrates are indigestible by human enzymes, but are broken down by intestinal bacteria. The amount of gas may not be as much as most people fear, however.
  Solution: Use rinsed canned beans or dried beans that are well cooked, because cooked carbohydrates are more readily digestible. Try enzyme drops or pills that can help break down the carbohydrate before it reaches the intestine.
- Air swallowed during eating or drinking can cause gas, as can the gas of carbonated beverages. Each swallow of a beverage can carry three times as much gas as fluid, which some people belch up.
  Solution: Slow down during eating and drinking, and don't chew gum or suck on hard candies that may cause you to swallow air. Limit carbonated beverages.
- Vegetables may or may not cause gas in some people, but research is lacking.
  Solution: If you feel certain vegetables cause gas, try eating small portions of the cooked products. Do try the vegetable again: the gas you experienced may have been a coincidence and unrelated to eating the vegetable.

Chapter 3 The Remarkable Body

Table 3-4

Definitions of Selected Common Digestive Problems

These conditions occur frequently in the U.S. population.

constipation infrequent, difficult bowel movements often caused by diet, inactivity, dehydration, or medication. Also defined in Chapter 4.

diarrhea frequent, watery bowel movements usually caused by diet, stress, or irritation of the colon. Severe, prolonged diarrhea robs the body of fluid and certain minerals, causing dehydration and imbalances that can be dangerous if left untreated.

gastroesophageal (GAS-tro-eh-SOFF-ahjeel) **reflux disease (GERD)** a severe and chronic splashing of stomach acid and enzymes into the esophagus, throat, mouth, or airway that causes injury to those organs. Untreated GERD may increase the risk of esophageal cancer; treatment may require surgery or management with medication.

heartburn a burning sensation in the chest (in the area of the heart) caused by backflow of stomach acid into the esophagus.

hemorrhoids (HEM-or-oids) swollen, hardened (varicose) veins in the rectum, usually caused by the pressure resulting from constipation.

hernia a protrusion of an organ or part of an organ through the wall of the body chamber that normally contains the organ. An example is a *hiatal* (high-AY-tal) *hernia*, in which part of the stomach protrudes up through the diaphragm into the chest cavity, which contains the esophagus, heart, and lungs.

hiccups spasms of both the vocal cords and the diaphragm, causing periodic, audible, short, inhaled coughs. Can result from irritation of the diaphragm, indigestion, or other causes. Hiccups usually resolve in a few minutes but can have serious effects if prolonged. Breathing into a paper bag (inhaling carbon dioxide) or dissolving a teaspoon of sugar in the mouth may stop them.

irritable bowel syndrome (IBS) intermittent disturbance of bowel function, especially diarrhea or alternating diarrhea and constipation, often with abdominal cramping or bloating; managed with diet, physical activity, or relief from psychological stress. The cause is uncertain, but inflammation is often involved, and a role for an altered intestinal microbiota is suspected. IBS does not permanently harm the intestines or lead to serious diseases.

ulcer an erosion in the topmost, and sometimes underlying, layers of cells that form a lining. Ulcers of the digestive tract commonly form in the esophagus, stomach, or upper small intestine.

Note: Other conditions, such as celiac disease and diverticulosis, are defined in later chapters—check the index at the back of the book.

before or after, but not during, meals; wear reasonably loose clothing; and relax after eating, but sit up (don't lie down). Don't smoke, and go easy on the alcohol and carbonated beverages, too—they all make heartburn likely.

Sometimes your food choices irritate me. Specifically, chemical irritants in foods, such as the "hot" component of chili peppers and the chemicals in coffee, as well as fat, chocolate, carbonated soft drinks, and alcohol, may worsen heartburn in some people. Avoid the ones that cause trouble. Above all, do not smoke. Smoking makes my heartburn worse—and you should hear your lungs bellyache about it.

By the way, I can tell you've been taking heartburn medicines again. You need to know that **antacids** are designed only to temporarily relieve pain caused by heartburn by neutralizing stomach acid for a while. But when the antacids reduce my normal stomach acidity, I respond by producing *more* acid to restore the normal acid condition. Also, the ingredients in antacids can interfere with my ability to absorb nutrients. Please check with our doctor if heartburn occurs more than just occasionally and certainly before you decide that we need to take the heavily advertised **acid reducers**; these restrict my normal ability to produce acid so much that my job of digesting food becomes harder.

Given a chance, my powerful stomach acid helps to fight off many bacterial infections—most disease-causing bacteria won't survive a bath in my caustic juices. Acid-reducing drugs reduce acid (I'll bet you knew that), so they allow more bacteria to pass through. And, even worse, self-prescribed heartburn medicine can mask

antacids medications that react directly and immediately with the acid of the stomach, neutralizing it. Antacids are most suitable for treating occasional heartburn.

acid reducers prescription and over-the-counter drugs that reduce the acid output of the stomach; effective for treating severe, persistent forms of heartburn but not for neutralizing acid already present. Side effects are frequent and include diarrhea, other gastrointestinal complaints, and reduction of the stomach's capacity to destroy alcohol, thereby producing higher-than-expected blood alcohol levels from each drink (see this chapter's Controversy section). Also called *acid controllers*.

Figure 3–14
Normal Swallowing and Choking

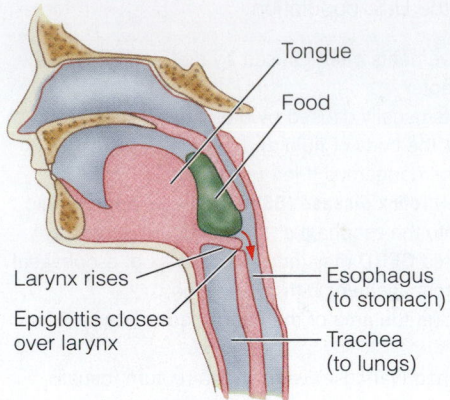
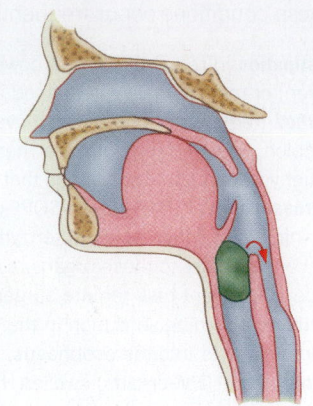

Tongue

Food

Larynx rises

Epiglottis closes over larynx

Esophagus (to stomach)

Trachea (to lungs)

A normal swallow. The epiglottis acts as a flap to seal the entrance to the lungs (trachea) and direct food to the stomach via the esophagus.

Choking. A choking person cannot speak or gasp because food lodged in the trachea blocks the passage of air. The red arrow points to where the food should have gone to prevent choking.

the symptoms of **ulcer**, **hernia**, or the destructive form of chronic heartburn known as **gastroesophageal reflux disease (GERD)**. This can be serious; the bacterium *H. pylori* that causes most ulcers responds to antibiotic drugs, but some ulcers have other causes, such as frequent use of certain painkillers—the *cause* of the ulcer must be treated, as well as its symptoms. A hernia can cause food to back up into the esophagus, so it can feel like heartburn, but many times hernias require corrective treatment by a physician, not antacids. GERD can feel like heartburn, too, but requires the correct drug therapy to prevent respiratory problems or damage to the esophagus that can lead to cancer.[8] So please don't wait too long to get medical help for chronic or severe heartburn—it may not be simple indigestion.

When you eat too quickly, I worry about choking (see Figure 3–14, above). Please take time to cut your food into small pieces and chew it until it is crushed and moistened with saliva. Also, refrain from talking or laughing before swallowing, and never attempt to eat when you are breathing hard. Also, for our sake and the sake of others, learn first aid for choking, as shown in Figure 3–15, p. 95.

When I'm suffering, you suffer, too, and when **constipation** or **diarrhea** strikes, neither of us is having fun. Slow, hard, dry bowel movements can be painful, and failing to have a movement for too long brings on headaches, backaches, stomachaches, and other ills; if chronic, constipation may cause **hemorrhoids**.[9] Most people suffer occasional harmless constipation, and laxatives may help, but too frequent use of laxatives and enemas can lead to dependency; can upset our fluid, salt, and mineral balances; and, in the case of mineral oil laxatives, can interfere with the absorption of fat-soluble vitamins. (Mineral oil, which is not absorbed, dissolves the vitamins and carries them out of the body with it.)

Instead of relying on laxatives, listen carefully for my signal that it is time to defecate, and make time for it even if you are busy. The longer you ignore my signal, the more time the colon has to extract water from the feces, hardening them. Also, please choose foods that provide enough fiber (some high-fiber foods are listed in Chapter 4, p. 123).‡ Fiber attracts water, creating softer, bulkier stools that stimulate my muscles to contract, pushing the contents along. Fiber helps my muscles to stay fit, too, making elimination easier. Be sure to drink enough water because dehydration causes

‡Rarely, a spastic, constricted bowel causes constipation; this condition requires medical attention, not fiber.

Figure 3–15

First Aid for Choking

First aid for choking relies on abdominal thrusts, sometimes called the Heimlich maneuver. If abdominal thrusts are not successful and the person loses consciousness, lower him to the floor, call 911, remove the object blocking the airway if possible, and begin CPR. Because there is no time for hesitation when called upon to perform this death-defying act, you would do well to take a life-saving course to learn these techniques.

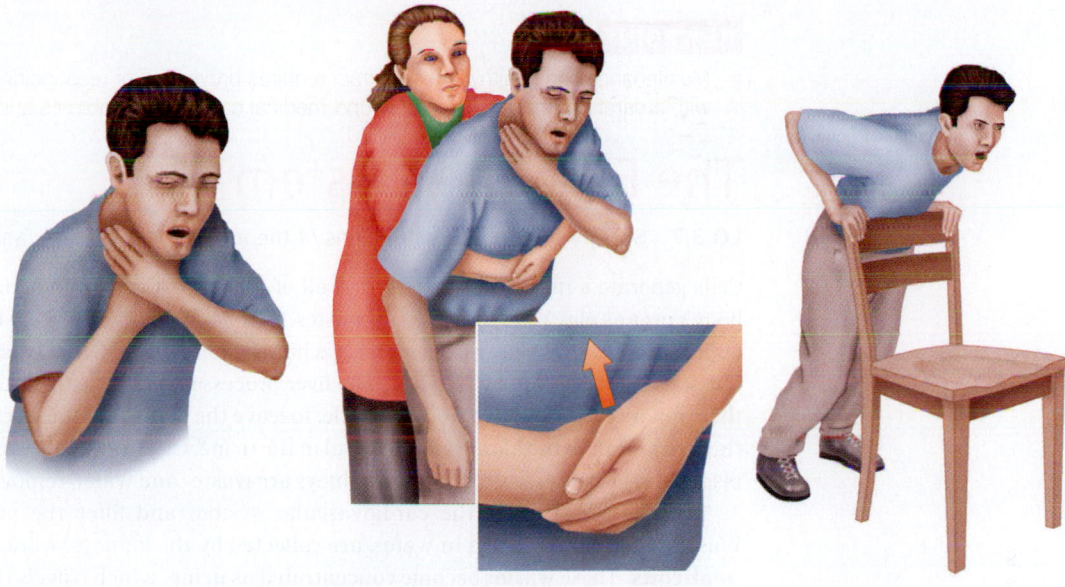

The universal signal for choking alerts others to the need for assistance.

Stand behind the person with your arms wrapped around him. Make a fist with one hand and place the thumb side snugly against the body, slightly above the navel and below the breastbone.

Grasp the fist with your other hand and make a quick upward and inward thrust. Repeat thrusts until the object is dislodged.

To perform abdominal thrusts on yourself, make a fist and place the thumb below your breastbone and above your navel. Grasp your fist with your other hand and press inward with a quick upward thrust. Alternatively, quickly thrust your upper body against a table edge, chair, or railing.

the colon to absorb all the water it can get from the feces. And please make time to be physically active; exercise strengthens not just the muscles of arms, legs, and torso but those of the colon, too.

When I have the opposite problem, diarrhea, my system will rob you of water and salts. In diarrhea, my intestinal contents have moved too quickly, drawing water and minerals from your tissues into the contents. When this happens, please rest a while and drink fluids (I prefer clear juices and broths). However, if diarrhea is bloody, or if it worsens or persists, call our doctor—severe diarrhea can be life-threatening.

To avoid diarrhea, try not to change my diet too drastically or quickly. I'm willing to work with you and learn to digest new foods, but if you suddenly change your diet, we're both in for it. I hate even to think of it, but one likely cause of diarrhea is foodborne illness. (*Please* read, and use, the tips in Chapter 12 to keep us safe.) Also, if diarrhea lasts longer than a day or two or if it alternates with constipation, it may be **irritable bowel syndrome (IBS)**, and you should see a physician. In IBS, strong contractions speed up the intestinal contents, causing gas, bloating, diarrhea, and frequent or severe abdominal pain.[10] Weakened and slowed contractions may then follow, causing constipation. When you're stressed out, so am I, and stress may contribute to IBS. Try eating smaller meals, avoiding onions or other irritating foods, and using relaxation techniques or exercise to relieve mental stress. If those don't work, by all means, call our doctor—IBS often responds to exercise, antibiotics, antispasmodic drugs, or even peppermint oil taken under medical supervision.[11]

By the way, I trust you not to believe false claims that health troubles can be solved by washing the colon with a powerful enema machine—in fact, this "colonic irrigation" is unnecessary and has caused illness and even some deaths from equipment contamination, electrolyte depletion, and intestinal perforation.

Thank you for listening. I know we'll both benefit from communicating like this because you and I are in this together for the long haul.

Affectionately,

Your Digestive Tract

KEY POINT

- Maintenance of a healthy digestive tract requires preventing or responding to symptoms with a carefully chosen diet and sound medical care when problems arise.

The Excretory System

LO 3.7 Specify the excretory functions of the lungs, liver, kidneys, and bladder.

Cells generate a number of wastes, and all of them must be eliminated. Many of the body's organs play roles in removing wastes. Carbon dioxide waste from the cells travels in the blood to the lungs, where it is exchanged for oxygen. Other wastes are pulled out of the bloodstream by the liver. The liver processes these wastes and either tosses them out into the digestive tract with bile, to leave the body with the feces, or prepares them to be sent to the kidneys for disposal in the urine. Organ systems work together to dispose of the body's wastes, but the kidneys are waste- and water-removal specialists.

The kidneys straddle the cardiovascular system and filter the passing blood. Waste materials, dissolved in water, are collected by the kidneys' working units, the **nephrons**. These wastes become concentrated as urine, which travels through tubes to the urinary **bladder**. The bladder collects the urine continuously and empties periodically, removing the wastes from the body. Thus, the blood is purified continuously throughout the day, and dissolved materials are excreted as necessary. One dissolved mineral, sodium, helps to regulate blood pressure, and its excretion or retention by the kidneys is a vital part of the body's blood pressure–controlling mechanism.

Though they account for just 0.5 percent of the body's total weight, the kidneys use up 10 percent of the body's oxygen supply, indicating intense metabolic activity. The kidney's waste-excreting function rivals breathing in its importance to life, but the kidneys act in other ways as well. By sorting among dissolved substances, retaining some, while excreting others, the kidneys regulate the fluid volume and concentrations of substances in the blood and extracellular fluid with great precision. Through these mechanisms, the kidneys help to regulate blood pressure (see Chapter 11 for details). As you might expect, the kidneys' work is regulated by hormones secreted by glands that respond to conditions in the blood (such as the sodium concentration). The kidneys also release certain hormones.

Because the kidneys remove toxins that could otherwise damage body tissues, whatever supports the health of the kidneys supports the health of the whole body. A strong cardiovascular system and an abundant supply of water are important to keep blood flushing swiftly through the kidneys. In addition, the kidneys need sufficient energy to do their complex sifting and sorting job, and many vitamins and minerals serve as the cogs of their machinery. Exercise and nutrition are vital to healthy kidney function.

KEY POINT

- The kidneys adjust the blood's composition in response to the body's needs, disposing of everyday wastes and helping remove toxins.

Storage Systems

LO 3.8 Explain how body tissues store excess nutrients.

The human body is designed to eat at intervals of about four to six hours, but cells need nutrients around the clock. Providing the cells with a constant flow of the

nephrons (NEFF-rons) the working units in the kidneys, consisting of intermeshed blood vessels and tubules.

bladder the sac that holds urine until time for elimination.

needed nutrients requires the cooperation of many body systems. These systems store and release nutrients to meet the cells' needs between meals. Among the major storage sites are the liver and muscles, which store carbohydrate, and the fat cells, which store fat and other fat-related substances.

When I Eat More Than My Body Needs, What Happens to the Extra Nutrients?

Nutrients collected from the digestive system sooner or later all move through a vast network of capillaries that weave among the liver cells. This arrangement ensures that liver cells have access to the newly arriving nutrients for processing.

Body tissues store excess energy-containing nutrients in two forms (details will follow in later chapters). The liver makes some of the excess into **glycogen** (a carbohydrate), and some is stored as body fat. Liver glycogen can sustain cell activities when the intervals between meals become long. Should no food be available, the liver's glycogen supply dwindles; it can be effectively depleted within as few as three to six hours. Muscle cells make and store glycogen, too, but selfishly reserve it for their own use.

Whereas the liver stores glycogen, it ships out fat in packages (see Chapter 5) to be picked up by cells that need it. All body cells may withdraw the fat they need from these packages, and the fat cells of the **adipose tissue** pick up the remainder and store it to meet long-term energy needs. Unlike the liver, fat tissue has virtually infinite storage capacity. It can continue to supply the body's cells with fat for days, weeks, or possibly even months when no food is eaten.

These storage systems for glucose and fat ensure that the body's cells will not go without energy even if the body is hungry for food. Body stores also exist for many other nutrients, each with a characteristic capacity. For example, liver and fat cells store many vitamins, and bones provide reserves of calcium and other minerals. Stores of nutrients are available to keep the blood levels constant and to meet cellular demands.

Variations in Nutrient Stores

Some nutrients are stored in the body in much larger quantities than others. For example, certain vitamins are stored without limit, even if they reach toxic levels within the body. Other nutrients are stored in only small amounts, regardless of the amount taken in, and these can readily be depleted. As you learn how the body handles various nutrients, pay particular attention to their storage so that you can know your tolerance limits. For example, you needn't eat fat at every meal because fat is stored abundantly. On the other hand, you normally do need to have a source of carbohydrate at intervals throughout the day because the liver stores less than one day's supply of glycogen.

KEY POINTS

- The body stores limited amounts of carbohydrate as glycogen in muscle and liver cells.
- The body stores large quantities of fat in fat cells
- Various nutrients are stored by the body in differing quantities.

Conclusion

In addition to the systems just described, the body has many more: bones, muscles, and reproductive organs, among others. All of these cooperate, enabling each cell to carry on its own life. For example, the skin and body linings defend other tissues against microbial invaders while being nourished and cleansed by tissues specializing in these tasks. Each system needs a continuous supply of many specific nutrients to maintain itself and carry out its work. Calcium is particularly important for bones, for example; iron for muscles; and glucose for the brain. But all systems need all nutrients, and every system is impaired by an undersupply or oversupply of them.

glycogen a storage form of carbohydrate energy (glucose); described more fully in Chapter 4.

adipose tissue the body's fat tissue, consisting of masses of fat-storing cells and blood vessels to nourish them.

Whereas external events clamor and vie for attention, the body quietly continues its life-sustaining work. Most of the body's work is directed automatically by the unconscious portions of the brain and nervous system, and this work is finely regulated to achieve a state of well-being. But you need to involve your brain's cortex—your conscious, thinking brain—to cultivate an understanding and appreciation of your body's needs. In doing so, attend to nutrition first. The rewards are liberating—ample energy to tackle life's tasks, a robust attitude, and the glowing appearance that comes from the best of health. Read on, and learn to let nutrition principles guide your food choices.

KEY POINT

■ To nourish a body's systems, nutrients from outside must be supplied through a human being's conscious food choices.

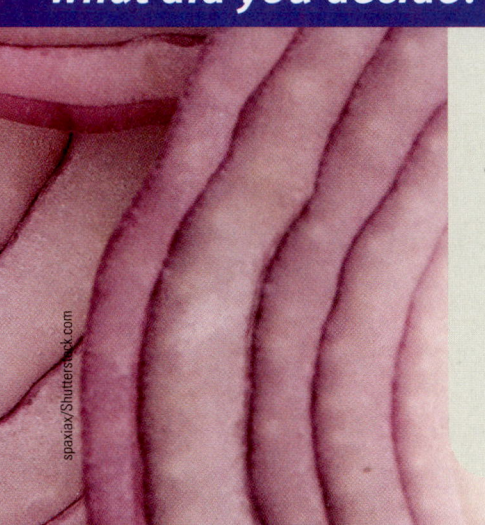

spaxiax/Shutterstock.com

what did you decide?

Can nutrition affect the workings of the immune system?

Is it true that "you are what you eat"?

How does food on the plate become nourishment for your body?

Should you take antacids to relieve heartburn?

Self Check

1. (LO 3.1) Cells
   a. are self-contained, living units.
   b. serve the body's needs but have few needs of their own.
   c. remain alive throughout a person's lifetime.
   d. b and c.

2. (LO 3.1) Each gene is a blueprint that directs the production of one or more of the body's organs.
   T   F

3. (LO 3.2) After circulating around the cells of the tissues, all extracellular fluid then
   a. evaporates from the body.
   b. becomes urine.
   c. returns to the bloodstream.
   d. a and b.

4. (LO 3.2) Blood carries nutrients absorbed from food
   a. from the intestine to the liver.
   b. from the lungs to the extremities.
   c. from the kidneys to the liver.
   d. Nutrients do not travel in blood.

5. (LO 3.3) Hormones
   a. are rarely involved in disease processes.
   b. are chemical messengers that travel from one system of cells to affect another.
   c. are produced and remain inside single cells for intracellular communications.
   d. are unaffected by nutrition status of the body.

6. (LO 3.3) The nervous system sends messages to the glands, telling them what to do.

   T   F

7. (LO 3.4) T-cells are immune cells that "read" and "remember" chemical messages to identify future invaders.

   T   F

8. (LO 3.4) White blood cells include all except the following:

   a. phagocytes
   b. killer T-cells
   c. B-cells
   d. antibodies

9. (LO 3.5) Chemical digestion of all nutrients mainly occurs in which organ?

   a. mouth
   b. stomach
   c. small intestine
   d. large intestine

10. (LO 3.5) Which of the following passes through the large intestine mostly unabsorbed?

    a. starch
    b. vitamins
    c. minerals
    d. fiber

11. (LO 3.5) Absorption of the majority of nutrients takes place across the mucus-coated lining of the stomach.

    T   F

12. (LO 3.6) Which of the following increases the production of intestinal gas?

    a. chewing gum
    b. drinking carbonated beverages
    c. eating or drinking hastily
    d. all of the above

13. (LO 3.6) Concerning ulcers, which of the following statements is *not* correct:

    a. They usually occur in the large intestine.
    b. Some are caused by a bacterium.
    c. If not treated correctly, they can lead to stomach cancer.
    d. Their symptoms can be masked by using antacids regularly.

14. (LO 3.7) The kidneys' working units are

    a. photons.
    b. genes.
    c. nephrons.
    d. villi.

15. (LO 3.7) The bladder straddles the cardiovascular system and filters the blood.

    T   F

16. (LO 3.8) The body's stores of _____ can sustain cellular activities when the intervals between meals become long.

    a. vitamins
    b. fat
    c. phytochemicals
    d. minerals

17. (LO 3.8) The body's adipose tissue has a virtually infinite capacity to store fats.

    T   F

18. (LO 3.9) A drinker may delay intoxication somewhat by

    a. eating plenty of snacks.
    b. quickly finishing drinks.
    c. drinking on an empty stomach.
    d. drinking undiluted drinks.

19. (LO 3.9) Alcohol is a natural substance and therefore does no real damage to body tissues.

    T   F

Answers to these Self Check questions are in Appendix G.

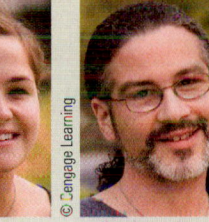

My Turn   watch it!

I Am What I Drink

What do college students think about drinking alcohol? Two students talk about their drinking habits—how much, how often, and where.

Visit www.cengagebrain.com to access MindTap, a complete digital course that includes these videos and other resources.

Ashley   Christopher

© Cengage Learning

© Cengage Learning

Alcohol: Do the Benefits Outweigh the Risks?

LO 3.9 Compare the effects of moderate and heavy alcohol consumption.

Virtually everyone has heard media reports about positive associations between moderate alcohol consumption and a number of potential health benefits. Equally widely known, however, are alcohol's destructive effects. In the United States, alcohol-related deaths top 88,000 each year, making alcohol a top contributor to illness and mortality.[1]*

Should nondrinkers take up drinking for their health's sake? Or should drinkers stop now to avoid problems? This Controversy presents evidence on both sides of the issue.

U.S. Alcohol Consumption

On a given day, adult drinkers consume about 16% of their total calorie intakes from alcoholic beverages, with men drinking more than women by far.[2] Each individual, however, usually follows a general drinking pattern: some people drink no alcohol at all, many take a glass of wine with meals, many others drink mainly at social functions, and still others take in large quantities of alcohol daily because of a life-shattering addiction.

Both heavy drinking and **heavy episodic drinking** (binge drinking) are common drinking patterns, particularly among college-age people, and pose serious health and social consequences for drinkers and nondrinkers alike.[3] Among U.S. adults, one in six is a binge drinker, a pattern accounting for more than half of the estimated 88,000 annual deaths attributable to alcohol consumption.[4] **Moderate drinkers**, in contrast, limit daily alcohol to one drink each day for women and two for men—no more—and there-

*Reference notes are found in Appendix F.

fore minimize their risks. Table C3–1 provides definitions concerning alcohol and drinking.

Does Moderate Alcohol Use Benefit Health?

Some studies report a positive association between moderate drinking (one drink a day for women, two for men) and reduced risk of heart attacks, strokes, and diabetes.[5] Indirect indicators of heart health, such as improved blood lipids and blood clotting factors, often link with moderate alcohol intake.[6] However, almost all of this evidence is epidemiological—that is, arising from studies that correlate drinking habits with heart disease or its risk factors. Such research can never say with certainty that alcohol *causes* a reduction in heart disease, only that the two conditions often occur together. It may be that moderate alcohol consumption is simply a marker for a higher socioeconomic status, together with better diet, more exercise, less smoking, and greater access to medical care. Researchers reporting in favor of alcohol may have also failed to distinguish between lifelong alcohol abstainers and those who made this choice because of a previous drinking problem or heart problem, skewing the results.[7] The nature of alcohol itself prevents the double-blind clinical studies that might otherwise help to uncover the truth.

Some research also suggests that light or moderate drinking may be associated with mental acuity in aging, but other findings are inconsistent.[8] Higher alcohol intakes are not associated with benefits of any kind, however.[9]

Age and Risk

Among teens and young adults, the highest mortality rates are not from heart disease but from car crashes, homicides, and other violence. Drinking—even light drinking—raises these risks. For these age groups, any slight potential of alcohol to benefit heart health would be insignificant because the risk of developing heart disease before middle age is low.

The Influence of Drinking Patterns

Curiously, in some countries, such as France, a light or moderate alcohol intake generally correlates with improved indicators of heart health and lower mortality. In other countries, though, no beneficial correlations can be found.[10]

One explanation may be that drinking *patterns*, not just total intake, influence alcohol's effects on the body.[11] In France, light and moderate daily drinking dispersed throughout the week is the norm. In other countries, people may consume the same amount of alcohol but drink it in heavy episodic patterns. Drinkers who abstain on many days but then consume four or five drinks or more each weekend night may be counted among light drinkers in surveys, but they are in fact heavy episodic drinkers who may be increasing their risk of heart disease and mortality.

Is Wine a Special Case?

Anyone you ask will probably tell you that red wine is good for health. Labels on wines sold in the United States often sport statements such as, "We encourage you to consult your family doctor about the health effects of wine consumption." Such statements seem

Table C3–1

Alcohol and Drinking Terms

- **acetaldehyde** (ass-et-AL-deh-hide) a substance to which ethanol is metabolized on its way to becoming harmless waste products that can be excreted.
- **alcohol dehydrogenase** (dee-high-DRAH-gen-ace) **(ADH)** an enzyme system that breaks down alcohol. The antidiuretic hormone listed below is also abbreviated ADH.
- **alcoholism** a dependency on alcohol marked by compulsive, uncontrollable drinking with negative effects on physical health, family relationships, and social health.
- **antidiuretic** (AN-tee-dye-you-RET-ick) **hormone (ADH)** a hormone produced by the pituitary gland in response to dehydration (or a high sodium concentration in the blood). It stimulates the kidneys to reabsorb more water and so to excrete less. (This hormone should not be confused with the enzyme alcohol dehydrogenase, which is also abbreviated ADH.)
- **beer belly** central-body fatness associated with alcohol consumption.
- **cirrhosis** (seer-OH-sis) advanced liver disease, often associated with alcoholism, in which liver cells have died, hardened, turned an orange color, and permanently lost their function.
- **drink** a dose of any alcoholic beverage that delivers half an ounce of pure ethanol.
- **ethanol** the alcohol of alcoholic beverages, produced by the action of microorganisms on the carbohydrates of grape juice or other carbohydrate-containing fluids.
- **euphoria** (you-FOR-ee-uh) an inflated sense of well-being and pleasure brought on by a moderate dose of alcohol and by some other drugs.
- **fatty liver** an early stage of liver deterioration seen in several diseases, including nonalcoholic and alcoholic liver diseases, in which fat accumulates in the liver cells.
- **fibrosis** (fye-BROH-sis) an intermediate stage of alcoholic liver deterioration. Liver cells lose their function and assume the characteristics of connective tissue cells (become fibrous).
- **formaldehyde** a substance to which methanol is metabolized on the way to being converted to harmless waste products that can be excreted.
- **heavy episodic drinking** a common pattern of excessive alcohol use that elevates blood alcohol to 0.08% or above; typically, five or more drinks for men, four for women, in about two hours' time. Also called *binge drinking*.
- **methanol** an alcohol produced in the body continually by all cells.
- **moderate drinkers** people who do not drink excessively and do not behave inappropriately because of alcohol. A moderate drinker's health may or may not be harmed by alcohol over the long term.
- **nonalcoholic** a term used on beverage labels, such as wine or beer, indicating that the product contains less than 0.5% alcohol. The terms *dealcoholized* and *alcohol removed* mean the same thing. *Alcohol free* means that the product contains no detectable alcohol.
- **problem drinkers** or **alcohol abusers** people who suffer social, emotional, family, job-related, or other problems because of alcohol. A problem drinker is on the way to alcoholism.
- **proof** a statement of the percentage of alcohol in an alcoholic beverage. Liquor that is 100 proof is 50% alcohol, 90 proof is 45%, and so forth.
- **Wernicke-Korsakoff** (VER-nik-ee KOR-sah-koff) **syndrome** a cluster of symptoms involving nerve damage arising from a deficiency of the vitamin thiamin in alcoholism. Characterized by mental confusion, disorientation, memory loss, jerky eye movements, and staggering gait.

---

to promise some good news about wine and health, but the science on wine and health is mixed. For example:

- The good news: in some (but not all) population studies, a glass or two of wine each day often correlates with a lower risk of heart attacks.[12] The high potassium content and phytochemicals of grape juice may help to maintain normal blood pressure and reduce inflammation, and both potassium and phytochemicals persist when grape juice is made into wine.[13]

- The bad news: alcohol in large amounts, even from wine, raises blood pressure and increases inflammation, effects detrimental to the heart.
- More good news: wine contains phytochemicals that could potentially reduce the risk of certain digestive tract cancers.[14]
- More bad news: such phytochemicals are poorly absorbed, so only tiny amounts reach body tissues. Additionally, alcohol, sometimes in amounts of less than one drink per day, raises the risk of many other forms of cancer, particularly breast cancer.

And so it goes.

As mentioned, most research evidence in support of health benefits of alcohol is indirect or observational, and other explanations, particularly genetic predispositions, are gaining momentum and cannot be entirely ruled out. The Dietary Guidelines for Americans recommend that no one begin drinking or drink more frequently in hopes of benefitting their health.[15] Later sections describe the well-established risks that follow alcohol consumption, and the next section provides some basic facts about alcohol.

What Is Alcohol?

In chemistry, the term *alcohol* refers to a class of chemical compounds whose names end in *-ol*. The glycerol molecule of a triglyceride is an example. Alcohols affect living things profoundly, partly because they act as lipid solvents. Alcohols can easily penetrate a cell's outer lipid membrane and, once inside, denature the cell's protein structures and kill the cell. Because some alcohols kill microbial cells, they make useful disinfectants and antiseptics.

The alcohol of alcoholic beverages, **ethanol**, is somewhat less toxic than others. Sufficiently diluted and taken in moderation, its action in the brain produces **euphoria**, a pleasant sensation that people seek. (More alcohol *impedes* social interactions and diminishes feelings of euphoria, however.) Used in this way, alcohol is a drug, and like many drugs, alcohol presents both benefits and hazards to the taker.

All beverages seem to ease conversation, whether they contain alcohol or not. For example, **nonalcoholic** beers and wines on the market also elevate mood and encourage social interaction, as do tea, coffee, or sodas. People in many circumstances should not drink alcohol at all (Table C3–2).

What Is a "Drink"?

Alcoholic beverages contain a great deal of water and some other substances, as well as the alcohol ethanol. In beer, wine, and wine coolers, alcohol contributes a relatively low percentage of the beverage's volume—about 5 percent in most beers to about 13 to 15 percent in many wines.[†] Malt beverages, even those with added sugar and fruity flavors, range from 5 to 10 percent ethanol. In contrast, about 50 percent of the volume of whiskey, vodka, rum, and brandy may be ethanol. The percentage of alcohol is stated as **proof**. Proof equals twice the percentage of alcohol; for example, 100-proof liquor is 50 percent alcohol.

[†] *Nonalcoholic beers and wines may contain a small amount of alcohol, up to 0.5 percent.*

Table C3–2

Who Should Not Drink Alcohol?

People in these circumstances should not drink alcoholic beverages at all:

- *People of any age who cannot restrict their drinking to moderate levels.* Examples include people recovering from alcoholism, problem drinkers, and people whose family members have alcohol problems.
- *Anyone younger than the legal drinking age.* Besides being illegal, alcohol consumption increases the risk of drowning, car accidents, and traumatic injury, which are common causes of death in children and adolescents.
- *Women who are pregnant or who may be pregnant.* No safe level of alcohol consumption during pregnancy has been established. (A breastfeeding woman should use caution; if she chooses to drink, she may consume a single alcoholic beverage if she waits at least four hours afterward to breastfeed.)
- *People taking medications that can interact with alcohol.* Alcohol alters the effectiveness or toxicity of many medications, and some drugs may increase blood alcohol levels.
- *People with certain specific medical conditions.* Examples are liver disease, high blood lipids, and pancreatitis.
- *People who plan to drive, operate machinery, or take part in other activities that require attention, skill, or coordination or who are in situations where impaired judgment could cause injury or death.* Examples are swimming, biking, and boating.

Source: Adapted from Dietary Guidelines for Americans 2010, reaffirmed in 2015, www.dietaryguidelines.gov.

A serving of an alcoholic beverage, commonly called a **drink**, delivers a little over ½ ounce of pure ethanol.[‡] Figure C3–1 depicts servings of alcoholic beverages that are considered to be one drink. These standard measures may have little in common with the drinks

[‡] *One drink contains 0.6 fluid ounces of alcohol.*

Figure C3–1

Servings of Alcoholic Beverages That Equal One Drink

Each of these beverage servings is one standard drink, containing 13.7 g (0.6 oz) of pure ethanol.

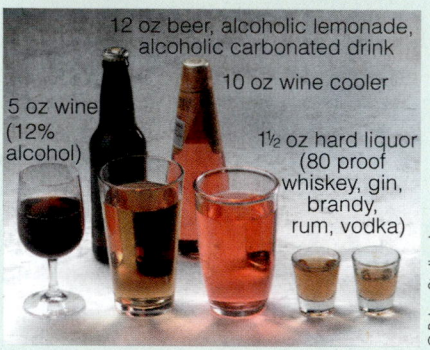

12 oz beer, alcoholic lemonade, alcoholic carbonated drink
10 oz wine cooler
5 oz wine (12% alcohol)
1½ oz hard liquor (80 proof whiskey, gin, brandy, rum, vodka)

© Polara Studios, Inc.

served by enthusiastic party hosts, however. Many wine glasses easily hold 6 to 8 ounces of wine; wine coolers may come packaged 12 ounces to a bottle; a large beer stein can hold 16, 20, or even more ounces; a strong liquor drink may contain 2 or 3 ounces of various liquors.

A powdered form of alcohol, branded *Palcohol*, was approved for sale nationally in 2015, but its sale is banned in some places primarily on concerns about increased availability to minors, and its ease of concealment at public events. The powder is made of tiny chemical spheres that hold minute droplets of alcohol and dissolve when mixed with water. One packet equals the alcohol in one drink.

What's on a Label?

Labels on alcoholic beverages specify the name of the product and its maker, the percentage of alcohol by volume, the fluid measure of the container, and a few other bits of information. The labels lack some important details, however. For instance, no one but the manufacturer can know all of the additives, preservatives, or flavoring agents that might be present in a beverage because federal regulations

Symptoms of Problem Drinking and Alcoholism

A health professional can diagnose and evaluate problem drinking or alcohol addiction with the answers to these questions. In the past year, have you:

- Ever ended up drinking more or for longer than you intended?
- Wanted to cut down or stop drinking, or tried to, but couldn't on more than one occasion?
- Felt a strong urge or craving for a drink?
- Endangered yourself more than once while or after drinking (such as driving, swimming, using machinery, walking in a dangerous area, or having unsafe sex)?
- Noticed that you need more than your regular number of drinks to feel the effect?
- Continued to drink even though it made you feel depressed, anxious, or physically ill?
- Spent a lot of time drinking, or being sick, or getting over other aftereffects?

- Continued to drink even though it was causing trouble with your family or friends?
- Found that drinking—or being sick from drinking—often interfered with taking care of your home or family? Or caused job troubles? Or school problems?
- Given up or cut back on activities that were important or interesting to you or that gave pleasure in order to drink?
- Found that, when the effects of alcohol were wearing off, you had withdrawal symptoms, such as trouble sleeping, shakiness, restlessness, nausea, sweating, racing heartbeat, or seizure? Or sensed things that were not there?
- Found yourself drinking to hold off withdrawal symptoms?

If you have any of these symptoms, or if people close to you are concerned about your drinking, then alcohol may be a cause for concern. The more symptoms you have and the more often you have them, the more urgent the need for change. See a health professional.

Note: These questions are based on symptoms for alcohol use disorders in the American Psychiatric Association's *Diagnostic and Statistical Manual of Mental Disorders, Fifth Edition*, 2013. The DSM is the most commonly used system in the United States for diagnosing mental health disorders.

require disclosure of just a few, such as sulfites (preservatives), some coloring agents, and two artificial sweeteners. Helpful manufacturers voluntarily list all of their ingredients on their websites.

All alcoholic beverages must bear these two warnings:

1. According to the surgeon general, women should not drink alcoholic beverages during pregnancy because of the risk of birth defects.

2. Consumption of alcoholic beverages impairs your ability to drive a car or operate machinery and may cause health problems.

Later sections make clear why these warnings should be taken seriously.

Drinking Patterns

When people congregate to enjoy conversation and companionship, alcoholic beverages may be part of the scene. How alcohol affects the picture depends on how (and whether) it is consumed.

Moderate Drinking

Moderation is not easily defined for an individual because tolerance to alcohol differs. In general, women cannot handle as much alcohol as can men, and women should never try to match drinks with men. Genetic makeup also affects tolerance: people of Asian and Native American descent often have lower-than-average tolerance to alcohol, for example.

To repeat, health authorities define moderation as:

- No more than two drinks in any one day for the average-sized, healthy man.
- No more than one drink in any one day for the average-sized, healthy woman.

Doubtless some people can safely consume slightly more than this; others, especially those prone to alcohol addiction, cannot handle nearly so much without significant risk.

These are not average amounts, as noted earlier, but 24-hour maximums. In other words, a person who drinks no alcohol during the week but has seven drinks on Saturday night is not a moderate drinker. Instead, that drinking pattern characterizes heavy episodic drinking—binge drinking.

Problem Drinkers and Alcoholism

In contrast to moderate drinking, the effect of alcohol on problem drinkers or people with **alcoholism** is overwhelmingly negative. For these people, drinking alcohol brings irrational and often dangerous behavior, such as driving a car while intoxicated, and regrettable human interactions, such as arguments, violence, or unplanned and risky sexual activity. With continued drinking, such people face psychological depression, physical illness, severe malnutrition, and demoralizing erosion of self-esteem. A tool for self-analysis for alcohol problems is found in Table C3–3. If you suspect that your own drinking may not be moderate or if alcohol has caused problems in your life, you should seek a professional evaluation.[§]

Heavy Episodic (Binge) Drinking

Young adults enjoy parties, sports events, and other social occasions, but

[§] If you need to talk with someone right away, call (24 hours a day) the federal Substances Abuse and Mental Health Services Administration: (800) 729–6686. For SAMHSA's National Directory of Drug and Alcohol Abuse Treatment Programs, go to http://findtreatment.samhsa.gov/. For a free hard copy, call 1-877-SAMHSA-7 (1-877-726-4727). Request inventory number SMA12-4675.

Table C3–4

Behaviors Typical of Moderate Drinkers and Problem Drinkers

Moderate Drinkers Typically	Problem Drinkers Typically
▪ Drink slowly, casually.	▪ Gulp or "chug" drinks.
▪ Eat food while drinking or beforehand.	▪ Drink on an empty stomach.
▪ Don't binge drink; know when to stop.	▪ Binge drink; drink to get drunk.
▪ Respect nondrinkers.	▪ Pressure others to drink.
▪ Avoid drinking when solving problems or making decisions.	▪ Turn to alcohol when facing problems or decisions.
▪ Do not admire or encourage drunkenness.	▪ Consider drunks to be funny or admirable.
▪ Remain peaceful, calm, and unchanged by drinking.	▪ Become loud, angry, violent, or silent when drinking.
▪ Cause no problems to others or themselves by drinking.	▪ Physically or emotionally harm themselves, family members, or others when drinking.

these settings often encourage heavy drinking. Emergency room nurses describe a condition in intoxicated people called "holiday heart syndrome," marked by dangerous, irregular heartbeats.[16] This syndrome can occur in people of any age who suddenly take more than a few drinks in a short time.

Binge drinking skews national statistics, making alcohol use on college campuses appear to be more common than it is. The median number of drinks consumed by all college students is 1.5 per week, but for heavy episodic drinkers, it is 14.5 per week. This destructive drinking pattern is observed among people aged 18 to 34 in the greatest numbers and is responsible for most of this group's alcohol-related problems.

Harms from Binge Drinking

Each day in the United States, six people, mostly men aged 35-64 years, die as a result of alcohol poisoning from binge drinking.[17] Compared with nondrinkers or moderate drinkers, binge drinkers are also more likely to damage property, to assault other people, to cause fatal automobile accidents, and to engage in, unprotected sexual intercourse, resulting in sexually transmitted diseases and unplanned pregnancies.[18] Female binge drinkers are more likely to be victims of rape.

Binge drinkers on and off campus may not recognize themselves as **problem drinkers** (refer to Table C3–4, above) until their drinking behavior

causes a crisis, such as a car crash, or until they are old enough to have caused substantial damage to their health. The World Health Organization has called for greater worldwide efforts to reduce the millions of annual deaths from heavy alcohol consumption.[19]

Caffeine and Alcohol

The dangers of binge drinking are amplified by the use of highly caffeinated beverages. In high doses, caffeine seems to mask internal cues of intoxication that might otherwise cause a person to stop drinking. In fact, drinking alcoholic beverages mixed with caffeine may create an urge to continue drinking, compared with drinking alcoholic beverages alone.[20] Unawares, the person drinks more and more, while intoxication builds up. The Food and Drug Administration (FDA) effectively banned sales of alcoholic beverages with added caffeine because they pose a hazard of alcohol poisoning, alcoholic blackouts, driving while intoxicated, and other dangerous outcomes of too much alcohol. It's a bad idea to mix alcohol with highly caffeinated beverages, such as "energy drinks," for the same reasons.

Immediate Effects of Alcohol

From the moment an alcoholic beverage is swallowed, the body gives it special attention. As alcohol passes through body tissues, it affects their functioning.

Alcohol Enters the Body

Unlike food, which requires digestion before it can be absorbed, tiny alcohol molecules start diffusing right through the stomach walls, and they reach the brain within a minute. Ethanol is a toxin, and a too-high dose in the stomach triggers one of the body's primary defenses against poison—vomiting. Many times, though, alcohol arrives gradually, diluted in enough fluid or food that the vomiting reflex is suppressed and the alcohol passes into the small intestine, which readily absorbs it.

A drinker can soon become intoxicated, especially when drinking on an empty stomach. When the stomach is full of food, molecules of alcohol have less chance of touching the stomach walls and diffusing through, so alcohol reaches the brain more gradually. Also, a full stomach delays alcohol's flow into the small intestine, allowing time for a stomach enzyme to destroy some of it. A person who wants to drink socially and not become intoxicated should eat the snacks provided by the host (but avoid the salty ones; they increase thirst and so may increase alcohol intake).

Alcohol Dehydrates the Tissues

Anyone who has had an alcoholic drink has experienced one of alcohol's physical effects: alcohol increases urine output because alcohol depresses the brain's production of the **antidiuretic hormone**. Loss of body water leads to thirst. The only fluid that relieves dehydration is water, so adding ice to alcoholic drinks to dilute them and alternating alcoholic beverages with nonalcoholic ones will quench thirst. Otherwise, each alcoholic drink may worsen the thirst, leading to more drinking.

The water lost due to hormone depression takes with it important minerals, such as magnesium, potassium, calcium, and zinc, depleting the body's reserves. These minerals are vital to fluid balance and to nerve and muscle coordination. When drinking results in mineral loss, minerals must be made up in subsequent meals to avoid deficiencies.

If a person drinks slowly enough, the liver will collect the alcohol after absorption and process it without much effect on other parts of the body. If a person drinks more rapidly, however, some of the alcohol bypasses the liver and flows for a while through the rest of the body and the brain.

Alcohol Arrives in the Brain

Some people use alcohol as a kind of social lubricant to help them enjoy social occasions. Many people use alcohol as a sort of medication to help them to relax or become less anxious. However, alcohol can do the opposite and prolong tension and stress.[21]

One drink relieves inhibitions, which gives people the impression that alcohol is a stimulant. In reality, alcohol acts as a depressant that sedates the inhibitory nerves, allowing excitatory nerves to take over. This effect is temporary, and when blood alcohol rises high enough, it sedates all of the nerve cells (see Figure C3–2).

A Lethal Dose of Alcohol

It is lucky that the brain centers respond to rising blood alcohol in the order shown in Figure C3–2 because a person usually passes out before drinking a lethal dose. If a person drinks fast enough, though, the alcohol continues to be absorbed, and both the blood alcohol level and its effects continue to accelerate after the person has gone to sleep. Figure C3–3 (p. 106) shows blood alcohol levels that correspond with progressively greater intoxication.

Alcohol Toxicity, Oxidative Stress, and the Brain

Brain cells are particularly sensitive to alcohol. The working brain tissue is made largely of lipid (fat) materials, and alcohol is a lipid solvent. With chronic alcohol exposure, brain cells die off,

---

Figure C3–2

Effects of Rising Blood Alcohol Levels on the Brain

The higher the blood alcohol, the more severe its effect on brain tissues. This is a typical progression, but individual responses vary to some degree.

Blood alcohol level (%)   Effects on the Brain

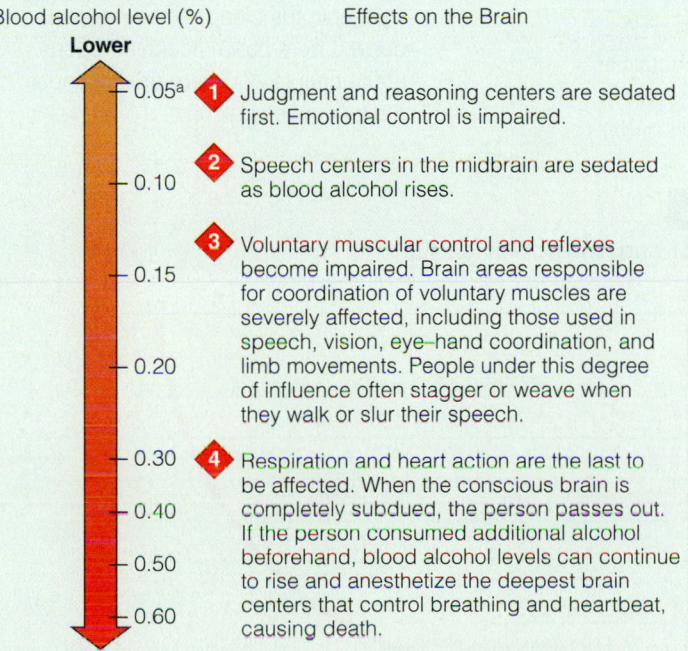

1 Judgment and reasoning centers are sedated first. Emotional control is impaired.

2 Speech centers in the midbrain are sedated as blood alcohol rises.

3 Voluntary muscular control and reflexes become impaired. Brain areas responsible for coordination of voluntary muscles are severely affected, including those used in speech, vision, eye–hand coordination, and limb movements. People under this degree of influence often stagger or weave when they walk or slur their speech.

4 Respiration and heart action are the last to be affected. When the conscious brain is completely subdued, the person passes out. If the person consumed additional alcohol beforehand, blood alcohol levels can continue to rise and anesthetize the deepest brain centers that control breathing and heartbeat, causing death.

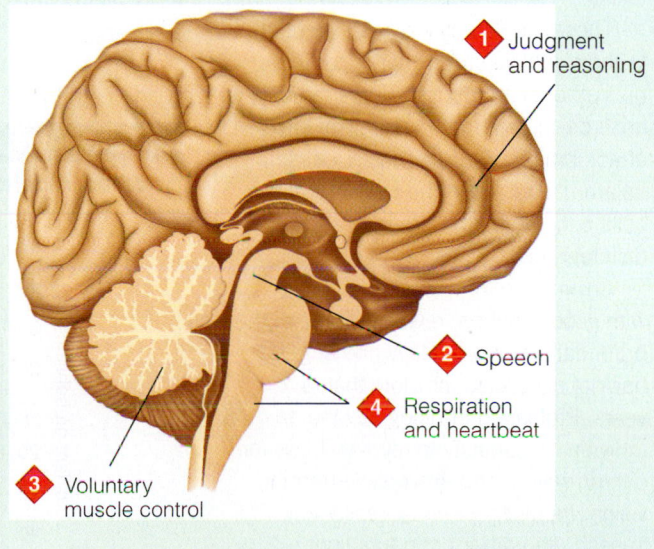

1 Judgment and reasoning

2 Speech

4 Respiration and heartbeat

3 Voluntary muscle control

aThe legal limit for intoxication is 0.08, according to most highway safety ordinances. Driving ability may be impaired at blood alcohol levels below this amount.

Figure C3–3

Alcohol Doses and Average Blood Level Percentages in Men and Women

A blood alcohol level of around 0.30% causes stupor and loss of consciousness; in the 0.40% to 0.50% range, it is most often a lethal dose.

Drinks[a]	Body Weight in Pounds—Men								
	100	120	140	160	180	200	220	240	
	00	00	00	00	00	00	00	00	ONLY SAFE DRIVING LIMIT
1	.04	.03	.03	.02	.02	.02	.02	.02	IMPAIRMENT BEGINS
2	.08	.06	.05	.05	.04	.04	.03	.03	
3	.11	.09	.08	.07	.06	.06	.05	.05	DRIVING SKILLS SIGNIFICANTLY AFFECTED
4	.15	.12	.11	.09	.08	.08	.07	.06	
5	.19	.16	.13	.12	.11	.09	.09	.08	
6	.23	.19	.16	.14	.13	.11	.10	.09	
7	.26	.22	.19	.16	.15	.13	.12	.11	LEGALLY INTOXICATED
8	.30	.25	.21	.19	.17	.15	.14	.13	
9	.34	.28	.24	.21	.19	.17	.15	.14	
10	.38	.31	.27	.23	.21	.19	.17	.16	

Drinks[a]	Body Weight in Pounds—Women									
	90	100	120	140	160	180	200	220	240	
	00	00	00	00	00	00	00	00	00	ONLY SAFE DRIVING LIMIT
1	.05	.05	.04	.03	.03	.03	.02	.02	.02	IMPAIRMENT BEGINS
2	.10	.09	.08	.07	.06	.05	.05	.04	.04	
3	.15	.14	.11	.10	.09	.08	.07	.06	.06	DRIVING SKILLS SIGNIFICANTLY AFFECTED
4	.20	.18	.15	.13	.11	.10	.09	.08	.08	
5	.25	.23	.19	.16	.14	.13	.11	.10	.09	
6	.30	.27	.23	.19	.17	.15	.14	.12	.11	
7	.35	.32	.27	.23	.20	.18	.16	.14	.13	LEGALLY INTOXICATED; DRIVING SKILLS SEVERELY AFFECTED
8	.40	.36	.30	.26	.23	.20	.18	.17	.15	
9	.45	.41	.34	.29	.26	.23	.20	.19	.17	
10	.51	.45	.38	.32	.28	.25	.23	.21	.19	

Note: In some states, driving under the influence is proved when an adult's blood contains 0.08% alcohol, and in others, 0.10%. Many states have adopted a "zero-tolerance" policy for drivers under age 21, using 0.02% as the limit.

[a] Taken within an hour or so: each drink equivalent to ½ ounce pure ethanol.

Source: National Clearinghouse for Alcohol and Drug Information.

and brain tissues shrink, with the extent of the shrinkage in proportion to the amount drunk. Alcohol addicts are prone to brain hemorrhages and strokes; postmortem examinations reveal brain cell loss and diminished functioning of the barrier that protects the brain from toxins.

These conditions may also be related to the oxidative stress that accompanies ethanol metabolism. Free radicals arise during ethanol metabolism and attack brain cell components, causing inflammation. Then the working brain cells become injured, die off, and disintegrate.

Abstinence from alcohol, together with good nutrition, reverses some of the brain damage from heavy drinking if it has not continued for more than a few years. Prolonged drinking beyond an individual's capacity to recover, however, can do severe and irreversible harm to vision, memory, learning, reasoning, speech, and other brain functions.

Alcohol and Accidents

Accidents constitute an immediate and often severe consequence of alcohol use, arising from its deleterious effects on the brain. Alcohol is involved in a large percentage of:

- Boating fatalities.
- Suicides.
- Traffic fatalities.
- Residential fire fatalities.
- Homicides.
- Intimate partner violence and sexual assaults.[22]

Figure C3–4 shows that the risk of having an auto accident rises precipitously with greater amounts of alcohol in the blood. The data were derived from police accident reports about people who were driving under the influence of alcohol.

Figure C3–4

Blood Alcohol and Traffic Accidents

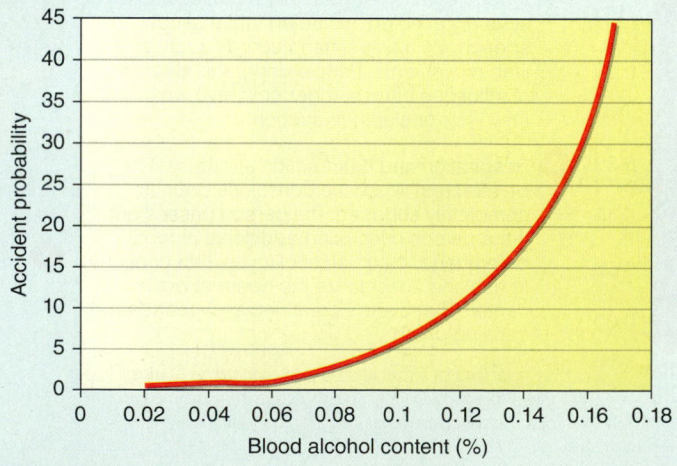

Chapter 3 The Remarkable Body

The major route of alcohol breakdown produces acetaldehyde, creates free radicals, and increases oxidative stress in the tissues.

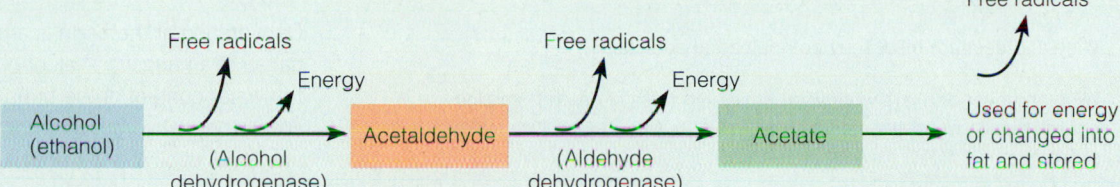

Alcohol Arrives in the Body

The capillaries that surround the digestive tract merge into veins that carry the alcohol-laden blood to the liver. The routing of blood through the liver allows the cells to go right to work detoxifying alcohol and other ingested toxins before they reach other sensitive body organs such as the heart and brain.

A Liver Enzyme for Alcohol Breakdown

The liver is the primary site of alcohol metabolism—it makes and maintains most of the body's equipment for metabolizing alcohol. Its primary tool is an enzyme that removes hydrogens from alcohol to break it down; the enzyme's name, **alcohol dehydrogenase (ADH)**, almost says what it does (see Figure C3–5).** This enzyme converts about 80 percent of the alcohol in the body to **acetaldehyde**, the major breakdown product of alcohol. Other alcohol-metabolizing enzymes help out, too, especially when alcohol levels exceed ADH capacity.

The maximum amount of blood alcohol a person's body can process in a given time is limited by the amount of ADH residing in the liver. If more alcohol arrives at the liver than the enzymes can handle, the extra alcohol circulates again and again through the brain, liver, and other organs until enzymes are available to degrade it.

**ADH exists in several variants.

Alcohol Breakdown in the Stomach

The stomach wall also produces ADH that breaks down some alcohol before it reaches the bloodstream. Research shows that women make less stomach ADH than do men.

Experts often warn that women should not try to keep up with male drinkers, and here are the reasons why: pound for pound of body weight, men have more lean tissue and therefore a greater volume in which to dilute a given amount of alcohol. In women, the same amount of alcohol becomes more concentrated. Also, with her lower stomach ADH levels, a woman absorbs more alcohol from each drink than does a man of equal body weight.

Excretion in Breath and Urine

About 10 percent of blood alcohol is not metabolized at all but is excreted as is, about half exhaled by the lungs in the breath and the other half excreted by the kidneys in urine. The alcohol in the breath is directly proportional to the alcohol in the blood, so the breathalyzer test that law enforcement officers administer to someone suspected of driving while intoxicated accurately reveals the person's degree of intoxication.

Rate of Alcohol Clearance

The liver can process about ½ ounce of blood ethanol (one drink's worth) per hour, depending on the person's body size, previous drinking experience, food intake, gender, and general health. Fasting for as little as one day causes degradation of body proteins, including ADH levels, and cuts the rate of alcohol metabolism by half.

The liver's maximum rate of alcohol clearance cannot be accelerated. This explains why only time restores sobriety. Walking doesn't help, because muscles cannot metabolize alcohol. Nor will drinking a cup of coffee be effective. Caffeine is a stimulant, but it won't speed up the metabolism of alcohol. The police say that a cup of coffee only makes a sleepy drunk into a wide-awake drunk. Table C3–5 (p. 108) presents other alcohol myths.

Alcohol Affects the Liver

Among energy sources, ethanol receives the body's highest priority for breakdown. Toxic ethanol cannot be stored in body tissues without first being converted to something safer. Along the way, however, *other* harmful chemicals arise. For example, alcohol's first breakdown product, acetaldehyde, can bind to enzymes and other structures, disrupting their functions. Also, as Figure C3–5 showed, alcohol metabolism generates damaging free radicals and increases oxidative stress, a condition linked with inflammation and the development of diabetes, cancer, and other serious diseases. Together, these factors are thought to contribute to the liver damage and other organ damage sustained from drinking ethanol.

Myths and Truths Concerning Alcohol

Myth:	A shot of alcohol warms you up.
Truth:	Alcohol diverts blood flow to the skin, making you feel warmer, but it actually cools the body.
Myth:	Wine and beer are mild; they do not lead to addiction.
Truth:	Wine and beer drinkers worldwide have high rates of death from alcohol-related illnesses. It's not what you drink but how much that makes the difference.
Myth:	Mixing drinks is what gives you a hangover.
Truth:	Too much alcohol in any form produces a hangover.
Myth:	Alcohol is a stimulant.
Truth:	Alcohol depresses the brain's activity.
Myth:	Alcohol is legal; therefore, it is not a drug.
Truth:	Alcohol is legal, but it alters body functions and is medically defined as a depressant drug.

Fatty Liver

When presented with alcohol, the liver speeds up its production of fats, which can build up in liver tissues. The first stage of liver deterioration seen in heavy drinkers is therefore known as **fatty liver**; the condition interferes with the distribution of nutrients and oxygen to the liver cells. Fat is known to accumulate in the livers of young men after a single night of heavy episodic drinking and to remain there for more than a day.

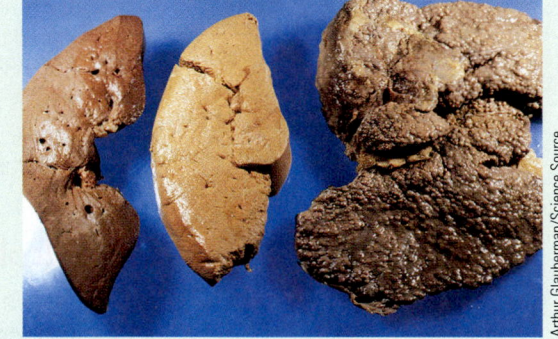

Left, normal liver; center, fatty liver; right, cirrhosis

Arthur Glauberman/Science Source

Liver Fibrosis and Cirrhosis

If heavy drinking continues for long enough, fibrous scar tissue invades the liver. This is the second stage of liver deterioration, called **fibrosis**. Fibrosis is reversible with good nutrition and abstinence from alcohol, but the next (last) stage, **cirrhosis**, is not. In cirrhosis, the liver cells harden, turn orange, and die, losing function forever. Cirrhosis

develops after 10 to 20 years from the cumulative effects of frequent episodes of heavy drinking.

The Hangover

The hangover—the awful feeling of headache, pain, unpleasant sensations in the mouth, and nausea the morning after drinking too much—is a mild form of drug withdrawal. (The worst form is a delirium with tremors that can kill the person and demands medical management.) Hangovers depress mood, disrupt sleep, increase anxiety, cause fatigue,

reduce cognitive ability and reaction time, and reduce the ability to cope with stress. Hangovers are caused by several factors.

Dehydration

Dehydration of the brain is a major cause of a hangover—alcohol reduces the water content of the brain cells. When they rehydrate the morning after and swell back to their normal size, nerve pain results.

Formaldehyde and Methanol

Another contributor to the hangover is **formaldehyde**, the smelly chemical laboratories use to preserve dead animals. Formaldehyde arises from **methanol**, another alcohol produced in tiny amounts by cellular metabolic processes. Occupational exposure to formaldehyde is known to raise the risk for certain cancers; no one knows whether formaldehyde generated from alcohol may do the same.

Normally, a set of liver enzymes converts methanol to formaldehyde, with a second set immediately converting the formaldehyde to carbon dioxide and water, harmless waste products that can be excreted. But these same two sets of liver enzymes are the very ones that process ethanol to its own intermediate (and highly toxic) waste product, acetaldehyde, and finally to carbon dioxide and water. The enzymes prefer ethanol 20 times over methanol. Normally, both alcohols are metabolized without delay, but when excess acetaldehyde monopolizes the second set of enzymes, formaldehyde must wait for later detoxification. At that point, formaldehyde starts accumulating, and the hangover begins.

The Sure Cure for Hangover

Time alone is the cure for a hangover. Taking vitamins, tranquilizers, or aspirin; drinking more alcohol; breathing pure oxygen; exercising; eating; and drinking something awful are all useless. Fluid replacement can help to normalize the body's chemistry and may provide a degree of relief. The headache, bad mood, nausea, and other effects of a hangover come simply from drinking too much alcohol. The best cure is prevention: drink less next time.

Alcohol's Long-Term Effects on the Body

A couple of drinks set in motion many destructive processes in the body. The next day's abstinence can reverse them only if the doses taken are moderate, the time between them is ample, and nutrition is adequate. If the doses of alcohol are heavy, however, and the time between them is short, complete recovery cannot take place, and repeated onslaughts of alcohol take a toll on the body.

Effects in Pregnancy
By far the longest-term effects of alcohol are those felt by the child of a woman who drinks during pregnancy. When a pregnant woman takes a drink, her fetus takes the same drink within minutes, and its body is defenseless against the effects. Pregnant women should not drink alcohol—this topic is so important that Chapter 13 devotes a section to it. The rest of this section concerns the effects on drinkers themselves.

Effects on Heart and Brain
Alcohol is directly toxic to skeletal and cardiac muscle, causing weakness and deterioration that increase as the dose becomes larger. Alcoholism makes heart disease likely, probably because chronic alcohol use raises blood pressure. At autopsy, the heart of a person with alcoholism appears bloated and weighs twice as much as a normal heart. In middle-aged populations, taking one to two drinks a day (moderate drinking) may benefit the heart, but more than this amount substantially *increases* the risk of cardiovascular diseases.

As described earlier, both alcohol and its metabolic products attack brain cells directly, and even moderate intakes slow production of certain brain cells. Heavy

drinking can result in dementia. Mental impairments of alcoholism remain evident even between drinking bouts, but abstinence from alcohol often brings a degree of recovery.

Cancer
Experts include daily ethanol exposure among cancer-causing substances for human beings. Even moderate drinking increases the chances of developing cancers of the breast, colon and rectum, esophagus, liver, mouth, throat, and, in smokers, lung.[23] Once cancer is established, alcohol seems to speed up its development. Alcohol's metabolic by-products contribute to cancer risk, as does ethanol itself.

A large body of evidence implicates alcohol in elevating the risk of breast cancer in women, even in young women whose risk is generally low.[24] Even one drink per day elevates the risk by as much as 10 percent, and with greater consumption, the risk rises accordingly.[25] In men, moderate drinking increases the risks of cancers at many sites, risks that increase substantially with increasing daily alcohol consumption. A popular myth holds that red wine is safer than other types—in reality, the alcohol in all colors of wine presents identical cancer risks.

Long-Term Effects of Alcohol Abuse
Some of the effects just mentioned may also affect people who drink moderately; however, the long-term effects of alcohol abuse and alcoholism can be devastating. They include the following:

- Bladder, kidney, pancreas, and prostate damage
- Bone deterioration and osteoporosis
- Brain disease, central nervous system damage, and stroke
- Deterioration of the testicles and adrenal glands
- Diabetes (type 2 diabetes)
- Disease of the muscles of the heart
- Feminization and sexual impotence in men

- Impaired immune response
- Impaired memory and balance
- Increased risks of death from all causes
- Lung damage and susceptibility to lung disease[26]
- Major psychological depression, possibly caused by alcohol
- Malnutrition
- Nonviral hepatitis
- Skin rashes and sores
- Ulcers and inflammation of the stomach and intestines

This list is by no means all-inclusive. Alcohol abuse exerts direct toxic effects on all body organs. Monetarily, alcoholism is estimated to cost our society hundreds of *billions* of dollars every year in medical services, lost wages, criminal offenses, auto crashes, and other losses.

Alcohol's Effects on Nutrition

Alcohol causes disturbances in nutrition. Its calories are often overlooked by drinkers. Alcohol also causes direct negative effects on nutrients that the body needs to function.

Alcohol and Appetite
Alcoholic beverages affect the appetite. Usually, they reduce it, making people unaware that they are hungry. But in people who are tense and unable to eat or in the elderly who have lost interest in food, a small dose of alcohol, such as a glass of wine, taken 20 minutes before meals may improve the appetite. Although beyond the scope of this discussion, alcohol affects neurotransmitters, hormones, and other signals in ways that modify food intake.

Another example of the beneficial use of alcohol comes from research showing that moderate use of wine in later life improves morale, stimulates social interaction, and promotes restful sleep. In nursing homes, improved patient and staff relations have been attributed to offering a moderate amount of wine or a cocktail to elderly patients who drink.

Alcohol and Body Weight

Alcohol's association with weight gain is complex. Alcohol itself is caloric, and alcoholic beverages can be high in calories. Ethanol yields 7 calories of energy per gram, and drink mixers often present many additional calories (examples are shown in Table C3–6). A small percentage of ethanol's calories escape from the body in breath and urine.

Metabolic interactions occur between fat and alcohol in the body. Presented with both fat and alcohol, the body stores the comparatively harmless fat and rids itself of the toxic alcohol by using it preferentially for energy.[27] Thus, alcohol is reported to promote overweight by increasing fat storage, particularly in the central abdominal area—the **"beer belly"** often seen in drinkers.

Alcohol's Effects on Vitamins

Alcohol has direct toxic effects on body organs, and its abuse damages them indirectly via malnutrition. Like pure sugar and pure fat, alcohol provides empty calories. The more alcohol a person drinks, the less likely it is that he or she will eat enough food to obtain the needed nutrients. Simply put, the greater the alcohol intake, the less nutritious the diet.

Alcohol abuse also disrupts every tissue's metabolism of nutrients. In the presence of alcohol, stomach cells oversecrete both acid and histamine, the latter an agent of the immune system that produces inflammation. Intestinal cells fail to absorb thiamin, folate, vitamin B_{12}, and other vitamins. Liver cells lose efficiency in activating vitamin D. Cells of the eye's retina, which normally process the alcohol form of vitamin A (retinol) to the form needed in vision (retinal), must process ethanol instead. Liver cells, too, suffer a reduced capacity to process and use vitamin A. The kidneys excrete needed minerals: magnesium, calcium, potassium, and zinc.

The inadequate food intake and impaired nutrient absorption of alcohol abuse frequently lead to a deficiency of the B vitamin thiamin. In fact, the cluster of thiamin-deficiency symptoms commonly seen in chronic alcoholism has its own name—the **Wernicke-Korsakoff syndrome**. This syndrome is characterized by paralysis of the eye muscles, poor muscle coordination, impaired memory, and damaged nerves. Thiamin supplements may help to repair some of the damage, especially if the person stops drinking.

Most dramatic is alcohol's effect on folate. When an excess of alcohol is present, the body actively expels folate from its sites of action and storage. The liver, which normally contains enough folate to meet all needs, leaks its folate into the blood. As blood folate rises, the kidneys excrete it, as if it were in excess. The intestine normally releases and retrieves folate continuously, but it becomes so damaged by folate deficiency and alcohol toxicity that it fails to absorb folate. Alcohol also interferes with the action of what little folate is left. This interference inhibits the production of new cells, especially the rapidly dividing cells of the intestine and the blood.

Nutrient deficiencies are thus an inevitable consequence of alcohol abuse not only because alcohol displaces food but also because alcohol interferes directly with the body's use of nutrients. People treated for alcohol addiction also need nutrition therapy to reverse deficiencies and to treat deficiency diseases rarely seen in others: night blindness, beriberi, pellagra, scurvy, and acute malnutrition.

The Final Word

This discussion has explored some of the ways alcohol affects health and nutrition. In the end, each person must decide individually whether or not to consume alcohol, a decision that can change at any time. Table C3–7 sums up both sides of selected issues.

Table C3–6

Calories in Alcoholic Beverages and Mixers

Labels of alcoholic beverage containers need not list calorie amounts, but calories in alcoholic drinks, such as cocktails, may soon appear on many restaurant menus.

Beverage	Amount (oz)	Energy (cal)
Malt beverage (sweetened, such as hard lemonade)	16[a]	350
Malt beverage (unsweetened)	16	175
Wine cooler	12	170
Pina colada mix (no alcohol)	4	160
Beer	12	150
Dessert wine	3½	140
Fruit-flavored soda, Tom Collins mix	8	115
Gin, rum, vodka, whiskey (86 proof)	1½	105
Cola, root beer, tonic, ginger ale	8	100
Margarita mix (no alcohol)	4	100
Light beer	12	100
Table wine	3½	85
Tomato juice, Bloody Mary mix (no alcohol)	8	45
Club soda, plain seltzer, diet drinks	8	1

[a]Typical container size, but up to 32-oz containers are common.

Table C3–7

Moderate Drinking: Point, Counterpoint

Many people debate the merits and demerits of drinking alcohol on many levels. This table outlines some of the arguments made for and against drinking.

Point: Arguments in Favor of Drinking Alcohol	Counterpoint: Arguments Against Drinking Alcohol
1. *Ease social interactions*. Alcohol removes inhibitions, making it easier to interact socially.	1. *Removes social inhibitions*. Alcohol removes inhibitions, permitting socially unacceptable behaviors and interactions.
2. *Relieve stress*. Drinking alcohol relieves stress and produces euphoria.	2. *Increased depression and anxiety*. Regular drinking can deepen depression and cause anxiety. Removing the source of stress provides more lasting relief.
3. *Heart health*. Population studies suggest that moderate drinking can benefit the heart in older adults.	3. *Correlation, not cause*. Controlled clinical trials are lacking to support the heart health theory. Other factors may confound these results, and even moderate drinking has been associated with heart damage in some people.
4. *Brain protection*. A small amount of preliminary research associates moderate drinking with less dementia and improved memory in aging.	4. *Brain cell destruction*. Research is inconclusive about dementia or memory in aging, but firmly concludes that, in quantity, alcohol kills brain cells, and heavy drinking causes dementia.
5. *Reduced mortality*. In large populations, moderate drinking is sometimes associated with reduced mortality.	5. *Increased mortality*. For young people, alcohol increases risks of car crashes and violence, negating any potential health benefits. *Increased cancer*. For women, even one drink a day raises breast cancer risks significantly. Other cancers may also be affected.
6. *Natural equals harmless*. Alcoholic beverages have been used for centuries as natural tonics to "fix what ails you."	6. *Natural toxin*. Alcohol is a toxin that can be lethal when overconsumed. Safe, effective medications achieve the same things with less risk.
7. *Phytochemicals*. Red wine provides beneficial phytochemicals.	7. *Not the only source*. Ordinary foods, such as grapes and whole grains, are also good sources.
8. *Taste*. Many people perceive alcoholic beverages to taste good; they like the flavors.	8. *Taste*. Safer beverages are equally tasty. Alcohol is addictive and causes massive harm to health and life for many people (see the text).
9. *Thirst quencher*. Cold beer, coolers, or malt beverages are thirst quenchers.	9. *Diuretic*. Alcohol is a diuretic that causes water loss. Other beverages hydrate more efficiently.
10. *Ubiquitous*. Everyone drinks.	10. *Not everyone*. More than a third of U.S. adults do not drink alcohol.
11. *Nutrient source*. Alcoholic beverages are claimed to "provide B vitamins and minerals."	11. *Nutrient poor*. The truth is that alcoholic beverages are generally poor nutrient sources, and alcohol in large doses causes nutrient losses from the body.

Sources: Point: J. H. O'Keefe and coauthors, Alcohol and cardiovascular health: The dose makes the poison…or the remedy, Mayo Clinic Proceedings 89 (2014): 382–393; E. Nova and coauthors, Potential health benefits of moderate alcohol consumption: Current perspectives in research, Proceedings of the Nutrition Society 71 (2012): 307–315; M. Krenz and R. J. Korthius, Moderate ethanol ingestion and cardiovascular protection: From epidemiologic associations to cellular mechanisms, Journal of Molecular and Cellular Cardiology 52 (2012): 93–104. Counterpoint: C. S. Knott and coauthors, All cause mortality for age specific alcohol consumption guidelines: Pooled analyses of up to 10 population based cohorts, British Medical Journal 350 (2015), epub, doi: 10.1136/bmj.h384; A. Gonçalves and coauthors, Relationship between alcohol consumption and cardiac structure and function in the elderly, Epidemiology (2015), epub ahead of print, doi:10.1161/circimaging.114.002846; B. Hansel, A. Kontush, and E. Bruckert, Is a cardioprotective action of alcohol a myth? Current Opinion in Cardiology 27 (2012): 550–555; M. Stahre and coauthors, Contribution of excessive alcohol consumption to deaths and years of potential life lost in the United States, Preventing Chronic Disease 11 (2014), epub, doi: http://dx.doi.org/10.5888/pcd11.130293; K. Gonzales and coauthors, Alcohol-attributable deaths and years of potential life lost—11 states, 2006–2010, Morbidity and Mortality Weekly Report 63 (2014): 213–216.

As for drinking wine or other alcoholic beverages for health's sake, most researchers conclude that, while people who drink moderately may gain some small benefits, far greater benefits come from engaging in regular physical activity and maintaining a healthy body weight. Alcohol also poses some serious risks, so nondrinkers should not start drinking with the thought of improving their health. If you do choose to drink, do so with care and strictly in moderation.

Critical Thinking

1. Moderate alcohol use has been credited with providing possible health benefits. Construct an argument for why moderate alcohol use to provide protection from heart disease or other health problems may not be a good idea.

2. Your daughter is leaving for college in the fall. Recently, there has been disturbing news about the excessive drinking on college campuses and even a report about the death of one student who had been drinking excessively at the college your daughter is planning to attend. Form a group of four or five people. Each group has an imaginary daughter who is leaving for college. Each member of the group will choose one of the topics listed below and prepare a short (one-minute) speech that attempts to educate your daughter on the dangers of excessive drinking.

To facilitate the speaker's delivery, a group member takes on the role of "daughter," rotating the role with each speaker. Be sure to emphasize facts as much as possible with your argument.

- Explain the physiology of the hangover, including dehydration, formaldehyde, and methanol.
- Discuss the role of alcohol in weight gain.
- Describe alcohol's effect on vitamins.
- Describe the effect of alcohol on the heart and brain.
- Describe alcohol's effect on the liver and other organs.

4

The Carbohydrates: Sugar, Starch, Glycogen, and Fiber

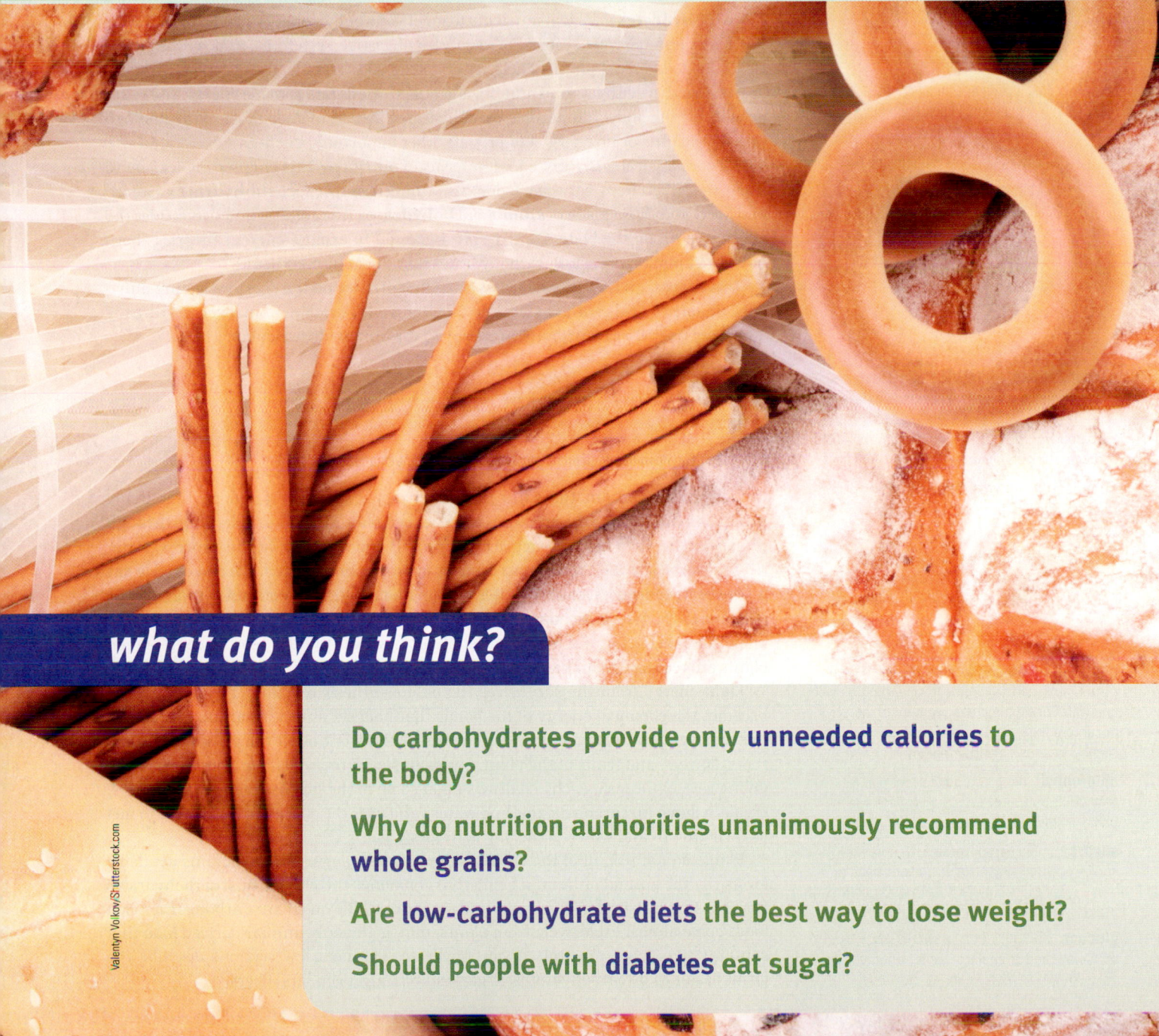

what do you think?

Do carbohydrates provide only **unneeded calories** to the body?

Why do nutrition authorities unanimously recommend **whole grains**?

Are **low-carbohydrate diets** the best way to lose weight?

Should people with **diabetes** eat sugar?

Learning Objectives

After completing this chapter, you should be able to accomplish the following:

LO 4.1 Explain how plants synthesize carbohydrates.

LO 4.2 Describe the need for carbohydrates in the diet.

LO 4.3 Explain how carbohydrates are converted to glucose in the human body.

LO 4.4 Discuss the body's use of glucose.

LO 4.5 Summarize the causes, consequences, and management of diabetes.

LO 4.6 Discuss hypoglycemia.

LO 4.7 Identify foods that are rich in carbohydrates.

LO 4.8 Recognize the effects of added sugars on health.

Carbohydrates are ideal nutrients to meet your body's energy needs, to feed your brain and nervous system, to keep your digestive system fit, and, within calorie limits, to help fuel physical activity and keep your body lean. Digestible carbohydrates, together with fats and protein, add bulk to foods and provide energy and other benefits for the body. Indigestible carbohydrates, which include most of the fibers in foods, yield little or no energy but provide other important benefits.

All carbohydrates are not equal in terms of nutrition. This chapter invites you to learn the differences between foods containing **complex carbohydrates** (starch and fiber) and those made of **simple carbohydrates** (the sugars) and to consider the effects of both on the body. Controversy 4 goes on to explore current theories about how consumption of certain carbohydrates may affect human health.

This chapter on the carbohydrates is the first of three on the energy-yielding nutrients. Chapter 5 deals with the fats and Chapter 6 with protein. Controversy 3 already addressed one other contributor of energy to the human diet, alcohol.

A Close Look at Carbohydrates

LO 4.1 Explain how plants synthesize carbohydrates.

Carbohydrates contain the sun's radiant energy, captured in a form that living things can use to drive the processes of life. Green plants make carbohydrate through **photosynthesis** in the presence of **chlorophyll** and sunlight. In this process, water (H_2O) absorbed by the plant's roots donates hydrogen and oxygen. Carbon dioxide gas (CO_2) absorbed into its leaves donates carbon and oxygen. Water and carbon dioxide combine to yield the most common of the **sugars**, the single sugar **glucose**. Scientists know the reaction in the minutest detail but have yet to fully reproduce it—green plants are required to make it happen (see Figure 4–1).

Light energy from the sun drives the photosynthesis reaction. The light energy becomes the chemical energy of the bonds that hold six atoms of carbon together in the sugar glucose. Glucose provides energy for the work of all the cells of the stem, roots, flowers, and fruits of the plant. For example, in the roots, far from the energy-giving rays of the sun, each cell draws upon some of the glucose made in the leaves, breaks it down (to carbon dioxide and water), and uses the energy thus released to fuel its own growth and water-gathering activities.

Plants do not use all of the energy stored in their sugars, so it remains available for use by the animal or human being that consumes the plant. Thus, carbohydrates form the first link in the food chain that supports all life on earth. Carbohydrate-rich foods come almost exclusively from plants; milk is the only animal-derived food that contains significant amounts of carbohydrate. The next few sections describe the forms assumed by carbohydrates: sugars, starch, glycogen, and fibers.

carbohydrates compounds composed of single or multiple sugars. The name means "carbon and water," and a chemical shorthand for carbohydrate is CHO, signifying carbon (C), hydrogen (H), and oxygen (O).

complex carbohydrates long chains of sugar units arranged to form starch or fiber; also called *polysaccharides*.

simple carbohydrates sugars, including both single sugar units and linked pairs of sugar units. The basic sugar unit is a molecule containing six carbon atoms, together with oxygen and hydrogen atoms.

photosynthesis the process by which green plants make carbohydrates from carbon dioxide and water using the green pigment chlorophyll to capture the sun's energy (*photo* means "light"; *synthesis* means "making").

chlorophyll the green pigment of plants that captures energy from sunlight for use in photosynthesis.

sugars simple carbohydrates; that is, molecules of either single sugar units or pairs of those sugar units bonded together. By common usage, *sugar* most often refers to sucrose.

glucose (GLOO-cose) a single sugar used in both plant and animal tissues for energy; sometimes known as blood sugar or *dextrose*.

Figure 4–1
Carbohydrate Is Made by Photosynthesis

The sun's energy becomes part of the glucose molecule—its calories, in a sense. In the molecule of glucose on the leaf here, black dots represent the carbon atoms; bars represent the chemical bonds that contain energy.

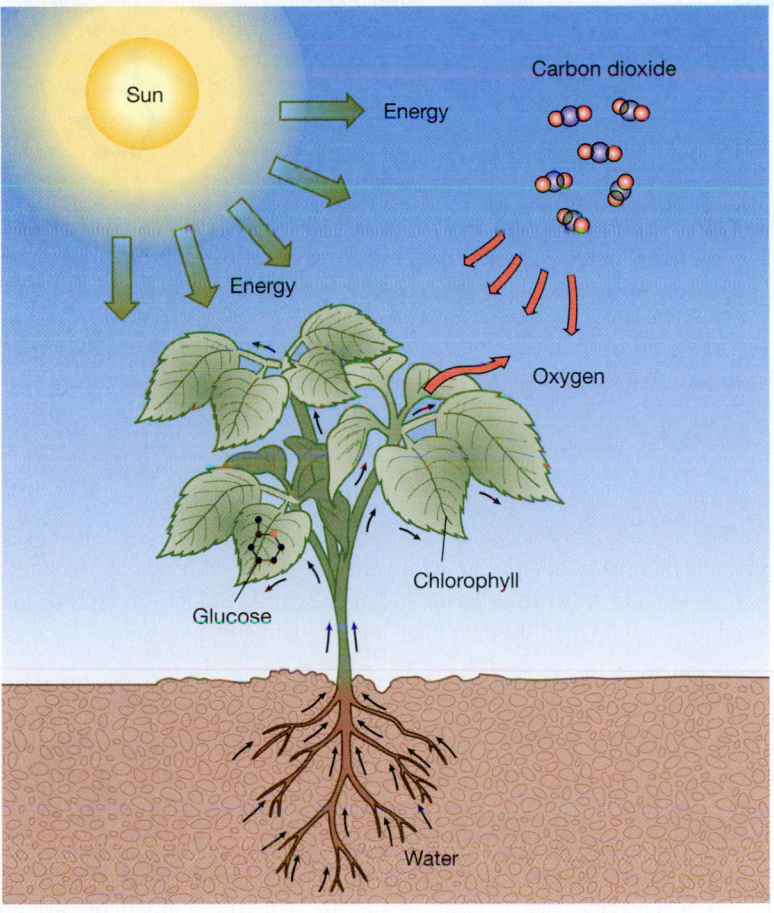

KEY POINTS

- Through photosynthesis, plants combine carbon dioxide, water, and the sun's energy to form glucose.
- Carbohydrates are made of carbon, hydrogen, and oxygen held together by energy-containing bonds: carbo means "carbon"; hydrate means "water."

Sugars

Six sugar molecules are important in nutrition. Three of these are single sugars, or **monosaccharides**. The other three are double sugars, or **disaccharides**. All of their chemical names end in *ose*, which means "sugar." Although they all sound alike at first, they exhibit distinct characteristics once you get to know them as individuals. Figure 4–2 (p. 116) shows the relationships among the sugars.

Monosaccharides   The three monosaccharides are glucose, **fructose**, and **galactose**. Fructose or fruit sugar, the intensely sweet sugar of fruit, is made by rearranging the atoms in glucose molecules. Fructose occurs naturally in fruits, in honey, and as part of table sugar. However, most fructose is consumed in sweet beverages, desserts, and other foods sweetened with **high-fructose corn syrup (HFCS)** or other **added sugars**.[1] Glucose and fructose are the most common monosaccharides in nature.

monosaccharides (mon-oh-SACK-ah-rides) single sugar units (*mono* means "one"; *saccharide* means "sugar unit").

disaccharides pairs of single sugars linked together (*di* means "two").

fructose (FROOK-tose) a monosaccharide; sometimes known as fruit sugar (*fruct* means "fruit"; *ose* means "sugar").

galactose (ga-LACK-tose) a monosaccharide; part of the disaccharide lactose (milk sugar).

high-fructose corn syrup (HFCS) a widely used commercial caloric sweetener made by adding enzymes to cornstarch to convert a portion of its glucose molecules into sweet-tasting fructose.

added sugars sugars and syrups added to a food for any purpose, such as to add sweetness or bulk or to aid in browning (baked goods). Also called *carbohydrate sweeteners*, they include concentrated fruit juice, glucose, fructose, high-fructose corn syrup, sucrose, and other sweet carbohydrates. Also defined in Chapter 2.

[1]Reference notes are found in Appendix F.

Figure 4–2

How Monosaccharides Join to Form Disaccharides

Single sugars are monosaccharides, while pairs of sugars are disaccharides.

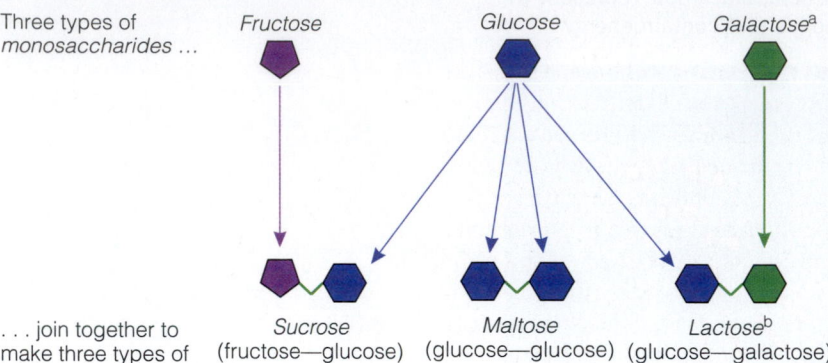

Three types of *monosaccharides* ...

Fructose   Glucose   Galactose[a]

... join together to make three types of *disaccharides*.

Sucrose (fructose—glucose)   Maltose (glucose—glucose)   Lactose[b] (glucose—galactose)

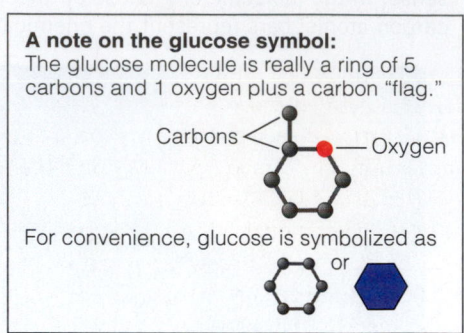

A note on the glucose symbol:
The glucose molecule is really a ring of 5 carbons and 1 oxygen plus a carbon "flag."

Carbons   Oxygen

For convenience, glucose is symbolized as   or

[a]*Galactose does not occur in foods singly but only as part of lactose.*
[b]*The chemical bond that joins the monosaccharides of lactose differs from those of other sugars and makes lactose hard for some people to digest—lactose intolerance (see later section, p. 134).*

The other monosaccharide, galactose, has the same number and kind of atoms as glucose and fructose but in another arrangement. Galactose is one of two single sugars that are bound together to make up the sugar of milk. Galactose rarely occurs free in nature but is tied up in milk sugar until it is freed during digestion.

Disaccharides   The three other sugars important in nutrition are disaccharides, which are linked pairs of single sugars. The disaccharides are **lactose**, **maltose**, and **sucrose**. All three contain glucose. In lactose, the milk sugar just mentioned, glucose is linked to galactose. Malt sugar, or maltose, has two glucose units. Maltose appears wherever starch is being broken down. It occurs in germinating seeds and arises during the digestion of starch in the human body.

The last of the six sugars, sucrose, is familiar table sugar, the product most people think of when they refer to *sugar*. In sucrose, fructose and glucose are bonded together. Table sugar is obtained by refining the juice from sugar beets or sugar cane, but sucrose also occurs naturally in many vegetables and fruits. It tastes sweet because it contains the sweetest of the monosaccharides, fructose.

When you eat a food containing monosaccharides, you can absorb them directly into your blood. When you eat disaccharides, though, you must digest them first. Enzymes in your intestinal cells must split the disaccharides into separate monosaccharides so that they can enter the bloodstream. The blood delivers all products of digestion first to the liver, which possesses enzymes to modify nutrients, making them useful to the body. Glucose is the monosaccharide used for energy by all the body's tissues, so the liver releases abundant glucose into the bloodstream for delivery inside the body. Galactose can be converted into glucose by the liver, adding to the body's supply. Fructose, however, is normally used for fuel by the liver or broken down to building blocks for fat or other needed molecules.

Although it is true that the energy of fruits and many vegetables comes from sugars, this doesn't mean that eating them is the same as eating concentrated sweets such as candy or drinking cola beverages. From the body's point of view, fruits are vastly different from purified sugars (as later sections make clear) except that both provide glucose in abundance.

KEY POINTS

- Glucose is the most important monosaccharide in the human body.
- Monosaccharides can be converted by the liver to other needed molecules.

lactose a disaccharide composed of glucose and galactose; sometimes known as milk sugar (*lact* means "milk"; *ose* means "sugar").

maltose a disaccharide composed of two glucose units; sometimes known as malt sugar.

sucrose (SOO-crose) a disaccharide composed of glucose and fructose; sometimes known as table, beet, or cane sugar and, often, as simply *sugar*.

Starch

In addition to occurring in sugars, the glucose in food occurs in long strands of thousands of glucose units. These are the **polysaccharides** (see Figure 4–3, p. 118). **Starch** is a polysaccharide, as are glycogen and most of the fibers.

Starch is a plant's storage form of glucose. As a plant matures, it not only provides energy for its own needs but also stores energy in its seeds for the next generation. For example, after a corn plant reaches its full growth and has many leaves manufacturing glucose, it links glucose together to form starch, stores packed clusters of starch molecules in **granules**, and packs the granules into its seeds. These giant starch clusters are packed side by side in the kernels of corn. For the plant, starch is useful because it is an insoluble substance that will stay with the seed in the ground and nourish it until it forms shoots with leaves that can catch the sun's rays. Glucose, in contrast, is soluble in water and would be washed away by the rains while the seed lay in the soil. The starch of corn and other plant foods is nutritive for people, too, because they can digest the starch to glucose and extract the sun's energy stored in its chemical bonds. A later section describes starch digestion in detail.

KEY POINT
- Starch is the storage form of glucose in plants and is also nutritive for human beings.

Glycogen

Just as plant tissues store glucose in long chains of starch, animal liver and muscle tissues store glucose in long chains of **glycogen**. Glycogen resembles starch in that it consists of glucose molecules linked together to form chains, but its chains are longer and more highly branched (see Figure 4–3). Unlike starch, which is abundant in grains, potatoes, and other foods from plants, glycogen is nearly undetectable in meats because it breaks down rapidly when the animal is slaughtered. A later section describes how the human body handles its own packages of stored glucose.

KEY POINT
- Glycogen is the storage form of glucose in animals and human beings.

Fibers

Some of the **fibers** of a plant form the supporting structures of its leaves, stems, and seeds. Other fibers play other roles; for example, they retain water and thus protect seeds from drying out. Like starch, most fibers are polysaccharides—chains of

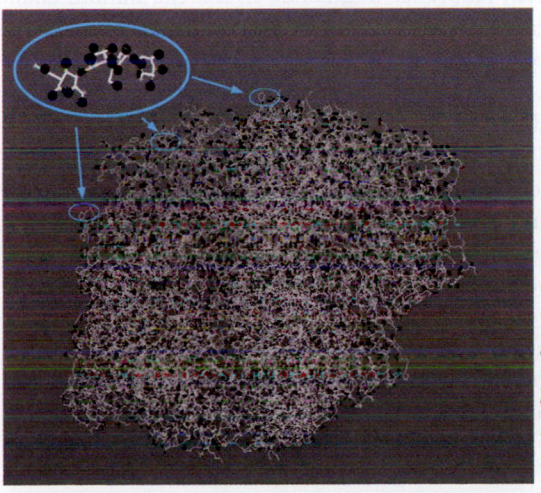

Jon Lomberg/Science Source

A glycogen molecule stores tens of thousands of glucose units nested in an easy-to-retrieve form. In this photo, individual glucose molecules are depicted as black balls linked together with white sticks.

polysaccharides another term for complex carbohydrates; compounds composed of long strands of glucose units linked together (*poly* means "many"). Also called *complex carbohydrates*.

starch a plant polysaccharide composed of glucose. After cooking, starch is highly digestible by human beings; raw starch often resists digestion.

granules small grains. Starch granules are packages of starch molecules. Various plant species make starch granules of varying shapes.

glycogen (GLY-co-gen) a highly branched polysaccharide that is made and stored by liver and muscle tissues of human beings and animals as a storage form of glucose. Glycogen is not a significant food source of carbohydrate and is not counted as one of the complex carbohydrates in foods.

fibers the indigestible parts of plant foods, largely nonstarch polysaccharides that are not digested by human digestive enzymes, although some are digested by resident bacteria of the colon. Fibers include cellulose, hemicelluloses, pectins, gums, mucilages, and a few non-polysaccharides such as lignin.

Figure 4–3
How Glucose Molecules Join to Form Polysaccharides

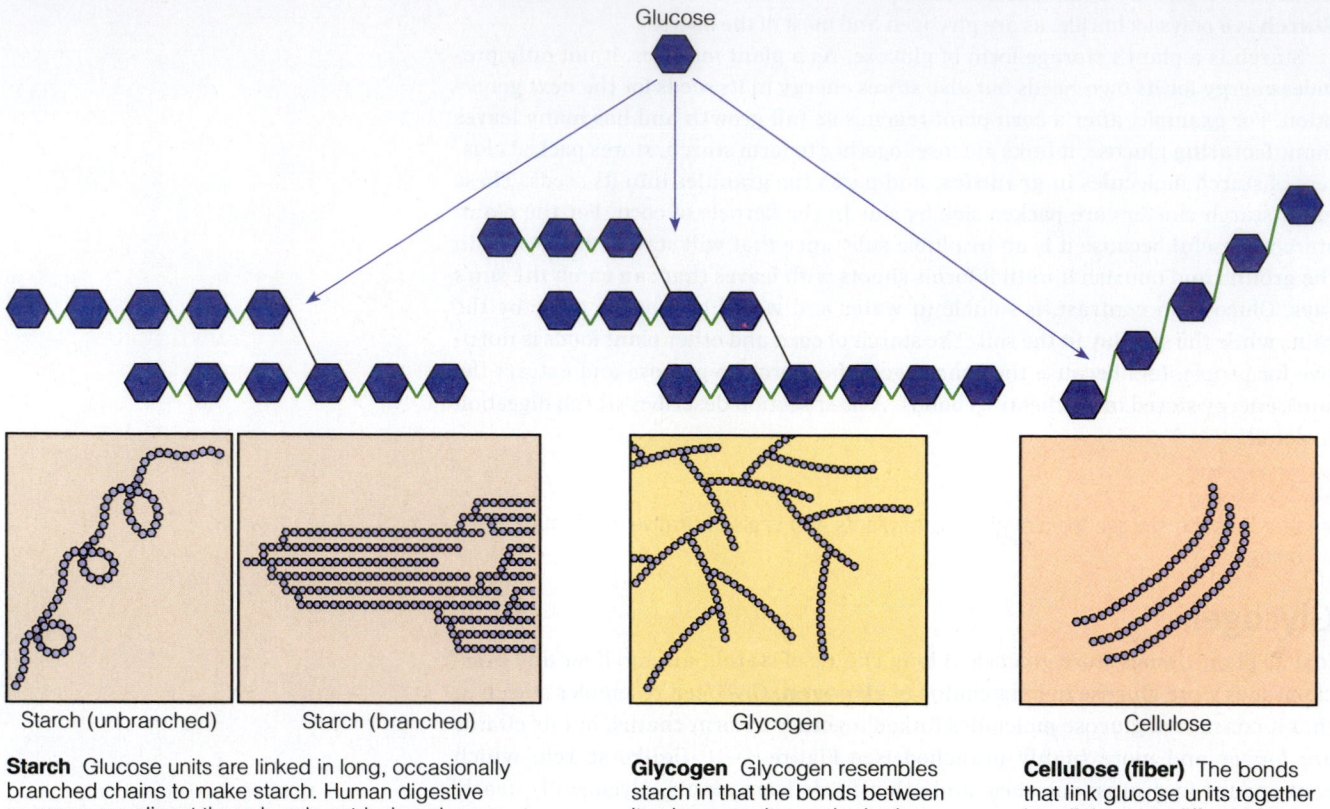

Starch Glucose units are linked in long, occasionally branched chains to make starch. Human digestive enzymes can digest these bonds, retrieving glucose. Real glucose units are so tiny that you can't see them, even with the highest-power light microscope.

Glycogen Glycogen resembles starch in that the bonds between its glucose units can be broken by human enzymes, but the chains of glycogen are more highly branched.

Cellulose (fiber) The bonds that link glucose units together in cellulose are different from the bonds in starch or glycogen. Human enzymes cannot digest them.

sugars—but they differ from starch in that the sugar units are held together by bonds that human digestive enzymes cannot break. Most fibers therefore pass through the human body intact, without providing energy for its use. A little energy arises, however, when certain fibers encounter the colon's bacterial colonies, which do possess fiber-digesting enzymes. This digestion involves **fermentation**, a form of breakdown that produces tiny products, mainly fat fragments, which the human colon absorbs. Many animals, such as cattle, depend heavily on their digestive system's bacteria to make the energy of glucose available from the abundant cellulose, a form of fiber, in their fodder. Thus, when we eat beef, we indirectly receive some of the sun's energy that was originally stored in the fiber of the plants. Beef itself, like other animal products, contains no fiber.

In summary, plants combine carbon dioxide, water, and the sun's energy to form glucose, which can be stored as the polysaccharide starch. Then animals or people eat the plants and retrieve the glucose. In the body, the liver and muscles may store the glucose as the polysaccharide glycogen, but ultimately it becomes glucose again. The glucose delivers the sun's energy to fuel the body's activities. In the process, glucose breaks down to the waste products carbon dioxide and water, which are excreted. Later, plants use these compounds again as raw materials to make carbohydrate. Fibers are plant constituents that are not digested directly by human enzymes, but intestinal bacteria ferment some fibers, and dietary fiber contributes to the health of the body.

fermentation the anaerobic (without oxygen) breakdown of carbohydrates by microorganisms that releases small organic compounds along with carbon dioxide and energy.

- Human digestive enzymes cannot break the chemical bonds of fiber.
- Some fiber is susceptible to fermentation by bacteria in the colon.

The Need for Carbohydrates

LO 4.2 Describe the need for carbohydrates in the diet.

Glucose from carbohydrate is an important fuel for most body functions. Only two other nutrients provide energy to the body: protein and fats.[†] Protein-rich foods are usually expensive and, when used to make fuel for the body, provide no advantage over carbohydrates. Moreover, excess dietary protein has disadvantages, as Chapter 6 explains. Fats normally are not used as fuel by the brain and central nervous system—these tissues prefer glucose, and red blood cells use glucose exclusively. Thus, glucose is a critical energy source, and whole foods that supply carbohydrates—particularly the fiber-rich ones—are the preferred source of glucose in the diet.

Carbohydrates also play vital roles in the functioning of body tissues. For example, sugars that dangle from protein molecules, once thought to be mere hitchhikers, are now known to dramatically alter the shape and function of certain proteins. Such a sugar-protein complex is responsible for the slipperiness of mucus, the watery lubricant that coats and protects the body's internal linings and membranes.[‡] Sugars also bind to the outsides of cell membranes, where they facilitate cell-to-cell communication and nerve and brain cell functioning. Clearly, the body needs carbohydrates for more than just energy.

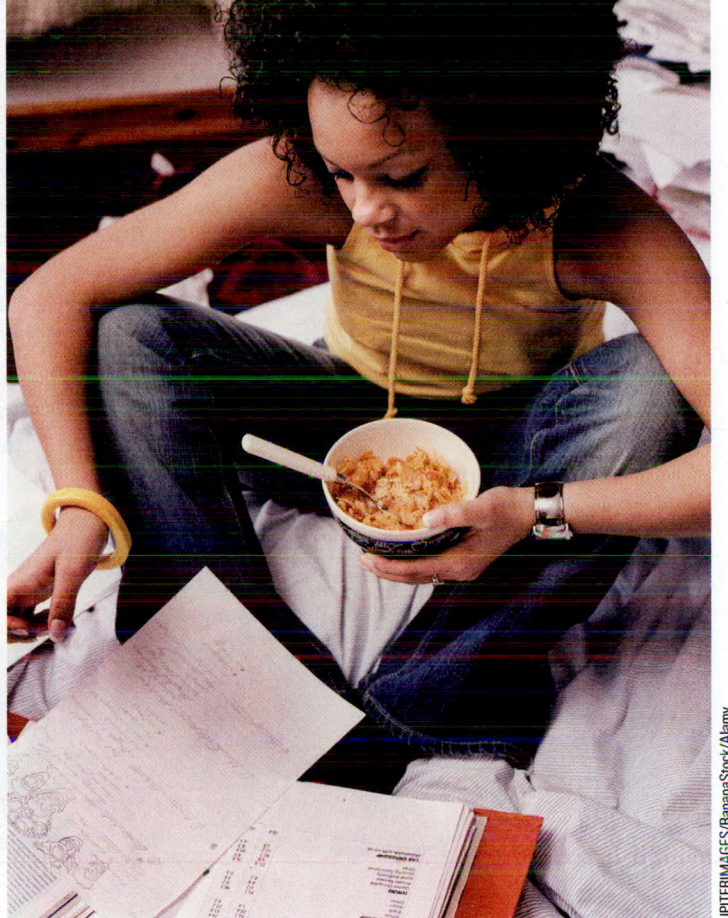

The brain uses glucose as its primary fuel.

JUPITERIMAGES/BananaStock/Alamy

If I Want to Lose Weight and Stay Healthy, Should I Avoid Carbohydrates?

Carbohydrates have been wrongly accused of being the "fattening" ingredient of foods, thereby misleading millions of weight-conscious people into eliminating nutritious carbohydrate-rich foods from their diets. In truth, people who wish to lose fat, maintain lean tissue, and stay healthy can do no better than to attend closely to portion sizes and calorie intakes, and to design an eating plan around carbohydrate-rich fruit, legumes, vegetables, and **whole grains**.

Lower in Calories Gram for gram, carbohydrates donate fewer calories than do dietary fats, and converting glucose into fat for storage is metabolically costly. Still, it is possible to consume enough calories of carbohydrate to exceed the need for energy, which reliably leads to weight *gain*. To lose weight, the

---

[†]Ethanol, the alcohol in alcoholic beverages, also supplies calories, but alcohol is toxic to body tissues.

[‡]Such combination molecules are known as *glycoproteins.*

whole grains grains or foods made from them that contain all the essential parts and naturally occurring nutrients of the entire grain seed (except the inedible husk).

dieter must plan to consume fewer total calories from all foods and beverages each day.

Empty Calories of Added Sugars   Recommendations to choose carbohydrate-rich foods do not extend to refined added sugars. Purified, refined sugars (mostly sucrose or fructose) contain no other nutrients—no protein, vitamins, minerals, or fiber—and thus are low in nutrient density. A person choosing 400 calories of sugar in place of 400 calories of whole-grain bread loses the nutrients, phytochemicals, and fiber of the bread. You can afford to do this only if you have already met all of your nutrient needs for the day and still have calories to spend.

Overuse of added sugars may have other effects as well. The Controversy section of this chapter considers evidence concerning added sugars, blood lipids, and chronic disease risks.

Guidelines   For health's sake, then, most people should increase their intakes of fiber-rich whole-food sources of carbohydrates and reduce their intakes of foods high in refined white flour and added sugars. Table 4–1 presents carbohydrate recommendations and guidelines from several authorities. This chapter's Consumer's Guide describes various whole-grain foods, and the Food Feature comes back to the sugars in foods. For weight loss, authorities do not recommend omitting carbohydrates. In fact, the opposite is true.

KEY POINTS

- The body tissues use carbohydrate for energy and other critical functions.
- The brain and nerve tissues prefer carbohydrate as fuel, and red blood cells can use nothing else.
- Intakes of refined carbohydrates should be limited.

Unlike the added sugars in concentrated sweets, the sugars in fruit are diluted with water and naturally packaged with vitamins, minerals, phytochemicals, and fiber.

iStockphoto.com/vgajic

Why Do Nutrition Experts Recommend Fiber-Rich Foods?

People who regularly eat fiber-rich fruit, legumes, vegetables, and whole grains are often reported to be healthier than those who do not, and the fiber in those foods deserves some of the credit.[2] This section introduces the fibers and explores their health effects.

Fibers in foods are complex and difficult to categorize. One way to group them is by whether they are soluble in water, although certain fibers possess both soluble and insoluble characteristics. Other ways are by the degree to which they form gels, add viscosity, or by their susceptibility to fermentation, also imperfect systems. For convenience, this chapter sorts them by solubility.

Soluble Fibers   Fibers that readily dissolve in water are the **soluble fibers**. In foods, soluble fibers add a pleasing consistency, such as the pectin that puts the gel in jelly and the gums that make bottled salad dressings more **viscous**. Soluble fibers

soluble fibers food components that readily dissolve in water, become viscous, and often impart gummy or gel-like characteristics to foods. An example is pectin from fruit, which is used to thicken jellies.

viscous (VISS-cuss) having a sticky, gummy, or gel-like consistency that flows relatively slowly.

Table 4-1

Recommendations for Carbohydrate Intakes

1. Total carbohydrate

Dietary Reference Intakes (DRI)

- At a minimum, adults and children need 130 g/day to provide glucose to the brain.
- For health, most people should consume between 45 and 65% of total calories from carbohydrate.

Dietary Guidelines for Americans

- Choose nutrient-dense grains, fruit, starchy vegetables, legumes, and milk to meet the day's total carbohydrate intake.

2. Added sugars

Dietary Guidelines for Americans

- Limit intakes of added sugars to a maximum of 10% of total calories.

American Heart Association

- A prudent daily upper limit is not more than 100 cal of added sugars for most women or 150 cal for most men.

World Health Organization (WHO)

- *Strong recommendation*[a] Both children and adults should aim for a reduced intake of free (added) sugars throughout the lifecourse.

- *Strong recommendation* Both adults and children should reduce the intake of added sugars to less than 10% of total energy intake.
- *Conditional recommendation*[b] Both children and adults should further reduce the intake of added sugars to below 5% of total energy intake.

3. Whole grains

Dietary Guidelines for Americans

- A healthy eating pattern includes grains, at least half of which are whole grains.

4. Fiber

Dietary Reference Intakes (DRI)

- 38 g of total fiber per day for men through age 50; 30 g for men 51 and older.
- 25 g of total fiber per day for women through age 50; 21 g for women 51 and older.

[a]*Strong recommendations indicate that desirable effects of adherence to the recommendation outweigh undesirable consequences. The recommendation can applied in most situations.*

[b]*Conditional recommendations are made with less certainty, but with some scientific support.*

are naturally abundant in oats, barley, legumes, okra, and citrus fruits. In addition to food sources, extracted single soluble fiber preparations are used as medications or as food additives.[†]

In the body, soluble fibers are best known for their ability to modulate blood glucose levels, lower blood cholesterol, and promote the health of the colon (details later on).[3] In addition, products of fiber fermentation may:

- maintain the health of the colon in ways that oppose colon cancer,

- oppose allergies,

- reduce inflammation, and

- support immunity.[4]

Clearly, an eating pattern that supplies ample soluble fibers helps to maintain the body's health.

KEY POINTS

- Soluble fibers dissolve in water, form viscous gels, and are easily fermented by colonic bacteria.
- Soluble fibers and products of their fermentation play roles in maintaining the body's health.

Insoluble Fibers Other fibers are **insoluble fibers** that do not dissolve in water, do not form gels, are not viscous, and are poorly fermented. Insoluble fibers, such as cellulose, form structures such as the outer layers of whole grains (bran), the strings of celery, the hulls of seeds, and the skins of corn kernels. These fibers retain their shape and rough texture even after hours of cooking. In the body, they aid the digestive system by easing elimination, as described later.

insoluble fibers the tough, fibrous structures of fruits, vegetables, and grains; indigestible food components that do not dissolve in water.

[†]Examples are pills of the fibers psyllium or methylcellulose used to relieve constipation; inulin, a slightly sweet-tasting fiber, is added to increase fiber in foods and reduce calories.

Figure 4–4

Characteristics, Sources, and Health Effects of Fibers

People who eat these foods...	obtain these types of fibers...	with these actions in the body...	and receive these probable health benefits.

Viscous, soluble, often fermentable and gel-forming

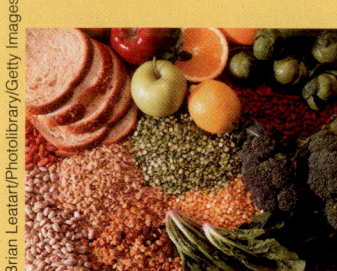

• Barley, oats, oat bran, rye, fruits (apples, citrus), legumes (especially young green peas and black-eyed peas), seaweeds, seeds, many vegetables, fibers used as food additives[b]	• Beta-glucans • Gums • Inulin[a] • Pectins • Psyllium[b] • Some hemicellulose	• Reduce blood cholesterol by binding bile • Slow glucose absorption • Slow transit of food through upper GI tract; delay nutrient absorption • Hold moisture in stools, softening them (less fermentable soluble fibers) • Nourish beneficial bacterial colonies in the colon • Yield small fat molecules after fermentation that the colon can use for energy • Increase satiety	• Alleviate constipation (less fermentable soluble fibers) • Lower risk of heart disease • Lower risk of diabetes • Lower risk of colon and rectal cancer • Increase satiety (improve weight management)

Nonviscous, insoluble, mostly unfermentable

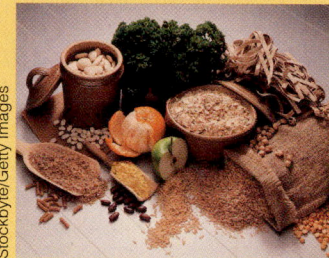

• Brown rice, fruits, legumes, seeds, vegetables (cabbage, carrots, brussels sprouts), wheat bran, whole grains, extracted fibers used as food additives	• Cellulose • Lignins • Resistant starch • Hemicellulose	• Stimulate colon lining, increase fecal weight, and speed fecal passage through colon • Provide bulk and feelings of fullness	• Alleviate constipation • Lower risk of hemorrhoids and appendicitis • Reduce complications from diverticulosis • Lower risk of colon and rectal cancer

[a]Inulin, a soluble and fermentable but nonviscous fiber, is found naturally in a few vegetables, but is also purified from chicory root for use as a food additive.
[b]Psyllium, a soluble fiber derived from seed husks, is used as a laxative and food additive.

Sources: Information from J. W. McRorie, Evidence-based approach to fiber supplements and clinically meaningful health benefits, Part I, Nutrition Today 50 (2015): 82–89; J. W. McRorie, Evidence-based approach to fiber supplements and clinically meaningful health benefits, Part II, Nutrition Today 50 (2015): 90–97.

Figure 4–4 shows the diverse effects of different fibers, and Figure 4–5 provides a brief guide to finding these fibers in foods (Appendix A lists the fiber contents of thousands of foods). Most unrefined plant foods contain a mix of fiber types.

KEY POINTS

- Insoluble fibers do not dissolve in water; they form structural parts of plants and are less readily fermented by colonic bacteria.
- Insoluble fibers benefit digestive tract health.

Heart Disease and Stroke Strong evidence suggests that diets rich in fruit, legumes, vegetables, and whole grains—and therefore rich in fibers and other complex carbohydrates—are protective against heart disease and stroke.[5] Such diets are also generally low in saturated fat and *trans* fat and high in nutrients and phytochemicals—all factors associated with a lower risk of heart disease. Oatmeal was first to be identified among cholesterol-lowering foods.[6] Apples, barley, carrots, and legumes are also rich in gel-forming fibers that can lower blood cholesterol. In contrast, diets high in refined grains and added sugars may push blood lipids toward elevate heart disease risk.

Soluble, gel-forming fibers may lower blood cholesterol by binding bile, a digestive juice that contains cholesterol compounds. Bile is made by the liver and secreted into the intestine (see Chapter 3). Normally, much of bile's cholesterol would be reabsorbed from the intestine for reuse, but the fiber carries some of it out with the feces

Figure 4–5
Fiber Composition of Common Foods

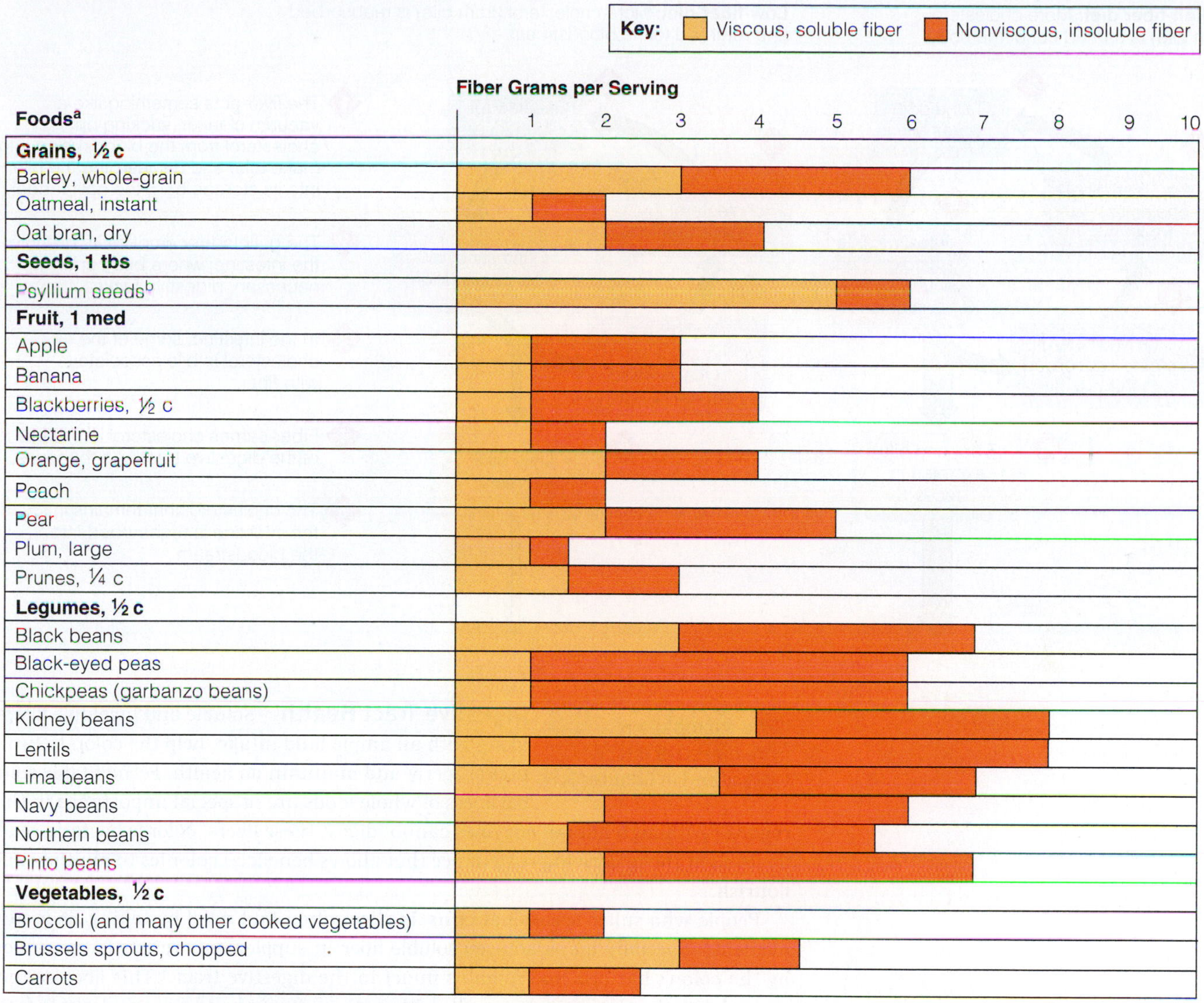

Key: ▮ Viscous, soluble fiber ▮ Nonviscous, insoluble fiber

Fiber Grams per Serving

Foods[a]	1	2	3	4	5	6	7	8	9	10
Grains, ½ c										
Barley, whole-grain										
Oatmeal, instant										
Oat bran, dry										
Seeds, 1 tbs										
Psyllium seeds[b]										
Fruit, 1 med										
Apple										
Banana										
Blackberries, ½ c										
Nectarine										
Orange, grapefruit										
Peach										
Pear										
Plum, large										
Prunes, ¼ c										
Legumes, ½ c										
Black beans										
Black-eyed peas										
Chickpeas (garbanzo beans)										
Kidney beans										
Lentils										
Lima beans										
Navy beans										
Northern beans										
Pinto beans										
Vegetables, ½ c										
Broccoli (and many other cooked vegetables)										
Brussels sprouts, chopped										
Carrots										

[a]Values are for cooked or ready-to-serve foods unless specified.
[b]Psyllium is used as a fiber laxative and fiber-rich food additive.

(Figure 4–6, p. 124). These bile compounds are needed in digestion, so the liver responds to their loss by drawing on the body's cholesterol stocks to synthesize more.

KEY POINT

■ Foods rich in soluble fibers help control blood cholesterol.

Blood Glucose Control High-fiber foods may play a role in reducing the risk of type 2 diabetes. The soluble fibers of foods such as oats and legumes help regulate blood glucose following a carbohydrate-rich meal.[7] Soluble fibers delay the transit of nutrients through the digestive tract, slowing glucose absorption and preventing the glucose surge and rebound often associated with diabetes onset. In people with established diabetes, high-fiber foods can modulate blood glucose and insulin levels, thus helping to prevent medical complications. A later section comes back to insulin in diabetes.

KEY POINT

■ Foods rich in soluble fibers help to modulate blood glucose concentrations.

Figure 4–6
One Way Fiber in Food May Lower Cholesterol in the Blood

High-fiber diet: More cholesterol (in bile) is carried out of the body.

Low-fiber diet: More cholesterol (from bile) is reabsorbed and returned to the bloodstream.

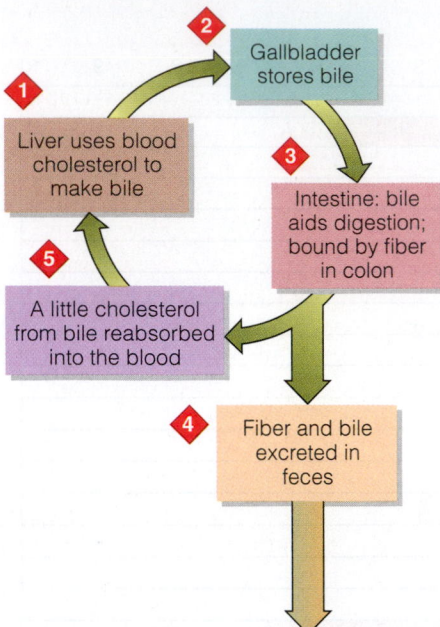

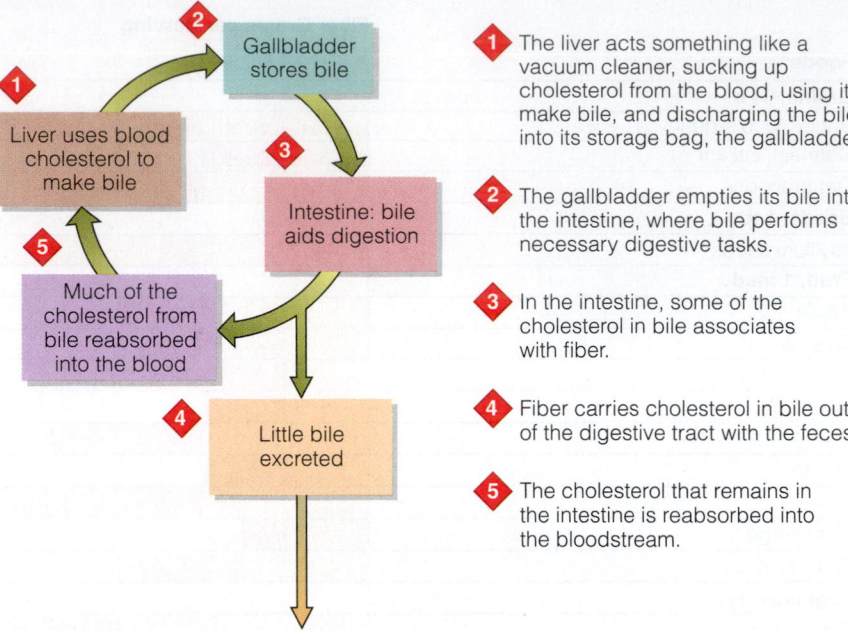

The liver acts something like a vacuum cleaner, sucking up cholesterol from the blood, using it to make bile, and discharging the bile into its storage bag, the gallbladder.

The gallbladder empties its bile into the intestine, where bile performs necessary digestive tasks.

In the intestine, some of the cholesterol in bile associates with fiber.

Fiber carries cholesterol in bile out of the digestive tract with the feces.

The cholesterol that remains in the intestine is reabsorbed into the bloodstream.

The microbiota of the digestive tract is described in **Chapter 3**.

Digestive Tract Health   Soluble and insoluble fibers, along with an ample fluid intake, help the colon to function properly and maintain its health. Fermentable soluble fibers of whole foods are of special importance in this regard.[8] Although human enzymes cannot digest these fibers, colonic bacteria readily ferment them, deriving sustenance that allows beneficial colonies to multiply and flourish.

People who suffer occasional **constipation** often find relief by taking fiber supplements. Specially manufactured soluble fiber in supplements resists fermentation by the colon's bacteria and remains intact in the digestive tract.* This fiber cannot nourish beneficial bacteria but swells with water, softening and giving weight to fecal matter, easing its passage from the system. Coarse insoluble fibers also relieve constipation by stimulating the colon lining to secrete mucus and water which enlarge and soften the stools.

Large, soft stools ease the task of elimination. Pressure is then reduced in the lower bowel (colon), making it less likely that rectal veins will swell (**hemorrhoids**). Fiber prevents compaction of the intestinal contents, which could obstruct the appendix and permit bacteria to invade and infect it (**appendicitis**). In addition, many people suffer from a weakness in the wall of the large intestine that leads portions of the wall to bulge out into pouches known as **diverticula** (illustrated in Figure 4–7). Ample dietary fiber may help to reduce complications of diverticula, but, contrary to long-held beliefs, it may not prevent them from forming.[9]

KEY POINTS

- Soluble fibers are particularly valuable for maintaining intestinal colonies of beneficial bacteria.
- Both soluble and insoluble fibers ease elimination by enlarging and softening stools, and maintain digestive tract health.

---

*The unfermentable manufactured fibers are methylcellulose (from wood pulp) and psyllium (from seed husk).

constipation   difficult, incomplete, or infrequent bowel movements associated with discomfort in passing dry, hardened feces from the body.

hemorrhoids   (HEM-or-oids) swollen, hardened (varicose) veins in the rectum, usually caused by the pressure resulting from constipation.

appendicitis   inflammation and/or infection of the appendix, a sac protruding from the intestine.

diverticula   (dye-ver-TIC-you-la) sacs or pouches that balloon out of the intestinal wall, caused by weakening of the muscle layers that encase the intestine. The painful inflammation of one or more of the diverticula is known as *diverticulitis*.

Digestive Tract Cancers   Cancers of the colon and rectum claim tens of thousands of lives each year.[10] The risk of these cancers is lower, however, among people with higher dietary fiber intakes. A recent European study of almost a half-million adults confirmed a strong, linear inverse association between dietary fiber and cancers of the colon and rectum.[11] Subjects who ate the most fiber (28 or more grams per day) reduced their risk of colon and rectal cancer by 17 percent, compared with those who ate the least. This study assessed fiber from grains, fruits, and vegetables but not supplements. Fiber supplements lack the nutrients and phytochemicals of whole foods that may also help to protect against cancers.

All plant foods—vegetables, fruits, and whole-grain products—have attributes that may reduce the risks of colon and rectal cancers. Their fiber dilutes, binds, and rapidly removes potential cancer-causing agents from the colon. In addition, small fat molecules arising from bacterial fermentation of fiber may activate cancer-destroying mechanisms and inhibit inflammation in the colon.[12] Many other daily choices influence colon cancer risks, and you can read about them in Chapter 11.

> **KEY POINTS**
> - Adequate dietary fiber may reduce the risks of colon and rectal cancers.
> - Plant foods supply fiber, nutrients and phytochemicals that may oppose cancers in many ways.

Healthy Weight Management   Foods rich in fibers tend to be low in fats, added sugars, and calories and can therefore help to prevent weight gain and promote weight loss by delivering less energy per bite. In addition, fibers absorb water from the digestive juices; as they swell, they create feelings of fullness, delay hunger, and reduce food intake. Fermentable fibers may be especially useful for appetite control. The small fat molecules formed during fiber fermentation may shift the body's hormones in ways that promote feelings of fullness.[13] By whatever mechanism, as populations eat more refined low-fiber foods and concentrated sweets, body fat stores creep up.

For fiber intakes, follow the eating patterns of the Dietary Guidelines for Americans—choose the recommended servings of whole, nutrient-dense fruit and vegetables, make at least half the grain choices whole grains, and choose legumes several times per week. That way, you'll obtain all of the benefits that plant foods have to offer. Eating a diet of highly refined foods and adding a fiber supplement is simply not the same.

Fiber Intakes and Excesses

Few people in the United States or Canada consume sufficient fiber. The DRI intake recommendation for fiber is 14 grams per 1,000 calories, or 25 grams per day for most women and 38 grams for most men—almost twice the average current intake of about 15 (women) and 18 (men) grams.[14] Fiber recommendations (inside front cover, p. A) are made in terms of total fiber with no distinction between fiber types because most fiber-rich foods supply a mixture of fibers.

An effective way to add fiber while lowering saturated fat is to substitute plant sources of protein (legumes) for some of the animal sources of protein (meats and cheeses) in the diet. Another way is to focus on consuming the recommended amounts of fruits, vegetables, legumes, and whole grains each day. You can make a quick approximation of a day's fiber intake by following the instructions in Table 4–2. People choosing high-fiber foods are also wise to drink extra fluids to help the fiber do its job.

Can My Diet Have Too Much Fiber?   No Tolerable Upper Intake Level has been established for fiber, but consuming purified fiber added to foods or supplements can be taken to extremes. One overly enthusiastic eater of oat bran muffins required emergency surgery for a blocked intestine; too much oat bran and too little fluid

---

Figure 4–7

Diverticula

Diverticula are abnormally bulging pockets in the colon wall. These pockets can entrap feces and become painfully infected and inflamed, requiring hospitalization, antibiotic therapy, or surgery.

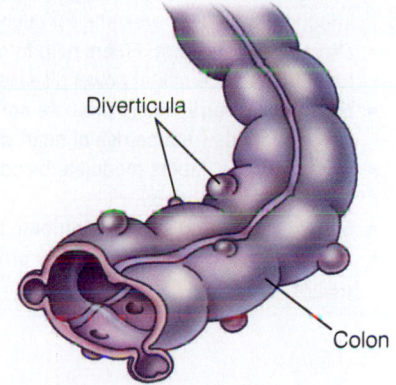

Diverticula

Colon

Table 4–2

A Quick Method for Estimating Fiber Intake

To quickly estimate fiber in a day's meals:

1. Multiply servings (½ c cut up or 1 medium piece) of any fruit or vegetable (excluding juice) by 1.5 g.[a]
   Example: 5 servings of fruits and vegetables × 1.5 = 7.5 g fiber

2. Multiply ½ c servings of refined grains by 1.0 g.
   Example: 4 servings of refined grains × 1.0 = 4.0 g fiber

3. Multiply ½ c servings of whole grains by 2.5 g.
   Example: 3 servings of whole grains × 2.5 = 7.5 g fiber

4. Add fiber values for servings of legumes, nuts, seeds, and high-fiber cereals and breads; look these up in Appendix A.
   Example: ½ c navy beans = 6.0 g fiber

5. Add up the grams of fiber from the previous lines.
   Example: 7.5 + 4.0 + 7.5 + 6.0 = 25 g fiber

Day's total fiber = 25 g fiber

[a]*Most cooked and canned fruits and vegetables contain about this amount, while whole raw fruits and some vegetables contain more.*

Table 4–3

Usefulness of Carbohydrates

Carbohydrates in the Body	Carbohydrates in Foods
■ *Energy source.* Sugars and starch from the diet provide energy for many body functions; they provide glucose, the preferred fuel for the brain and nerves.	■ *Flavor.* Sugars provide sweetness.
■ *Glucose storage.* Muscle and liver glycogen store glucose.	■ *Browning.* When exposed to heat, sugars undergo browning reactions, lending appealing color, aroma, and taste.
■ *Raw material.* Sugars are converted into other compounds, such as amino acids (the building blocks of proteins), as needed.	■ *Texture.* Sugars help make foods tender. Cooked starch lends a smooth, pleasing texture.
■ *Structures and functions.* Sugars interact with protein molecules, affecting their structures and functions.	■ *Gel formation.* Starch molecules expand when heated and trap water molecules, forming gels. The fiber pectin forms the gel of jellies when cooked with sugar and acid from fruit.
■ *Digestive tract health.* Fibers help to maintain healthy bowel function (reduce risk of bowel diseases).	■ *Bulk and viscosity (thickness).* Carbohydrates lend bulk and increased viscosity to foods. Soluble, viscous fibers lend thickness to foods such as salad dressings.
■ *Blood cholesterol.* Fibers promote normal blood cholesterol concentrations (reduce risk of heart disease).	■ *Moisture.* Sugars attract water and keep foods moist.
■ *Blood glucose.* Fibers modulate blood glucose concentrations (help control diabetes).	■ *Preservative.* Sugar in high concentrations dehydrates bacteria and preserves the food.
■ *Satiety.* Fibers and sugars contribute to feelings of fullness.	■ *Fermentation.* Carbohydrates are fermented by yeast, a process that causes bread dough to rise and beer to brew, among other uses.
■ *Body weight.* A fiber-rich diet may promote a healthy body weight.	

overwhelmed his digestive system. Approach bran and other purified fibers with an attitude of moderation, and be sure to drink an extra beverage with them.

Fiber makes food bulky and takes up space in the stomach, so a person who eats only small amounts of food at a time may not meet energy or nutrient needs when the diet presents too much high-fiber food. The malnourished, the elderly, and young children adhering to all-plant (vegan) diets are especially vulnerable to this problem.

A by-product of fiber fermentation can be any of several odorous gases, an effect most noticeable with sudden increases in fiber intake. Don't give up on high-fiber foods if they cause gas. Instead, start with small servings and gradually increase the serving size over several weeks; chew foods thoroughly to break up hard-to-digest lumps that can ferment in the intestine; and try a variety of fiber-rich foods until you find some that do not cause the problem. Some people also find relief from excessive gas by using commercial enzyme preparations sold for use with beans. Such products contain enzymes that help to break down some of the indigestible fibers in foods before they reach the colon.

The Binders in Fiber   Binders in some fibers act as **chelating agents**. This means that they link chemically with important nutrient minerals (iron, zinc, calcium, and others) and then carry them out of the body. The mineral iron is mostly absorbed at the beginning of the intestinal tract, and excess insoluble fibers may limit its absorption by speeding foods through the upper part of the digestive tract. Chelating agents are often sold by supplement vendors to "remove toxins" from the body. Some valid medical uses exist, such as the treatment of lead poisoning, but most chelating agents sold over the counter are unnecessary.

A later section focuses on the handling of carbohydrates by the digestive system. Table 4–3 sums up the points made so far concerning the functions of carbohydrates in the body and in foods.

KEY POINTS

- Few people consume sufficient fiber.
- The best fiber sources are whole foods, and fluid intake should increase along with fiber.
- Very-high-fiber all-plant diets can pose nutritional risks for some people.

chelating agents molecules that attract or bind with other molecules and are therefore useful in either preventing or promoting movement of substances from place to place.

Table 4-4

Terms That Describe Grain Foods

- **bran** the protective fibrous coating around a grain; the chief fiber donator of a grain.
- **brown bread** bread containing ingredients such as molasses that lend a brown color; may be made with any kind of flour, including white flour.
- **endosperm** the bulk of the edible part of a grain, the starchy part.
- **enriched, fortified** refers to the addition of nutrients to a refined food product. As defined by U.S. law, these terms mean that specified levels of thiamin, riboflavin, niacin, folate, and iron have been added to refined grains and grain products. The terms *enriched* and *fortified* can refer to the addition of more nutrients than just these five; read the label.[a]
- **germ** the nutrient-rich inner part of a grain.
- **husk** the outer, inedible part of a grain.
- **multi-grain** a term used on food labels to indicate a food made with more than one kind of grain. Not an indicator of a whole-grain food.
- **refined** refers to the process by which the coarse parts of food products are removed. For example, the refining of wheat into white enriched flour involves removing three of the four parts of the kernel—the chaff, the bran, and the germ—leaving only the endosperm, composed mainly of starch and a little protein.
- **refined grains** grains and grain products from which the bran, germ, or other edible parts of whole grains have been removed; not a whole grain. Many refined grains are low in fiber and are enriched with vitamins, as required by U.S. regulations.
- **stone ground** refers to a milling process using limestone to grind any grain, including refined grains, into flour.
- **unbleached flour** a beige-colored refined endosperm flour with texture and nutritive qualities that approximate those of regular white flour.
- **wheat bread** bread made with any wheat flour, including refined enriched white flour.
- **wheat flour** any flour made from wheat, including refined white flour.
- **white flour** an endosperm flour that has been refined and bleached for maximum softness and whiteness.
- **white wheat** a wheat variety developed to be paler in color than common red wheat (most familiar flours are made from red wheat). White wheat is similar to red wheat in carbohydrate, protein, and other nutrients, but it lacks the dark and bitter, but potentially beneficial, phytochemicals of red wheat.
- **100% whole grain** a label term for food in which the grain is entirely whole grain, with no added refined grains.
- **whole-wheat flour** flour made from whole-wheat kernels; a whole-grain flour. Also called *graham flour.*

[a]*Formerly, enriched and fortified carried distinct meanings with regard to the nutrient amounts added to foods, but a change in the law has made these terms virtually synonymous.*

Whole Grains

The Dietary Guidelines for Americans urge everyone to make at least half of their daily grain choices *whole* grains, an amount equal to at least three 1-ounce equivalents of whole grains a day. To do this, you must distinguish among grain foods that are **refined**, **enriched**, **fortified**, and whole grain (see Table 4–4). This chapter's Consumer's Guide section (p. 130) explains how to find whole-grain foods.

Flour Types   The part of a typical grain plant, such as wheat, that is made into flour (and then into bread, cereals, and pasta) is the seed, or kernel. The kernel has four main parts: the **germ**, the **endosperm**, the **bran**, and the **husk**, as shown in Figure 4–8. The germ is the part that grows into a new plant, in this case wheat, and therefore contains concentrated food to support the new life—it is especially rich in oils, vitamins, and minerals. The endosperm is the soft, white inside portion of the kernel, containing starch and proteins that help nourish the seed as it sprouts. The kernel is encased in the bran, a protective coating that is similar in function to the shell of a nut; the bran is also rich in nutrients and fiber. The husk, commonly called chaff, is the dry outermost layer that is inedible by human beings but can be used in animal feed.

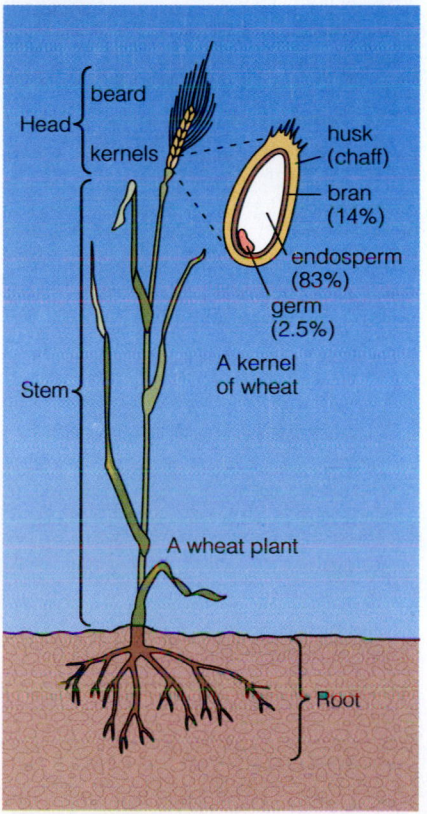

Figure 4–8

A Wheat Plant and a Single Kernel of Wheat

Head { beard, kernels }

Stem

A wheat plant

Root

husk (chaff)

bran (14%)

endosperm (83%)

germ (2.5%)

A kernel of wheat

In earlier times, people milled wheat by grinding it between two stones, blowing or sifting out the tough outer chaff, but retaining all the nutrient-rich bran and germ, as well as the endosperm. With advances in milling machinery, it became possible to remove the dark, heavy bran and germ, leaving a whiter, smoother-textured flour with a higher starch content and far less fiber. An advantage of this flour, besides producing soft, white baked goods, is its durability—white flour "keeps" much longer than whole-grain flour because the nutrient-rich, oily germ of whole grains turns rancid over time. As food production became more industrialized, suppliers realized that customers also favored this refined, soft, white flour over the crunchy, dark brown, "old-fashioned" flour.

KEY POINT

- Whole-grain flours retain all edible parts of grain kernels.

Enrichment of Refined Grains   In turning to highly refined grains, many people suffered deficiencies of iron, thiamin, riboflavin, and niacin—nutrients formerly obtained from whole grains. To reverse this tragedy, Congress passed the U.S. Enrichment Act of 1942, requiring that iron, niacin, thiamin, and riboflavin be added to all refined grain products before they were sold. In 1996, the vitamin folate (often called *folic acid* on labels) was added to the list. Today, all refined grain products are enriched with at least the nutrients mandated by the Act.

A single serving of enriched grain food is not "rich" in the enrichment nutrients, but people who eat several servings a day obtain significantly more of these nutrients than they would from unenriched refined products, as the bread example of Figure 4–9 shows.

Enriched grain foods are nutritionally comparable to whole-grain foods only with respect to their added nutrients; whole grains provide greater amounts of vitamin B_6 and the minerals magnesium and zinc that refined grains lack. Whole grains also provide substantial fiber (see Table 4–5), along with a wide array of potentially beneficial phytochemicals in the bran and the essential oils of the germ.

KEY POINT

- Refined grain products are less nutritious than whole grains.

Health Effects of Whole Grains   Whole-grain intakes provide health benefits beyond just nutrients and fiber. People who take in just three daily servings of whole grains often have healthier body weights and less body fatness than other people.[15] It could be that whole grains fill up the stomach, slow down digestion, or promote longer-lasting feelings of fullness than refined grains. The same three daily servings of whole grains also correlate with lower risks of heart disease and type 2 diabetes. Finally, people who make whole grains a habit have lower risks of certain cancers, particularly of the colon. It may be that the fiber, phytochemicals, or nutrients of whole grains improve body tissue health, but these issues need clarification.

Refined grains in amounts of up to one-half of the daily grain intake (without added sugars, fats, or sodium) seem to pose little risk to health.[16] Clearly, however, those who choose to ignore the Dietary Guidelines for Americans recommendation to consume sufficient whole grains do so at their peril.

KEY POINT

- A diet rich in whole grains is associated with reduced risks of overweight and certain chronic diseases.

From Carbohydrates to Glucose

LO 4.3   Explain how carbohydrates are converted to glucose in the human body.

You may eat bread or a baked potato, but the body's cells cannot use foods or even whole molecules of lactose, sucrose, or starch for energy. They need the glucose in those molecules. The various body systems must make glucose available to the cells, not all at once when it is eaten but at a steady rate all day.

Table 4–5
Grams of Fiber in One Cup of Flour
Dark rye, 31 g
Barley flour, 15 g
Whole wheat, 13 g
Buckwheat, 12 g
Whole-grain cornmeal, 9 g
Light rye, 8 g
Enriched white, 3 g

Figure 4-9

Nutrients in Whole-Grain, Enriched White, and Unenriched White Breads

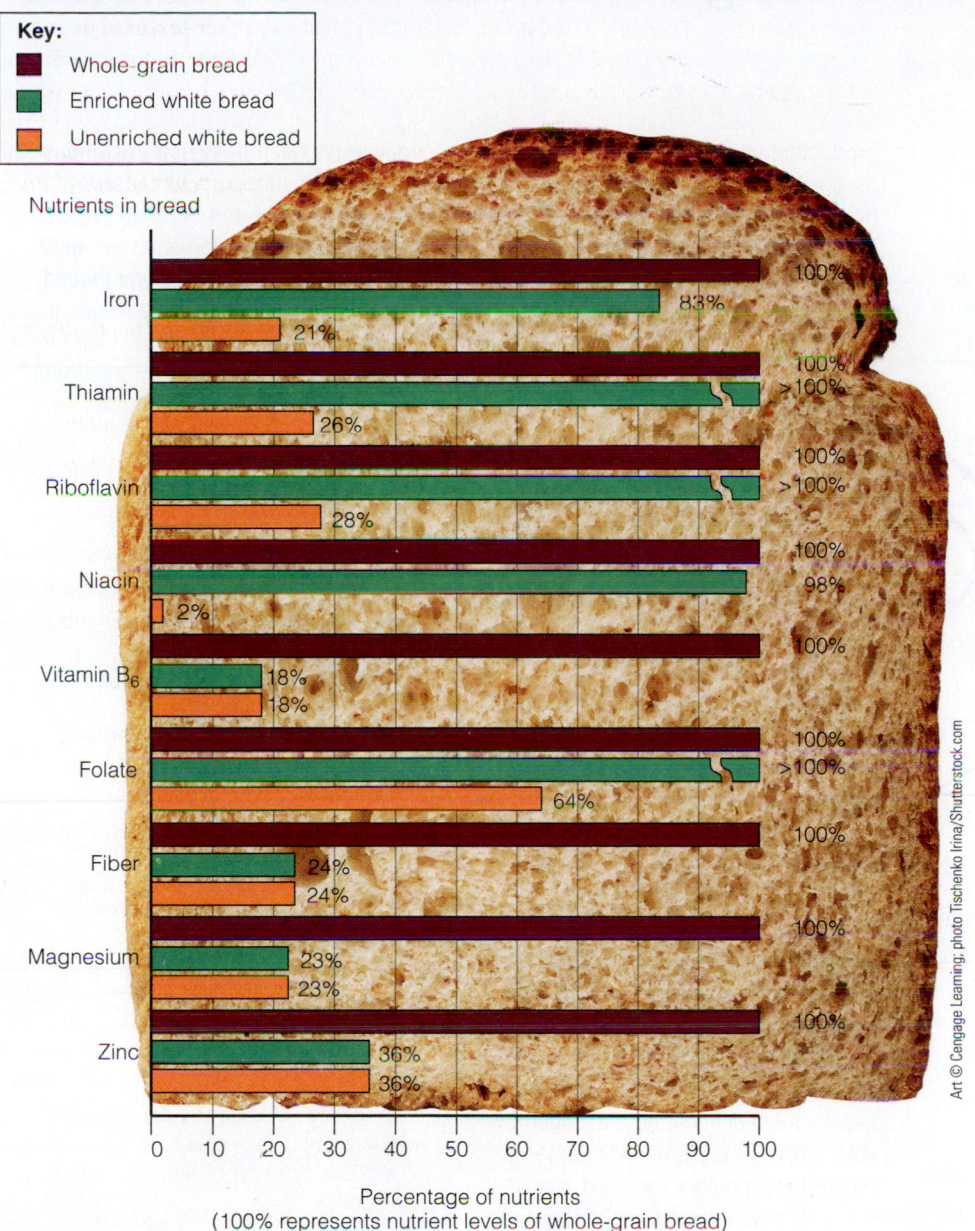

Key:
- Whole-grain bread
- Enriched white bread
- Unenriched white bread

Nutrients in bread

Iron — 100% / 83% / 21%

Thiamin — 100% / >100% / 26%

Riboflavin — 100% / >100% / 28%

Niacin — 100% / 98% / 2%

Vitamin B₆ — 100% / 18% / 18%

Folate — 100% / >100% / 64%

Fiber — 100% / 24% / 24%

Magnesium — 100% / 23% / 23%

Zinc — 100% / 36% / 36%

0 10 20 30 40 50 60 70 80 90 100

Percentage of nutrients
(100% represents nutrient levels of whole-grain bread)

Art © Cengage Learning; photo Tischenko Irina/Shutterstock.com

Digestion and Absorption of Carbohydrate

To obtain glucose from newly eaten food, the digestive system must first render the starch and disaccharides from the food into monosaccharides that can be absorbed through the cells lining the small intestine. The largest of the digestible carbohydrate molecules, starch, requires the most extensive breakdown. Disaccharides, in contrast, need be split only once before they can be absorbed.

Starch Digestion of most starch begins in the mouth, where an enzyme in saliva mixes with food and begins to split starch into shorter units. While chewing a bite of bread, you may notice that a slightly sweet taste develops—the disaccharide maltose is being liberated from starch by the enzyme. The salivary enzyme continues to act on the starch in the bite of bread while it remains tucked in the stomach's upper storage area. As each chewed lump is pushed downward and mixed with the stomach's acid and other juices, the salivary enzyme (made

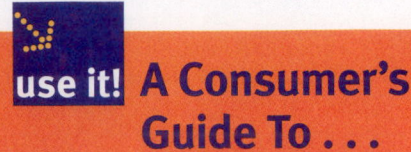
Finding Whole-Grain Foods

"OK, it's time to take action." A consumer, ready to switch to some whole-grain foods, may find these good intentions derailed in the tricky terrain of the grocery store. Even an experienced shopper may feel bewildered in store-length aisles bulging with breads that range from light-as-a-feather, refined enriched white loaves to the heaviest, roughest-textured whole-grain varieties. A baffling array of label claims vies for our shopper's attention, too—and while some are trustworthy, others are not.

Not Every Choice Must Be 100 Percent Whole Grain

If you are just now starting to include whole grains in your diet, keep in mind that various combinations of whole and refined grains can meet the Dietary Guidelines recommendation that half of the day's grains be whole grains.[1]* Until your taste buds adjust, you may prefer breads, cereals, pastas, and other grain foods made from a half-and-half blend of whole and refined grains for all of your day's choices. The addition of some refined enriched white flour smoothes the texture of whole grain foods and provides a measure of folate, an important enrichment vitamin in the U.S. diet. Alternatively, you might choose 100 percent whole grains half of the time and refined grains for the other half, or any other combination to meet the need. Research shows that no harm comes from consuming up to half of the day's grains as refined grains.[2]

In addition to whole-grain blends, a variety of white durum wheat has been developed to mimic the taste and appearance of ordinary enriched refined white flour while offering nutrients similar to those of whole grains. Such **white wheat** products lack the dark-colored and strong-flavored phytochemicals associated with ordinary whole-wheat

*Reference notes are found in Appendix F.

products, however, and research has not established whether its effects on the health of the body are equivalent.** (See Table 4–4, p. 127, for definitions.)

High Fiber Does Not Equal Whole Grain

An important distinction exists between foods labeled "high-fiber" and those made of whole grains. High-fiber breads or cereals may derive their fiber from the addition of wheat bran or even purified cellulose, and not from whole grains. Label readers can differentiate one kind from the other by scanning the food's ingredients list for words like *bran, cellulose, methylcellulose, gums,* or *psyllium.* Such high-fiber foods may be nutritious and useful in their own way, but they cannot substitute for whole-grain foods in the diet.

Brown Color Does Not Equal Whole Grain

"**Brown bread**" may sound healthy, and white bread less so, but the term *brown* simply refers to color that may derive from brown ingredients, such as molasses. Similarly, whole-grain rice, commonly called brown rice, cannot be judged by color alone. Whole-grain rice comes in red and other colors, too. Also, many rice dishes appear brown because they contain brown-colored ingredients, such as soy sauce, beef broth, or seasonings. Pasta comes in a rainbow of colors, and whole-grain noodles and blends are increasingly available—just read the ingredients list on the label to check that any descriptors on the outside of the package accurately reflect the food inside.

Label Subtleties

A label proclaiming "Multi-Grain Goodness" or "Natural Wheat Bread"

**In 2005, ConAgra began marketing white wheat as UltraGrain.

may imply healthfulness but can mislead uninformed shoppers, who assume, falsely, that such terms mean "whole grain." Like descriptors such as **multi-grain**, **wheat bread**, and **stone ground**, these terms do not indicate whole grains. To find the real whole grains, look for the words *whole* or *whole grain* preceding the name of a grain in the ingredients list. Learn to recognize individual whole grains by name, too. Many are listed in Table 4–6.

Table 4–6
A Sampling of Whole Grains
If a food has at least 8 grams of whole grains per ounce, it is at least half whole grains.

- Amaranth, a grain of the ancient Aztec people.[a]
- Barley (hulled but not pearled).[b]
- Buckwheat.[a]
- Bulgur wheat.
- Corn, including whole cornmeal and popcorn.
- Millet.
- Oats, including oatmeal.
- Quinoa (KEEN-wah), a grain of the ancient Inca people.[a]
- Rice, including brown, red, and others.
- Rye.
- Sorghum (also called milo), a drought-resistant grain.
- Teff, popular in Ethiopia, India, and Australia.
- Triticale, a cross of durum wheat and rye.
- Wheat, in many varieties such as spelt, emmer, farro, einkorn, durum; and forms such as bulgur, cracked wheat, and wheatberries.
- Wild rice.[a]

[a]Although not botanical grains, these foods are similar to grains in nutrient contents, preparation, and use.

[b]Hulling removes only inedible husk; pearling removes beneficial bran.

Look at the bread labels in Figure 4–10 below, and recall from Chapter 2 that ingredients must be listed in descending order of prominence on an ingredients list. It's easy to see from the label of the "Natural Wheat Bread" in the figure that this bread contains no whole grains whatsoever. This loaf is made entirely of refined enriched wheat flour, another name for white flour. The word "Natural" in the name is a marketing gimmick and has no meaning in nutrition.

Now read the label of "Multi-Grain, Honey Fiber Bread." It does contain multiple whole grains, but the major ingredient is still unbleached enriched wheat flour. The key here is the refinement of the wheatberries to yield refined "white" flour that requires enrichment, a flour called "enriched wheat flour" on labels. The bleaching status is irrelevant. Most of the fiber of this bread's name comes from added cellulose and not

from its tiny amounts of "multi-grains." Now focus on the bread labeled "Whole Grain, Whole Wheat." This, at last, is a 100 percent whole-grain food.

After the Salt

Here's a trick: a loaf of bread generally contains about one teaspoon of salt. Therefore, if an ingredient is listed *after* the salt, you'll know that the entire loaf contains less than a teaspoonful of that ingredient, not enough to make a significant contribution to the eater's whole-grain intake. In the "Multi-Grain" bread of the figure, all of the whole grains are listed after the salt.

A Word about Cereals

Ready-to-eat breakfast cereals, from toasted oat rings to granola, are a pleasant way to include whole grains in almost anyone's diet. Like breads, cereals vary widely in their contents

of whole grains, but, also like breads, they can be evaluated by reading their ingredients, lists.

Oatmeal in all its forms—old-fashioned, quick cooking, and even microwavable instant—qualifies as whole grain, but be careful: some instant oatmeal packets contain more sugar than grain. Limit intake of any cereal, hot or cold, with a high sugar, sodium, or saturated fat content, even if it touts "whole grains" on the label.

Moving Ahead

"I've tried buckwheat pancakes, and they're pretty tasty. But what on earth is quinoa?" Admittedly, certain whole grains may be unavailable in mainstream grocery stores. It may take a trip to a "health-food" store to find quinoa, for example. In a welcome trend, larger chain stores are responding to increased consumer demand and

---

Figure 4–10
Bread Labels Compared

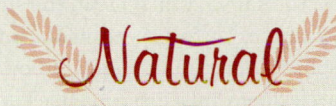

Natural Wheat Bread

Nutrition Facts

Serving size 1 slice (30g)
Servings Per Container 15

Amount per serving	
Calories 90	Calories from Fat 14
	% Daily Value*
Total Fat 1.5g	2%
Trans Fat 0g	
Sodium 220mg	9%
Total Carbohydrate 15g	5%
Dietary fiber less than 1g	2%
Sugars 2g	
Protein 4g	

INGREDIENTS: UNBLEACHED ENRICHED WHEAT FLOUR [MALTED BARLEY FLOUR, NIACIN, REDUCED IRON, THIAMIN MONONITRATE (VITAMIN B1), RIBOFLAVIN (VITAMIN B2), FOLIC ACID], WATER, HIGH FRUCTOSE CORN SYRUP, MOLASSES, PARTIALLY HYDROGENATED SOYBEAN OIL, YEAST, CORN FLOUR, SALT, GROUND CARAWAY, WHEAT GLUTEN, CALCIUM PROPIONATE (PRESERVATIVE), MONOGLYCERIDES, SOY LECITHIN.

Multi-Grain Honey Fiber

Nutrition Facts

Serving size 1 slice (43g)
Servings Per Container 18

Amount per serving	
Calories 120	Calories from Fat 15
	% Daily Value*
Total Fat 1.5g	2%
Trans Fat 0g	
Sodium 170mg	7%
Total Carbohydrate 9g	3%
Dietary fiber 4g	16%
Sugars 2g	
Protein 5g	

INGREDIENTS: UNBLEACHED ENRICHED WHEAT FLOUR, WATER, WHEAT GLUTEN, CELLULOSE, YEAST, SOYBEAN OIL, HONEY, SALT, BARLEY, NATURAL FLAVOR PRESERVATIVES, MONOCALCIUM PHOSPHATE, MILLET, CORN, OATS, SOYBEAN FLOUR, BROWN RICE, FLAXSEED.

Whole Grain Whole Wheat

Nutrition Facts

Serving size 1 slice (30g)
Servings Per Container 18

Amount per serving	
Calories 90	Calories from Fat 14
	% Daily Value*
Total Fat 1.5g	2%
Trans Fat 0g	
Sodium 135mg	6%
Total Carbohydrate 15g	5%
Dietary fiber 2g	8%
Sugars 2g	
Protein 4g	

MADE FROM: UNBROMATED STONE GROUND 100% WHOLE WHEAT FLOUR, WATER, CRUSHED WHEAT, HIGH FRUCTOSE CORN SYRUP, PARTIALLY HYDROGENATED VEGETABLE SHORTENING (SOYBEAN AND COTTONSEED OILS), RAISIN JUICE CONCENTRATE, WHEAT GLUTEN, YEAST, WHOLE WHEAT FLAKES, UNSULPHURED MOLASSES, SALT, HONEY, VINEGAR, ENZYME MODIFIED SOY LECITHIN, CULTURED WHEY, UNBLEACHED WHEAT FLOUR AND SOY LECITHIN.

From Carbohydrates to Glucose

stocking more brown rice, wild rice, bulgur, and other whole-grain goodies on their shelves.

Once a person begins to enjoy the added taste dimensions of whole grains, he or she may be less drawn to the bland refined foods formerly eaten out of habit. More than 90 percent of Americans are stuck in this rut, failing to eat the whole grains they need. Be adventurous with health in mind, and give the hearty flavors of a variety of whole-grain foods a try.

These memory joggers can remind you to choose whole grains during the day:

1. Morning, choose a whole-grain cereal breakfast.
2. Noon, choose whole-grain bread for lunch.
3. Night, choose whole-grain pasta or rice for supper.

Vary your choices, and remember to make at least half of your grain foods whole grains.

Review Questions†

1. When searching for whole-grain bread, a consumer should search the labels _____.

   a. for words like *multi-grain, wheat bread, brown bread,* or *stone ground*
   b. for the order in which whole grains appear on the ingredients list
   c. for the word "unbleached," which indicates that the food is primarily made from whole grains
   d. b and c

†Answers to Consumer's Guide review questions are found in Appendix G.

2. Whole-grain rice, often called brown rice, _____.

   a. can be recognized by its characteristic brown color
   b. cannot be recognized by color alone
   c. is often more refined than white rice
   d. b and c

3. A bread labeled "high-fiber" _____.

   a. may not be a whole-grain food
   b. is a good substitute for whole-grain bread
   c. is required by law to contain whole grains
   d. may contain the dangerous chemical cellulose

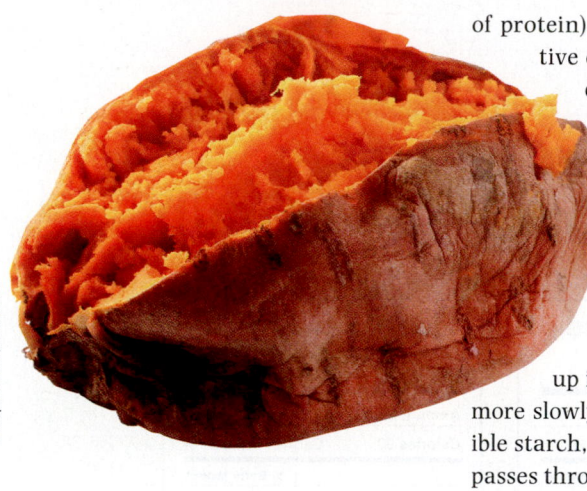

istockphoto.com/NRedmond

of protein) is deactivated by the stomach's protein-digesting acid. Not all digestive enzymes are susceptible to digestion in the stomach—one enzyme that digests protein works best in the stomach. Its structure protects it from the stomach's acid.

With the breakdown of the salivary enzyme in the stomach, starch digestion ceases, but it resumes at full speed in the small intestine, where another starch-splitting enzyme is delivered by the pancreas. This enzyme breaks starch down into disaccharides and small polysaccharides. Other enzymes liberate monosaccharides for absorption.

Most forms of starch are easily digested. The starch of refined white flour, for example, breaks down rapidly to glucose that is absorbed high up in the small intestine. Other starch, such as that of cooked beans, digests more slowly and releases its glucose later in the digestion process. The least digestible starch, called **resistant starch**, is technically a kind of fiber because much of it passes through the small intestine undigested into the colon.[17] Some resistant starch may be digested, but slowly, and most remains intact until the bacteria of the colon eventually ferment it. Barley, raw or chilled cooked potatoes, cooked dried beans and lentils, oatmeal, intact seeds and kernels, and under-ripe bananas all contain resistant starch.

Sugars Sucrose and lactose from food, along with maltose and small polysaccharides freed from starch, undergo one more split to yield free monosaccharides before they are absorbed. This split is accomplished by digestive enzymes attached to the cells of the lining of the small intestine. The conversion of a bite of bread to nutrients for the body is completed when monosaccharides cross these cells and are washed away in a rush of circulating blood that carries them to the waiting liver. Figure 4–11 presents a quick review of carbohydrate digestion.

The absorbed carbohydrates (glucose, galactose, and fructose) travel in the bloodstream to the liver, which can convert fructose and galactose to glucose. The circulatory system transports the glucose and other products to the cells. Liver and muscle cells store circulating glucose as glycogen; all cells split glucose for energy.

resistant starch the fraction of starch in a food that is digested slowly, or not at all, by human enzymes.

Figure 4–11

How Carbohydrate in Food Becomes Glucose in the Body

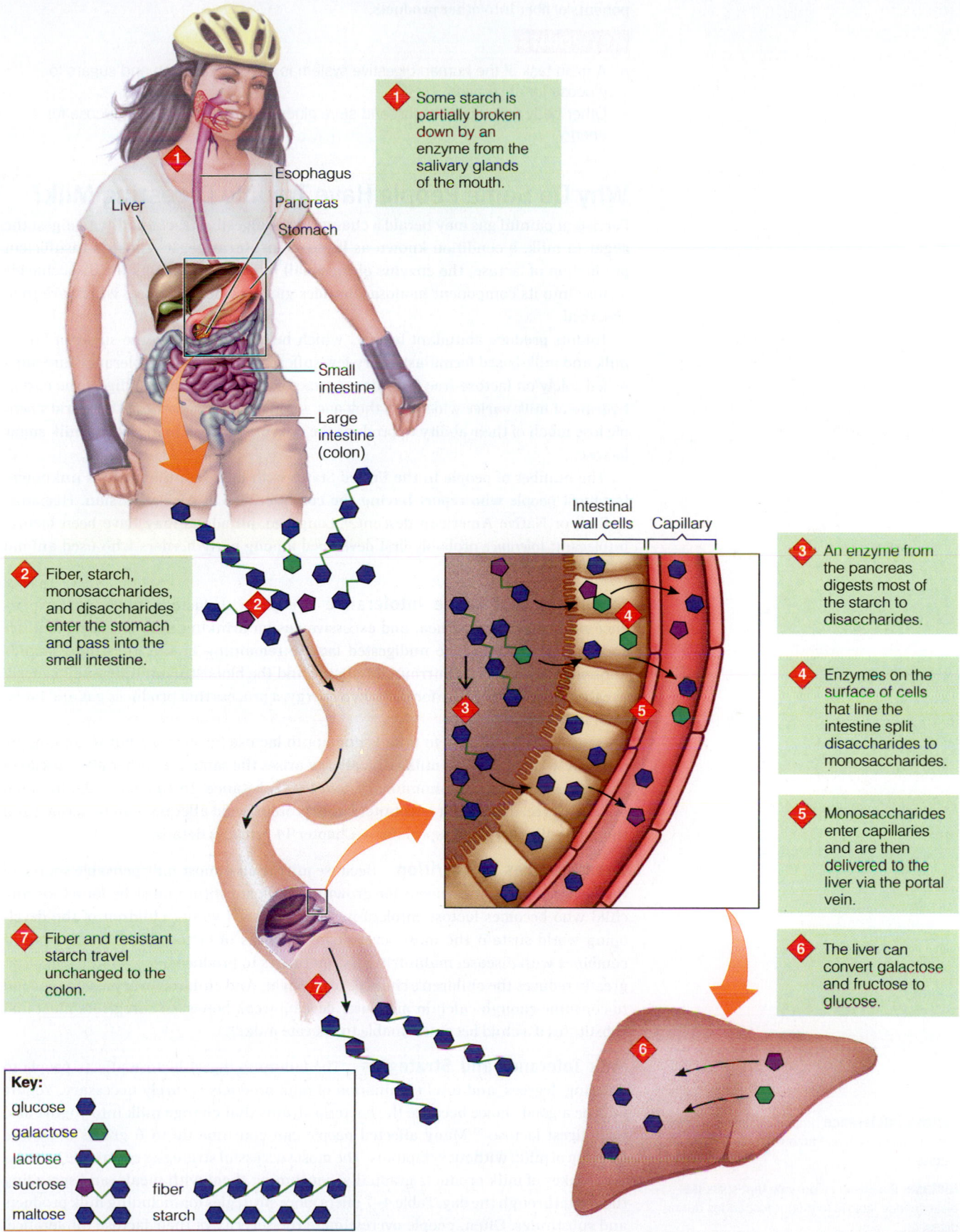

Liver

Esophagus

Pancreas

Stomach

Small intestine

Large intestine (colon)

Intestinal wall cells

Capillary

1 Some starch is partially broken down by an enzyme from the salivary glands of the mouth.

2 Fiber, starch, monosaccharides, and disaccharides enter the stomach and pass into the small intestine.

3 An enzyme from the pancreas digests most of the starch to disaccharides.

4 Enzymes on the surface of cells that line the intestine split disaccharides to monosaccharides.

5 Monosaccharides enter capillaries and are then delivered to the liver via the portal vein.

6 The liver can convert galactose and fructose to glucose.

7 Fiber and resistant starch travel unchanged to the colon.

Key:

glucose

galactose

lactose

sucrose   fiber

maltose   starch

Fiber As explained earlier, although molecules of most fibers are not changed by human digestive enzymes, many of them can be fermented by the bacterial inhabitants of the human colon. The fermentation process breaks down carbohydrate components of fiber into other products.

Why Do Some People Have Trouble Digesting Milk?

Persistent painful gas may herald a change in the digestive tract's ability to digest the sugar in milk, a condition known as **lactose intolerance**. Its cause is insufficient production of lactase, the enzyme of the small intestine that splits the disaccharide lactose into its component monosaccharides glucose and galactose, which are then absorbed.

Infants produce abundant lactase, which helps them absorb the sugar of breast milk and milk-based formulas; a very few suffer inborn lactose intolerance and must be fed solely on lactose-free formulas. Among adults, the ability to digest the carbohydrate of milk varies widely. As they age, upward of 75 percent of the world's people lose much of their ability to produce the enzyme **lactase** to digest the milk sugar lactose.

The number of people in the United States with lactose intolerance is unknown, but most people who report having the condition are of African, Asian, Hispanic, Indian, or Native American descent.[18] Long ago, all adults may have been lactose intolerant; *tolerance* probably first developed among early herders who used animal milk as food and thrived.

Symptoms of Lactose Intolerance
People with lactose intolerance experience nausea, pain, diarrhea, and excessive gas on drinking milk or eating lactose-containing products. The undigested lactose remaining in the intestine demands dilution with fluid from surrounding tissue and the bloodstream. Intestinal bacteria use the undigested lactose for their own energy, a process that produces gas and intestinal irritants.

Sometimes sensitivity to milk is due not to lactose intolerance but to an allergic reaction to the protein in milk. Milk allergy arises the same way other allergies do—from sensitization of the immune system to a substance. In this case, the immune system overreacts when it encounters milk protein. Food allergies can be serious and should be diagnosed by a specialist—Chapter 14 provides details.

Consequences to Nutrition
Because milk is an almost indispensable source of the calcium every child needs for growth, a milk substitute must be found for any child who becomes lactose intolerant. Disadvantaged young children of the developing world sustain the most severe consequences of lactose intolerance when it combines with disease, malnutrition, or parasites to produce a loss of nutrients that greatly reduces the children's chances of survival. And children everywhere who fail to consume enough calcium may later develop weak bones, so caregivers must find substitutes if a child becomes unable to tolerate milk.[19]

Milk Tolerance and Strategies
The failure to digest lactose affects people to differing degrees, and total elimination of milk products is rarely necessary. Yogurt may be a good choice because the bacteria strains that change milk into yogurt also help digest lactose.[20] Many affected people can consume up to 6 grams of lactose (1/2 cup of milk) without symptoms. The most successful strategies seem to be increasing intakes of milk products gradually, consuming them with meals, and spreading them out through the day. Table 4–7 offers more strategies for including milk products and substitutes. Often, people overestimate the severity of their lactose intolerance,

lactose intolerance impaired ability to digest lactose due to reduced amounts of the enzyme lactase.

lactase the intestinal enzyme that splits the disaccharide lactose to monosaccharides during digestion.

Table 4–7

Lactose Intolerance Strategies

People with lactose intolerance can experiment with milk-based foods to find a strategy that works for them. The trick is to find ways of splitting lactose to glucose and galactose before a food is consumed, rather than providing a lactose feast for colonic bacteria.

Product	Effects/Strategies
Aged cheeses	Bacteria or molds used to create cheeses ferment lactose during the aging process. Use in moderation.
Lactase pills and drops	Lactase added to milk products by consumers or pills taken before milk product consumption split lactose molecules in the digestive tract. Harmless when used as directed by the manufacturer.
Lactase-treated milk products	Lactase added to milk products during manufacturing splits lactose before purchase. Use freely in place of ordinary milk products.
Milk substitutes (soy, nut, or grain-based beverages), cheese and yogurt substitutes	Nonmilk replacments for milk products may or may not be fortified with the nutrients of milk. Compare Nutrition Facts panels for calcium, protein, and vitamin D in particular.
Yogurt (live culture type)	Yogurt-making bacteria can survive in the human digestive tract; the bacteria possess an enzyme to split lactose.
Yogurt (with added milk solids listed on the label)	These contain *extra* lactose and can overwhelm the system.

blaming it for symptoms most probably caused by something else—a mistake that could cost them the health of their bones (details in Chapter 8).

KEY POINTS

- In lactose intolerance, the body fails to produce sufficient amounts of the enzyme needed to digest the sugar of milk, leading to uncomfortable symptoms.
- People with lactose intolerance or milk allergy need alternatives that provide the nutrients of milk.

The Body's Use of Glucose

LO 4.4 Discuss the body's use of glucose.

Glucose is the basic carbohydrate unit used for energy by each of the body's cells. The body handles its glucose judiciously—maintaining an internal store to be used when needed and tightly controlling its blood glucose concentration to ensure a steady supply. Recall that carbohydrates serve functional roles, too, such as forming part of mucus, but they are best known for providing energy.

Splitting Glucose for Energy

Glucose fuels the work of every cell in the body to some extent, but the cells of the brain and nervous system depend almost exclusively on glucose, and the red blood cells use glucose alone. When a cell splits glucose for energy, it performs an intricate sequence of maneuvers that are of great interest to the biochemist—and of no interest at all to most people who eat bread and potatoes. What everybody needs to understand, though, is that there is no good substitute for carbohydrate. Carbohydrate is *essential*, as the following details illustrate.

The Point of No Return   At a certain point in the process of splitting glucose for energy, glucose itself is forever lost to the body. First, glucose is broken in half, releasing some energy. Then two pathways open to these glucose halves. They can be put

Figure 4–12

The Breakdown of Glucose Yields Energy and Carbon Dioxide

Cell enzymes split the bonds between the carbon atoms in glucose, liberating the energy stored there for the cell's use. **1** The first split yields two 3-carbon fragments. The two-way arrows mean that these fragments can also be rejoined to make glucose again. **2** Once they are broken down further into 2-carbon fragments, however, they cannot rejoin to make glucose. **3** The carbon atoms liberated when the bonds split are combined with oxygen and released into the air, via the lungs, as carbon dioxide. Although not shown here, water is also produced at each split.

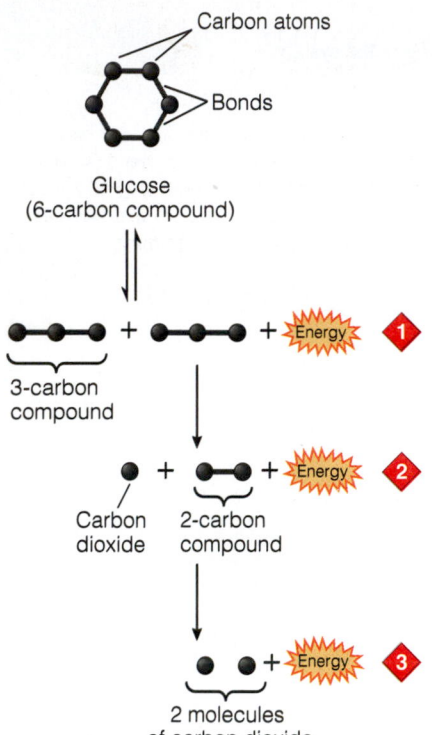

Carbon atoms

Bonds

Glucose
(6-carbon compound)

3-carbon compound + 3-carbon compound + Energy **1**

Carbon dioxide + 2-carbon compound + Energy **2**

2 molecules of carbon dioxide + Energy **3**

protein-sparing action the action of carbohydrate and fat in providing energy that allows protein to be used for purposes it alone can serve.

ketone (kee-tone) **bodies** acidic, water-soluble compounds that arise during the breakdown of fat when carbohydrate is not available.

ketosis (kee-TOE-sis) an undesirable high concentration of ketone bodies, such as acetone, in the blood or urine.

back together to make glucose again, or they can be broken into smaller molecules. If they are broken further, they cannot be reassembled to form glucose.

The smaller molecules can also take different pathways. They can continue along the breakdown pathway to yield still more energy and eventually break down completely to just carbon dioxide and water. Or they can be formed into building blocks of protein or be hitched together into units of body fat.[21] Figure 4–12 shows how glucose is broken down to yield energy and carbon dioxide.

Below a Healthy Minimum Although glucose can be converted into body fat, body fat cannot be converted into glucose to feed the brain adequately. When the body faces a severe carbohydrate deficit, it has two problems. Having no glucose, it must turn to protein to make some (the body has this ability), diverting protein from its own critical functions, such as maintaining immune defenses. When body protein is used, it is taken from blood, organ, or muscle proteins; no surplus of protein is stored specifically for such emergencies. Protein is indispensable to body functions, and carbohydrate should be kept available precisely to prevent the use of protein for energy. This is called the **protein-sparing action** of carbohydrate. As for fat, it regenerates a small amount of glucose—but not enough to feed the brain and nerve tissues.

Ketosis The second problem with an inadequate supply of carbohydrate concerns a precarious shift in the body's energy metabolism. Instead of producing energy by following its main metabolic pathway, fat takes another route in which fat fragments combine with each other. This shift causes an accumulation of normally scarce acidic products called **ketone bodies**.

Ketone bodies can accumulate in the blood, causing **ketosis**. When they reach high levels, they can disturb the normal acid-base balance, a life-threatening situation. People eating diets that produce ketosis may develop deficiencies of vitamins and minerals, loss of bone minerals, elevated blood cholesterol, impaired mood, and other adverse outcomes. In addition, glycogen stores become too scanty to meet a metabolic emergency or to support vigorous muscular work.

Ketosis isn't all bad, however. Ketone bodies provide a fuel alternative to glucose for brain and nerve cells when glucose is lacking, such as in starvation or very-low-carbohydrate diets. Not all brain tissues can use ketones, however—some rely exclusively on glucose, so the body must still sacrifice some protein to provide it—but at a slower rate. A therapeutic ketogenic diet in addition to medication has substantially reduced seizures in many children and adults with hard-to-treat epilepsy, although many find the diet difficult to follow for long periods.[22]

The DRI Minimum Recommendation for Carbohydrate The minimum amount of digestible carbohydrate determined by the DRI committee to adequately feed the brain and reduce ketosis has been set at 130 grams a day for an average-sized person.[23] Several times this minimum is recommended to maintain health and glycogen stores (explained in the next section). The recommended amounts of vegetables, fruits, legumes, grains, and milk presented in Chapter 2 deliver abundant carbohydrates.

KEY POINTS

- Without glucose, the body is forced to alter its uses of protein and fat.
- To help supply the brain with glucose, the body breaks down its protein to make glucose and converts its fats into ketone bodies, incurring ketosis.

How Is Glucose Regulated in the Body?

Should your blood glucose ever climb abnormally high, you might become confused or have difficulty breathing. Should your glucose supplies ever fall too low, you would feel dizzy and weak. The healthy body guards against both conditions with two safeguard activities:

- Siphoning off excess blood glucose into the liver and muscles for storage as glycogen and into the adipose tissue for storage as body fat.
- Replenishing diminished blood glucose from liver glycogen stores.

Two hormones prove critical to these processes. The hormone **insulin** stimulates glucose storage as glycogen, while the hormone **glucagon** helps to release glucose from its glycogen nest.

Insulin After a meal, as blood glucose rises, the pancreas is the first organ to respond. It releases insulin, which signals body tissues to take up glucose from the blood. Muscle tissue responds to insulin by taking up excess blood glucose and using it to build the polysaccharide glycogen. The liver takes up excess blood glucose, too, but it needs no help from insulin to do so. Instead, liver cells respond to insulin by speeding up their glycogen production. Adipose tissue also responds to insulin by taking up excess blood glucose. Simply put, insulin regulates blood glucose by:

- Facilitating blood glucose uptake by the muscles and adipose tissue.
- Stimulating glycogen synthesis in the liver.

Figure 4–13 (p. 138) provides an overview of these relationships.

Tissue Glycogen Stores The muscles hoard two-thirds of the body's total glycogen to ensure that glucose, a critical fuel for physical activity, is available for muscular work. The brain stores a tiny fraction of the total as an emergency reserve to fuel the brain for an hour or two in severe glucose deprivation. The liver stores the remainder and is generous with its glycogen, releasing glucose into the bloodstream for the brain or other tissues when the supply runs low. Without carbohydrate from food to replenish it, the glycogen stores in the liver can be depleted in less than a day.

The Release of Glucose from Glycogen The glycogen molecule is highly branched, with hundreds of ends bristling from each molecule's surface (review this structure in Figure 4–3 on p. 118). When blood glucose starts to fall too low, the hormone glucagon floods the bloodstream and triggers the breakdown of liver glycogen to single glucose molecules. Enzymes in liver cells respond to glucagon by attacking a multitude of glycogen ends simultaneously to release a surge of glucose into the blood for use by all the body's cells. Thus, the highly branched structure of glycogen uniquely suits the purpose of releasing glucose on demand.

Be Prepared: Eat Carbohydrate Another hormone, epinephrine, also triggers the breakdown of liver glycogen as part of the body's defense mechanism to provide extra glucose for quick action in times of danger.[§] To store glucose for emergencies, we are well advised to eat carbohydrate at each meal.

You may be asking, "What kind of carbohydrate?" Candy, "energy bars," and sugary beverages are quick sources of abundant sugar energy, but they are not the best choices. Balanced meals and snacks, eaten on a regular schedule, help the body to maintain its blood glucose. Meals with starch and soluble fiber combined with some protein and a little fat slow digestion so that glucose enters the blood gradually in an ongoing, steady rate.

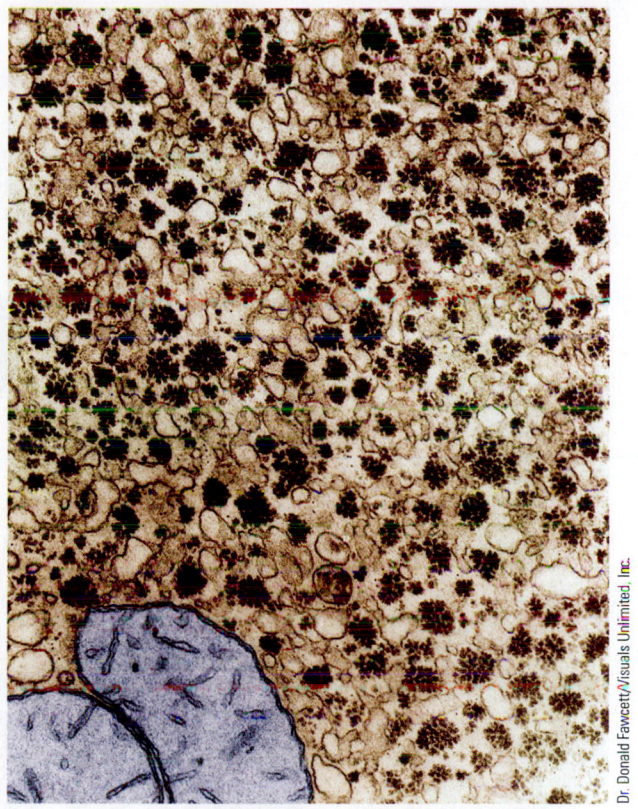

This photo peeks inside of a single liver cell after a meal (magnified over 100,000 times). The clusters of dark-colored dots are glycogen granules. (The blue structures at the bottom are cellular organelles.)

Dr. Donald Fawcett/Visuals Unlimited, Inc.

KEY POINTS

- The muscles and liver store glucose as glycogen; the liver can release glucose from its glycogen into the bloodstream.
- The hormones insulin and glucagon regulate blood glucose concentrations.

Excess Glucose and Body Fatness

Suppose you have eaten dinner and are now sitting on the couch, munching pretzels and drinking cola as you watch a ball game on television. Your digestive tract is delivering molecules of glucose to your bloodstream, and your blood is carrying these molecules to your liver and other body cells. The body cells use as much glucose as they

---
[§]Epinephrine is also called adrenaline.

insulin a hormone secreted by the pancreas in response to a high blood glucose concentration. It assists cells in drawing glucose from the blood.

glucagon (GLOO-cah-gon) a hormone secreted by the pancreas that stimulates the liver to release glucose into the blood when blood glucose concentration dips.

Figure 4–13

Blood Glucose Regulation—An Overview

The pancreas monitors blood glucose (shown as blue hexagons) and adjusts its concentration by way of its two opposing hormones, insulin and glucagon. When glucose is high, the pancreas releases insulin; when glucose is low, it releases glucagon. When glucose is restored to the normal range, the pancreas slows its hormone output in an elegant feedback system operating in a healthy body. Many more details about this system are known.

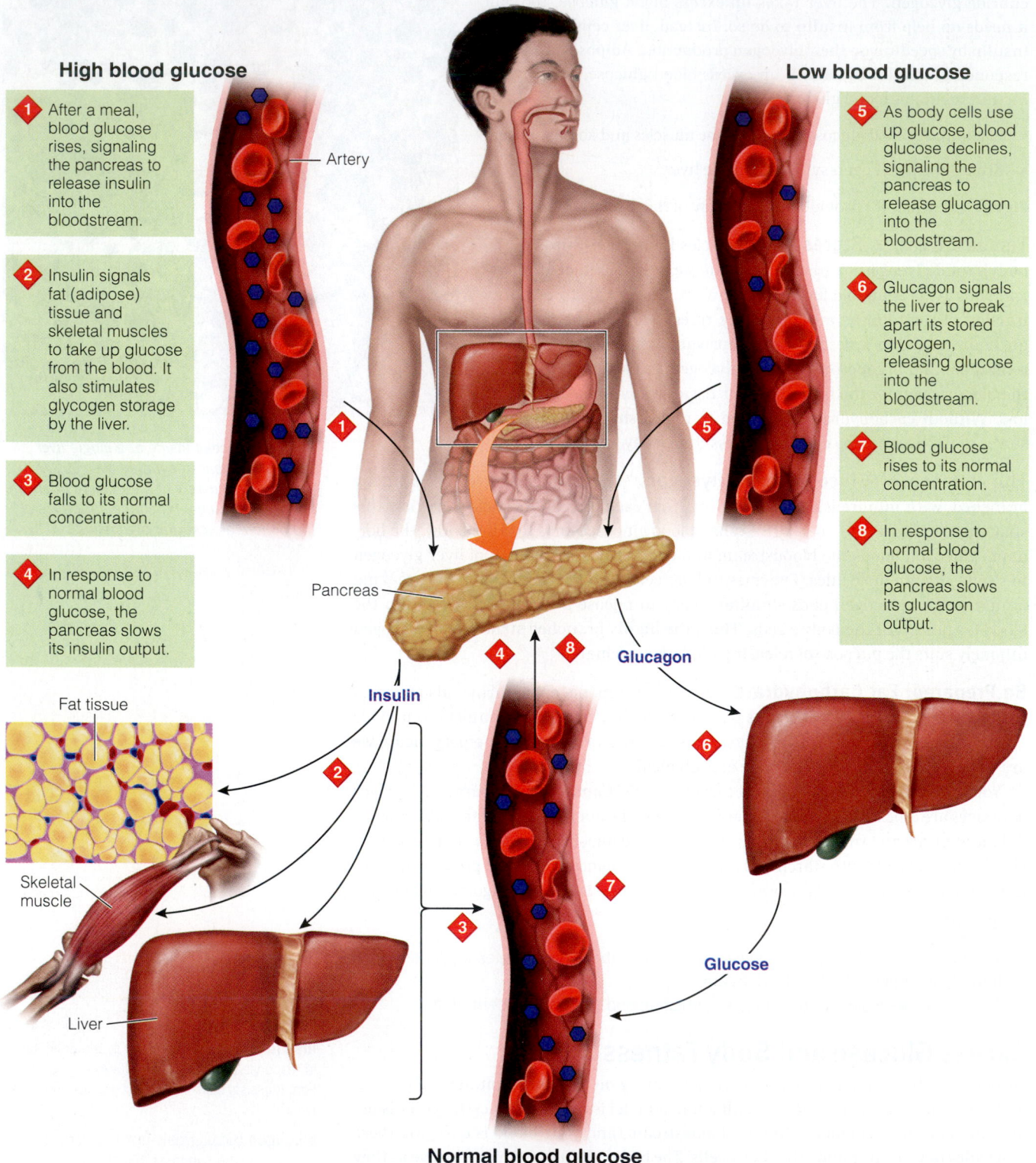

High blood glucose

1. After a meal, blood glucose rises, signaling the pancreas to release insulin into the bloodstream.

2. Insulin signals fat (adipose) tissue and skeletal muscles to take up glucose from the blood. It also stimulates glycogen storage by the liver.

3. Blood glucose falls to its normal concentration.

4. In response to normal blood glucose, the pancreas slows its insulin output.

Low blood glucose

5. As body cells use up glucose, blood glucose declines, signaling the pancreas to release glucagon into the bloodstream.

6. Glucagon signals the liver to break apart its stored glycogen, releasing glucose into the bloodstream.

7. Blood glucose rises to its normal concentration.

8. In response to normal blood glucose, the pancreas slows its glucagon output.

Artery

Pancreas

Fat tissue

Skeletal muscle

Liver

Insulin

Glucagon

Glucose

Normal blood glucose

A working body needs carbohydrate fuel to replenish glycogen, and when it runs low, physical activity can seem more difficult. If your workouts seem to drag and never get easier, take a look at your eating pattern. Are your meals regularly timed? Do they provide abundant carbohydrate from nutritious whole foods to fill up glycogen stores so they last through a workout?

Here's a trick: at least an hour before your workout, eat a small snack of about 300 calories of foods rich in complex carbohydrates and drink some extra fluid (see Chapter 10 for ideas). Remember to cut back your intake at other meals by an equivalent amount to prevent unwanted weight gain. The snack provides glucose at a steady rate to spare glycogen, and the fluid helps to maintain hydration.

start now! ⟶ Choose a one-week period and have a healthy carbohydrate-rich snack of about 300 calories, along with a bottle of water, about an hour before you exercise. Be sure to track your diet in Diet & Wellness Plus during this period so that you can accurately determine your total calorie intake. Did you have more energy for exercise after you changed your eating plan?

---

can for their energy needs of the moment. Excess glucose is linked together and stored as glycogen until the muscle and liver stores are full to overflowing with glycogen. Still, the glucose keeps coming.

To handle the excess, body tissues shift to burning more glucose for energy in place of fat. As a result, more fat is left to circulate in the bloodstream until it is picked up by the fatty tissues and stored there. If these measures still do not accommodate all of the incoming glucose, the liver has no choice but to handle the excess because excess glucose left circulating in the blood can harm the tissues.

Carbohydrate Stored as Fat   The liver possesses enzymes to break the extra glucose into smaller molecules, which can then be assembled into durable energy-storage compounds—fatty acids. Newly made fatty acids travel in the blood to the adipose tissues, where they are combined into larger fat molecules and stored. Unlike the liver cells, which store only about 2,000 calories of glycogen, the fat cells of an average-size person store over 70,000 calories of fat, and their capacity to store fat is almost limitless. Moral: you had better play the game if you are going to eat the food. (The Think Fitness feature offers tips to help you play.)

Carbohydrate and Weight Maintenance   A balanced eating pattern that provides the recommended complex carbohydrates can help to control body weight and maintain lean tissue. Bite for bite, such carbohydrate-rich foods contribute less to the body's available energy than do fat-rich foods, and they best support physical activity to promote a lean body. Thus, if you want to stay healthy and remain lean, you should make every effort to follow a calorie-appropriate eating pattern providing 45 to 65 percent of its calories from mostly unrefined sources of complex carbohydrates.

This chapter's Food Feature provides the first set of tools required for the job of choosing such a diet. Once you have learned to identify the food sources of various carbohydrates, you must then set about learning which fats are which (Chapter 5) and how to obtain adequate protein without overdoing it (Chapter 6). By Chapter 9, you can put it all together with the goal of achieving and maintaining a healthy body weight.

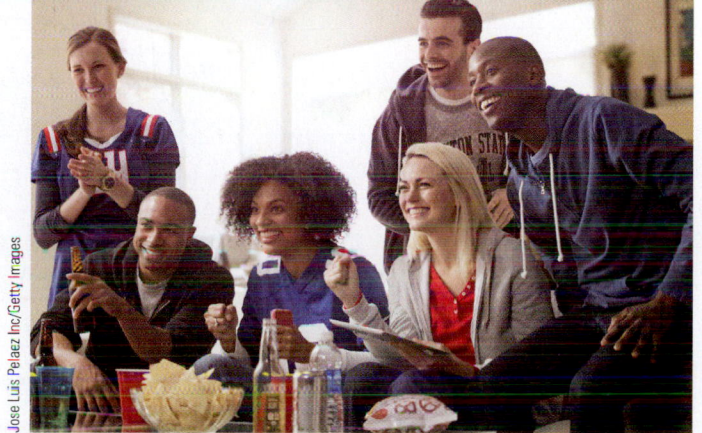

You had better play the game if you are going to eat the food.

KEY POINT

- The liver has the ability to convert glucose into fat, but under normal conditions, most excess glucose is stored as glycogen or used to meet the body's immediate needs for fuel.

The Glycemic Index of Food

Carbohydrate-rich foods vary in the degree to which they elevate both blood glucose and insulin concentrations. A food's average effect in laboratory tests can be ranked on a scale known as the **glycemic index (GI)**. It can then be compared with the score of a standard food, usually glucose, taken by the same person. A food's ranking may surprise you. For example, baked potatoes rank higher than ice cream, partly because ice cream contains sucrose, made of equal parts fructose and glucose. Fructose only slightly raises blood glucose. In contrast, the starch of the potatoes is all glucose. The milk fat of ice cream also slows digestion and glucose absorption, factors that lower its GI ranking. Table 4–8 shows generally where foods have been ranked, but test results often vary widely between laboratories, depending on food ripeness, processing, and seasonal and varietal differences.

In addition to food factors, an individual's own metabolism affects the body's insulin response to carbohydrate. The glycemic response to any one food often varies widely among individual people.

Diabetes and the Glycemic Index The GI, and its mathematical offshoot, **glycemic load (GL)**, may be of interest to people with diabetes who must regulate their blood glucose to protect their health. Overall, however, little difference in blood glucose control or cardiovascular disease risk is reported between low-GI diets and high-GI diets.[24] Researchers often report no effect or sometimes even the opposite effect—unexpectedly *higher* fasting blood glucose concentrations—in people fed a low-GI or -GL diet.[25] Also under study are potential links among the GI and GL of the diet and blood lipids, inflammation, and body weight.[26] However, experimental diets used to test these ideas almost always differ not only in GI or GL but also in fiber,

---

Table 4–8

Glycemic Index of Selected Common Foods

Glycemic Index	Grains	Fruits	Vegetables	Milk Products	Protein Foods[a]	Other
Low	Barley, chapati, corn tortilla, rice noodles, rolled oats, udon noodles, spaghetti	Apple, apple juice, banana, dates, mango, orange, orange juice, peaches (canned), strawberry jam	Carrots, corn	Ice cream, milk, soy milk, yogurt	Legumes	Chocolate
Medium	Brown rice, couscous	Pineapple	Potatoes (French fries), sweet potatoes			Popcorn, potato chips, soft drinks
High	Breads, breakfast cereals, white rice	Watermelon	Potatoes (boiled)			Rice crackers

Note: Using the glucose reference scale, foods are classified as low (55 or less), medium (56 to 69), or high (70 or greater).

[a]Protein foods that contain little or no carbohydrate (such as meats, poultry, fish, and eggs) do not raise blood glucose, and therefore do not have a glycemic index.

Source: Adapted from F. S. Atkinson, K. Foster-Powell, and J. C. Brand-Miller, International tables of glycemic index and glycemic load values: 2008, Diabetes Care 31 (2008): 2281–2283.

---

glycemic index (GI) a ranking of foods according to their potential for raising blood glucose relative to a standard food such as glucose.

glycemic load (GL) a mathematical expression of both the glycemic index and the carbohydrate content of a food, meal, or diet.

Chapter 4 The Carbohydrates: Sugar, Starch, Glycogen, and Fiber

calories, nutrients, phytochemicals, and other confounding factors that often prevent meaningful conclusions.[27]

Nutrition Concerns   Choosing foods by GI alone is often not the best choice nutritionally—chocolate candy, for example, has a lower GI than does nutritious brown rice. For people with diabetes, the glycemic index is not of primary concern.[28] In fact, research suggests it may be unnecessary in the context of a diet that follows the eating patterns of the Dietary Guidelines for Americans, and is based on whole grains, legumes, vegetables, fruits, low-fat protein foods, and milk and milk products.[29]

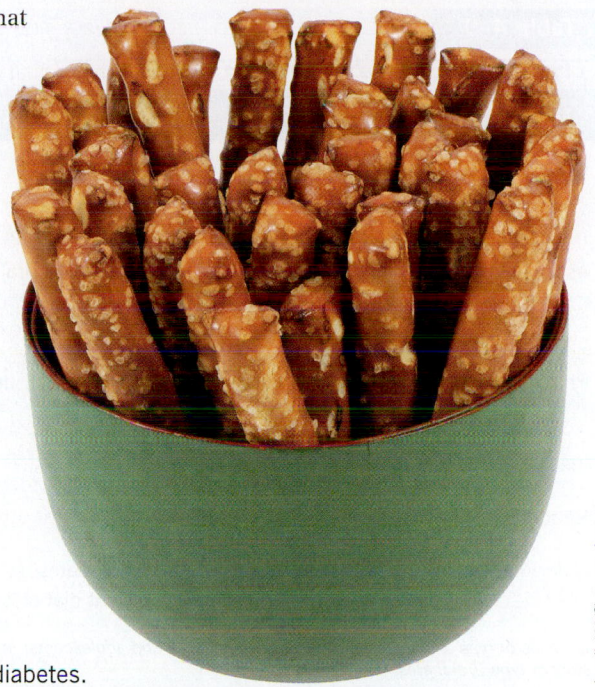

Louella938/Shutterstock.com

KEY POINTS

- The glycemic index reflects the degree to which a food raises blood glucose.
- The concept of good and bad foods based solely on the glycemic response is an oversimplification.

Diabetes

LO 4.5   Summarize the causes, consequences, and management of diabetes.

What happens if the body cannot handle carbohydrates normally? One result is **diabetes**. Diabetes afflicts a rapidly growing number of U.S. adults and has reached record numbers in children. Over 29 million people in the United States now have diabetes.[30] Of these, over 8 million are unaware of it and so go untreated. In addition, well over one-third of U.S. adults, or 86 million more people, have **prediabetes**—their blood glucose is elevated but not yet high enough to be classified as having diabetes.

The Dangers of Diabetes

Diabetes is a leading cause of death in the United States. For people with diabetes, the risk of heart disease, stroke, and dying on any particular day is doubled. Diabetes is also the leading cause of amputations, fatal kidney failure, and permanent blindness. Each year, diabetes costs an estimated $174 billion in U.S. health-care services, disability, lost work, and other costs.

The common forms of diabetes are type 1 and type 2. Both disorders involve abnormalities of insulin and blood glucose, and they share some similar risks to health. As later sections explain, however, type 1 and type 2 diabetes are very different diseases (Table 4–9, p. 142).

Toxicity of Excess Blood Glucose   Chronically elevated blood glucose associated with diabetes alters metabolism in virtually every cell of the body. Some cells convert excess glucose to toxic alcohols, causing the cells to swell. Other cells respond by attaching excess glucose to protein molecules in abnormal ways; these altered proteins cannot function, causing many problems.

Chronic inflammation of body tissues accompanies uncontrolled diabetes and may contribute to eye, kidney, heart, and other associated problems. The structures of the blood vessels and nerves become damaged, leading to loss of circulation and nerve function.

Circulation Problems   Loss of blood flow to the kidneys damages them, often resulting in the need to cleanse the blood by means of kidney **dialysis** or, in later stages, to undergo kidney transplant. Poor circulation also increases the likelihood of infections. With loss of both circulation and nerve function, undetected injury and infection may lead to death of tissue (gangrene), necessitating amputation of the limbs (most often the legs or feet).

diabetes (dye-uh-BEET-eez) metabolic diseases characterized by elevated blood glucose and inadequate or ineffective insulin, which impair a person's ability to regulate blood glucose. The technical name is *diabetes mellitus* (*mellitus* means "honey-sweet" in Latin, referring to sugar in the urine).

prediabetes condition in which blood glucose levels are higher than normal but not high enough to be diagnosed as diabetes; a major risk factor for diabetes and cardiovascular diseases.

dialysis (die-AL-ih-sis) in kidney disease, treatment of the blood to remove toxic substances or metabolic wastes; more properly, *hemodialysis*, meaning "dialysis of the blood."

Table 4–9

Type 1 and Type 2 Diabetes Compared

	Type 1	Type 2
Percentage of cases	5–10%	90–95%
Age of onset	<30 years	>45 years[a]
Associated characteristics	Autoimmune diseases, viral infections, family history	Aging, overweight or obesity, family history, heart disease, elevated blood lipids, hypertension, psychological depression, some medications
Primary problems	Destruction of pancreatic beta cells; insulin deficiency	Insulin resistance, insulin deficiency (relative to needs)
Insulin secretion	Little or none	Varies; may be normal, increased, or decreased
Requires insulin	Always	Sometimes
Older names	Juvenile-onset diabetes Insulin-dependent diabetes mellitus (IDDM)	Adult-onset diabetes Non-insulin-dependent diabetes mellitus (NIDDM)

[a]Incidence of type 2 diabetes is increasing in children and adolescents; in more than 90% of these cases, it is associated with overweight or obesity and a family history of type 2 diabetes.

- Diabetes is a major threat to health and life, and its prevalence is increasing.
- Diabetes involves the body's abnormal handling of glucose and the toxic effects of excess glucose.

Prediabetes and the Importance of Testing

Prediabetes, a fasting blood glucose level just slightly higher than normal, presents few or none of the warning signs of diabetes (see Table 4–10), but tissue damage may progress silently, and type 2 diabetes often soon develops.[31] Of the millions of people in the United States with prediabetes, few are aware of it.

Diagnosis of diabetes or prediabetes can be made using one of several tests, such as a **fasting plasma glucose test** or a nonfasting **A1C test**.[32]** In a fasting plasma glucose test, a clinician draws a patient's blood after a night of fasting to determine whether the blood glucose level falls within the normal range on the day of the test (values are listed in Table 4–11). In a nonfasting A1C test, a blood indicator reveals how well blood glucose has been controlled over the past few months.[33] A registered dietitian nutritionist, a Certified Diabetes Educator, or a physician can help those with prediabetes or diabetes learn to manage their condition.

- Prediabetes silently threatens the health of tens of millions of people in the United States.
- Medical tests can reveal current plasma glucose concentrations and can detect markers of blood glucose control over previous months.

Type 1 Diabetes

Type 1 diabetes is responsible for 5 to 10 percent of diabetes cases. It usually occurs in childhood and adolescence but can occur at any age, even late in life. Its incidence among children and adolescents seems to be on the rise, both in the United States and overseas.[34] Often an **autoimmune disorder** influenced by genetic inheritance, type 1 diabetes arises when the person's own immune system misidentifies the protein insulin as an enemy and attacks the cells of the pancreas that produce it. Soon the

fasting plasma glucose test a blood test that measures the current blood glucose concentration in a person who has not eaten or consumed caloric beverages for at least 8 hours; the test can detect both diabetes and prediabetes. *Plasma* is the fluid part of whole blood.

A1C test a blood test for type 2 diabetes that measures the percentage of hemoglobin (a blood protein) with glucose attached to it. The test reflects blood glucose control over the previous few months. Also called *glycosylated hemoglobin test* or *HbA1C test* (*Hb* stands for *hemoglobin*).

type 1 diabetes the type of diabetes in which the pancreas produces no or very little insulin; often diagnosed in childhood, although some cases arise in adulthood. Formerly called *juvenile-onset* or *insulin-dependent diabetes*.

autoimmune disorder a disease in which the body develops antibodies to its own proteins and then proceeds to destroy cells containing these proteins. Examples are type 1 diabetes and lupus.

**Another test for diabetes is the oral glucose tolerance test.

damaged pancreas no longer produces enough insulin. Then, after each meal, glucose concentration builds up in the blood, while body tissues are simultaneously starving for glucose, a life-threatening situation. The person must receive insulin from an external source to assist the cells in taking up the glucose they need from the bloodstream, which is carrying too much.

Insulin is a protein, and if it were taken orally, the digestive system would digest it. Insulin must therefore be taken as daily injections, inhaled in powder form, or pumped from an insulin pump that delivers it through a tiny tube implanted under the skin. Some insulin pumps also monitor blood glucose and report its levels throughout the day. Fast-acting and long-lasting forms of insulin allow more flexibility in managing meals and treatments, but users must still plan ahead to balance blood insulin and glucose consumption.

Doing so can make a difference to health—those who control their blood glucose suffer fewer cardiovascular and other diseases than those who do not. Experimental treatments such as surgical transplants of insulin-producing pancreatic cells and a vaccine to prevent type 1 diabetes are under development.[35]

Type 2 Diabetes

Recent decades have seen a sharp rise in the rate of the predominant type of diabetes mellitus, **type 2 diabetes** (responsible for 90 to 95 percent of cases) in both adults and children. In type 2 diabetes, body tissues lose their sensitivity to insulin. The insulin-resistant muscle and adipose tissues no longer respond to insulin by increasing their uptake of glucose from the blood. As blood glucose climbs higher, the pancreas compensates by producing larger and larger amounts of insulin. Blood insulin may rise abnormally high—but to no avail. Eventually, the overtaxed cells of the pancreas begin to fail and reduce their insulin output, while blood glucose spins further out of control.

Type 2 Diabetes and Obesity Obesity underlies a great many cases of type 2 diabetes and constitutes a major risk factor for its development. In many people, the greater the degree of body fatness, particularly around the waistline, the more insulin-resistant the cells become, and the higher the blood glucose rises. Even moderate weight gain, particularly among middle-aged people, increases diabetes risk, as do physical inactivity and genetic inheritance.[36]

Exactly how obesity leads to diabetes is a topic of research, but evidence suggests roles for elevated fatty acids in the bloodstream.[37] When normal fat storage sites are full to overflowing with lipid, some excess lipid from the bloodstream may be deposited

Table 4–10

Warning Signs of Diabetes

These signs appear reliably in type 1 diabetes and often in the later stages of type 2 diabetes.

- Excessive urination and thirst
- Glucose in the urine
- Weight loss with nausea, easy tiring, weakness, or irritability
- Cravings for food, especially for sweets
- Frequent infections of the skin, gums, vagina, or urinary tract
- Vision disturbances; blurred vision
- Pain in the legs, feet, or fingers
- Slow healing of cuts and bruises
- Itching
- Drowsiness
- Abnormally high glucose in the blood

Table 4–11

Diabetes Tests

Plasma glucose is measured in milligrams per deciliter (mg/dL). Other tests or repeated testing, may also be used to diagnose diabetes.

Test	Prediabetes	Diabetes
Fasting plasma glucose	100-125 mg/dL	≥126 mg/dL
A1C	5.7–6.4%	≥6.5%

Source: American Diabetes Association Position Statement: Standards of Medical Care in Diabetes—2015, Diabetes Care 38 (2015): S1–S94.

type 2 diabetes the type of diabetes in which the pancreas makes plenty of insulin but the body's cells resist insulin's action; often diagnosed in adulthood. Formerly called *adult-onset* or *non-insulin-dependent diabetes*.

in other tissues, such as the liver and muscle. This fat, or molecules traveling with it, may trigger changes in complex metabolic processes involving inflammation, immune system responses, and insulin signaling within the cells.[38] These disruptions may ultimately foster **insulin resistance** and type 2 diabetes.

Preventing Type 2 Diabetes   Once in the grip of type 2 diabetes, the body struggles to control blood glucose and often fails to stop its damage, even with the best of medical care. Prevention, however, is not only possible but also likely when individuals take action. In research, these three lifestyle factors consistently and dramatically reduce people's risk of developing diabetes:

1. A healthy body weight.
2. A nutritious eating pattern (moderate in calories; low in saturated fat; high in vegetables, legumes, fruit, fish, poultry, and whole grains).
3. Regular physical activity.[39]

Even people with prediabetes or diabetes can often change their fate by losing weight, exercising, choosing a nutritious diet, and, if necessary, faithfully using prescribed medications. It's never too late—even older adults can lower their diabetes risk by changing their lifestyles.

KEY POINT

- Type 2 diabetes risk factors make the disease likely to develop, but prevention is possible.

Medical Nutrition Therapy

Many people with type 2 diabetes urgently need to lose weight because overweight worsens type 2 diabetes and its associated conditions—generally, a loss of 5 to 7 percent of body weight is enough to improve well-being. For some obese people, weight-loss surgery becomes necessary and can often resolve their diabetes, but relapses are common, and surgery imposes serious risks of its own (see Chapter 9).[40] In making treatment decisions, a person-centered approach that respects the individual's needs, preferences, and values often works best.[41]

How Much Carbohydrate Is Best?   Controlling carbohydrate intake plays a central role in controlling blood glucose. A common misconception is that people with diabetes need only to avoid sugary foods, but as far as blood glucose is concerned, the *amount* of carbohydrate often matters more than its *source*.

The amount of daily carbohydrate recommended for people with diabetes varies with an individual's glucose tolerance. Proper timing of carbohydrate intake helps to hold blood glucose levels steady. Eating too much carbohydrate at one time can raise blood glucose too high, whereas eating too little can lead to abnormally low glucose levels (**hypoglycemia**). A low-carbohydrate diet (less than 130 grams of

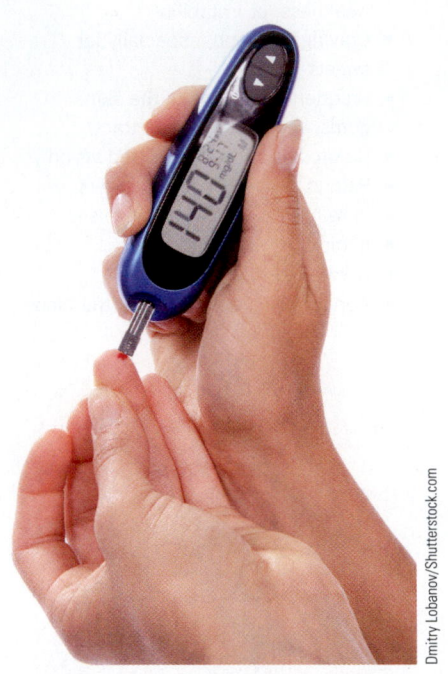

Monitoring is critical to controlling blood glucose.

insulin resistance   a condition in which a normal or high level of circulating insulin produces a less-than-normal response in muscle, liver, and adipose tissues; thought to be a metabolic consequence of obesity.

hypoglycemia   (HIGH-poh-gly-SEE-mee-ah) an abnormally low blood glucose concentration, often accompanied by symptoms such as anxiety, rapid heartbeat, and sweating.

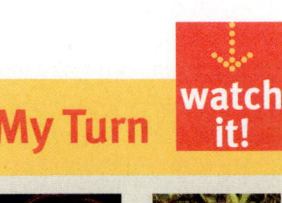

My Turn   **watch it!**

21st-Century Epidemic?

Two young people talk about living with diabetes.

Visit www.cengagebrain.com to access MindTap, a complete digital course that includes these videos and other resources.

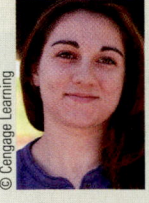

Liz

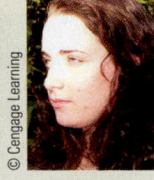

Ariela

Figure 4–14

Sugar Alcohols Replace Added Sugars in Foods

The sugar alcohol erythritol lends a sugary texture and sweetness to this sugar replacement product (Wholesome Zero). The product provides about 1 calorie of energy in a teaspoon serving, but labeling laws specify that less than 5 calories per serving may be listed as "0."

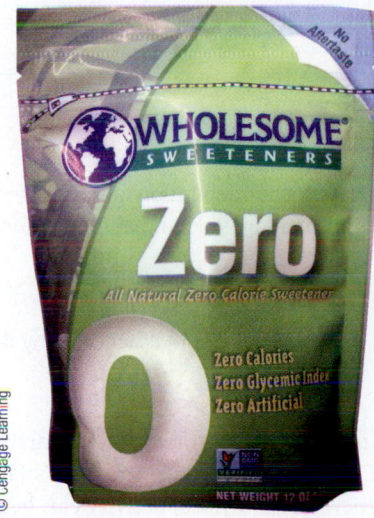

Nutrition Facts		
Serving Size about 1 teaspoon (4g)		
Serving Per Container 57		
Amount Per Serving		
Calories 0 Calories from Fat 0		
		% Daily Vaue
Total Fat 0g		0%
Saturated Fat 0g		0%
Trans Fat 0g		
Cholesterol 0mg		0%
Sodium 0mg		0%
Total Carbohydrate 6g		>2%
Erythritol 6g		>2%
Sugars 0g		
Protein 0g		
*Percent Daily Values are based on a 2,000 calorie diet. • Ingredients: Erythritol, Xylitol		

carbohydrate per day) is not recommended. Instead, an eating pattern that derives carbohydrates from fruit, vegetables, legumes, whole grains, and low-fat milk, spaced throughout the day, best serves the goals of diabetes treatment. Many people with diabetes learn to count their carbohydrate grams with the food list system developed for this purpose (see Appendix D).

Sugar Alcohols and Nonnutritive Sweeteners   Sugar substitutes are often useful to people wishing to control calorie or sugar intakes. Products sweetened with **sugar alcohols**, such as cookies, sugarless gum, hard candies, and jams and jellies, are safe in moderation. Sugar alcohols provide about half the calories of sugars and produce a lower glycemic response. One exception, erythritol, cannot be metabolized by human enzymes and so is calorie-free. The label of Figure 4–14 illustrates that sugar alcohols can replace the sugar in foods, and Table 4–12 names some common sugar alcohols.

Sugar alcohols are safer for teeth than sugars, making them useful in chewing gums, breath mints, toothpaste, and other products that people keep in their mouths for a while. Mouth bacteria rapidly metabolize regular sugars into acids that cause **dental caries**; sugar alcohols resist such metabolism. Side effects such as gas, abdominal discomfort, and diarrhea arise from ingesting large quantities of sugar alcohols.

Noncaloric, **nonnutritive sweeteners** sweeten foods without calories, but people have concerns about their use. Their nature and safety are topics of Chapter 12.

Diet Recommendations in Summary   Effective nutrition therapy can help to stabilize blood glucose, control blood lipids, achieve a healthy body weight, and normalize blood pressure in people with diabetes.[42] For an individualized approach, the person's preferences and cultural patterns should be honored; factors such as insulin use or high blood pressure must be considered. Anyone with diabetes should pay strict attention to the Dietary Guidelines for Americans, particularly concerning

Table 4–12

Sugar Alcohols

These common sugar alcohols may be listed on food labels:

- Erythritol
- Isomalt
- Lactitol
- Maltitol
- Mannitol
- Sorbitol
- Xylitol

sugar alcohols sugarlike compounds in the chemical family *alcohol* derived from fruits or manufactured from sugar dextrose or other carbohydrates; sugar alcohols are absorbed more slowly than sugars, are metabolized differently, and do not elevate the risk of dental caries. Also called *polyols*.

dental caries decay of the teeth (*caries* means "rottenness"). Dental caries are a topic of Chapter 14.

nonnutritive sweeteners sugar substitutes that provide negligible, if any, energy. Also defined in Chapter 12.

intakes of nutrient-dense foods, sodium, added fats, and added sugars. In addition, these characteristics apply:

- Moderate amounts of carbohydrate should be delivered in well-timed meals in amounts sufficient to balance the body's available insulin. (No additional benefit is seen with low-carbohydrate diets.)

- Carbohydrate from controlled portions of whole foods, such as vegetables, fruit, whole grains, legumes, and dairy products, is preferable to sources with added fats, sugars, or sodium. (Avoid sugar-sweetened beverages.)

- Protein should be consumed in adequate amounts. (Excess protein can worsen diabetic kidney disease.)

- Alcohol intake, if any, should be moderate. (Those using insulin or insulin-releasing drugs must take alcohol only with food.)

- Vitamin or mineral supplements are not advised for those without nutrient deficiencies. (Herbal, spice, or other unproven supplements are not recommended.)

A wide range of meal plans can meet these and other recommendations for diabetes. The person at risk for diabetes can do no better than to adopt such a diet long before symptoms appear.

KEY POINT

- Diet plays a central role in controlling diabetes and the illnesses that accompany it.

Physical Activity

The role of regular physical activity in preventing and controlling diabetes, particularly type 2 diabetes, cannot be overstated.[43] Exercise helps reduce the body's fatness and heightens tissue sensitivity to insulin. Increasing physical activity can help to delay onset of type 2 diabetes and to regulate blood glucose in established cases, sometimes to the degree that medication can be reduced or eliminated. People with type 1 diabetes should check with a physician because physical activity can bring on hypoglycemia. Like a juggler who keeps three balls in motion, the person with diabetes must constantly balance three factors—diet, exercise, and medication—to control the blood glucose level.

KEY POINT

- Regular physical activity, in addition to diet and medication, helps to control blood glucose in diabetes.

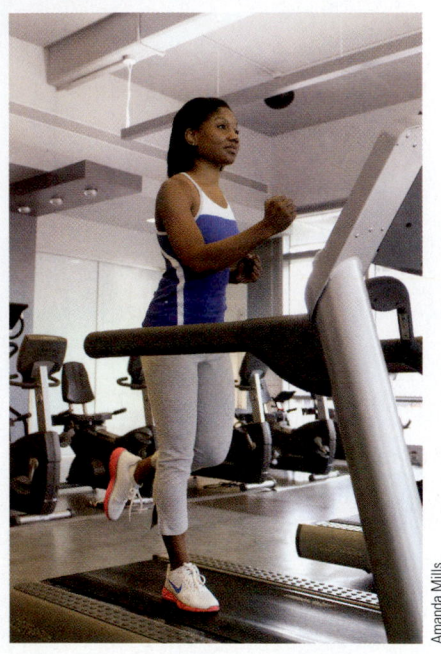

Amanda Mills

Physical activity is a key player in controlling diabetes.

If I Feel Dizzy between Meals, Do I Have Hypoglycemia?

LO 4.6 Discuss hypoglycemia.

In healthy people, blood glucose rises after eating and then gradually falls back into the normal range. The transition occurs without notice. Should blood glucose drop below normal, a person would experience the symptoms of hypoglycemia: weakness, rapid heartbeat, sweating, anxiety, hunger, and trembling. Most commonly, hypoglycemia is a consequence of poorly managed diabetes: too much insulin, strenuous physical activity, inadequate food intake, or illness that causes blood glucose levels to plummet.

Hypoglycemia is rare as a true disease, but many people believe they experience its symptoms at times. Most people who experience hypoglycemia need only adjust their diets by replacing refined carbohydrates with fiber-rich whole-food sources of carbohydrate and eating adequate protein at each meal. In addition, smaller meals eaten more frequently may help. Hypoglycemia caused by certain medications, pancreatic tumors, overuse of insulin, alcohol abuse, uncontrolled diabetes, or other illnesses requires medical intervention.

- In hypoglycemia, blood glucose falls too low; it arises mainly in people with diabetes or other conditions or as a result of medications and is rare among healthy people.

Conclusion

Part of eating right is choosing wisely among the many foods available. Largely without your awareness, the body responds to the carbohydrates supplied by your diet. Now you take the controls by learning how to integrate carbohydrate-rich foods into an eating pattern that meets your body's needs.

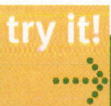

try it!

Food Feature

Finding the Carbohydrates in Foods

LO 4.7   Identify foods that are rich in carbohydrates.

To support optimal health, an eating pattern must supply enough of the right kinds of carbohydrate-rich foods. Dietary recommendations for a health-promoting 2,000-calorie diet suggest that carbohydrates provide in the range of 45 to 65 percent of calories, or total between 225 and 325 grams, each day. This amount more than meets the minimum DRI amount of 130 grams needed to feed the brain and ward off ketosis. People needing more or less energy require proportionately more or less carbohydrate.

If you are curious about your own carbohydrate need, find your DRI estimated energy requirement (see the inside front cover of this text), and multiply by 45 percent to obtain the bottom of your carbohydrate intake range and then by 65 percent for the top; then divide both answers by 4 calories per gram (see the example in the margin).

Breads and cereals, starchy vegetables, fruits, and milk are all good contributors of starch and dilute sugars. Many foods also provide fiber in varying amounts, as Figure 4–15 (p. 148) demonstrates. Concentrated sweets provide sugars but little else, as the last section demonstrates.

Fruits

A fruit portion of ½ cup of juice, a small banana or apple or orange, ½ cup of most canned or fresh fruit, or ¼ cup of dried fruit supplies an average of about 15 grams of carbohydrate, mostly as sugars, including the fruit sugar fructose. Fruits vary greatly in their water and fiber contents and in their sugar concentrations. Juices should contribute no more than one-half of a day's intake of fruit. Except for avocados and olives, which are high in fat, fruits contain insignificant amounts of fat and protein.

Vegetables

Starchy vegetables are major contributors of starch in the diet. Just one small white or sweet potato or ½ cup of cooked dry beans, corn, peas, plantain, or winter squash provides 15 grams of carbohydrate, as much as in a slice of bread, though as a mixture of sugars and starch. One-half cup of carrots, okra, onions, tomatoes, cooked greens, or most other nonstarchy vegetables or a cup of salad greens provides about 5 grams as a mixture of starch and sugars.

Grains

Breads and other starchy foods are famous for their carbohydrate. Nutrition authorities encourage people to reduce intakes of refined grains and to make at least half of the grain choices whole grains. A slice of bread, half an English muffin, a 6-inch tortilla, ⅓ cup of rice or pasta, or ½ cup of cooked cereal provides about 15 grams of carbohydrate, mostly as starch. Ready-to-eat cereals, particularly those that children prefer, can derive over half their weight from added sugars, so consumers must read labels.

Do the Math

The carbohydrate intake recommended in a 2,700-calorie eating pattern ranges between about 300 and 440 grams per day.

Example for 45% of calories in a 2,700-calorie diet:

- 2,700 cal × 0.45 = 1,215 cal
- 1,215 cal ÷ 4 cal/g = 304 g

Example for 65% of calories in a 2,700-calorie diet:

- 2,700 cal × 0.65 = 1,755 cal
- 1,775 cal ÷ 4 cal/g = 439 g

Using the information above, find the carbohydrate range for a 1,600-calorie diet.

Figure 4–15

Fiber in the Food Groups

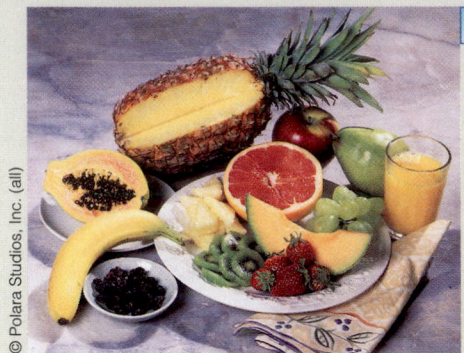

Fruits

Food[a]	Fiber (g)	Food	Fiber (g)
Pear, raw, 1 medium	5	Other berries, raw, 1/2 c	2
Blackberries/raspberries, raw, 1/2 c	4	Peach, raw, 1 medium	2
Prunes, cooked, 1/4 c	4	Strawberries, sliced, 1/2 c	2
Figs, dried, 3	3	Cantaloupe, raw, 1/2 c	1
Apple, 1 medium	3	Cherries, raw, 1/2 c	1
Apricots, raw, 4	3	Fruit cocktail, canned, 1/2 c	1
Banana, raw, 1	3	Peach half, canned	1
Orange, 1 medium	3	Raisins, dry, 1/4 c	1
		Orange juice, 3/4 c	<1

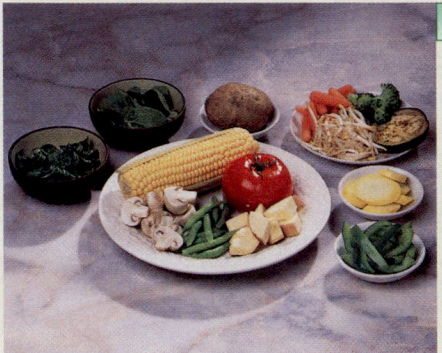

Vegetables

Food	Fiber (g)	Food	Fiber (g)
Baked potato with skin, 1	4	Mashed potatoes, home recipe, 1/2 c	2
Broccoli, chopped, 1/2 c	3	Bell peppers, 1/2 c	1
Brussels sprouts, 1/2 c	3	Broccoli, raw, chopped, 1/2 c	1
Spinach, 1/2 c	3	Carrot juice, 1/2 c	1
Asparagus, 1/2 c	2	Celery, 1/2 c	1
Baked potato, no skin, 1	2	Dill pickle, 1 whole	1
Cabbage, red, 1/2 c	2	Eggplant, 1/2 c	1
Carrots, 1/2 c	2	Lettuce, romaine, 1 c	1
Cauliflower, 1/2 c	2	Onions, 1/2 c	1
Corn, 1/2 c	2	Tomato, raw, 1 medium	1
Green beans, 1/2 c	2	Tomato juice, canned, 3/4 c	1

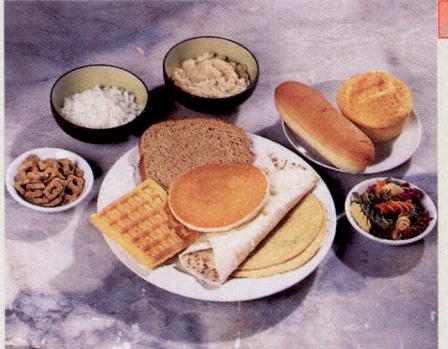

Grains

Food	Fiber[a] (g)	Food	Fiber (g)
100% bran cereal, 1 oz	10	Pumpernickel bread, 1 slice	2
Barley, pearled, 1/2 c	3	Shredded wheat, 1 large biscuit	2
Cheerios, 1 oz	3	Cornflakes, 1 oz	1
Whole-wheat bread, 1 slice	3	Muffin, blueberry, 1	1
Whole-wheat pasta,[b] 1/2 c	3	Puffed wheat, 1 1/2 c	1
Wheat flakes, 1 oz	3	White pasta,[b] 1/2 c	1
Brown rice, 1/2 c	2	Cream of Wheat, 1/2 c	<1
Light rye bread, 1 slice	2	White bread, 1 slice	<1
Muffin, bran, 1 small	2	White rice, 1/2 c	<1
Oatmeal, 1/2 c	2		
Popcorn, 2 c	2		

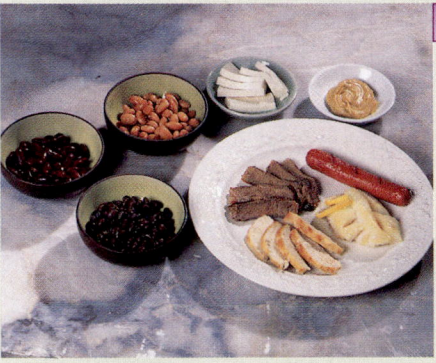

Protein Foods

Food	Fiber (g)	Food	Fiber (g)
Lentils, 1/2 c	8	Soybeans, 1/2 c	5
Kidney beans, 1/2 c	8	Almonds or mixed nuts, 1/4 c	4
Pinto beans, 1/2 c	8	Peanuts, 1/4 c	3
Black beans, 1/2 c	7	Peanut butter, 2 tbs	2
Black-eyed peas, 1/2 c	6	Cashew nuts, 1/4 c	1
Lima beans, 1/2 c	5	Meat, poultry, fish, and eggs	0

[a]All values are for ready-to-eat or cooked foods unless otherwise noted. Fruit values include edible skins. All values are rounded values.
[b]Pasta includes spaghetti noodles, lasagna, and other noodles.

© Polara Studios, Inc. (all)

Most grain choices should also be low in solid fats and added sugar. When extra calories are required to meet energy needs, some selections higher in unsaturated fats (see Chapter 5) and added sugar can supply needed calories and provide pleasure in eating. These choices might include biscuits, cookies, croissants, muffins, ready-to-eat sweetened cereals, and snack crackers.

Protein Foods

With two exceptions, foods of this group provide almost no carbohydrate to the diet. The exceptions are nuts, which provide a little starch and fiber along with their abundant fat, and legumes (dried beans), revered by diet-watchers as high-protein, low-fat sources of both starch and fiber that can reduce feelings of hunger. Just ½ cup of cooked beans, peas, or lentils provides 15 grams of carbohydrate, an amount equaling the richest carbohydrate sources. Among sources of fiber, legumes are peerless, providing as much as 8 grams in ½ cup.

Milk and Milk Products

A cup of milk or plain yogurt is a generous contributor of carbohydrate, donating about 12 grams. Cottage cheese provides about 6 grams of carbohydrate per cup, but most other cheeses contain little, if any, carbohydrate. These foods also contribute high-quality protein (a point in their favor), as well as several important vitamins and minerals. Calcium-fortified soy beverages (soy milk) and soy yogurts approximate the nutrients of milk, providing some amount of added calcium and 14 grams of carbohydrate. Milk and soy milk products vary in fat content, an important consideration in choosing among them. Sweetened milk and soy products contain added sugars.

Butter and cream cheese, though dairy products, are not equivalent to milk because they contain little or no carbohydrate and insignificant amounts of the other nutrients important in milk. They are appropriately associated with the solid fats.

Oils, Solid Fats, and Added Sugars

Oils and solid fats are devoid of carbohydrate, but added sugars provide almost pure carbohydrate. Most people enjoy sweets, so it is important to learn something of their nature and to account for them in an eating pattern. First, the definitions of "sugar" come into play (Table 4–13 defines sugar terms).

Table 4–13
Terms That Describe Sugar

Note: The term *sugars* here refers to all of the monosaccharides and disaccharides. On a label's ingredients list, the term *sugar* means sucrose. See Chapter 12 for terms related to noncaloric, nonnutritive sweeteners.

- **added sugars** sugars and syrups added to a food for any purpose, such as to add sweetness or bulk or to aid in browning (baked goods). Also called carbohydrate sweeteners, they include glucose, fructose, corn syrup, concentrated fruit juice, and other sweet carbohydrates.
- **agave syrup** a carbohydrate-rich sweetener made from a Mexican plant; a higher fructose content gives some agave syrups a greater sweetening power per calorie than sucrose.
- **brown sugar** white sugar with molasses added, 95% pure sucrose.
- **coconut sugar** a granulated sugar composed of sucrose, glucose, and fructose; made by evaporating the sap of flower buds of coconut palm trees.
- **concentrated fruit juice sweetener** a concentrated sugar syrup made from dehydrated, deflavored fruit juice, commonly grape juice; used to sweeten products that can then claim to be "all fruit."
- **confectioner's sugar** finely powdered sucrose, 99.9% pure.
- **corn sweeteners** corn syrup and sugar solutions derived from corn.
- **corn syrup** a syrup, mostly glucose, partly maltose, produced by the action of enzymes on cornstarch. Includes corn syrup solids.
- **dextrose, anhydrous dextrose** forms of glucose.
- **evaporated cane juice** raw sugar from which impurities have been removed.
- **fructose, galactose, glucose** the monosaccharides.
- **granulated sugar** common table sugar, crystalline sucrose, 99.9% pure.
- **high-fructose corn syrup** a commercial sweetener used in many foods, including soft drinks. Composed almost entirely of the monosaccharides fructose and glucose, its sweetness and caloric value are similar to sucrose.
- **honey** a concentrated solution primarily composed of glucose and fructose, produced by enzymatic digestion of the sucrose in nectar by bees.
- **invert sugar** a mixture of glucose and fructose formed by the splitting of sucrose in an industrial process. Sold only in liquid form and sweeter than sucrose, invert sugar forms during certain cooking procedures and works to prevent crystallization of sucrose in soft candies and sweets.
- **lactose, maltose, sucrose** the disaccharides.
- **levulose** an older name for fructose.
- **malt syrup** a sweetener made from sprouted barley.
- **maple syrup** a concentrated solution of sucrose derived from the sap of the sugar maple tree. This sugar was once common but is now usually replaced by sucrose and artificial maple flavoring.
- **molasses** a thick brown syrup left over from the refining of sucrose from sugar cane. The major nutrient in molasses is iron, a contaminant from the machinery used in processing it.
- **naturally occurring sugars** sugars that are not added to a food but are present as its original constituents, such as the sugars of fruit or milk.
- **nectars** concentrated peach nectar, pear nectar, or others.
- **raw sugar** the first crop of crystals harvested during sugar processing. Raw sugar cannot be sold in the United States because it contains too much filth (dirt, insect fragments, and the like). Sugar sold as "raw sugar" is actually evaporated cane juice.
- **turbinado (ter-bih-NOD-oh) sugar** raw sugar from which the filth has been washed; legal to sell in the United States.
- **white sugar** granulated sucrose, produced by dissolving, concentrating, and recrystallizing raw sugar. Also called *table sugar*.

All sugars originally develop by way of photosynthesis in a plant. A sugar molecule inside a grape (one of the **naturally occurring sugars**) is chemically indistinguishable from one extracted from sugar beets, sugar cane, grapes, or corn and added to sweeten strawberry jam. Honey added to food is also an added sugar with similar chemical makeup. All arise naturally and, through processing, are purified of most or all of the original plant material—bees process honey and machines process the other types. The body handles all the sugars in the same way, whatever their source.

Added sugars, when consumed in large amounts, may be linked with health problems (see the Controversy section), and they bring only empty calories into the diet, with no other significant nutrients. Conversely, the naturally occurring sugars of, say, an orange provide calories but also the vitamins, minerals, fiber, and phytochemicals of oranges. Added sugars can contribute to nutrient deficiencies by displacing nutritious food from the diet. Most people can afford only a little added sugar in their diets if they are to meet nutrient needs within calorie limits. The Dietary Guidelines for Americans suggest a limit of about 8 teaspoons of sugar, or almost one soft drink's worth, in a nutrient-dense 2,200-calorie eating pattern. Table 4–14 provides some tips for taking in less added sugar while still enjoying its sweet taste.

The Nature of Sugar

Each teaspoonful of any sweet can be assumed to supply about 16 calories

Table 4–14
Tips for Reducing Intakes of Added Sugars

These tricks can help reduce added sugar intake by changing old habits.

- A good use of sugar is to make nutrient-dense but bland or sharp-tasting foods (such as oatmeal or grapefruit) more palatable. Use the least amount possible to do the job.
- Add sweet spices such as cinnamon, nutmeg, allspice, or clove.
- Add a tiny pinch of salt; it will make food taste sweeter.
- Nonnutritive sweeteners add sweetness without calories. Read about them in Chapter 12.
- Choose fruit for dessert most often.
- Choose smaller portions of cake, cookies, ice cream, other desserts, and candy, or skip them.
- Compare sugar contents of similar foods on their Nutrition Facts panels, and choose those with less sugar.
- Reduce sugar added to recipes or foods at the table by a third—the difference in taste generally isn't noticeable.
- Replace empty-calorie-rich regular sodas, sports drinks, energy drinks, and fruit drinks with water, fat-free milk, 100% fruit juice, or unsweetened tea or coffee.
- Warm up sweet foods before serving (heat enhances sweet tastes).

and 4 grams of carbohydrate. An exception is honey, which packs more calories into each teaspoon because its crystals are dissolved in water; the dry crystals of sugar take up more space. If you use ketchup liberally, remember that each tablespoon of it contains a teaspoon of sugar. And for the soft-drink user, a 12-ounce can of sugar-sweetened cola contains at least 8 teaspoons of added sugar.

What about the nutritional value of a product such as molasses or concentrated fruit juice sweetener compared to white sugar? Molasses contains 1 milligram of iron per tablespoon, so, if used frequently, it can contribute some of this important nutrient. Molasses is less sweet than the other sweeteners, however, so more molasses is needed to provide the same sweetness as sugar. Also, its iron comes from the machinery in which molasses is made and is in the form of an iron salt not easily absorbed by the body.

As for concentrated juice sweeteners, such as the concentrated grape or pear "juice" used to sweeten foods and beverages, these are highly refined and have lost virtually all of the beneficial nutrients and phytochemicals of the original fruit. A child's fruit punch sweetened with grape juice concentrate, for example, may claim to be "100 percent fruit juice" and sounds nutritious but can contain as much sugar as punches sweetened with sucrose or high-fructose corn syrup. No form of sugar, even honey, is any "more healthy" than white sugar, as Table 4–15, page 151, shows.

Finally, enjoy whatever sugar you do eat. Sweetness is one of life's great sensations, so enjoy it in moderation.

Table 4–15

The Empty Calories of Sugar

These data demonstrate the absurdity of trying to rely on any added sugar for nutrient contributions. The 64 calories of honey (1 tablespoon) listed bring 0.1 mg of iron into the diet, but it would take 11,500 calories of honey (180 tablespoons) to provide the needed 18 mg of iron for a young woman. The nutrients of added sugars do not add up as fast as their calories.

Food	Energy (cal)	Protein (g)	Fiber (g)	Calcium (mg)	Iron (mg)	Magnesium (mg)	Potassium (mg)	Zinc (mg)	Vitamin A (µg)	Thiamin (mg)	Riboflavin (mg)	Niacin (mg)	Vitamin B_6 (mg)	Folate (µg)	Vitamin C (mg)
Sugar (1 tbs)	46	0	0	0	0	0	0	0	0	0	0	0	0	0	0
Honey (1 tbs)	64	0	0	1	0.1	0	11	0	0	0	0	0	0	<1	0
Molasses (1 tbs)	55	0	0	42	1.0	50	300	0.1	0	0	0	0.2	0.1	0	0
Concentrated grape or fruit juice sweetener (1 tbs)	30	0	0	0	0	0	0	0	0	0	0	0	0	0	
Jelly (1 tbs)	49	0	0	1	0	1	12	0	0	0	0	0	0	0	<1
Brown sugar (1 tbs)	54	0	0	8	0.2	3	31	0	0	0	0	0	0	0	0
Cola beverage (12 fl oz)	153	0	0	11	0.1	4	4	0	0	0	0	0	0	0	0
Daily Values	2,000	56	25	1,000	18	400	3,500	15	1,000	1.5	1.7	20	2	400	60

Food Feature   151

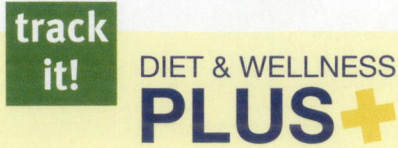

Analyze Your Carbohydrate Intake

The purpose of this chapter's exercise is to help you examine the carbohydrate-rich foods in your diet, compare your intakes with recommendations, and help you obtain the recommended daily intake of carbohydrates and soluble and insoluble fiber.

1. In the D&W+ program, select the Reports tab, and then select the Macronutrient Ranges. Using your three-day diet records, choose Day Two and choose all meals. Did your intake meet the recommendation to consume between 45 and 65 percent of total calories as carbohydrate?

2. Determine the distribution of carbohydrate among the day's foods. Select Reports, then Source Analysis, and then Carbohydrate from the drop-down box. Which foods were the greatest carbohydrate contributors?

3. Did your fiber intake fall within the recommended range (25–35 grams per day)? From the Reports tab, select Intake vs. Goals. Choose Day One, choose all. Did you meet your fiber need?

4. From Reports, select Source Analysis. Using Day Three, choose all meals. Which foods provided the greatest amounts of fiber for the day's intake? If you are short

on fiber, take a look at Figure 4–4 (p. 122), Figure 4–5 (p. 123), and Figure 4–15 (p. 148), and suggest fiber-rich foods to increase your intake of both soluble and insoluble fibers.

5. Whole-grain foods add more than just fiber to the diet. From Track Diet, create a new day (do not alter your three-day record). Enter two food items as a snack: 2.5 cups Froot Loops cereal and 0.5 cup granola (these amounts are about equal in calories). Select Reports, Source Analysis, and the mineral magnesium from the drop-down box. Which was the better magnesium source?

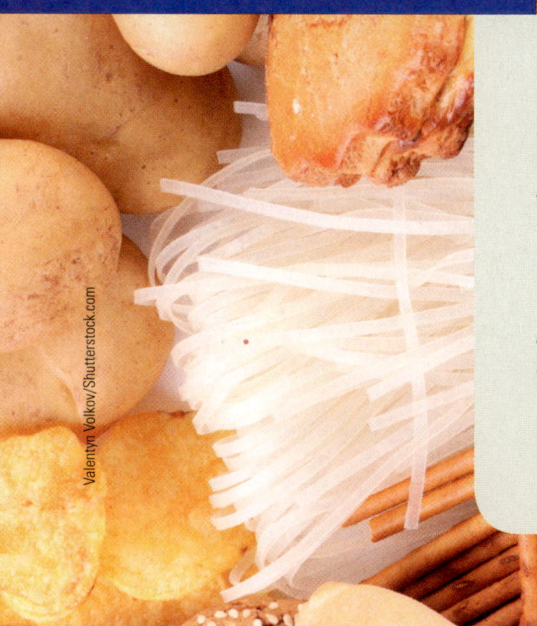

Valentyn Volkov/Shutterstock.com

what did you decide?

Do carbohydrates provide only unneeded calories to the body?

Why do nutrition authorities unanimously recommend whole grains?

Are low-carbohydrate diets the best way to lose weight?

Should people with diabetes eat sugar?

Self Check

1. (LO 4.1) The dietary monosaccharides include _____.
   a. sucrose, glucose, and lactose
   b. fructose, glucose, and galactose
   c. galactose, maltose, and glucose
   d. glycogen, starch, and fiber

2. (LO 4.1) The polysaccharide that helps form the supporting structures of plants is _____.
   a. cellulose
   b. maltose
   c. glycogen
   d. sucrose

3. (LO 4.2) Foods rich in soluble fiber lower blood cholesterol.
   T   F

4. (LO 4.2) The fiber-rich portion of the wheat kernel is the bran layer.
   T   F

5. (LO 4.3) Digestible carbohydrates are absorbed as _____ through the small intestinal wall and are delivered to the liver, which releases _____ into the bloodstream.
   a. disaccharides; sucrose
   b. glucose; glycogen
   c. monosaccharides; glucose
   d. galactose; cellulose

6. (LO 4.3) Around the world, most people are lactose intolerant.
   T   F

7. (LO 4.4) When blood glucose concentration rises, the pancreas secretes _____, and when blood glucose levels fall, the pancreas secretes _____.
   a. glycogen; insulin
   b. insulin; glucagon
   c. glucagon; glycogen
   d. insulin; fructose

8. (LO 4.4) The body's use of fat for fuel without the help of carbohydrate results in the production of _____.
   a. ketone bodies
   b. glucose
   c. starch
   d. galactose

9. (LO 4.5) For people with diabetes, the risk of heart disease, stroke, and dying on any particular day is cut in half.
   T   F

10. (LO 4.5) Type 1 diabetes is most often controlled by successful weight-loss management.
    T   F

11. (LO 4.5) Type 2 diabetes often improves with a diet that is
    a. low in carbohydrates (less than 130 g per day).
    b. as low in fat as possible.
    c. controlled in carbohydrates and calories.
    d. a and b

12. (LO 4.5) For managing type 2 diabetes, regular physical activity can help by redistributing the body's fluids.
    T   F

13. (LO 4.6) Fasting hypoglycemia may be caused by all except
    a. pancreatic tumors.
    b. poorly controlled diabetes.
    c. overuse of alcohol.
    d. lactose intolerance.

14. (LO 4.6) Hypoglycemia as a disease is relatively common.
    T   F

15. (LO 4.7) Protein foods provide almost no carbohydrate to the U.S. diet, with these two exceptions:
    a. chicken and turkey
    b. beef and pork
    c. fish and eggs
    d. nuts and legumes

16. (LO 4.7) Fruit punch sweetened with grape juice concentrate can contain as much sugar as fruit punch sweetened with high-fructose corn syrup.
    T   F

17. (LO 4.8) In the United States, diets high in refined carbohydrate intakes, particularly added sugars from soft drinks, are often associated with increased body fatness.
    T   F

18. (LO 4.8) When added sugar is consumed in excess of calorie need,
    a. it alters blood lipids in potentially harmful ways.
    b. it suppresses the insulin response and so is more fattening.
    c. it provides more calories per gram than fat and so is more fattening.
    d. its metabolism in the body diminishes chronic disease risks.

Answers to these Self Check questions are in Appendix G.

Are Added Sugars "Bad" for You?

LO 4.8   Recognize the effects of added sugars on health.

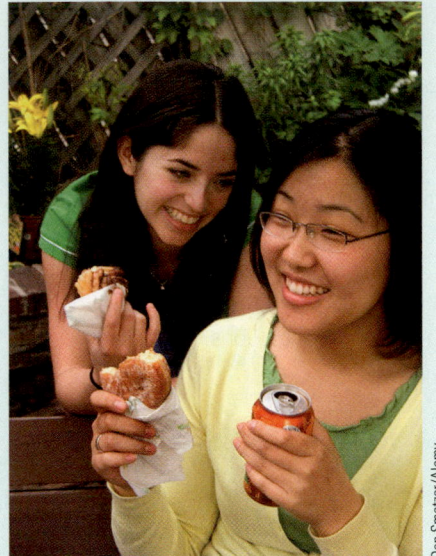

Don Smetzer/Alamy

Authorities around the world urge people to strictly limit their intakes of added sugars.[1]* Does this mean that sugary soft drinks and snack cakes constitute a health hazard? This Controversy addresses some of the accusations made against added sugars and demonstrates a scientific response via peer-reviewed, published research.

Do Added Sugars Cause Obesity?

Over the past several decades, people in the United States have grown dramatically fatter (Figure C4–1). At the same time, their intakes of calories from carbohydrates have jumped from 42 percent in the 1970s to 49 percent today, with much of the additional energy coming from refined grains and

*Reference notes are found in Appendix F.

added sugars.[2] In fact, sugary desserts, such as snack cakes, cookies, and doughnuts, are the number one source of calories for people age 2 years and older.[3] Sugar-sweetened soft drinks follow closely behind for adolescents and young adults.

During the same period, total calorie intakes climbed sharply. The increase, estimated at over 300 calories a day (see Figure C4–2), was more than enough to cause a nationwide weight gain of two pounds *every month*.[†] In addition, as calorie intakes went up, physical activity declined, and most people were not active enough to use up those extra calories.[4] Not surprisingly, then, the average body weight for adults increased significantly at the same time. This is important because excess body weight

[†] *Based on a gain of 1 lb of body weight per 3,500 excess calories; actual amounts vary widely among individuals.*

Figure C4–2

Daily Energy Intake over Time

Carbohydrates, and mostly added sugars, account for almost all of the increase in energy intakes during this period. The recent dip in calorie intakes parallels a slight reduction in added sugars intakes and a slowing of the rate of increase in obesity prevalence.

Figure C4–1

Increases in Adult Body Weight over Time

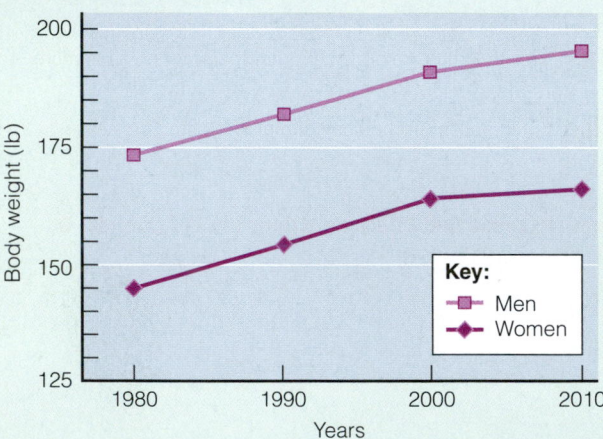

Key:
■ Men
◆ Women

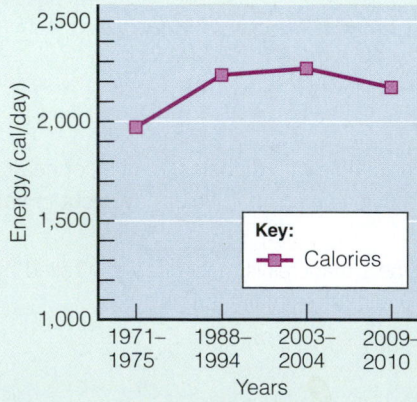

Key:
■ Calories

Source: Anthropometric reference data for children and adults: United States, 2007–2010, National Center for Health Statistics, 2013, available at www.cdc.gov/nchs/data/series/sr_11/sr11_252.pdf.

Source: E. S. Ford and W. H. Dietz, Trends in energy intake among adults in the United States: Findings from NHANES, American Journal of Clinical Nutrition 97 (2013): 848–853.

raises a person's risk of harm from chronic diseases.

Intakes of Added Sugars

In past centuries, the only concentrated sweetener was honey, a rare treat. Today, thanks to farming and manufacturing advances, added sugars of many kinds are commonplace in the U.S. diet, and average sugar consumption weighs in at about double the recommended upper limit.[5] In an encouraging trend, sugar intakes have declined somewhat in recent years, but they are still high. Table C4–1 shows that adolescent boys, the top sugar consumers, take in more than a half cup of added sugars in foods and beverages each day, or almost 90 pounds of sugar per year. At adulthood, intake has dropped a bit, but it still amounts to over 80 pounds a year. Although girls and women take in less than their male counterparts, their sugar intakes also exceed recommendations.

All kinds of sugary foods and beverages taste delicious, cost little money, and are constantly available, making overconsumption extremely likely. More than 95 percent of the sugars in the U.S. diet are now added to foods and beverages by manufacturers (Figure C4–3 depicts sugar sources). In comparison, very little sugar is added from the sugar bowl at home. Because sugar is pre-packaged into foods, most consumers fail to realize just how much added sugar they take in each day.

Sugars or Calories?

In the United States, observational studies often link intakes of added sugars, particularly from soft drinks, with increased body fatness.[6] At the same time, studies of other cultures report an *inverse* relationship between total carbohydrate intake and body weight. For example, the world's leanest peoples are often those eating traditional low-sugar diets that are high in carbohydrate-rich rice or root vegetables, such as Japanese, Chinese, or Africans. When such people abandon their traditional diets in favor of "Western" style foods and beverages, they take in far more sugars and calories, and

their rates of obesity and chronic diseases soar.[7] In addition, as a society gains wealth, its people also consume more meat, grains, and cooking fats, making it difficult to tease apart the effects of sugars from the other dietary constituents in causation of obesity and its associated diseases.

Does Sugar Cause Diabetes?

Diabetes involves blood sugar, so people once believed that eating sugar *caused* diabetes by "overstraining the pancreas." Now we know that this is not the case. Excess body fatness is more closely related to type 2 diabetes than is diet composition.

Still, type 2 diabetes often gains ground in populations as they take in more added sugars. A striking example is the profound increase in diabetes observed among some Native American tribes when added sugars and refined flour replaced traditional roots, gourds, whole corn, and seeds as staple foods in their diets.[8] No simple cause-and-effect conclusion about sugar is possible, however, because at the same time these people ate more processed meats and fats, increased total calorie intakes, and gained body fatness, too.[9] Conversely, groups with an eating pattern of mostly nutrient-dense whole foods are much less likely to develop type 2 diabetes, a finding that has been repeated many times. Overall, when *calorie* intakes do not exceed the daily need, links between sugar intakes and obesity, and between sugar and type 2 diabetes, evaporate.[10]

Table C4–1 Who Takes in the Most Added Sugars? U.S. Average Daily Intakes				
	Age 12–19	Age 20–39	Age 40–59	Age 60+
Male	28 tsp	25 tsp	21 tsp	14 tsp
Female	20 tsp	17 tsp	15 tsp	11 tsp

Sources: NCHS Data Brief 122, May 2013; NCHS Data Brief 87, March 2012.

Figure C4–3
Sources of Added Sugars in the U.S. Diet

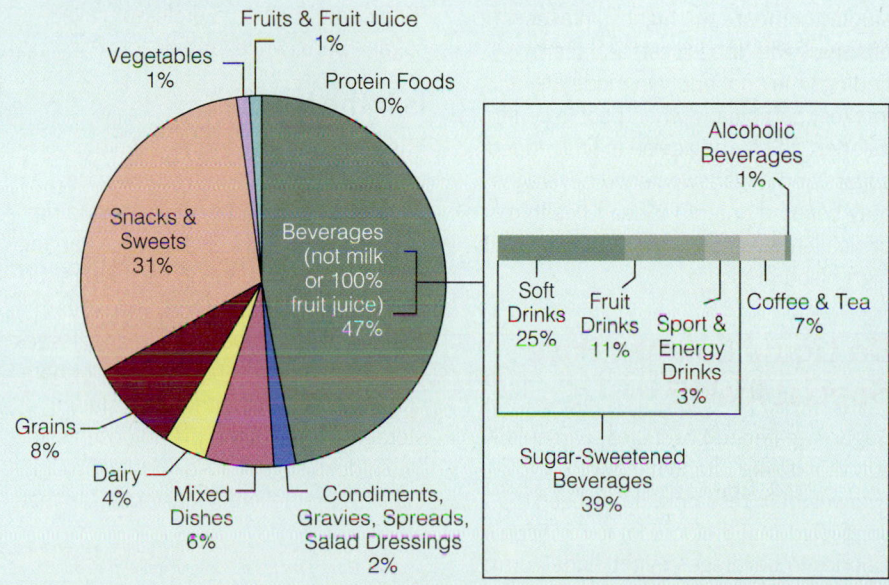

Sources: U.S. Department of Health and Human Services and U.S. Department of Agriculture, 2015–2020 Dietary Guidelines for Americans, 8th edition (2015), available at http://health.gov/dietaryguidelines/2015/guidelines/.

It is impossible to say, given this evidence alone, whether or not sugar causes diabetes—the evidence is observational and therefore circumstantial. The best conclusion may be that maintaining a healthy body weight and eating according to the Dietary Guidelines for Americans reduces diabetes risk; in addition, the person who is physically active, limits alcohol, and doesn't smoke reduces those risks dramatically.[11] Limiting sugar intake is part of a healthy lifestyle.

Do Added Sugars Cause High Blood Pressure?

Added sugars may affect blood pressure, and blood pressure plays a critical role in the health of the heart. Body weight reliably affects blood pressure—the higher the weight, the greater the risk. However, even when body weight was taken into account, a recent systematic review exposed a significant link between higher sugar intakes and higher blood pressure.[12] Another review revealed a trend toward increasing blood pressure with increasing intakes of sugar-sweetened beverages, such as soft drinks, punches, and fruit drinks.[13] More evidence, this time in children, adds to the story: sugar was positively associated with increased blood pressure, even in the very young.[14] However, most studies compare the highest intakes of sugars with the lowest, and their findings may not apply to moderate intakes, particularly when people control calories.[15] Still, the advice to limit added sugars and sugar-sweetened beverages may become urgent for heart health if clinical studies confirm a causal link with high blood pressure.

Do Liquid Calories Pose Special Risks?

Sugar-sweetened beverages, particularly soft drinks, are often linked with overweight in research. It has been suggested that the liquid nature of sugar calories in beverages might elude normal appetite control mechanisms. To test this idea, subjects were given jelly beans (solid sugar) before a meal. At mealtime, they automatically compensated by eating fewer calories of food. When liquid sugar was substituted for the jelly beans, subjects did not compensate—they ate the full meal. These results seem to indicate that liquid sugars may be particularly fattening, but subsequent studies have yielded only mixed results.[16]

It may be that people's expectations modify their intakes: if they do not expect a clear, caloric liquid to make them feel full, that expectation may influence their subsequent eating.[17] In addition, the liquid sugars of fruit punches and soft drinks are easily gulped down—no chewing required. Few people realize that a sugary 16-ounce soft drink can easily deliver 200 calories, and many young people drink several each day. When overweight people substituted water or diet beverages for caloric beverages, they dropped significant amounts of weight with no other dietary changes.[18]

Hints of Metabolic Mayhem

It may be tempting to close the book on added sugars in foods and beverages as just calorie sources—but before you do, consider some metabolic links among added sugars, obesity, and chronic diseases.[19] Such links have held researchers' attention since the mid-20th century, when a professor called sugar, "pure, white, and deadly."[‡]

Is It the Insulin?

The hormone insulin has been a target of investigation in this regard. All digestible carbohydrates, including sugars, elevate blood glucose to varying degrees, and blood glucose triggers the release of insulin into the bloodstream. Then insulin interacts with many tissues to regulate fat metabolism and promote storage of energy nutrients, including storage of body fat in the adipose tissue.

So does sugar cause obesity through insulin's promotion of fat storage? In fact,

[‡] The professor was the late John Yudkin, as reported in G. A. Bray, Fructose: Pure, white, and deadly? Fructose, by any other name, is a health hazard, Journal of Diabetes Science and Technology 4 (2010): 1003–1007.

in healthy, normal-weight people who eat a reasonable diet, insulin works in balance with other hormones and mechanisms to dampen the appetite and maintain a normal body weight. In people with insulin resistance, however, cells fail to respond to insulin's effects, upsetting the normal balance. (Insulin resistance was defined earlier in the chapter.) In healthy people, insulin itself is unlikely to trigger obesity. Other metabolic mechanisms involving the monosaccharide fructose, however, may be in play.

Is It the Fructose?

Fructose makes up about half of all sweet sugars (see Figure C4–4). Some people, particularly young people, consume up to 140 grams of fructose a day, the vast majority coming from added sugars. Note that chemically, most added sugars are similar to each other. The exception is regular corn syrup, made by separating the glucose molecules that compose cornstarch to yield a glucose syrup. High fructose corn syrup (HFCS) is also made from cornstarch, but some of its glucose is chemically converted into fructose to increase its sweet taste.

Glucose and fructose, despite both being monosaccharides, are handled differently in the body.[20] In digestion, the intestine avidly absorbs glucose, but restricts absorption of fructose to half or less. Inside the body, all the cells pick up glucose from the bloodstream and use it as such. In contrast, the liver soaks up almost all the absorbed fructose and quickly converts it into other compounds.

Fructose and Appetite

Glucose and fructose affect appetite differently, too. Glucose and the insulin it triggers help to suppress the appetite. Fructose, in contrast, does not raise blood insulin by much and does not suppress appetite through this mechanism.[21] Also, circulating glucose itself acts on the brain directly in ways that may reduce desire for high-calorie foods. Fructose cannot enter the brain's tissues and so cannot suppress the appetite directly.

Fructose, Sugars, and Fatness

In rodents, a diet high in fructose or sucrose often leads to obesity, diabetes, and blood lipid disturbances. For example, when groups of rats are given solutions of glucose, fructose, or sucrose in addition to their chow, all reliably gain body fatness, but the fructose-fed rats gain the most. Fructose-fed rats also reliably develop insulin resistance and other ills. In studies of people, when calories are held constant and fructose is *substituted* for other carbohydrates, no effect on body weight is observed.[22] However, most people do not reduce calories from other foods when they have a sweet treat, particularly a sugary beverage. The calories of the sugar are extra.

Fructose intake bears a connection with obesity.[23] In experiments, intake of fructose stimulates the liver to synthesize new fat molecules that can be stored in adipose tissue. Whether this occurs in people consuming fructose in a mixed diet is unknown.

Two properties of fructose could also oppose obesity. Recall that some portion of ingested fructose is not absorbed by the intestine, and fructose metabolism by the liver is energy costly. However, these factors clearly do not prevent weight gain from excess added sugars in the diet.

Fructose and Blood Lipids

Added sugars influence the balance between the body's fat-making and fat-clearing mechanisms, a balance that plays critical roles in the development of heart disease.[24] Fructose stimulates the body's fat-making pathways and impairs its fat-clearing pathways in ways that could lead to an unhealthy buildup of blood lipids (triglycerides; see Chapter 5). This effect was first noted in people given large experimental doses of purified fructose—about a third of their daily calories. Few people eat pure fructose, particularly in such large amounts, however. They eat added sugars that contain fructose.

To determine whether added sugars, as sources of fructose, raise blood lipids, researchers reviewed 15 studies of added sugars intake. They observed that people with higher intakes had blood lipid values indicating an increased risk of heart disease.[25] This unhealthy blood lipid shift is evident in both children and adults who receive daily beverages sweetened with HFCS in experiments.[26] It may not take an unrealistic amount of added sugars to cause this effect. As little as the equivalent of one or two HFCS-sweetened soft drinks a day consumed for only two weeks significantly changes blood lipids in ways that may pose risks to the heart and arteries.[27] The greater the intake, the greater the change in blood lipids.

Fructose and Fatty Liver

In animal studies, when fructose enters the liver in large amounts, it produces fat that can accumulate and progress to a condition known as nonalcoholic fatty liver disease (NAFLD). NAFLD ranges in severity from lipid droplets in liver cells to inflammation, cell death, damaging fibrosis, and even liver cancer.[28] NAFLD often marks the onset of type 2 diabetes, and both conditions are increasing among overweight people of all ages. Insulin resistance, known to accompany overweight and foreshadow diabetes, may cause liver tissues to produce excess fats, resulting in NAFLD.[29] Does fructose *cause* NAFLD, as some claim? Scientists have yet to untangle these relationships, but both excess calories and sugary beverage intakes may be culpable.[30]

Moderate amounts of fructose consumed by healthy people in the context of an adequate, calorie-controlled, nutrient-dense diet, are likely to be safe.[31] In people with obesity, insulin resistance, or diabetes, evidence is insufficient to assess the effects of the current average intakes of fructose.

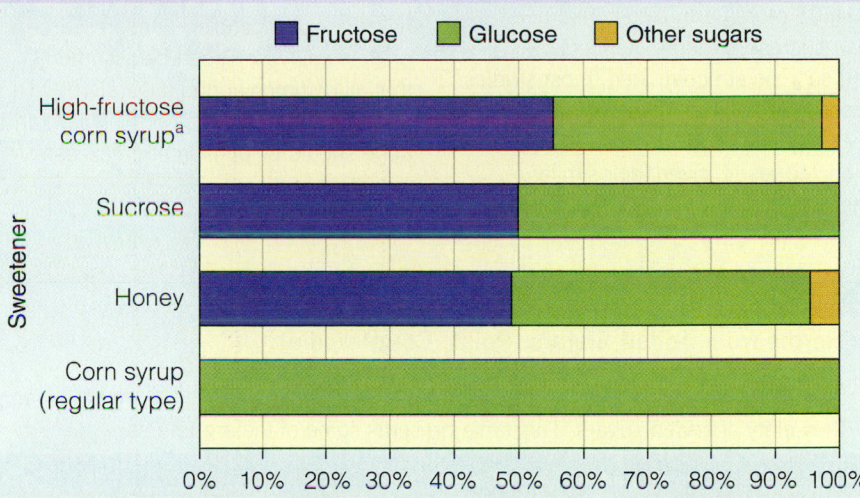

Figure C4–4

Glucose and Fructose in Common Added Sugars

Legend: ■ Fructose ■ Glucose ■ Other sugars

Sweetener (y-axis):
- High-fructose corn syrup[a]
- Sucrose
- Honey
- Corn syrup (regular type)

x-axis: 0% 10% 20% 30% 40% 50% 60% 70% 80% 90% 100%

[a]A typical mixture; others exist.

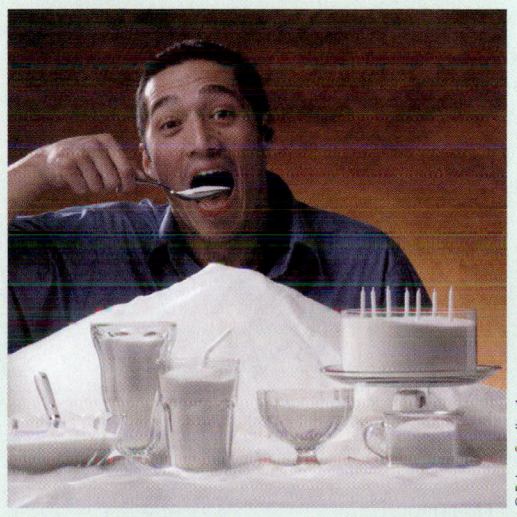

Most people are unaware of how much added sugar they consume.

© Polara Studios, Inc.

Is High-Fructose Corn Syrup Hazardous?

Is HFCS more harmful to consumers than sucrose? When the effects of HFCS and sucrose are compared, most studies observe virtually identical metabolic effects of HFCS and sucrose—an expected result, given their similar chemical makeup. The 2015 Dietary Guidelines committee concludes that U.S. intakes of all types of added sugars are too high, and are increasing health risks for many people.[32] Until research proves otherwise, it can be assumed that all common added sugars are similar from the body's point of view, and none should be consumed in excess of recommendations.

Conclusion

Investigation into the potential health effects of carbohydrates is ongoing. The idea that complex problems, such as obesity or diabetes, might be easily resolved by removing a single ingredient, such as added sugars, from the diet is inviting but simplistic. Table C4–2 provides a sampling of the

---

Table C4–2

Harms from Added Sugars: Point, Counterpoint

Scientists, politicians, food and beverage manufacturers, sugar industry representatives, and others debate issues surrounding the safety of added sugars. This table presents some of the arguments.

Point: Added Sugars Cause Harm	Counterpoint: Added Sugars Are Safe
1. *Increased obesity risk.* Obesity rates are growing rapidly throughout the world. This trend parallels dramatic increases in world intakes of added sugars.	1. *Correlation, not cause.* World meat, oil, and grain intakes have also increased. It could be calories or another factor causing obesity, not sugars.
2. *Sugars and gain of body weight.* When sugars are added to the diet, they appear to cause weight gain, particularly in the abdomen.	2. *Caloric substitution, not addition.* When sugars replace other calorie sources instead of being added to the diet, no effect on weight is observed; excess calories from any source cause weight gain.
3. *Dental caries.* No doubt remains that added sugars cause dental caries, particularly when consumed in excess of 10% of calories.	3. *Dental caries.* True, added sugars can cause dental caries, but this harm can be minimized by brushing the teeth after consuming sugary foods and drinking fluoridated water.
4. *Less satiety value.* Fructose fails to trigger the body's appetite control mechanisms, but glucose suppresses the appetite.	4. *No real-life application.* People rarely consume isolated fructose or glucose. Most sugars are half glucose.
5. *Increased disease risks.* In populations, greater intakes of added sugars correlate with higher rates of metabolic diseases, such as diabetes, heart disease, high blood pressure, metabolic syndrome, and fatty liver.	5. *Correlation, not cause.* Population studies can reveal associations, but not causes. Some other factor, such as obesity or excess calorie intakes, may be causing these ills, not added sugars.
6. *Metabolic disturbances.* Fructose, in large quantities, has negative effects on lipid and glucose metabolism, causes fatty liver disease, and has other damaging effects.	6. *Safe moderate intakes.* Agree, but fructose in small amounts is harmless to health.
7. *Fat deposits in tissues.* Fructose, but not glucose, causes increased fat deposits in the abdomen, liver, and muscles.	7. *No real-life application.* Few people consume isolated fructose or glucose.
8. *Nutrient lack.* Sugar provides only empty calories, displacing nutritious foods and beverages from the diet and increasing the risk of nutrient deficiencies.	8. *Deficiency diseases rare.* Nutrient deficiency diseases are not common in the United States; even many sugary foods and beverages are fortified with certain vitamins and minerals.
9. *Too much sugar.* U.S. added-sugars intakes exceed most guidelines, particularly among young people.	9. *Too much sugar.* Average U.S. intakes have leveled off in the past decade, but experts agree that intakes are too high.

Sources: Point: World Health Organization, *Guideline: Sugars Intake for Adults and Children* (Geneva: World Health Organization, 2015), available at http://who.int/nutrition/publications/guidelines/sugars_intake/en/; USDA, *Scientific Report of the 2015 Dietary Guidelines Advisory Committee* (2015): D-6, 20–23, available at www.health.gov; G. A. Bray and B. M. Popkin, Dietary sugar and body weight: Have we reached a crisis in the epidemic of obesity and diabetes? Health be damned! Pour on the sugar, *Diabetes Care* 37 (2014): 950–956; G. A. Bray, Energy and fructose from beverages sweetened with sugar or high-fructose corn syrup pose a health risk for some people, *Advances in Nutrition* 4 (2013): 220–225; R. H. Lustig, Fructose: It's "alcohol without the buzz," *Advances in Nutrition* 4 (2013): 226–235; A. Rebollo and coauthors, Way back for fructose and liver metabolism: Bench side to molecular insights, *World Journal of Gastroenterology* 18 (2012): 6552–6559. *Counterpoint:* J. M. Rippe, The metabolic and endocrine response and health implications of consuming sugar-sweetened beverages: Findings from recent randomized controlled trials, *Advances in Nutrition* 4 (2013): 677–686; J. S. White, Challenging the fructose hypothesis: New perspectives on fructose consumption and metabolism, *Advances in Nutrition* 4 (2013): 246–256.

Read about nonnutritive sweeteners and other sugar replacers in **Chapter 12**.

ongoing scientific debates about the health effects of added sugars.

What is clear is that the *source* of sugars matters to disease risks. Fruits and vegetables package their naturally occurring sugars with fiber, vitamins, minerals, and protective phytochemicals. Any advice to eliminate fruits and vegetables from the diet may harm otherwise healthy people and should be ignored. In fact, for optimal health, most people need to seek out more fruits and vegetables to meet the recommendations of the Dietary Guidelines for Americans.

The pleasure of sweet foods and beverages is part of the enjoyment of life. Just remember to keep them in their place—as occasional treats in the context of a nutritious diet, not as staple foods or drinks at every meal.

Critical Thinking

1. This controversy addresses accusations launched against sugars in foods and beverages as causes of health problems. Break into groups of five. Each person in the group takes one accusation from the list below and presents a one-minute argument in support of the accuracy of that accusation. When each person has completed his or her argument, vote as a group to determine which is most likely to cause health problems.

   - Added sugars are making us fat.
   - Added sugars cause diabetes.
   - Added sugars cause obesity and illness.
   - High-fructose corn syrup harms health.
   - Blood insulin is to blame.

2. Recommendations about carbohydrate intake can seem to be contradictory. On one hand, it is recommended that the bulk of the diet be carbohydrates (fruit, vegetables, and whole grains), yet some research indicates that certain carbohydrates may be bad for you. Explain this discrepancy in three paragraphs. Use one paragraph to explain why the bulk of the diet should be carbohydrates, including a description of the type of foods that should be eaten. The second paragraph should explain in detail why carbohydrates can be bad for you (give at least three examples). Finally, use the third paragraph to summarize how carbohydrates should be consumed in a way that makes them part of a healthy diet.

5

The Lipids: Fats, Oils, Phospholipids, and Sterols

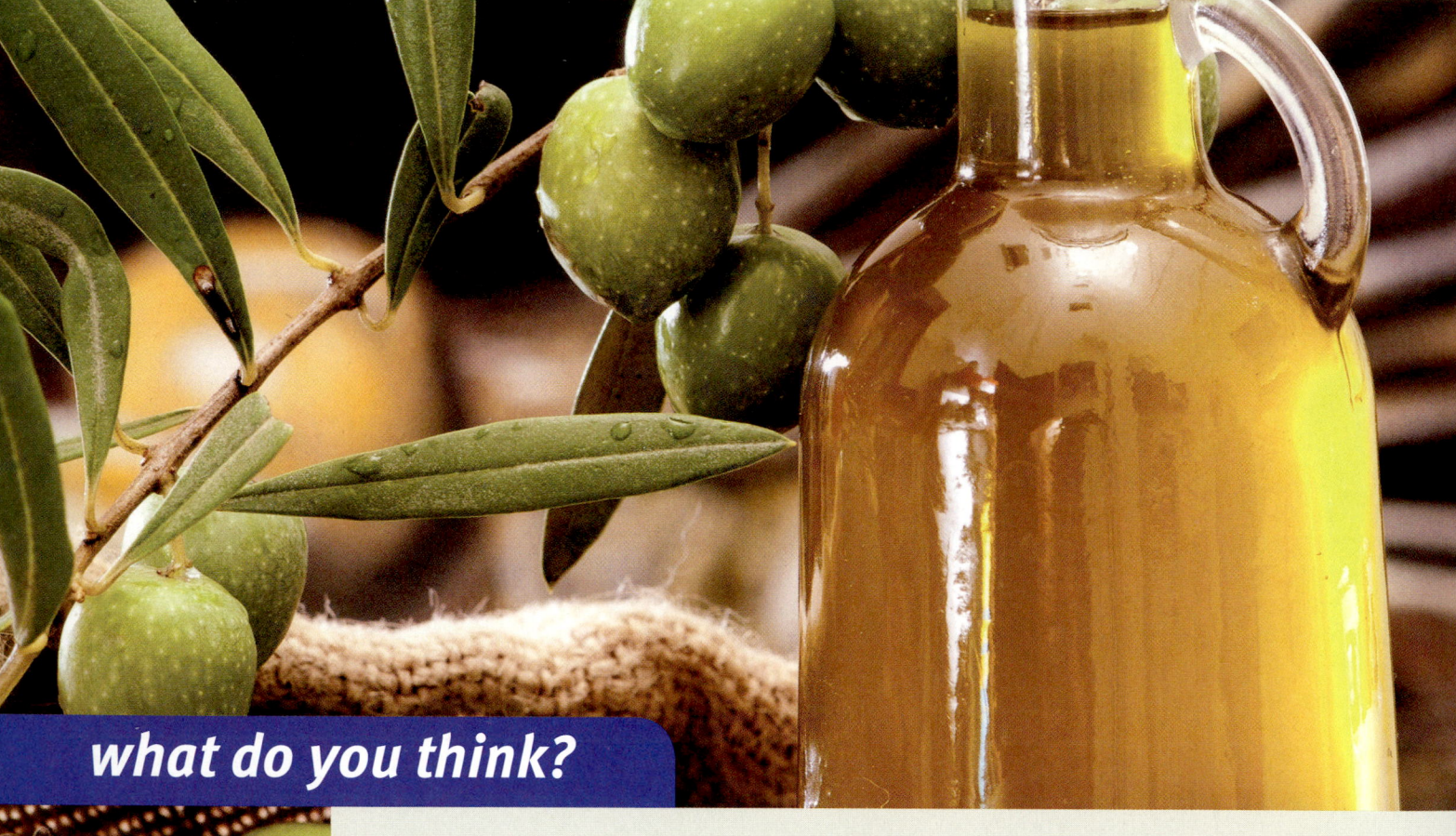

what do you think?

Are **fats** unhealthy food constituents that are best eliminated from the diet?

What are the differences between **"bad"** and **"good" cholesterol**?

Why is choosing **fish** recommended in a healthy diet?

If you trim all **visible fats** from foods, will your diet meet lipid recommendations?

Learning Objectives

After completing this chapter, you should be able to accomplish the following:

LO 5.1 Explain the usefulness of lipids in the body and in food.

LO 5.2 Compare the physical and chemical properties and the functions of the three categories of lipids.

LO 5.3 Explain the processes of digestion, absorption, and transportation of lipids in the body.

LO 5.4 Discuss how fats are stored and used by the body.

LO 5.5 State the health implications of blood lipoproteins and dietary fats.

LO 5.6 Summarize the functions of essential fatty acids.

LO 5.7 Outline the process of hydrogenation and its effects on health.

LO 5.8 Discuss the sources of fats among the food groups.

LO 5.9 Identify the ways to reduce solid fats in an average diet.

LO 5.10 Discuss both sides of the scientific debate about current lipid guidelines.

Your bill from a medical laboratory reads "Blood **lipid** profile—$250." A health-care provider reports, "Your blood **cholesterol** is high." Your physician advises, "You must cut down on the saturated **fats** in your diet and replace them with **oils** to lower your risk of **cardiovascular disease (CVD)**." Blood lipids, cholesterol, saturated fats, and oils—what are they, and how do they relate to health?

No doubt you are expecting to hear that fats have the potential to harm your health, but lipids are also valuable. In fact, lipids are absolutely necessary, and the diet recommended for health is by no means a "no-fat" diet. Luckily, at least traces of fats and oils are present in almost all foods, so you needn't make an effort to eat any extra. The trick is to choose the right ones.

Introducing the Lipids

LO 5.1 Explain the usefulness of lipids in the body and in food.

The lipids in foods and in the human body, though many in number and diverse in function, generally fall into three classes. About 95 percent are **triglycerides**. The other major classes of the lipid family are the **phospholipids** (of which **lecithin** is one) and the **sterols** (cholesterol is the best known of these). Some of these names may sound unfamiliar, but most people will recognize at least a few functions of lipids in the body and in the foods that are listed in Table 5–1 (p. 162). More details about each class of lipids follow later.

How Are Fats Useful to the Body?

When people speak of fat, they are usually talking about triglycerides. The term *fat* is more familiar, though, and we will use it in this discussion.

Fuel Stores Fat provides the majority of the energy needed to perform much of the body's muscular work. Fat is also the body's chief storage form for the energy from food eaten in excess of need. The storage of fat is a valuable survival mechanism for people who live a feast-or-famine existence: stored during times of plenty, fat enables them to remain alive during times of famine.

Most body cells can store only limited fat, but some cells are specialized for fat storage. These fat cells seem able to expand almost indefinitely—the more fat they store, the larger they grow. An obese person's fat cells may be many times the size of a thin person's. Far from being a collection of inert sacks of fat, adipose (fat) tissue secretes hormones that help to regulate appetite and influence other body functions in ways critical to health. A fat cell is shown in Figure 5–1 (p. 163).

lipid (LIP-id) a family of organic (carbon-containing) compounds soluble in organic solvents but not in water. Lipids include triglycerides (fats and oils), phospholipids, and sterols.

cholesterol (koh-LESS-ter-all) a member of the group of lipids known as sterols; a soft, waxy substance made in the body for a variety of purposes and also found in animal-derived foods.

fats lipids that are solid at room temperature (70°F or 21°C).

oils lipids that are liquid at room temperature (70°F or 21°C).

cardiovascular disease (CVD) disease of the heart and blood vessels; disease of the arteries of the heart is called *coronary heart disease (CHD)*. Also defined in Chapter 11.

triglycerides (try-GLISS-er-ides) one of the three main classes of dietary lipids and the chief form of fat in foods and in the human body. A triglyceride is made up of three units of fatty acids and one unit of glycerol (*fatty acids* and *glycerol* are defined later). In research, triglycerides are often called *triacylglycerols* (try-ay-seal-GLISS-er-ols).

phospholipids (FOSS-foh-LIP-ids) one of the three main classes of dietary lipids. These lipids are similar to triglycerides, but each has a phosphorus-containing acid in place of one of the fatty acids. Phospholipids are present in all cell membranes.

lecithin (LESS-ih-thin) a phospholipid manufactured by the liver and also found in many foods; a major constituent of cell membranes.

sterols (STEER-alls) one of the three main classes of dietary lipids. Sterols have a structure similar to that of cholesterol.

Table 5–1
The Usefulness of Fats

Fats in the Body	Fats in Food
■ *Energy fuel*. Fats provide 80 to 90 percent of the resting body's energy and much of the energy used to fuel muscular work. ■ *Energy stores*. Fats are the body's chief form of stored energy. ■ *Emergency reserve*. Fats serve as an emergency fuel supply in times of illness and diminished food intake. ■ *Padding*. Fats protect the internal organs from shock, cushioning them with fat pads inside the body cavity. ■ *Insulation*. Fats insulate against temperature extremes by forming a fat layer under the skin. ■ *Cell membranes*. Fats form the major material of cell membranes. ■ *Raw materials*. Lipids are converted to other compounds, such as hormones, bile, and vitamin D, as needed.	■ *Nutrients*. Food fats provide essential fatty acids, fat-soluble vitamins, and other needed compounds. ■ *Transport*. Fats carry fat-soluble vitamins A, D, E, and K along with some phytochemicals and assist in their absorption. ■ *Energy*. Food fats provide a concentrated energy source. ■ *Sensory appeal*. Fats contribute to the taste and smell of foods. ■ *Appetite*. Fats stimulate the appetite. ■ *Texture*. Fats make fried foods crisp and other foods tender. ■ *Satiety*. Fats contribute to feelings of fullness.

Efficiency of Fat Stores   You may be wondering why the carbohydrate glucose is not the body's major form of stored energy. As mentioned in Chapter 4, glucose is stored in the form of glycogen. Because glycogen holds a great deal of water, it is quite bulky and heavy, and the body cannot store enough to provide energy for very long. Fats, however, pack tightly together without water and can store much more energy in a small space. Gram for gram, fats provide more than twice the energy of carbohydrate or protein, making fat the most efficient storage form of energy. The body fat found on a normal-weight person contains more than enough energy to fuel an entire marathon run or to battle disease, should the person become ill and stop eating for a while.

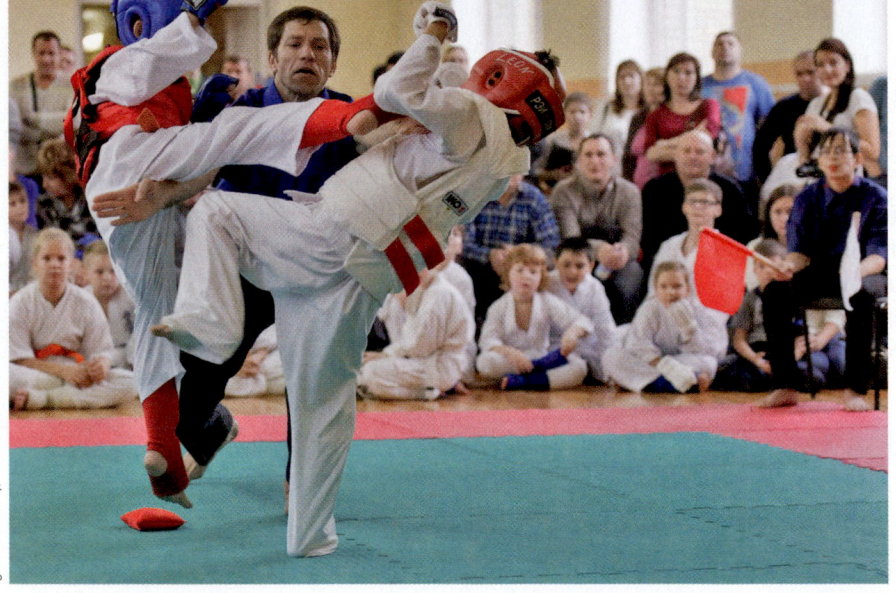

Igor Simanovskiy/Shutterstock.com

Internal fat pads help to cushion vital organs from shock.

Cushions, Climate, and Cell Membranes
Fat serves many other purposes in the body. Pads of fat surrounding the vital internal organs serve as shock absorbers. Thanks to these fat pads, you can play sports or ride a motorcycle for many hours with no serious internal injuries. A fat blanket under the skin also insulates the body from extremes of temperature, thus assisting with internal climate control. Lipids also play critical roles in all of the body's cells as part of their surrounding envelopes, the cell membranes.

Transport and Raw Material   Lipids move around the body in association with other lipids, as described in later sections. Once a lipid arrives at its destination, it may serve as raw material for making any of a number of needed products, such as vitamin D, which helps build and maintain the bones, or bile, which assists in digestion, or lipid hormones, which regulate tissue functions.

KEY POINT

■ Lipids provide and store energy, cushion vital organs, insulate against temperature extremes, form cell membranes, transport fat-soluble substances, and serve as raw materials.

Figure 5–1

A Fat Cell

Within the fat cell, lipid is stored in a droplet. This droplet can greatly enlarge, and the fat cell membrane will expand to accommodate its swollen contents. More about fat tissue (also called *adipose tissue*) and body functions in Chapter 9.

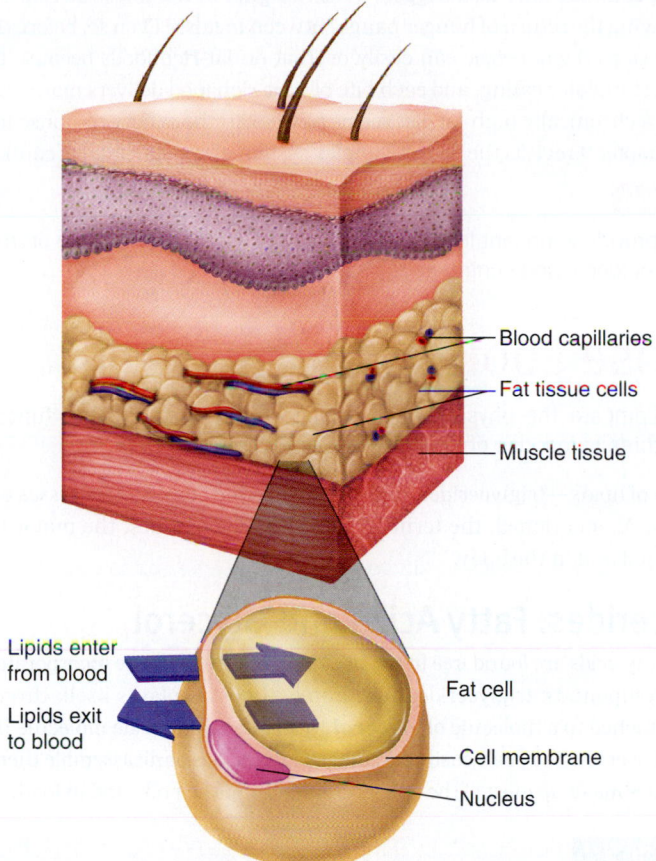

Blood capillaries

Fat tissue cells

Muscle tissue

Lipids enter from blood

Lipids exit to blood

Fat cell

Cell membrane

Nucleus

How Are Fats Useful in Food?

Fats in foods are valuable in many ways. They provide concentrated energy and needed substances to the body, and they are notoriously tempting to the palate.

Concentrated Calorie Source Energy-dense fats are uniquely valuable in many situations. A hunter or hiker must consume a large amount of food energy to travel long distances or to survive in intensely cold weather. An athlete must meet often enormous energy needs to avoid weight loss that could impair performance. As Figure 5–2 (p. 164) demonstrates, for such a person fat-rich foods most efficiently provide the needed energy in the smallest package. But for a person who is not expending much energy in physical work, those same high-fat foods may deliver many unneeded calories in only a few bites.

Fat-Soluble Nutrients and Their Absorption Some essential nutrients are lipid in nature and therefore soluble in fat. They often occur in foods that contain fat, and some amount of fat in the diet is necessary for their absorption. These nutrients are the fat-soluble vitamins: A, D, E, and K. Other lipid nutrients are **fatty acids** themselves, including the **essential fatty acids**. Fat also aids in the absorption of some phytochemicals, plant constituents that may be of benefit to health.

Sensory Qualities People naturally like high-fat foods. Fat carries with it many dissolved compounds that give foods enticing aromas and flavors, such as the aroma of frying bacon or French fries. In fact, when a sick person refuses food, dietitians offer foods flavored with some fat to spark the appetite and tempt that person to eat

Do the Math

Fats are energy-dense nutrients:

- 1 g fat = 9 cal
- 1 g carbohydrate = 4 cal
- 1 g protein = 4 cal

Following the general formula given on page 34, find the percentage of calories from fat in a day's meals providing 1,950 calories and 80 g fat.

fatty acids organic acids composed of carbon chains of various lengths. Each fatty acid has an acid end and hydrogens attached to all of the carbon atoms of the chain.

essential fatty acids fatty acids that the body needs but cannot make and so must be obtained from the diet.

Figure 5-2

Two Lunches

Both lunches contain the same number of calories, but the fat-rich lunch takes up less space and weighs less.

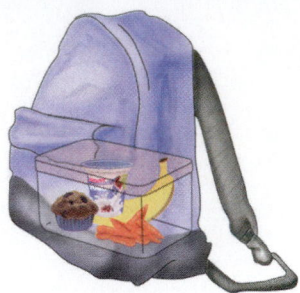

Carbohydrate-rich lunch
1 low-fat muffin
1 banana
2 oz carrot sticks
8 oz fruit yogurt

calories = 550
weight (g) = 500

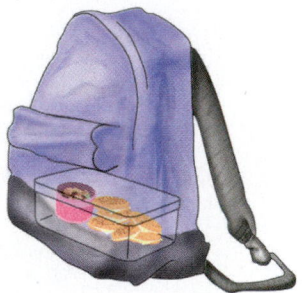

Fat-rich lunch
6 butter-style crackers
1½ oz American cheese
2 oz trail mix with candy

calories = 550
weight (g) = 115

again. Fat also lends crispness to fried foods and tenderness to foods such as meats and baked goods. Around the world, as fats becomes less expensive and more available in a given food supply, people consistently choose fatty foods more often.

A Role in Satiety Fat also contributes to **satiety**, the satisfaction of feeling full after a meal.[1*] The fat of swallowed food triggers a series of physiological events that slows down the movement of food through the digestive tract and eventually promotes satiety. In addition, a common fatty acid triggers a nerve signal in the intestine that travels to the brain, delaying the return of hunger pangs between meals.[2†] Even so, before the sensation of fullness stops them, people can easily overeat on fat-rich foods because the delicious taste of fat stimulates eating, and each bite of a fat-rich food delivers many calories. Also, over time, a chronically high-fat diet seems to weaken the satiety response to fat, at least in rats.[3] Chapter 9 revisits the body's complex system of appetite and its control.

KEY POINT

- Lipids provide abundant food energy in a small package, enhance aromas and flavors of foods, and contribute to satiety.

A Close Look at Lipids

LO 5.2 Compare the physical and chemical properties and the functions of the three categories of lipids.

Each class of lipids—triglycerides, phospholipids, and sterols—possesses unique characteristics. As mentioned, the term *fat* refers to triglycerides, the major form of lipid found in food and in the body.

Triglycerides: Fatty Acids and Glycerol

Very few fatty acids are found free in the body or in foods; most are incorporated into large, complex compounds: triglycerides. The name almost explains itself: three fatty acids (*tri*) are attached to a molecule of **glycerol** to form a triglyceride molecule (Figure 5–3). Tissues all over the body can easily assemble triglycerides or disassemble them as needed. Triglycerides make up most of the lipid present both in the body and in food.

Figure 5-3

Triglyceride Formation

Glycerol, a small, water-soluble carbohydrate derivative, plus three fatty acids equals a triglyceride.

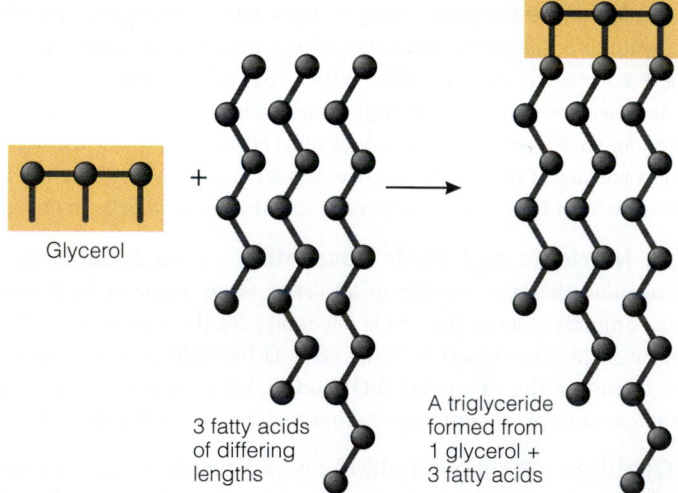

Glycerol

3 fatty acids of differing lengths

A triglyceride formed from 1 glycerol + 3 fatty acids

satiety (sat-EYE-uh-tee) the feeling of fullness or satisfaction that people experience after meals.

glycerol (GLISS-er-all) an organic compound, three carbons long, of interest here because it serves as the backbone for triglycerides.

*Reference notes are found in Appendix F.
†The fatty acid that forms this hunger-suppressing compound is oleic acid.

Fatty acids can differ from one another in two ways: in chain length and in degree of saturation (explained next). Triglycerides usually include mixtures of various fatty acids. Depending on which fatty acids are incorporated into a triglyceride, the resulting fat will be softer or harder at room temperature. Triglycerides containing mostly the shorter-chain fatty acids or the more unsaturated ones are softer and melt more readily at lower temperatures.

Each species of animal (including people) makes its own characteristic kinds of triglycerides, a function governed by genetics. Fats in the diet, though, can affect the types of triglycerides made because dietary fatty acids are often incorporated into triglycerides in the body. For example, many animals raised for food can be fed diets containing specific triglycerides to give the meat the types of fats that consumers demand.

> More details about lipid chemical structures are found in **Appendix I.**

KEY POINTS

- The body combines three fatty acids with one glycerol to make a triglyceride, its storage form of fat.
- Fatty acids in food influence the composition of fats in the body.

Saturated vs. Unsaturated Fatty Acids

Saturation refers to whether or not a fatty acid chain is holding all of the hydrogen atoms it can hold. If every available bond from the carbons is holding a hydrogen, the chain forms a **saturated fatty acid**; it is filled to capacity with hydrogen. The zigzag structure on the left in Figure 5–4 represents a saturated fatty acid.

Saturation of Fatty Acids Sometimes, especially in the fatty acids of plants and fish, the chain has a place where hydrogens are missing: an "empty spot," or **point of unsaturation**.[‡] A fatty acid carbon chain that possesses one or more points

---

Figure 5–4

Three Types of Fatty Acids

The more carbon atoms in a fatty acid, the longer it is. The more hydrogen atoms attached to those carbons, the more saturated the fatty acid is.

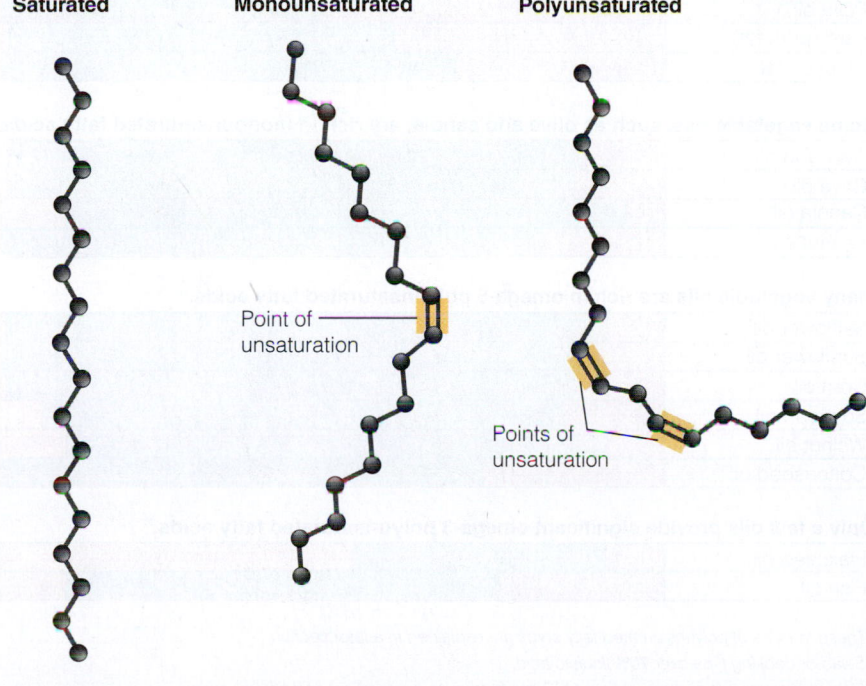

Saturated   **Monounsaturated**   **Polyunsaturated**

Point of unsaturation

Points of unsaturation

[‡]These points of unsaturation can also be referred to as double bonds.

> **saturated fatty acid** a fatty acid carrying the maximum possible number of hydrogen atoms (having no points of unsaturation). A saturated fat is a triglyceride that contains three saturated fatty acids.
>
> **point of unsaturation** a site in a molecule where the bonding is such that additional hydrogen atoms can easily be attached.

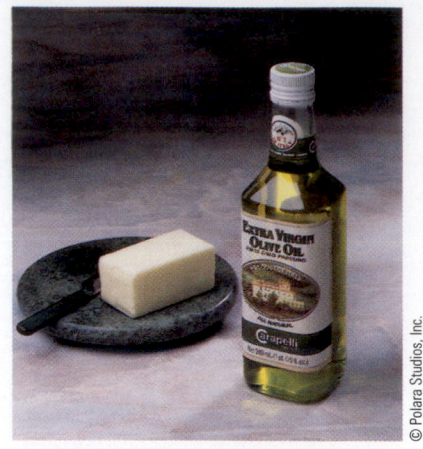

The more unsaturated a fat, the more liquid it is at room temperature. The more saturated a fat, the more solid it is at room temperature.

of unsaturation is an **unsaturated fatty acid**. With one point of unsaturation, the fatty acid is a **monounsaturated fatty acid** (see the second structure in Figure 5–4, on the previous page). With two or more points of unsaturation, it is a **polyunsaturated fatty acid**, often abbreviated **PUFA** (see the third structure in Figure 5–4; other examples are given later in the chapter). Often, a single triglyceride contains both saturated and unsaturated fatty acids of varying lengths, making it a mixed triglyceride.

Melting Point and Fat Hardness   The degree of saturation of the fatty acids in a fat affects the temperature at which the fat melts. Generally, the more unsaturated the fatty acids, the more liquid the fat will be at room temperature. Conversely, the more saturated the fatty acids, the more solid the fat will be at room temperature. Thus, looking at three fats—beef tallow (a type of beef fat), chicken fat, and safflower oil—beef tallow is the most saturated and the hardest; chicken fat is less saturated and somewhat soft; and safflower oil, which is the most unsaturated, is a liquid at room temperature.

If a health-care provider recommends replacing **solid fats**, **saturated fats**, and **trans fats** with **monounsaturated fats** and **polyunsaturated fats** to protect your health, you can generally judge by the hardness of the fats which ones to choose. Figure 5–5 compares the percentages of saturated, monounsaturated, and

unsaturated fatty acid   a fatty acid that lacks some hydrogen atoms and has one or more points of unsaturation. An unsaturated fat is a triglyceride that contains one or more unsaturated fatty acids.

monounsaturated fatty acid   a fatty acid containing one point of unsaturation.

polyunsaturated fatty acid   a fatty acid with two or more points of unsaturation.

solid fats   fats that are high in saturated fatty acids and are usually solid at room temperature. Solid fats are found naturally in most animal foods but also can be made from vegetable oils through hydrogenation. Also defined in Chapter 2.

saturated fats   triglycerides in which most of the fatty acids are saturated.

trans fats   fats that contain any number of unusual fatty acids—trans-fatty acids—formed during processing.

monounsaturated fats   triglycerides in which most of the fatty acids have one point of unsaturation (are monounsaturated).

polyunsaturated fats   triglycerides in which most of the fatty acids have two or more points of unsaturation (are polyunsaturated).

Figure 5–5
Fatty Acid Composition of Common Food Fats

Most fats are a mixture of saturated, monounsaturated, and polyunsaturated fatty acids.

Key:
- Saturated fatty acids
- Monounsaturated fatty acids
- Polyunsaturated, omega-6 fatty acids[a]
- Polyunsaturated, omega-3 fatty acids[a]

Tropical oils (coconut and palm) and animal fats contain mostly saturated fatty acids.

Coconut oil	
Butter	
Beef tallow (beef fat)	
Palm oil	
Lard (pork fat)	
Chicken fat	

Some vegetable oils, such as olive and canola, are rich in monounsaturated fatty acids.

Avocado oil	
Olive oil	
Canola oil	
Peanut oil	

Many vegetable oils are rich in omega-6 polyunsaturated fatty acids.[a]

Safflower oil[b]	
Sunflower oil	
Corn oil	
Soybean oil	
Walnut oil	
Cottonseed oil	

Only a few oils provide significant omega-3 polyunsaturated fatty acids.[a]

Flaxseed oil	
Fish oil[c]	

[a]These families of polyunsaturated fatty acids are explained in a later section.
[b]Salad or cooking type over 70% linoleic acid.
[c]Fish oil average values derived from USDA data for salmon, sardine, and herring oils.
Note: The USDA Nutrient Database (http://ndb.nal.usda.gov) lists the fatty acid contents of many other foods.

polyunsaturated fatty acids in various fats and oils. To determine the degree of saturation of the fats in the oil you use, place it in a clear container in the refrigerator and watch how solid it becomes. The least saturated oils, such as polyunsaturated vegetable oils, remain clear. Olive oil, mostly monounsaturated fat, may turn cloudy when chilled, but olive oil is still an excellent choice from the standpoint of the health of the heart, as a later section reveals.

Another exception is the solid fat of homogenized milk. Highly saturated milk fat normally collects and floats as a layer of cream (butterfat) on top of the watery milk fluids. Once skimmed from the milk and churned into butter, the solid fat is revealed and quickly hardens in the refrigerator. During **homogenization**, heated milk and cream are forced under high pressure through tiny nozzle openings to finely divide and disperse the fat droplets evenly throughout the milk. Thus, fluid milk can be a source of solid fat that remains liquid at cold temperatures.

Where the Fatty Acids Are Found   Most vegetable and fish oils are rich in polyunsaturated fatty acids. Some vegetable oils are also rich in monounsaturated fatty acids. Animal fats are generally the most saturated. But you have to know your oils—it is not enough to choose foods with plant oils over those containing animal fats. Coconut oil comes from a plant, for example, but it disobeys the rule that plant oils are less saturated than animal fats; the fatty acids of coconut oil—even the heavily advertised "virgin" types—are more saturated than those of cream.[4] By the way, no solid evidence supports claims made by advertisers for special curative powers of coconut oil. Palm oil, a vegetable oil used in food processing, is also highly saturated. Likewise, shortenings, stick margarine, and commercially fried or baked products may claim to be or use "all vegetable fat," but much of their fat may be saturated, as a later section makes clear.

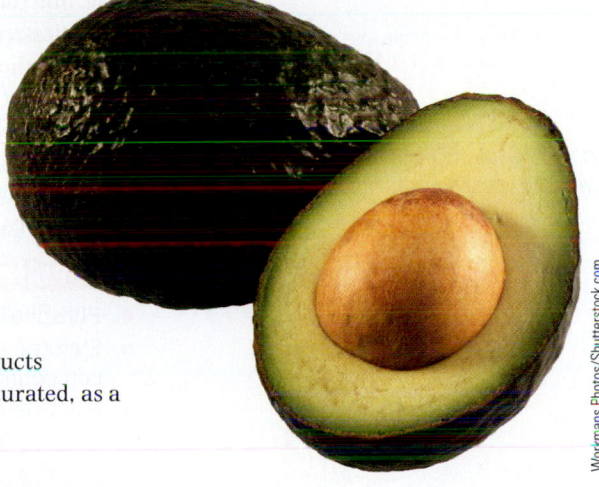

Workmans Photos/Shutterstock.com

Phospholipids and Sterols

Thus far, we have dealt with the largest of the three classes of lipids—the triglycerides and their component fatty acids. The other two classes—phospholipids and sterols—play important structural and regulatory roles in the body.

Phospholipids   A phospholipid, like a triglyceride, consists of a molecule of glycerol with fatty acids attached, but it contains two, rather than three, fatty acids. In place of the third is a molecule containing phosphorus, which makes the phospholipid soluble in water, while its fatty acids make it soluble in fat. This versatility permits any phospholipid to play a role in keeping fats dispersed in water—it can serve as an **emulsifier**.

Food manufacturers blend fat with watery ingredients by way of **emulsification**. Some salad dressings separate to form two layers—vinegar on the bottom, oil on top. Other dressings, such as mayonnaise, are also made from vinegar and oil, but they never separate. The difference lies in a special ingredient of mayonnaise, the emulsifier lecithin in egg yolks. Lecithin, a phospholipid, blends the vinegar with the oil to form the stable, spreadable mayonnaise.

Health-promoting properties, such as the ability to lower blood cholesterol, are sometimes attributed to lecithin, but the people making the claims profit from selling supplements. Lecithin supplements have no special ability to promote health—the body makes all of the lecithin it needs.

homogenization a process by which milk fat is evenly dispersed within fluid milk; under high pressure, milk is passed through tiny nozzles to reduce the size of fat droplets and reduce their tendency to cluster and float to the top as cream.

emulsifier a substance that mixes with both fat and water and permanently disperses the fat in the water, forming an emulsion.

emulsification the process of mixing lipid with water by adding an emulsifier.

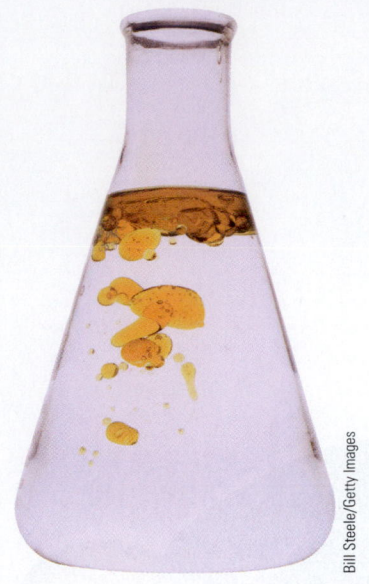

Oil and water. Without help from emulsifiers, fats and water separate into layers.

Phospholipids also play key structural and regulatory roles in the cells. Phospholipids bind together in a strong double layer that forms the membranes of cells. Because phospholipids have both water-loving and fat-loving characteristics, they help fats travel back and forth across the lipid membranes of cells into the watery fluids on both sides. In addition, some phospholipids generate signals inside the cells in response to hormones, such as insulin, to help modulate body conditions.

Sterols   Sterols such as cholesterol are large, complicated molecules consisting of interconnected *rings* of carbon atoms with side chains of carbon, hydrogen, and oxygen attached. Cholesterol serves as the raw material for making emulsifiers in **bile** (see the next section for details), important to fat digestion. Cholesterol is also important in the structure of the cell membranes of every cell, making it necessary to the body's proper functioning. Like lecithin, cholesterol can be made by the body, so it is not an essential nutrient. Other sterols include vitamin D, which is made from cholesterol, and the familiar steroid hormones, including the sex hormones.

Cholesterol forms the major part of the plaques that narrow the arteries in atherosclerosis, the underlying cause of heart attacks and strokes. Sterols other than cholesterol exist in plants. These plant sterols resemble cholesterol in structure and can inhibit cholesterol absorption in the human digestive tract, lowering the cholesterol concentration in the blood.[5] Plant sterols occur naturally in nuts, seeds, legumes, whole grains, vegetables, and fruits and are added to margarine that makes a "heart healthy" claim on the label.

KEY POINTS

- Phospholipids play key roles in cell membranes.
- Sterols play roles as part of bile, vitamin D, the sex hormones, and other important compounds.
- Plant sterols in foods inhibit cholesterol absorption.

Lipids in the Body

LO 5.3   Explain the processes of digestion, absorption, and transportation of lipids in the body.

From the moment they enter the body, lipids affect the body's functioning and condition. They also demand special handling because fat separates from water and body fluids consist largely of water.

How Are Fats Digested and Absorbed?

A bite of food in the mouth first encounters the enzymes of saliva. An enzyme produced by the tongue plays a major role in digesting milk fat in infants but is of little importance to lipid digestion in adults.

Fat in the Stomach   After being chewed and swallowed, the food travels to the stomach, where droplets of fat separate from the watery components and tend to float as a layer on top. Even the stomach's powerful churning cannot completely disperse the fat, so little fat digestion takes place in the stomach.

Fat in the Small Intestine   As the stomach contents empty into the small intestine, the digestive system faces a problem: how to thoroughly mix fats, which are now separated, with its own watery fluids. The solution is an emulsifier: bile. Bile, made by the liver, is stored in the gallbladder and released into the small intestine when it is needed for fat digestion. Bile contains compounds made from cholesterol that work as emulsifiers; one end of each molecule attracts and holds fat, while the other end is attracted to and held by water.

By the time fat enters the small intestine, the gallbladder, which stores the liver's output of bile, has contracted and squirted its bile into the intestine. Bile emulsifies and suspends fat droplets within the watery fluids (see Figure 5–6) until the fat-digesting enzymes contributed by the pancreas can split them into smaller molecules

bile   an emulsifier made by the liver from cholesterol and stored in the gallbladder. Bile does not digest fat as enzymes do but emulsifies it so that enzymes in the watery fluids may contact it and split the fatty acids from their glycerol for absorption.

Figure 5-6

The Action of Bile in Fat Digestion

Bile and detergents are both emulsifiers and work the same way, which is why detergents are effective in removing grease spots from clothes. Molecule by molecule, the grease is dissolved out of the spot and suspended in the water, where it can be rinsed away.

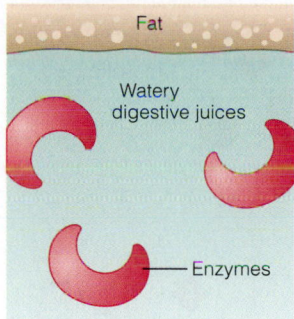 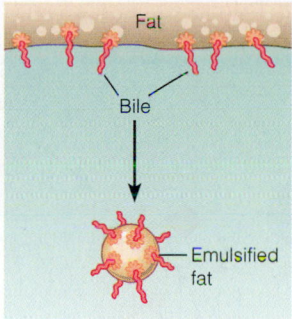 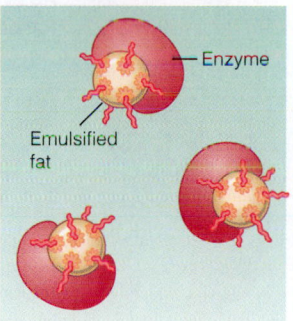

In the stomach, the fat and watery digestive juices tend to separate. Enzymes are in the water and can't get at the fat.

When fat enters the small intestine, the gallbladder secretes bile. Bile compounds have an affinity for both fat and water, so bile can mix the fat into the water.

After emulsification, more fat is exposed to the enzymes, and fat digestion proceeds efficiently.

for absorption. These fat-splitting enzymes act on triglycerides to split fatty acids from their glycerol backbones. Free fatty acids, phospholipids, and **monoglycerides** all cling together in balls surrounded by bile emulsifiers.

To review: first, the digestive system mixes fats with bile-containing digestive juices to emulsify the fats. Then fat-digesting enzymes break the fats down into absorbable pieces. The pieces then assemble themselves into balls that remain emulsified by bile.

People sometimes wonder how a person without a gallbladder can digest food. The gallbladder is just a storage organ. Without it, the liver still produces bile but delivers it into a duct that conducts it into the small intestine instead of into the gallbladder.

Fat Absorption Once split and emulsified, the fats face another barrier: the watery layer of mucus that coats the absorptive lining of the digestive tract. Fats must traverse this layer to enter the cells of the digestive tract lining. The solution again depends on bile, this time in the balls of digested lipids. The bile shuttles the lipids across the watery mucus layer to the waiting absorptive surfaces on cells of the intestinal villi. The cells then extract the lipids. The bile may be absorbed and reused by the body, or it may flow back into the intestinal contents and exit with the feces, as was shown in Figure 4–6 (p. 124).

The digestive tract absorbs triglycerides from a meal with remarkable efficiency: up to 98 percent of fats consumed are absorbed. Very little fat is excreted by a healthy system. The process of fat digestion takes time, though, so the more fat taken in at a meal, the slower the digestive system action becomes. The efficient series of events just described is depicted in Figure 5–7 (p. 170).

KEY POINTS

- In the stomach, fats separate from other food components.
- In the small intestine, bile emulsifies the fats, enzymes digest them, and the intestinal cells absorb them.

Transport of Fats

Glycerol and shorter-chain fatty acids pass directly through the cells of the intestinal lining into the bloodstream, where they travel unassisted to the liver. The larger lipids, however, present a problem for the body. As mentioned, fat floats in water. Without some mechanism to keep them dispersed, large lipid globules would separate out

monoglycerides (mon-oh-GLISS-er-ides) products of the digestion of lipids; a monoglyceride is a glycerol molecule with one fatty acid attached (*mono* means "one"; *glyceride* means "a compound of glycerol").

Figure 5–7

The Process of Lipid Digestion and Absorption

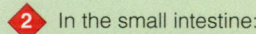

1 In the mouth and stomach:

Little fat digestion takes place.

2 In the small intestine:

Digestive enzymes accomplish most fat digestion in the small intestine. There, bile emulsifies fat, making it available for enzyme action. The enzymes cleave triglycerides into free fatty acids, glycerol, and monoglycerides.

3 At the intestinal lining:

The parts are absorbed by intestinal villi. Glycerol and short-chain fatty acids enter directly into the bloodstream.

4 The cells of the intestinal lining convert large lipid fragments, such as monoglycerides and long-chain fatty acids, back into triglycerides and combine them with protein, forming chylomicrons (a type of lipoprotein) that travel in the lymph vessels to the bloodstream.

5 In the large intestine:

A small amount of cholesterol trapped in fiber exits with the feces.

Note: In this diagram, molecules of fatty acids are shown as large objects, but, in reality, molecules of fatty acids are too small to see even with a powerful microscope, while villi are visible to the naked eye.

Liver · Esophagus · Pancreas · Stomach · Small intestine · Large intestine (colon)

Emulsified lipids · Capillary network · Lymph · Villi · Chylomicrons · Small artery · Small vein · Lymph travels to blood · Bloodstream

of the watery blood as it circulates around the body, disrupting the blood's normal functions. The solution to this problem lies in an ingenious use of proteins: many fats travel from place to place in the watery blood as passengers in **lipoproteins**, assembled packages of lipid and protein molecules.

The larger digested lipids, monoglycerides and long-chain fatty acids, must form lipoproteins before they can be released into the lymph in vessels that lead to the bloodstream. Inside the intestinal cells, these lipids re-form into triglycerides and cluster together with proteins and phospholipids to form **chylomicrons** that can safely carry lipids from place to place in the watery blood. Chylomicrons form one type of lipoprotein (shown in Figure 5–7) and are part of the body's efficient lipid transport system. Other lipoproteins are discussed later with regard to their profound effects on health.

KEY POINTS

- Glycerol and short-chain fatty acids travel in the bloodstream unassisted.
- Other lipids need special transport vehicles—the lipoproteins—to carry them in watery body fluids.

lipoproteins (LYE-poh-PRO-teens, LIH-poh-PRO-teens) clusters of lipids associated with protein, which serve as transport vehicles for lipids in blood and lymph. The major lipoproteins include chylomicrons, VLDL, LDL, and HDL.

chylomicrons (KYE-low-MY-krons) lipoproteins formed when lipids from a meal cluster with carrier proteins in the cells of the intestinal lining. Chylomicrons transport food fats through the watery body fluids to the liver and other tissues.

Storing and Using the Body's Fat

LO 5.4 Discuss how fats are stored and used by the body.

Methodically, the body conserves fat molecules not immediately required for energy. Stored fat serves as a sort of "rainy day" fund to fuel the body's activities at times when food is unavailable, when illness impairs the appetite, or when energy expenditures increase.

The Body's Fat Stores Many triglycerides eaten in foods are transported by the chylomicrons to the fat depots—the external fat layer under the skin, the internal fat pads of the abdomen, the breasts, and others—where they are stored by the body's fat cells for later use. When a person's body starts to run out of available fuel from food, it begins to retrieve this stored fat to use for energy. (It also draws on its stored glycogen, as the last chapter described.)

With sufficient food energy, the body can convert excess carbohydrate to fat, but this conversion is not energy-efficient. Figure 5–8 illustrates a simplified series of conversion steps from carbohydrate to fat. Before excess glucose can be stored as fat, it must first be broken into tiny fragments by enzymes and then reassembled into fatty acids, steps that require energy to perform. The body also possesses enzymes to convert excess protein to fat or to glucose, but these processes are even less efficient.[6] Storing fat itself is most efficient; fat requires fewer chemical steps before storage. This does not mean that excess calories from carbohydrate- and protein-rich foods do not contribute to energy stores in the body, however—far from it. Excess calorie intakes reliably lead to weight gain, and overfatness often correlates with diets high in sweets and meats.

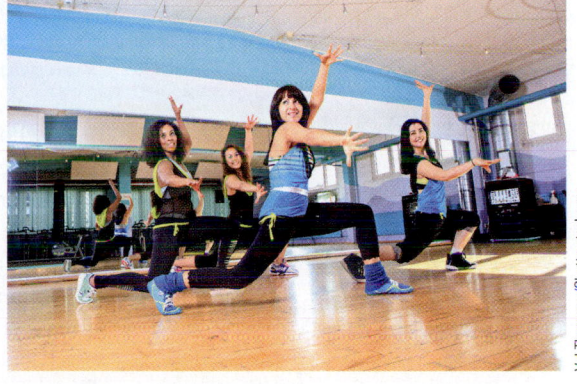

Body fat supplies much of the fuel these muscles need to do their work.

What Happens When the Tissues Need Energy? Fat cells respond to the call for energy by dismantling stored fat molecules (triglycerides) and releasing fatty acids into the blood. Upon receiving these fatty acids, the energy-hungry cells break them down further into small fragments. Finally, each fat fragment is combined with a fragment derived from glucose, and the energy-releasing process continues, liberating energy, carbon dioxide, and water. The way to use more of the energy stored as body fat, then, is to create a greater demand for it in the tissues by decreasing the intake of food energy, by increasing the body's expenditure of energy, or both.

Carbohydrate in Fat Breakdown When fat is broken down to provide cellular energy, carbohydrate helps the process run most efficiently. Without carbohydrate, products of incomplete fat breakdown (ketones) build up in the tissues and blood, and they spill out into the urine.

Carbohydrate's role in fat metabolism is discussed on page 136.

Figure 5–8

Glucose to Fat

Glucose can be used for energy, or it can be changed into fat and stored.

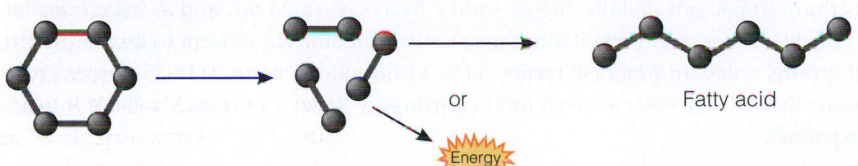

or

Fatty acid

Glucose is broken down into fragments.

The fragments can provide immediate energy for the tissues.

Energy

Or, if the tissues need no more energy, the fragments can be reassembled, not back into glucose but into fatty acid chains.

For weight-loss dieters who want to use their body fat for energy, knowing these details of energy metabolism is less important than remembering what research and common sense tell us: successful weight loss depends on taking in less energy than the body needs—not on the proportion of energy nutrients in the diet (Chapter 9 provides details). For the body's health, however, the proportions of certain lipids in the diet matter greatly, as the next section makes clear.

KEY POINTS

- The body draws on its stored fat for energy.
- Carbohydrate is necessary for the complete breakdown of fat.

Dietary Fat, Cholesterol, and Health

LO 5.5 State the health implications of blood lipoproteins and dietary fats.

High intakes of saturated and *trans* fats are associated with serious diseases, and particularly with heart and artery disease (cardiovascular disease, or CVD), the number-one cause of death among adults in the United States and Canada.[7] So much research is focused on the links between diet and diseases that an entire chapter, Chapter 11, is devoted to presenting the details of these connections.

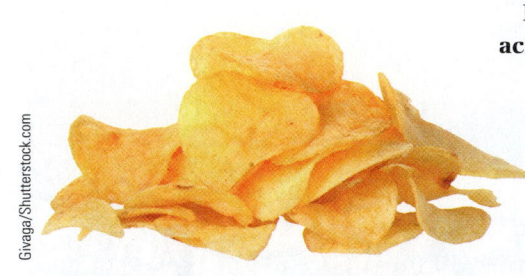

People who center their diets on foods rich in saturated fatty acids and ***trans*-fatty acids** often have blood lipid profiles that indicate higher risk of developing CVD. When they replace these foods with those rich in polyunsaturated or monounsaturated fat, their blood lipids often shift toward a profile associated with good health.[8] Even greater benefits may be expected from an eating pattern that includes protein-rich nuts, seafood, and soy foods; soluble fiber–rich legumes, barley, and oatmeal; and a variety of fruit, vegetables, and other whole foods.

Reducing saturated fats is important, but what replaces them in the diet matters, too. When added sugars and refined carbohydrates take the place of saturated or *trans* fats, little benefit to health is observed.

If you are a woman, take note: these observations apply to you. Heart disease kills more women in the United States than any other cause, and the old myth that heart disease is a "man's disease" should be forever put to rest.

Recommendations for Lipid Intakes

As mentioned, some fat is essential to good health. The Dietary Guidelines for Americans recommend that a portion of each day's total fat intake come from a few teaspoons of raw oil, such as found in nuts, avocados, olives, or vegetable oils. A little peanut butter on toast or mayonnaise in tuna salad, for example, can easily meet this need. In addition, the DRI committee sets specific recommended intakes for the essential fatty acids, **linoleic acid** and **linolenic acid**, and they are listed in Table 5–2.

A Healthy Range of Fat Intakes Defining an upper limit—the exact gram amount of fat, saturated fat, or *trans* fat that begins to harm people's health—is difficult, so no Tolerable Upper Intake Level for the lipids is set. Instead, the DRI committee suggests an intake range of 20 to 35 percent of daily energy from total fat and less than 10 percent of daily energy intake from saturated fat, and as little *trans* fat as possible. Older recommendations also limited dietary cholesterol to less than 300 milligrams a day. In practical terms, for a 2,000-calorie diet, 20 to 35 percent represents 400 to 700 calories from total fat (roughly 45 to 75 grams, or about 9 to 15 teaspoons).

U.S. Fat Intakes According to surveys, the average U.S. diet provides about 34 percent of total energy from fat, with saturated fat contributing more than 11 percent of the total.[9] The solid fats in cheese, burgers, and grain-based desserts are top providers of saturated fat (see Figure 5–9 for details), but chicken and

***trans*-fatty acids** fatty acids with unusual shapes that can arise when hydrogens are added to the unsaturated fatty acids of polyunsaturated oils (a process known as *hydrogenation*).

linoleic (lin-oh-LAY-ic) **acid** an essential polyunsaturated fatty acid of the omega-6 family.

linolenic (lin-oh-LEN-ic) **acid** an essential polyunsaturated fatty acid of the omega-3 family. The full name of linolenic acid is *alpha-linolenic acid*.

Table 5–2

Lipid Intake Recommendations for Healthy People

1. Total fat[a]

Dietary Reference Intakes

- An acceptable range of fat intake is estimated at 20 to 35% of total calories.

2. Saturated fat

American Heart Association

- For adults who would benefit from lowering blood LDL cholesterol:
  - Reduce percentage of calories from saturated fat to 5 to 6%.

Dietary Reference Intakes

- Keep saturated fat intake low, less than 10% of calories, within the context of an adequate diet.

Dietary Guidelines for Americans[b]

- Consume less than 10% of calories per day from saturated fats.

3. *Trans* fat

American Heart Association

- For adults who would benefit from lowering blood LDL cholesterol:
  - Reduce percentage of calories from *trans* fat.

Dietary Guidelines for Americans[b]

- A healthy eating pattern limits *trans* fats.

4. Polyunsaturated fatty acids

Dietary Reference Intakes[c]

- Linoleic acid (5 to 10% of total calories):
  17 g/day for young men.
  12 g/day for young women.
- Linolenic acid (0.6 to 1.2% of total calories):
  1.6 g/day for men.
  1.1 g/day for women.

Dietary Guidelines for Americans

- A healthy eating pattern includes oils.

5. Cholesterol

Dietary Reference Intakes[c]

- Minimize cholesterol intake within the context of a healthy diet.

[a]*Includes monounsaturated fatty acids.*

[b]*The Dietary Guidelines for Americans 2015 use the term solid fats to describe sources of saturated and trans-fatty acids. Solid fats include milk fat, fats of high-fat meats and cheeses, hard margarines, butter, lard, and shortening.*

[c]*For DRI values set for various life stages, see the inside front cover. Linoleic and linolenic acids are defined on page 172.*

Figure 5–9

Sources of Saturated Fats in the U.S. Diet

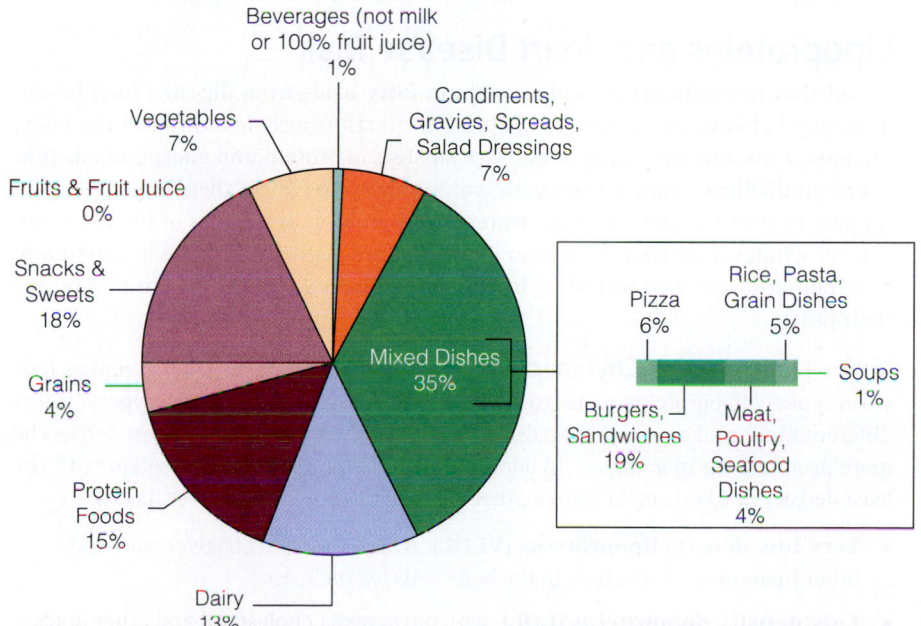

Beverages (not milk or 100% fruit juice) 1%
Vegetables 7%
Fruits & Fruit Juice 0%
Snacks & Sweets 18%
Grains 4%
Protein Foods 15%
Dairy 13%
Condiments, Gravies, Spreads, Salad Dressings 7%
Mixed Dishes 35%

Pizza 6%
Rice, Pasta, Grain Dishes 5%
Burgers, Sandwiches 19%
Meat, Poultry, Seafood Dishes 4%
Soups 1%

Source: U.S. Department of Health and Human Services and U.S. Department of Agriculture, 2015–2020 Dietary Guidelines for Americans, 8th edition (2015), available at http://health.gov/dietaryguidelines/2015/guidelines/.

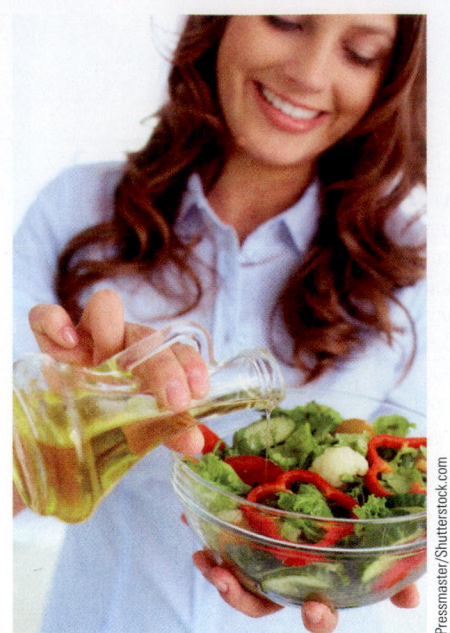

People who eat the Mediterranean way rely on olive oil, olives, nuts, and seeds for most of their fats.

chicken dishes, dairy desserts, fried potatoes, red meats of all kinds, and fast foods all contribute substantially as well.

Traditional Mediterranean Fat Intakes   In the mid-20th century, people eating the traditional diets of the Mediterranean Sea regions were observed to achieve a rare feat: they consumed a relatively large amount of dietary fat (about 40 percent of calories) while having low rates of cardiovascular diseases.[10] Their diets also provided abundant nutrients from vegetables, legumes, nuts and seeds, fruits, whole grains, fish, other seafood, and some cheeses and yogurt, but little red meat, few added sugars, and no ultra-processed foods. Today, the Dietary Guidelines for Americans recommend this healthy Mediterranean-style eating pattern for meeting nutrient needs and lowering disease risks.

The fats of healthy Mediterranean-style diets derive mostly from **extra virgin olive oil**, olives, nuts, and seeds. These foods are rich in monounsaturated fatty acids and phytochemicals, and when they replace the solid fats of butter, stick margarine, coconut and palm oil, or meats, improvements in markers of heart disease risks, such as factors related to blood clotting and inflammation, often follow.[11] Research hints that such diets may also lower risks of diabetes, breast cancer, and mental decline in aging, but more evidence is needed in these areas.[12]

Eating the Mediterranean way involves more than just adding olives to your taco salads and nuts to desserts, or drizzling olive oil like a magic potion on cheesy sausage pizzas (Appendix E provides some details). Adding nuts or oils instead of replacing solid fats can add many hundreds of calories to a day's intake, with weight gain and worsened disease risks the likely result.

Too Little Lipid   A very few people manage to eat too little fat to support health. Among them are people with eating disorders who eat too little of all foods and misguided athletes hoping to improve performance. When fat intake falls short of the 20 percent minimum, energy, vitamins, and essential fatty acids, may also be lacking, and the eater's health may suffer.

Some points about lipids and heart health are presented next because they form the foundation of lipid intake recommendations. The lipoproteins take center stage because they play important roles concerning the heart.

KEY POINTS

- A small amount of raw oil is recommended each day.
- Energy from fat should provide 20 to 35 percent of the total energy in the diet.

Lipoproteins and Heart Disease Risk

Recall that monoglycerides and long-chain fatty acids from digested food fat depend on chylomicrons, a type of lipoprotein, to transport them around the body. Chylomicrons and other lipoproteins are clusters of protein and phospholipids that act as emulsifiers—they attract both water and fat to enable their large lipid passengers to travel dispersed in the watery body fluids. The tissues of the body can extract whatever fat they need from chylomicrons passing by in the bloodstream. The remnants are then picked up by the liver, which dismantles them and reuses their parts.

Major Lipoproteins: Chylomicrons, VLDL, LDL, HDL   The body makes four main types of lipoproteins, distinguished by their size and density. Each type contains different kinds and amounts of lipids and proteins: the more lipids, the less dense; the more proteins, the more dense. In addition to chylomicrons, the lipoprotein with the least density, the body makes three other types of lipoproteins to carry its fats:

- **Very-low-density lipoproteins (VLDL)**, which transport triglycerides and other lipids made in the liver to the body cells for their use.

- **Low-density lipoproteins (LDL)**, which transport cholesterol and other lipids to the tissues for their use. LDL are made from VLDL after they have donated many of their triglycerides to body cells.

extra virgin olive oil minimally processed olive oil produced by mechanical means, such as pressing (not chemical extraction), to preserve phytochemicals, green color, and flavor from the original olives. The highest grade of olive oil.

very-low-density lipoproteins (VLDL) lipoproteins that transport triglycerides and other lipids from the liver to various tissues in the body.

low-density lipoproteins (LDL) lipoproteins that transport lipids from the liver to other tissues such as muscle and fat; contain a large proportion of cholesterol.

Figure 5–10

Lipoproteins

As the graph shows, the density of a lipoprotein is determined by its lipid-to-protein ratio. All lipoproteins contain protein, cholesterol, phospholipids, and triglycerides in varying amounts. An LDL has a high ratio of lipid to protein (about 80 percent lipid to 20 percent protein) and is especially high in cholesterol. An HDL has more protein relative to its lipid content (about equal parts lipid and protein).

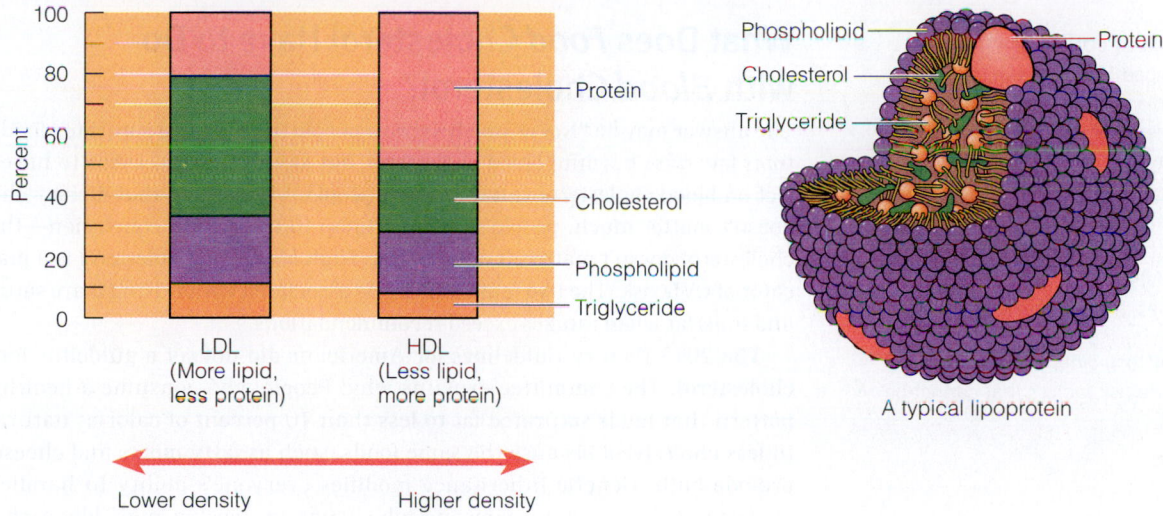

A typical lipoprotein

- **High-density lipoproteins (HDL)**, which pick up cholesterol from body cells and carry it away to the liver for disposal.[13]**

Figure 5–10 depicts typical lipoproteins and demonstrates how a lipoprotein's density changes with its lipid and protein contents.

The LDL and HDL Difference   The separate functions and effects of LDL and HDL are worth a moment's attention because they carry important implications for the health of the heart and blood vessels.

- Both LDL and HDL carry lipids in the blood, but LDL are larger, lighter, and richer in cholesterol; HDL are smaller, denser, and packaged with more protein.

- LDL deliver cholesterol to the tissues; HDL scavenge excess cholesterol and other lipids from the tissues, transport them via the bloodstream, and deposit them in the liver for disposal.

- When LDL cholesterol is too high, it contributes to lipid buildup in tissues, particularly in the linings of the arteries, that can trigger **inflammation** and lead to heart disease; HDL cholesterol opposes these effects, and when HDL in the blood drops below the recommended level, heart disease risks rise in response.

Both LDL and HDL carry cholesterol, but high blood LDL concentrations warn of an increased risk of heart attack, whereas *low* HDL concentrations are associated with a greater risk (Chapter 11 has details). Thus, some people refer to LDL as "bad" cholesterol and HDL as "good" cholesterol—yet they carry the same kind of cholesterol. The key difference to health between LDL and HDL lies in the proportions of lipids they contain and the tasks they perform, not in the *type* of cholesterol they carry.

The Importance of Cholesterol Testing   The importance of blood cholesterol concentrations to heart health cannot be overstated.†† The blood lipid profile, a medical

high-density lipoproteins (HDL) lipoproteins that return cholesterol from the tissues to the liver for dismantling and disposal; contain a large proportion of protein.

inflammation (in-flam-MAY-shun) an immune defense against injury, infection, or allergens marked by heat, fever, and pain. Chronic, low-grade inflammation is associated with many disease states. Also defined in Chapter 3.

**HDL are also under study for roles in immunity, inflammation, glucose metabolism, and blood clotting.

††*Blood*, *plasma*, and *serum* all refer to about the same thing; this book uses the term *blood* cholesterol. Plasma is blood with the cells removed; in serum, the clotting factors are also removed. The concentration of cholesterol is not much altered by these treatments.

Table 5–3

Modifiable Lifestyle Factors in Heart Disease Risk

The more of these factors present in a person's life, the more urgent the need for changes in diet and lifestyle to reduce heart disease risk:

- High blood LDL cholesterol
- Low blood HDL cholesterol
- High blood pressure (hypertension)
- Diabetes (insulin resistance)
- Obesity
- Physical inactivity
- Cigarette smoking
- A diet high in saturated fats, including *trans* fats, and low in fish, vegetables, legumes, fruit, and whole grains

Family history, older age, and male gender are risk factors that cannot be changed.

Table 5–4

Normal Blood Lipids

These numbers (in milligrams per deciliter) represent a desirable blood lipid profile:

- Total cholesterol: <200
- LDL cholesterol: <100
- HDL cholesterol: ≥60
- Triglycerides: <150

---

test mentioned at the beginning of this chapter, tells much about a person's blood cholesterol and the lipoproteins that carry it.[14] High blood LDL cholesterol and low blood HDL cholesterol account for two major risk factors for CVD (see Table 5–3). Table 5–4 lists the standards for blood lipid profile testing.

KEY POINTS

- The chief lipoproteins are chylomicrons, VLDL, LDL, and HDL.
- High blood LDL and low blood HDL are major heart disease risk factors.

What Does *Food* Cholesterol Have to Do with *Blood* Cholesterol?

The answer may be "Not as much as most people think." Most saturated food fats and *trans* fats raise harmful blood cholesterol, but food *cholesterol* seems to have little effect on blood cholesterol values in most people.[15] When told that dietary cholesterol doesn't matter much, people may then jump to the wrong conclusion—that blood cholesterol doesn't matter. It does matter. High *blood* LDL cholesterol is a major indicator of CVD risk. The two main food lipids associated with raising it are saturated fat and *trans* fat when intakes exceed recommendations.

The 2015 Dietary Guidelines for Americans did not set a guideline for dietary cholesterol. The committee explains why: People who consume a healthy eating pattern that holds saturated fat to less than 10 percent of calories naturally take in less cholesterol because the same foods, such as fatty meats and cheeses, often provide both. Genetic inheritance modifies everyone's ability to handle dietary cholesterol, however, so someone who tends to develop high blood cholesterol should follow the advice of a physician.[16]

KEY POINTS

- Saturated fat and *trans* fat intakes raise blood cholesterol.
- Dietary cholesterol seems to have little effect on blood cholesterol in most people.

Recommendations Applied

In a welcome trend, fewer people in the United States have high blood cholesterol than in past decades. Even so, a large number—more than a quarter of adults—still test too high for LDL cholesterol.[17] In addition, blood HDL cholesterol often measures too low, and the combination poses a threat to the heart and arteries.[18] To repeat, dietary saturated fat and *trans* fat can trigger a rise in LDL cholesterol in the blood. Conversely, trimming the saturated fat and *trans* fat from foods and replacing them with monounsaturated and polyunsaturated fats while keeping calories reasonable can lower LDL levels.

Lowering LDL Cholesterol   A step toward improving blood lipids is to identify sources of saturated fat—that is, solid fats—in the diet and reduce their intakes. Figure 5–11 shows that, when food is trimmed of solid fat, it also loses saturated fat and energy. A pork chop trimmed of its border of fat drops almost 70 percent of its saturated fat and 220 calories. A plain baked potato has no saturated fat and contains about 40 percent of the calories of one with butter and sour cream. Choosing fat-free milk over whole milk provides large savings of saturated fat and calories. Then, with solid fats identified and eliminated, the diner is free to replace them with unsaturated fats, as a later section demonstrates.

Nutritionists know this: the best diet for health not only replaces saturated fats with polyunsaturated and monounsaturated oils but also is adequate, balanced, calorie-controlled, varied, and based mostly on nutrient-dense whole foods. The overall eating pattern is important, too.

Raising HDL   As for blood HDL cholesterol, dietary measures are generally ineffective at raising its concentration. Regular physical activity raises it most effectively and reduces heart disease risks, as the Think Fitness feature points out.

Why Exercise the Body for the Health of the Heart?

Every leading authority recommends physical activity to promote and maintain the health of the heart. The blood, arteries, heart, and other body tissues respond to exercise in these ways:

- Blood lipids shift toward higher HDL cholesterol.
- The muscles of the heart and arteries strengthen and circulation improves, easing delivery of blood to the lungs and tissues.
- A larger volume of blood is pumped with each heartbeat, reducing the heart's workload.
- The body grows leaner, reducing overall risk of cardiovascular disease.
- Blood glucose regulation is improved, reducing the risk of diabetes.

start now! ···} Ready to make a change? Set a goal of exercising 30 minutes per day at least five days per week, then track your activity in Diet & Wellness Plus.

Figure 5–11

Cutting Solid Fats Cuts Calories and Saturated Fat

The solid fats in these foods are easy to spot—you can see much of the solid fat on a pork chop and in a butter pat, and you can read about it on a milk label.

Savings:
110 cal, 10 g solid fat, 4 g saturated fat

Savings:
150 cal, 14 g solid fat, 10 g saturated fat

Savings:
60 cal, 8 g solid fat, 5 g saturated fat

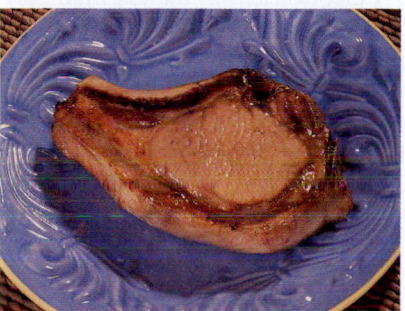

Pork chop with fat
- 340 cal
- 19 g solid fat
- 7 g saturated fat

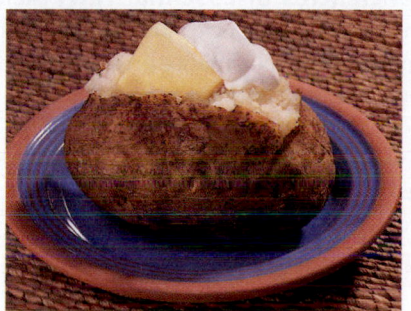

Potato with 1 tbs butter and 1 tbs sour cream
- 350 cal
- 14 g solid fat
- 10 g saturated fat

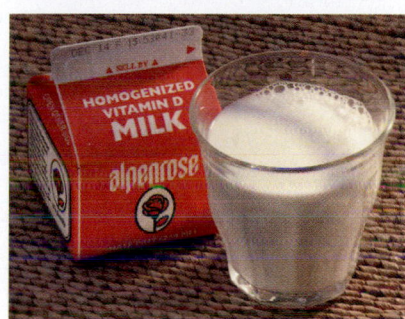

Whole milk, 1 c
- 150 cal
- 8 g solid fat
- 5 g saturated fat

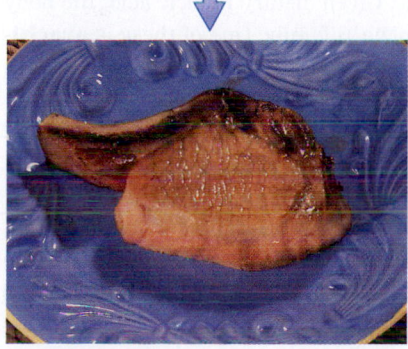

Pork chop trimmed of fat
- 230 cal
- 9 g solid fat
- 3 g saturated fat

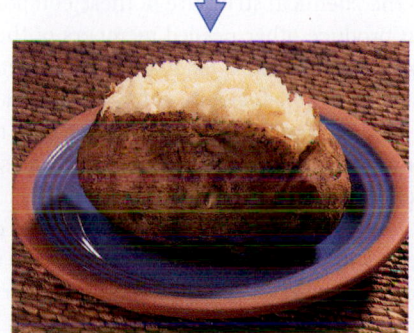

Plain potato
- 200 cal
- 0 g solid fat
- 0 g saturated fat

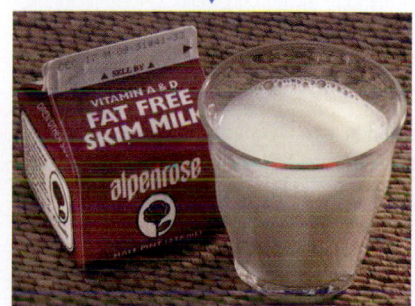

Fat-free milk, 1 c
- 90 cal
- 0 g solid fat
- 0 g saturated fat

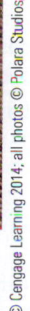

Art © Cengage Learning 2014; all photos © Polara Studios, Inc.

Table 5–5

Functions of the Essential Fatty Acids

These roles for the essential fatty acids are known, but others are under investigation.

- Provide raw material for eicosanoids.
- Serve as structural and functional parts of cell membranes.
- Contribute lipids to the brain and nerves.
- Promote normal growth and vision.
- Maintain outer structures of the skin, thus protecting against water loss.
- Help regulate genetic activities affecting metabolism.
- Participate in immune cell functions.

Having enough HDL in the blood is an important indicator of heart health, but raising HDL to higher-than-normal levels by medical means provides no extra protection against heart disease.[19] The physically active person also reaps many other benefits, as Chapter 10 makes clear.

KEY POINTS

- To lower LDL in the blood, follow a healthy eating pattern that replaces dietary saturated fat and *trans* fat with polyunsaturated and monounsaturated oils.
- To raise HDL in the blood and lower heart disease risks, be physically active.

Essential Polyunsaturated Fatty Acids

LO 5.6 Summarize the functions of essential fatty acids.

The human body needs fatty acids, and it can use carbohydrate, fat, or protein to synthesize nearly all of them. Two are well-known exceptions: linoleic acid and linolenic acid. Body cells cannot make these two polyunsaturated fatty acids from scratch, nor can the cells convert one to the other.

Why Do I Need Essential Fatty Acids?

Because the body cannot make linoleic or linolenic acids, they must be supplied by the diet and are therefore essential nutrients. For this reason, the DRI committee set recommended intake levels for them (see the inside front cover). Table 5–5 summarizes their many established roles in the body, but new functions continue to emerge.

Deficiencies of Essential Fatty Acids A diet deficient in the essential polyunsaturated fatty acids produces symptoms such as skin abnormalities and poor wound healing. In infants, growth is retarded, and vision is impaired. The body stores some essential fatty acids, so deficiencies are seldom seen except when intentionally induced in research or on rare occasions when inadequate diets have been provided to infants or hospital patients by mistake. In the United States and Canada, such deficiencies are almost unknown among otherwise healthy adults. The story doesn't end there, however.

KEY POINT

- Deficiencies of the essential fatty acids are virtually unknown in the United States and Canada.

Omega-6 and Omega-3 Fatty Acid Families

Linoleic acid is the "parent" member of the **omega-6 fatty acid** family, so named for the chemical structure of these compounds. Given dietary linoleic acid, the body can produce other needed members of the omega-6 family. One of these is **arachidonic acid**, notable for its role as a starting material from which the body makes a number of biologically active lipids, known as **eicosanoids**. Somewhat like hormones, eicosanoids arise in tissues where they help regulate body functions and then are quickly destroyed. Omega-6 fatty acids are supplied abundantly in the U.S. diet in vegetable oils.

Linolenic acid is the parent member of the **omega-3 fatty acid** family. Given dietary linolenic acid, the body can make other members of the omega-3 series. Two family members of great interest to researchers are **EPA** and **DHA**. The body makes only limited amounts of EPA and even less DHA, but they are found abundantly in the oils of certain fish. U.S. intakes of these oils are limited.

EPA (omega-3) forms its own eicosanoids that often oppose those from arachidonic acid (omega-6). For example, an omega-3 eicosanoid relaxes blood vessels and lowers the blood pressure, whereas an omega-6 eicosanoid constricts the vessels

---

omega-6 fatty acid a polyunsaturated fatty acid with its endmost double bond six carbons from the end of the carbon chain. Linoleic acid is an example.

arachidonic (ah-RACK-ih-DON-ik) **acid** an omega-6 fatty acid derived from linoleic acid.

eicosanoids (eye-COSS-ah-noyds) biologically active compounds that regulate body functions.

omega-3 fatty acid a polyunsaturated fatty acid with its endmost double bond three carbons from the end of the carbon chain. Linolenic acid is an example.

EPA, DHA eicosapentaenoic (EYE-cossa-PENTA-ee-NO-ick) acid, docosahexaenoic (DOE-cossa-HEXA-ee-NO-ick) acid; omega-3 fatty acids made from linolenic acid in the tissues of fish.

and increases pressure.[20] A balance between EPA and arachidonic acid therefore promotes normal blood pressure.

- The essential fatty acids fall into two chemical families: omega-6 or omega-3 fatty acids.
- The omega-6 family of polyunsaturated fatty acids includes linoleic acid and arachidonic acid.
- The omega-3 family includes linolenic acid, EPA, and DHA.

Health Effects of Omega-3 Fatty Acids

An area of active research concerns links between intakes of omega-3 fatty acids and reduced risks of certain diseases. This section describes some of the findings.

Heart Health Years ago, someone thought to ask why the native peoples of the extreme north, who eat a diet very high in animal fat, were reported to have low rates of heart disease. The trail led to their abundant intake of fish and marine foods, then to the oils in fish, and finally to EPA and DHA in fish oils. EPA and DHA each play important roles in regulating heartbeats, regulating blood pressure, reducing blood clot formation, reducing blood triglycerides, stabilizing plaques in the arteries, and reducing inflammation—all factors associated with heart health.[21]

Research often links higher EPA and DHA in the blood and greater intakes of fish in the diet with fewer deaths from heart attacks and strokes.[22] Not every study reports lower cardiovascular risks with higher EPA and DHA intakes, however, partly because genetic inheritance influences the degree to which a person may benefit from consuming EPA and DHA.[23]

Cancer Prevention Consuming seafood that provides omega-3 fatty acids is associated with lower rates of some cancers, possibly because they suppress inflammation, a factor in cancer development, or through other mechanisms.[24] However, in a surprising twist, some studies seem to link higher EPA and DHA intakes with an *increased* risk of certain cancers in some people.[25] So little is known about the relationships between cancers and omega-3 fatty acids that people are wise to eat fish, not take supplements, to provide them.

Cell Membranes EPA and DHA tend to collect in cell membranes. Unlike straight-backed saturated fatty acids, which physically stack closely together, the kinked shape of unsaturated fatty acids demands more elbow room (look back at Figure 5–4, p. 165).†† When the highly unsaturated EPA and DHA amass in cell membranes, they profoundly change cellular activities and structures in ways that may promote healthy tissue functioning.

Brain Function and Vision The brain is a fatty organ with a quarter of its dry weight as lipid. Its cell membranes avidly collect DHA in their structures.[26] Once there, DHA may assist in the brain's communication processes and reduce inflammation associated with aging.[27] Likewise, the retina of the eye selectively gathers up and holds DHA for its use. In infants, breast milk and fortified formula provide abundant DHA, associated with normal growth, visual acuity, immune system functioning, and brain development.[28] Many more details about these remarkable lipids are known; Table 5–6 summarizes their best-known functions.[29]

- EPA and DHA may play roles in disease prevention, brain communication and human development.

---

††Triglyceride structures are depicted in Appendix I.

Table 5–6

Potential Health Benefits of Fish Oils

These benefits from fish or fish oil are well established, but researchers are investigating many others.

Against heart disease
- Shifts in eicosanoid activities, with normalized blood clotting, regular heartbeats, and less inflammation in many body tissues, including the arteries of the heart.
- Reduced blood triglycerides. (In some studies, fish oil supplements elevated blood LDL cholesterol, an opposing, detrimental outcome.)
- Stabilization of plaques in the arteries (atherosclerosis).
- Relaxation of blood vessels, mildly reducing blood pressure.

In infant growth and development
- Normal brain development in infants. DHA concentrates in the brain's cortex, the conscious thinking part.
- Normal vision development in infants. DHA helps to form the eye's retina, the seat of normal vision.

Table 5–7

Food Sources of Omega-6 and Omega-3 Fatty Acids

Omega-6	
Linoleic acid	Vegetable oils (corn, cottonseed, safflower, sesame, soybean, sunflower); margarines made from these oils Nuts and seeds (cashews, walnuts, sunflower seeds, others) Poultry fat

Omega-3	
Linolenic acid[a]	Vegetable oils (canola, flaxseed, soybean, walnut, wheat germ; liquid or soft margarine made from canola or soybean oil) Nuts and seeds (chia seeds, flaxseeds, walnuts, soybeans) Vegetables (soybeans)
EPA and DHA	Human milk Fish and seafood: *500–1,800 mg/3.5 oz serving.* Barramundi, European seabass (bronzini), herring (Atlantic and Pacific), mackerel,[b] oyster (Pacific wild), salmon (wild and farmed), sardines, shark,[b] swordfish,[b] tilefish,[b] toothfish (includes Chilean seabass), lake trout (freshwater, wild and farmed) *150–500 mg/3.5 oz serving.* Black bass, catfish (wild and farmed), clam, crab (Alaskan king), croakers, flounder, haddock, hake, halibut, oyster (eastern and farmed), perch, scallop, shrimp (mixed varieties), sole *25–150 mg/3.5 oz serving.* Cod (Atlantic and Pacific), grouper, lobster, mahi-mahi, monkfish, orange roughy,[c] red snapper, skate, tilapia, triggerfish, tuna, wahoo

[a]Alpha-linolenic acid. Also found in the seed oil of the herb evening primrose.

[b]King mackerel, shark, swordfish, and tilefish are highest in mercury and should not be consumed by children or pregnant or lactating women (see the Consumer's Guide section, p. 182).

[c]Orange roughy tends to be high in mercury.

Where Are the Omega-3 Fatty Acids in Foods?

No DRI recommended intake for EPA or DHA has yet been established for healthy people, but authorities recommend choosing 8 to 12 ounces of a variety of seafood each week to provide an average of 250 mg of EPA and DHA per day.[30] Very few people in the United States regularly meet this recommendation, however.[31] They seldom choose fish, and when they do, they prefer species low in EPA and DHA. Many of the richest species are harvested from cold water; for example, salmon provides about 1,800 milligrams of EPA and DHA in just an ounce and a half of fish. It would take a pound and a half of popular warm water species, such as grouper and tilapia, to provide the same 1,800 milligrams. Grouper and tilapia are tasty, low-fat, nutritious, high-protein foods—just don't rely on them alone for EPA and DHA. Common foods that provide essential fatty acids are listed in Table 5–7. The Food Feature (p. 189) suggests ways to include seafood in the diet.

What about Fish Oil Supplements? Fish, not fish oil supplements, is the preferred source of omega-3 fatty acids for most healthy people. Evidence is mixed for people with heart disease—several studies show improvements in blood lipids and prevention of further heart disease, whereas others reveal no benefits or even increased metabolic risks from supplements.[32]

For people with specific forms of heart disease, however, the American Medical Association recommends 1,000 milligrams (1 gram) or more a day of EPA and DHA. (Figure 5–12 illustrates how to read a fish oil supplement label.) Supplements can help such people to meet this goal, but in large doses they may bring risks, such as increased bleeding, delayed wound healing, and immune suppression. The benefits and risks from EPA and DHA illustrate an important concept in nutrition: too much of a nutrient is often as harmful as too little.

Omega-3 Enriched Foods Manufacturers cannot simply add fish oil to staple foods such as milk, juice, or bread because it adds a fishy taste and quickly undergoes **oxidation**, becoming rancid. Food products may be enriched with omega-3 fatty

oxidation interaction of a compound with oxygen; in this case, a damaging effect by a chemically reactive form of oxygen. Chapter 7 provides details.

Figure 5–12

Fish Oil Supplement Label

A capsule of this supplement offers 180 mg of EPA and 120 mg of DHA, for a total of 300 mg of omega-3 oils—not the same as the 1,000 mg of fish oil weight listed on the front of the bottle. The balance is made up of other fats, as the Supplement Facts panel makes clear. Check the supplement's expiration date, too: EPA and DHA are destroyed by oxidation over time.

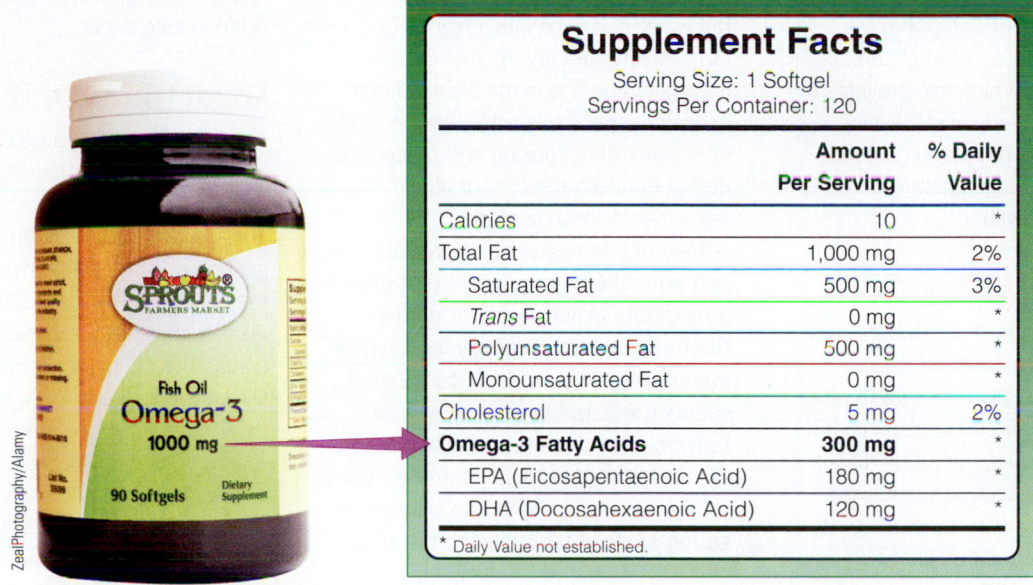

Supplement Facts

Serving Size: 1 Softgel
Servings Per Container: 120

	Amount Per Serving	% Daily Value
Calories	10	*
Total Fat	1,000 mg	2%
Saturated Fat	500 mg	3%
Trans Fat	0 mg	*
Polyunsaturated Fat	500 mg	*
Monounsaturated Fat	0 mg	*
Cholesterol	5 mg	2%
Omega-3 Fatty Acids	**300 mg**	*
EPA (Eicosapentaenoic Acid)	180 mg	*
DHA (Docosahexaenoic Acid)	120 mg	*

* Daily Value not established.

acids indirectly, but rarely do labels identify which fatty acids do the enriching. For example, eggs can be enriched with EPA and DHA by feeding laying hens grains laced with fish oil or algae oil, but most "omega-3 enriched eggs" on the market come from chickens fed on flaxseed. The hens do convert some of the linolenic acid of the flaxseed to DHA and transfer it to the egg yolk, but you'd have to eat two or three such eggs daily to obtain the suggested 250 milligrams of DHA.

An alarming depletion of the world's fish stocks has spurred a search for more sustainable sources of omega-3 fatty acids. Krill, a small, abundant, shrimplike crustacean, is rich in EPA and DHA, making it a promising choice. Marine algae and their oils provide vegetarian sources of DHA, and soybean and yeast sources are under development.[33] The Consumer's Guide (p. 182) addresses other concerns.

KEY POINTS

- Many people should increase their seafood consumption.
- Supplements of omega-3 fatty acids are not recommended.

The Effects of Processing on Unsaturated Fats

LO 5.7 Outline the process of hydrogenation and its effects on health.

Vegetable oils make up most of the added fat in the U.S. diet because fast-food chains use them for frying, food manufacturers add them to processed foods, and consumers tend to choose margarine over butter. Consumers of vegetable oils may feel safe in choosing them because they are generally less saturated than animal fats. If consumers choose a liquid oil, they may be justified in feeling secure. If the choice is a processed food, however, their security may be questionable, especially if the words *hydrogenated* or *partially hydrogenated* appear on the label's ingredient list.

Weighing Seafood's Risks and Benefits

Do you ever stand at a seafood counter or sit in a restaurant imagining a healthy fish dinner but wondering what to choose? These days, seafood comes with some questions: Which fish provides the needed essential fatty acids? Which fish is lowest in toxins or microorganisms that may pose risks to health? Which is best—farmed or wild?

Finding the EPA and DHA

Fish in many forms—fresh, frozen, and canned—makes a nutritious choice because EPA and DHA, along with other key nutrients, survive most cooking and processing. However, the *type* of fish is critical—among frozen selections, for example, pre-fried fish sticks and fillets are most often cod, a nutritious fish but one that provides little EPA and DHA (look again at the bottom of Table 5–7, p. 180).

In fast-food places, fried fish sand-wiches are generally cod. These fried fillets derive more of their calories from their oily breading or batter than from the fish itself, and more still from fatty sauces that flavor the bun. Cod, like any fish, provides little solid fat when served grilled, baked, poached, or broiled. And if it displaces fatty meats from the diet, it provides a benefit to the heart—just don't count on cod for EPA and DHA. In sit-down restaurants, diners can almost always find EPA- and DHA-rich species, such as salmon, on menus—but only if they know which is which.

Concerns about Toxins

Analyses of seafood samples have revealed widespread contamination by toxins, raising concerns about seafood safety, particularly regarding the heavy metal mercury. Mercury escapes from many industries, power

methylmercury any toxic compound of mercury to which a characteristic chemical structure, a methyl group, has been added, usually by bacteria in aquatic sediments. Methyl-mercury is readily absorbed from the intestine and causes nerve damage in people.

plants, and natural sources into the earth's waterways, where bacteria in the water convert it into a highly toxic form, **methylmercury**. Methylmercury then concentrates in the flesh of large predatory species of both saltwater and freshwater fish. Cooking and processing do not diminish mercury or other industrial toxins in seafood.

Mercury damages living tissues, and animal studies suggest that even a moderate exposure might damage the heart.[1]* Encouragingly, an average mercury exposure in U.S. consumers seems unrelated to the risk of hyper-tension.[2] For diabetes, research results are mixed, and studies continue.[3] Cur-rently, for most people, the benefits of eating seafood far outweigh the risks.[4]

Special Populations

Children and pregnant and lactating women have a critical need for EPA and DHA, but they are also most susceptible to harm from the mercury that contaminates many food fish species. For children, the U.S. Food and Drug Administration (FDA) suggests two or three age-appropriate weekly servings of a variety of lower-mercury seafood.[5] For women who are pregnant or breastfeeding, 8 to 12 ounces weekly of a variety of lower-mercury seafood, including some EPA- and DHA-rich species, is compatible with good health. However, intakes of white albacore tuna, a high-mercury fish, should be limited to no more than 6 ounces per week, and tilefish, shark, swordfish, and king mackerel should be off the menu entirely because their mercury content is too high for children and pregnant and nursing women.

Cooked vs. Raw

Many people love sushi, but authorities never recommend eating raw fish and shellfish—doing so causes many cases of serious or fatal bacterial, viral, and other illnesses each year (Chapter 12 provides

*Reference notes are found in Appendix F.

many details). Cooking easily kills off all illness-causing microorganisms, making seafood safe to eat.

Fresh from the Farm

Are farm-raised fish safer? Compared with wild fish, farm-raised fish do tend to collect somewhat less methylmercury in their flesh, and the levels of other harmful pollutants generally test below the maximums set by the FDA. However, fish "farms" are often giant ocean cages, exposed to whatever contaminants float by in the water. Farmed fish vary in EPA and DHA, too, because they are fed manufactured fish chow that varies in omega-3 fatty acid content.[6] The contamination of fish serves as a reminder that our health is inextricably linked with the health of our planet (details in Chapter 15).

Moving Ahead

Keep these pointers in mind:

- Choose a variety of fish and shellfish (prepared without the addition of solid fats) instead of red meat several times a week—people who do generally stay healthier than those who don't.
- Apply the dietary principles of ade-quacy, moderation, and variety to obtain the benefits of seafood while minimizing risks.
- Avoid eating raw seafood.

In conclusion, use a variety of seafood to meet your needs—just don't go overboard.

Review Questions**

1. Methylmercury is a toxic industrial pollutant that is easily destroyed by cooking. T F

2. Children and pregnant or lac-tating women should definitely not consume fish because of contamination. T F

3. Cod is one of the richest sources of the beneficial fatty acids, EPA and DHA. T F

**Answers to Consumer's Guide review questions are found in Appendix G.

Figure 5–13

Hydrogenation Yields Both Saturated and *Trans*-Fatty Acids

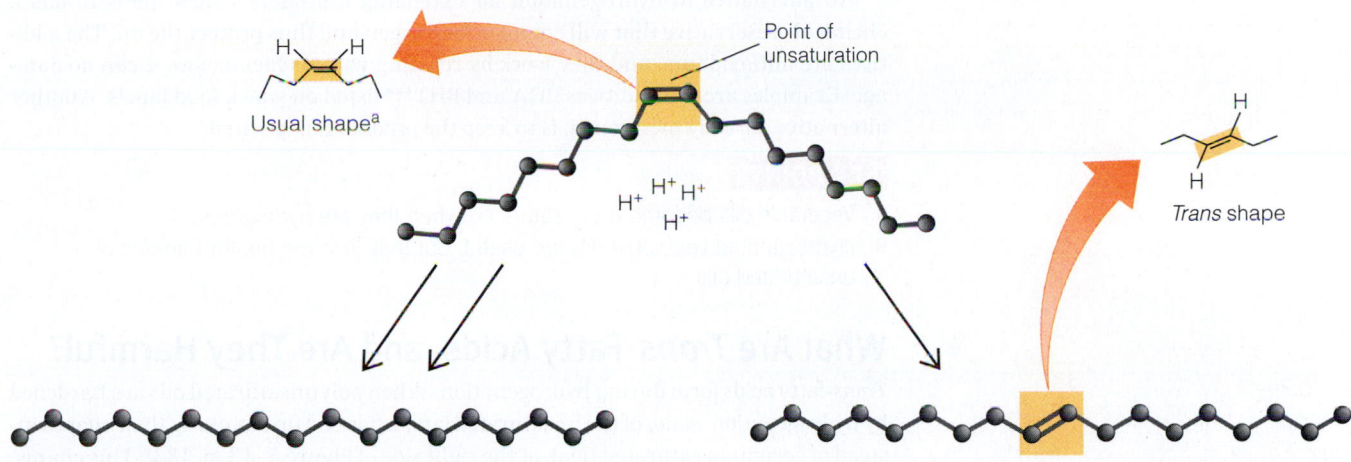

Unsaturated fatty acid
Points of unsaturation are places on fatty acid chains where hydrogen is missing. The bonds that would normally be occupied by hydrogen in a saturated fatty acid are shared, reluctantly, as a double bond between two carbons that both carry a slightly negative charge.

Usual shape[a]

Point of unsaturation

Trans shape

Hydrogenated fatty acid (now fully saturated)
When a positively charged hydrogen is made available to an unsaturated bond, it readily accepts the hydrogen and, in the process, becomes saturated. The fatty acid no longer has a point of unsaturation.

***Trans*-fatty acid**
The hydrogenation process also produces some *trans*-fatty acids. The *trans*-fatty acid retains its double bond but takes a twist instead of becoming fully saturated. It resembles a saturated fatty acid both in its shape and in its effects on health.

[a] The usual shape of the double bond structure is known as a cis (pronounced sis) formation.

What Is "Hydrogenated Vegetable Oil," and What's It Doing in My Chocolate Chip Cookies?

When manufacturers process foods, they often alter the fatty acids in the fat (triglycerides) the foods contain through a process called **hydrogenation**. Hydrogenation of fats makes them stay fresher longer and also changes their physical properties.

Hydrogenation of Oils   Points of unsaturation in fatty acids are weak spots that are vulnerable to attack by oxygen damage. When the unsaturated points in the oils of food are oxidized, the oils become rancid and the food tastes "off." This is why cooking oils should be stored in tightly covered containers that exclude air. If stored for long periods, they need refrigeration to retard oxidation.

One way to prevent spoilage of unsaturated fats and also to make them harder and more stable when heated to high temperatures is to change their fatty acids chemically by hydrogenation, as shown on the left side of Figure 5–13. When food producers want to use a polyunsaturated oil such as soybean oil to make a spreadable margarine, for example, they hydrogenate it by forcing hydrogen into the liquid oil. Some of the unsaturated fatty acids become more saturated as they accept the hydrogen, and the oil hardens. The resulting product is more saturated and more spreadable than the original oil. It is also more resistant to damage from oxidation or breakdown from high cooking temperatures. Hydrogenated oil has a high **smoking point**, so it is suitable for frying foods at high temperatures in restaurants.

Hydrogenated oils are thus easy to handle and easy to spread, and they store well. Makers of peanut butter often replace a small quantity of the liquid oil from the ground peanuts with hydrogenated vegetable oils to create a creamy paste that does

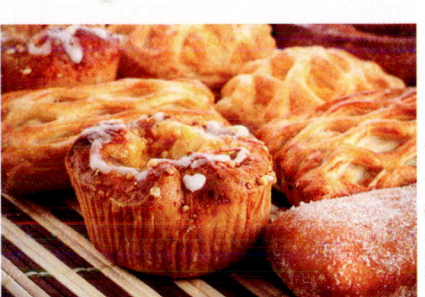

Baked goods with no trans *fat may still contain a great deal of saturated fat from shortening.*

Petr Malyshev/Shutterstock.com

hydrogenation (high-dro-gen-AY-shun) the process of adding hydrogen to unsaturated fatty acids to make fat more solid and resistant to the chemical change of oxidation.

smoking point the temperature at which fat gives off an acrid blue gas.

not separate into layers of oil and peanuts as the "old-fashioned" types do. Neither type of peanut butter is high in saturated fat, however.

Nutrient Losses   Once fully hydrogenated, oils lose their unsaturated character and the health benefits that go with it. Hydrogenation may affect not only the essential fatty acids in oils but also vitamins, such as vitamin K, decreasing their activity in the body. If you, the consumer, are looking for health benefits from polyunsaturated oils, hydrogenated oils such as those in shortening or stick margarine will not meet your need.

An alternative to hydrogenation for extending a product's shelf life is to add a chemical preservative that will compete for oxygen and thus protect the oil. The additives are antioxidants, and they work by reacting with oxygen before it can do damage. Examples are the additives BHA and BHT*** listed on snack food labels. Another alternative, already mentioned, is to keep the product refrigerated.

KEY POINTS

- Vegetable oils become more saturated when they are hydrogenated.
- Hydrogenated vegetable oils are useful, but they lose the health benefits of unsaturated oils.

What Are *Trans*-Fatty Acids, and Are They Harmful?

Trans-fatty acids form during hydrogenation. When polyunsaturated oils are hardened by hydrogenation, some of the unsaturated fatty acids end up changing their shapes instead of becoming saturated (look at the right side of Figure 5–13, p. 183). This change in chemical structure creates *trans* unsaturated fatty acids that are similar in shape to saturated fatty acids. The change in shape changes their effects in the body.

Health Effects of *Trans*-Fatty Acids   Consuming manufactured *trans* fat poses a risk to the heart and arteries by raising blood LDL cholesterol, worsening atherosclerosis, causing heart cell toxicity, and increasing tissue inflammation.[34] In addition, when hydrogenation changes essential fatty acids into their saturated or *trans* counterparts, the consumer loses the health benefits of the original raw oil. The risk to health from *trans* fat is similar to or slightly greater than that from saturated fat, so guidelines suggest that people avoid *trans* fats as much as possible. A small amount of naturally occurring *trans* fat also comes from animal sources, such as milk and lean beef, but these *trans* fats have little effect on blood lipids and are under study for potential health benefits.[†††35]

In the past decade, the level of manufactured *trans* fats in the U.S. diet has been reduced by an impressive 70 percent.[36] Following this trend, blood *trans*-fatty acid

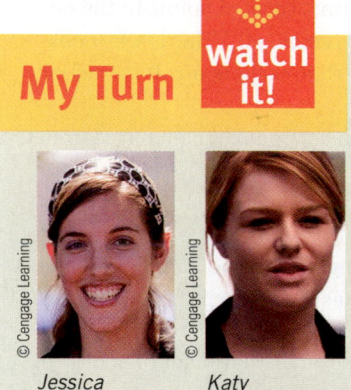

My Turn   **watch it!**   Heart to Heart

Jessica   *Katy*

How often do you think about the consequences of your food choices now on your heart health later in life? Two people talk about planning heart-healthy meals.

Visit www.cengagebrain.com to access MindTap, a complete digital course that includes these videos and other resources.

***BHA and BHT are butylated hydroxyanisole and butylated hydroxytoluene.
†††The natural *trans* fats of milk are conjugated linoleic acids.

levels are dropping, too.[37] *Trans* fats can still be found in some processed foods, such as desserts, microwave popcorn, frozen pizza, some margarines, and coffee creamers.

Swapping *Trans* Fats for Saturated Fats?   In the past, most commercially fried foods, from doughnuts to chicken, delivered a sizeable load of *trans* fats to consumers. Today, newly formulated commercial oils and fats perform the same jobs as the old hydrogenated fats but with fewer *trans*-fatty acids.[38]

If a fatty food lacks *trans* fats, is it safe for the heart? It might be, but some new fats merely substitute saturated fat for *trans* fat—and the risk to the heart and arteries from saturated fats is well established.[39] In addition, label information may not be ideal. A food listing 0 grams of either *trans* fat or saturated fat may actually contain up to 0.5 grams in a serving, an amount that can add up significantly with many servings in a day.

KEY POINTS

- The process of hydrogenation creates *trans*-fatty acids.
- *Trans* fats act like saturated fats in the body.

Fat in the Diet

LO 5.8   Discuss the sources of fats among the food groups.

The remainder of this chapter and its Controversy show you how to choose fats wisely, with the goals of providing optimal health and pleasure in eating. A column of Appendix A, entitled *Fat Breakdown (g)*, makes fascinating reading when evaluating the fat contents of foods.

Get to Know the Fats in Foods

Fats, naturally occurring or added, are widely distributed among foods. Learning their sources can help you to choose wisely among them.

Essential Fats   Everyone needs the essential fatty acids and vitamin E provided by such foods as fish, nuts, and vegetable oils. Infants receive them indirectly via breast milk, but all others must choose the foods that provide them. Luckily, the amount of fat needed to provide these nutrients is small—just a few teaspoons of raw oil a day and two servings of seafood a week are sufficient. Most people consume more than this minimum amount, however. The goal is to choose unsaturated fats in liquid oils instead of saturated solid fats as often as possible.

Visible vs. Invisible Solid Fats   The solid fat of some foods, such as the rim of fat on a steak, is visible (and therefore identifiable and removable). Other solid fats, such as those in candy, cheeses, coconut, hamburger, homogenized milk, and lunchmeats, are invisible (and therefore easily missed or ignored). Equally hidden are the solid fats blended into biscuits, cakes, cookies, chip dips, ice cream, mixed dishes, pastries, sauces, and creamy soups and in fried foods and spreads. Invisible fats supply the majority of the solid fats in the U.S. diet.

Replace, Don't Add   Keep in mind that, whether solid or liquid, essential or nonessential, all fats bring the same abundant calories to the diet and excesses contribute to body fat stores. Each of these provides about 5 grams of fat, 45 calories, and negligible protein and carbohydrate:

- 1 teaspoon oil or shortening
- 1½ teaspoons mayonnaise, butter, or margarine
- 1 tablespoon regular salad dressing, cream cheese, or heavy cream
- 1½ tablespoons sour cream

Remember to replace and not add. No benefits can be expected when oil is added to an already fat-rich diet.

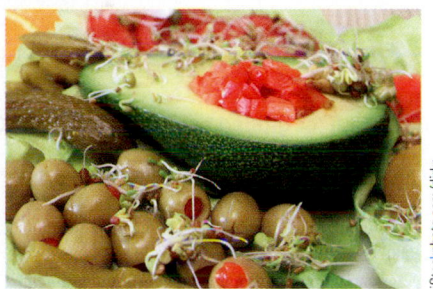

A serving of 10 small olives or a sixth of an avocado each provides about 5 grams of mostly monounsaturated fat, along with essential nutrients and potentially beneficial phytochemicals.

iStockphoto.com/dirkr

Fats in Protein Foods

The marbling of meats and the fat ground into lunchmeat, chicken products, and hamburger conceal a hefty portion of the solid fat that people consume. All meats contain about equal amounts of protein, but their fat, saturated fat, and calorie amounts vary significantly. Figure 5–14 shows the fat and calorie data on packages of ground meats, and it depicts the amount of solid fat provided by a 3-ounce serving of each kind. Nutrition Facts panels list the fat contents of many packaged meats.

> Definitions of terms relating to the fat contents of meats were provided in **Chapter 2**.

The USDA Eating Patterns (see Chapter 2) suggest that most adults limit their intake of protein foods to about 5 to 7 ounces a day. For comparison, the smallest fast-food hamburger weighs about 3 ounces. Steaks served in restaurants often run 8, 12, or 16 ounces, more than a whole day's meat allowance. You may have to weigh a serving or two of meat to see how much you are eating.

Meat: Mostly Protein or Fat?   People recognize meat as a protein-rich food, but a close look at some nutrient data reveals a surprising fact. A big (4-ounce) fast-food hamburger sandwich contains 23 grams of protein and 23 grams of fat, more than 8 of them saturated fat.[40] Because protein offers 4 calories per gram and fat offers 9, the meat of the sandwich provides 92 calories from protein but 207 calories from fat. Hot dogs, fried chicken sandwiches, and fried fish sandwiches also provide hundreds of mostly invisible calories of solid fat. Because so much meat fat is hidden from view, meat eaters can easily and unknowingly consume a great many grams of solid fat from this source.

Clues to Lower-Fat Meats   When choosing beef or pork, look for lean cuts named *loin* or *round* from which the fat can be trimmed, and eat small portions. Chicken and

Do the Math

A ground beef label may state "85% lean," but this number refers to *weight*. To calculate the percentage of *calories* from fat, use the general equation of Chapter 2 (p. 34 margin).

For a quarter pound of beef hamburger with 328 calories and 24 grams of fat:

24×9 cal/g = 216 cal from fat
$(216 \div 328) \times 100 = 66\%$

This hamburger patty derives almost two-thirds of its *calories* from fat. What percentage of calories from fat does a hamburger with 425 calories and 30 grams of fat provide?

Figure 5–14

Calories, Fat, and Saturated Fat in Cooked Ground Meat Patties[a]

Only the ground round, at 10 percent fat by raw weight, qualifies to bear the word *lean* on its label. To be called "lean," products must contain fewer than 10 grams of fat and 4 grams of saturated fat per 100 grams of food. The red labels on these packages list rules for safe meat handling, explained in Chapter 12.

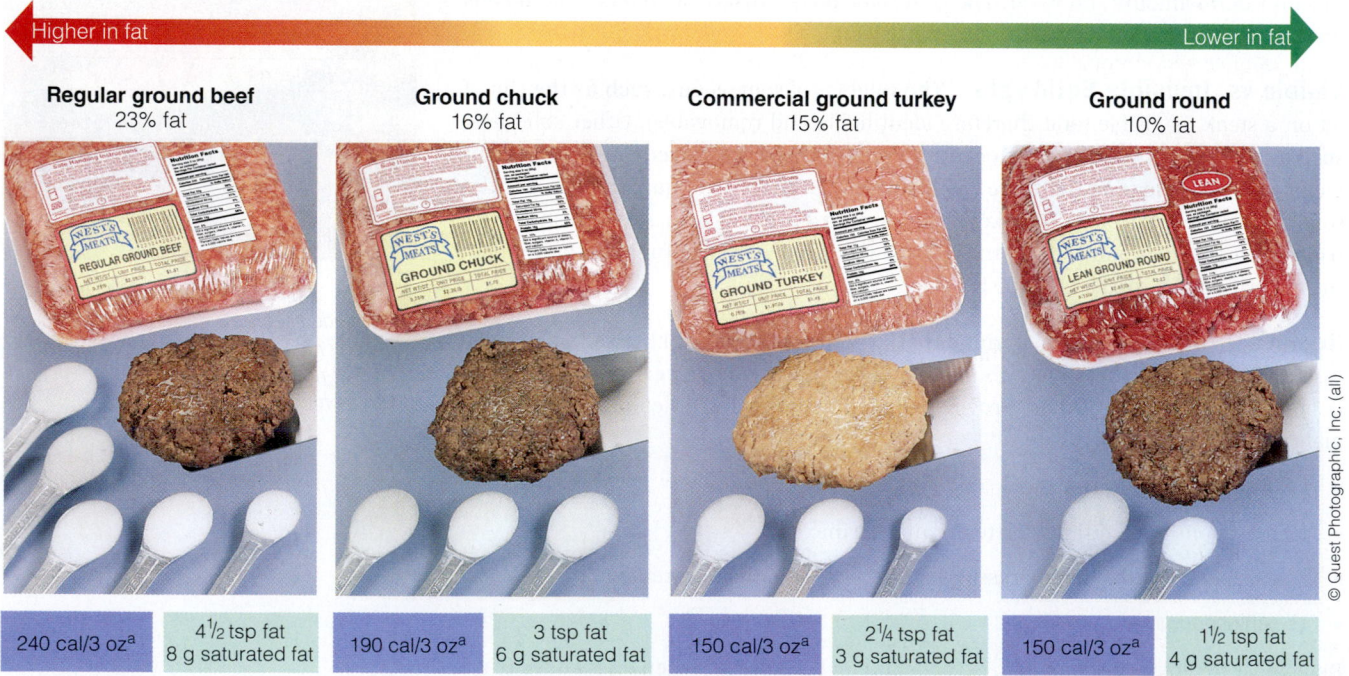

Higher in fat → Lower in fat

| **Regular ground beef** 23% fat | **Ground chuck** 16% fat | **Commercial ground turkey** 15% fat | **Ground round** 10% fat |

© Quest Photographic, Inc. (all)

| 240 cal/3 oz[a] | 4½ tsp fat 8 g saturated fat | 190 cal/3 oz[a] | 3 tsp fat 6 g saturated fat | 150 cal/3 oz[a] | 2¼ tsp fat 3 g saturated fat | 150 cal/3 oz[a] | 1½ tsp fat 4 g saturated fat |

[a]All patties weigh three ounces, cooked. Larger servings will, of course, provide more fat, saturated fat, and calories than the values listed here.

Figure 5–15

Lipids in Milk and Milk Products

Red boxes below indicate foods with higher lipid contents that warrant moderation in their use. Green indicates lower-fat choices.

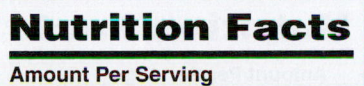

Nutrition Facts

Amount Per Serving

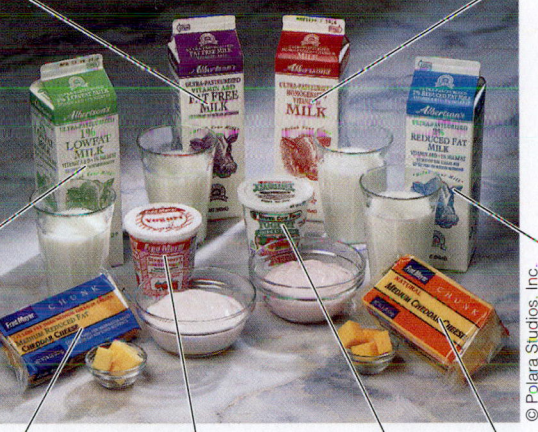

© Polara Studios, Inc.

Fat-free, skim, zero-fat, no-fat, or nonfat milk, 8 oz (<0.5% fat by weight)

Calories 80	Calories from Fat 0
	% Daily Value*
Total Fat 0g	**0%**
Saturated Fat 0g	**0%**

Low-fat milk, 8 oz (1% fat by weight)

Calories 105	Calories from Fat 20
	% Daily Value*
Total Fat 2g	**3%**
Saturated Fat 1.5g	**8%**

Low-fat cheddar cheese, 1.5 oz

Calories 70	Calories from Fat 30
	% Daily Value*
Total Fat 3g	**5%**
Saturated Fat 2g	**10%**

Strawberry yogurt, 8 oz

Calories 250	Calories from Fat 45
	% Daily Value*
Total Fat 5g	**8%**
Saturated Fat 3g	**15%**

Whole milk, 8 oz (3.3% fat by weight)

Calories 150	Calories from Fat 70
	% Daily Value*
Total Fat 8g	**12%**
Saturated Fat 5g	**25%**

Reduced-fat, less-fat milk, 8 oz (2% fat by weight)

Calories 120	Calories from Fat 45
	% Daily Value*
Total Fat 5g	**8%**
Saturated Fat 2g	**10%**

Cheddar cheese, 1.5 oz

Calories 165	Calories from Fat 130
	% Daily Value*
Total Fat 14g	**22%**
Saturated Fat 9g	**45%**

Low-fat strawberry yogurt, 8 oz

Calories 240	Calories from Fat 20
	% Daily Value*
Total Fat 2.5g	**4%**
Saturated Fat 2g	**10%**

turkey flesh are naturally lean, but commercial processing and frying add solid fats, especially to "patties," "nuggets," "fingers," and wings. Watch out for ground turkey or chicken products. The skin is often ground in to add pleasing moistness, but the food ends up with more solid fat than the amount found in many cuts of lean beef. Also, some people (even famous chefs) misinterpret Figure 5–5 (p. 166), reasoning that, if poultry or pork fat is less saturated than beef fat, it must be harmless to the heart. Nutrition authorities emphatically state, however, that all sources of saturated fat pose a risk and that even the skin of poultry should be removed before eating the food.

KEY POINT

■ Meats account for a large proportion of the hidden solid fat in many people's diets.

Milk and Milk Products

Milk products go by many names that reflect their varying fat contents, as Figure 5–15 shows. A cup of homogenized whole milk contains the protein and carbohydrate of fat-free milk, but in addition, it contains about 80 extra calories from butterfat, a solid fat. A cup of reduced-fat (2 percent fat) milk falls between whole and fat-free, with 45 calories of fat. The fat of whole milk occupies only a teaspoon or two of the volume but nearly doubles the calories in the milk.

Milk and yogurt appear together in the Milk and Milk Products group, but cream and butter do not. Milk and yogurt are rich in calcium and protein, but cream and butter are not. Cream and butter are solid fats, as are whipped cream, sour cream, and cream cheese, and they are properly grouped together with other fats. Other cheeses, grouped with milk products, vary in their fat contents and are major contributors of saturated fat in the U.S. diet.

Figure 5–16

Lipids in Grains

Red boxes below indicate foods with higher lipid contents that warrant moderation in their use. Green indicates lower-fat choices.

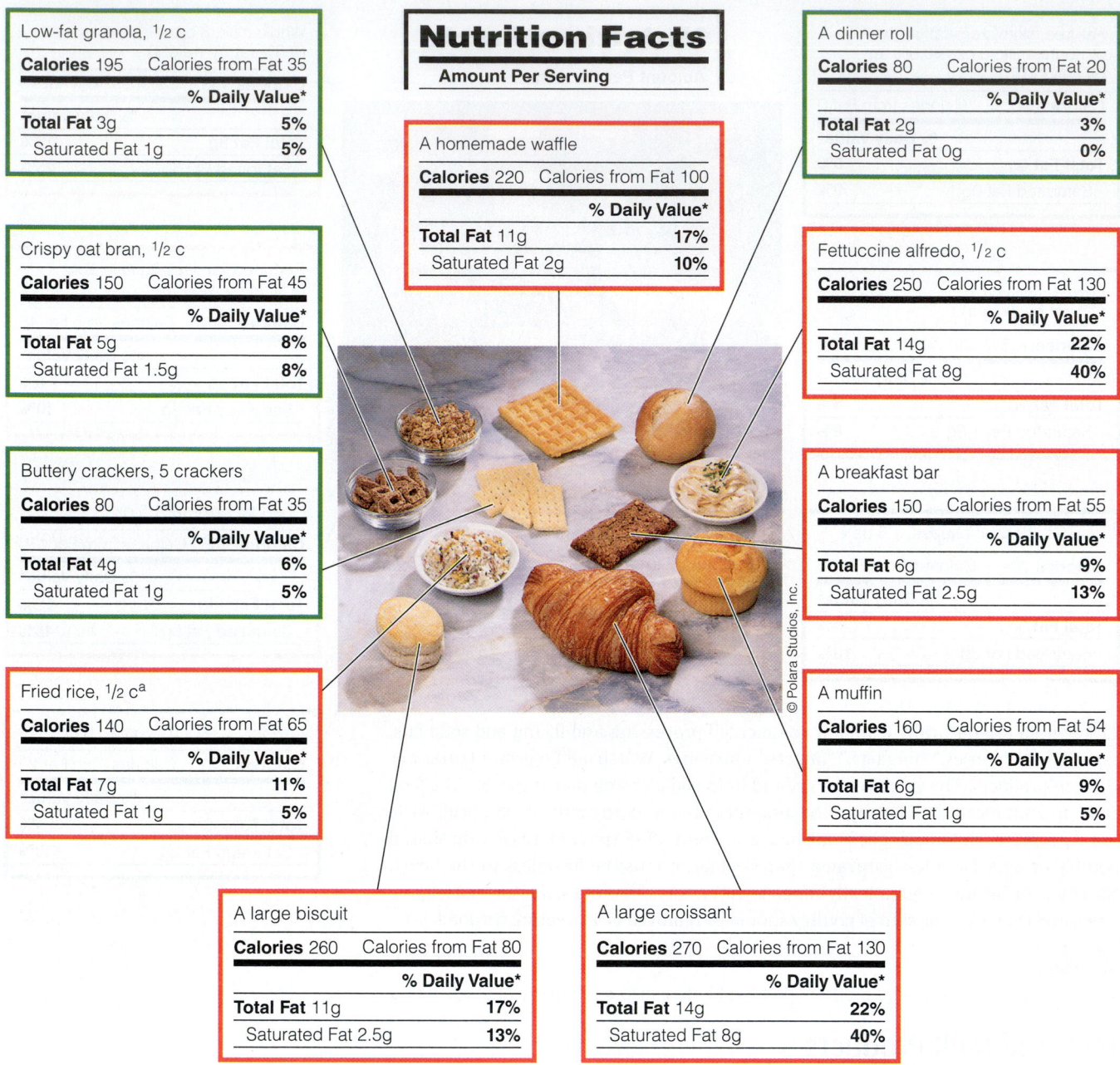

Low-fat granola, 1/2 c	
Calories 195	Calories from Fat 35
	% Daily Value*
Total Fat 3g	**5%**
Saturated Fat 1g	**5%**

Crispy oat bran, 1/2 c	
Calories 150	Calories from Fat 45
	% Daily Value*
Total Fat 5g	**8%**
Saturated Fat 1.5g	**8%**

Buttery crackers, 5 crackers	
Calories 80	Calories from Fat 35
	% Daily Value*
Total Fat 4g	**6%**
Saturated Fat 1g	**5%**

Fried rice, 1/2 c^a	
Calories 140	Calories from Fat 65
	% Daily Value*
Total Fat 7g	**11%**
Saturated Fat 1g	**5%**

Nutrition Facts

Amount Per Serving

A homemade waffle	
Calories 220	Calories from Fat 100
	% Daily Value*
Total Fat 11g	**17%**
Saturated Fat 2g	**10%**

A dinner roll	
Calories 80	Calories from Fat 20
	% Daily Value*
Total Fat 2g	**3%**
Saturated Fat 0g	**0%**

Fettuccine alfredo, 1/2 c	
Calories 250	Calories from Fat 130
	% Daily Value*
Total Fat 14g	**22%**
Saturated Fat 8g	**40%**

A breakfast bar	
Calories 150	Calories from Fat 55
	% Daily Value*
Total Fat 6g	**9%**
Saturated Fat 2.5g	**13%**

A muffin	
Calories 160	Calories from Fat 54
	% Daily Value*
Total Fat 6g	**9%**
Saturated Fat 1g	**5%**

A large biscuit	
Calories 260	Calories from Fat 80
	% Daily Value*
Total Fat 11g	**17%**
Saturated Fat 2.5g	**13%**

A large croissant	
Calories 270	Calories from Fat 130
	% Daily Value*
Total Fat 14g	**22%**
Saturated Fat 8g	**40%**

© Polara Studios, Inc.

^a The calorie and fat values of fried rice vary with preparation.

KEY POINT

- Milk products bear names that identify their fat contents.

Grains

Grain foods in their natural state are very low in fat, but fats of all kinds may be added during manufacturing, processing, or cooking (see Figure 5–16). In fact, today's leading single contributor of solid fats to the U.S. diet is grain-based desserts, such as cookies, cakes, and pastries, foods often prepared with butter, margarine, or hydrogenated shortening. Other grain foods made with solid fats include biscuits, cornbread, granola and other ready-to-eat cereals, croissants, doughnuts, fried rice, pasta with creamy or oily sauces, quick breads, snack and party crackers, muffins, pancakes, and homemade waffles. Packaged breakfast bars often resemble vitamin-fortified candy bars in their solid fat and added sugar contents.

Now that you know where the fats in foods are found, how can you reduce or eliminate the harmful ones? The Food Feature provides some pointers.

KEY POINT

- Solid fat in grain foods can be well hidden.

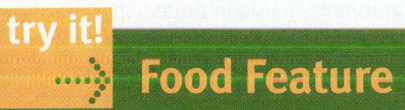

Defensive Dining

LO 5.9 Identify the ways to reduce solid fats in an average diet.

Following today's lipid guidelines can be tricky. To reduce intakes of saturated and *trans*-fatty acids, for example, you need to identify food sources of these fatty acids in your diet—that is, foods rich in solid fats (see Table 5–8). Then, to replace them appropriately you need to identify food sources of unsaturated oils and do something about all of them in your own eating pattern. Here are some tips to help simplify these feats:

1. Select the most nutrient-dense foods from all food groups. Solid fats and high-calorie choices lurk in every group.
2. Consume fewer and smaller portions of foods and beverages that contain solid fats.
3. Replace solid fats with liquid oils whenever possible.

Table 5–8

Solid Fat Ingredients Listed on Labels

- Beef fat (tallow)
- Butter
- Chicken fat
- Coconut oil
- Cream
- Hydrogenated oil
- Margarine
- Milk fat
- Palm kernel oil; palm oil
- Partially hydrogenated oil
- Pork fat (lard)
- Shortening

4. Check Nutrition Facts labels and select foods with little saturated fat and no *trans* fat.

Such advice is easily dispensed but not easily followed, however. This Food Feature provides some guidance for doing so.

In the Grocery Store

The right choices in the grocery store can save you many grams of saturated and *trans* fats. Armed with label information, you can decide whether to use a food often as a staple item or limit it to an occasional treat. For example, plain frozen vegetables without butter or other high-fat sauces are a staple food—they are high in nutrient density and devoid of solid fats. Within calorie limits, vegetables with olive oil or other unsaturated oils are also low in solid fats.

Make the same distinctions among precooked meats. Avoid those that are coated and fried or prepared in fatty gravies. Try rotisserie chicken from the deli section—rotisserie cooking lets much of the solid fat drain away. Removing the skin leaves only the chicken—a nutrient-dense food.

Choosing Seafood

Grocery stores offer many kinds and forms of seafood, such as salmon (fresh, canned, or broiled in the deli), canned tuna, and many frozen fillets, scallops, or shrimp that can help meet your need for the omega-3 fatty acids. Look back at Table 5–7, p. 180, for a list of good sources. Limit fried fish

sticks and breaded fillets, as well as seafood prepared in butter or creamy sauces. Stock pantry shelves with canned salmon, sardines, or tuna for a quick lunch; keep plain frozen fillets and seafood in the freezer for a week or two to sauté or bake from frozen (no defrosting necessary); and use up fresh fish within a day or two after purchasing it. Twice a week, try one of these quick meals:

- Tuna salad sandwich on whole-grain bread
- Tuna melt on a whole-wheat English muffin with low-fat cheddar cheese
- Grilled fish tacos with shredded coleslaw mix and salsa
- Crab cakes or salmon cakes with Greek yogurt, capers, and dill mixed for a sauce
- Smoked or grilled salmon or other fish as a main dish or in pasta salad
- Manhattan-style clam chowder or other broth-based seafood soups for lunch or supper
- Sardines on crackers for a snack
- Shrimp marinated in Italian dressing or lime juice tossed with black beans, onion, and corn for a delicious salad
- Sushi made with cooked seafood

Choosing among Margarines

Soft or liquid margarines made from unhydrogenated vegetable oils are mostly unsaturated, so they make better choices than the saturated solid fats of butter or stick margarines. Some margarines are made with extra virgin olive oil or omega-3 fatty acids, which may provide extra benefits.

Diet margarines contain fewer calories than regular varieties because water, air, or fillers have been added. A few margarines advertised to "support heart health" contain added plant sterols, phytochemicals known to lower blood LDL cholesterol somewhat, but whether they are safe for children is not known.[‡‡‡] Bottom line: read the Nutrition Facts panels. Choose margarines made with oils (but not hydrogenated oils) that have little saturated fat and no *trans* fats.

Choosing Unsaturated Oils

When choosing oils, trade off among different types to obtain the benefits different oils offer. Peanut and safflower oils are especially rich in vitamin E. Olive oil presents naturally occurring antioxidant phytochemicals (see the following paragraph), and canola oil is rich with monounsaturated and essential fatty acids. High temperatures, such as those used in frying, destroy some omega-3 acids and other beneficial constituents, so treat your oils gently. Take care to *substitute* oils for saturated fats in the diet; do not add oils to an already fat-rich diet.

Some oils are valued for their pleasing flavors or their phytochemicals believed to support health.[41] Virgin or extra virgin olive oils are mechanically pressed from olives, a process that retains the phytochemicals that confer a characteristic green color and full flavor. Less colorful "light" or regular olive oils may be extracted with chemicals or processed to remove some of the bitter-tasting phytochemicals to

[‡‡‡]The brand name of the margarine is Benecol.

fat replacers ingredients that replace some or all of the functions of fat and may or may not provide energy.

artificial fats zero-energy fat replacers that are chemically synthesized to mimic the sensory and cooking qualities of naturally occurring fats but that are totally or partially resistant to digestion.

olestra a noncaloric artificial fat made from sucrose and fatty acids; formerly called *sucrose polyester*. A trade name is *Olean*.

please consumer palates. These less costly, lower-quality oils lack many phytochemicals but are as rich in monounsaturated fatty acids as the more expensive kinds, so they still make good substitutes for saturated fats. Many people enjoy the interesting flavors of avocado oil, grape seed oil, sesame oil, and walnut oil, each with its own array of phytochemicals; research about their health effects is ongoing.

Adding Nuts

Little doubt remains about the value of nuts for heart health—people who include nuts and peanuts in the diet often have lower risks of chronic diseases.[42] Try some traditional Mediterranean uses for nuts: grind, chop, sliver, and shave almonds and walnuts into savory sauces, as toppings for vegetables and salads, for crunch in grain dishes, and for richness for desserts. Use restraint, however: a quarter cup of nuts can deliver between 130 to 200 calories.[43]

Fat-Free Products and Artificial Fats

Keep in mind that "fat-free" versions of normally high-fat foods, such as cakes or cookies, do not necessarily provide fewer calories than the original and may not provide a health advantage if added sugars take the place of fats. Some foods contain **fat replacers**—ingredients made from carbohydrate or protein that provide some of the taste and texture of solid fats but with fewer calories and less saturated fat. Others contain **artificial fats**, synthetic compounds offering the sensory properties of fat but none of the calories or fat. For example, "lite" potato chips and other snack foods contain **olestra**, an artificial fat. Chapter 12 comes back to the topic of artificial fats and other food additives.

Revamp Recipes

Once at home, minimize solid fats used as seasonings. This means enjoying the natural flavor of steamed or roasted vegetables, seasoned with lemon pepper, garlic, and herbs or a squeeze of lemon, lime, or other citrus. You might also like

vegetables with a teaspoon or two of tasty oils: olive oil or liquid margarine, sesame seed oil, nut oils, or some toasted nuts or seeds. Seek out recipes that replace solid shortening with liquid vegetable oil such as canola oil and that provide replacements for meat gravies and cheese or cream sauces. To prepare seafood, use tomatoes, onions, peppers, herbs, and other flavorful, nutrient-dense ingredients; frying in butter, shortening, or other solid fats negates some of the benefit that seafood offers.

Figure 5–17 illustrates how saturated fats are affected by some simple substitutions. Here are some other tips to help revise recipes:

- Grill, roast, broil, boil, bake, stir-fry, microwave, or poach foods. Don't fry in solid fats, such as shortening, lard, or butter. Try pan frying in a few teaspoons of olive or vegetable oil instead of deep frying.

- Reduce or eliminate food "add-ons" such as buttery, cheesy, or creamy sauces; sour cream dressings; and bacon bits that drive up the calories and saturated fat. Instead, add a small amount of olives, nuts, hummus (a tangy chickpea paste), or avocado for rich flavor.

- Cut recipe amounts of meat in half; use only lean meats. Fill in the lost bulk with soy meat replacers, shredded vegetables, legumes, pasta, or whole grains.

- Refrigerate meat pan drippings and broth, and lift off the fat when it solidifies. Add the defatted broth to flavor a casserole, cooked vegetables, or soup, or use it as a gravy.

- Make prepared mixes, such as rice or potato mixtures, by substituting liquid oils for the solid fats called for on the label. Avoid processed, refrigerated potato and other mixtures with high saturated fat contents.

For snacks, replace commercial "buttery" popcorn with the plain kind, and season it yourself with fat-free butter-flavored sprinkles, liquid or spray margarine, or a little grated parmesan cheese. The fats used in most popcorn

Figure 5–17

Fat Substitution in a Grilled Meal

These two meals are similar in total fat and calories and are equally delicious, but look at the graph to see what happens to saturated fat when olive oil, fish, and seeds replace butter, meat, and cheese. Importantly, the calories remain the same.

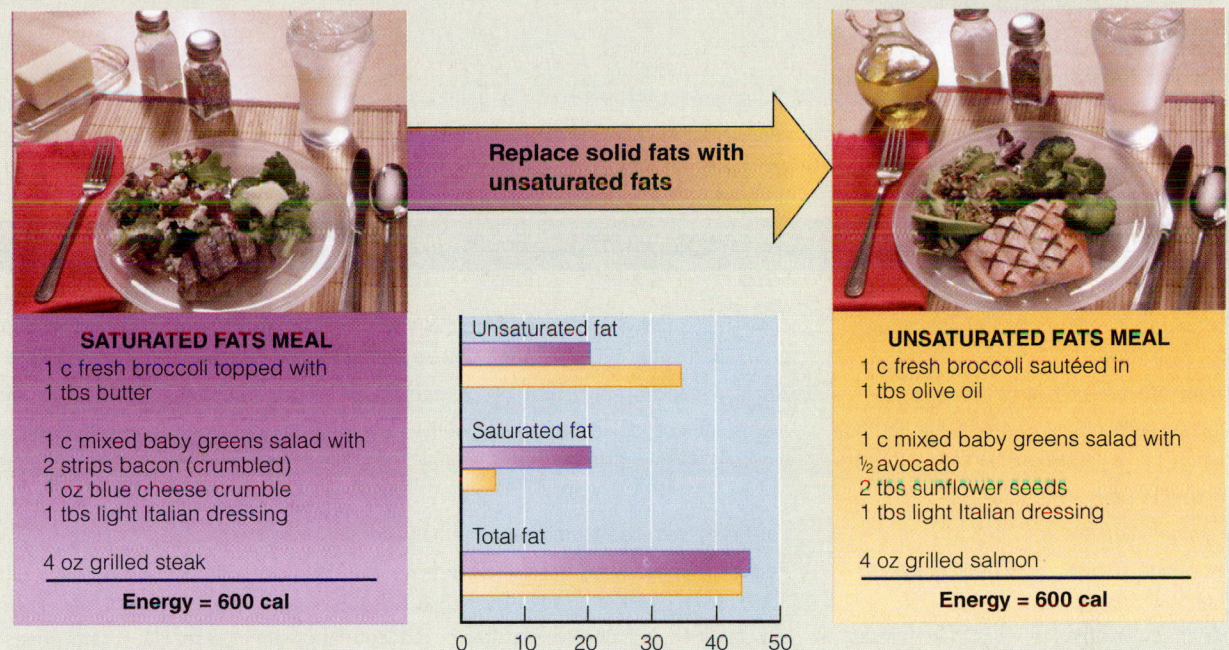

Replace solid fats with unsaturated fats

SATURATED FATS MEAL
1 c fresh broccoli topped with
1 tbs butter

1 c mixed baby greens salad with
2 strips bacon (crumbled)
1 oz blue cheese crumble
1 tbs light Italian dressing

4 oz grilled steak

Energy = 600 cal

UNSATURATED FATS MEAL
1 c fresh broccoli sautéed in
1 tbs olive oil

1 c mixed baby greens salad with
½ avocado
2 tbs sunflower seeds
1 tbs light Italian dressing

4 oz grilled salmon

Energy = 600 cal

Unsaturated fat / Saturated fat / Total fat — GRAMS (0, 10, 20, 30, 40, 50)

brands are extraordinarily high in saturated fats.

Table 5–9 (p. 192) lists practical ways to cut down on solid fats and replace them with liquid oils in foods. These replacements don't change the taste or appearance much, but they dramatically lower the saturated fat contents of the foods.

Feast on Fast Foods

All of these suggestions work well when a person plans and prepares each meal at home. But in the real world, people fall behind schedule and don't have time to shop or cook, so they eat fast food. Figure 5–18 (p. 193) compares some fast-food choices and offers tips to reduce the calories and saturated fat to make fast-food meals healthier.

Keep these facts about fast food in mind:

- Salads are a good choice, but beware of toppings such as fried noodles, bacon bits, grease-soaked croutons, sour cream, or shredded cheese that can drive up the calories and solid fat contents.

- If you are really hungry, order a small hamburger, broiled chicken sandwich, or "veggie burger" and a side salad. Hold the cheese (usually full-fat in fast-food restaurants); use mustard or ketchup as condiments.

- A small bowl of chili (hold the cheese and sour cream) poured over a plain baked potato can also satisfy a bigger appetite. Top it with chopped raw onions or hot sauce for spice, and pair it with a small salad and fat-free milk for a complete meal.

- Chicken or fish tacos, bean burritos, and other Mexican treats are delicious topped with salsa and onions instead of cheese and sour cream.

- Fast-food fried fish or fried chicken sandwiches can provide as much solid fat as hamburgers. Broiled chicken and fish sandwiches are far less fatty if you order them without cheese, bacon, or mayonnaise sauces.

- Chicken wings are mostly fatty skin, and the tastiest wing snacks are fried in cooking fat (often a saturated type), smothered with

a buttery, spicy sauce, and then dipped in blue cheese dressing, making wings an extraordinarily high-fat, high-calorie food. If you snack on wings, plan on eating more nutrient-dense foods at several other meals to balance them out.

Because fast foods are short on variety, let them be part of a lifestyle in which they complement the other parts. Eat differently, often, elsewhere.

Change Your Habits

The lipid guidelines offered in this chapter do not occur in isolation—they accompany recommendations to achieve and sustain a healthy body weight, to keep calories under control, and to eat a nutrient-dense diet with adequate fruits, vegetables, whole grains, and legumes, which provide cholesterol-lowering soluble fiber as well. By this time, you may be wondering if you can realistically make all the changes recommended for your diet.

Be assured that even small changes can yield big dividends in terms of reducing solid fats intake, and most such changes can become habits after a few repetitions. You do not have to give up all high-fat treats, even chicken wings, nor should you strive to eliminate all fats. You decide what the treats should be and then choose them in moderation, just for pure pleasure. Meanwhile, make sure that your everyday, ordinary choices are those whole, nutrient-dense foods suggested throughout this book. That way you'll meet all your body's needs for nutrients and never feel deprived.

Table 5–9

Solid Fat Replacements

Select foods that replace solid fats with polyunsaturated or monounsaturated fats. Avoid foods that replace fats with refined white flour or added sugars, as these may present risks of their own. Remember that "light" on a label can refer to color or texture, so always compare the Nutrition Facts panel with the regular product.

Instead of these ...	... try choosing these
Solid Fats and Oils	
Regular margarine and butter for spreading, cooking, or baking	Olive, nut, seed, and other vegetable oils; reduced-fat, diet, liquid, or spray margarine; granulated butter replacers; fruit butters, hummus, nut butters, or avocado for spreading
Shortening or lard in cooking	Nonstick cooking spray, olive oil, or vegetable oil for frying; applesauce or oil for baking
Solid fats as seasonings: bacon, bacon fat, butter; fried onion or greasy crouton salad toppers	Herbs, lemons, spices, liquid smoke flavoring, ham-flavored bouillon cubes, broth, wine; olive oil; olives; toasted nut or toasted whole-grain crouton toppers
Milk Products/Dairy Products	
Whole milk; half and half	Fat-free or reduced-fat milk; fat-free half and half
Regular ricotta cheese; mozzarella cheese; yogurt or sour cream	Part-skim ricotta or fat-free cottage cheese; part-skim mozzarella; fat-free sour cream, "zero" plain Greek-style yogurt[a]
Regular cheddar, American, or other cheeses; cream cheese	Low-fat or fat-free cheeses; fat-free or reduced-fat cream cheese, Neufchatel cheese
Large amounts of mild cheeses	Small amounts of strong-flavored aged cheeses (sharp cheddar; grated Asiago, Romano, or Parmesan)
Ice cream, mousse, cream custards	"Light" ice cream, frozen yogurt, or other frozen desserts; low-sugar sherbet or sorbet; skim milk low-sugar puddings
Protein Foods	
Bologna, salami, other sliced sandwich meats; hot dogs	Low-fat sandwich meats and hot dogs (95–97% lean, or "light")
Breakfast sausage or bacon	Canadian bacon, lean ham, or soy-based sausage or bacon-like products
High-fat beef, pork, or lamb; ground beef	Leaner cuts trimmed of fat, broiled salmon or other seafood; ground turkey breast (98% lean), soy-based "ground beef" crumbles; legume main dishes
Poultry with skin	Skinless poultry
Commercial fish sticks, breaded fried fish fillets	Plain fish fillets, broiled or rolled in seasoned whole-wheat breadcrumbs and pan sautéed in oil
Grains and Desserts	
Chips, such as tortilla or potato; appetizer crackers	Baked or "light" chips; reduced-fat crackers and cookies, saltine-type crackers; nut, seed, or whole-grain crackers low in saturated and *trans* fat
Cakes, cookies; doughnuts, pastries, other desserts	Fresh and dried fruit; whole-grain muffins, quick breads, or cakes made with oil (not shortening)
Granola, other cereals with saturated fat or hydrogenated fat	Cereals low in saturated fat, with no *trans* fat (compare the Nutrition Facts panel information)
Macaroni and cheese	Spaghetti and marinara sauce
Ramen-type noodles[b]	Soba noodles or other whole-grain noodles cooked in broth, with Asian seasonings
Other	
Frozen or canned main dishes with more than 2 or 3 g saturated fat per serving	Similar foods with less saturated fat per serving (compare the Nutrition Facts panel information)
Cream-based, cheese, or "loaded" soups	Broth-based, vegetable, or bean soups; poultry-based, meatless, or other low-fat chili

[a]If the food must be boiled, stabilize the cottage cheese or yogurt with a small amount of cornstarch or flour.
[b]Ramen noodles are often fried in saturated oils during processing.

Chapter 5 The Lipids: Fats, Oils, Phospholipids, and Sterols

Figure 5–18

Making Fast-Food Choices

Scan fast-food menus for lower-calorie options, and then make substitutions like these. Chapter 9 revisits calorie information on menus.

Key: ■ Calories ■ Grams saturated fat ■ % Daily Value (DV=20 g saturated fat)

Indulgent Choices

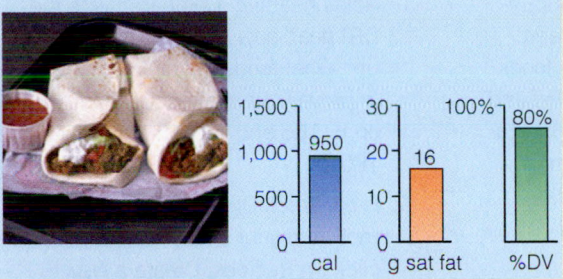

1,500 — 30 — 100% — 80%
1,000 — 950 — 20 — 16
500 — 10
0 — 0
cal — g sat fat — %DV

2 "grande" burritos with beef, beans, cheese, and sour cream; salsa

Burrito choices
- Enjoy beans, cheese, and salsa.
- Omit beef and sour cream.

Enlightened Choices

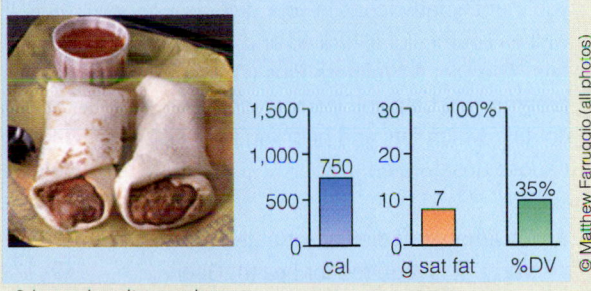

1,500 — 30 — 100%
1,000 — 750 — 20
500 — 10 — 7 — 35%
0 — 0
cal — g sat fat — %DV

© Matthew Farruggio (all photos)

2 bean burritos; salsa

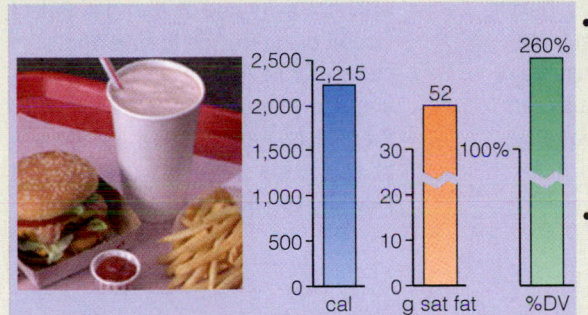

2,500 — 2,215 — 260%
2,000 — 52
1,500 — 30 — 100%
1,000 — 20
500 — 10
0 — 0
cal — g sat fat — %DV

Big double cheeseburger, large fries, regular milkshake

Sandwich choices
- Choose grilled (not fried) chicken with spicy mustard, lettuce, onion, and tomato; milk; and a crunchy side salad with reduced-calorie dressing.
- Omit beef, mayonnaise sauce, fries, and shake.

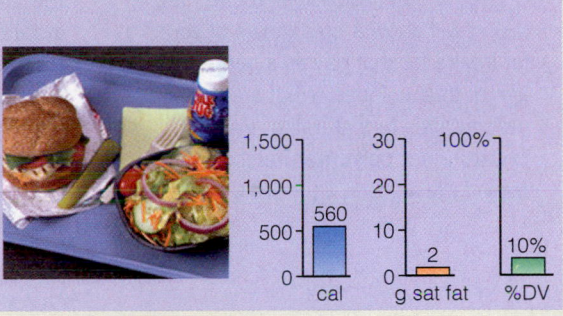

1,500 — 30 — 100%
1,000 — 20
560 — 10
500 — 2 — 10%
0 — 0
cal — g sat fat — %DV

Big grilled chicken breast sandwich, pickle, side salad with reduced-calorie dressing, fat-free milk

---

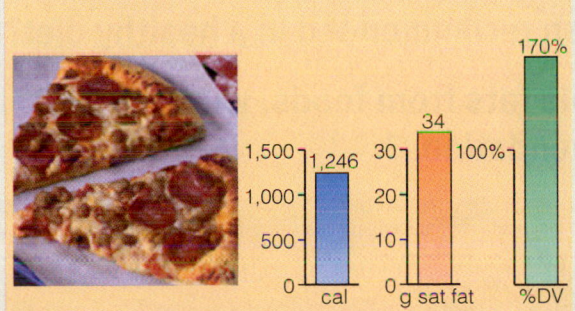

1,500 — 30 — 100% — 80%
1,000 — 910 — 20 — 16
500 — 10
0 — 0
cal — g sat fat — %DV

Taco salad with chili, cheese, sour cream, salsa, and taco chips

Salad choices
- Enjoy chili, onions, salsa, and a few chips on crispy salad vegetables. Use half the dressing.
- Omit cheese and sour cream.

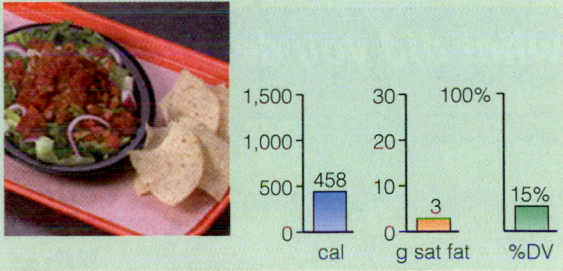

1,500 — 30 — 100%
1,000 — 20
500 — 458 — 10 — 3 — 15%
0 — 0
cal — g sat fat — %DV

Taco salad with chili, salsa, and taco chips

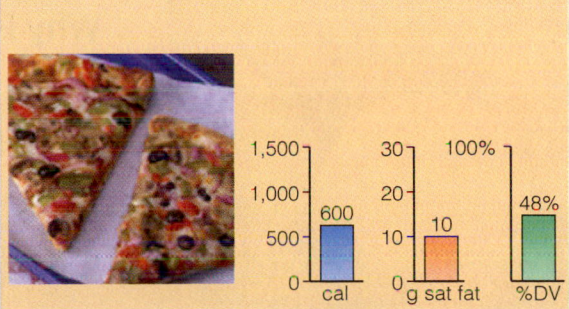

Pizza choices
- Top with mushrooms, bell and hot peppers, onions, olives, artichokes, sun-dried tomatoes, and the regular amount of cheese.
- Omit fatty meats and extra cheese.

1,500 — 1,246 — 34 — 170%
30 — 100%
1,000 — 20
500 — 10
0 — 0
cal — g sat fat — %DV

Two slices extra cheese pizza with sausage and pepperoni

1,500 — 30 — 100%
1,000 — 20
600 — 10 — 10 — 48%
500
0 — 0
cal — g sat fat — %DV

Two slices cheese pizza with mushrooms, olives, onions, and peppers

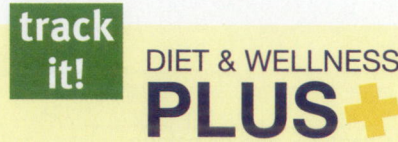

DIET & WELLNESS PLUS+ Concepts in Action

Analyze Your Lipid Intake

The purpose of this exercise is to help you identify fatty foods in your diet, as well as sources of saturated and *trans* fats. The Diet & Wellness Plus (D&W+) program will help you learn which foods contain which fats and help you to choose unsaturated fats.

1. No amount of dietary saturated or *trans* fat is required for health. Open the D&W+ Home page. From the Reports tab, select Fat Breakdown. Choose a date, choose all meals. Your report will show a breakdown of your fat intake for that day as a percentage of total calories. What are the percentages for saturated, mono-unsaturated, polyunsaturated, and *trans*-fatty acids in your day's intake?

2. Which foods provide the most fat to your diet? Select Source Analysis from the Report tab. Select a date and choose all meals. Select Save as PDF. Do the same for monoun-saturated, polyunsaturated, and *trans*-fatty acids. What three foods contributed the most saturated and monounsaturated fats? Polyunsatu-rated and *trans* fats? Which of your foods are listed as solid fat contributors in Figure 5–9 (p. 173)?

3. The Macronutrient Ranges re-port compares your intakes to the recommended intake ranges. Select a date, click on the Macronutrient Range report, select the entire day's food intake. Did your intake for fats fall within the recommended range? What percentage of your calories came from fat?

4. To study your intake of essential fatty acids, select Reports, Intake vs. Goals, and then select day one, all meals. Look for the Essential Fatty Acids heading. Compared with the DRI goal, how did your intake stack up? What foods might you change to improve your intake (see Figure 5–5 on p. 166 and Table 5–7 on page 180)?

5. From Track Diet, select a new day (not from your 3-day record) and click on Recipes, Create a New Recipe. Invent an appealing, heart-healthy salad by adding ingredients with little saturated or *trans* fat. Select Done Editing Recipe to save and close your recipe. Select Track Diet, and find your salad below. Click on the "i" icon next to the recipe name to display the nutrients in the salad. How did you do?

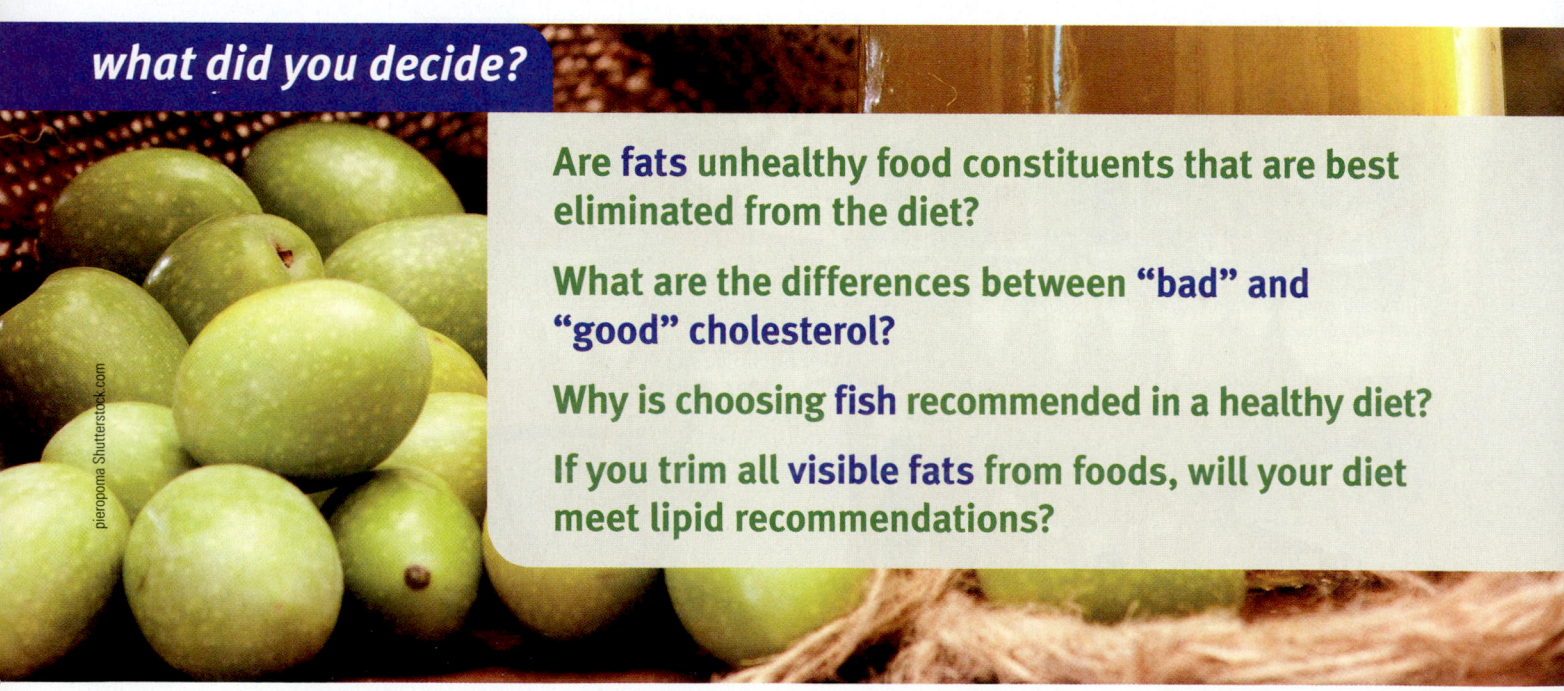

what did you decide?

Are **fats** unhealthy food constituents that are best **eliminated** from the diet?

What are the differences between **"bad"** and **"good" cholesterol**?

Why is choosing **fish** recommended in a healthy diet?

If you trim all **visible fats** from foods, will your diet meet **lipid recommendations**?

pieropoma Shutterstock.com

Self Check

1. (LO 5.1) Which of the following is *not* one of the ways fats are useful in foods?
   a. Fats contribute to the taste and smell of foods.
   b. Fats carry fat-soluble vitamins.
   c. Fats provide a low-calorie source of energy compared to carbohydrates.
   d. Fats provide essential fatty acids.

2. (LO 5.1) Fats play few roles in the body, apart from providing abundant fuel in the form of calories.
   T   F

3. (LO 5.2) Saturation refers to
   a. the ability of a fat to penetrate a barrier, such as paper.
   b. whether or not a fatty acid chain is holding all of the hydrogen atoms it can hold.
   c. the characteristic of pleasing flavor and aroma.
   d. the fattening power of fat.

4. (LO 5.2) Generally speaking, vegetable and fish oils are rich in saturated fat.
   T   F

5. (LO 5.2) A benefit to health is seen when _____ is used in place of _____ in the diet.
   a. saturated fat/monounsaturated fat
   b. saturated fat/polyunsaturated fat
   c. polyunsaturated fat/saturated fat
   d. triglycerides/cholesterol

6. (LO 5.3) Little fat digestion takes place in the stomach.
   T   F

7. (LO 5.3) Bile is essential for fat digestion because it
   a. splits triglycerides into fatty acids and glycerol.
   b. emulsifies fats in the small intestine.
   c. works as a hormone to suppress appetite.
   d. emulsifies fat in the stomach.

8. (LO 5.4) When energy from food is in short supply, the body
   a. dismantles its glycogen and releases triglycerides for energy.
   b. dismantles its cholesterol and releases glucose for energy.
   c. converts its glucose to fat for more efficient energy.
   d. dismantles its stored triglycerides and releases fatty acids for energy.

9. (LO 5.4) Fat breakdown without carbohydrate causes ketones to build up in the tissues and blood and be excreted in the urine.
   T   F

10. (LO 5.5) LDL, a class of lipoprotein, delivers triglycerides and cholesterol from the liver to the body's tissues.
    T   F

11. (LO 5.5) Chylomicrons, a class of lipoprotein, are produced in the liver.
    T   F

12. (LO 5.5) Consuming large amounts of saturated fatty acids lowers LDL cholesterol and thus lowers the risk of heart disease and heart attack.
    T   F

13. (LO 5.6) The roles of the essential fatty acids include
    a. forming parts of cell membranes.
    b. supporting infant growth and vision development.
    c. supporting normal blood pressure.
    d. all of the above.

14. (LO 5.6) Taking supplements of fish oil is recommended for those who don't like fish.
    T   F

15. (LO 5.6) Fried fish from fast-food restaurants and frozen fried fish products are often low in omega-3 and high in solid fats.
    T   F

16. (LO 5.7) A way to prevent spoilage of unsaturated fats and make them harder is to change their fatty acids chemically through
    a. acetylation.
    b. hydrogenation.
    c. oxidation.
    d. mastication.

17. (LO 5.7) *Trans*-fatty acids arise when unsaturated fats are
    a. used for deep frying.
    b. hydrogenated.
    c. baked.
    d. used as preservatives.

18. (LO 5.8) An eating pattern with sufficient essential fatty acids includes
    a. nuts and vegetable oils.
    b. ¼ cup of raw oil each day.
    c. two servings of seafood a week.
    d. a and c.

19. (LO 5.8) The majority of solid fats in the U.S. diet are supplied by invisible fats.
    T   F

20. (LO 5.9) Solid fats and high-calorie choices lurk in every food group.
    T   F

21. (LO 5.10) Which is true of very low-fat diets?
    a. They may lack essential fatty acids and certain vitamins.
    b. They may be high in carbohydrate calories.
    c. They are difficult to maintain over time.
    d. All of the above.

Answers to these Self Check questions are in Appendix G.

Is Butter Really Back? The Lipid Guidelines Debate

LO 5.10 Discuss both sides of the scientific debate about current lipid guidelines.

drbimages/Getty Images

To consumers, advice about dietary fats appears to change almost daily. "Eat less fat—choose more margarine." "Give up butter and margarine—use soft margarine." "Forget soft margarine—replace it with olive oil." Then headlines seem to turn all the previous advice on its head. To researchers, however, the evolution of advice about fats reflects decades of research that built a foundation of knowledge about the health effects of dietary fats.

This Controversy explores these changing guidelines and the arguments both for and against current lipid guidelines. It ends with the current opinion that, while specific lipids are associated with disease risks, a person's repetitive daily food choices—that is, their entire eating pattern—seems to have the greatest impact.

Shifting Guidelines

In years past, Dietary Guidelines urged all healthy people, not just those with heart disease, to cut their total fat intakes in everything from hot dogs to salad dressings to preserve their good health. This advice was straightforward: cut the fat and improve your health. Did this strategy work? Yes, but only for those few who consistently replaced all high-fat foods with whole grains, vegetables, fruit, fat-free milk products, and small portions of low-fat fish and poultry.[1]*

In response to total fat guidelines, food manufacturers flooded market shelves with an abundance of fat-free (but sugar-laden) cookies, candies, and ice cream and low-fat (but high-calorie) main courses. In the mistaken belief that "fat-free" means "no limits," consumers

*Reference notes are found in Appendix F.

gobbled them up, often in addition to their regular diets. Calorie intakes from carbohydrates, mainly from added sugars and refined starches, climbed, and so did rates of obesity and heart disease.[2] In the end, most consumers gave up in frustration after a few weeks or months and went back to their old ways of eating.

Research Revelations

A classic study, the Seven Countries Study, initially published in the 1960s, helped to nudge national guidelines away from the total fat approach to heart health.[3] In the study, researchers compared death rates from cardiovascular diseases (CVD) with intakes of total fat and saturated fat in seven countries of the world. Study subjects reported their diet histories to dietitians who interviewed them at home, in the presence of the person who prepared their food, and then cross-checked the information with records of the food purchased by that family during the week—a valid approach for assessing intakes. The researchers also collected personal, medical, and lifestyle information, and then repeated all of these processes 5 and 10 years

afterward. Later phases of the study continued to yield data for decades.

The results were, at the time, remarkable. Two of the seven countries, Finland and the Greek island of Crete, emerged as having the highest intake of total fat—40 percent of calories. What the researchers discovered next was unexpected: Finland also had the highest CVD death rate by far of all the countries, but Crete had the lowest. These findings suggested that total fat intake alone could not account for differences in risks of CVD—something else had to be responsible. When they examined the two diets more closely, the researchers found that the Finns ate diets high in saturated fats (18 percent of calories). Conversely, diets in Crete were low in saturated fat (less than 10 percent of calories) but high in unsaturated fat from olive oil, an eating pattern still linked with relatively low risks of CVD today.

Soon, nutrition guidelines had singled out saturated fats for restriction to address soaring rates of heart disease. Again, food manufacturers acted quickly, replacing lard and butter in their formulations with partially hydrogenated vegetable shortenings and margarines. No one knew it at the time, but these replacements for saturated fats were rich in *trans*-fatty acids, now known to be as bad or worse than saturated fatty acids with regard to CVD risk.[4] As you might expect, heart disease rates remained high during this period.

Dietary Guidelines for Americans 2015

Many studies in the decades that followed, including clinical, epidemiological, and animal studies, have largely supported the saturated fat theory.[5] After reviewing available evidence, the Dietary Guidelines 2015 committee concluded that saturated fat is a nutrient of concern for public health, because:

- Strong, consistent evidence shows that replacing saturated fats with unsaturated fats, especially polyunsaturated fats, significantly reduces total and LDL cholesterol in the blood.
- Strong, consistent evidence shows that replacing saturated fats with polyunsaturated fats reduces the risk of developing CVD and of dying of heart disease (see Figure C5–1).[6]

Figure C5–1

Saturated Fatty Acids and CVD Risk

Replacing saturated fat with unsaturated fat reduces in CVD risk. The reverse is also true: increasing saturated fat intakes increases the risk.

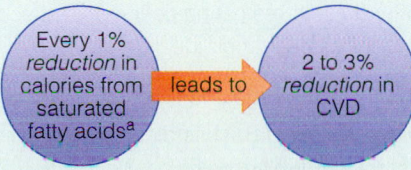

Every 1% *reduction* in calories from saturated fatty acids[a] — leads to — 2 to 3% *reduction* in CVD

[a] When replaced by polyunsaturated fat; the effect of carbohydrate is not clear and may depend on the type and source of carbohydrate.

Source: U.S. Department of Agriculture and U.S. Department of Health and Human Services, Scientific Report of the 2015 Dietary Guidelines Advisory Committee (2015): D-6-12-17, available at www.health.gov.

They also state that:

- Partially hydrogenated oils containing *trans* fat should be avoided.

The committee based these conclusions on multiple recent high-quality systematic reviews and meta-analyses comparing saturated fat intake with factors such as:

- Blood lipids,
- Blood pressure,
- CVD development,
- Heart attacks,
- Strokes, and
- Death.

Taken together, the evidence supports replacing saturated fatty acids in the diet with unsaturated fats, rather than restricting total fat intakes. Replacing saturated fats with carbohydrates also reduces total and LDL cholesterol but significantly *increases* blood triglycerides and reduces HDL cholesterol, two indicators of elevated CVD risk. These effects may depend on the form of the carbohydrate—for example, added sugars may raise CVD risk, but fiber-rich legumes reduce it (details in Controversy 4).

The results of some studies on consumption of saturated fat and risk of CVD suggest no relationship between reducing saturated fat intake and heart disease or mortality. The problem, however, is that some of these studies failed to specify what, exactly, took the place of the saturated fat in the diet. Typically, when people reduce saturated fats, they increase carbohydrates. The Dietary Guidelines committee concluded that simply reducing saturated fat and replacing it with unspecified types of carbohydrate, which could be refined starches and added sugars, is not effective in reducing CVD risk.[7]

You can read more about the research that the committee used in setting the guidelines on the Internet—open a free copy of the *Scientific Report of the 2015 Dietary Guidelines*

Advisory Committee.[1] For the committee's current advice to the nation, turn back to Table 5–2 (p. 173) in the preceding chapter.

The American Heart Association and American College of Cardiologists Concur

In 2014, two venerable medical organizations, the American Heart Association and the American College of Cardiologists (AHA/ACC), on reviewing similar research, reasserted with their strongest level of confidence that people who need to lower their blood LDL cholesterol should reduce their intake of saturated fat. In addition to raising blood LDL cholesterol, these experts say, high intake of one saturated fatty acid (**palmitic acid**; see Table C5–1) may worsen a dangerous form of irregular heartbeat.[8] The AHA/ACC intake goal for saturated fat in this population is therefore set at no more than 5–6 percent of total calories, a reduction from their earlier goal of 7 percent.[9]

The ultimate goal of the Dietary Guidelines for Americans is to reduce the likelihood of a heart attack or other CVD event, and this outcome is supported by research.[10] A thorough review indicated that people who replace saturated fats in the diet with unsaturated fats can expect a substantial (up to 14 percent) drop in their risk of a major CVD event.

Table C5–1

Saturated Fatty Acid Terms

palmitic acid a 16-carbon saturated fatty acid found in tropical palm oil, among other foods. Palmitic acid intake is associated with atrial fibrillation, a dangerous form of irregular heartbeat.

stearic acid an 18-carbon saturated fatty acid found in most animal fats. Unlike most other saturated fatty acids, it does not raise blood LDL cholesterol.

[1] Available at www.health.gov.

So What's the Debate?

Most scientists generally agree with current lipid intake guidelines, but others argue that saturated fat is irrelevant to heart health.[11] They offer the following lines of research to defend their position.

Missing Mechanism

First, they correctly argue that no biological mechanism has been firmly established to explain how, exactly, saturated fat leads to the formation of atherosclerosis, the hardening of the arteries that underlies CVD.[12] Before condemning saturated fat by association with CVD, they want to find the smoking gun, so to speak—the physiological mechanism by which these fats may cause the disease.

Actions of Genes

Second, they point out that a person's genetic inheritance strongly influences how his or her body handles fatty acids. Some people are more susceptible to forming particularly harmful types of LDL cholesterol or inefficient types of HDL cholesterol, changing their CVD risks independently of diet.

Differing Actions of Saturated Fatty Acids

Third, the effects of individual saturated fatty acids vary with regard to CVD risk. Most saturated fatty acids elevate blood LDL, but **stearic acid**, a saturated fatty acid found in meats, milk products, chocolate, and other foods, is exceptional—it does not raise blood LDL cholesterol.[13] In addition, other saturated fatty acids in milk products are under study to determine their effects on LDL cholesterol.

Is Butter Really Back?

In 2014, opposing arguments appeared in a broad range of stories and articles in the media. Gleeful headlines proclaiming "Butter Is Back," shocked (and often delighted) consumers with stories urging them to ignore the Dietary Guidelines for Americans and eat all the ice cream,

marbled steaks, and butter that they desire. Research, the journalists said, had vindicated saturated fat of its role in causing heart disease.[14]

These claims were spawned by the publication of a scientific meta-analysis (a study that combines prior published data and reanalyzes them) that did, in fact, fail to find a correlation between dietary saturated fat intakes and elevated CVD risk.[15] This study included data from many previous observational studies—that is, studies that asked people what they ate and then tracked their health over time.

Authorities Weigh In

Challenges to this meta-analysis were immediate and vigorous.[16] One objection arose from the kinds of data that were included in the study. The data were drawn from observational research that relies on what people *say* they eat, which most often differs from what those people *actually* eat. Apparently, something about human nature, perhaps memory lapse or fear of embarrassment, impedes an accurate accounting of food consumption, so the best studies verify intakes.

Another objection concerned the studies chosen for inclusion. The Dietary Guidelines committee pointed out that the analysis was based on a limited number of certain kinds of studies.[17] A summary of the arguments surrounding these issues is presented in Table C5–2.

Research Continues

Today, in the normal pace of science, studies are quietly probing into the roles of saturated and *trans* fats in CVD risk. For example, a recent study reported no association between saturated fat intake and heart attack or death in people already suffering from heart disease.[18] Another reported that diets high in unsaturated fat reduced the most harmful type of LDL cholesterol.[19] No one now knows what future research might uncover, but informed readers should engage their critical thinking skills when evaluating media accounts of new findings.

The Power of Eating Patterns

While debates continue, researchers note that people choose foods, not individual nutrients such as saturated fat, and their choices form habitual eating patterns that affect health.[20] For this reason, an eating pattern approach was used to set the 2015 Dietary Guidelines for Americans.[21] Following an eating pattern that meets the ideals of the Dietary Guidelines (see Chapter 2) reliably improves health in many ways, including controlling body fatness and reducing CVD risk factors, such as diabetes and hypertension. The individual components of such a pattern have synergistic and cumulative effects—that is, they work in harmony over decades to improve health beyond the effects of fats alone.

Figure C5–2 (p. 200) presents two meals that characterize two very different eating patterns—one associated with lower chronic disease risks and the other with increased risks. If most of your meals resemble the dinner on the left, you can be assured of obtaining the nutrients you need within a pattern that supports health superbly. Conversely, if most of your meals resemble the commercially prepared fried chicken fingers and french fries in the other meal, without a fruit or nonstarchy vegetable in sight, you may want to reconsider your choices for your health's sake. This is not to say that an occasional treat of chicken fingers and fries or a corndog and cola can never fit into your diet, but if your choices follow this pattern on most days, disease risks climb.

The Dietary Guidelines for Americans offer these three eating patterns as effective for meeting their ideals:

- A healthy vegetarian diet,
- A healthy U.S.-style diet, and
- A healthy Mediterranean diet.

Details about all three are in Appendix E. Following any of these eating patterns can help to both meet nutrient needs and keep the risks of chronic diseases low.

Table C5–2

Saturated Fat Debate: Point, Counterpoint

The left column below presents some points made by leading agencies and medical experts in support of guidelines to limit saturated fat intakes. The right column presents dissenting opinions.

Point	Counterpoint
1. *Long-established research.* Saturated fat raises serum LDL cholesterol, and high LDL cholesterol signals increased risk for heart disease. Hundreds of trials over many decades confirm these findings.	1. *Missing mechanism.* High intakes of saturated fat raise serum LDL cholesterol, but how, exactly, does saturated fat cause heart and artery disease to ensue? The underlying mechanism is not known.
2. *Clinical human trials.* Human clinical studies that change one condition but control everything else can help determine cause, not just association. Experiments that replace saturated fat from butter and cheese or meat with polyunsaturated fat from corn, soy, or seed oils consistently show a reduction in blood LDL cholesterol and CVD risk.	2. *Flawed studies.* Even the best clinical trials cannot control everything. Genetic predisposition (some people make more- or less-efficient HDL and more- or less-damaging varieties of LDL cholesterol, among other things), food preparation methods, and other factors can skew results.
3. *Reducing LDL cholesterol reduces risks.* Reducing LDL cholesterol by way of diet or drugs reduces diseases of the heart and arteries in real people; these data are observable, not hypothetical.	3. *Genes raise LDL cholesterol.* True, drugs that oppose blood LDL cholesterol reduce disease risk, but elevated blood LDL is probably workings of the genes than to the diet.
4. *A mixture of fatty acids.* Individual saturated fatty acids pose differing degrees of CVD risk, but food fats are mixtures of fatty acids. It's impossible to limit intakes of only the most harmful ones, so people must limit all saturated fat intakes.	4. *Individual fatty acids.* Stearic acid, a saturated fatty acid, doesn't raise LDL cholesterol. Why burden people with ridding the diet of all saturated fatty acids when some are clearly more harmful than others?
5. *Voice of authority.* After reviewing all the evidence, the American Heart Association and American College of Cardiology, with their highest level of confidence, recommend reducing saturated fat to lower LDL cholesterol. For those who would benefit from reducing LDL cholesterol, an intake of 5–6% of energy from saturated fat is prudent.	5. *Mystifying advice.* Advice to lower intakes of all sources of saturated fat is "irrational," given that not all fatty acids carry the same risk. Some evidence also suggests that certain short-chain saturated fatty acids found in dairy and tropical oils may be less harmful than most other saturated fatty acids.
6. *Unintentional misinformation.* Errors in methodology account for reports by recent studies that there is no higher risk of CVD with high saturated fat intakes. A meta-analysis cannot correct previous scientific errors in methodology.	6. *Expected scientific limitations.* Data from observational studies in a meta-analysis revealed no association between lipid intakes and CVD. All scientists acknowledge the shortcomings of their studies.
7. *Conclusion.* Why throw away a landslide of previous science in support of reducing saturated fat intakes because of some inconclusive study results?	7. *Conclusion.* Why waste resources distracting people with saturated fat recommendations when they should be concentrating on eating a calorie-controlled, adequate diet of whole foods?

Sources: Point: L. C. Blekkenhorst and coauthors, Dietary saturated fat intake and atherosclerotic vascular disease mortality in elderly women: A prospective cohort study, American Journal of Clinical Nutrition (2015), epub ahead of print, doi: 10.3945/ajcn.114.102392; Katan, world-renowned expert on diet and CVD, as interviewed in B. Liebman, Fat under fire: New findings or shaky science? Nutrition Action Healthletter, May 2014, pp. 3–7; R. H. Eckel and coauthors, 2013 AHA/ACC Guideline on Lifestyle Management to Reduce Cardiovascular Risk, Circulation 129 (2014): 576–599; A. M. Fretts and coauthors, Plasma phospholipid saturated fatty acids and incident atrial fibrillation: The Cardiovascular Health Study, Journal of the American Heart Association 3 (2014), epub, doi: 10.1161/JAHA.114.000889. Counterpoint: G. D. Lawrence, Dietary fats and health: Dietary recommendations in the context of scientific evidence, Advances in Nutrition 4 (2013): 294–302; U. Ravnskov and coauthors, The questionable benefits of exchanging saturated fat with polyunsaturated fat, Mayo Clinic Proceedings 89 (2014): 451–453.

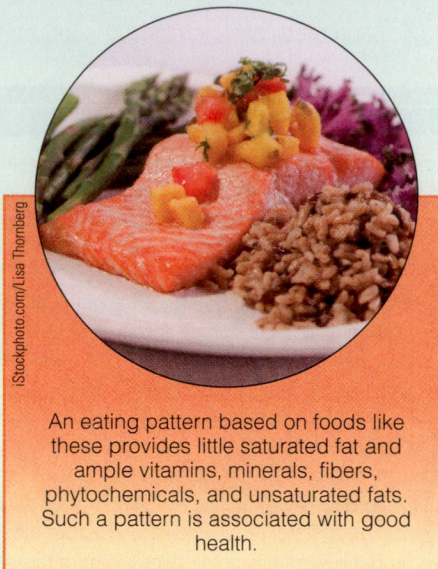

An eating pattern based on foods like these provides little saturated fat and ample vitamins, minerals, fibers, phytochemicals, and unsaturated fats. Such a pattern is associated with good health.

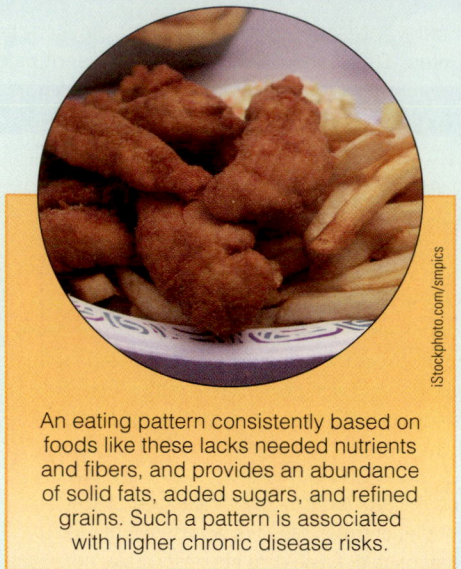

An eating pattern consistently based on foods like these lacks needed nutrients and fibers, and provides an abundance of solid fats, added sugars, and refined grains. Such a pattern is associated with higher chronic disease risks.

Conclusion

It's easy for consumers to become confused when headlines howl for attention, particularly when they say what people want to hear. Keep in mind that no one study is sufficient to reverse decades of previous findings and that the best action may be no action while you wait and watch for other studies to examine the issue. Meanwhile, don't take chances with your health—follow the advice of the Dietary Guidelines for Americans.

Critical Thinking

1. Find an article in a newspaper or magazine or on the Internet that makes claims about saturated fat, particularly one that extols the safety of high intakes of butter, fatty meats, and cheeses. Based on what you know about the science behind national recommendations, analyze the article's talking points, and come to a conclusion about its veracity.

2. Discuss whether you believe that an eating pattern approach to dietary guidelines is best, or that specific nutrient limits, such as percentages of calories from fats, are most helpful. Defend your opinion.

6 The Proteins and Amino Acids

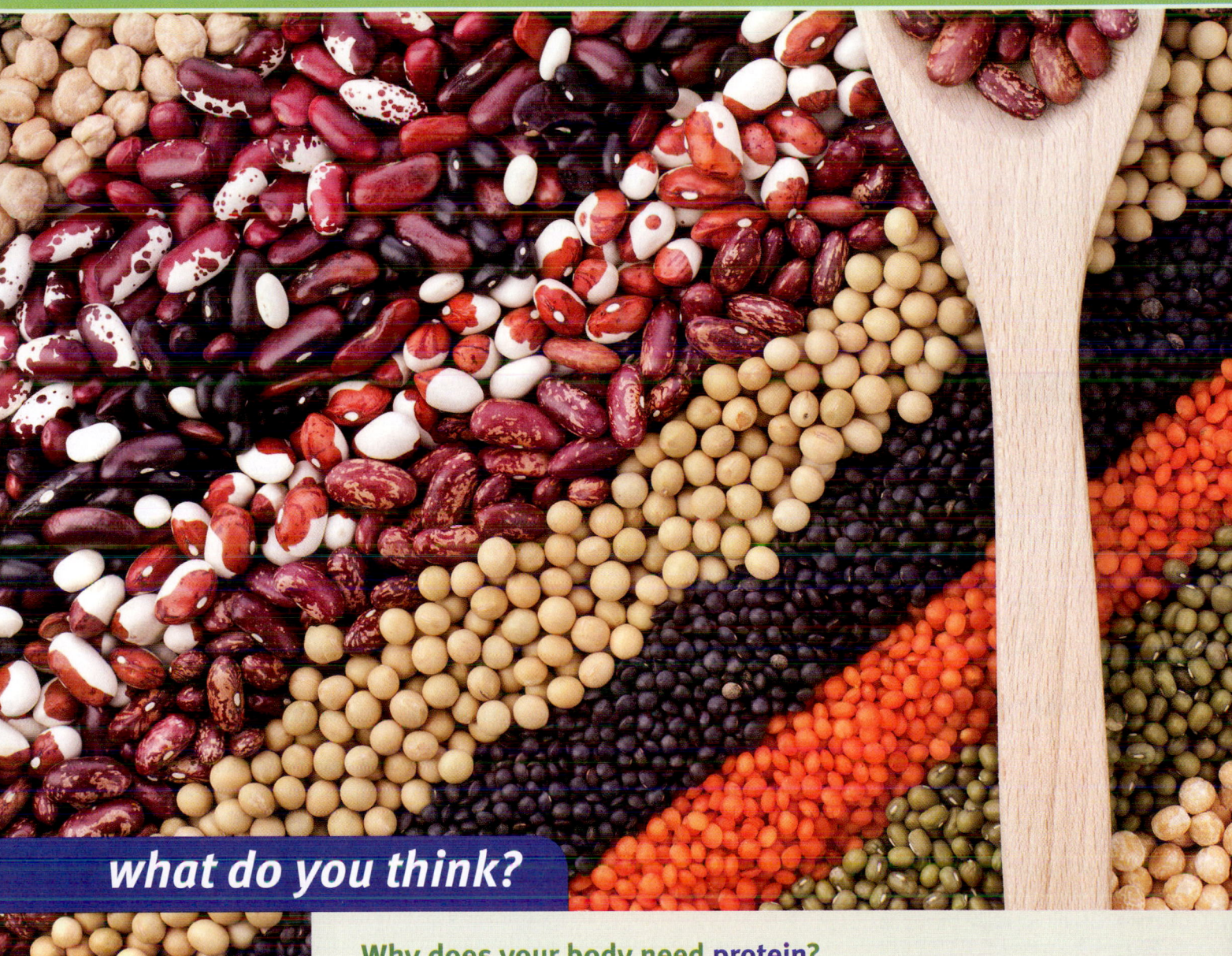

what do you think?

Why does your body need protein?

How does heating an egg change it from a liquid to a solid?

Do protein or amino acid supplements bulk up muscles?

Will your diet lack protein if you don't eat meat?

Learning Objectives

After completing this chapter, you should be able to accomplish the following:

LO 6.1   Discuss the nature of proteins and amino acids.

LO 6.2   Explain the processes of protein digestion and absorption of amino acids.

LO 6.3   Discuss the roles of proteins and amino acids in the body.

LO 6.4   List the factors that determine the daily protein needs of an individual.

LO 6.5   Discuss the potential health problems from an eating plan that is too low or too high in protein.

LO 6.6   Identify the benefits and drawbacks of protein-rich foods in the diet.

LO 6.7   Compare the advantages and disadvantages of the vegetarian diet and the meat eater's diet.

The proteins are amazing, versatile, and vital molecules. Without them, life would not exist. First named 150 years ago after the Greek word *proteios* (meaning "of prime importance"), **proteins** have revealed countless secrets of the processes of life and have helped to answer many questions in nutrition: How do we grow? How do our bodies replace the materials they lose? How does blood clot? What gives us immunity? What makes one person different from another? Understanding the nature of the proteins helps to solve these mysteries.

The Structure of Proteins

LO 6.1   Discuss the nature of proteins and amino acids.

The structure of proteins enables them to perform many vital functions. One key difference from carbohydrates and fats is that proteins contain nitrogen atoms in addition to the carbon, hydrogen, and oxygen atoms that all three energy-yielding nutrients contain. These nitrogen atoms give the name *amino* (which means "nitrogen containing") to the **amino acids**, the building blocks of proteins. Another key difference is that in contrast to the carbohydrates—whose repeating units, glucose molecules, are identical—the amino acids in a strand of protein are different from one another. A strand of amino acids that makes up a protein may contain 20 *different* kinds of amino acids.

Amino Acids

All amino acids have the same simple chemical backbone consisting of a single carbon atom with both an **amine group** (the nitrogen-containing part) and an acid group attached to it. Each amino acid also has a distinctive chemical **side chain** attached to the center carbon of the backbone (see Figure 6–1). This side chain gives each amino acid its identity and chemical nature. About 20 amino acids, each with its own different side chain, make up most of the proteins of living tissue.[1]* Other rare amino acids appear in a few proteins.

The side chains make the amino acids differ in size, shape, and electrical charge. Some are negative, some are positive, and some have no charge (are neutral). The first part of Figure 6–2 is a diagram of three amino acids, each with a different side chain attached to its backbone. The rest of the figure shows how amino acids link to form protein strands. Long strands of amino acids form large protein molecules, and the side chains of the amino acids ultimately help to determine the protein's molecular shape and behavior.

---

*Reference notes are found in Appendix F.

Figure 6–1

An Amino Acid

The "backbone" is the same for all amino acids. The side chain differs from one amino acid to the next. The nitrogen is in the amine group.

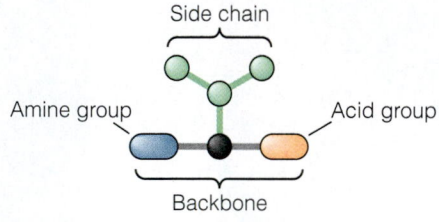

Side chain

Amine group · · · Acid group

Backbone

proteins compounds composed of carbon, hydrogen, oxygen, and nitrogen and arranged as strands of amino acids. Some amino acids also contain the element sulfur.

amino (a-MEEN-o) **acids** the building blocks of protein. Each has an amine group at one end, an acid group at the other, and a distinctive side chain.

amine (a-MEEN) **group** the nitrogen-containing portion of an amino acid.

side chain the unique chemical structure attached to the backbone of each amino acid that differentiates one amino acid from another.

Figure 6–2

Different Amino Acids Join Together

This is the basic process by which proteins are assembled.

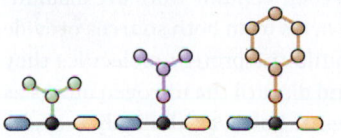 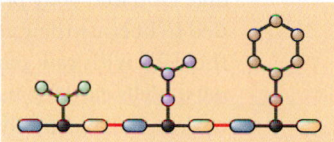

Valine   Leucine   Tyrosine

Single amino acids with different side chains …   can bond to form …   a strand of amino acids, part of a protein.

Essential Amino Acids The body can make about half of the 20 amino acids for itself, given the needed parts: fragments derived from carbohydrate or fat to form the backbones and nitrogen from other sources to form the amine groups. The healthy adult body cannot make some amino acids or makes them too slowly to meet its needs. These are the **essential amino acids** (listed in Table 6–1). Without these essential nutrients, the body cannot make the proteins it needs to do its work. Because the essential amino acids can be replenished only from foods, a person must frequently eat the foods that provide them.

Under special circumstances, a nonessential amino acid can become essential. For example, the body normally makes tyrosine (a nonessential amino acid) from the essential amino acid phenylalanine. If the diet fails to supply enough phenylalanine or if the body cannot make the conversion for some reason (as happens in the inherited disease

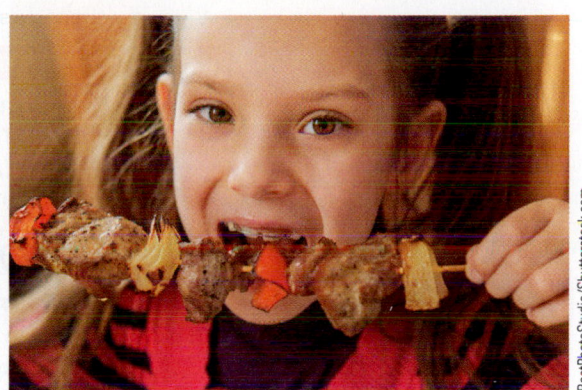

Hair, skin, eyesight, and the health of the whole body depend on proteins from food.

Table 6–1

Amino Acids Important in Nutrition

The left-hand column lists amino acids that are essential for human beings—the body cannot make them, and they must be provided in the diet. The right-hand column lists other, nonessential amino acids—the body can make these for itself. In special cases, some nonessential amino acids may become conditionally essential (see the text).

Essential Amino Acids (pronunciation)	Nonessential Amino Acids (pronunciation)
Histidine (HISS-tuh-deen)	Alanine (AL-ah-neen)
Isoleucine (eye-so-LOO-seen)	Arginine (ARJ-ih-neen)
Leucine (LOO-seen)	Asparagine (ah-SPAR-ah-geen)
Lysine (LYE-seen)	Aspartic acid (ah-SPAR-tic acid)
Methionine (meh-THIGH-oh-neen)	Cysteine (SIS-the-een)
Phenylalanine (fen-il-AL-ah-neen)	Glutamic acid (GLU-tam-ic acid)
Threonine (THREE-oh-neen)	Glutamine (GLU-tah-meen)
Tryptophan (TRIP-toe-fan, TRIP-toe-fane)	Glycine (GLY-seen)
Valine (VAY-leen)	Proline (PRO-leen)
	Serine (SEER-een)
	Tyrosine (TIE-roe-seen)

essential amino acids amino acids that either cannot be synthesized at all by the body or cannot be synthesized in amounts sufficient to meet physiological need. Also called *indispensable amino acids.*

phenylketonuria; see Chapter 3, p. 72), then tyrosine becomes a **conditionally essential amino acid**.

Recycling Amino Acids　The body not only makes some amino acids but also breaks protein molecules apart and reuses those amino acids. Both food proteins after digestion and body proteins when they have finished their cellular work are dismantled to liberate their component amino acids. Amino acids from both sources provide the cells with raw materials from which they can build the protein molecules they need. Cells can also use the amino acids for energy and discard the nitrogen atoms as wastes. By reusing intact amino acids to build proteins, however, the body recycles and conserves a valuable commodity while easing its nitrogen disposal burden.

This recycling system also provides access to an emergency fund of amino acids in times of fuel, glucose, or protein deprivation. At such times, tissues can break down their own proteins, sacrificing working molecules before the ends of their normal lifetimes, to supply energy and amino acids to the body's cells.

KEY POINTS

- Proteins are unique among the energy nutrients in that they possess nitrogen-containing amine groups and are composed of 20 different amino acid units.
- Of the 20 amino acids, some are essential and some are essential only in special circumstances.

How Do Amino Acids Build Proteins?

In the first step of making a protein, each amino acid is hooked to the next (as was shown in Figure 6–2, p. 203). A chemical bond, called a **peptide bond**, is formed between the amine group end of one amino acid and the acid group end of the next. A string of 10 or more amino acids is known as a **polypeptide**. The side chains bristle out from the backbone of the structure, giving the protein molecule its unique character. Figure 6–2 shows only the first step in making all proteins—the linking of amino acid units with peptide bonds until the strand contains from several dozen to as many as 300 amino acids.

The strand of protein does not remain a straight chain. Amino acids at different places along the strand are chemically attracted to each other, and this attraction can cause some segments of the strand to coil, somewhat like a metal spring. Also, each spot along the strand is attracted to, or repelled from, other spots along its length (demonstrated in Figure 6–3). These interactions often cause the entire protein coil to fold this way and that to form a globular structure, as shown in Figure 6–4 (p. 206). Other strands link together in other ways to form different structures that perform specific functions.

The amino acids whose side chains are electrically charged are attracted to water. Therefore, in the body's watery fluids, they orient themselves on the outside of the protein structure. The amino acids whose side chains are neutral are repelled by water and are attracted to one another; these tuck themselves into the center away from the body fluids. All these interactions among the amino acids and the surrounding fluids fold each protein into a unique architecture, a form to suit its function.

One final detail may be needed for the protein to become functional. Several strands may cluster together into a functioning unit, or a metal ion (mineral), a vitamin, or a carbohydrate molecule may join to the unit and activate it.

KEY POINT

- Amino acids link into long strands that make a wide variety of different proteins.

The Variety of Proteins

The particular shapes of proteins enable them to perform different tasks in the body. Those of globular shape, such as some proteins of blood, are water-soluble. Some form hollow balls, which can carry and store materials in their interiors. Some proteins, such as those of tendons, are more than 10 times as long as they are wide, forming stiff, rodlike structures that are somewhat insoluble in water and very strong. A form of the protein **collagen** acts somewhat like glue between cells. The hormone insulin,

conditionally essential amino acid　an amino acid that is normally nonessential but must be supplied by the diet in special circumstances when the need for it exceeds the body's ability to produce it.

peptide bond　a bond that connects one amino acid with another, forming a link in a protein chain.

polypeptide (POL-ee-PEP-tide)　protein fragments of many (more than 10) amino acids bonded together (*poly* means "many"). A peptide is a strand of amino acids.

collagen (KAHL-ah-jen)　a type of body protein from which connective tissues such as scars, tendons, ligaments, and the foundations of bones and teeth are made.

Figure 6–3

The Coiling and Folding of a Protein Molecule

1 The first shape of a strand of amino acids is a chain, which can be very long. This shows just a portion of the strand.

2 Coiling the strand. The strand of amino acids takes on a springlike shape as the side chains variously attract and repel each other.

3 Folding the coil. The coil then folds and flops over on itself to take a functional shape.

4 Once coiled and folded, the protein may be functional as is, or it may need to join with other proteins or to add a carbohydrate molecule or a vitamin or mineral, as the iron of the protein hemoglobin demonstrates in Figure 6-4 (p. 206).

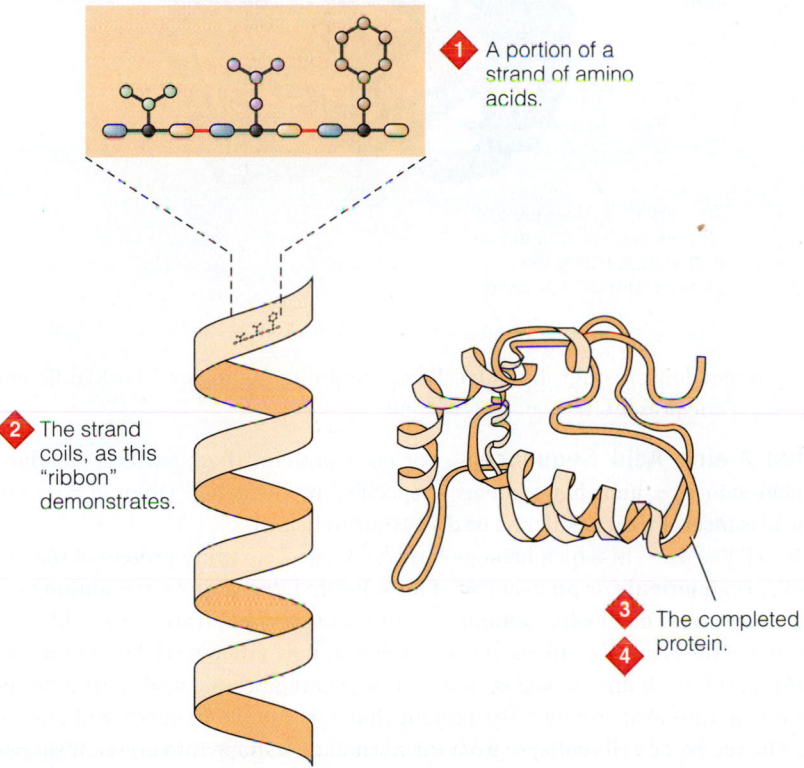

1 A portion of a strand of amino acids.

2 The strand coils, as this "ribbon" demonstrates.

3 **4** The completed protein.

a protein, helps to regulate blood glucose. Among the most fascinating proteins are the **enzymes**, which act on other substances to change them chemically. More roles of the body's proteins are discussed in a later section.

Some protein strands work alone, while others must associate in groups of strands to become functional. One molecule of **hemoglobin**—the large, globular protein molecule that is packed into the red blood cells by the billions and carries oxygen—is made of four associated protein strands, each holding the mineral iron (see Figure 6–4).

The great variety of proteins in the world is possible because an essentially infinite number of sequences of amino acids can be formed. To understand how so many different proteins can be designed from only 20 or so amino acids, think of how many words are in an unabridged dictionary—all of them constructed from just 26 letters. If you had only the letter "G," all you could write would be a string of Gs: G–G–G–G–G–G–G. But with 26 different letters available, you can create poems, songs, or novels. Similarly, the 20 amino acids can be linked together in a huge variety of sequences—many more than are possible for letters in a word, which must alternate consonant and vowel sounds. Thus, the variety of possible sequences for amino acid

enzymes (EN-zimes) proteins that facilitate chemical reactions without being changed in the process; protein catalysts.

hemoglobin the globular protein of red blood cells, whose iron atoms carry oxygen around the body via the bloodstream (more about hemoglobin in Chapter 8).

Figure 6–4

The Structure of Hemoglobin

Four highly folded protein strands form the globular hemoglobin protein.

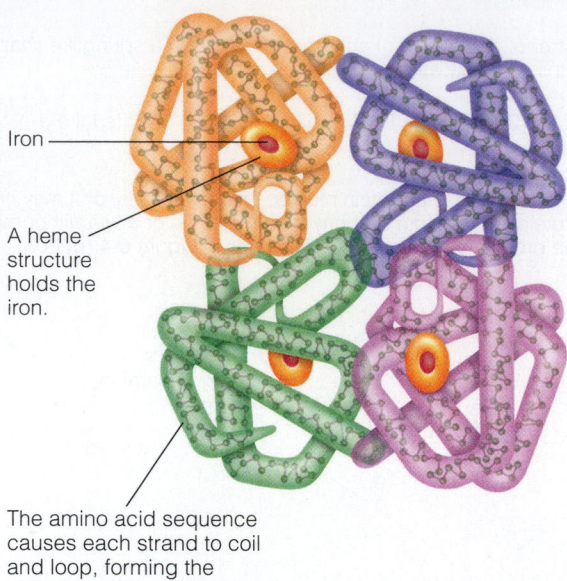

Iron

A heme structure holds the iron.

The amino acid sequence causes each strand to coil and loop, forming the globular protein structure.

strands is tremendous. A single human cell may contain as many as 10,000 different proteins, each one present in thousands of copies.

Inherited Amino Acid Sequences   For each protein, there exists a standard amino acid sequence, and that sequence is specified by the genes. Often, if a wrong amino acid is inserted, the result can be disastrous to health.

Sickle-cell disease—in which hemoglobin, the oxygen-carrying protein of the red blood cells, is abnormal—is an example of an inherited variation in the amino acid sequence. Normal hemoglobin contains two kinds of protein strands. In sickle-cell disease, one of the strands is an exact copy of that in normal hemoglobin, but in the other strand, the sixth amino acid is valine rather than glutamic acid. This replacement of one amino acid so alters the protein that it is unable to carry and release oxygen. The red blood cells collapse from the normal disk shape into crescent shapes (see Figure 6–5). If too many crescent-shaped cells appear in the blood, the result is abnormal blood clotting, strokes, bouts of severe pain, susceptibility to infection, and early death.[2]

You are unique among human beings because of minute differences in your body proteins that establish everything from eye color and shoe size to susceptibility to certain diseases. These differences are determined by the amino acid sequences of your proteins, which are written into the genetic code you inherited from your parents and they from theirs. Ultimately, the genes determine the sequence of amino acids in each finished protein, and some genes are involved in making more than one protein (how DNA directs protein synthesis and **RNA** molecules perform it is described in Figure 6–6, p. 208). As scientists completed the identification of the human genome, they recognized a still greater task that lies ahead: the identification of every protein made by the human body.[†]

Nutrients and Gene Expression   When a cell makes a protein, as shown in Figure 6–6, scientists say that the gene for that protein has been "expressed." Every

RNA (ribonucleic acid) cellular nucleic acids that play key roles in the process and control of protein synthesis.

[†] The identification of the entire collection of human proteins, the *human proteome* (PRO-tee-ohme), is a work in progress.

Figure 6–5

Normal Red Blood Cells and Sickle Cells

Normal red blood cells are disk-shaped. In sickle-cell disease, one amino acid in the protein strands of hemoglobin takes the place of another, causing the red blood cell to change shape and lose function.

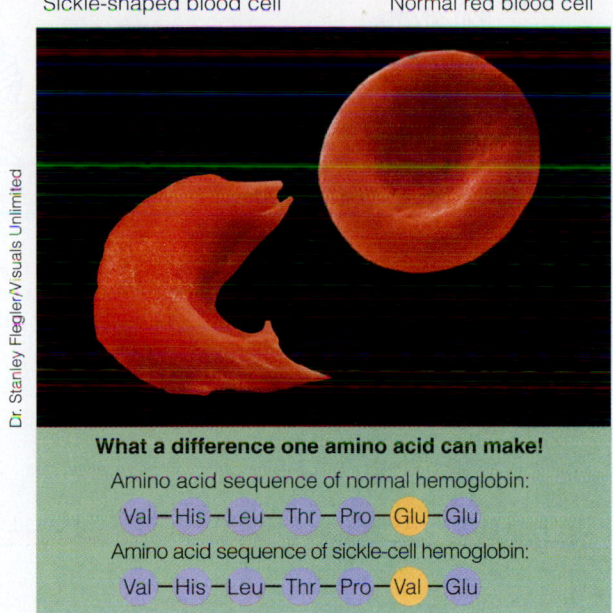

Sickle-shaped blood cell   Normal red blood cell

Dr. Stanley Flegler/Visuals Unlimited

What a difference one amino acid can make!

Amino acid sequence of normal hemoglobin:

Val —His —Leu—Thr —Pro—Glu—Glu

Amino acid sequence of sickle-cell hemoglobin:

Val —His —Leu—Thr —Pro—Val —Glu

cell nucleus contains the DNA for making every human protein, but cells do not make them all. Some cells specialize in making certain proteins; for example, cells of the pancreas express the gene for the protein hormone insulin. The gene for making insulin exists in all other cells of the body, but it is idle or silenced.

Nutrients, including amino acids and proteins, do not change DNA structure, but they greatly influence genetic expression.[3] As research in **nutritional genomics** advances, researchers hope to one day use nutrients to influence a person's genes in ways that reduce chronic disease risks, but for now, that day is firmly in the future. The Controversy section of Chapter 11 comes back to nutritional genomics. The Think Fitness feature (p. 209) addresses a related concern of exercisers and athletes about whether extra dietary protein or amino acids can trigger the synthesis of muscle tissue and increase strength.

KEY POINTS

- Each type of protein has a distinctive sequence of amino acids and so has great functional specificity.
- Often, cells specialize in synthesizing particular types of proteins in addition to the proteins necessary to all cells.
- Nutrients can greatly affect genetic expression.

Denaturation of Proteins

Proteins can be denatured (distorted in shape) by heat, radiation, alcohol, acids, bases, or the salts of heavy metals. The **denaturation** of a protein is the first step in its destruction; thus, these agents are dangerous because they can disrupt a protein's folded structure, making it unable to function in the body. In digestion, however, denaturation is useful to the body.

During the digestion of a food protein, the stomach acid opens up the protein's structure, permitting digestive enzymes to make contact with the peptide bonds and cleave them. Denaturation also occurs during the cooking of foods. Cooking an egg

nutritional genomics the science of how food components, such as nutrients, interact with the body's genetic material.

denaturation the irreversible change in a protein's folded shape brought about by heat, acids, bases, alcohol, salts of heavy metals, or other agents.

Figure 6–6
Protein Synthesis

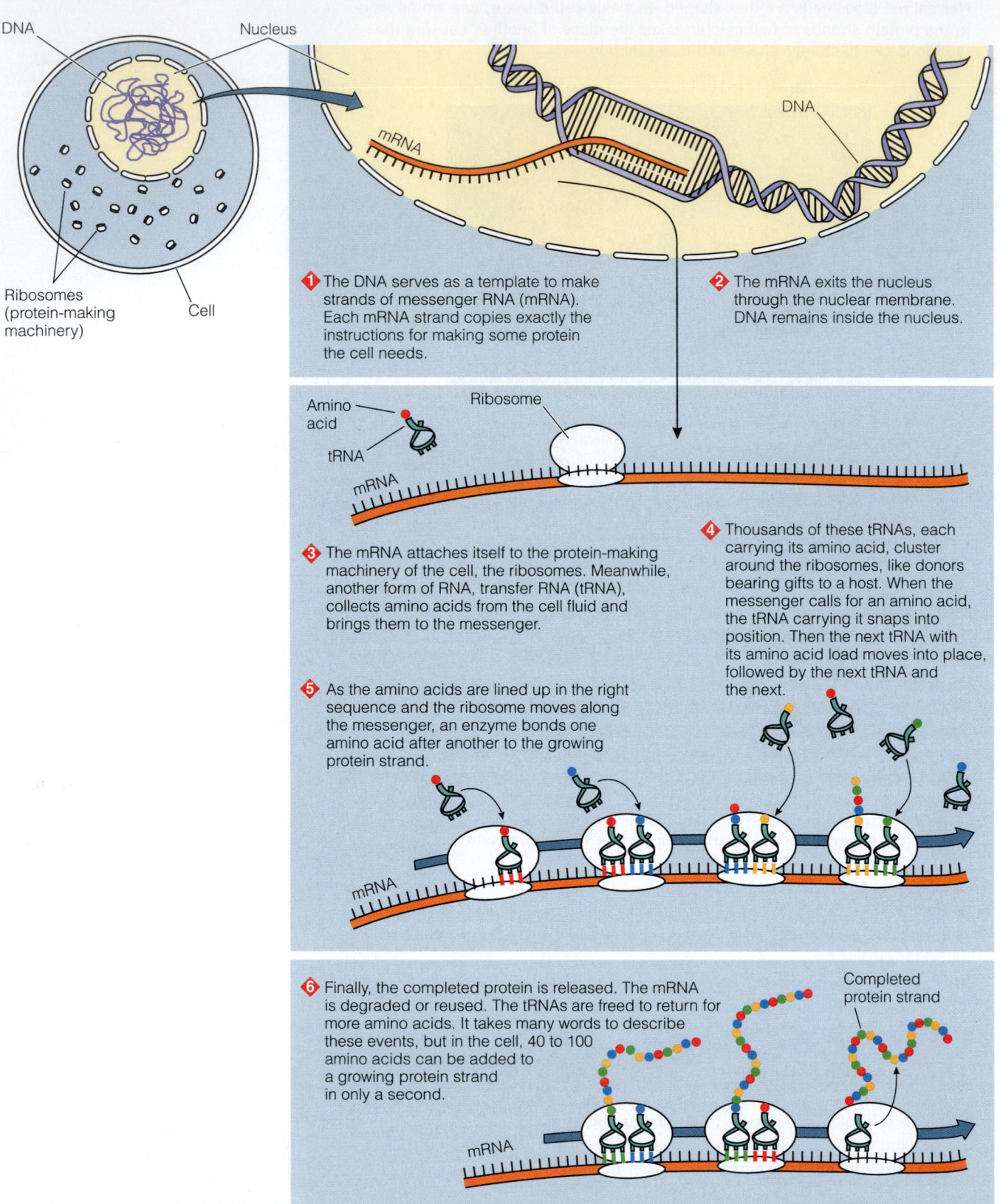

DNA

Nucleus

Ribosomes (protein-making machinery)

Cell

DNA

mRNA

1 The DNA serves as a template to make strands of messenger RNA (mRNA). Each mRNA strand copies exactly the instructions for making some protein the cell needs.

2 The mRNA exits the nucleus through the nuclear membrane. DNA remains inside the nucleus.

Amino acid

Ribosome

tRNA

mRNA

3 The mRNA attaches itself to the protein-making machinery of the cell, the ribosomes. Meanwhile, another form of RNA, transfer RNA (tRNA), collects amino acids from the cell fluid and brings them to the messenger.

4 Thousands of these tRNAs, each carrying its amino acid, cluster around the ribosomes, like donors bearing gifts to a host. When the messenger calls for an amino acid, the tRNA carrying it snaps into position. Then the next tRNA with its amino acid load moves into place, followed by the next tRNA and the next.

5 As the amino acids are lined up in the right sequence and the ribosome moves along the messenger, an enzyme bonds one amino acid after another to the growing protein strand.

mRNA

6 Finally, the completed protein is released. The mRNA is degraded or reused. The tRNAs are freed to return for more amino acids. It takes many words to describe these events, but in the cell, 40 to 100 amino acids can be added to a growing protein strand in only a second.

Completed protein strand

mRNA

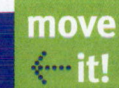
The answer is mostly "no" but also a qualified "yes." Athletes and fitness seekers cannot stimulate their muscles to gain size and strength simply by consuming more protein or amino acids. Hard work is necessary to trigger the genes to build more of the muscle tissue needed for sport. The "yes" part of the answer reflects research suggesting that well-timed protein intakes can often further stimulate muscle growth. Protein intake cannot replace exercise in this regard, however, as many supplement sellers would have people believe. Exercise generates cellular messages that stimulate the DNA to begin synthesizing the muscle proteins needed to perform the work. A protein-rich snack—say, a glass of skim milk or soy milk—consumed shortly after strength-building exercise (such as weight lifting) also stimulates muscle protein synthesis, but evidence is lacking for a benefit to athletic performance.

Athletes may need somewhat more dietary protein than other people do, and exercise authorities recommend higher protein intakes for athletes pursuing various activities (see Chapter 10 for details).[4] Amino acid or protein supplements, however, offer no advantage over food, and amino acid supplements are more likely to cause problems (as this chapter's Consumer's Guide, p. 218, makes clear). Bottom line: the path to bigger muscles is well-planned, consistent physical training with adequate energy and nutrients from balanced, well-timed meals, snacks, and beverages. Research findings concerning dietary protein and muscles are interesting and important, but this truth remains: extra protein and amino acids without physical work add nothing but excess calories.

start now! ⋯⟩ Ready to make a change? Go to Diet & Wellness Plus and generate an Intake Report for your three-day dietary tracking. What is your protein intake level? If it is low, create an alternate profile and substitute one 8-oz glass of skim or low-fat milk at two meals (or one meal and one snack). What is the effect on your protein intake?

denatures its proteins and makes them firm, as the margin photo demonstrates. More important for nutrition is that heat denatures two proteins in raw eggs: one binds the B vitamin biotin and the mineral iron, and the other slows protein digestion. Thus, cooking eggs liberates biotin and iron and aids digestion.

Many well-known poisons are salts of heavy metals like mercury and silver; these poisons denature protein strands wherever they touch them. The common first-aid antidote for swallowing a heavy-metal poison is to drink milk. The poison then acts on the protein of the milk rather than on the protein tissues of the mouth, esophagus, and stomach. Later, vomiting can be induced to expel the poison that has combined with the milk.

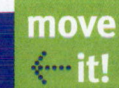

Heat denatures protein, making it firm.

KEY POINTS

- Proteins can be denatured by heat, acids, bases, alcohol, or the salts of heavy metals.
- Denaturation begins the process of digesting food protein and can also destroy body proteins.

Digestion and Absorption of Dietary Protein

LO 6.2 Explain the processes of protein digestion and absorption of amino acids.

Each protein performs a special task in a particular tissue of a specific kind of animal or plant. When a person eats food proteins, whether from cereals, vegetables, beef, fish, or cheese, the body must first alter them by breaking them down into amino acids; only then can it rearrange them into specific human body proteins.

Protein Digestion

Other than being crushed and torn by chewing and moistened with saliva in the mouth, nothing happens to protein until it reaches the stomach. Then the action begins.

In the Stomach   Strong hydrochloric acid produced by the stomach denatures proteins in food. This acid helps to uncoil the protein's tangled strands so that molecules of the stomach's protein-digesting enzyme can attack the peptide bonds. You might expect that the stomach enzyme, being a protein itself, would be denatured by the stomach's acid. Unlike most enzymes, though, the stomach enzyme functions best in an acid environment. Its job is to break *other* protein strands into smaller pieces. The stomach lining, which is also made partly of protein, is protected against attack by acid and enzymes by its coat of mucus, secreted by its cells.

The whole process of digestion is an ingenious solution to a complex problem. Proteins (enzymes), activated by acid, digest proteins from food, denatured by acid. Digestion and absorption of other nutrients, such as iron, also rely on the stomach's ability to produce strong acid. The acid in the stomach is so strong (pH 1.5) that no food is acidic enough to make it stronger; for comparison, the pH of vinegar is about 3.

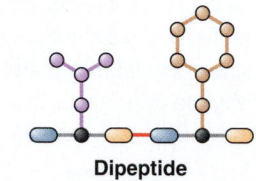

pH was defined in **Chapter 3** on page 85.

In the Small Intestine   By the time most proteins slip from the stomach into the small intestine, they are denatured and cleaved into smaller pieces. A few are single amino acids, but the majority remain in large strands—polypeptides. In the small intestine, alkaline juice from the pancreas neutralizes the acid delivered by the stomach. The pH rises to about 7 (neutral), enabling the next enzyme team to accomplish the final breakdown of the strands. Protein-digesting enzymes from the pancreas and intestine continue working until almost all pieces of protein are broken into single amino acids or into strands of two or three amino acids, **dipeptides** and **tripeptides**, respectively (see Figure 6–7). Figure 6–8 summarizes the whole process of protein digestion.

Common Misconceptions   Consumers who fail to understand the basic mechanism of protein digestion are easily misled by advertisers of books and other products who urge, "Take enzyme A to help digest your food" or "Don't eat foods containing enzyme C, which will digest cells in your body." The writers of such statements fail to realize that enzymes (proteins) are digested before they are absorbed, just as all proteins are. Even the stomach's digestive enzymes are denatured and digested when their jobs are through. Similar false claims suggest that predigested proteins (amino acid supplements) are "easy to digest" and can therefore protect the digestive system from "overworking." Of course, the healthy digestive system is superbly designed to digest whole proteins with ease. In fact, it handles whole proteins better than predigested ones because it dismantles and absorbs the amino acids at rates that are optimal for the body's use.

> **KEY POINT**
> - Digestion of protein involves denaturation by stomach acid and enzymatic digestion in the stomach and small intestine to amino acids, dipeptides, and tripeptides.

What Happens to Amino Acids after Protein Is Digested?

The cells all along the small intestine absorb single amino acids. As for dipeptides and tripeptides, enzymes on the cells' surfaces split most of them into single amino acids, and the cells absorb them, too. Dipeptides and tripeptides are also absorbed as-is into the cells, where they are split into amino acids and join with the others to be released into the bloodstream. A few larger peptide molecules can escape the digestive process altogether and enter the bloodstream intact. Scientists believe these larger particles may act as hormones to regulate body functions and provide the body with information about the external environment. The larger molecules may also stimulate an immune response and thus play a role in food allergy.

The cells of the small intestine possess separate sites for absorbing different types of amino acids. Amino acids of the same type compete for the same absorption sites.

Figure 6–7

A Dipeptide and Tripeptide

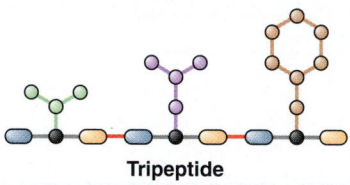

Dipeptide

Tripeptide

dipeptides (dye-PEP-tides) protein fragments that are two amino acids long (*di* means "two").

tripeptides (try-PEP-tides) protein fragments that are three amino acids long (*tri* means "three").

Figure 6–8

How Protein in Food Becomes Amino Acids in the Body

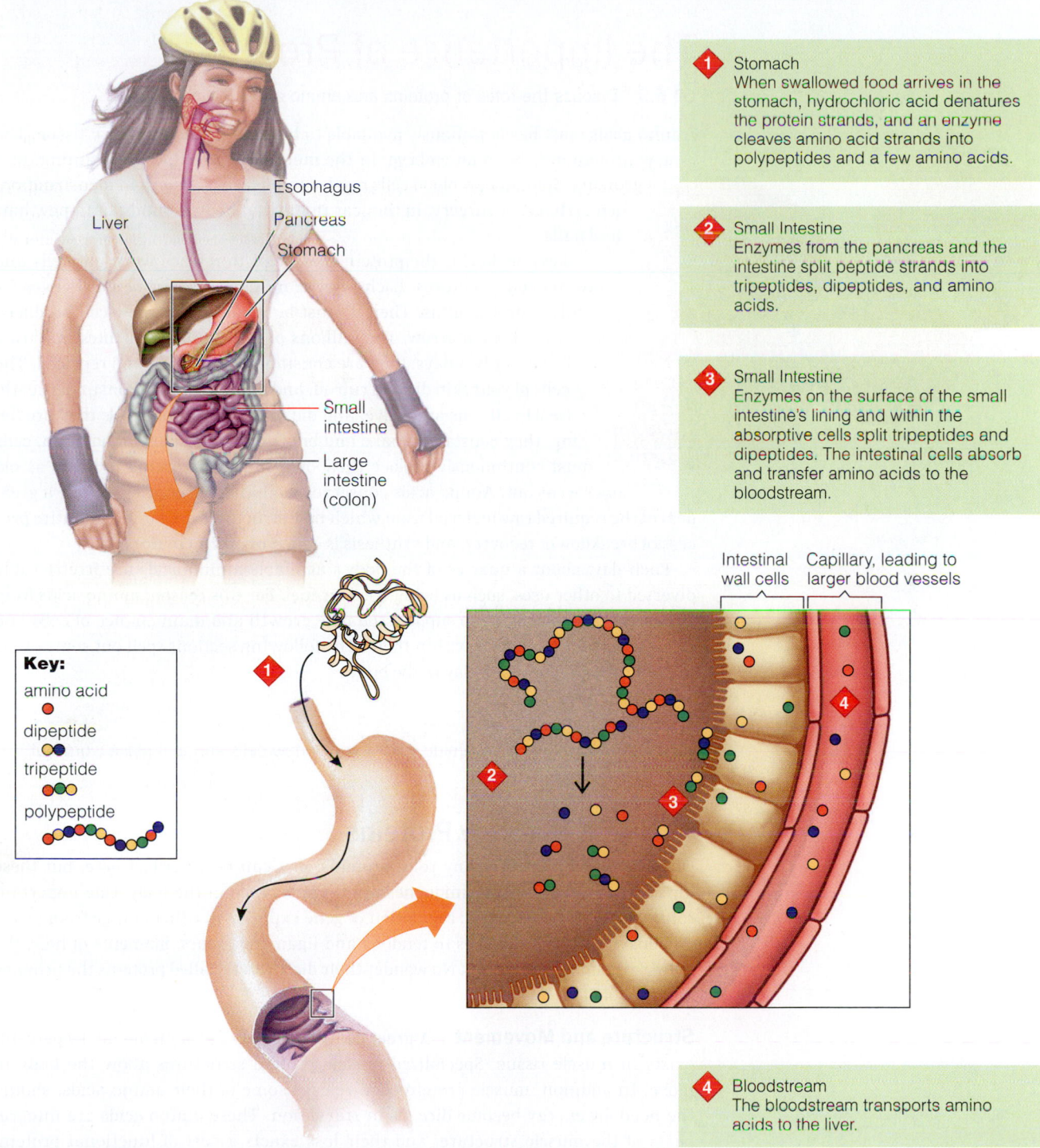

1 Stomach
When swallowed food arrives in the stomach, hydrochloric acid denatures the protein strands, and an enzyme cleaves amino acid strands into polypeptides and a few amino acids.

2 Small Intestine
Enzymes from the pancreas and the intestine split peptide strands into tripeptides, dipeptides, and amino acids.

3 Small Intestine
Enzymes on the surface of the small intestine's lining and within the absorptive cells split tripeptides and dipeptides. The intestinal cells absorb and transfer amino acids to the bloodstream.

4 Bloodstream
The bloodstream transports amino acids to the liver.

Esophagus
Liver
Pancreas
Stomach
Small intestine
Large intestine (colon)

Intestinal wall cells   Capillary, leading to larger blood vessels

Key:
amino acid
dipeptide
tripeptide
polypeptide

Consequently, when a person ingests a large dose of any single amino acid, that amino acid may limit absorption of others of its general type. The Consumer's Guide (p. 218) cautions against taking single amino acids as supplements partly for this reason.

Once amino acids are circulating in the bloodstream, they are carried to the liver, where they may be used or released into the blood to be taken up by other cells of the body. The cells can then link the amino acids together to make proteins that they keep for their own use or liberate them into lymph or blood for other uses. When necessary, the body's cells can also use amino acids for energy.

- The cells of the small intestine complete digestion, absorb amino acids and some larger peptides, and release them into the bloodstream for use by the body's cells.

The Importance of Protein

LO 6.3 Discuss the roles of proteins and amino acids in the body.

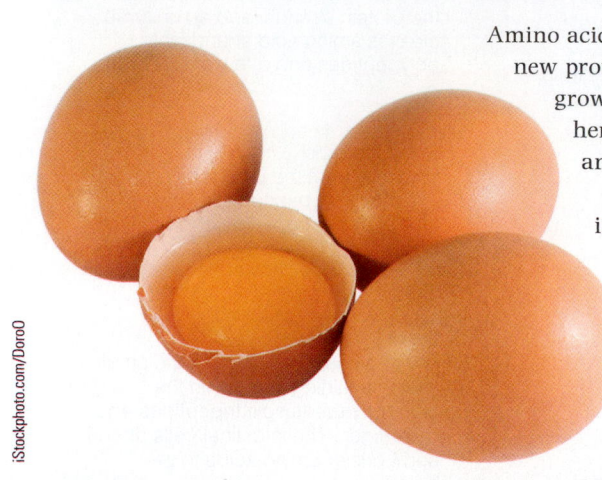

iStockphoto.com/Doro0

Amino acids must be continuously available to build the proteins of new tissue. The new protein may be in an embryo; in the muscles of an athlete in training; in a growing child; in new blood cells needed to replace blood lost in menstruation, hemorrhage, or surgery; in the scar tissue that heals wounds; or in new hair and nails.

Less obvious is the protein that helps to replace worn-out cells and internal cell structures. Each of your millions of red blood cells lives for only 3 or 4 months. Then it must be replaced by a new cell produced by the bone marrow. The millions of cells lining your intestinal tract live for only 3 days; they are constantly being shed and replaced. The cells of your skin die and rub off, and new ones grow from underneath. Nearly all cells arise, live, and die in this way, and while they are living, they constantly make and break down proteins. In addition, cells must continuously replace their own internal working proteins as old ones wear out. Amino acids conserved from these processes provide a great deal of the required raw material from which new structures are built. The entire process of breakdown, recovery, and synthesis is called **protein turnover**.

Each day, about a quarter of the body's available amino acids are irretrievably diverted to other uses, such as being used for fuel. For this reason, amino acids from food are needed each day to support the new growth and maintenance of cells and to make the working parts within them. The following sections spell out some of the critical roles that proteins play in the body.

KEY POINT

- The body needs dietary amino acids to grow new cells and to replace worn-out ones.

The Roles of Body Proteins

Only a sampling of the many roles proteins play can be described here, but these illustrate their versatility, uniqueness, and importance in the body. One important role was already mentioned: regulation of gene expression. Others range from digestive enzymes and antibodies to tendons and ligaments, scars, filaments of hair, the materials of nails, and more. No wonder their discoverers called proteins the primary material of life.

Structure and Movement   A great deal of the body's protein (about 40 percent) exists in muscle tissue. Specialized muscle protein structures allow the body to move. In addition, muscle proteins can release some of their amino acids, should the need for energy become dire, as in starvation. These amino acids are integral parts of the muscle structure, and their loss exacts a cost of functional protein. Other structural proteins confer shape and strength on bones, teeth, skin, tendons, cartilage, blood vessels, and other tissues. All are important to the workings of a healthy body.

Enzymes, Hormones, and Other Compounds   Among proteins formed by living cells, enzymes are metabolic workhorses. An enzyme acts as a **catalyst**: it speeds up a reaction that would happen anyway, but much more slowly. Thousands of enzymes reside inside a single cell, and each one facilitates a specific chemical reaction. Figure 6–9 shows how a hypothetical enzyme works—this one synthesizes a

protein turnover the continuous breakdown and synthesis of body proteins involving the recycling of amino acids.

catalyst a substance that speeds the rate of a chemical reaction without itself being permanently altered in the process. All enzymes are catalysts.

Figure 6–9
Enzyme Action

Compounds A and B are attracted to the enzyme's active site and park there for a moment in the exact position that makes the reaction between them most likely to occur. They react by bonding together and leave the enzyme as a new compound, AB.

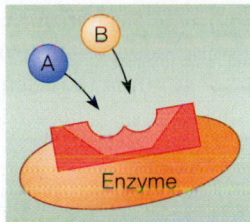

Enzyme plus two
compounds A and B

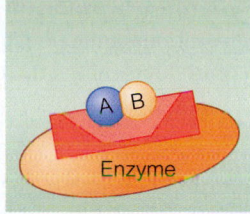

Enzyme complex
with A and B

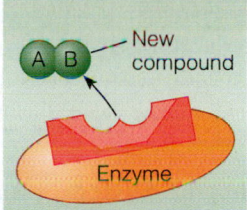

Enzyme plus new
compound AB

compound from two chemical components. Other enzymes break compounds apart into two or more products or rearrange the atoms in one kind of compound to make another. A single enzyme can facilitate several hundred reactions in a second.

The body's **hormones** are messenger molecules, and many of them are made from amino acids. Various body glands release hormones when changes occur in the internal environment; the hormones then elicit tissue responses necessary to restore normal conditions. For example, the familiar pair of hormones, insulin and glucagon, oppose each other to maintain blood glucose levels. Both are built of amino acids. For interest, Figure 6–10 shows how many amino acids are linked in sequence to form human insulin. It also shows how certain side groups attract one another to complete the insulin molecule and make it functional.

In addition to serving as building blocks for proteins, amino acids perform other tasks in the body. For example, the amino acid tyrosine forms parts of the neurotransmitters epinephrine and norepinephrine, which relay messages throughout the nervous system. The body also uses tyrosine to make the brown pigment melanin, which is responsible for skin, hair, and eye color. In addition, tyrosine is converted into the thyroid hormone **thyroxine**, which regulates the body's metabolism. Another amino acid, tryptophan, serves as starting material for the neurotransmitter **serotonin** and the vitamin niacin.

Antibodies Of all the proteins in living organisms, the **antibodies** best demonstrate that proteins are specific to one organism. Antibodies distinguish foreign

Figure 6–10

Amino Acid Sequence of Human Insulin

This picture shows a refinement of protein structure not mentioned in the text. The amino acid cysteine (Cys) has a sulfur-containing side group. The sulfur groups on two cysteine molecules can bond together, creating a bridge between two protein strands or two parts of the same strand. Insulin contains three such bridges.

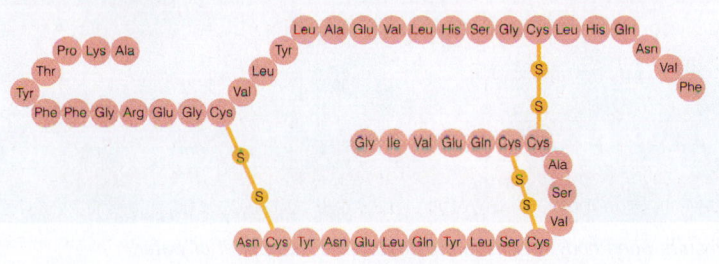

hormones chemical messengers secreted by a number of body organs in response to conditions that require regulation. Each hormone affects a specific organ or tissue and elicits a specific response. Also defined in Chapter 3.

thyroxine (thigh-ROX-in) a principal peptide hormone of the thyroid gland that regulates the body's rate of energy use.

serotonin (SARE-oh-TONE-in) a compound related in structure to (and made from) the amino acid tryptophan. It serves as one of the brain's principal neurotransmitters.

antibodies (AN-te-bod-ees) large proteins of the blood, produced by the immune system in response to an invasion of the body by foreign substances (antigens). Antibodies combine with and inactivate the antigens. Also defined in Chapter 3.

particles (usually proteins) from all the proteins that belong in "their" body. When they recognize an intruder, they mark it as a target for attack. The foreign protein may be part of a bacterium, a virus, or a toxin, or it may be present in a food that causes an allergic reaction.

Each antibody is designed to help destroy one specific invader. An antibody active against one strain of influenza is of no help to a person ill with another strain. Once the body has learned how to make a particular antibody, it remembers. The next time the body encounters that same invader, it destroys the invader even more rapidly. In other words, the body develops **immunity** to the invader. This molecular memory underlies the principle of immunizations, injections of drugs made from destroyed and inactivated microbes or their products that activate the body's immune defenses. Some immunities are lifelong; others, such as that to tetanus, must be "boosted" at intervals.

Transport System   A large group of proteins specializes in transporting other substances, such as lipids, vitamins, minerals, and oxygen, around the body. To do their jobs, such substances must travel within the bloodstream, into and out of cells, or around the cellular interiors. Two familiar examples are the protein hemoglobin that carries oxygen from the lungs to the cells and the lipoproteins that transport lipids in the watery blood.

Fluid and Electrolyte Balance   Proteins help to maintain the **fluid and electrolyte balance** by regulating the quantity of fluids in the compartments of the body. To remain alive, cells must contain a constant amount of fluid. Too much can cause them to rupture; too little makes them unable to function. Although water can diffuse freely into and out of cells, proteins cannot, and proteins attract water.

By maintaining stores of internal proteins and also of some minerals, cells retain the fluid they need. By the same mechanism, fluid is kept inside the blood vessels by proteins too large to move freely across the capillary walls. The proteins attract water and hold it within the vessels, preventing it from freely flowing into the spaces between the cells. Should any part of this system begin to fail, too much fluid will soon collect in the spaces between the cells of tissues, causing **edema**.

Not only is the quantity of the body fluids vital to life but so also is their composition. Transport proteins in the membranes of cells also help to maintain this composition by continuously transferring substances into and out of cells (see Figure 6–11). For example, sodium is concentrated outside the cells, and potassium is concentrated inside.

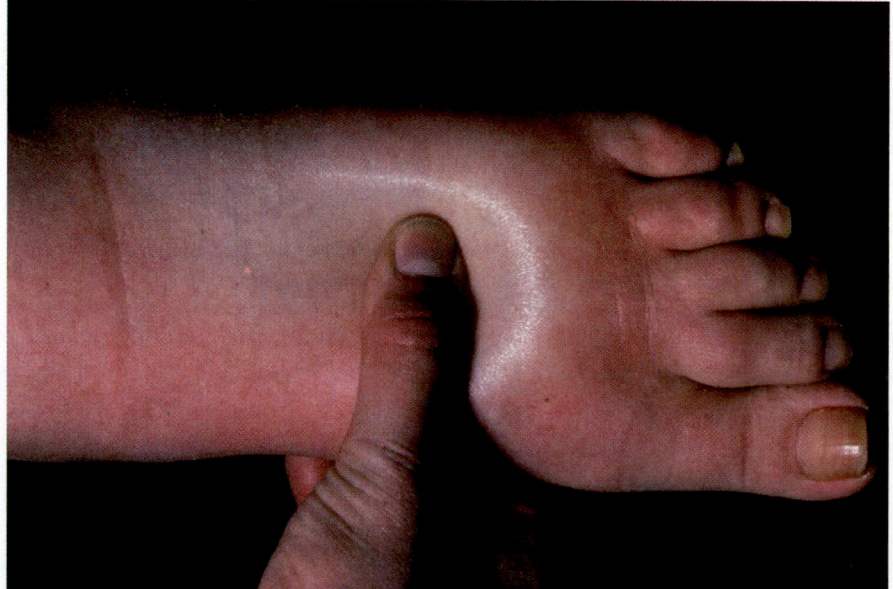

Edema results when body tissues fail to control the movement of water.

immunity protection from or resistance to a disease or infection by the development of antibodies and by the actions of cells and tissues in response to a threat.

fluid and electrolyte balance the distribution of fluid and dissolved particles among body compartments (see also Chapter 8).

edema (eh-DEEM-uh) swelling of body tissue caused by leakage of fluid from the blood vessels; seen in protein deficiency (among other conditions).

Chapter 6 The Proteins and Amino Acids

Figure 6–11

Proteins Transport Substances into and out of Cells

A transport protein within the cell membrane acts as a sort of two-door passageway—substances enter on one side and are released on the other, but the protein never leaves the membrane. The protein differs from a simple passageway in that it actively escorts the substances in and out of cells; therefore, this form of transport is often called active transport.

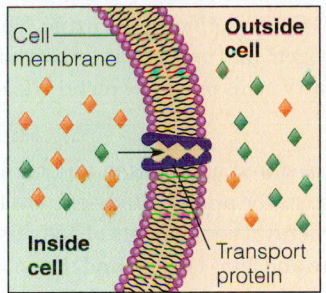

Molecule enters protein from inside cell.

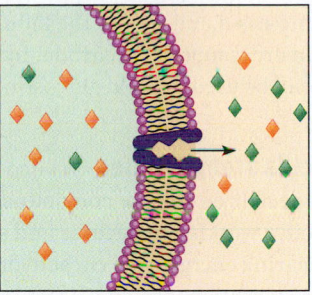

Protein changes shape; molecule exits protein outside the cell.

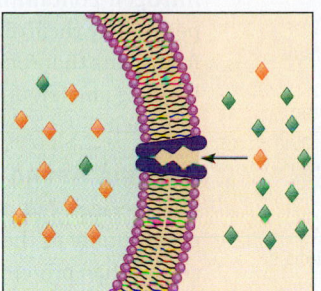

Molecule enters protein from outside cell.

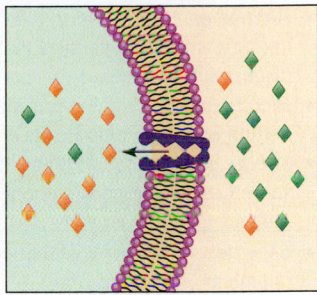

Molecule exits protein; proper balance restored.

A disturbance of this balance can impair the action of the heart, lungs, and brain, triggering a major medical emergency. Cell proteins avert such a disaster by holding fluids and electrolytes in their proper chambers.

Acid-Base Balance   Normal processes of the body continually produce **acids** and their opposite, **bases**, that must be carried by the blood to the organs of excretion. The blood must do this without allowing its own **acid-base balance** to be affected. This feat is another trick of the blood proteins, which act as **buffers** to maintain the blood's normal pH. The protein buffers pick up hydrogens (acid) when there are too many in the bloodstream and release them again when there are too few. The secret is that negatively charged side chains of amino acids can accommodate additional hydrogens, which are positively charged.

Blood pH is one of the most rigidly controlled conditions in the body. If blood pH changes too much, **acidosis** or the opposite basic condition, **alkalosis**, can cause coma or death. These conditions constitute medical emergencies because of their effect on proteins. When the proteins' buffering capacity is filled—that is, when they have taken on all the acid hydrogens they can accommodate—additional acid pulls them out of shape, denaturing them and disrupting many body processes.

Blood Clotting   To prevent dangerous blood loss, special blood proteins respond to an injury by clotting the blood. In an amazing series of chemical events, these proteins form a stringy net that traps blood cells to form a clot. The clot acts as a plug to stem blood flow from the wound. Later, as the wound heals, the protein collagen finishes the job by replacing the clot with scar tissue.

The final function of protein, providing energy, depends on some metabolic adjustments, as described in the next section. Table 6–2 (p. 216) provides a summary of the functions of proteins in the body.

KEY POINT

- Proteins help regulate gene expression; provide structure and movement; serve as enzymes, hormones, and antibodies; provide molecular transport; help regulate fluid and electrolyte balance; buffer the blood; contribute to blood clotting; and provide energy.

Providing Energy and Glucose

Only protein can perform all the functions just described, but protein will be surrendered to provide energy if need be. Under conditions of inadequate carbohydrate or energy, protein breakdown speeds up.

acids compounds that release hydrogens in a watery solution.

bases compounds that accept hydrogens from solutions.

acid-base balance equilibrium between acid and base concentrations in the body fluids.

buffers compounds that help keep a solution's acidity or alkalinity constant.

acidosis (acid-DOH-sis) the condition of excess acid in the blood, indicated by a below-normal pH (*osis* means "too much").

alkalosis (al-kah-LOH-sis) the condition of excess base in the blood, indicated by an above-normal blood pH (*alka* means "base"; *osis* means "too much").

Amino Acids to Glucose   The body must have energy to live from moment to moment, so obtaining that energy is a top priority. Not only can amino acids supply energy, but also many of them can be converted to glucose, as fatty acids can never be. Thus, if the need arises, protein can help to maintain a steady blood glucose level and serve the glucose need of the brain.

When amino acids are degraded for energy or converted into glucose, their nitrogen-containing amine groups are stripped off and used elsewhere or are incorporated by the liver into **urea** and sent to the kidneys for excretion in the urine. The fragments that remain are composed of carbon, hydrogen, and oxygen, as are carbohydrate and fat, and can be used to build glucose or fatty acids or can be metabolized like them.

Drawing Amino Acids from Tissues   Glucose is stored as glycogen and fat as triglycerides, but no specialized storage compound exists for protein. Body protein is present only as the active working molecular and structural components of body tissues. When protein-sparing energy from carbohydrate and fat is lacking and the need becomes urgent, as in starvation, prolonged fasting, or severe calorie restriction, the body must dismantle its tissue proteins to obtain amino acids for building the most essential proteins and for energy. Each protein is taken in its own time: first, small proteins from the blood, then proteins from the muscles. The body guards the structural proteins of the heart and other organs until forced, by dire need, to relinquish them. Thus, energy deficiency (starvation) always incurs wasting of lean body tissue as well as loss of fat.

Using Excess Amino Acids   When amino acids are oversupplied, the body cannot store them. It has no choice but to remove and excrete their amine groups and then use the residues in one of three ways: to meet immediate energy needs, to make glucose for storage as glycogen, or to make fat for energy storage. The body readily converts amino acids to glucose. The body also possesses enzymes to convert amino acids into fatty acids. An indirect contribution of amino acids to fat stores also exists—the body speeds up its use of excess amino acids for fuel, burning them instead of fat, making fat more abundantly available for storage in the fat tissue.

The similarities and differences of the three energy-yielding nutrients should now be clear. Carbohydrate offers energy; fat offers concentrated energy; and protein can offer energy plus nitrogen (see Figure 6–12).

Figure 6–12

Three Different Energy Sources

Carbohydrate offers energy; fat offers concentrated energy; and protein, if necessary, can offer energy plus nitrogen. The compounds at the left yield the 2-carbon fragments shown at the right. These fragments oxidize quickly in the presence of oxygen to yield carbon dioxide, water, and energy.

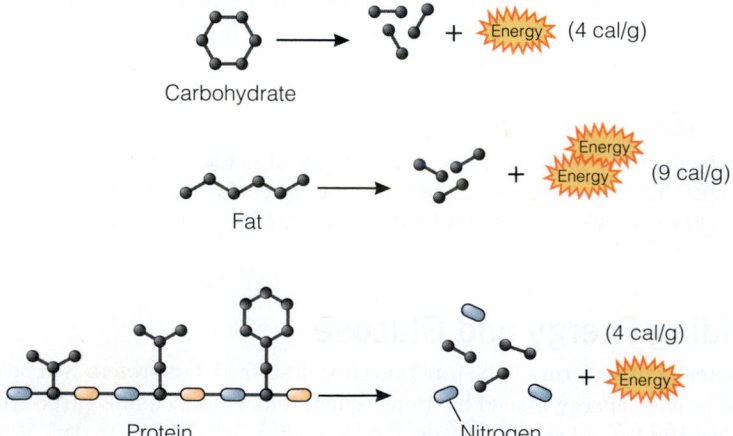

Carbohydrate + Energy (4 cal/g)

Fat + Energy Energy (9 cal/g)

Protein → Nitrogen + Energy (4 cal/g)

urea (yoo-REE-uh) the principal nitrogen-excretion product of protein metabolism; generated mostly by removal of amine groups from unneeded amino acids or from amino acids being sacrificed for energy.

The Fate of an Amino Acid

To review the body's handling of amino acids, let us follow the fate of an amino acid that was originally part of a protein-containing food. When the amino acid arrives in a cell, it can be used in one of several ways, depending on the cell's needs at the time:

- The amino acid can be used as-is to build part of a growing protein.

- The amino acid can be altered somewhat to make another needed compound, such as the vitamin niacin.

- The cell can dismantle the amino acid in order to use its amine group to build a different amino acid. The remainder can be used for fuel or, if fuel is abundant, converted to glucose or fat.

When a cell is starved for energy and has no glucose or fatty acids, it strips the amino acid of its amine group (the nitrogen part) and uses the remainder of its structure for energy. The amine group is excreted from the cell and then from the body in the urine. In a cell that has a surplus of energy and amino acids, the cell takes the amino acid apart, excretes the amine group, and uses the rest to meet immediate energy needs or converts it to glucose or fat for storage.

When not used to build protein or make other nitrogen-containing compounds, amino acids are "wasted" in a sense. This wasting occurs under any of four conditions:

1. When the body lacks energy from other sources.
2. When the diet supplies more protein than the body needs.
3. When the body has too much of any single amino acid, such as from a supplement.
4. When the diet supplies protein of low quality, with too few essential amino acids, as described in the next section.

To prevent the wasting of dietary protein and permit the synthesis of needed body protein, the dietary protein must be of adequate quality: it must supply all essential amino acids in the proper amounts. It must also be accompanied by enough energy-yielding carbohydrate and fat to permit the dietary protein to be used as such.

To review, amino acids in a cell can be:

- Used to build protein.

- Converted to other amino acids or small nitrogen-containing compounds.

Stripped of their nitrogen, amino acids can be:

- Burned as fuel.

- Converted to glucose or fat.

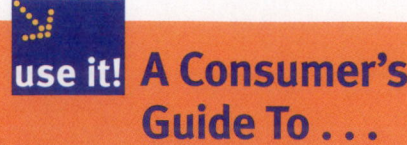
Evaluating Protein and Amino Acid Supplements

Nature provides protein abundantly in foods, but many people become convinced that they need extra protein and amino acids from supplements. Sorting truth from wishful thinking in advertisements can be tricky: "Take this protein supplement to build muscle," "This one will help you lose weight," "Take an amino acid to get to sleep, grow strong fingernails, cure herpes, build immunity . . ." Can these products really do these things?

Protein Supplements

Athletes often take protein supplements, but most well-fed athletes probably do not need them. True, protein is necessary for building muscle tissue, and, true, consuming protein in conjunction with resistance exercise helps build new muscle proteins. But protein from supplements is not "muscle in a bottle," as advertisers claim. A "couch potato" who takes protein supplements cannot expect gains of muscle tissue or athletic performance. Also, if the supplements create a surplus of nitrogen, it must be metabolized and excreted, placing a burden on the kidneys, particularly if they are already weak. Much more information about athletes and supplements is found in Chapter 10.

What a boon it would be to people on weight-loss diets if they could take the right protein or amino acids in a milkshake and effortlessly lose weight. Adding extra protein from bars and shakes is unlikely to produce this effect, however, and these products add many calories to the diet. A grain of truth is present in the claims of advertisers, however. Sufficient protein in a meal may help to expend a small amount of energy after eating and help increase satiety.[1]* Take note: ordinary protein-rich foods, such as fat-free Greek-style yogurt, offer just as much

Reference notes are found in Appendix F.

protein as do many "protein drinks"— but with far fewer calories and at a much lower cost. Evidence does not support taking protein supplements to lose weight, and common sense opposes it.

Amino Acid Supplements

Enthusiastic popular reports of benefits of amino acid supplements boost their sales. One such amino acid is lysine, touted to prevent or relieve the infections that cause herpes sores on the mouth or genital organs. Lysine does not cure herpes infections. Whether it reduces outbreaks or even whether it is safe is unknown; scientific studies are lacking.

Supplements containing amino acids are often sold to athletes with promises of greater blood flow to muscles or increased muscle protein synthesis. It's true that the essential amino acid leucine is necessary for normal protein synthesis regulation, but all complete protein sources, even a turkey sandwich or a glass of milk, supply plenty of leucine. No clear benefit to muscle tissue has been demonstrated for leucine supplements, and their safety is under review.[2]

Millions of people take amino acid supplements hoping to strengthen soft, dry, weak, easily breakable nails. Nails are sensitive to nutrition. Made largely of protein, nails depend on sulfur bonds between amino acids (this was shown in Figure 6–10) for flexible strength, fatty acids for water resistance, and sufficient water for proper hydration.[3] In addition, nails need many minerals and vitamins to metabolize it all into place. Pills of amino acids or even the protein gelatin, often sold as a nail supplement, cannot provide the complex array of nutrients needed for nail strength. Only a nutritious diet can do so.

Pills of the amino acid tryptophan are sold to relieve pain, depression, and insomnia. Tryptophan provides raw

material for making the brain neurotransmitter serotonin, an important regulator of sleep, appetite, mood, and sensory perception. High doses of tryptophan (up to 5 grams per day) may induce sleepiness, but may also cause nausea and other unpleasant but short-lived side effects.[4]

What Scientists Say

The body handles whole proteins best. It breaks them into manageable pieces (dipeptides and tripeptides) and then splits these, a few at a time, simultaneously releasing them into the blood. This slow, bit-by-bit assimilation is ideal because groups of chemically similar amino acids compete for the carriers that absorb them into the blood. An excess of one amino acid can tie up a carrier and disturb amino acid absorption, creating a temporary imbalance.

Deep in the cells' nuclei, amino acids play key roles in gene regulation, and amino acid imbalances may alter these processes in unpredictable ways. In mice, for example, feeding excess methionine causes the buildup of an amino acid associated with heart disease (homocysteine), accelerates atherosclerosis in the heart's main artery, and increases inflammation in the liver.[5] No one knows if the same is true in people. Many supplement takers experience digestive disturbances because a high concentration of amino acids causes excess water to flow into the digestive tract from body tissues, resulting in diarrhea and dehydration. Recently, some takers of sports supplements with added amino acids developed a serious liver condition known as toxic hepatitis that reversed when they stopped taking the supplements.[6] Others have ended up in hospital emergency rooms with racing heartbeats and other serious symptoms.

In cases of disease or malnutrition, particularly among the elderly, a registered dietitian nutritionist may employ a special protein or amino acid supplement to help treat the condition.[7] Not every patient is a candidate for such therapy, however, because supplemental amino acids can stimulate inflammation, which can worsen some diseases. In addition, protein or amino acid supplements can interfere with the actions of certain medications, allowing disease conditions to advance.[8]

A lack of research prevents the DRI committee from setting Tolerable Upper Intake Levels for amino acids.[9] Therefore, no level of amino acid supplementation can be assumed safe. The people most likely to be harmed are listed in Table 6–3. Take heed: much is still unknown, and the taker of amino acid supplements cannot be certain of their safety or effectiveness, despite convincing marketing materials.

Moving Ahead

Even with all that we've learned from science, it is hard to improve on nature. In almost every case, the complex balance of amino acids and other nutrients found together in whole foods is best for nutrition. Keep it safe and simple: select a variety of protein-rich foods that are low in saturated fat each day, and avoid unnecessary protein and amino acid supplements.

Review Questions*

1. Commercial shakes and energy bars have proven to be the best protein sources to support weight-loss efforts. T F

2. Lysine does not cure herpes infections. T F

3. In high doses, tryptophan can improve nausea and skin disorders. T F

*Answers to Consumer's Guide review questions are found in Appendix G.

Food Protein: Need and Quality

LO 6.4 List the factors that determine the daily protein needs of an individual.

A person's use of and need for dietary protein depend on many factors. To know whether, say, 60 grams of a particular protein is enough to meet a person's daily needs, one must consider the effects of factors discussed in this section, some pertaining to the body and some to the nature of the protein.

How Much Protein Do People Need?

The DRI recommendation for protein intake is designed to cover the need to replace protein-containing tissue that healthy adults lose and wear out every day. Therefore, it depends on body size: larger people have a higher protein need. For adults of healthy body weight, the DRI recommended intake is set at 0.8 grams for each kilogram (or 2.2 pounds) of body weight (see inside front cover). The minimum amount is set at 10 percent of total calories, although some evidence suggests that certain groups of people, such as the elderly, may need more than this minimum for optimal health.[5] Athletes may need slightly more protein—1.2–1.7 grams per kilogram per day—but even this amount is provided by a well-chosen eating pattern with enough energy for an athlete (see Chapter 10).

For infants and growing children, the protein recommendation, like all nutrient recommendations, is higher per unit of body weight. The DRI committee set an upper limit for protein intake of no more than 35 percent of total calories, an amount significantly higher than average intakes. The margin provides a method for determining

Do the Math

The DRI recommended intake for protein (adult) = 0.8 g/kg. To figure out your protein need:

1. Look up the healthy weight for a person of your height (inside back cover). If your weight falls within the range, use it; if outside the range, use the midpoint of the range.
2. Convert pounds to kilograms (by dividing pounds by 2.2).
3. Multiply kilograms by 0.8 to find total grams of protein recommended.

For example:

Weight = 130 lb

130 lb ÷ 2.2 = 59 kg

59 kg × 0.8 = 47 g

Table 6–4
Protein Intake Recommendations for Healthy Adults

DRI Recommended Intake[a]

- 0.8 g protein/kg body weight/day.
- Women: 46 g/day; men: 56 g/day.
- Acceptable intake range: 10 to 30% of calories from protein.

Dietary Guidelines for Americans 2015–2020

- A healthy eating pattern includes a variety of protein foods, including seafood, lean meats and poultry, eggs, legumes (peas and beans), and nuts, seeds and soy products.

[a] *Protein recommendations for infants, children, and pregnant and lactating women are higher; see inside front cover, page B.*

---

your own protein need, and Table 6–4 reviews recommendations for protein intake. The following factors also modify protein needs.

The Body's Health   Malnutrition or infection may greatly increase the need for protein while making it hard to eat even normal amounts of food. In malnutrition, secretion of digestive enzymes slows as the tract's lining degenerates, impairing protein digestion and absorption. When infection is present, extra protein is needed for enhanced immune functions.

Other Nutrients and Energy   The need for ample energy, carbohydrate, and fat has already been emphasized. To be used efficiently by the cells, protein must also be accompanied by the full array of vitamins and minerals.

Protein Quality   The remaining factor, protein quality, helps determine how well a diet supports the growth of children and the health of adults. Protein quality becomes crucial for people in areas where food is scarce, as described in a later section.

DRI protein intake recommendations assume a normal mixed diet—that is, an eating pattern that provides sufficient nutrients and protein from a combination of animal and plant sources. Because not all proteins are used with 100 percent efficiency, the recommendation is generous. Many healthy people can consume less than the recommended amount and still meet their bodies' protein needs. What this means in terms of food selections is presented in this chapter's Food Feature.

KEY POINTS

- The protein intake recommendation depends on size and stage of growth.
- The DRI recommended intake for adults is 0.8 grams of protein per kilogram of body weight.
- Factors concerning both the body and food sources modify an individual's protein need.

Nitrogen Balance

Underlying the protein recommendation are **nitrogen balance** studies, which compare nitrogen lost by excretion with nitrogen eaten in food.[6] In healthy adults, nitrogen-in (consumed) must equal nitrogen-out (excreted). Scientists measure the body's daily nitrogen losses in urine, feces, sweat, and skin under controlled conditions and then estimate the amount of protein needed to replace these losses.[‡]

Under normal circumstances, healthy adults are in nitrogen equilibrium, or zero balance; that is, they have the same amount of total protein in their bodies at all times. When nitrogen-in exceeds nitrogen-out, people are said to be in positive nitrogen balance; somewhere in their bodies more proteins are being built than are being broken down and lost. When nitrogen-in is less than nitrogen-out, people are said to be in negative nitrogen balance; they are losing protein. Figure 6–13 illustrates these different states.

Positive Nitrogen Balance   Growing children add new blood, bone, and muscle cells to their bodies every day, so children have more protein, and therefore more nitrogen, in their bodies at the end of each day than they had at the beginning. A growing child is therefore in positive nitrogen balance. Similarly, when a woman is pregnant, she must be in positive nitrogen balance until after the birth, when she once again reaches equilibrium.

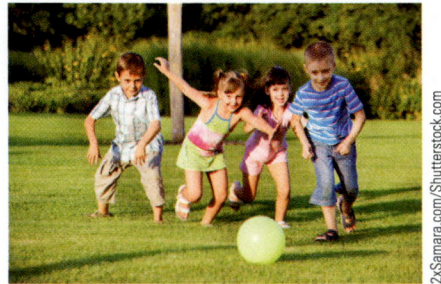

Growing children end each day with more bone, blood, muscle, and skin cells than they had at the beginning of the day.

---

nitrogen balance   the amount of nitrogen consumed compared with the amount excreted in a given time period.

[‡] The average protein is 16 percent nitrogen by weight; that is, each 100 grams of protein contain 16 grams of nitrogen. Scientists can estimate the general amount of protein in a sample of food, body tissue, or other material by multiplying the weight of the nitrogen in it by 6.25.

Figure 6–13

Nitrogen Balance

Nitrogen in ● Nitrogen out ●

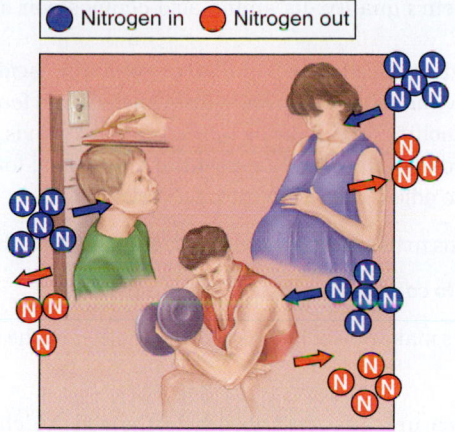

Positive Nitrogen Balance
These people—a growing child, a person building muscle, and a pregnant woman—are all retaining more nitrogen than they are excreting.

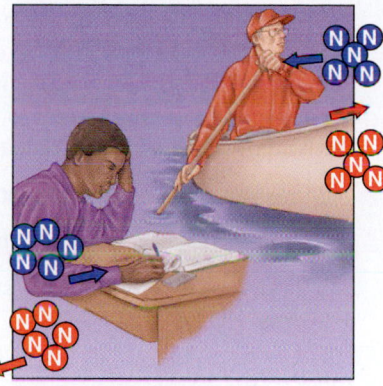

Nitrogen Equilibrium
These people—a healthy college student and a young retiree—are in nitrogen equilibrium.

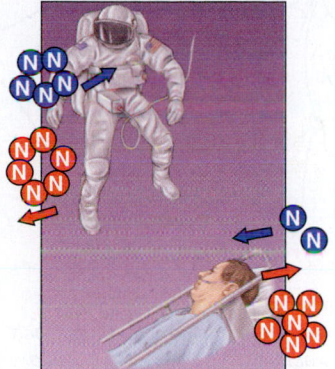

Negative Nitrogen Balance
These people—an astronaut and a surgery patient—are losing more nitrogen than they are taking in.

Negative Nitrogen Balance

Negative nitrogen balance occurs when muscle or other protein tissue is broken down and lost: nitrogen excretion increases. Illness or injury triggers the release of powerful messengers that signal the body to break down some of the less vital proteins, such as those of the blood, skin, and muscle.[§] This action floods the blood with amino acids, which are then stripped of their nitrogen and used for energy to fuel the body's defenses and fight the illness. The result is greater nitrogen excretion and negative nitrogen balance. Astronauts, too, experience negative nitrogen balance. In the stress of space flight and with no need to support the body's weight against gravity, the astronauts' muscles waste and weaken. To minimize the inevitable loss of muscle tissue, the astronauts must do special exercises in space.

KEY POINT

- Protein recommendations are based on nitrogen balance studies, which compare nitrogen excreted from the body with nitrogen ingested in food.

My Turn watch it! **Veggin' Out**

Joshua

© Cengage Learning

Have you ever considered not eating meat? Listen to Joshua discuss how becoming vegetarian affected his social life.

Visit www.cengagebrain.com to access MindTap, a complete digital course that includes this video and other resources.

[§]The messengers are cytokines.

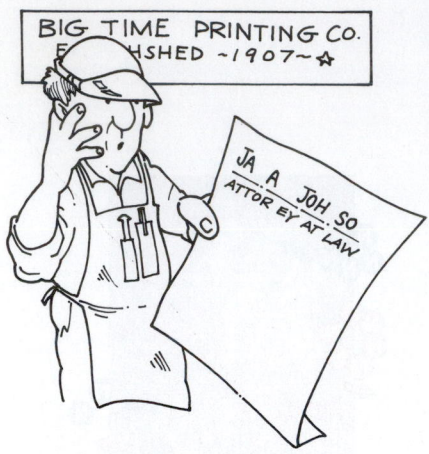

Just as each letter of the alphabet is important in forming whole words, each amino acid must be available to build finished proteins.

Protein Quality

Put simply, **high-quality proteins** provide enough of all the essential amino acids needed by the body to create its own working proteins, whereas low-quality proteins don't. Two factors influence a protein's quality: its amino acid composition and its digestibility.

In making their required proteins, the cells need a full array of amino acids. If a nonessential amino acid (that is, one the cells can make) is unavailable from food, the cells synthesize it and continue attaching amino acids to the protein strands being manufactured. If the diet fails to provide enough of an essential amino acid (one the cells cannot make), the cells begin to adjust their activities. The cells:

- Break down more internal proteins to liberate the needed essential amino acid, and
- Limit their synthesis of proteins to conserve the essential amino acid.

As the deprivation continues, tissues make one adjustment after another in the struggle to survive.

Limiting Amino Acids   The measures just described help the cells to channel the available **limiting amino acid** to its wisest use: making new proteins. Even so, the normally fast rate of protein synthesis slows to a crawl as the cells make do with the proteins on hand. When the limiting amino acid once again becomes available in abundance, the cells resume their normal protein-related activities. If the shortage becomes chronic, however, the cells begin to break down their protein-making machinery. Consequently, when protein intakes become adequate again, protein synthesis lags behind until the needed machinery can be rebuilt. Meanwhile, the cells function less and less effectively as their proteins wear out and are only partially replaced.

Thus, a diet that is short in any of the essential amino acids limits protein synthesis. An earlier analogy likened amino acids to letters of the alphabet. To be meaningful, words must contain all the right letters. For example, a print shop that has no letter "N" cannot make personalized stationery for Jana Johnson. No matter how many Js, As, Os, Hs, and Ss are in the printer's possession, the printer cannot use them to replace the missing Ns. Likewise, in building a protein molecule, no amino acid can fill another's spot. If a cell that is building a protein cannot find a needed amino acid, synthesis stops, and the partial protein is released.

Partially completed proteins are not held for completion at a later time when the diet may improve. Rather, they are dismantled, and the component amino acids are returned to the circulation to be made available to other cells. If they are not soon inserted into protein, their amine groups are removed and excreted, and the residues are used for other purposes. The need that prompted the call for that particular protein will not be met. Since the other amino acids are wasted, the amine groups are excreted, and the body cannot resynthesize the amino acids later.

Complementary Proteins   It follows that, if a person does not consume all the essential amino acids in proportion to the body's needs, the body's pools of essential amino acids will dwindle until body organs are compromised. Consuming the essential amino acids presents no problem to people who regularly eat proteins containing ample amounts of all of the essential amino acids, such as those of meat, fish, poultry, cheese, eggs, milk, and most soybean products.

An equally sound choice is to eat a variety of protein foods from plants so that amino acids that are low in some foods will be supplied by the others. The combination of such protein-rich foods yields **complementary proteins** (see Figure 6–14), or proteins containing all the essential amino acids in amounts sufficient to support health. This concept, often employed by vegetarians, is illustrated in Figure 6–15. The figure demonstrates that the amino acids of **legumes** and grains balance each other to provide all of the needed amino acids. The complementary proteins need not be eaten together, so long as the day's meals supply all of them, along with sufficient energy and enough total protein from a variety of sources.

high-quality proteins dietary proteins containing all the essential amino acids in relatively the same amounts that human beings require. They may also contain nonessential amino acids.

limiting amino acid an essential amino acid that is present in dietary protein in an insufficient amount, thereby limiting the body's ability to build protein.

complementary proteins two or more proteins whose amino acid assortments complement each other in such a way that the essential amino acids missing from one are supplied by the other.

legumes (leg-GOOMS, LEG-yooms) plants of the bean, pea, and lentil family that have roots with nodules containing special bacteria. These bacteria can trap nitrogen from the air in the soil and make it into compounds that become part of the plant's seeds. The seeds are rich in protein compared with those of most other plant foods. Also defined in Chapter 1.

Figure 6–14

Complementary Protein Combinations

Healthful foods like these contribute substantial protein (42 grams total) to this day's meals without meat. Additional servings of nutritious foods, such as milk, bread, and eggs, can easily supply the remainder of the day's need for protein (14 additional grams for men and 4 for women).

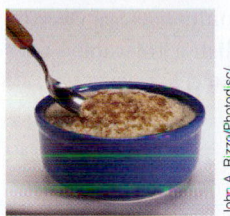

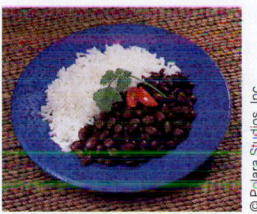

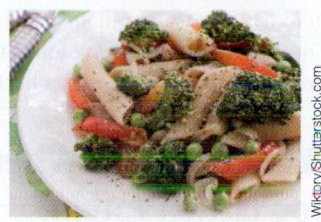

¾ c oatmeal =	5 g
Protein total	5 g

1 c rice =	4 g
1 c beans =	16 g
Protein total	20 g

1½ c pasta	= 11 g
1 c vegetables	= 2 g
2 tbs Parmesan cheese =	4 g
Protein total	17 g

Protein Digestibility In measuring a protein's quality, digestibility is also important. Simple measures of the total protein in foods are not useful by themselves—even animal hair and hooves would receive a top score by those measures alone. They are made of protein, but the protein is not in a form that people can use.

The digestibility of protein varies from food to food and bears profoundly on protein quality. The protein of oats, for example, is less digestible than that of eggs. In general, proteins from animal sources, such as chicken, beef, and pork, are most easily digested and absorbed (over 90 percent). Those from legumes are next (about 80 to 90 percent). Those from grains and other plant foods vary (from 70 to 90 percent). Cooking with moist heat improves protein digestibility, whereas dry heat methods can impair it.

KEY POINT

- Digestibility of protein varies from food to food, and cooking can improve or impair it.

Perspective on Protein Quality Concern about the quality of individual food proteins is of only theoretical interest in settings where food is abundant. Healthy adults in these places would find it next to impossible *not* to meet their protein needs, even if they were to eat no meat, fish, poultry, eggs, or cheese products at all. They need not pay attention to balancing amino acids so long as they follow an eating pattern that is varied, nutritious, and adequate in energy and other nutrients—not made up of, say, just cookies, crackers, potato chips, and juices. Protein sufficiency follows effortlessly behind a balanced, nutritious eating pattern.

For people in areas where food sources are less reliable, protein quality can make the difference between health and disease. When food energy is restricted, where malnutrition is widespread, or when the variety of available foods is severely limited (where a single low-protein food, such as **fufu** made from cassava root,** provides 90 percent of the calories), the primary food source of protein must be checked because its quality is crucial.

KEY POINTS

- A protein's amino acid assortment greatly influences its usefulness to the body.
- Food proteins that lack essential amino acids can be used by the body only if those amino acids are present from other sources.
- Protein quality becomes more important whenever food supplies are limited.

**Cassava is also called *manioc* or *yucca*.

Figure 6–15

How Complementary Proteins Work Together

Legumes provide plenty of the amino acids isoleucine (Ile) and lysine (Lys) but fall short in methionine (Met) and tryptophan (Trp). Grains have the opposite strengths and weaknesses, making them a perfect match for legumes.

	Ile	Lys	Met	Trp
Legumes	✓	✓		
Grains			✓	✓
Together	✓	✓	✓	✓

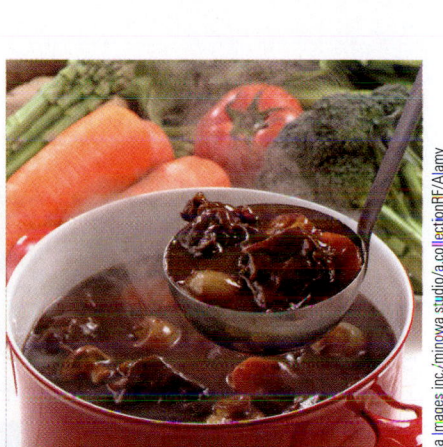

Cooking with moist heat improves protein digestibility, whereas frying makes protein harder to digest.

fufu a low-protein staple food that provides abundant starch energy to many of the world's people; fufu is made by pounding or grinding root vegetables or refined grains and cooking them to a smooth, semisolid consistency.

Protein Deficiency and Excess

LO 6.5 Discuss the potential health problems from an eating plan that is too low or too high in protein.

When diets lack sufficient protein from food or sufficient amounts of any of the essential amino acids, symptoms of malnutrition become evident. In contrast, the health effects of protein excess are less well established, but high-protein diets, and particularly high-meat diets, have been implicated in several chronic diseases (see the Controversy section). Evidence is currently insufficient to establish a Tolerable Upper Intake Level for protein, but both deficiency and excess are of concern.

What Happens When People Consume Too Little Protein?

In protein deficiency, when the diet supplies too little protein or lacks a specific essential amino acid relative to the others (a limiting amino acid), the body slows its synthesis of proteins while increasing its breakdown of body tissue protein to liberate the amino acids it needs to build other proteins of critical importance. Without these critical proteins to perform their roles, many of the body's life-sustaining activities would come to a halt. The most recognizable consequences of protein deficiency include slow growth in children, impaired brain and kidney functions, weakened immune defenses, and impaired nutrient absorption from the digestive tract.

In clinical settings, the term *protein-energy malnutrition* has been used to describe the condition that develops when the diet delivers too little protein, too little energy, or both. However, such malnutrition reflects insufficient food intake, with not only too little protein and energy but also too few vitamins, too few minerals, and, in fact, too little of most of the nutrients needed for health and growth. The severe malnutrition of starvation and its clinical manifestations are a focus of Chapter 15's discussion of world hunger.

Is It Possible to Consume Too Much Protein?

Overconsumption of protein-rich foods offers no benefits and may pose a health risk for people with weakened kidneys. This section explores current protein intakes and considers the potential for harm from excesses.

How Much Protein Do People Take In? Most people suspect that Americans eat far too much protein. In fact, the average protein intake for U.S. men is about 16 percent of total calories, with women consuming slightly less at 15.5 percent.[7] These amounts are well within the DRI suggested range of between 10 and 35 percent of calories. Stated another way, the DRI range for protein intake in a 2,000-calorie diet is 50 to 175 grams; the average U.S. daily intake of protein amounts to about 78 grams.

Weight-Loss Dieting Some popular weight-loss diet advice suggests 65 percent or more of calories from protein as a way to lose weight. True, meeting protein recommendations during weight loss is critical for preserving the body's working lean tissues, such as liver and muscles. Also, evidence suggests that protein may help control the appetite, and may cost some extra energy for its metabolism.[8] However, as Chapter 9 explains, it is calorie intake reduction alone and not the proportion of energy nutrients in the diet that brings about long-term weight loss.

Protein Sources in Heart Disease Protein itself is not known to contribute to heart disease and mortality, but some of its food sources may do so.[9] Selecting too many animal-derived protein-rich foods, such as fatty red meats, processed meats, and fat-containing milk products, adds a burden of saturated fat to the diet and crowds out fruits, vegetables, legumes, nuts, and whole grains.[10] Consequently, it is not surprising that people who habitually take in a great deal of animal protein,

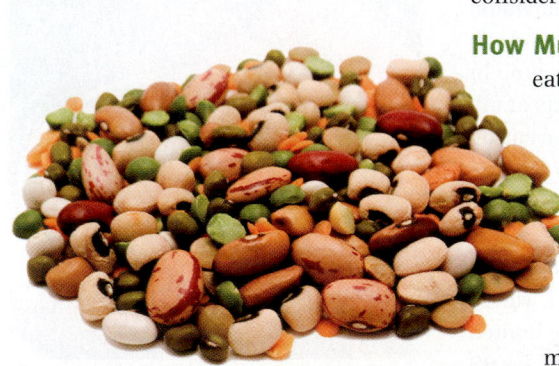

Malnutrition: too little food causes deficiencies of protein and many other nutrients. See Chapter 15.

Margaret Prout/Associated Press

iStockphoto.com/Only_fabrizio

and particularly processed meat such as lunchmeats and hot dogs, have higher body weights and a greater risk of chronic diseases than those who take in less.[11] The Controversy section explores how substituting vegetable protein for at least some of the animal protein in the diet may improve risk factors for chronic diseases and mortality.[12]

Kidney Disease Animals fed experimentally on high-protein diets often develop enlarged kidneys or livers. In human beings, a high-protein diet increases the kidneys' workload, but this alone does not appear to damage healthy kidneys or to cause kidney disease.[13] In people with kidney stones or other kidney diseases, however, a high-protein diet may speed the kidneys' decline, and increase the risk of stone formation.[14] For people with established kidney problems, a lower protein intake often improves the symptoms of their disease.

Adult Bone Loss When human subjects are given increasing doses of purified protein, they spill larger and larger amounts of calcium from the body into the urine. This finding raised concerns that high-protein diets may harm the bones. However, research now suggests that higher protein intakes from whole food such as legumes, meats, or milk may not increase calcium loss from the bones and, when consumed in the context of an otherwise adequate diet, may help to prevent the crippling bone-loss disease **osteoporosis** in some people.[15] The two groups most likely to have osteoporosis, elderly women and adolescents with the eating disorder anorexia nervosa, typically do not meet the DRI recommendation for protein.

Cancer The risk of cancer does not appear to increase with greater protein intakes. However, eating a diet high in red meats and **processed meats** often does correlate with certain cancers, particularly colon cancer.[16] Being overweight, being physically inactive, smoking, and drinking alcohol also raise cancer risks significantly. In contrast, people who eat just three servings of protein-rich legumes each week may lower their cancer risks. Chapter 11 discusses the known links between diet and cancer.

Is a Gluten-Free Diet Best for Health?

Gluten, a protein that forms in grain foods, is best known for providing a pleasing stretchy texture to yeast breads. It also provides bulk and texture to many other foods made from wheat, triticale, barley, rye, and related grains.

Celiac Disease In people with **celiac disease**, gluten triggers an abnormal immune response that inflames the small intestine and erodes the intestinal villi, severely limiting nutrient absorption. The result is a lifelong battle against extreme weight loss with vitamin, mineral, and other nutrient deficiencies.[17] Symptoms often include chronic diarrhea or constipation, vomiting, bloating, and pain; alternatively, the person may develop anemia, fatigue, aches and pains, bone loss, depression, anxiety, infertility, mouth sores, or an itchy, blistering skin rash.

A blood test revealing high levels of certain antibodies confirms the diagnosis of celiac disease or the similar problem of gluten allergy. To heal their intestines, people with these conditions must eliminate all gluten-containing foods from their diet and then continue avoiding them for the rest of their lives. This may be easier said than done because gluten can hide in foods that contain wheat-based additives, such as modified food starch and preservatives. Even corn and rice, naturally gluten-free foods, can be contaminated with gluten if they are milled in machines that also process wheat. The U.S. Food and Drug Administration requires food labels to clearly identify ingredients containing wheat and related grains; foods labeled "gluten-free" are held to strict standards.[††]

[††] A food labeled "gluten-free" may not contain gluten-containing grains or ingredients derived from them (unless processed to remove gluten).

osteoporosis (OSS-tee-oh-pore-OH-sis) a disease of older persons characterized by porous and fragile bones that easily break, leading to pain, infirmity, and death. Also defined in Chapter 8.

processed meats a general term for meat products preserved by smoking, curing, salting, or adding chemical preservatives—for example, ham, bacon, jerky, hot dogs (including chicken and turkey), luncheon meats, salami and other sausages, SPAM, and Vienna sausages.

gluten (GLOO-ten) a type of protein in certain grain foods that is toxic to the person with celiac disease.

celiac (SEE-lee-ack) **disease** a disorder characterized by an abnormal immune response, weight loss, and intestinal inflammation on exposure to the dietary protein gluten; also called *gluten-sensitive enteropathy* or *celiac sprue*.

Non-Celiac Gluten Sensitivity Physicians increasingly report a group of symptoms called **non-celiac gluten sensitivity** (NCGS).[18] The patient suffers from digestive symptoms resembling those of celiac disease or a gluten allergy, but tests negative for these conditions. Some people with NCGS find relief when they eat a gluten-free diet, although the reasons why are not clear.[19]

> More on food allergies in **Chapter 13**.

Gluten-Free Hype Recently, popular media have blamed gluten for causing headaches, insomnia, obesity, and even cancer and Alzheimer's disease, but no evidence supports these accusations. Gluten-free diets have no special power to spur weight loss either, despite noisy claims made by diet sellers. In fact, the opposite is often true: many gluten-sensitive people become overweight when they begin eating a gluten-free diet that relieves their symptoms.[20] Manufactured gluten-free foods are often higher in fats, added sugars, and calories than their regular counterparts, making overconsumption of calories likely.

Most people with celiac disease are never diagnosed, and without treatment, they continue to suffer needlessly. Ironically, most people following a gluten-free diet may not have celiac disease, NCGS, or gluten allergy.[21] They eat expensive, high-calorie, processed specialty foods and unnecessarily omit nutritious whole grains because they believe the false claims of faddists.

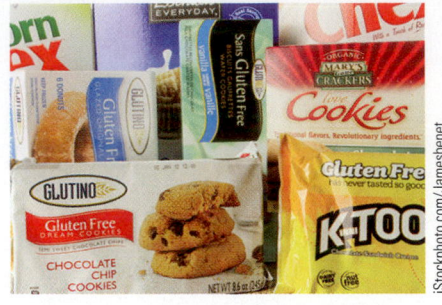

A gluten-free diet can bring relief to people with celiac disease.

iStockphoto.com/Jamesbenet

non-celiac gluten sensitivity a poorly defined collection of digestive symptoms that improves with elimination of gluten from the diet.

KEY POINTS

- Most U.S. protein intakes fall within the DRI recommended protein intake range of 10 to 35 percent of calories.
- No Tolerable Upper Intake Level exists for protein, but health risks may follow the overconsumption of protein-rich foods.
- Gluten-free diets often relieve symptoms of celiac disease, non-celiac gluten sensitivity, or gluten allergy, but no evidence supports claims that they cure other ills.

---

try it! ⟩⟩⟩ **Food Feature**

Getting Enough but Not Too Much Protein

LO 6.6 Identify the benefits and drawbacks of protein-rich foods in the diet.

Most foods contribute at least some protein to the diet. The most nutrient-dense selections among them are generally best for nutrition.

Protein-Rich Foods

Foods in the Protein Foods group (meat, poultry, fish, dry peas and beans, eggs, and nuts) and in the Milk and Milk Products group (milk, yogurt, and cheese) contribute an abundance of high-quality protein. Two others, the Vegetables group and the Grains group, contribute smaller amounts of protein,

but they can add up to significant quantities. What about the Fruits group? Don't rely on fruit for protein; fruit contains only small amounts. Figure 6–16 (p. 227) demonstrates that a wide variety of foods contribute protein to the diet. Figure 6–17 (p. 228) lists the top protein contributors in the U.S. diet.

Protein is critical in nutrition, but too many protein-rich foods can displace other important foods from the diet. Foods richest in protein carry with them a characteristic array of vitamins and minerals, including vitamin B_{12} and iron,

but they lack others—vitamin C and folate, for example. In addition, many protein-rich foods such as meat are high in calories, and to overconsume them is to invite obesity.

Because American consumption of protein is ample, you can plan meatless or reduced-meat meals with pleasure. Meats are not always the best, or even the most desirable, sources of protein in a balanced, nutritious diet. Of the many interesting, protein-rich meat equivalents available, one has already been mentioned: the legumes.

Chapter 6 The Proteins and Amino Acids

Figure 6–16

Finding the Protein in Foods[a]

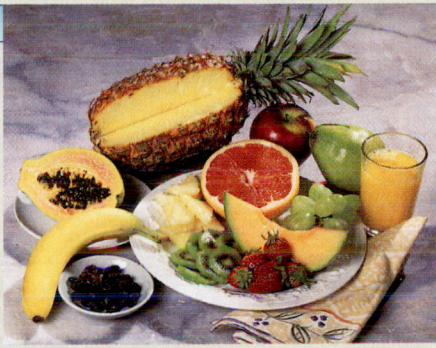

Fruits

Food		Protein g	%DV[b]
Avocado	1/2 c	2	4
Cantaloupe	1/2 c	1	2
Orange sections	1/2 c	1	2
Strawberries	1/2 c	1	2

Vegetables

Food		Protein g	%DV[b]
Corn	1/2 c	3	6
Broccoli	1/2 c	2	4
Collard greens	1/2 c	2	4
Sweet potato	1/2 c	2	4
Baked potato	1/2 c	1	2
Bean sprouts	1/2 c	1	2
Winter squash	1/2 c	1	2

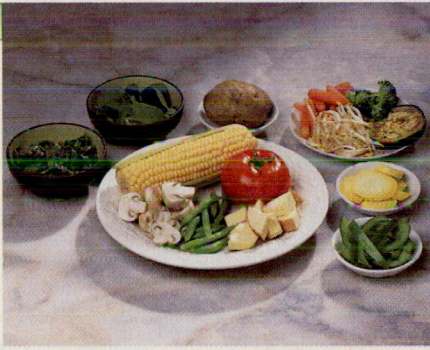

Grains

Food		Protein g	%DV[b]
Pancakes	2 sm	6	12
Bagel	1/2	4	8
Brown rice	1/2 c	3	6
Whole-grain bread	1 sl	3	6
Noodles, pasta	1/2 c	3	6
Oatmeal	1/2 c	3	6
Barley	1/2 c	2	4
Cereal flakes	1 oz	2	4

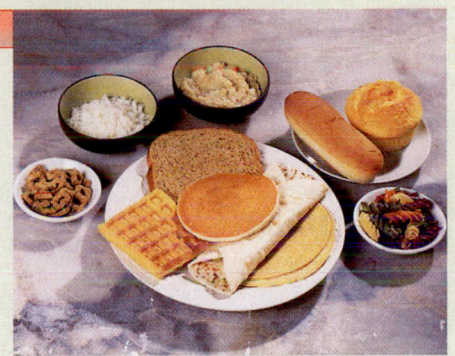

Protein Foods

Food		Protein g	%DV[b]
Roast beef	2 oz	19	33
Turkey leg	2 oz	16	32
Chicken breast	2 oz	15	30
Pork meat	2 oz	15	30
Tuna	2 oz	14	28
Lentils, beans, peas	1/2 c	9	18
Peanut butter	2 tbs	8	16
Almonds	1/4 c	8	16
Hot dog	1 reg	7	14
Lunchmeat	2 oz	6	12
Egg	1 lg	6	12
Cashew nuts	1/4 c	5	10

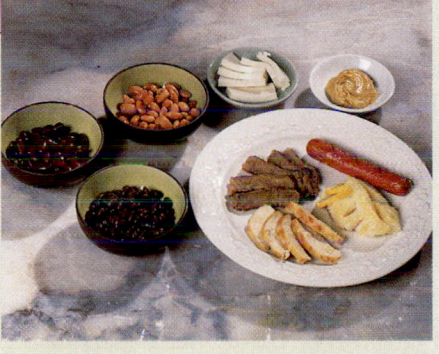

Milk and Milk Products

Food		Protein g	%DV[b]
Cheese, processed	2 oz	13	26
Milk, yogurt	1 c	10	20
Pudding	1 c	5	10

Oils, Solid Fats, and Added Sugars

Not a significant source

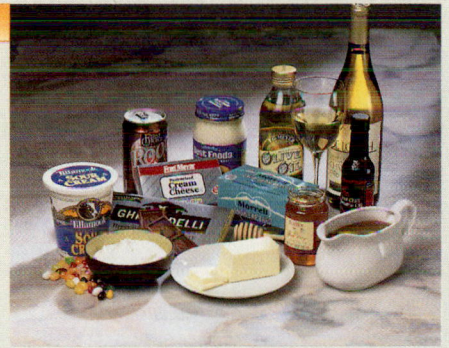

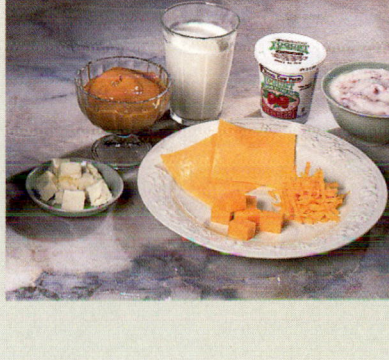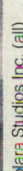

© Polara Studios Inc. (all)

[a]All foods are prepared and ready to eat.
[b]The Daily Value (DV) for protein is 50 g, based on an energy intake of 2,000 cal/day.

Figure 6–17

Top Contributors of Protein to the U.S. Diet[a]

In recent decades, poultry (largely chicken) intakes have been rising steadily, while beef intakes have been declining.

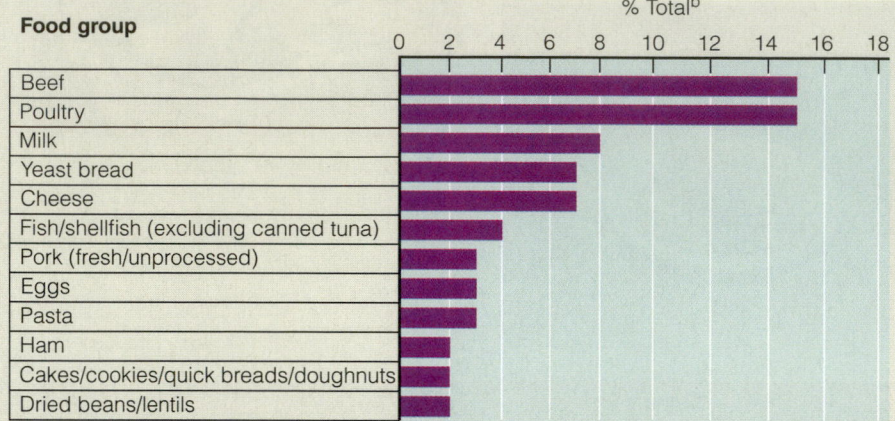

Food group	% Total[b]
Beef	
Poultry	
Milk	
Yeast bread	
Cheese	
Fish/shellfish (excluding canned tuna)	
Pork (fresh/unprocessed)	
Eggs	
Pasta	
Ham	
Cakes/cookies/quick breads/doughnuts	
Dried beans/lentils	

[a]These foods supply about 70 percent of the protein in the U.S. diet. The remainder comes from foods contributing less than 2 percent of the total.
[b]Rounded values.

The Advantages of Legumes

The protein of some legumes, and soybeans in particular, is of a quality almost comparable to that of meat, an unusual trait in a fiber-rich vegetable. Figure 6–18 shows a legume plant's special root system that enables it to make abundant protein by obtaining nitrogen from the soil. Legumes are also excellent sources of many B vitamins, iron, and other minerals, making them exceptionally nutritious foods. On average, a cup of cooked legumes contains about 30 percent of the Daily Values for both protein and iron. Like meats, though, legumes do not offer every nutrient, and they do not make a complete meal by themselves. They contain no vitamin A, vitamin C, or vitamin B_{12}, and their balance of amino acids can be much improved by using grains and other vegetables with them.

Soybeans are versatile legumes, and many nutritious products are made from them. Heavy use of soy products in place of meat, however, inhibits iron absorption. The effect can be alleviated by using small amounts of meat and/or foods rich in vitamin C in the same meal with soy products.

Vegetarians and others sometimes use convenience foods made from **textured vegetable protein** (soy protein) formulated to look and taste like hamburgers or breakfast sausages. Many of these are intended to match the known nutrient contents of animal protein foods, but they often fall short.[‡‡] A wise vegetarian uses such foods in combination with whole foods to supply an entire array of needed nutrients. The nutrients of soybeans are also available as bean curd, or **tofu**, a staple used in many Asian dishes. Thanks to the use of calcium salts when some tofu is made, it can be high in calcium. Check the Nutrition Facts panel on the label.

textured vegetable protein processed soybean protein used in products formulated to look and taste like meat, fish, or poultry.

tofu (TOE-foo) a curd made from soybeans that is rich in protein, often enriched with calcium, and variable in fat content; used in many Asian and vegetarian dishes in place of meat. Also defined in Controversy 2.

[‡‡] In Canada, regulations govern the nutrient contents of such products.

Figure 6–18

A Legume

The legumes include such plants as the kidney bean, soybean, green pea, lentil, black-eyed pea, and lima bean. Bacteria in the root nodules can "fix" nitrogen from the air, contributing it to the beans. Ultimately, thanks to these bacteria, the plant accumulates more nitrogen than it can get from the soil and also contributes more nitrogen to the soil than it takes out. The legumes are so efficient at trapping nitrogen that farmers often grow them in rotation with other crops to fertilize fields. Legumes are included with meat in the protein foods group in Figure 6–16.

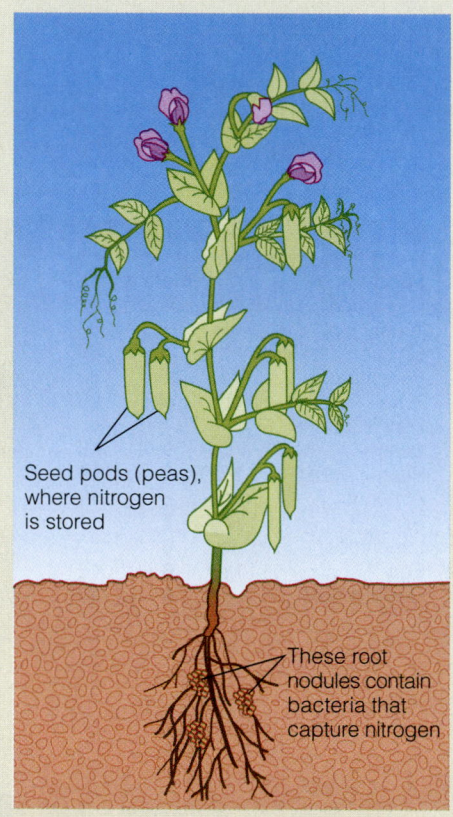

Seed pods (peas), where nitrogen is stored

These root nodules contain bacteria that capture nitrogen

Food Label Trickery

Protein has become a marketing buzzword, and everything from cereal to supplements now sports the word *protein* on the label. Oftentimes, however, "protein" bars, cereals, and beverages would be more accurately

Figure 6–19

Greek-Style Yogurt: A Protein-Rich Food

Plain, nonfat Greek yogurt provides more protein with fewer calories than most products that tout "protein" on the label. Adding berries adds nutrients, phytochemicals, and a touch of sweetness.

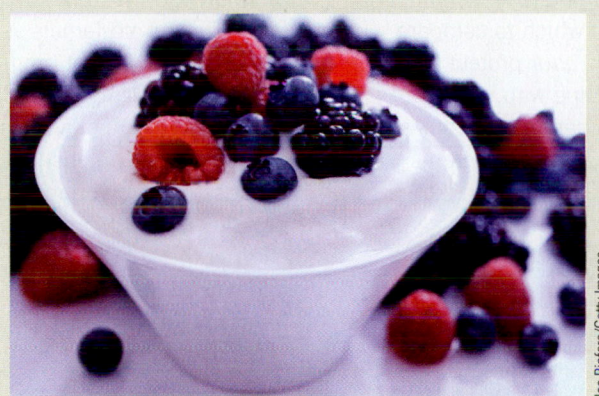

Joe Biafore/Getty Images

Greek Yogurt

Nutrition Facts

Serving Size 6 ounces (168 g)
Serving Per Container 1

Amount Per Serving

Calories 100	Calories from Fat 6

	% Daily Value
Total Fat 0.7g	1%
Cholesterol 9 mg	3%
Sodium 61 mg	2%
Potassium 240 mg	6%
Total Carbohydrate 6 g	2%
Dietary fiber 0 g	0%
Sugar 6 g	
Protein 17 g	34%

Vitamin A	0%	•	Vitamin C	0%
Calcium	18%	•	Iron	0%
Vitamin D	0%	•	Vitamin B6	5%
Vitamin B12	21%	•	Magnesium	4%

*Percent Daily Values are based on a 2,000 calorie diet.

labeled "sugar." A cereal bar named "Protein," for example, offers just 4 grams of protein per bar, not enough to qualify as a "good source," but provides added sugars in abundance: 14 grams per bar.* A serving of a "protein" beverage with 15 grams (60 calories) of protein also delivers more than 120 calories of added sugars. In contrast, plain, nonfat Greek yogurt (6-ounce container, see Figure 6–19) provides 17 grams of protein but with just 100 calories and no added sugar. Another trick of marketing: a package

*A food is a "good source" if it provides ≥10% of a nutrient's Daily Value in a serving.

banner may claim that a serving of cereal provides as much as 12 grams of protein, but this amount includes the protein in a half-cup of milk, typically added to a serving of cereal. The cereal itself provides less than half this amount. The moral of the story: ignore trendy labels and banners, and turn to the Nutrition Facts panel for the real story about protein, sugars, and calories in foods.

Conclusion

The Food Features presented so far show that the recommendations for the three energy-yielding nutrients

occur in balance with each other. The diets of most people, however, supply too little fiber, too much fat, too many calories, and abundant protein. To bring their diets into line with recommendations, then, requires changing the bulk of intake from calorie-rich fried foods, fatty meats, and sweet treats to lower-calorie complex carbohydrates and fiber-rich choices, such as whole grains, legumes, and vegetables. With these changes, protein totals remain adequate, while other constituents automatically fall into place in a healthier eating pattern.

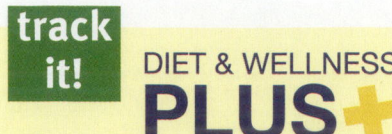

track it! DIET & WELLNESS PLUS+ Concepts in Action

Analyze Your Protein Intake

The purpose of this exercise is to make you aware of the effects of choosing protein-rich foods in balancing the three energy-yielding nutrients while planning a nutritious diet.

1. Do you take in adequate protein? From the D&W+ Home page, select Reports and then Macronutrient Ranges, choose Day Three, include the entire day's meals. Is your protein intake within the recommended 10 to 35 percent of total energy intake range, as recommended by the DRI? What percent of your caloric intake consists of protein? If your protein intake is higher than 35 percent, what foods could you choose less often to bring you within range? If your intake is lower than 10 percent of calories, what foods would you add to your eating pattern to meet your protein need?

2. From the Reports tab, select Intake vs. Goals report; choose all Day Two, all meals. Table 6–4 (p. 220) provides protein intake recommendations against which to compare your intake. Did your protein gram values fall into line with your DRI recommended intake (multiply your healthy weight in kilograms by 0.8 grams, as demonstrated on p. 219)?

3. Which foods in your meals provide the greatest amounts of protein? From the Reports tab, select Source Analysis, choose all meals for Day Two, select protein in the drop-down box. This report will help you determine your protein sources. Which foods were your top providers?

4. Using Figure 6–14 (p. 223), Figure 6–16 (p. 227), and the Controversy section, create a vegan meal that provides one-third of the daily requirement for protein for a 19-year-old female vegan. Select the Track Diet program, a new date, and input the foods in your meal; then generate a report on the Intake Spreadsheet. How successful were you in achieving protein adequacy? If the meal fell short of the goal, what vegan foods can you change or add to the meal to more closely match this person's protein need?

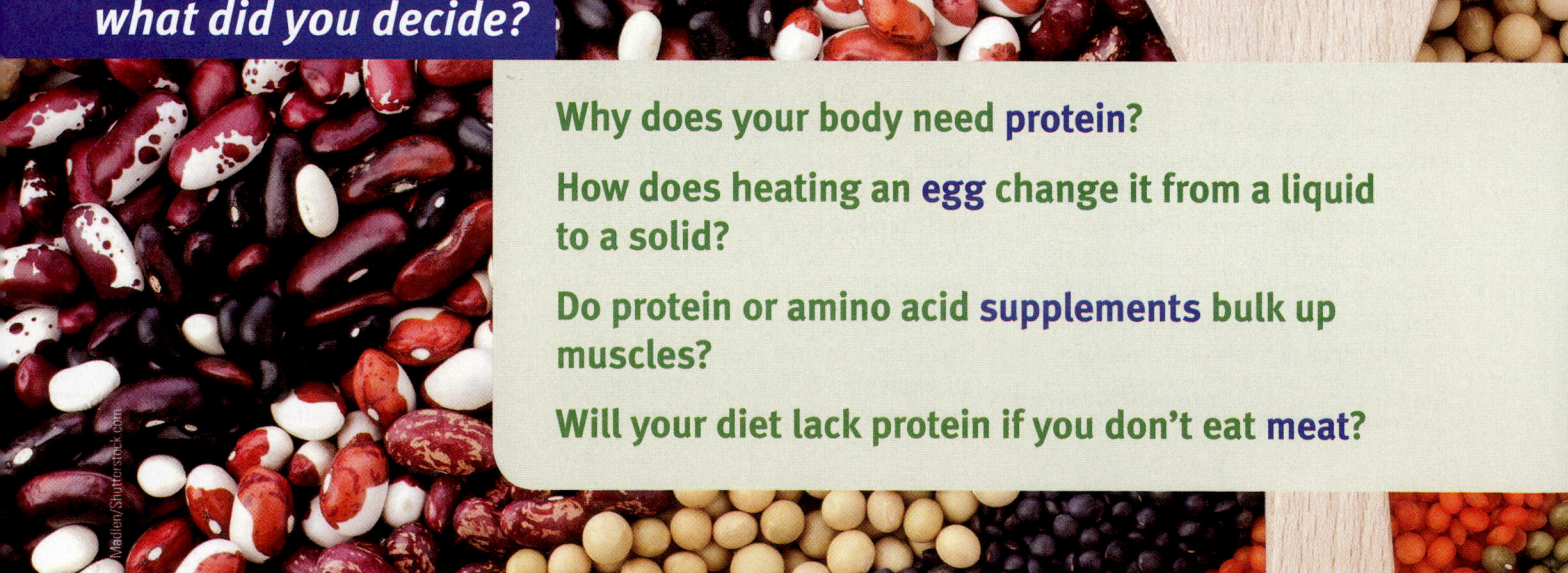

what did you decide?

Why does your body need protein?

How does heating an egg change it from a liquid to a solid?

Do protein or amino acid supplements bulk up muscles?

Will your diet lack protein if you don't eat meat?

Self Check

1. (LO 6.1) The basic building blocks for protein are
   a. glucose units.
   b. amino acids.
   c. side chains.
   d. saturated bonds.

2. (LO 6.1) The roles of protein in the body include all but
   a. blood clot formation.
   b. tissue repair.
   c. gas exchange.
   d. immunity.

3. (LO 6.1) Amino acids are linked together to form a protein strand by
   a. peptide bonds.
   b. essential amino acid bonds.
   c. side chain attraction.
   d. super glue.

4. (LO 6.1) Some segments of a protein strand coil, somewhat like a metal spring, because
   a. amino acids at different places along the strand are chemically attracted to each other.
   b. the protein strand has been denatured by acid.
   c. the protein strand is missing one or more essential amino acids.
   d. a coil structure allows access by enzymes for digestion.

5. (LO 6.2) Protein digestion begins in the
   a. mouth.
   b. stomach.
   c. small intestine.
   d. large intestine.

6. (LO 6.2) In the intestine, amino acids of the same general type compete for the same absorption sites, so a large dose of any one amino acid can limit absorption of another.
   T   F

7. (LO 6.3) Under certain circumstances, amino acids can be converted to glucose and so serve the energy needs of the brain.
   T   F

8. (LO 6.3) To prevent wasting of dietary protein, which of the following conditions must be met?
   a. Dietary protein must be adequate in quantity.
   b. Dietary protein must supply all essential amino acids in the proper amounts.
   c. The diet must supply enough carbohydrate and calories.
   d. All of the above.

9. (LO 6.4) For healthy adults, the DRI recommended intake for protein has been set at
   a. 0.8 grams per kilogram of body weight.
   b. 2.2 pounds per kilogram of body weight.
   c. 12 to 15 percent of total calories.
   d. 100 grams per day.

10. (LO 6.4) An example of a person in positive nitrogen balance is a pregnant woman.
    T   F

11. (LO 6.4) Partially completed proteins are not held for completion at a later time when the diet may improve.
    T   F

12. (LO 6.4) The following are complementary proteins:
    a. pot roast and chicken
    b. pot roast and carrots
    c. rice and French fries
    d. peanut butter on whole-wheat bread

13. (LO 6.5) Insufficient dietary protein can have severe consequences, but excess dietary protein cannot cause harm.
    T   F

14. (LO 6.5) Insufficient dietary protein can cause
    a. slowed protein synthesis.
    b. hepatitis.
    c. accelerated growth in children.
    d. all of the above.

15. (LO 6.5) The critical diagnostic criterion for celiac disease is
    a. high levels of blood antibodies.
    b. high levels of blood gluten.
    c. weight gain.
    d. none of the above.

16. (LO 6.6) Two tablespoons of peanut butter offer about the same amount of protein as a hot dog.
    T   F

17. (LO 6.6) Legumes are a particularly nutritious choice among protein-rich foods because they also provide
    a. vitamin C and vitamin E.
    b. fiber.
    c. B vitamins, iron, and other minerals.
    d. b and c.

18. (LO 6.7) Blood LDL values of people eating typical, meat-rich Western diets are generally higher than LDL values of vegetarians.
    T   F

19. (LO 6.7) A vegetarian diet planner should be sure to include sources of
    a. carbohydrate.
    b. vitamin C.
    c. vitamin B_{12}.
    d. vitamin E.

20. (LO 6.7) Fried banana or vegetable snack chips make a healthy everyday snack choice for vegetarians.
    T   F

Answers to these Self Check questions are in Appendix G.

Vegetarian and Meat-Containing Diets: What Are the Benefits and Pitfalls?

LO 6.7 Compare the advantages and disadvantages of the vegetarian diet and the meat eater's diet.

In affluent countries, where heart disease and cancer claim many lives, people who eat well-planned **vegetarian** diets often have lower risks of chronic diseases, and a lower risk of dying from all causes, than people whose diets center on meat.[1]* Should everyone consider using a vegetarian eating pattern, then? If so, is it enough to simply omit meat, or is more demanded of the vegetarian diet planner? What positive contributions do animal products make to the diet? (Table C6–1 defines some vegetarian terms.) This Controversy looks at these issues and ends with some practical advice for the vegetarian diet planner.

A vegetarian lifestyle may be immediately associated with a particular cultural, religious, political, or other belief system, but there are many reasons why people might choose it, as Table C6–2 makes clear. Vegetarians are categorized not by motivation but by the foods they choose to eat. Distinctions among vegetarian diets

are useful academically, but they do not represent uncrossable lines. Some people use meat or broth as a condiment or seasoning for vegetable or grain dishes. Some people eat meat only once a week and use plant protein foods the rest of the time. Others rely mostly on milk products and eggs for protein but will eat fish, too, and so forth. To force people into the categories of "vegetarians" and "meat eaters" leaves out all those with in-between eating styles (aptly named *flexitarian* by the press) that have much to recommend them.

Positive Health Aspects of Vegetarian Diets

Today, nutrition authorities state with confidence that a well-chosen vegetarian diet can meet nutrient needs while supporting health superbly.[2] Although much evidence supports this choice, such evidence is not easily obtained. It would be easy if vegetarians differed from others only in the absence of meat, but they often have *increased* intakes of whole grains, legumes, nuts, fruits, and vegetables as well. Such eating patterns are rich contributors of carbohydrates, fiber, vitamins, minerals, and phytochemicals that also correlate with low disease risks.[3] For example, in one study, as servings of fruit and vegetables increased from less than one to more than five per day, overall risk of death decreased by 36 percent, risk from cancers decreased by 25 percent, and risk from heart disease decreased by 20 percent, regardless of meat consumption.[4]

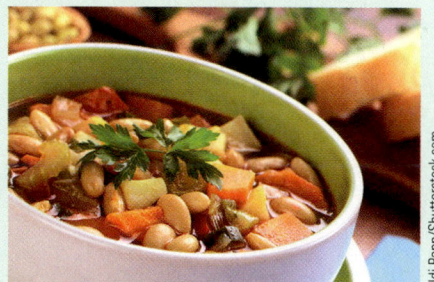

Can an eating pattern without animal products supply the needed nutrients?

*Reference notes are found in Appendix F.

Table C6–1

Terms Used to Describe Vegetarian Diets

Some of the terms below are in common usage, but others are useful only to researchers.

- **fruitarian** includes only raw or dried fruits, seeds, and nuts in the diet.
- **lacto-ovo vegetarian** includes dairy products, eggs, vegetables, grains, legumes, fruits, and nuts; excludes flesh and seafood.
- **lacto-vegetarian** includes dairy products, vegetables, grains, legumes, fruits, and nuts; excludes flesh, seafood, and eggs.
- **macrobiotic diet** a vegan diet composed mostly of whole grains, beans, and certain vegetables; taken to extremes, macrobiotic diets can compromise nutrient status.
- **ovo-vegetarian** includes eggs, vegetables, grains, legumes, fruits, and nuts; excludes flesh, seafood, and milk products.
- **partial vegetarian** a term sometimes used to mean an eating style that includes seafood, poultry, eggs, dairy products, vegetables, grains, legumes, fruits, and nuts; excludes or strictly limits certain meats, such as red meats. Also called *flexitarian*.
- **vegan** includes only food from plant sources: vegetables, grains, legumes, fruits, seeds, and nuts; also called strict vegetarian.
- **vegetarian** includes plant-based foods and eliminates some or all animal-derived foods.

Table C6–2

Reasons for Choosing Eating Styles

Why Some People Are Vegetarians	Why Some People Eat Meat
■ *Health concerns.* Vegetarian diets are often high in whole grains, fruits, vegetables, and legumes and often low in saturated fats, diet characteristics associated with good health.	■ *Convenience.* Some people find that a hamburger or chicken salad sandwich makes a convenient lunch.
■ *Moral objections.* Some believe that animals should not be killed for food; others object to use of any animal products, such as milk, cheese, eggs, or honey, or to use of items made from leather, wool, feathers, or silk.	■ *Nutrients.* Some people rely on animal products for the energy and key nutrients they supply.
■ *Humane treatment of animals.* Many people object to inhumane treatment of livestock and food-producing animals.	■ *Taste.* Others enjoy the taste of roasted chicken, barbecued ribs, or a grilled steak.
■ *Environmental concerns.* Producing meat protein requires a much greater input of resources than does an equal amount of vegetable protein.	■ *Familiarity.* Some people wouldn't know what to eat without meat; they are accustomed to seeing it on the plate.
■ *Weight-control efforts.* Some people mistakenly believe that simply eliminating meat will produce weight loss (it doesn't if high-calorie vegetarian foods and treats are consumed in excess of the daily energy need).	■ *Weight-control efforts.* Some people believe that eating meat instead of whole grains, fruits and vegetables, and legumes speeds weight loss (it doesn't).
■ *Cover-Up.* Some adolescents may hide an eating disorder under the guise of being "vegetarian" (Chapter 9 takes up the issues of weight-loss dieting and eating disorders).	

Sources: C. Leitzmann, Vegetarian nutrition: Past, present, future, American Journal of Clinical Nutrition *100 (2014): 496S–502S*; A. M. Bardone-Cone, The interrelationships between vegetarianism and eating disorders among females, Journal of the Academy of Nutrition and Dietetics *112 (2012): 12-47-1252.*

Also, many vegetarians live a healthy lifestyle: they avoid tobacco, use alcohol in moderation, if at all, and are more physically active than other adults. When researchers take into account people's lifestyle on disease development, the evidence still often weighs in favor of vegetarian eating patterns, as the next sections make clear.

Defense against Obesity

Among both men and women and across many ethnic groups, vegetarians more often maintain a healthier body weight than nonvegetarians.[5] The converse is also true: meat consumption correlates with increased energy intake and increased obesity. The reason for this is not clear but may reflect that many vegetarians make health a high priority.

Defense against Heart and Artery Disease

Vegetarians die less often from heart disease and related illnesses than do meat-eating people, although not all

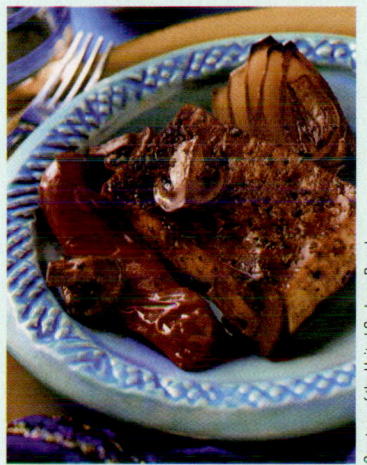

When consumed in sufficient quantity, soy foods, such as this roasted tofu, may improve the health of the heart.

indicators of heart health are consistently improved in vegetarians.[6]

When vegetarians choose the unsaturated fats of soybeans, seeds, avocados, nuts, olives, and vegetable oils and shun the saturated fats of cheese, sour cream, butter, shortening,

and other sources, their risks of heart disease are reduced. If their diet also contains nuts and legumes, as most vegetarian diets do, then LDL cholesterol typically falls, and heart benefits compound.

Defense against High Blood Pressure

Vegetarians tend to have lower blood pressure and lower rates of hypertension than average.[7] Often, vegetarians maintain a healthy body weight, and appropriate body weight helps to maintain healthy blood pressure. So does eating enough fiber, fruit, vegetables, low-fat milk products, and soy protein, often amply supplied by a vegetarian diet. The mineral sodium promotes high blood pressure, but vegetarian diets are not always low-sodium diets. Other lifestyle factors such as not smoking, moderating alcohol intake, and being physically active all work together to keep blood pressure normal.

Defense against Cancer

Questions about diet and cancers are not easily answered, but the World Health Organization has concluded that high intakes of red meats, such as beef, goat, lamb, pork, veal, and non-bird game meat, are likely to raise the risk of colon and rectal cancers.[8] The group also lists processed meats, such as lunchmeats and hot dogs, among human carcinogens and concludes that eating about two ounces daily increases colon and rectal cancer risks by 18 percent.

In a study of over 60,000 people in the United Kingdom, those who ate fish or vegetables but not red meats had the lowest overall cancer rates—a finding that agrees with many other studies.[9] Accounting for smoking, exercise, and other lifestyle factors, the overall cancer risk (compared to meat eaters) was:

- 19 percent lower in **vegans**,
- 12 percent lower in fish eaters, and
- 11 percent lower in **lacto-ovo vegetarians**.

Other researchers, however, report no difference in cancer risks between meat eaters and vegetarians.[10] Such conflicts may stem partly from wide variations in eating patterns within groups—some meat eaters also love legumes, fish, and vegetables and eat them often, while some vegetarians may base their diets on fried foods, refined grains, cheeses, sweets, and daily alcohol (see Controversy 3). Such factors may influence cancer risks.

More details about diet and cancer appear in **Chapter 11.**

Other Health Benefits

In addition to obesity, heart disease, high blood pressure, and cancer, vegetarian eating patterns may help prevent cataracts, diabetes, diverticular disease, gallstones, high blood pressure, and osteoporosis. However, these effects may arise more from

what vegetarians include in their diet—abundant fruit, legumes, vegetables, and whole grains—than from omission of meat. Table C6–3 spells out some arguments for and against eliminating meat from the diet.

Positive Health Aspects of the Meat Eater's Diet

With prudent choices, both meat eaters and lacto-ovo vegetarians can rely on their diets to support health during critical times of life. In contrast, a vegan eating pattern poses challenges. Protein is critical for building new tissues during growth, for fighting illnesses, for building bone during youth, and for maintaining bone and muscle in old age. While protein from plant sources can meet most people's needs, very young children and very elderly people with small appetites may not consume enough legumes, whole grains, or nuts to supply the protein they need.

The chapter made clear that protein from meat, fish, milk, and eggs is the clear winner in tests of digestibility and availability to the body, with soy protein a close second. Also, animal-derived foods provide abundant iron, zinc, vitamin D, calcium, and vitamin B_{12}, needed by everyone but particularly by pregnant women, infants, children, adolescents, and the elderly (details about these needs appear in later chapters).

Iron and zinc are less readily absorbed from vegan sources, such as grains and legumes, than from meat, but iron and zinc from supplements or fortified foods can help prevent deficiencies. Vegans must also find and regularly consume alternate sources of vitamin D, calcium, vitamin B_{12}, and the omega-3 fatty acids EPA and DHA.

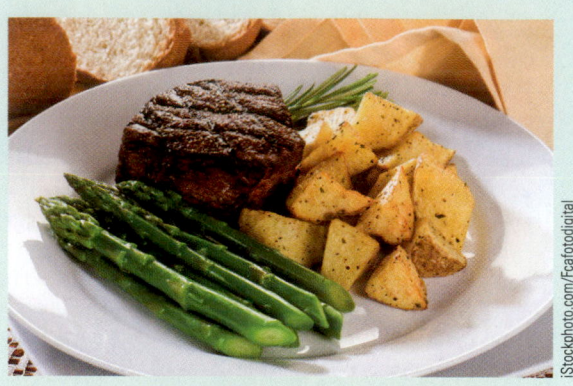

This 5-ounce steak provides almost all of the meat recommended for an entire day's intake in a 2,000-calorie diet.

iStockphoto.com/Fcafotodigital

In Pregnancy and Infancy

Women who eat seafood, eggs, or milk products can be sure of receiving enough energy, vitamin B_{12}, vitamin D, calcium, iron, and zinc, as well as protein, to support pregnancy and breastfeeding. A woman following a well-planned lacto-ovo vegetarian eating pattern can also relax in the knowledge that she is superbly supplied with energy and all necessary nutrients. A vegan woman who doesn't meet her nutrient needs, however, may enter pregnancy too thin and with scant nutrient stores to draw on as the nutrient demands of the fetus grow larger.

Of particular concern is vitamin B_{12}, a vitamin abundant in foods of animal origin but absent from vegetables. Obtaining enough vitamin B_{12} poses a challenge to vegans of all ages, who often test low in the vitamin.[11] For pregnant and lactating women, obtaining vitamin B_{12} is critical to prevent serious deficiency-related disorders in infants who do not receive sufficient vitamin B_{12}.[12]

In Childhood

Children who eat eggs, milk, and fish receive abundant protein, iron, zinc, vitamin D, calcium, and vitamin B_{12}; such foods are reliable, convenient sources of nutrients needed for growth.[13] Likewise, children eating well-planned lacto-ovo vegetarian diets receive

Table C6–3

Should Meat Be Eliminated from the Diet? Point, Counterpoint

Arguments can be made for and against eliminating meats on all points, save one: animal kindness. Many people choose a vegetarian diet on this point alone.

Point: Eliminating meat	Counterpoint: Including meat
1. *Reduced heart disease risk.* Vegetarians have reduced risks of developing heart disease and dying from heart disease.	1. *Reduced heart disease risk.* People who follow the Dietary Guidelines, and eat small portions of lean meat, fish, and poultry, have low rates of heart disease.
2. *Reduced cancer risks.* Vegetarians have reduced risks of developing certain cancers and dying from cancer. High intakes of red and processed meats may increase the risks of colon and rectal cancers.	2. *Reduced cancer risks.* Small daily intakes of meats, poultry, fish, and seafood are not associated with increased cancer risks, particularly when a diet follows the Dietary Guidelines for Americans.
3. *Reduced mortality risk.* Vegetarians have a reduced risk of early death from all causes.	3. *Reduced mortality risk.* Ample fruit and vegetable intakes, regular physical activity, not smoking, and other healthy lifestyle choices reduce mortality risk without eliminating meat.
4. *Reduced obesity and diabetes risks.* Vegetarians are less likely to develop obesity or diabetes.	4. *Reduced obesity and diabetes risks.* A calorie-controlled diet of whole foods reduces the likelihood of developing obesity or diabetes without eliminating meat.
5. *Normal blood pressure.* Vegetarians have reduced risk of hypertension.	5. *Normal blood pressure.* Normal blood pressure can be maintained with a healthy eating pattern such as DASH (Chapter 8) that includes moderate amounts of meat.
6. *Ample nutrients.* Vegetarian diets reliably provide fiber, vitamin A, vitamin C, vitamin K, folate, and magnesium. Protein is generally sufficient.	6. *Ample nutrients.* Diets with meats, fish, poultry, eggs, and milk products reliably provide protein, EPA and DHA (fish), vitamin B_{12}, vitamin D (milk fortification), calcium, iron, and zinc.
7. *Honored traditions.* Vegetarianism is often part of religious, family, and cultural traditions.	7. *Honored traditions.* Hunting and fishing are often family and cultural traditions. Holiday traditions often center on meat-containing meals, such as turkey at Thanksgiving.
8. *Ecological sustainability.* Nutrient-dense vegetarian diets require much less land, water, fuel, and other resources to produce than diets high in meats, cheeses, and highly processed foods. They also generate far less waste and pollution.	8. *Ecological sustainability.* Three eating patterns—Healthy U.S.-style, Healthy Mediterranean-style, and Healthy Vegetarian—are named by the Dietary Guidelines committee as having less environmental impact than the current U.S. diet. Two of the three contain significant amounts of meat.
9. *Animal kindness.* Vegetarian diets are obtained without cruelty to or death of animals.	9. *Animal kindness.* Cruelty-free animal products are becoming more available as consumer demand increases.

Sources: Position of the Academy of Nutrition and Dietetics: Vegetarian diets, Journal of the Academy of Nutrition and Dietetics *115 (2015): 801–810*; USDA, Scientific Report of the 2015 Dietary Guidelines Advisory Committee (2015): D-5, 49–52, available at www.health.gov; M. J. Orlich and G. E. Frasier, Vegetarian diets in the Adventist Health Study 2: A review of initial published findings, American Journal of Clinical Nutrition *100 (2014): 353S–358S*; N. S. Rizzo and coauthors, Nutrient profiles of vegetarian and nonvegetarian dietary patterns, Journal of the Academy of Nutrition and Dietetics *114 (2014): 1610–1619*; X. Wang and coauthors, Fruit and vegetable consumption and mortality from all causes, cardiovascular disease, and cancer: Systematic review and dose-response meta-analysis of prospective cohort studies, British Medical Journal *349 (2014), epub, doi: 10.1136/bmj.g4490*; O. Oyebode and coauthors, Fruit and vegetable consumption and all-cause, cancer and CVD mortality: Analysis of Health Survey for England data, Journal of Epidemiology and Community Health *68 (2014): 856–862*.

adequate nutrients and grow as well as their meat-eating peers. Child-sized servings of vegan foods, however, can fail to provide sufficient energy or several key nutrients needed for normal growth. A child's small stomach can hold only so much food, and the vegan child may feel full before eating enough to meet his or her nutrient needs.

Small, frequent meals of fortified breads, cereals, or pastas with legumes, nuts, nut butters, and sources of unsaturated fats can help to meet protein and energy needs in a smaller volume at each sitting. Because vegan children derive protein only from plant foods, their daily protein requirement may be higher than the DRI indicates for the general meat-eating population. Also, vegan children who rely on whole grains and vegetables for the minerals iron and zinc receive them, but in less absorbable forms, so a supplement or fortified foods may be needed.[14] Other nutrients of concern for vegan children include vitamin B_{12}, vitamin D, vitamin C, and calcium.

In Adolescence

The healthiest vegetarian adolescents choose balanced diets that are heavy in fruits and vegetables but light on the sweets, fast foods, and salty snacks that tempt the teenage palate. These healthy vegetarian teens often meet the goals of the Dietary Guidelines for Americans—a rare accomplishment in the United States.

Other teens, however, adopt poorly planned vegetarian eating patterns that provide too little energy and too few nutrients for health. Omissions of protein, calcium, and vitamin D, for example, lead to weak bone development at precisely the time when bones must develop strength to protect bone health through later life. If a vegetarian child or teen refuses sound dietary advice, a registered dietitian nutritionist can help to identify problems, dispense appropriate guidance, and put unwarranted parental worries to rest.

In Aging and in Illness

For elderly people with diminished appetites or impaired digestion, too little dietary protein compromises both bone and muscle strength, leading to bone fractures and infirmity. Providing frequent meals with high-quality protein, such as low-fat cheese, fish, or soft-cooked ground poultry or meat, may reduce these risks.[15] Vegetarians, and particularly vegans, may be at greater risk for weakened bones and fractures than nonvegetarians.[16]

People battling life-threatening diseases may encounter testimonial stories of cures attributed to restrictive eating plans, such as **macrobiotic diets**. However, such diets often severely limit food selections and can fail to deliver the energy and nutrients needed for recovery.

Planning a Vegetarian Diet

Eating a nutritious vegetarian diet requires more than just omitting certain foods and food groups—any eating pattern that omits key foods omits essential nutrients. Grains, fruits, and vegetables are naturally abundant in the vegetarian's diet and provide adequate amounts of the nutrients of plant foods: carbohydrate, fiber, thiamin, folate, and vitamins B_6, C, A, and E. Nutrients in animal-derived foods may be of concern, however—particularly zinc, along with protein, iron, calcium, vitamin B_{12}, vitamin D, and omega-3 fatty acids.[17] Table C6–4 (p. 237) presents vegetarian sources for these nutrients.

Choosing within the Food Groups

When selecting from the Vegetables and Fruits groups, vegetarians should emphasize sources of calcium and iron. Green leafy vegetables provide both calcium and iron. Similarly, dried fruits deserve special notice in the Fruits group because they can deliver more iron than other fruits. The Protein Foods group emphasizes legumes, soy products, nuts, and seeds. The Dietary Guidelines encourage the use of vegetable oils, nuts, and seeds rich in unsaturated fats and omega-3 fatty acids. To ensure adequate nutrient intakes, vegans need to select fortified foods or use supplements daily.

Milk Products and Protein Foods

It takes a little planning to ensure adequate intakes from a variety of vegetarian foods in the Milk and Milk Products group and the Protein Foods group. Figure C6–1 (p. 238) turns a spotlight on these food groups, and Appendix E provides the USDA Healthy Vegetarian Eating Pattern in full for many calorie levels. The USDA Eating Pattern also specifies weekly amounts that vegetarians should obtain from the Protein Foods subgroups. Note that the Milk and Milk Products group features fortified soy milk and yogurt for vegans. Protein-rich soy products are often fortified and match many of the nutrients of milk products. Other "milk" beverages and yogurts, based on almonds, coconuts, hemp, oats, or rice, generally lack protein and other nutrients. Smart shoppers compare the nutrients of substitutes with those of milk and dairy foods before choosing.

Convenience Foods

Prepared frozen or packaged vegetarian foods make food preparation quick and easy—just be sure to scrutinize each label's Nutrition Facts panel when choosing among them. Some products constitute a nutritional bargain, such as vegetarian "hot dogs" or "veggie burgers." Made of soy, these foods look and taste like the original meat product but contain much less fat and saturated fat. Some brands may be high in sodium or added sugars, however (read the labels). Soybeans in other forms, such as plain tofu (bean curd), edamame (cooked green soybeans, pronounced *ed-eh-MAH-may*), or soy flour, offer protein with fewer additives.

Among snack foods, banana or vegetable chips, often sold as "healthy" foods, are no bargain: a quarter cup of banana chips fried in saturated coconut oil provides 150 calories with 7 grams of saturated fat (a big hamburger has 8 grams). A plain banana has 100 calories and practically no fat. Look for freeze-dried fruit and vegetable "chips"—they

Table C6–4
Vegetarian Sources of Key Nutrients

NUTRIENTS	Grains	Vegetables	Fruits	Legumes and Other Protein-Rich Foods	Milk or Soy Milk	Oils
PROTEIN	Whole grains[a]			Legumes, seeds, nuts, soy products (tempeh, tofu, veggie burgers);[a] eggs (for ovo-vegetarians)	Milk, cheese, yogurt (for lacto-vegetarians); soy milk, soy yogurt, soy cheeses	
IRON	Fortified cereals, enriched and whole grains	Dark green, leafy vegetables (spinach, turnip greens)	Dried fruits (apricots, prunes, raisins)	Legumes (black-eyed peas, kidney beans, lentils), soy products		
ZINC	Fortified cereals, whole grains			Legumes (garbanzo beans, kidney beans, navy beans), nuts, seeds (pumpkin seeds)	Milk, cheese, yogurt (for lacto-vegetarians); soy milk, soy yogurt, soy cheeses	
CALCIUM	Fortified cereals	Dark green, leafy vegetables (bok choy, broccoli, collard greens, kale, mustard greens, turnip greens, watercress)	Fortified juices, figs	Fortified soy products, nuts (almonds), seeds (sesame seeds)	Milk, cheese, yogurt (for lacto-vegetarians); fortified soy milk, fortified soy yogurt, fortified soy cheese	
VITAMIN B$_{12}$	Fortified cereals			Eggs (for ovo-vegetarians); fortified soy products	Milk, cheese, yogurt (for lacto-vegetarians); fortified soy milk, fortified soy yogurt, fortified soy cheese	
VITAMIN D	Fortified cereals				Milk, cheese, yogurt (for lacto-vegetarians); fortified soy milk, fortified soy yogurt, fortified soy cheese	
OMEGA-3 FATTY ACIDS		Marine algae and their oils		Chia seeds, flaxseed, walnuts, soybeans, fortified margarine;[b] fortified eggs (for ovo-vegetarians)		Algae oil, flaxseed oil, walnut oil, soybean oil

FOOD GROUPS

[a] Many plant proteins lack certain essential amino acids or contain them in insufficient amounts for human health. A variety of daily plant protein sources, such as grains and legumes, can meet protein needs when energy intake is sufficient.

[b] Fortification sources of EPA and DHA may be fish oil or marine algae oil; read the ingredients list on the label.

Controversy 6 Vegetarian and Meat-Containing Diets: What Are the Benefits and Pitfalls?

237

Each day, in a 2,000-calorie diet, both vegans and lacto-ovo vegetarians require 3 cups of Milk and Milk Product equivalents and 5½ ounces of Protein Foods. (For details and for other calorie levels, see Appendix E.)

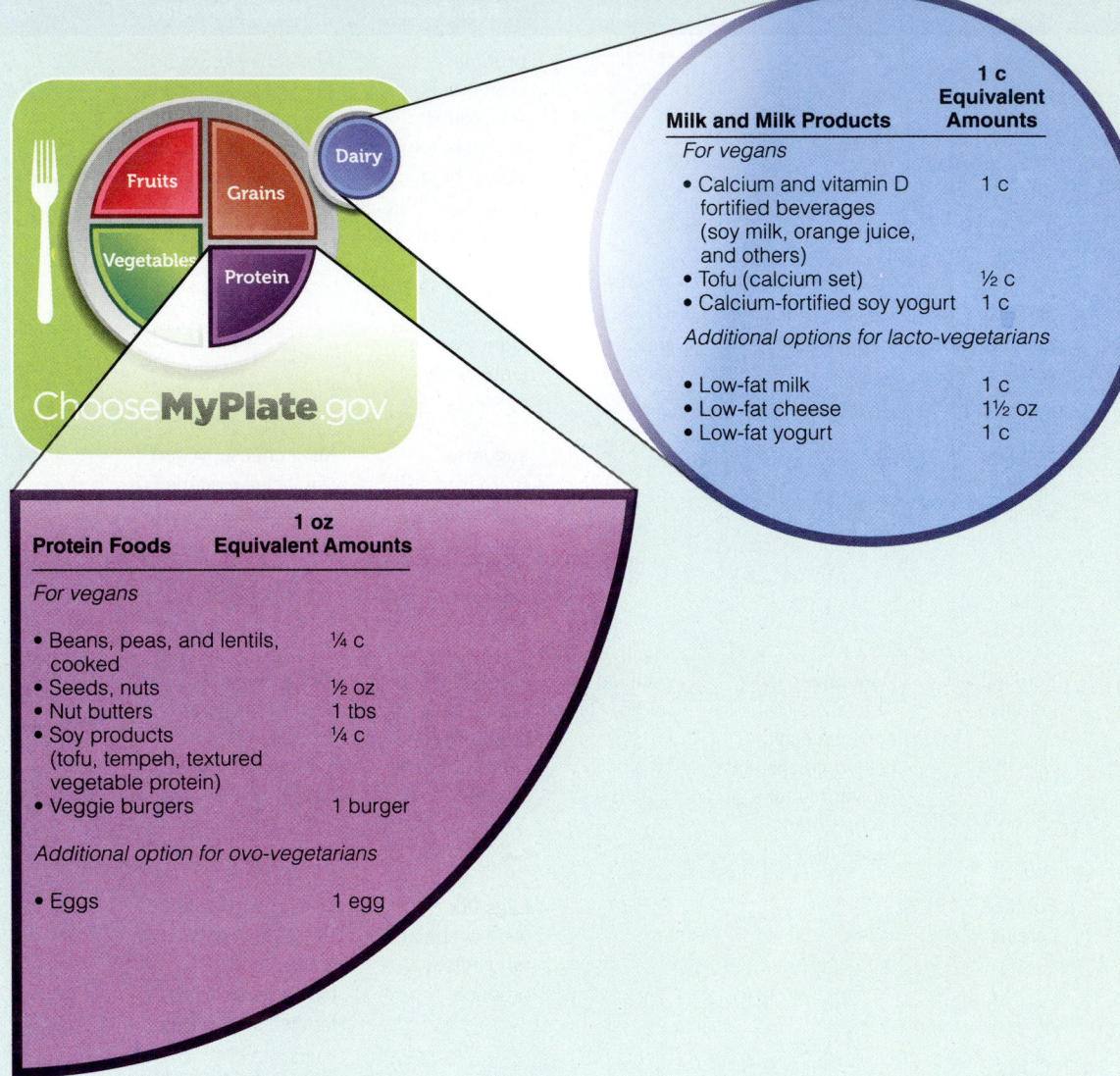

Milk and Milk Products	1 c Equivalent Amounts
For vegans	
• Calcium and vitamin D fortified beverages (soy milk, orange juice, and others)	1 c
• Tofu (calcium set)	½ c
• Calcium-fortified soy yogurt	1 c
Additional options for lacto-vegetarians	
• Low-fat milk	1 c
• Low-fat cheese	1½ oz
• Low-fat yogurt	1 c

Protein Foods	1 oz Equivalent Amounts
For vegans	
• Beans, peas, and lentils, cooked	¼ c
• Seeds, nuts	½ oz
• Nut butters	1 tbs
• Soy products (tofu, tempeh, textured vegetable protein)	¼ c
• Veggie burgers	1 burger
Additional option for ovo-vegetarians	
• Eggs	1 egg

have no added fats, but the freeze-drying process creates a pleasing crunch and preserves most nutrients.

Conclusion

This comparison has shown that both a meat-eater's diet and a vegetarian's diet are best approached scientifically. If you are just beginning to study nutrition, consider adopting the attitude that the choice to make is not whether to be a meat eater or a vegetarian but where along the spectrum to locate yourself. Your preferences should be honored with these caveats: that you plan your own diet and the diets of those in your care to be adequate, balanced, controlled in calories, and varied and that you limit intakes of foods high in sodium, solid fats, and added sugars. Whatever your eating style or reasons for choosing it, choose carefully: the foods that you eat regularly make an impact on your health.

Critical Thinking

1. Becoming a vegan takes a strong commitment and significant education to know how to combine foods and in what quantities to meet nutrient requirements. Most of us will not choose to become vegetarians, but many of us would benefit from a diet of less meat. Identify ways you could alter your diet so that you eat less meat.

2. Identify two critical periods of life that demand high nutrient intakes, and defend the use of a vegetarian diet during those times. Discuss specific nutrient challenges and solutions for both life stages.

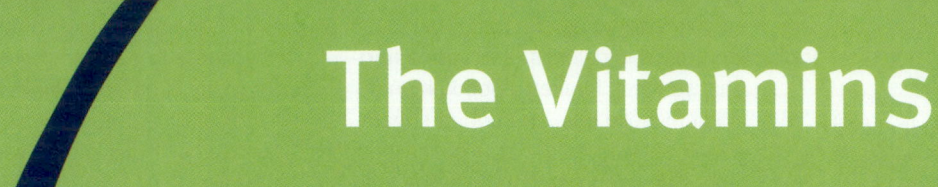

7 The Vitamins

Maximilian Stock Ltd./Getty Images

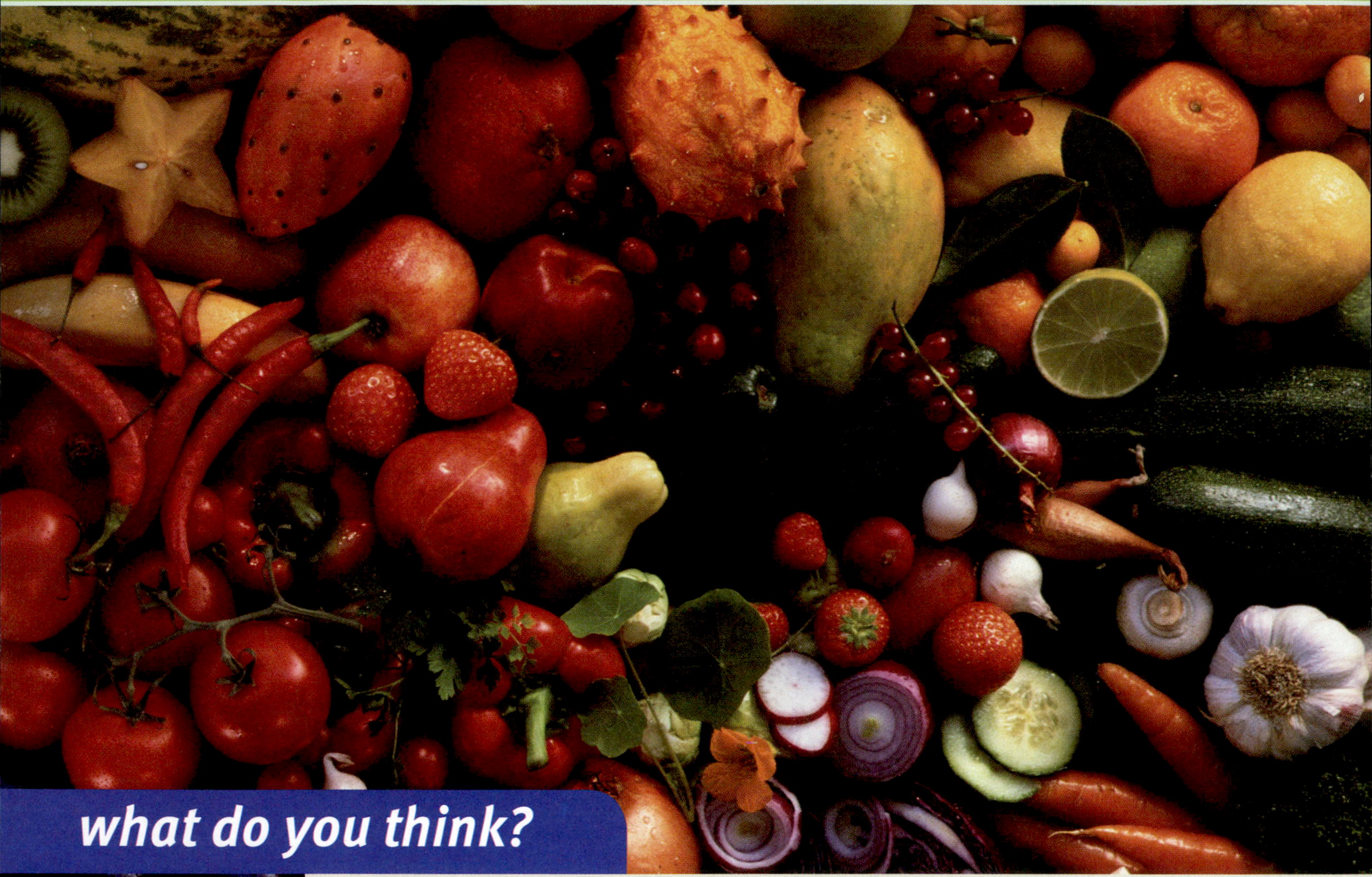

what do you think?

How do **vitamins** work in the body?

Why is **sunshine** associated with good health?

Can **vitamin C tablets** ward off a cold?

Should you choose **vitamin-fortified foods** and take **supplements** for "insurance"?

Learning Objectives

After completing this chapter, you should be able to accomplish the following:

LO 7.1 Compare fat-soluble vitamins with water-soluble vitamins.

LO 7.2 Discuss the characteristics and functions of fat-soluble vitamins.

LO 7.3 Discuss the roles, food sources, and precursor of vitamin A, and the effects of vitamin A deficiency and toxicity.

LO 7.4 Discuss the roles of vitamin D, its sources, and the consequences of its deficiency and toxicity.

LO 7.5 Discuss the roles, food sources, and effects of deficiency and toxicity of vitamin E.

LO 7.6 Discuss the roles of vitamin K, its food sources, and the effects of its deficiency and toxicity.

LO 7.7 Summarize the characteristics of water-soluble vitamins.

LO 7.8 Discuss the roles of vitamin C, effects of its deficiency and toxicity, and its food sources.

LO 7.9 Discuss the collective roles of B vitamins in metabolism and the effects of their deficiencies.

LO 7.10 Discuss the roles, the effects of deficiencies and toxicities, and food sources of each of the eight B vitamins.

LO 7.11 Describe how to choose foods to meet vitamin needs.

LO 7.12 Debate for and against taking vitamin supplements.

At the beginning of the 20th century, the thrill of the discovery of the first **vitamins** captured the world's imagination as seemingly miraculous cures took place. In the usual scenario, a whole group of people was becoming unable to walk (or going blind or bleeding profusely) until an alert scientist stumbled onto the substance missing from their diets. The scientist confirmed the discovery by feeding vitamin-deficient chow to laboratory animals, which responded by becoming unable to walk (or going blind or bleeding profusely). When the missing ingredient was restored to their diet, they soon recovered. People, too, were quickly cured from such conditions when they received the vitamins they lacked.

In the decades that followed, advances in chemistry, biology, and genetics allowed scientists to isolate the vitamins, define their chemical structures, and reveal their functions in maintaining health and preventing deficiency diseases. Today, research hints that certain vitamins may be linked with the development of two major scourges of humankind: cardiovascular disease (CVD) and cancer. Many other conditions, from infections to cracked skin, bear relation to vitamin nutrition, details that unscrupulous sellers of vitamin supplements often use to market their wares (see the Controversy section).

Can foods rich in vitamins protect us from life-threatening diseases? What about vitamin pills? For now, we can say this with certainty: the only disease a vitamin can *cure* is the one caused by a deficiency of that vitamin. As for chronic disease *prevention*, research is ongoing, but evidence so far supports the conclusion that vitamin-rich *foods*, but not vitamin supplements, are protective. The DRI recommended intakes for vitamins are listed on the inside front cover pages.

According to the Dietary Guidelines 2015 committee, today's U.S. intakes of these vitamins may fall below recommended intakes:

- Vitamin A
- Vitamin D
- Vitamin E
- Vitamin C
- Folate

These vitamins and others play critical roles in the body.

vitamins organic compounds that are vital to life and indispensable to body functions but that are needed only in minute amounts; essential, noncaloric nutrients.

[a]Vitamin names established by the International Union of Nutritional Sciences Committee on Nomenclature. Other names are listed in Tables 7–9 and 7–10 (pp. 276–280).

Definition and Classification of Vitamins

LO 7.1 Compare fat-soluble vitamins with water-soluble vitamins.

A child once defined a vitamin as "what, if you don't eat, you get sick." Although the grammar left something to be desired, the definition was accurate. Less imaginatively, a vitamin is defined as an essential, noncaloric, organic nutrient needed in tiny amounts in the diet. The role of many vitamins is to help make possible the processes by which other nutrients are digested, absorbed, and metabolized or built into body structures. Although small in size and quantity, the vitamins accomplish mighty tasks.

As each vitamin was discovered, it was given a name, and some were given letters and numbers—vitamin A came before the B vitamins, then came vitamin C, and so forth. This led to the confusing variety of vitamin names that still exists today. This chapter uses the names in Table 7–1; alternative names are given in Tables 7–9 and 7–10 at the end of the chapter (pp. 276–280).

The Concept of Vitamin Precursors

Some of the vitamins occur in foods in a form known as **precursors**. Once inside the body, these are transformed chemically to one or more active vitamin forms. Thus, to measure the amount of a vitamin found in food, we often must count not only the amount of the true vitamin but also the vitamin activity potentially available from its precursors. Tables 7–9 and 7–10 specify which vitamins have precursors.

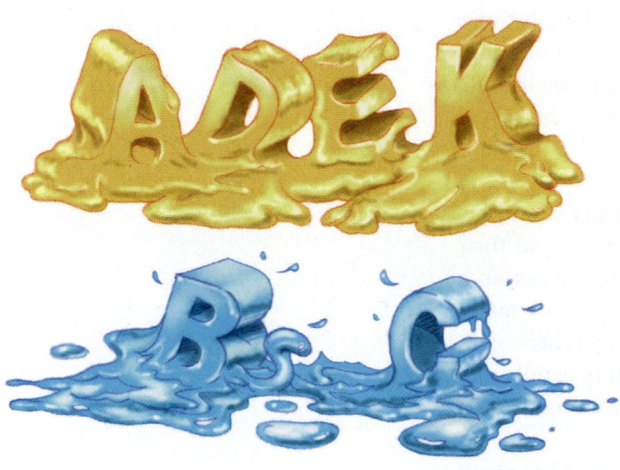

Vitamins fall into two classes—fat-soluble and water-soluble.

Two Classes of Vitamins: Fat-Soluble and Water-Soluble

The vitamins fall naturally into two classes: fat-soluble and water-soluble (listed in Table 7–1). Solubility confers on vitamins many of their characteristics. It determines how they are absorbed into and transported around by the bloodstream, whether they can be stored in the body, and how easily they are lost from the body.

Like other lipids, fat-soluble vitamins are mostly absorbed into the lymph, and they travel in the blood in association with protein carriers.[1]* Fat-soluble vitamins can be stored in the liver or with other lipids in fatty tissues, and some can build up to toxic concentrations. The water-soluble vitamins are absorbed directly into the bloodstream, where they travel freely. Most are not stored in tissues to any great extent; rather, excesses are excreted in the urine. Thus, the risks of immediate toxicities are not as great as for fat-soluble vitamins.

Table 7–2 outlines the general features of the fat-soluble and water-soluble vitamins. The chapter then goes on to provide important details first about the fat-soluble vitamins and then about the water-soluble ones. At the end of the chapter, two summary tables (Tables 7–9 and 7–10) summarize the basic facts about all of them.

KEY POINTS

- Vitamins are essential, noncaloric nutrients that are needed in tiny amounts in the diet and help to drive cellular processes.
- Vitamin precursors in foods are transformed into active vitamins by the body.
- The fat-soluble vitamins are vitamins A, D, E, and K.
- The water-soluble vitamins are vitamin C and the B vitamins.

---

precursors compounds that can be converted into active vitamins. Also called *provitamins*.

*Reference notes are found in Appendix F.

Table 7–2

Characteristics of the Fat-Soluble and Water-Soluble Vitamins

While each vitamin has unique functions and features, a few generalizations about the fat-soluble and water-soluble vitamins can aid understanding.

	Fat-Soluble Vitamins: Vitamins A, D, E, and K	Water-Soluble Vitamins: B Vitamins and Vitamin C
Absorption	Absorbed like fats, first into the lymph and then into the blood.	Absorbed directly into the blood.
Transport and Storage	Must travel with protein carriers in watery body fluids; stored in the liver or fatty tissues.	Travel freely in watery fluids; most are not stored in the body.
Excretion	Not readily excreted; tend to build up in the tissues.	Readily excreted in the urine.
Toxicity	Toxicities are likely from supplements but occur rarely from food.	Toxicities are unlikely but possible with high doses from supplements.
Requirements	Needed in periodic doses (perhaps weeks or even months) because the body can draw on its stores.	Needed in frequent doses (perhaps 1 to 3 days) because the body does not store most of them to any extent.

The Fat-Soluble Vitamins

LO 7.2   Discuss the characteristics and functions of fat-soluble vitamins.

The fat-soluble vitamins—A, D, E, and K—are found in the fats and oils of foods and require bile for absorption. Once absorbed, these vitamins are stored in the liver and fatty tissues until the body needs them.

Storage   Because they are stored, you need not eat foods containing each fat-soluble vitamin every day. If an eating pattern provides sufficient amounts of the fat-soluble vitamins on average over time, the body can survive for weeks without consuming them. This capacity to be stored also sets the stage for toxic buildup if you take in too much. Excess vitamin A from supplements and highly fortified foods is especially likely to reach toxic levels.

Deficiencies   Deficiencies of the fat-soluble vitamins occur when the diet is consistently low in them. They also occur in people who undergo intestinal surgery for obesity treatment, which decreases nutrient absorption by design. We also know that any disease that produces fat malabsorption (such as liver disease, which prevents bile production) can cause the loss of vitamins dissolved in undigested fat and so bring on deficiencies. In the same way, a person who uses mineral oil (which the body cannot absorb) as a laxative risks losing fat-soluble vitamins because they readily dissolve into the oil and are excreted. Deficiencies are also likely when people follow eating patterns that are extraordinarily low in fat because a little fat is necessary for absorption of these vitamins.

Roles   Fat-soluble vitamins play diverse roles in the body. Vitamins A and D act somewhat like hormones, directing cells to convert one substance to another, to store this, or to release that. They also directly influence the genes, thereby regulating protein production. Vitamin E flows throughout the body, guarding the tissues against harm from destructive oxidative reactions. Vitamin K is necessary for blood to clot and for bone health. Each is worth a book in itself.

Vitamin A

LO 7.3 Discuss the roles, food sources, and precursor of vitamin A, and the effects of vitamin A deficiency and toxicity.

Vitamin A has the distinction of being the first fat-soluble vitamin to be recognized. Today, after a century of scientific investigation, vitamin A and its plant-derived precursor, **beta-carotene**, are still very much a focus of research.

Three forms of vitamin A are active in the body. One of the active forms, **retinol**, is stored in specialized cells of the liver. The liver makes retinol available to the bloodstream and thereby to the body's cells. The cells convert retinol to its other two active forms, retinal and retinoic acid, as needed.

Foods derived from animals provide forms of vitamin A that are readily absorbed and put to use by the body. Foods derived from plants provide beta-carotene, which must be converted to active vitamin A before it can be used as such.[2]

Roles of Vitamin A and Consequences of Deficiency

Vitamin A is a versatile vitamin, with roles in gene expression, vision, maintenance of body linings and skin, immune defenses, growth of the body, and normal development of cells.[3] It is of critical importance for both male and female reproductive functions and for normal development of an embryo and fetus.[4] In short, vitamin A is needed everywhere (its chief functions in the body are listed in Snapshot 7–1 on page 248). The following sections provide some details.

Eyesight   The most familiar function of vitamin A is to sustain normal eyesight. Vitamin A plays two indispensable roles: in the process of light perception at the **retina** and in the maintenance of a healthy, crystal-clear outer window, the **cornea** (see Figure 7–1).

When light falls on the eye, it passes through the clear cornea and strikes the cells of the retina, bleaching many molecules of the pigment **rhodopsin** that lie within those cells. Vitamin A is a part of the rhodopsin molecule. When bleaching occurs, the vitamin is broken off, initiating the signal that conveys the sensation of sight to the optic center in the brain. The vitamin then reunites with the pigment, but a little vitamin A is destroyed each time this reaction takes place, and fresh vitamin A must replenish the supply.

Night Blindness   If the vitamin A supply begins to run low, a lag occurs before the eye can see again after a flash of bright light at night (see Figure 7–2). This lag in the recovery of night vision, termed **night blindness**, often indicates a vitamin A deficiency.[5] A bright flash of light can temporarily blind even normal, well-nourished eyes, but if you experience a long recovery period before vision returns, your healthcare provider may want to check your vitamin A intake.

Xerophthalmia and Blindness   A more profound deficiency of vitamin A is exhibited when the protein **keratin** accumulates and clouds the eye's outer vitamin A–dependent part, the cornea. The condition is known as **keratinization**, and if the deficiency of vitamin A is not corrected, it can worsen to **xerosis** (drying) and then progress to thickening and permanent blindness, **xerophthalmia**.[6] Tragically, a half million of the world's vitamin A–deprived children become blind each year from this often preventable condition; about half die within a year after losing their sight. Vitamin A supplements given early to children developing vitamin A deficiency can reverse the process and save both eyesight and lives.[7] Better still, a child fed a variety of fruits and vegetables regularly is virtually assured protection.

Gene Regulation   Hundreds of genes are regulated by the retinoic acid form of vitamin A.[8] Genes direct the synthesis of proteins, including enzymes that perform the metabolic work of the tissues. Hence, through its influence on gene expression, vitamin A affects the metabolic activities of a vast array of tissues and, in turn, the health of the body.

Figure 7–1

An Eye (Sectioned)

This eye is sectioned to reveal its inner structures.

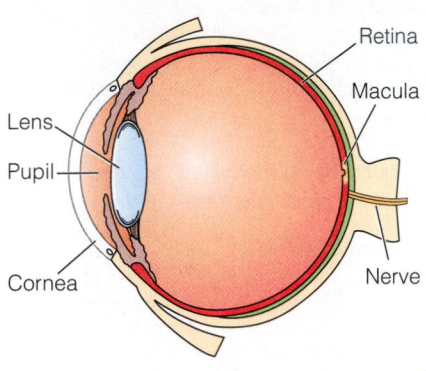

Retina
Macula
Lens
Pupil
Cornea
Nerve

---

beta-carotene an orange pigment with antioxidant activity; a vitamin A precursor made by plants and stored in human fat tissue.

retinol one of the active forms of vitamin A made from beta-carotene in animal and human bodies; an antioxidant nutrient. Other active forms are *retinal* and *retinoic acid*.

retina (RET-in-uh) the layer of light-sensitive nerve cells lining the back of the inside of the eye.

cornea (KOR-nee-uh) the hard, transparent membrane covering the outside of the eye.

rhodopsin (roh-DOP-sin) the light-sensitive pigment of the cells in the retina; it contains vitamin A (*opsin* means "visual protein").

night blindness slow recovery of vision after exposure to flashes of bright light at night; an early symptom of vitamin A deficiency.

keratin (KERR-uh-tin) the normal protein of hair and nails.

keratinization accumulation of keratin in a tissue; a sign of vitamin A deficiency.

xerosis (zeer-OH-sis) drying of the cornea; a symptom of vitamin A deficiency.

xerophthalmia (ZEER-ahf-THALL-me-uh) progressive hardening of the cornea of the eye in advanced vitamin A deficiency that can lead to blindness (*xero* means "dry"; *ophthalm* means "eye").

Cell Differentiation Vitamin A is needed by all **epithelial tissue** (external skin and internal linings). The cornea of the eye, already mentioned, is such a tissue; so are skin and all of the protective linings of the lungs, intestines, vagina, urinary tract, and bladder. These tissues serve as barriers to infection and other threats.

An example of vitamin A's health-supporting work is the process of **cell differentiation**, in which each type of cell develops to perform a specific function. For example, when goblet cells (cells that populate the linings of internal organs) mature, they specialize in synthesizing and releasing mucus to protect delicate tissues from toxins or bacteria and other harmful elements.

If vitamin A is deficient, cell differentiation is impaired, and goblet cells fail to mature, fail to make protective mucus, and eventually die off. Goblet cells are then displaced by cells that secrete keratin, mentioned earlier with regard to the eye. Keratin is the same protein that provides toughness in hair and fingernails, but in the wrong place, such as skin and body linings, keratin makes the tissue surfaces dry, hard, and cracked. As dead cells accumulate on the surface, the tissue becomes vulnerable to infection (see Figure 7–3, p. 246). In the cornea, keratinization leads to xerophthalmia; in the lungs, the displacement of mucus-producing cells makes respiratory infections likely; in the urinary tract, the same process leads to urinary tract infections.

Immune Function Vitamin A has gained a reputation as an "anti-infective" vitamin because so many of the body's defenses against infection depend on an adequate supply.[9] Much research supports the need for vitamin A in the regulation of the genes involved in immunity. Without sufficient vitamin A, these genetic interactions produce an altered response to infection that weakens the body's defenses.

When the defenses are weak, especially in vitamin A–deficient children, an illness such as measles can become severe. A downward spiral of malnutrition and infection can set in. The child's body must devote its scanty store of vitamin A to the immune system's fight against the measles virus, but this destroys the vitamin. As vitamin A dwindles further, the infection worsens. Measles takes the lives of more than 330 of the world's children *every day*.[10] Even if the child survives the infection, permanent blindness is likely to occur. The corneas, already damaged by the chronic vitamin A shortage, degenerate rapidly as their meager supply of vitamin A is diverted to the immune system.

Reproduction and Growth Vitamin A is essential for normal reproductive processes. In men, vitamin A participates in sperm development, and in women, it supports normal fetal development during pregnancy. In the developing embryo, vitamin A is crucial for the formation of the spinal cord, heart, and other organs.[11]

Vitamin A is also indispensable for growth in children. Normal children's bones grow longer, and the children grow taller, by remodeling each old bone into a new, bigger version. To do so, the body dismantles the old bone structures and replaces them with new, larger bone parts. Growth cannot take place just by adding on to the original small bone; vitamin A must be present for critical bone dismantling steps.[11] Failure to grow is one of the first signs of poor vitamin A status in a child. Restoring vitamin A to such children is imperative, but correcting dietary deficiencies may be more effective than giving vitamin A supplements alone because many other nutrients from nutritious foods are also needed for children to grow normally.

KEY POINTS

- Three active forms of vitamin A and one precursor are important in nutrition.
- Vitamin A plays major roles in gene regulation, eyesight, reproduction, cell differentiation, immunity, and growth.

Vitamin A Deficiency around the World Vitamin A deficiency presents a vast problem worldwide, placing a heavy burden on society. An estimated 5 million of the

Figure 7–2

Night Blindness

This is one of the earliest signs of vitamin A deficiency.

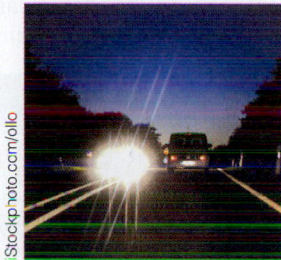

In dim light, you can see what's ahead on the road.

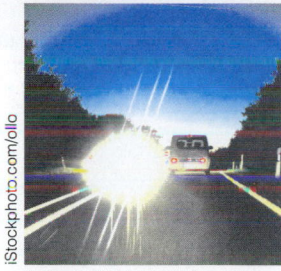

A flash of bright light, such as headlights, momentarily blinds you as the pigment in the retina is bleached.

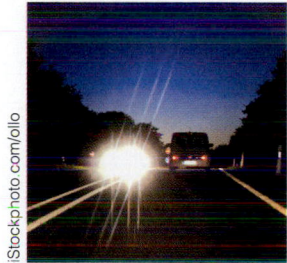

Normally, you quickly recover and can see the details again in a few seconds.

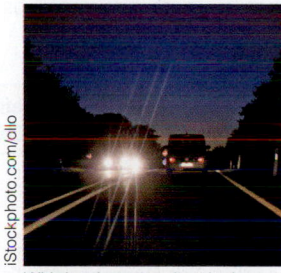

With inadequate vitamin A, you do not recover but remain blind for many seconds or minutes. This is night blindness.

epithelial (ep-ith-THEE-lee-ull) **tissue** the layers of the body that serve as selective barriers to environmental factors. Examples are the cornea, the skin, the respiratory tract lining, and the lining of the digestive tract.

cell differentiation (dih-fer-en-she-AY-shun) the process by which immature cells are stimulated to mature and gain the ability to perform functions characteristic of their cell type.

Figure 7–3

The Skin in Vitamin A Deficiency

The hard lumps on the skin of this person's arm reflect accumulations of keratin in the epithelial cells.

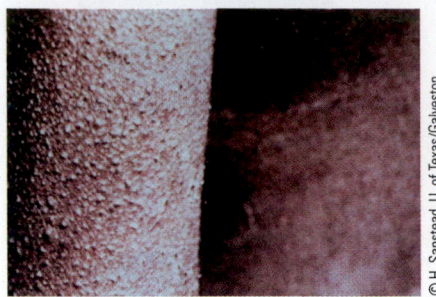

© H. Sanstead, U. of Texas/Galveston

world's preschool children suffer from obvious signs of vitamin A deficiency—not only night blindness but diarrhea, appetite loss, and reduced food intake that can rapidly worsen their condition. In addition, a staggering 190 million preschool children suffer from a milder deficiency that impairs immunity, leaving them open to infections.[12]

In countries where such children receive vitamin A supplements, childhood rates of blindness, disease, and death have declined dramatically. Even in the United States, vitamin A supplements are recommended for children with measles to ward off deficiency.[13] The World Health Organization (WHO) and United Nations International Children's Emergency Fund (UNICEF) are working to eliminate vitamin A deficiency around the world; achieving this goal would greatly improve child survival.

KEY POINT

- Vitamin A deficiency causes blindness, sickness, and death and is a major problem worldwide.

Vitamin A Toxicity

For people who take excess active vitamin A in supplements or fortified foods, toxicity is a real possibility. Figure 7–4 shows that toxicity compromises the tissues just as deficiency does and is equally damaging. Symptoms of vitamin A toxicity are many, and they vary depending partly on whether a sudden overdose occurs or too much of the vitamin is taken over time. The figure lists the best-known toxicity symptoms of both kinds. Hair loss, rashes, and a host of uncomfortable general symptoms are possible.

Ordinary vitamin supplements taken in the context of today's fortified food supply can add up to small daily excesses of vitamin A.[14] Substantial amounts can be found in fortified cereals, water beverages, energy bars, and even chewing gum (see Table 7–3).

Figure 7–4

Vitamin A Deficiency and Toxicity

Danger lies both above and below a normal range of intake of vitamin A.

Vitamin A intake, µg/day	Deficient 0–500		Normal 500–3,000		Toxic 3,000 and over	
	Effects on cells	**Health consequences**	**Effects on cells**	**Health consequences**	**Effects on cells**	**Health consequences**
	Decreased cell division and deficient cell development	Night blindness	Normal cell division and development	Normal body functioning	Overstimulated cell division	Skin rashes
		Keratinization				Hair loss
		Xerophthalmia				Hemorrhages
		Impaired immunity				Bone abnormalities
		Reproductive and growth abnormalities				Birth defects
		Exhaustion				Fractures
		Death				Liver failure
						Death

Pregnant women, especially, should be wary—excessive vitamin A during pregnancy can injure the spinal cord and other tissues of the developing fetus, causing birth defects.[15] Even a single, massive vitamin A dose (100 times the need) can do so. Children, too, can be easily hurt by vitamin A excesses when they mistake chewable vitamin pills and vitamin-laced gum for treats. Even misinformed adolescents put themselves at risk when they take high doses of vitamin A in misguided attempts to cure acne. Some effective remedies for acne are *derived* from vitamin A but they are chemically altered—vitamin A itself has no effect on acne.[16]

KEY POINT
- Vitamin A overdoses and toxicity are possible and cause many serious symptoms.

Vitamin A Recommendations and Sources

The DRI vitamin A intake recommendation is based on body weight. A typical man needs a daily average of about 900 micrograms of active vitamin A; a typical woman, who weighs less, needs about 700 micrograms. During lactation, her need is higher. Children need less.

The ability of vitamin A to be stored in the tissues means that, although the DRI recommendation is stated as a daily amount, you need not consume vitamin A every day. An intake that meets the daily need when averaged over several months is sufficient.

As for vitamin A supplements, the DRI committee warns against exceeding the Tolerable Upper Intake Level of 3,000 micrograms (for adults older than age 18). The best way to ensure a safe intake of vitamin A is to steer clear of supplements that contain it and to rely on food sources instead.

Food Sources of Vitamin A   Active vitamin A is present in foods of animal origin. The richest sources are liver and fish oil, but milk and milk products and other vitamin A–fortified foods such as enriched cereals can also be good sources. Even butter and eggs provide some vitamin A. The vitamin A precursor beta-carotene is naturally present in many vegetable and fruit varieties and may be added to cheeses for its yellow color. The definitive fast-food meal—a hamburger, fries, and cola—lacks vitamin A, but most fast-food places also offer fortified milk, or salads with cheese and carrots that provide it.

Liver: A Lesson in Moderation   Foods naturally rich in vitamin A pose little risk of toxicity, with the possible exception of liver. When young laboratory pigs eat daily chow made from salmon parts, including the livers, their growth halts, and they fall ill from vitamin A toxicity. Inuit people and Arctic explorers know that polar bear livers are a dangerous food source because the bears eat whole fish (with the livers) and, in turn, concentrate large amounts of vitamin A in their own livers.

An *ounce* of ordinary beef or pork liver delivers three times the DRI recommendation for vitamin A intake, and a common portion is 4 to 6 ounces. An occasional serving of liver can provide abundant nutrients and boost nutrient status, but daily use may invite vitamin A toxicity, especially in young children and pregnant women who also routinely take supplements. Snapshot 7–1 shows a sampling of foods that provide more than 10 percent of the Daily Value for a vitamin in a standard-size portion and that therefore qualify as "good sources."

KEY POINTS
- Vitamin A's active forms are supplied by foods of animal origin.
- Fruits and vegetables provide beta-carotene.

Table 7–3
Sources of Active Vitamin A

Vitamin A from highly fortified foods and other rich sources can add up. The UL for vitamin A is 3,000 micrograms (μg) per day.

High-potency vitamin pill	3,000 μg
Calf's liver, 1 oz cooked	2,300 μg
Regular multivitamin pill	1,500 μg
Vitamin gumball, 1	1,500 μg
Chicken liver, 1 oz cooked	1,400 μg
"Complete" liquid supplement drink, 1 serving	350–1,500 μg
Instant breakfast drink, 1 serving	600–700 μg
Cereal breakfast bar, 1	350–400 μg
"Energy" candy bar, 1	350 μg
Milk, 1 c	150 μg
Vitamin-fortified cereal, 1 serving	150 μg
Margarine, 1 tsp	55 μg

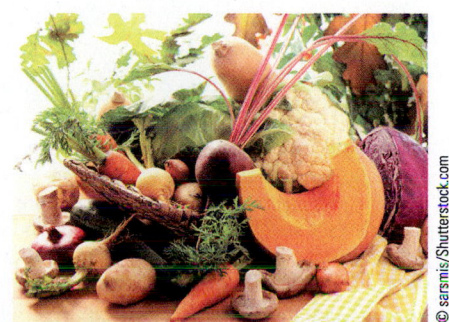

Colorful foods are often rich in vitamins.

© sarsmis/Shutterstock.com

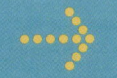
DRI Recommended Intakes
Men: 900 µg/day[a]
Women: 700 µg/day[a]

Tolerable Upper Intake Level
Adults: 3,000 µg vitamin A/day

Chief Functions
Vision; maintenance of cornea, epithelial cells, mucous membranes, skin; growth; regulation of gene expression; reproduction; immunity

Deficiency
Night blindness, corneal drying (xerosis), and blindness (xerophthalmia); impaired growth; keratin lumps on the skin; impaired immunity

Toxicity

Vitamin A:
Acute (single dose or short-term): nausea, vomiting, headache, vertigo, blurred vision, uncoordinated muscles, increased pressure inside the skull, birth defects
Chronic: birth defects, liver abnormalities, bone abnormalities, brain and nerve disorders
Beta-carotene: Harmless yellowing of skin

*These foods provide 10% or more of the vitamin A Daily Value in a serving. For a 2,000-cal diet, the DV is 900 µg/day.
[a]Vitamin A recommendations are expressed in retinol activity equivalents (RAE).
[b]This food contains preformed vitamin A.
[c]This food contains the vitamin A precursor, beta-carotene.

Good Sources*

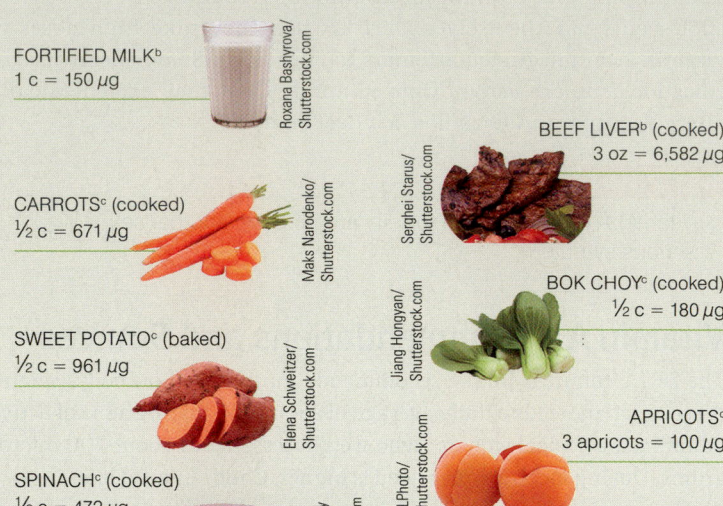

FORTIFIED MILK[b]
1 c = 150 µg
Roxana Bashyrova/ Shutterstock.com

CARROTS[c] (cooked)
½ c = 671 µg
Maks Narodenko/ Shutterstock.com

SWEET POTATO[c] (baked)
½ c = 961 µg
Elena Schweitzer/ Shutterstock.com

SPINACH[c] (cooked)
½ c = 472 µg
Daniel Gilbey Photography-My portfolio/ Shutterstock.com

BEEF LIVER[b] (cooked)
3 oz = 6,582 µg
Serghei Starus/ Shutterstock.com

BOK CHOY[c] (cooked)
½ c = 180 µg
Jiang Hongyan/ Shutterstock.com

APRICOTS[c]
3 apricots = 100 µg
HLPhoto/ Shutterstock.com

Beta-Carotene

In plants, vitamin A exists only in its precursor forms. Beta-carotene, the most abundant of these **carotenoid** precursors, has the highest vitamin A activity. Other carotenoids, although not vitamins, may play other roles in human health.[17] Beta-carotene is one of many **dietary antioxidants** present in foods—others include vitamin E, vitamin C, the mineral selenium, and many phytochemicals (see Table 7–4).

Does Eating Carrots Really Promote Good Vision? Bright orange fruits and vegetables derive their color from beta-carotene and are so colorful that they decorate the plate. Carrots, sweet potatoes, pumpkins, mango, cantaloupe, and apricots are all rich sources of beta-carotene—and therefore contribute vitamin A to the eyes and to the rest of the body—so, yes, eating carrots does promote good vision. Another colorful group, *dark* green vegetables, such as spinach, other greens, and broccoli, owes its deep dark green color to the blending of orange beta-carotene with the green leaf pigment chlorophyll.

Eating patterns lacking in dark green, leafy vegetables and orange vegetables are associated with the most common form of age-related blindness, **macular degeneration**.[†18] The macula, a yellow spot of pigment at the focal center of the retina (identified in Figure 7–1, p. 244), loses integrity, impairing the most important field of vision, the central focus. In some studies, supplements of carotenoids and several

carotenoid (CARE-oh-ten-oyd) a member of a group of pigments in foods that range in color from light yellow to reddish orange and are chemical relatives of beta-carotene. Many have a degree of vitamin A activity in the body. Also defined in Controversy 2.

dietary antioxidants compounds typically found in plant foods that significantly decrease the adverse effects of oxidation on living tissues. The major antioxidant vitamins are vitamin E, vitamin C, and beta-carotene. Many phytochemicals are also antioxidants.

macular degeneration a common, progressive loss of function of the part of the retina that is most crucial to focused vision (the macula was shown in Figure 7–1). This degeneration often leads to blindness.

---
†The carotenoids associated with protection from macular degeneration are lutein (LOO-tee-in) and its close chemical relative zeaxanthin (zee-ZAN-thin).

Table 7–4

Functional Group of Antioxidants

Key antioxidant vitamins:
- Beta-carotene
- Vitamin E
- Vitamin C

A key antioxidant mineral:
- Selenium

Many antioxidant phytochemicals

other nutrients have proven ineffective in preventing this cause of blindness, while in other studies this approach has been shown to be modestly effective.[19]

Measuring Beta-Carotene The conversion of beta-carotene to retinol in the body entails losses, so vitamin A activity for precursors is measured in **retinol activity equivalents (RAE)**. It takes about 12 micrograms of beta-carotene from food to supply the equivalent of 1 microgram of retinol to the body. Some food tables and supplement labels express beta-carotene and vitamin A contents using **IU (international units)**. When comparing vitamin A in foods, be careful to notice whether a food table or supplement label uses micrograms or IU. To convert one to the other, use the factor provided in Appendix C.

Toxicity Beta-carotene from food is not converted to retinol efficiently enough to cause vitamin A toxicity. A steady diet of abundant pumpkin, carrots, or carrot juice, however, has been known to turn light-skinned people bright yellow because beta-carotene builds up in the fat just beneath the skin and imparts a harmless yellow cast (see Figure 7–5). Likewise, red-colored carotenoids confer a rosy glow on those who consume the fruits and vegetables that contain them.[20] Food sources of the carotenoids are safe, but concentrated supplements may have adverse effects of their own.

Food Sources of Beta-Carotene Plants contain no active vitamin A, but many vegetables and fruits provide the vitamin A precursor, beta-carotene. Snapshot 7–1 shows good sources of beta-carotene. Other colorful vegetables, such as red beets, red cabbage, and yellow corn, can fool you into thinking they contain beta-carotene, but these foods derive their colors from other pigments and are poor sources of beta-carotene. As for "white" plant foods such as grains and potatoes, they have none. Some confusion exists concerning the term *yam*. A white-fleshed Mexican root vegetable called "yam" is devoid of beta-carotene, but the orange-fleshed sweet potato called "yam" in the United States is one of the richest beta-carotene sources known.

KEY POINTS
- The vitamin A precursor in plants, beta-carotene, is an effective antioxidant in the body.
- Many brightly colored plant foods are rich in beta-carotene.

Vitamin D

LO 7.4 Discuss the roles of vitamin D, its sources, and the consequences of its deficiency and toxicity.

Vitamin D is unique among nutrients in that, with the help of sunlight, the body can synthesize all it needs. In this sense, vitamin D is not an *essential* nutrient—given sufficient sun each day, most people can make enough to meet their need from this source.

Figure 7–5

Excess Beta-Carotene Symptom: Discoloration of the Skin

The hand on the right shows skin discoloration from excess beta-carotene. Another person's normal hand (left) is shown for comparison.

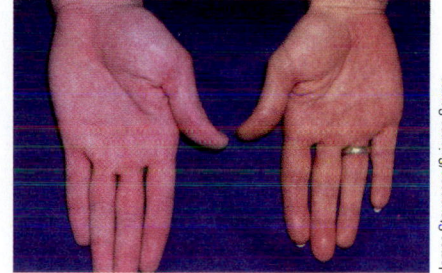

James Stevenson/Science Source

retinol activity equivalents (RAE) a new measure of the vitamin A activity of beta-carotene and other vitamin A precursors that reflects the amount of retinol that the body will derive from a food containing vitamin A precursor compounds.

IU (international units) a measure of fat-soluble vitamin activity sometimes used in food composition tables and on supplement labels.

Table 7–5

Functional Group for Bone Health

Key vitamins:
- Vitamin D
- Vitamin K
- Vitamin C

Key minerals:
- Calcium
- Phosphorus
- Magnesium
- Fluoride

Key energy nutrient:
- Protein

Do the Math

Vitamin D is measured in micrograms (μg) in research or international units (IU) on nutrient and supplement fact panels.

- To convert vitamin D amounts from micrograms (μg) to IU, multiply by 40:

  $1\mu g = 40$ IU vitamin D

If a vitamin D pill contains 50 micrograms, how many IU does it provide?

rickets the vitamin D–deficiency disease in children; characterized by abnormal growth of bone and manifested in bowed legs or knock-knees, outward-bowed chest, and knobs on the ribs.

As simple as it sounds to obtain vitamin D, many people may border on insufficiency.[21] The Dietary Guidelines 2015 report lists vitamin D among its nutrients of concern because most people's dietary intake falls short of the DRI recommendation. Even so, well over half of the U.S. population has normal blood concentrations, presumably put there by sunshine.

Roles of Vitamin D

Once in the body, whether made from sunlight or obtained from the diet, vitamin D must undergo a series of chemical transformations in the liver and kidneys to activate it. Once activated, vitamin D has profound effects on the tissues.

Calcium Regulation   Vitamin D is the best-known member of a large cast of nutrients and hormones that interact to regulate blood calcium and phosphorus levels—and thereby maintain bone integrity.[22] Table 7–5 lists nutrients, including vitamin D, that are important for bone health. Calcium is indispensable to the proper functioning of cells in all body tissues, including muscles, nerves, and glands, which draw calcium from the blood as they need it.

To replenish blood calcium, vitamin D acts at three body locations to raise the calcium level. First, the skeleton serves as a vast warehouse of stored calcium that can be tapped when blood calcium begins to fall. Only two other organs can act to increase blood calcium: the digestive tract, which can increase absorption of calcium from food, and the kidneys, which can recycle calcium that would otherwise be lost in urine.

Vitamin D and calcium are inextricably linked in nutrition—no matter how much vitamin D you take in, it cannot make up for a chronic shortfall of calcium. The reverse is also true: excess calcium cannot take the place of sufficient vitamin D for bone health.[23]

Other Vitamin D Roles   Activated vitamin D functions as a hormone—that is, a compound manufactured by one organ of the body that acts on other organs, tissues, or cells. Inside cells, for example, vitamin D acts at the genetic level to affect how cells grow, multiply, and specialize. Vitamin D exerts its effects all over the body, from hair follicles, to reproductive system cells, to cells of the immune system.

Research is hinting (sometimes strongly) that to incur a deficit of vitamin D may be to invite problems of many kinds, including cardiovascular diseases and risk factors, some cancers, respiratory infections such as tuberculosis or flu, inflammatory conditions, multiple sclerosis, and a higher risk of death.[24] Table 7–6 offers some evidence in this regard. Even so, research does not support taking vitamin D supplements to prevent diseases except those caused by deficiency.[25] The well-established vitamin D roles concern calcium balance and the bones during growth and throughout life, and these form the basis of the DRI intake recommendations.

KEY POINTS

- Low and borderline vitamin D levels are not uncommon in the United States.
- When exposed to sunlight, the skin makes vitamin D.
- Vitamin D helps regulate blood calcium and influences other body tissues.

Too Little Vitamin D—A Danger to Bones

Although vitamin D insufficiency is relatively common in the population, overt signs of vitamin D deficiency are rarely reported.[26] The most obvious sign occurs in early life—the abnormality of the bones in the disease **rickets** is shown in Figure 7–6. Children with rickets develop bowed legs because they are unable to mineralize newly forming bone material, a rubbery protein matrix. As gravity pulls their body weight against these weak bones, the legs bow. Many such children also have a protruding belly because of lax abdominal muscles.

Preventing Rickets   As early as the 1700s, rickets was known to be curable with cod-liver oil, now recognized as a rich source of vitamin D. More than a hundred

Table 7–6

Vitamin D in Disease: State of the Evidence

Optimal vitamin D nutrition has been associated with low rates of diseases, but fundamental knowledge gaps and conflicting evidence prevent conclusions about the nature of these associations. This table's long reference list is just a sampling of today's research.

Cancers

Low serum vitamin D levels have sometimes been associated with increased risk of bladder, breast, colon, prostate, and thyroid cancers. Very high intakes of supplemental vitamin D have also been linked with *higher* rates of breast cancer. No causal role has been established between vitamin D and cancers.

Cardiovascular Disease (CVD)

In hospital patients, low blood vitamin D levels have been associated with atherosclerosis, altered blood lipid profiles, hypertension, and inflammation. In the general population, higher blood vitamin D levels may be associated with lower risks of these conditions, but vitamin D supplements have not proved effective in this regard. Conflicting evidence prevents conclusions from being drawn.

Diabetes

Vitamin D deficiency has been associated with harm from diabetes, including damage to the eyes and poor glucose control; vitamin D supplements have been reported to improve blood glucose control in some people. Researchers disagree about the usefulness of supplements in diabetes prevention.

Multiple Sclerosis (MS)

Low blood vitamin D has been associated with increased risk of MS, while adequacy has been associated with a lower risk of MS and relapse.

Infectious Diseases, Other Conditions

Low vitamin D levels may increase susceptibility to respiratory infections, although not all studies support this finding. Potential links with obesity, inflammatory bowel disease, asthma, allergies, and many other conditions are also topics of research.

Sources: **Cancers:** *Y. Liao and coauthors, Impact of serum vitamin D level on risk of bladder cancer: A systematic review and meta-analysis,* Tumour Biology *(2014), epub ahead of print, doi:10.1007/s13277-014-2728-9; L. Hargrove, T. Francis, and H. Francis, Vitamin D and GI cancers: Shedding some light on dark diseases,* Annals of Translational Medicine *2 (2014), epub, doi:10.3978/j.issn.2305-5839.2013.03.04; C. J. Narvaez and coauthors, The impact of vitamin D in breast cancer: Genomics, pathways, metabolism,* Frontiers in Physiology *5 (2014), epub, doi:10.3389/fphys.2014.00213.* **Cardiovascular disease:** *M. Witham and coauthors, Effect of vitamin D supplementation on blood pressure: A systematic review and meta-analysis incorporating individual patient data,* JAMA Internal Medicine *175 (2015): 745–754; I. Mozos and O. Marginean, Links between vitamin D deficiency and cardiovascular diseases,* BioMed Research International *(2015), epub, doi:10.1155/2015/109275; K. T. Khaw, R. Luben, and N. Wareham, Serum 25-hydroxyvitamin D, mortality, and incident cardiovascular disease, respiratory disease, cancers, and fractures: A 13-y prospective population study,* American Journal of Clinical Nutrition *100 (2014): 1361–1370; U. Canpolat and coauthors, Impaired cardiac autonomic functions in apparently healthy subjects with vitamin D deficiency,* Annals of Noninvasive Electrocardiology *(2014), epub, doi: 10.1111/anec.12233; P. G. Weyland, W. B. Grant, and J. Howie Esquivel, Does sufficient evidence exist to support a causal association between vitamin D status and cardiovascular risk? An assessment using Hill's criteria for causality,* Nutrients *6 (2014): 3403–3430.* **Diabetes:** *C. Mathieu, Vitamin D and diabetes: Where do we stand? Diabetes Research and Clinical Practice 108 (2015): 201–209; R. Jorde and G. Grimes, Vitamin D and health: The need for more randomized controlled trials,* Journal of Steroid Biochemistry and Molecular Biology *148 (2015): 269-274; H. Nasri and coauthors, Efficacy of supplementary vitamin D on improvement of glycemic parameters in patients with type 2 diabetes mellitus: A randomized double blind clinical trial,* Journal of Renal Injury Prevention *3 (2013): 31–34; N. Shimo and coauthors, Vitamin D deficiency is significantly associated with retinopathy in young Japanese type 1 diabetic patients,* Diabetes Research and Clinical Practice *106 (2014), epub, doi:10.1016/j.diabres.2014.08.005; B. A. Laway, S. K. Kotwal, and Z. A. Shah, Pattern of 25 hydroxy vitamin D status in North Indian people with newly detected type 2 diabetes: A prospective case control study,* Indian Journal of Endocrinology and Metabolism *18 (2014): 726–730.* **Multiple Sclerosis:** *S. Duan and coauthors, Vitamin D status and the risk of multiple sclerosis: A systematic review and meta-analysis,* Neuroscience Letters *570 (2014): 108–113; T. F. Runia and coauthors, Lower serum vitamin D levels are associated with a higher relapse risk in multiple sclerosis,* Neurology *79 (2012): 261–266; J. Salzer and coauthors, Vitamin D as a protective factor in multiple sclerosis,* Neurology *79 (2012): 2140–2145; C. Pierrot-Deseilligny, Relationship between 25-OH-D serum level and relapse rate in multiple sclerosis patients before and after vitamin D supplementation,* Therapeutic Advances in Neurological Disorders *5 (2012): 187–198.* **Infectious diseases:** *M. D. Kerns and coauthors, Impact of vitamin D on infectious disease: A systematic review of controlled trials,* American Journal of the Medical Sciences *349 (2015); 245–262; H. Korf, B. Decallonne, and C. Mathieu, Vitamin D for infections,* Current Opinion in Endocrinology, Diabetes, and Obesity *21 (2014): 431–436.*

years later, a Polish physician linked sunlight exposure to prevention and cure of rickets.

Today, in some areas of the world, such as Mongolia, Tibet, and the Netherlands, more than half of the children suffer the bowed legs, knock-knees, beaded ribs, and protruding (pigeon) chests of rickets. In the United States, rickets is uncommon but not unknown.[27] Many adolescents abandon vitamin D–fortified milk in favor of soft drinks and punches; they may also spend little time outdoors during daylight hours. Soon, their vitamin D values decline, and they may fail to develop the bone mineral density needed to offset bone loss in later life. To prevent rickets and support optimal bone health, the DRI committee recommends that all infants, children, and adolescents consume the recommended amounts of vitamin D each day.

Figure 7–6

Rickets

This child has the bowed legs of the vitamin D–deficiency disease, rickets.

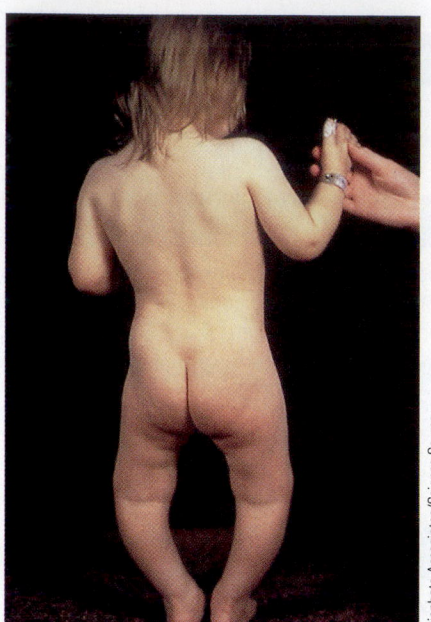

This child displays beaded ribs, a symptom of rickets.

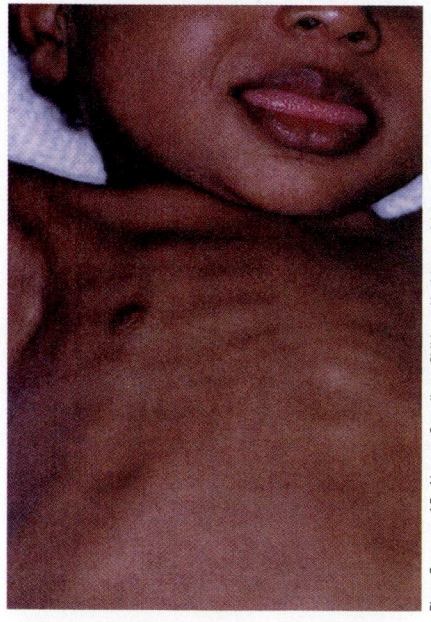

osteomalacia (OS-tee-o-mal-AY-shuh) the adult expression of vitamin D–deficiency disease, characterized by an overabundance of unmineralized bone protein (*osteo* means "bone"; *mal* means "bad"). Symptoms include bending of the spine and bowing of the legs.

osteoporosis a weakening of bone mineral structures that occurs commonly with advancing age. Also defined in Chapter 8.

Deficiency in Adults In adults, poor mineralization of bone results in the painful bone disease **osteomalacia**.[28] The bones become increasingly soft, flexible, weak, and deformed. Older people can suffer painful joints if their vitamin D levels are low, a condition easily misdiagnosed as arthritis during examinations. Inadequate vitamin D also sets the stage for a loss of calcium from the bones, which can result in fractures from **osteoporosis**. Vitamin D supplements themselves may not prevent fractures, but they may help to prevent falls in people with low levels of vitamin D. The simple act of taking a vitamin D supplement could easily save the life of an elderly person who might otherwise suffer bone fractures from falls.[29]

Who Should Be Concerned? People who restrict intakes of fish and dairy foods may not obtain enough vitamin D from food to meet recommendations. Strict vegetarians and people with milk allergies or lactose intolerance in particular must seek out other enriched foods or take supplements to be certain of obtaining enough vitamin D. People living in northern areas of North America; anyone lacking exposure to sunlight, such as office workers or institutionalized older people; and dark-skinned people, their breastfed infants, and their adolescent children often lack vitamin D. Some medications can also compromise vitamin D status.

Levels of circulating blood vitamin D have been falling among U.S. adults, particularly in those who are overweight.[30]§ Similar results have also been observed in overweight children.[31] While vitamin sellers use this information to tout vitamin D pills as "obesity cures," scientists suggest that the opposite may be true: *obesity* may cause a decrease in vitamin D status and, therefore, weight loss may help to correct the apparent deficiency.[32]

How can excess fat in the body cause low vitamin D in the blood? Two mechanisms have been suggested. First, extra fat tissue requires a great deal of extra blood flow, so vitamin D, even if amply consumed, may become diluted in the overweight person's larger blood volume, producing below-normal test results. Second, fat-soluble vitamin D may be taken up and sequestered in the fat tissue of the overweight person, making it less available to the bloodstream, thus lowering test results.[33] In the end, a combination of low intakes, greater blood volume, and sequestering may be responsible for low vitamin D values in many overweight people.

KEY POINTS

- A vitamin D deficiency causes rickets in childhood, low bone density in adolescence, and osteomalacia in later life.
- Vitamin D deficiency is likely in overweight people, those in northern climates, those who lack sun exposure, and among adults, breastfed infants, and adolescents with darker skin.

Too Much Vitamin D—A Danger to Soft Tissues

Vitamin D is the most potentially toxic among the vitamins. Vitamin D intoxication raises the concentration of blood calcium by withdrawing bone calcium, which can then collect in the soft tissues and damage them. With chronic high vitamin D intakes, kidney and heart function decline, blood calcium spins further out of control, and death ensues when the kidneys and heart ultimately fail.

High doses of vitamin D may bring on high blood calcium, nausea, fatigue, back pain, irregular heartbeat, and increased urination and thirst.[34] Several reports of patients with high blood calcium have emerged as more and more people self-prescribe high-dose vitamin D supplements in response to preliminary reports of potential health benefits.[35]

KEY POINTS

- Vitamin D is the most potentially toxic vitamin.
- Overdoses raise blood calcium and damage soft tissues.

---

§Standard used to determine vitamin D status: ≥ 20 μg/mL = sufficient.

Vitamin D from Sunlight

Sunlight supplies the needed vitamin D for most of the world's people. Sunlight presents no risk of vitamin D toxicity because after a certain amount of vitamin D collects in the skin, the sunlight itself begins breaking it down.

Vitamin D Synthesis and Activation   When ultraviolet (UV) light rays from the sun reach a cholesterol compound in human skin, the compound is transformed into a vitamin D precursor and is absorbed directly into the blood. Slowly, over the next day and a half, the liver and kidneys finish converting the inactive precursor to the active form of vitamin D. Diseases that affect either the liver or the kidneys can impair this conversion and therefore produce symptoms of vitamin D deficiency.

Like natural sunscreen, the pigments of dark skin protect against UV radiation. To synthesize several days' worth of vitamin D, dark-skinned people require up to 3 hours of direct sun (depending on the climate). Light-skinned people need much less time (an estimated 5 minutes without sunscreen or 10 to 30 minutes with sunscreen). Vitamin D deficiency is especially prevalent if sunlight is weak, such as in the winter months and in the extreme northern regions of the world.[36] The factors listed in Table 7–7 can all interfere with vitamin D synthesis.

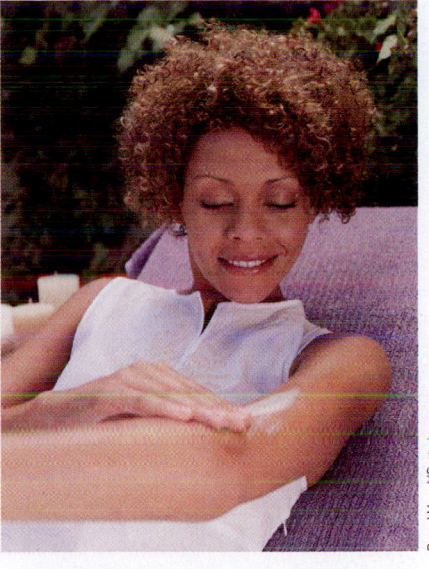

The sunshine vitamin: vitamin D.

> **KEY POINT**
>
> - Ultraviolet light from sunshine acts on a cholesterol compound in the skin to make vitamin D.

Table 7–7

Factors Affecting Vitamin D Synthesis

The more of these factors present in a person's life, the more critical it becomes to obtain vitamin D from food or supplements.

Factor	Effect on Vitamin D Synthesis
Advanced age	With age, the skin loses some of its capacity to synthesize vitamin D.
Air pollution	Particles in the air screen out the sun's rays.
City living	Tall buildings block sunlight.
Clothing	Most clothing blocks sunlight.
Cloudy skies	Heavy cloud cover reduces sunlight penetration.
Geography	Sunlight exposure is limited: - October through March at latitudes above 43 degrees (most of Canada) - November through February at latitudes between 35 and 43 degrees (many U.S. locations) In locations south of 35 degrees (much of the southern United States), direct sun exposure is sufficient for vitamin D synthesis year-round.
Homebound	Living indoors prevents sun exposure.
Season	Warmer seasons of the year bring more direct sun rays.
Skin pigment	Darker-skinned people synthesize less vitamin D per minute than lighter-skinned people.
Sunscreen	Proper use reduces or prevents skin exposure to sun's rays.
Time of day	Midday hours bring maximum direct sun exposure.

Bernd Vogel/Getty Images

Snapshot 7–2 →→→ Vitamin D

DRI Recommended Intakes
Adults: 15 µg (600 IU)/day (19–70 yr)
             20 µg (700 IU)/day (> 70 yr)

Tolerable Upper Intake Level
Adults: 100 µg (4,000 IU)/day

Chief Functions
Mineralization of bones and teeth (raises blood calcium and phosphorus by increasing absorption from digestive tract, withdrawing calcium from bones, stimulating retention by kidneys)

Deficiency
Abnormal bone growth resulting in rickets in children, osteomalacia in adults; malformed teeth; muscle spasms

Toxicity
Elevated blood calcium; calcification of soft tissues (blood vessels, kidneys, heart, lungs, tissues of joints), excessive thirst, headache, nausea, weakness

*These foods provide 10% or more of the vitamin D Daily Value in a serving. For a 2,000-cal diet, the DV is 20 µg/day.
[a]Average value.
[b]Avoid prolonged exposure to sun.

Good Sources*

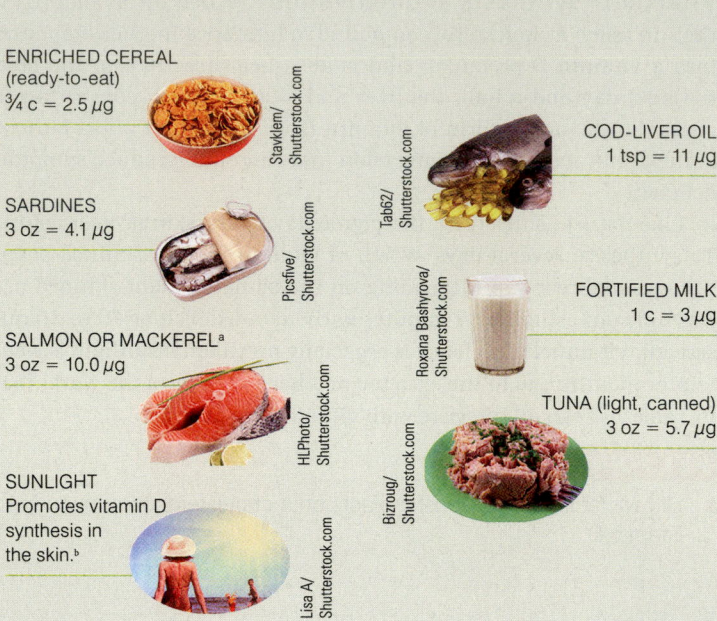

ENRICHED CEREAL (ready-to-eat)
¾ c = 2.5 µg
Stavklem/Shutterstock.com

SARDINES
3 oz = 4.1 µg
Picsfive/Shutterstock.com

SALMON OR MACKEREL[a]
3 oz = 10.0 µg
HLPhoto/Shutterstock.com

SUNLIGHT
Promotes vitamin D synthesis in the skin.[b]
Lisa A/Shutterstock.com

COD-LIVER OIL
1 tsp = 11 µg
Tab62/Shutterstock.com

FORTIFIED MILK
1 c = 3 µg
Roxana Bashyrova/Shutterstock.com

TUNA (light, canned)
3 oz = 5.7 µg
Bizroug/Shutterstock.com

Vitamin D Intake Recommendations

The need for vitamin D remains remarkably steady throughout most of life. People ages 1–70 years old need 15 micrograms of vitamin D daily. For those 71 and older, the need jumps to 20 micrograms per day because this group faces an increased threat of bone fractures. The Tolerable Upper Intake Level for vitamin D for adults of all ages is 100 micrograms (4,000 IU), above which the risk of harm increases.

Vitamin D from the sun, while substantial, varies widely among people of different ages and living in different locations. Measuring the contribution of vitamin D from sunlight is difficult, and sun exposure increases skin cancer risks, so the DRI committee set its recommendations in terms of dietary vitamin D alone, with no contribution from the sun.[37] The recommendations do assume an adequate intake of calcium because vitamin D and calcium each alter the body's handling of the other.

The recommendations are set high enough to maintain blood vitamin D levels known to support healthy bones throughout life, but some research suggests that recommendations for some people should be set even higher.[38] The Consumer's Guide provides some details about obtaining vitamin D.

KEY POINT

- The DRI recommended intake for dietary vitamin D varies little through most of life.

Vitamin D Food Sources

Snapshot 7–2 shows the few significant naturally occurring food sources of vitamin D. In addition, egg yolks provide small amounts, along with butter and cream. Milk, whether fluid, dried, or evaporated, is fortified with vitamin D, so it constitutes a major food source for the United States. Yogurt and cheese products may lack vitamin D, however, whereas orange juice, cereals, margarines, and other foods may be fortified with it, so read the labels.

Young adults who drink 3 cups of milk a day receive half of their daily requirement from this source; the other half comes from exposure to sunlight and other foods and supplements. Without adequate sunshine, enriched foods, or supplementation, strict vegetarians cannot meet their vitamin D needs. Certain mushrooms produce significant vitamin D upon brief exposure to ultraviolet light; such mushrooms are labeled and offered for sale in many stores.[39] Vegans can also rely on vitamin D–fortified foods, such as cereals and beverages, along with supplements, to supply their vitamin D. Importantly, feeding infants and young children unfortified "health beverages" instead of milk or infant formula can create severe nutrient deficiencies, including rickets.

KEY POINT

- Food sources of vitamin D include a few naturally rich sources and many fortified foods.

Vitamin E

LO 7.5 Discuss the roles, food sources, and effects of deficiency and toxicity of vitamin E.

Almost a century ago, researchers discovered a compound in vegetable oils essential for reproduction in rats. This compound was named **tocopherol** from *tokos*, a Greek word meaning "offspring." A few years later, the compound was named vitamin E.

Four tocopherol compounds have long been known to be of importance in nutrition, and each is designated by one of the first four letters of the Greek alphabet: alpha, beta, gamma, and delta. Of these, alpha-tocopherol is the gold standard for vitamin E activity, and the DRI intake recommendations are expressed as alpha-tocopherol. Additional forms of vitamin E have also been identified and are of interest to researchers for potential roles in health.**[40]

Roles of Vitamin E

Vitamin E is an antioxidant and thus acts as a bodyguard against oxidative damage. Such damage occurs when highly unstable molecules known as **free radicals**, formed during normal cell metabolism, run amok. Left unchecked, free radicals create a destructive chain reaction that can damage the polyunsaturated lipids in cell membranes and lipoproteins, the DNA in genetic material, and the working proteins of cells. This creates inflammation and cell damage associated with aging processes, cancer development, heart disease, and other diseases.[41] Vitamin E, by being oxidized itself, quenches free radicals and reduces inflammation. Figure 7–7 (p. 257) provides an overview of the antioxidant activity of vitamin E and its potential role in disease prevention.[42]

The antioxidant protection of vitamin E is crucial, particularly in the lungs, where high oxygen concentrations would otherwise disrupt vulnerable membranes. Red blood cell membranes also need vitamin E's protection as they transport oxygen from the lungs to other tissues. White blood cells that fight diseases equally depend on vitamin E's antioxidant nature, as do blood vessel linings, sensitive brain tissues, and even bones.[43] Tocopherols also perform some nonantioxidant tasks that support the body's health.

Vitamin E Deficiency

A deficiency of vitamin E produces a wide variety of symptoms in laboratory animals, but these are almost never seen in otherwise healthy human beings. Deficiency of vitamin E, which dissolves in fat, may occur in people with diseases that cause fat malabsorption or in infants born prematurely. Disease or injury of the liver (which makes bile, necessary for digestion of fat), the gallbladder (which delivers bile into the intestine), or the pancreas (which makes fat-digesting enzymes) makes vitamin E deficiency likely. In people without diseases, low blood levels of vitamin E are most likely when diets extremely low in fat are consumed for years.

**The other forms of Vitamin E are tocotrienols: alpha, beta, gamma, and delta.

tocopherol (tuh-KOFF-er-all) a kind of alcohol. The active form of vitamin E is alpha-tocopherol.

free radicals atoms or molecules with one or more unpaired electrons that make the atom or molecule unstable and highly reactive.

Sources of Vitamin D

Anyone who complains of feeling tired, or achy, or sleepless may hear this advice: "You're probably low in vitamin D and you need to take a supplement." These days, this bit of counsel has become more and more common from sellers of supplements and some medical professionals as well. Consumers aiming for optimal vitamin D blood levels while minimizing health risks have just three options: food, supplements, or sunshine.

Vitamin D in Food

Meeting vitamin D needs with unenriched foods can be tricky because just a few foods are naturally richly endowed: fatty fish, fish liver oil, beef liver, and eggs yolks. Just 3 ounces of salmon or mackerel provides one-half to three-quarters of a day's vitamin D need for most adults; the next-richest sources, egg yolk and beef liver, provide a little over 10 percent of the day's need per serving.

Today, more and more foods and beverages are fortified with vitamin D. Fortified milk, fruit juices, cereals, and breakfast or "energy" bars, are convenient sources of vitamin D, and they effectively contribute to the body's vitamin D supply.[1]* A caution is in order, however. A single serving of some highly fortified beverages or bars can meet an entire day's need, and when combined with a daily supplement, the day's vitamin D intake can mount up. Read the Nutrition Facts panel of vitamin D–enriched foods and compare the total provided with your need. Do not exceed the Tolerable Upper Intake Level of 4,000 IU (100 micrograms) per day except on the advice of a physician.

Supplement Speed Bumps

Going by the false theory that "more is better," some supplement manufacturers have increased the vitamin D in their pills to high levels, and the body readily absorbs a wide range of doses.[2] The toxic effects of large overdoses are well defined, but no one knows what consequences may follow mildly elevated vitamin D over time.[3] Women in particular, who often take calcium plus vitamin D pills, may also take a daily multivitamin pill, drink vitamin-fortified beverages, and eat highly enriched cereals or bars that push the day's intake beyond the upper levels of safety.

Sunshine—It's Free, but Is It Safe?

Supplements and enriched foods cost money, but sunshine is freely available to all and, in sunny seasons, can provide much of the vitamin D a person needs. But there's a catch: synthesis of vitamin D requires exposure to the same form of UV radiation that contributes to about a million skin cancers each year in the United States alone.[4] Even small daily exposures to intense sunlight can increase skin cancer risk.* Medical authorities therefore warn against too much sun exposure, but following their advice to use sunscreen or wear sun-protective clothing can reduce blood vitamin D concentrations.[5]

Tanning booths are not a safe sun alternative for vitamin D. Tanning booths may or may not promote vitamin D synthesis, but like the sun, they deliver UV radiation that promotes skin cancer and prematurely wrinkles the skin.

*For complete information about sun exposure and cancer risk, access the American Cancer Society website: www.cancer.org.

Moving Ahead

For vitamin D, then, nutrient-dense foods and beverages, such as vitamin D–fortified milk, yogurt, or soy milk, enriched whole grain cereals, and fatty fish are preferred sources because they pose virtually no risk and provide other nutrients that the body needs.[6] People who consume too few of such foods to meet their vitamin D requirements and who test low for vitamin D can often improve their vitamin D status by taking a supplement. If you choose to take a supplement, use the principles set forth in this chapter's Controversy section. Even with careful selection, however, supplements may or may not contain the substances or amounts listed on the labels because regulation and oversight are lax.

As for the sun exposure, if you live in a southern climate or spend time outdoors in sunny weather, your skin's own vitamin D will contribute to your supply as well. For safety's sake, however, protect your skin from the strong midday sun with sunscreen, wear sun-protective clothing, and take along a big hat.

Review Questions[†]

1. A daily regimen of supplements and vitamin D–enriched foods increases the risk of vitamin D toxicity. T F

2. Just 3 ounces of salmon, a naturally rich source of vitamin D, provides most of an adult's daily need for vitamin D. T F

3. The best and safest source of vitamin D for people in the United States is exposure to sunshine. T F

*Reference notes are found in Appendix F.

†Answers to Consumer's Guide review questions are found in Appendix G.

Figure 7–7

Free-Radical Damage and Antioxidant Protection

Free-radical formation occurs during metabolic processes, and it accelerates when diseases or other stresses strike.

Free radicals cause chain reactions that damage cellular structures.

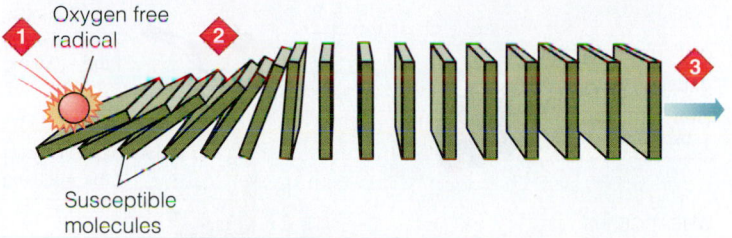

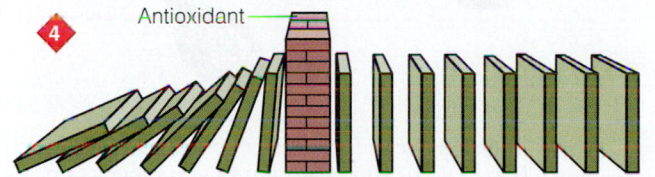

Antioxidants quench free radicals and protect cellular structures.

1. A chemically reactive oxygen free radical attacks fatty acid, DNA, protein, or cholesterol molecules, which form other free radicals in turn.

2. This initiates a rapid, destructive chain reaction.

3. The result is:
   - Cell membrane lipid damage.
   - Cellular protein damage.
   - DNA damage.
   - Oxidation of LDL cholesterol.
   - Inflammation.
   These changes may initiate steps leading to diseases such as heart disease, cancer, macular degeneration, and others.

4. Antioxidants, such as vitamin E, stop the chain reaction by changing the nature of the free radical.

A classic vitamin E deficiency occurs in premature babies born before the transfer of the vitamin from the mother to the fetus, which takes place late in pregnancy. Without sufficient vitamin E, the infant's red blood cells rupture (**erythrocyte hemolysis**), and the infant becomes anemic. The few symptoms of vitamin E deficiency observed in adults include loss of muscle coordination and reflexes and impaired vision and speech. Vitamin E corrects all of these symptoms.

Toxicity of Vitamin E

Vitamin E in foods is safe to consume, and reports of vitamin E toxicity symptoms are rare across a broad range of intakes. However, vitamin E in supplements augments the effects of anticoagulant medication used to oppose unwanted blood clotting, so people taking such drugs risk uncontrollable bleeding if they also take vitamin E. Supplemental doses of vitamin E prolong blood clotting times and increase the risk of brain hemorrhages, a form of stroke that has been noted among people taking supplements of vitamin E.[44]

The pooled results from 78 experiments involving over a quarter-million people suggested that taking vitamin E supplements may increase mortality in both healthy and sick people.[45] Other studies find no effect or a slight decrease in mortality among certain groups.[46] To err on the safe side, people who use vitamin E supplements should probably keep their dosages low, not to exceed the Tolerable Upper Intake Level of 1,000 milligrams of alpha-tocopherol per day.

Vitamin E Recommendations and U.S. Intakes

The DRI recommended intake (inside front cover) for vitamin E is 15 milligrams a day for adults. This amount is sufficient to maintain healthy, normal blood values for vitamin E for most people. On average, U.S. intakes of vitamin E fall substantially below the recommendation (see Figure 7–8).[47] The need for vitamin E rises as people consume more polyunsaturated oil because the oil requires antioxidant protection by the vitamin. Luckily, most raw oils also contain vitamin E, so people who eat raw oils also receive the vitamin. Smokers may have higher needs.

Vitamin E Food Sources

Vitamin E is widespread in foods (see Snapshot 7–3). Much of the vitamin E that people consume comes from vegetable oils and products made from them, such as

Figure 7–8

Vitamin E Recommendations and Intakes Compared

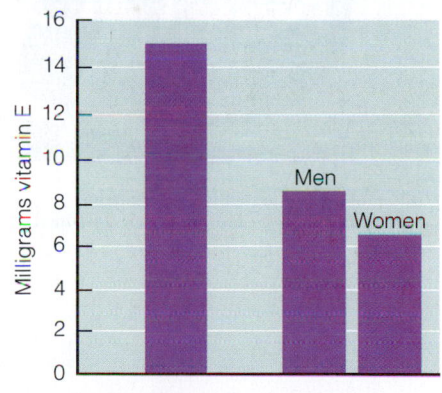

DRI recommendation   U.S. intakes

erythrocyte (eh-REETH-ro-sight) **hemolysis** (HEE-moh-LIE-sis, hee-MOLL-ih-sis) rupture of the red blood cells that can be caused by vitamin E deficiency (*erythro* means "red"; *cyte* means "cell"; *hemo* means "blood"; *lysis* means "breaking"). The anemia produced by the condition is *hemolytic* (HEE-moh-LIT-ick) *anemia.*

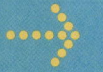
DRI Recommended Intake
Adults: 15 mg/day

Tolerable Upper Intake Level
Adults: 1,000 mg/day

Chief Functions
Antioxidant (protects cell membranes, regulates oxidation reactions, protects polyunsaturated fatty acids)

Deficiency
Red blood cell breakage, nerve damage

Toxicity
Augments the effects of anticlotting medication

* These foods provide 10% or more of the vitamin E Daily Value in a serving. For a 2,000-cal diet, the DV is 22 IU or 15 mg/day.
ᵃCooking destroys vitamin E.

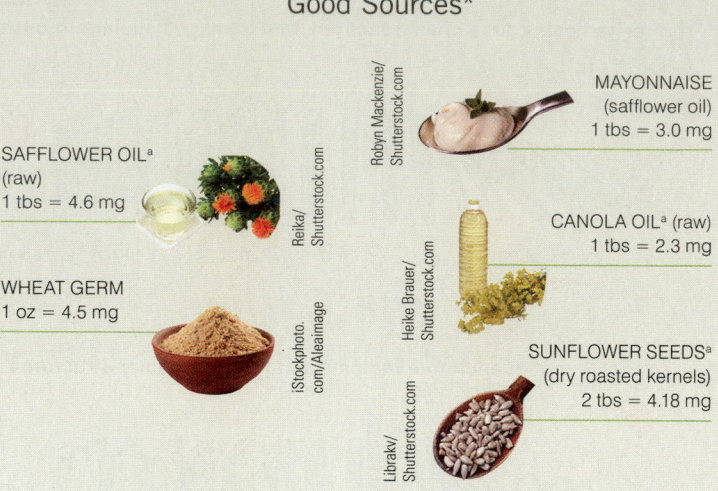

Good Sources*

SAFFLOWER OILᵃ (raw)
1 tbs = 4.6 mg

WHEAT GERM
1 oz = 4.5 mg

MAYONNAISE (safflower oil)
1 tbs = 3.0 mg

CANOLA OILᵃ (raw)
1 tbs = 2.3 mg

SUNFLOWER SEEDSᵃ (dry roasted kernels)
2 tbs = 4.18 mg

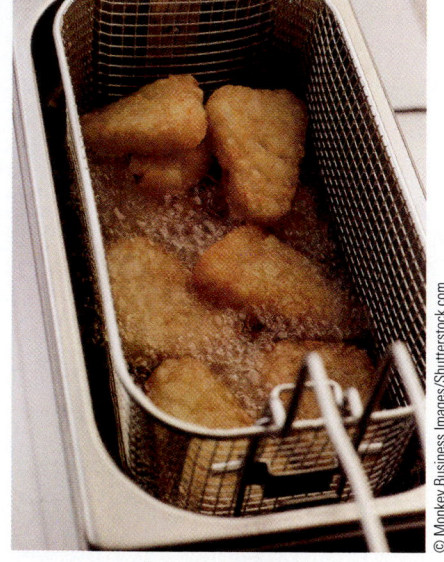

Raw vegetable oils contain substantial vitamin E, but high temperatures destroy it.

margarine and salad dressings. Wheat germ oil is especially rich in vitamin E. Animal fats have almost none.

Vitamin E is readily destroyed by heat and oxidation—thus, fresh, raw oils and lightly processed vitamin E–rich foods are the best sources. As people choose more ultra-processed foods, fried fast foods, or "convenience" foods, they lose vitamin E because little vitamin E survives the heating and other processes used to make these foods.

KEY POINTS

- Vitamin E acts as an antioxidant in cell membranes.
- Average U.S. intakes fall short of DRI recommendations.
- Vitamin E–deficiency disease occurs rarely in newborn premature infants.
- Toxicity is rare, but supplements may carry risks.

Vitamin K

LO 7.6   Discuss the roles of vitamin K, its food sources, and the effects of its deficiency and toxicity.

Have you ever thought about how remarkable it is that blood can clot? The liquid turns solid in a life-saving series of reactions—if blood did not clot, wounds would just keep bleeding, draining the blood from the body.

Roles of Vitamin K

The main function of vitamin K[††] is to help activate proteins that help clot the blood. Hospitals measure the clotting time of a person's blood before surgery and, if needed, administer vitamin K to reduce bleeding during the operation. Vitamin K is of value only if a vitamin K deficiency exists. Vitamin K does not improve clotting in those with other bleeding disorders, such as the inherited disease hemophilia.

Some people with heart problems need to *prevent* the formation of clots within their circulatory system—this is popularly referred to as "thinning" the blood. One of the best-known medicines for this purpose is warfarin (pronounced WAR-fuh-rin), which interferes with vitamin K's clot-promoting action. Vitamin K therapy may be needed for people on warfarin if uncontrolled bleeding should occur.[48] People taking

---

[††]K stands for the Danish word koagulation ("clotting").

warfarin who self-prescribe vitamin K supplements risk causing dangerous clotting of their blood; those who suddenly stop taking vitamin K risk causing excess bleeding.

Vitamin K is also necessary for the synthesis of key bone proteins. With low blood vitamin K, the bones produce an abnormal protein that cannot effectively bind the minerals that normally form bones.[49] People who consume abundant vitamin K in the form of green leafy vegetables suffer fewer hip fractures than those with lower intakes.[50] Vitamin K supplements, however, seem ineffective against bone loss, and more research is needed to clarify the links between vitamin K and bone health.[51]

Vitamin K Deficiency

Few U.S. adults are likely to experience vitamin K deficiency, even if they seldom eat vitamin K–rich foods. This is because, like vitamin D, vitamin K can be obtained from a nonfood source—in this case, the intestinal bacteria. Billions of bacteria normally reside in the intestines, and some of them synthesize vitamin K.

Newborn infants present a unique case with regard to vitamin K because they are born with a sterile intestinal tract and the vitamin K–producing bacteria take weeks to establish themselves. To prevent hemorrhage, the newborn is given a single dose of vitamin K at birth.[52] In an alarming trend, the number of parents who refuse vitamin K treatment for newborns has recently increased. This has led to increases in vitamin K deficiency–related vomiting, lethargy, and even bleeding, including bleeding of the brain, in such babies.[53] Prospective parents should be informed that vitamin K injections at birth pose almost no risk but can avert major problems in newborns.

People who have taken antibiotics that have killed the bacteria in their intestinal tracts also may develop vitamin K deficiency. In other medical conditions, bile production falters, making lipids, including all of the fat-soluble vitamins, unabsorbable. Supplements of the vitamin are needed in these cases because a vitamin K deficiency can be fatal.

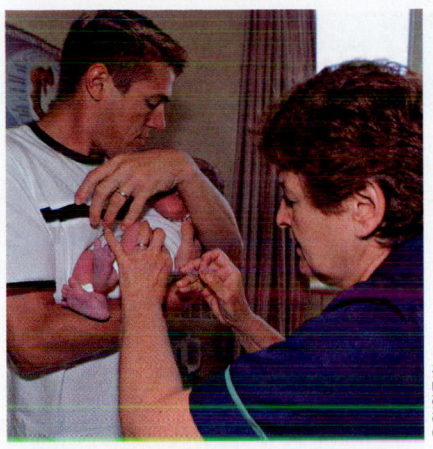

Soon after birth, newborn infants receive a dose of vitamin K.

Vitamin K Toxicity

Reports of vitamin K toxicity among healthy adults are rare, and the DRI committee has not set a Tolerable Upper Intake Level. For infants and pregnant women, however, vitamin K toxicity can result when supplements of a synthetic version of vitamin K are given too enthusiastically.[‡‡] Toxicity induces breakage of the red blood cells and release of their pigment, which colors the skin yellow. A toxic dose of synthetic vitamin K causes the liver to release the blood cell pigment (bilirubin) into the blood (instead of excreting it into the bile) and leads to **jaundice**.

Vitamin K Requirements and Sources

The vitamin K requirement for men is 120 micrograms a day; women require 90 micrograms. As Snapshot 7–4 shows, vitamin K's richest plant food sources include dark green, leafy vegetables such as cooked spinach and other greens, which provide an average of 300 micrograms per half-cup serving. Lettuces, broccoli, brussels sprouts, and other members of the cabbage family are also good sources.

Among protein foods, soybeans, green and black-eyed peas, and split pea soup are rich sources. Canola and soybean oils (unhydrogenated liquid oils) provide smaller but still significant amounts; fortified cereals can also be rich sources of added vitamin K. Tables of food composition now include the vitamin K contents of many foods, thanks to improved methods of analysis.

---

‡‡The version of vitamin K responsible for this effect is menadione.

jaundice (JAWN-dis) yellowing of the skin due to spillover of the bile pigment bilirubin (bill-ee-ROO-bin) from the liver into the general circulation.

DRI Recommended Intakes
Men: 120 µg/day
Women: 90 µg/day

Chief Functions
Synthesis of blood-clotting proteins and bone proteins

Deficiency
Hemorrhage; abnormal bone formation

Toxicity
Opposes the effects of anticlotting medication

* These foods provide 10% or more of the vitamin K Daily Value in a serving. For a 2,000-cal diet, the DV is 120 µg/day.
ᵃAverage value.

Good Sources*

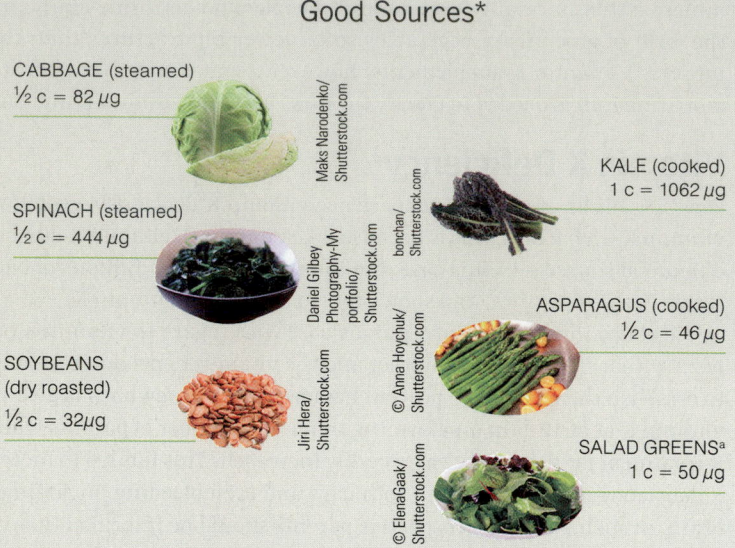

CABBAGE (steamed)
½ c = 82 µg

Maks Narodenko/ Shutterstock.com

SPINACH (steamed)
½ c = 444 µg

Daniel Gilbey Photography-My portfolio/ Shutterstock.com

SOYBEANS (dry roasted)
½ c = 32µg

Jiri Hera/ Shutterstock.com

KALE (cooked)
1 c = 1062 µg

bonchan/ Shutterstock.com

ASPARAGUS (cooked)
½ c = 46 µg

© Anna Hoychuk/ Shutterstock.com

SALAD GREENSᵃ
1 c = 50 µg

© ElenaBaak/ Shutterstock.com

The Water-Soluble Vitamins

LO 7.7   Summarize the characteristics of water-soluble vitamins.

Vitamin C and the B vitamins dissolve in water, which has implications for their handling in food and by the body. In food, water-soluble vitamins easily dissolve and drain away with cooking water, and some are destroyed on exposure to light, heat, or oxygen during processing. Later sections examine vitamin vulnerability and provide tips for retaining vitamins in foods. Recall characteristics of water-soluble vitamins from Table 7–2, earlier.

In the body, water-soluble vitamins are easily absorbed and just as easily excreted in the urine. A few of the water-soluble vitamins can remain in the lean tissues for a month or more, but these tissues actively exchange materials with the body fluids all the time—no real storage tissues exist for any water-soluble vitamins. At any time, the vitamins may be picked up by the extracellular fluids, washed away by the blood, and excreted in the urine.

Advice for meeting the need for these nutrients is straightforward: choose foods rich in water-soluble vitamins to achieve an average intake that meets the recommendation over a few days' time. The Snapshots in this section can help to guide your choices. Foods never deliver toxic doses of the water-soluble vitamins, and their easy excretion in the urine protects against toxicity from all but the largest supplemental doses.

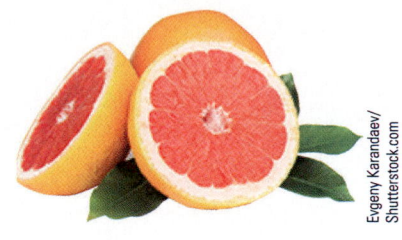

Evgeny Karandaev/ Shutterstock.com

KEY POINTS

- Water-soluble vitamins are easily absorbed and excreted from the body, and foods that supply them must be consumed frequently.
- Water-soluble vitamins are easily lost or destroyed during food preparation and processing.

Vitamin C

LO 7.8   Identify the roles of vitamin C, effects of its deficiency and toxicity, and its food sources.

More than 200 years ago, any man who joined the crew of a seagoing ship knew he had only half a chance of returning alive—not because he might be slain by

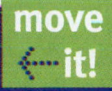
Do athletes who strive for top performance need more vitamins than foods can supply? Competitive athletes who choose their diets with reasonable care almost never need nutrient supplements. The reason is elegantly simple. The need for energy to fuel exercise requires that people eat extra calories of food, and if that extra food is of the kind shown in this chapter's Snapshots—fruits, vegetables, milk, eggs, whole or enriched grains, lean meats, and some oils—then the extra vitamins needed to support the activity flow naturally into the body. Chapter 10 comes back to the roles of vitamins in physical activity.

start now! ⟶ If you haven't already done so, go to Diet & Wellness Plus and track your diet for three days, including one weekend day. After you have recorded your foods for three days, create an Intake Report to see how close you come to meeting the nutrient recommendations for a person of your age, weight, and level of physical activity.

---

pirates or die in a storm but because he might contract **scurvy**, a disease that often killed many of a ship's crew on a long voyage. Ships that sailed on short voyages, especially around the Mediterranean Sea, were safe from this disease. The special hazard of long ocean voyages was that the ship's cook used up the perishable fresh fruits and vegetables early and relied on cereals and live animals for the duration of the voyage.

The first nutrition experiment to be conducted on human beings was devised more than 250 years ago to find a cure for scurvy. A physician divided some British sailors with scurvy into groups.[§§] Each group received a different test substance: vinegar, sulfuric acid, seawater, oranges, or lemons. Those receiving the citrus fruits were cured within a short time. Sadly, it took 50 years for the British navy to make use of the information and require all its vessels to provide lime juice to every sailor daily. British sailors were mocked with the term *limey* because of this requirement. The name later given to the vitamin that the fruit provided, **ascorbic acid**, literally means "no-scurvy acid." It is more commonly known today as vitamin C.

Long voyages without fresh fruits and vegetables spelled death by scurvy for the crew.

The Roles of Vitamin C

Vitamin C performs a variety of functions in the body. It is best known for two of them: its work in maintaining the connective tissues and as an antioxidant.

Connective Tissue　The enzymes involved in the formation and maintenance of the protein **collagen** depend on vitamin C for their activity, as do many other enzymes of the body. Collagen forms the base for all of the connective tissues: bones, teeth, skin, and tendons. Collagen forms the scar tissue that heals wounds, the reinforcing structure that mends fractures, and the supporting material of capillaries that prevents bruises. Vitamin C also participates in other synthetic reactions, such as in the production of carnitine, an important compound for transporting fatty acids within the cells, and in the creation of certain hormones.

Antioxidant Activity　Vitamin C also acts in a more general way as an antioxidant.[54] Vitamin C protects substances found in foods and in the body from oxidation by being oxidized itself. For example, cells of the immune system maintain high levels of vitamin C to protect themselves from free radicals that they generate to use during assaults on bacteria and other invaders. After use, some oxidized vitamin C is degraded irretrievably and must be replaced by the diet. Most of the vitamin, however, is not lost but efficiently recycled back to its active form for reuse.

In the intestines, vitamin C protects iron from oxidation and so promotes its absorption. Once in the blood, vitamin C protects sensitive blood constituents from oxidation, reduces tissue inflammation, and helps to maintain the body's supply of vitamin E by

---

[§§]The physician was James Lind.

scurvy　the vitamin C–deficiency disease.

ascorbic acid　one of the active forms of vitamin C (the other is *dehydroascorbic* acid); an antioxidant nutrient.

collagen (COLL-a-jen)　the chief protein of most connective tissues, including scars, ligaments, and tendons, and the underlying matrix on which bones and teeth are built.

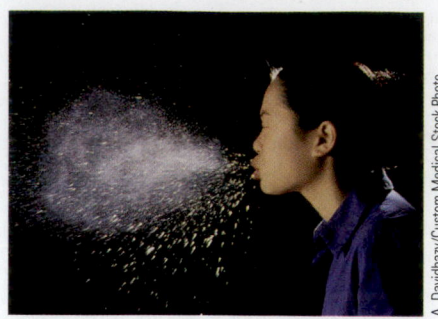

Can vitamin C ease the suffering of a person with a cold?

protecting it and recycling it to its active form. The antioxidant roles of vitamin C are the focus of extensive study, especially in relation to chronic disease prevention. So far, research has yielded only disappointing results: oral vitamin C supplements are useless against heart disease, cancer, and other diseases unless they are prescribed to treat a deficiency.

In test tubes, a high concentration of vitamin C has the opposite effect from antioxidants; that is, it acts as a **prooxidant** by activating oxidizing elements, such as iron and copper.[55] This might happen in people who take high doses, too. The opposing effects of vitamin C suggest that adequate vitamin C, but not excess, may be best for chronic disease prevention.[56]

Can Vitamin C Supplements Cure a Cold?

Many people hold that vitamin C supplements can prevent or cure a common cold, but research most often fails to support this long-lived belief.[57] In 29 trials of over 11,300 people, no relationship emerged between routine vitamin C supplementation and cold prevention. A few studies do report other modest potential benefits—fewer colds, fewer ill days, and shorter duration of severe symptoms, especially for those exposed to physical and environmental stresses. *Sufficient* vitamin C intake is critically important to certain white blood cells of the immune system that act as primary defenders against infection.[58]

Experimentally, supplements of at least 1 gram of vitamin C per day and often closer to 2 grams (the Tolerable Upper Intake Level and not recommended) seem to reduce blood histamine. Anyone who has ever had a cold knows the effects of histamine: sneezing, a runny or stuffy nose, and swollen sinuses. In drug-like doses, vitamin C may mimic a weak antihistamine drug, but studies vary in dosing and conditions; drawing conclusions is therefore difficult.

One other effect of taking pills might also provide relief. In one vitamin C study, some experimental subjects received a placebo but were told they were receiving vitamin C. These subjects reported having fewer colds than the group who had in fact received the vitamin but who thought they were receiving the placebo. At work was the healing effect of faith in a medical treatment—the placebo effect.

Deficiency Symptoms and Intakes

Figure 7–9

Scurvy Symptoms—Gums and Skin

Vitamin C deficiency causes the breakdown of collagen, which supports the teeth.

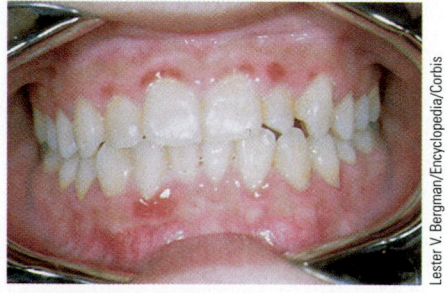

Small pinpoint hemorrhages (red spots) appear in the skin, indicating that invisible internal bleeding may also be occurring.

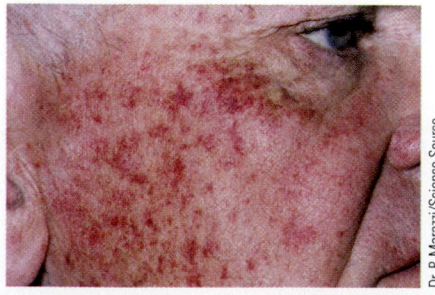

Most of the symptoms of scurvy can be attributed to the breakdown of collagen in the absence of vitamin C: loss of appetite, growth cessation, tenderness to touch, weakness, bleeding gums (shown in Figure 7–9), loose teeth, swollen ankles and wrists, and tiny red spots in the skin where blood has leaked out of capillaries (also shown in the figure). One symptom, anemia, reflects an important role worth repeating—vitamin C helps the body to absorb and use iron. Table 7–11 at the end of the chapter summarizes deficiency symptoms and other information about vitamin C.

Vitamin C is listed among the nutrients of national concern because U.S. intakes may fall short of the DRI recommendations. Especially people who smoke or have low incomes are at risk for deficiency. The disease scurvy is seldom seen today except in a few elderly people, people addicted to alcohol or other drugs, sick people in hospitals, and a few infants who are fed only cow's milk.[59] Breast milk and infant formula supply enough vitamin C, but infants who are fed cow's milk and receive no vitamin C in formula, fruit juice, or other outside sources are at risk. As for the elderly, poor appetites and low intakes of fruits and vegetables often lead to low vitamin C intakes.

Vitamin C Toxicity

The easy availability of vitamin C in pill form and the publication of books recommending vitamin C to prevent and cure colds and cancer have led thousands of people to take huge doses of vitamin C. These "volunteer" subjects enabled researchers to study potential adverse effects of large vitamin C doses. One effect observed with a 2-gram dose is alteration of the insulin response to carbohydrate in people with otherwise normal glucose tolerances. People taking anticlotting medications may unwittingly counteract the drug's effect if they also take massive doses of vitamin C. Those with kidney disease, a tendency toward gout, or abnormal vitamin C metabolism are prone to forming

prooxidant a compound that triggers reactions involving oxygen.

kidney stones if they take large doses of vitamin C.[60] Vitamin C supplements in any dosage may be unwise for people with an overload of iron in the body because vitamin C increases iron absorption from the intestine and releases iron from storage. Other adverse effects are mild, including digestive upsets, such as nausea, abdominal cramps, excessive gas, and diarrhea.

The safe range of vitamin C intakes seems to be broad, from the absolute minimum of 10 milligrams a day to the Tolerable Upper Intake Level of 2,000 milligrams (2 grams), as Figure 7–10 demonstrates. Doses approaching 10 grams can be expected to be unsafe. Vitamin C from food is always safe.

Vitamin C Recommendations

The adult DRI intake recommendation for vitamin C is 90 milligrams for men and 75 milligrams for women. These amounts are far higher than the 10 or so milligrams per day needed to prevent the symptoms of scurvy. In fact, they are close to the amount at which the body's pool of vitamin C is full to overflowing: about 100 milligrams per day.

Tobacco use introduces oxidants that deplete the body's vitamin C. Thus, smokers generally have lower blood vitamin C levels than nonsmokers. Even "passive smokers" who live and work with smokers and those who regularly chew tobacco need more vitamin C than others. Intake recommendations for smokers are set high, at 125 milligrams for men and 110 milligrams for women, in order to maintain blood levels comparable to those of nonsmokers. Importantly, vitamin C cannot reverse other damage caused by tobacco use. Physical stressors, including infections, burns, fever, toxic heavy metals such as lead, and certain medications, also increase the body's use of vitamin C.

Vitamin C Food Sources

Fruits and vegetables are the foods to remember for vitamin C, as Snapshot 7–5 shows. A cup of orange juice at breakfast, a salad for lunch, and a stalk of broccoli and a potato at dinner easily provide 300 milligrams, making pills unnecessary. People commonly identify orange juice as a source of vitamin C, but they often overlook other rich sources that may be lower in calories.

Vitamin C is vulnerable to heat and destroyed by oxygen, so for maximum vitamin C consumers should treat their fruits and vegetables gently. Losses occurring when a food is cut, processed, and stored may be large enough to reduce vitamin C's activity in the body. Fresh, raw, and quickly cooked fruits, vegetables, and juices retain the most vitamin C, and they should be stored properly and consumed within a week after purchase. Table 7–8 (p. 264) gives tips for maximizing vitamin retention in foods.

Because of their enormous popularity, white potatoes contribute significantly to vitamin C intakes, despite providing less than 10 milligrams per half-cup serving. The sweet potato, often ignored in favor of its paler cousin, is a gold mine of nutrients: a single half-cup serving provides about a third of many people's recommended intake for vitamin C, in addition to its lavish contribution of vitamin A.

KEY POINTS

- Vitamin C maintains collagen, protects against infection, acts as an antioxidant, and aids iron absorption.
- Ample vitamin C can be easily obtained from foods.

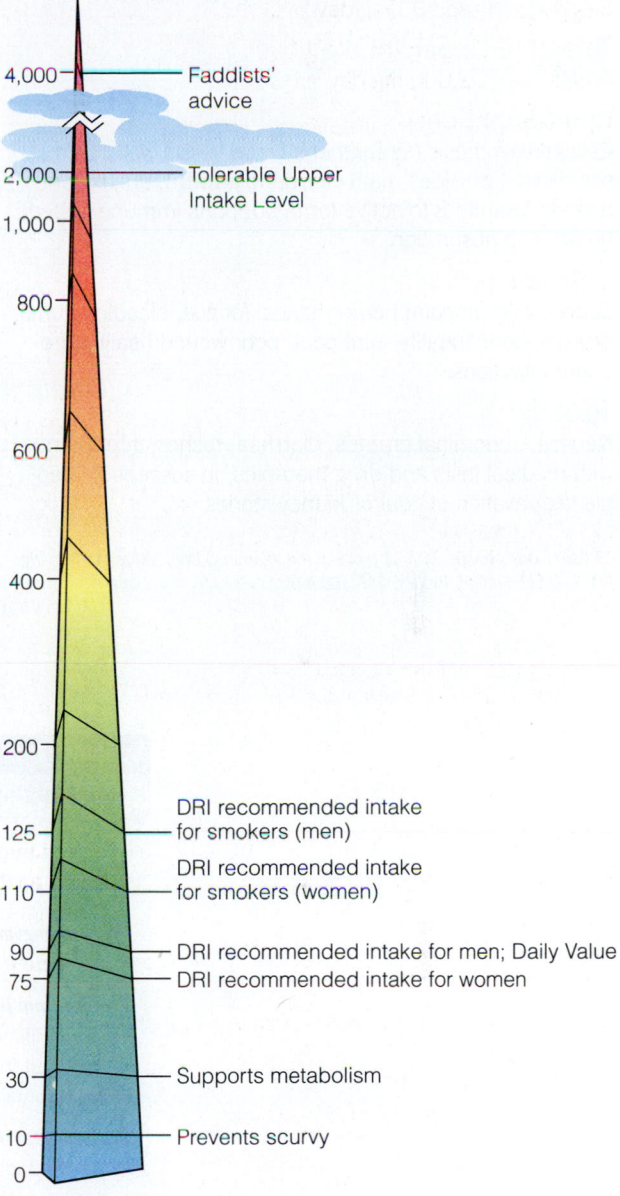

Figure 7–10

Vitamin C Tower of Recommendations

The DRI Tolerable Upper Intake Level for vitamin C is set at 2,000 mg (2 g)/day. Only 10 mg/day prevents scurvy.

4,000 — Faddists' advice

2,000 — Tolerable Upper Intake Level

1,000

800

600

400

200

125 — DRI recommended intake for smokers (men)

110 — DRI recommended intake for smokers (women)

90 — DRI recommended intake for men; Daily Value

75 — DRI recommended intake for women

30 — Supports metabolism

10 — Prevents scurvy

0

DRI Recommended Intakes
Men: 90 mg/day
Women: 75 mg/day
Smokers: add 35 mg/day

Tolerable Upper Intake Level
Adults: 2,000 mg/day

Chief Functions
Collagen synthesis (strengthens blood vessel walls, forms scar tissue, provides matrix for bone growth), antioxidant, restores vitamin E to active form, supports immune system, boosts iron absorption

Deficiency
Scurvy, with pinpoint hemorrhages, fatigue, bleeding gums, bruises; bone fragility, joint pain; poor wound healing, frequent infections

Toxicity
Nausea, abdominal cramps, diarrhea; rashes; interference with medical tests and drug therapies; in susceptible people, aggravation of gout or kidney stones

These foods provide 10% or more of the vitamin C Daily Value in a serving. For a 2,000-cal diet, the DV is 90 mg/day.

Good Sources*

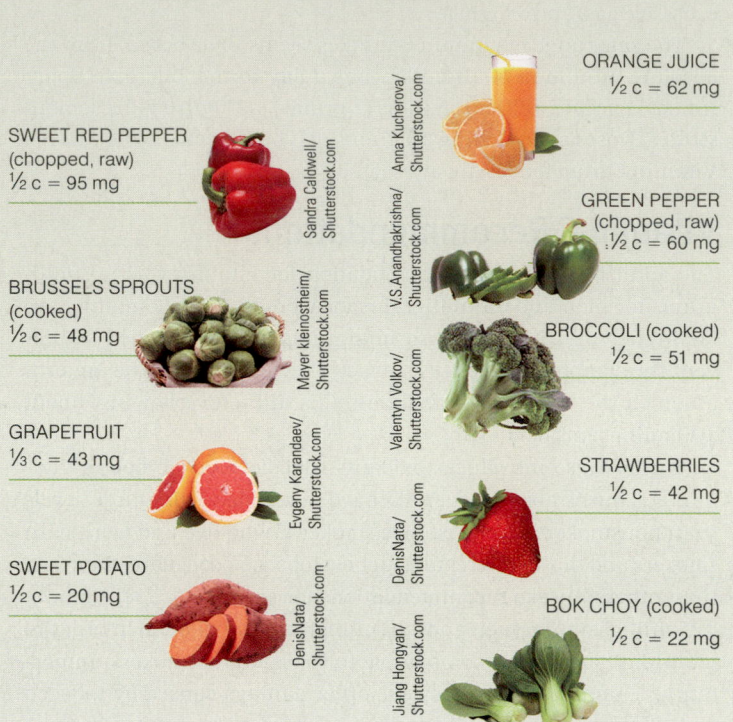

SWEET RED PEPPER (chopped, raw)
½ c = 95 mg
Sandra Caldwell//Shutterstock.com

BRUSSELS SPROUTS (cooked)
½ c = 48 mg
Mayer Kleinostheim/Shutterstock.com

GRAPEFRUIT
⅓ c = 43 mg
Evgeny Karandaev/Shutterstock.com

SWEET POTATO
½ c = 20 mg
DenisNata/Shutterstock.com

ORANGE JUICE
½ c = 62 mg
Anna Kucherova/Shutterstock.com

GREEN PEPPER (chopped, raw)
½ c = 60 mg
V.S. Anandhakrishna/Shutterstock.com

BROCCOLI (cooked)
½ c = 51 mg
Valentyn Volkov/Shutterstock.com

STRAWBERRIES
½ c = 42 mg
DenisNata/Shutterstock.com

BOK CHOY (cooked)
½ c = 22 mg
Jiang Hongyan/Shutterstock.com

Table 7–8
Minimizing Vitamin Losses

Each of these tactics saves a small percentage of the vitamins in foods but, repeated each day, can add up to a significant amount over time.

Prevent enzymatic destruction:
- Refrigerate most fruits, vegetables, and juices to slow breakdown of vitamins.

Protect from light and air:
- Store milk and enriched grain products in opaque containers to protect riboflavin.
- Store cut fruits and vegetables in the refrigerator in airtight wrappers; reseal opened juice containers before refrigerating.

Prevent heat destruction or losses in water:
- Wash intact fruits and vegetables before cutting or peeling to prevent vitamin losses during washing.
- Cook fruits and vegetables in a microwave oven, or quickly stir fry, or steam them over a small amount of water to preserve heat-sensitive vitamins and to prevent vitamin loss in cooking water. Recapture dissolved vitamins by using cooking water for soups, stews, or gravies.
- Avoid high temperatures and long cooking times.

The B Vitamins in Unison

LO 7.9   Discuss the collective roles of B vitamins in metabolism and the effects of their deficiencies.

The B vitamins function as part of coenzymes. A **coenzyme** is a small molecule that combines with an enzyme (described in Chapter 6) and activates it. Figure 7–11

coenzyme (co-EN-zime) a small molecule that works with an enzyme to promote the enzyme's activity. Many coenzymes have B vitamins as part of their structure (*co* means "with").

shows how a coenzyme enables an enzyme to do its job. Sometimes the vitamin part of a coenzyme forms the active site of the enzyme where the chemical reaction takes place. The substance to be worked on is attracted to the active site and snaps into place, enabling the reaction to proceed instantaneously. The shape of each enzyme predestines it to accomplish just one kind of job. Without its coenzyme, however, the enzyme is as useless as a car without wheels.

Each of the B vitamins has its own special nature, and the amount of detail known about each one is overwhelming. To simplify things, this introduction describes the teamwork of the B vitamins and emphasizes the consequences of deficiencies. Many of these nutrients are so interdependent that it is sometimes difficult to tell which vitamin deficiency is the cause of which symptom; the presence or absence of one affects the absorption, metabolism, and excretion of others. Later sections present a few details about these vitamins as individuals.

B Vitamin Roles in Metabolism

Figure 7–12 shows some body organs and tissues in which the B vitamins help the body metabolize carbohydrates, lipids, and amino acids. The purpose of the figure is not to present a detailed account of metabolism but to give you an impression of where the B vitamins work together with enzymes in the metabolism of energy nutrients and in the creation of new cells.

Many people mistakenly believe that B vitamins supply the body with energy. They do not, at least not directly. The B vitamins are "helpers." The energy-yielding nutrients—carbohydrate, fat, and protein—give the body fuel for energy; the B vitamins *help* the body to use that fuel. More specifically, active forms of five of the B vitamins—thiamin, riboflavin, niacin, pantothenic acid, and biotin—participate in the release of energy from carbohydrate, fat, and protein. Vitamin B_6 helps the body use amino acids to synthesize proteins; the body then puts the protein to work in many ways—to build new tissues, to make hormones, to fight infections, or to serve as fuel for energy, to name only a few.

Folate and vitamin B_{12} help cells to multiply, which is especially important to cells with short life spans that must replace themselves rapidly. Such cells include both the red blood cells (which live for about 120 days) and the cells that line the digestive tract (which replace themselves every 3 days). These cells absorb and deliver energy to all the others. In short, each and every B vitamin is involved, directly or indirectly, in energy metabolism.

B Vitamin Deficiencies

As long as B vitamins are present, their presence is not felt. Only when they are missing does their absence manifest itself in a lack of energy and a multitude of other symptoms, as you can imagine after looking at Figure 7–12. The reactions by which B vitamins facilitate energy release take place in every cell, and no cell can do its work without energy. Thus, in a B vitamin deficiency, every cell is affected. Among the symptoms of B vitamin deficiencies are nausea, severe exhaustion, irritability, depression, forgetfulness, loss of appetite and weight, pain in muscles, impairment of the immune response, loss of control of the limbs, abnormal heart action, severe skin problems, swollen red tongue, cracked skin at the corners of the mouth, and teary or bloodshot eyes. Figure 7–13 (p. 267) shows two of these signs. Because cell renewal depends on energy and protein, which, in turn, depend on the B vitamins, the digestive tract and the blood are invariably damaged. In children, full recovery may be impossible. In the case of a thiamin deficiency during growth, permanent brain damage can result.

In academic discussions of the B vitamins, different sets of deficiency symptoms are given for each one. Such clear-cut sets of symptoms are found only in laboratory animals that have been fed fabricated diets that lack just one vitamin. In real life, a deficiency of any one B vitamin seldom shows up by itself because people don't eat nutrients singly; they eat foods that contain mixtures of nutrients. A diet low in one B vitamin is likely low in other nutrients, too. If treatment involves giving wholesome

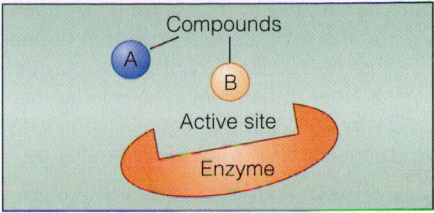
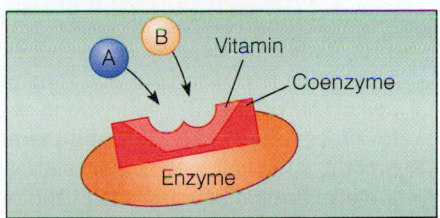
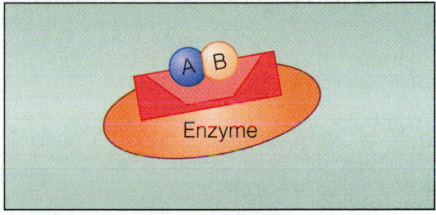
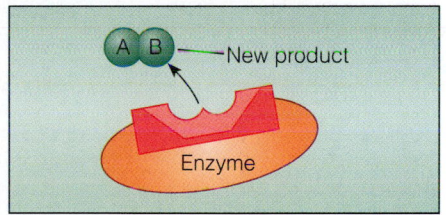

Figure 7–11

Coenzyme Action

Without the coenzyme, compounds A and B don't respond to the enzyme.

With the coenzyme in place, compounds A and B are attracted to the active site on the enzyme, and they react.

The reaction is completed with the formation of a new product. In this case, the product is AB.

The product AB is released.

Figure 7–12

Some Roles of the B Vitamins in Metabolism: Examples

The purpose of this figure is to show a few of the many tissue functions that depend on a host of B vitamin–containing enzymes working together in harmony. The B vitamins work in every cell, and this figure displays less than a thousandth of what they actually do.

Every B vitamin is part of one or more coenzymes that make possible the body's chemical work. For example, the niacin, thiamin, and riboflavin coenzymes are important in the energy pathways. The folate and vitamin B_{12} coenzymes are necessary for making RNA and DNA and thus new cells. The vitamin B_6 coenzyme is necessary for processing amino acids and therefore protein. Although many other relationships are also critical to metabolism, this figure does not attempt to teach intricate biochemical pathways or names of B vitamin–containing enzymes.

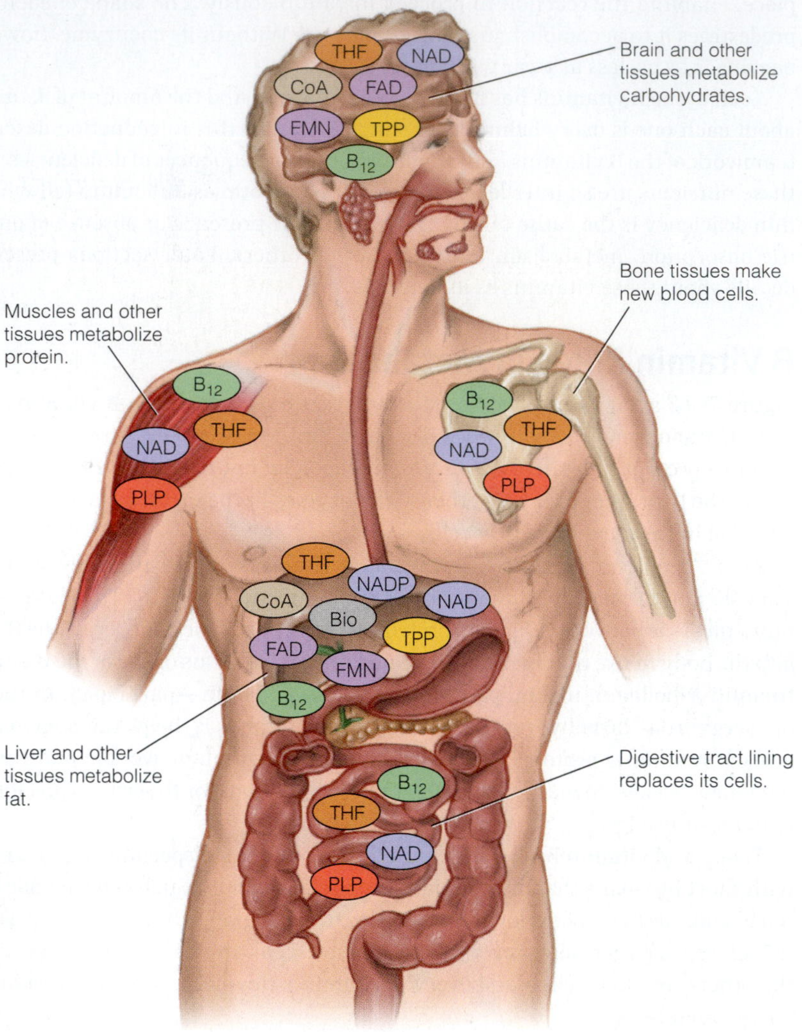

Key:

Coenzyme		Vitamin
TPP	=	thiamin
FAD FMN	=	riboflavin
NAD NADP	=	niacin
PLP	=	vitamin B_6
THF	=	folate
CoA	=	pantothenic acid
Bio	=	biotin
B_{12}	=	vitamin B_{12}

Brain and other tissues metabolize carbohydrates.

Bone tissues make new blood cells.

Muscles and other tissues metabolize protein.

Liver and other tissues metabolize fat.

Digestive tract lining replaces its cells.

food rather than a single supplement, subtler deficiencies and impairments will be corrected along with the major one. The symptoms of B vitamin deficiencies and toxicities are listed in Table 7–10 at the end of the chapter.

KEY POINTS

- As part of coenzymes, the B vitamins help enzymes in every cell do numerous jobs.
- B vitamins help metabolize carbohydrate, fat, and protein.

The B Vitamins as Individuals

LO 7.10 Discuss the roles, the effects of deficiencies and toxicities, and food sources of each of the eight B vitamins.

Although the B vitamins all work as part of coenzymes and share other characteristics, each B vitamin has special qualities. The next sections provide a few details.

Thiamin

Thiamin plays a critical role in the energy metabolism of all cells. Thiamin also occupies a special site on nerve cell membranes. Consequently, nerve processes and their responding tissues, the muscles, depend heavily on thiamin.

thiamin (THIGH-uh-min) a B vitamin involved in the body's use of fuels.

beriberi (berry-berry) the thiamin-deficiency disease; characterized by loss of sensation in the hands and feet, muscular weakness, advancing paralysis, and abnormal heart action.

Thiamin Deficiency The classic thiamin-deficiency disease, **beriberi**, was first observed in East Asia, where rice provided 80 to 90 percent of the total calories most people consumed and was therefore their principal source of thiamin. When the custom of polishing rice (removing its brown coat, which contained the thiamin) became widespread, beriberi swept through the population like an epidemic. Scientists wasted years of effort hunting for a microbial cause of beriberi before they realized that the cause was not something present in the environment but something absent from it. Figure 7–14 (p. 268) depicts beriberi and describes its two forms.

Just before the year 1900, an observant physician working in a prison in East Asia discovered that beriberi could be cured with proper diet. The physician noticed that the chickens at the prison had developed a stiffness and weakness similar to that of the prisoners who had beriberi. The chickens were being fed the rice left on prisoners' plates. When the rice bran, which had been discarded in the kitchen, was given to the chickens, their paralysis was cured. The physician met resistance when he tried to feed the rice bran, the "garbage," to the prisoners, but it worked—it produced a miracle cure like those described at the beginning of the chapter. Later, extracts of rice bran were used to prevent infantile beriberi; still later, thiamin was identified.

In developed countries today, alcohol abuse often leads to a severe form of thiamin deficiency, Wernicke-Korsakoff syndrome, defined in Controversy 3. Alcohol contributes energy but carries almost no nutrients with it and often displaces food from the diet. In addition, alcohol impairs absorption of thiamin from the digestive tract and hastens its excretion in the urine, tripling the risk of deficiency. The syndrome is characterized by symptoms almost indistinguishable from alcohol abuse itself: apathy, irritability, mental confusion, disorientation, memory loss, jerky eye movements, and a staggering gait (listed in Snapshot 7–6).[61] Unlike alcohol toxicity, the syndrome responds quickly to an injection of thiamin.

Recommended Intakes and Food Sources The DRI committee set the thiamin intake recommendation at 1.2 milligrams per day for men and at 1.1 milligrams per day for women. Pregnancy and lactation demand somewhat more thiamin

Figure 7–13.
B Vitamin–Deficiency Symptoms: Tongue and Mouth

The normally rough and bumpy tongue becomes smooth and swollen, and the corners of the mouth become inflamed and cracked.

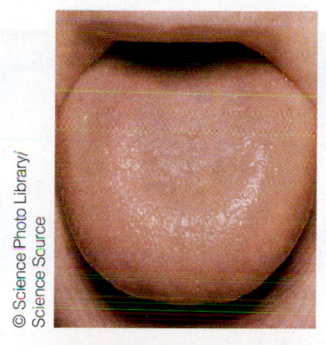

© Science Photo Library/ Science Source

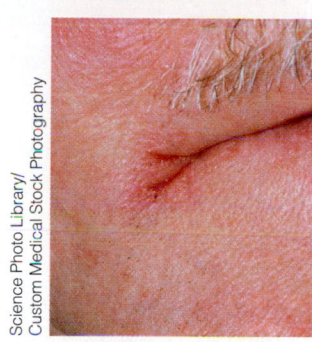

Science Photo Library/ Custom Medical Stock Photography

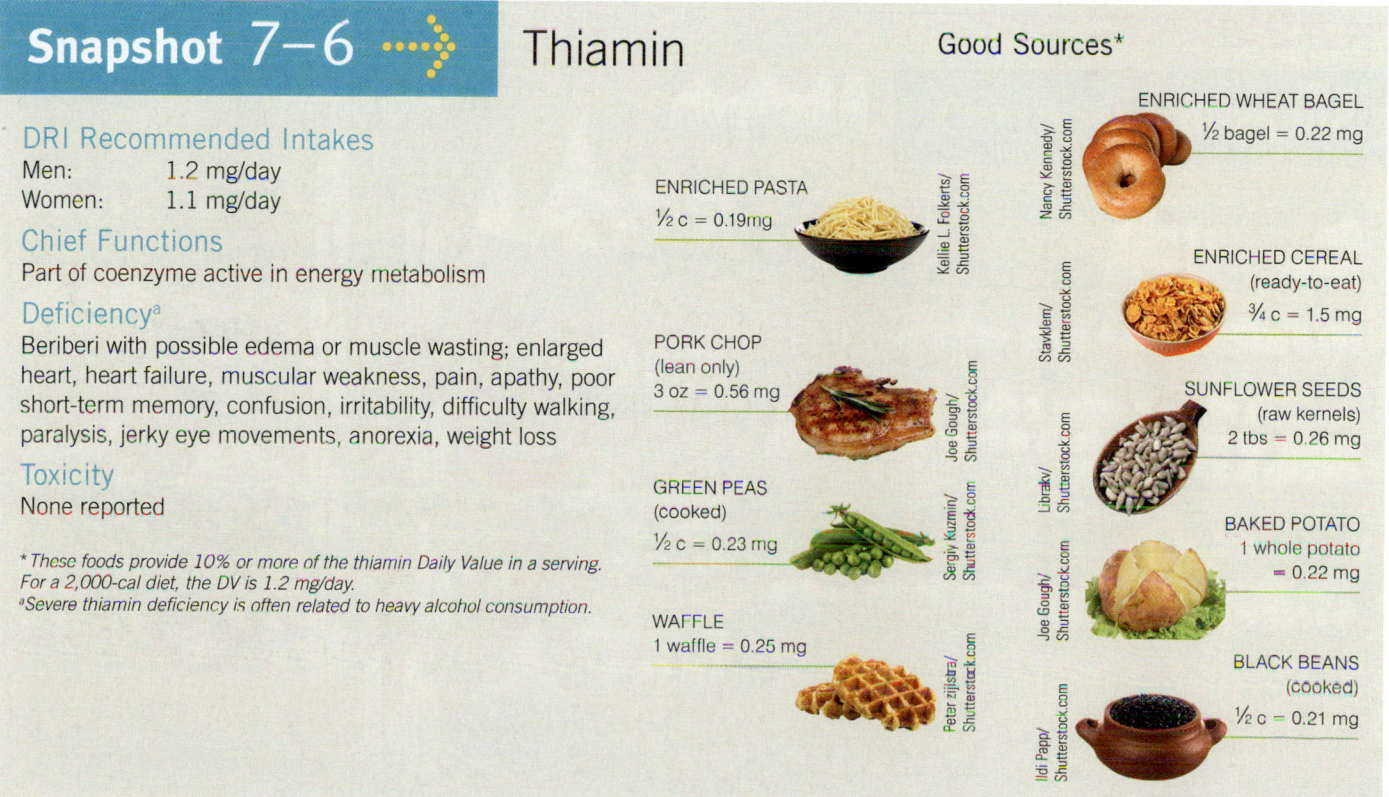

Snapshot 7–6 ···⟶ Thiamin

Good Sources*

DRI Recommended Intakes
Men: 1.2 mg/day
Women: 1.1 mg/day

Chief Functions
Part of coenzyme active in energy metabolism

Deficiency[a]
Beriberi with possible edema or muscle wasting; enlarged heart, heart failure, muscular weakness, pain, apathy, poor short-term memory, confusion, irritability, difficulty walking, paralysis, jerky eye movements, anorexia, weight loss

Toxicity
None reported

*These foods provide 10% or more of the thiamin Daily Value in a serving. For a 2,000-cal diet, the DV is 1.2 mg/day.
[a]Severe thiamin deficiency is often related to heavy alcohol consumption.

ENRICHED PASTA
½ c = 0.19mg
Kellie L. Folkerts/ Shutterstock.com

PORK CHOP (lean only)
3 oz = 0.56 mg
Joe Gough/ Shutterstock.com

GREEN PEAS (cooked)
½ c = 0.23 mg
Sergiy Kuzmin/ Shutterstock.com

WAFFLE
1 waffle = 0.25 mg
Peter zijlstra/ Shutterstock.com

ENRICHED WHEAT BAGEL
½ bagel = 0.22 mg
Nancy Kennedy/ Shutterstock.com

ENRICHED CEREAL (ready-to-eat)
¾ c = 1.5 mg
Stavklem/ Shutterstock.com

SUNFLOWER SEEDS (raw kernels)
2 tbs = 0.26 mg
Librakv/ Shutterstock.com

BAKED POTATO
1 whole potato = 0.22 mg
Joe Gough/ Shutterstock.com

BLACK BEANS (cooked)
½ c = 0.21 mg
Ildi Papp/ Shutterstock.com

Figure 7–14
Beriberi

Beriberi takes two forms: wet beriberi, characterized by edema (fluid accumulation), and dry beriberi, without edema. This person's ankle retains the imprint of the physician's thumb, showing the edema of wet beriberi.

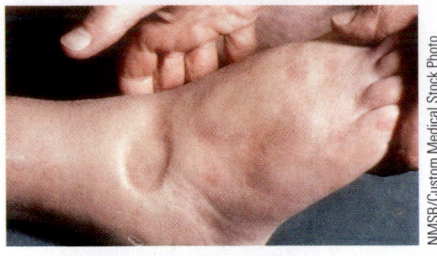

NMSB/Custom Medical Stock Photo

riboflavin (RIBE-o-flay-vin) a B vitamin active in the body's energy-releasing mechanisms.

(see the DRI, inside front cover, page B). Thiamin occurs in small amounts in many nutritious foods. Ham and other pork products, sunflower seeds, enriched and whole-grain cereals, and legumes are especially rich in thiamin. If you keep empty-calorie foods to a minimum and focus your meals on nutritious foods each day, you will easily meet your thiamin needs.

KEY POINTS

- Thiamin works in energy metabolism and in nerve cells.
- The thiamin deficiency disease is beriberi.
- Many foods supply small amounts of thiamin.

Riboflavin Roles

Like thiamin, **riboflavin** plays a role in the energy metabolism of all cells.[62] When thiamin is deficient, riboflavin may be lacking, too, but its deficiency symptoms, such as cracks at the corners of the mouth, sore throat, or hypersensitivity to light, may go undetected because those of thiamin deficiency are more severe. Worldwide, riboflavin deficiency has been documented among children whose eating patterns lack milk products and meats, and researchers suspect that it occurs among some U.S. elderly as well. An eating pattern that remedies riboflavin deficiency invariably contains some thiamin and so clears up both deficiencies.

Riboflavin recommendations are listed in Snapshot 7–7. People in this country obtain over a quarter of their riboflavin from enriched breads, cereals, pasta, and other grain products, while milk and milk products supply another 20 percent. Certain vegetables, eggs, and meats contribute most of the rest (see Snapshot 7–7). Ultraviolet light and irradiation destroy riboflavin. For these reasons, milk is sold in cardboard or opaque plastic containers, and precautions are taken if milk is processed by irradiation. Riboflavin is heat stable, so cooking does not destroy it.

KEY POINTS

- Riboflavin works in energy metabolism.
- Riboflavin is destroyed by ordinary light.

Snapshot 7–7   Riboflavin

Good Sources*

DRI Recommended Intakes
Men: 1.3 mg/day
Women: 1.1 mg/day

Chief Functions
Part of coenzyme active in energy metabolism

Deficiency
Cracks and redness at corners of mouth; painful, smooth, purplish red tongue; sore throat; inflamed eyes and eyelids, sensitivity to light; skin rashes

Toxicity
None reported

*These foods provide 10% or more of the riboflavin Daily Value in a serving. For a 2,000-cal diet, the DV is 1.3 mg/day.

BEEF LIVER (cooked)
3 oz = 2.9 mg
Serghei Starus/Shutterstock.com

COTTAGE CHEESE
1 c = 0.38 mg
Africa Studio/Shutterstock.com

ENRICHED CEREAL (ready-to-eat)
½ c = 1.7 mg
StockHem/Shutterstock.com

SPINACH (cooked)
½ c = 0.21 mg
Daniel Gilbey Photography-My portfolio/Shutterstock.com

MILK
1 c = 0.45 mg
Roxana Bashyrova/Shutterstock.com

YOGURT (plain)
1 c = 0.57 mg
Gyorgy Barna/Shutterstock.com

PORK CHOP (lean only)
3 oz = 0.23 mg
Joe Gough/Shutterstock.com

MUSHROOMS (cooked)
½ c = 0.23 mg
Yasonya/Shutterstock.com

Niacin

The vitamin **niacin**, like thiamin and riboflavin, participates in the energy metabolism of every cell. Its absence causes serious illness.

Niacin Deficiency The niacin-deficiency disease **pellagra** appeared in Europe in the 1700s when corn from the New World became a staple food. During the early 1900s in the United States, pellagra was devastating lives throughout the South and Midwest. Hundreds of thousands of pellagra victims were thought to be suffering from a contagious disease until this dietary deficiency was identified. The disease still occurs among poorly nourished people living in urban slums and particularly among those with alcohol addiction.[63] Pellagra is also still common in parts of Africa and Asia.[64] Its symptoms are known as the four "Ds": diarrhea, dermatitis, dementia, and, ultimately, death.

Figure 7–15 shows the skin disorder (dermatitis) associated with pellagra. For comparison, Figure 7–3 (p. 246) and Figure 7–18 (p. 274) show skin disorders associated with vitamin A and vitamin B$_6$ deficiencies, respectively. These figures serve as reminders that any nutrient deficiency affects the skin as well as all other cells; the skin just happens to be the organ you can see. Table 7–10 at the end of the chapter lists the symptoms of niacin deficiency.

Niacin Toxicity and Pharmacology For over 50 years, large doses of a form of niacin have been prescribed to help improve blood lipids associated with cardiovascular disease.[65]*** Its use is limited, however, by the most common side effect of large doses of niacin, the "niacin flush," a dilation of the capillaries of the skin with perceptible tingling that can be painful.[66] Today, effective, well-tolerated drugs are often used instead, and scientists question the effectiveness of niacin and debate its utility.[67] Reported risks from large doses of niacin include liver injury, digestive upset, impaired glucose tolerance, serious infection, muscle weakness, and, rarely, vision disturbances.[68] Anyone considering taking large doses of niacin on their own should instead consult a physician who can prescribe safe, effective alternatives.[69]

Niacin Recommendations and Food Sources Niacin recommendations are listed in Snapshot 7–8 (p. 270). The key nutrient that prevents pellagra is niacin, but any protein containing sufficient amounts of the amino acid tryptophan will serve in its place. Tryptophan, which is abundant in almost all proteins (but is limited in the protein of corn), is converted to niacin in the body, and it is possible to cure pellagra by administering tryptophan alone. Thus, a person eating adequate protein (as most people in developed nations do) will not be deficient in niacin. The amount of niacin in a diet is stated in terms of **niacin equivalents (NE)**, a measure that takes available tryptophan into account.

Early workers seeking the cause of pellagra observed that well-fed people never got it. From there, the researchers defined an eating pattern that reliably produced the disease—one of cornmeal, salted pork fat, and molasses. Corn not only is low in protein but also lacks tryptophan. Salt pork is almost pure fat and contains too little protein to compensate, and molasses is virtually protein-free. Snapshot 7–8 shows some good food sources of niacin.

KEY POINTS

- Niacin deficiency causes the disease pellagra, which can be prevented by adequate niacin intake or adequate dietary protein.
- The amino acid tryptophan can be converted to niacin in the body.

Folate

To make new cells, tissues must have the vitamin **folate**. Each new cell must be equipped with new genetic material—copies of the parent cell's DNA—and folate

***The form of niacin is nicotinic acid.

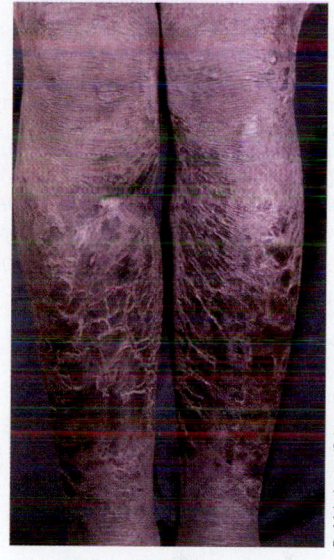

niacin a B vitamin needed in energy metabolism. Niacin can be eaten preformed or made in the body from tryptophan, one of the amino acids. Other forms of niacin are *nicotinic acid*, *niacinamide*, and *nicotinamide*.

pellagra (pell-AY-gra) the niacin-deficiency disease (*pellis* means "skin"; *agra* means "rough"). Symptoms include the "4 Ds": diarrhea, dermatitis, dementia, and, ultimately, death.

niacin equivalents (NE) the amount of niacin present in food, including the niacin that can theoretically be made from its precursor tryptophan that is present in the food.

folate (FOH-late) a B vitamin that acts as part of a coenzyme important in the manufacture of new cells. The form added to foods and supplements is *folic acid*.

DRI Recommended Intakes
Men: 16 mg/day[a]
Women: 14 mg/day

Tolerable Upper Intake Level
Adults: 35 mg/day

Chief Functions
Part of coenzymes needed in energy metabolism

Deficiency
Pellagra, characterized by flaky skin rash (dermatitis) where exposed to sunlight; mental depression, apathy, fatigue, loss of memory, headache; diarrhea, abdominal pain, vomiting; swollen, smooth, bright red or black tongue

Toxicity
Painful flush, hives, and rash ("niacin flush"); excessive sweating; blurred vision; liver damage, impaired glucose tolerance

* These foods provide 10% or more of the niacin Daily Value in a serving. For a 2,000-cal diet, the DV is 16 mg/day. The DV values are for preformed niacin, not niacin equivalents.
[a]Niacin DRI recommended intakes are expressed in niacin equivalents (NE); the Tolerable Upper Intake Level refers to preformed niacin.

Good Sources*

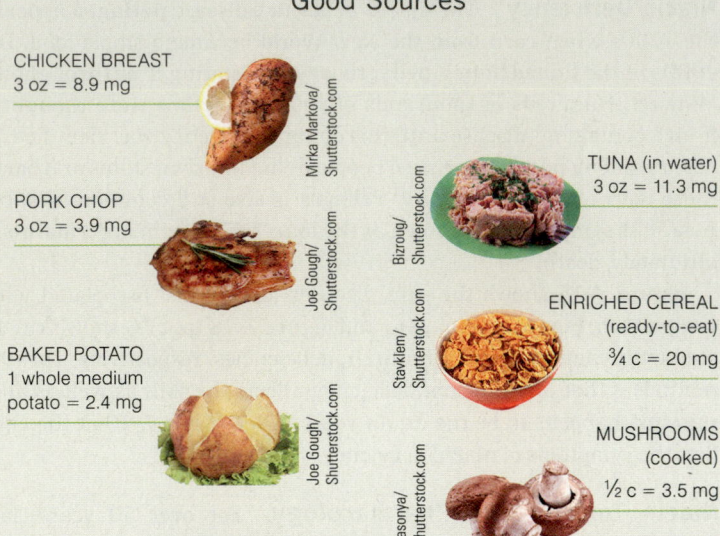

CHICKEN BREAST
3 oz = 8.9 mg
Mirka Markova/Shutterstock.com

PORK CHOP
3 oz = 3.9 mg
Joe Gough/Shutterstock.com

BAKED POTATO
1 whole medium potato = 2.4 mg
Joe Gough/Shutterstock.com

TUNA (in water)
3 oz = 11.3 mg
Bizroug/Shutterstock.com

ENRICHED CEREAL
(ready-to-eat)
¾ c = 20 mg
Stawklem/Shutterstock.com

MUSHROOMS
(cooked)
½ c = 3.5 mg
Yasonya/Shutterstock.com

helps to synthesize DNA. Folate also participates in the metabolism of vitamin B$_{12}$ and several amino acids.[70]

Folate Deficiency   Folate deficiencies may result from following an eating pattern that is too low in folate or from experiencing illnesses that impair folate absorption, increase folate excretion, require medication that interacts with folate, or otherwise increase the body's folate need. However it occurs, folate deficiency has wide-reaching effects.

Immature red and white blood cells and the cells of the digestive tract divide most rapidly and therefore are most vulnerable to folate deficiency. Deficiencies of folate cause anemia, diminished immunity, and abnormal digestive function. The anemia of folate deficiency is related to the anemia of vitamin B$_{12}$ malabsorption because the two vitamins work as teammates in producing red blood cells. Research links a chronic deficiency of folate with greater risks for developing breast cancer (particularly among women who drink alcohol), prostate cancer, and other cancers; research also suggests that high doses of folic acid from supplements may speed up cancer progression.[71]

Of all the vitamins, folate is most likely to interact with medications. Many drugs, including antacids and aspirin and its relatives, have been shown to interfere with the body's use of folate. Occasional use of these drugs to relieve headache or upset stomach presents no concern, but frequent users may need to pay attention to their folate intakes. These include people with chronic pain or ulcers who rely heavily on aspirin or antacids, as well as those who smoke or take oral contraceptives or anticonvulsant medications.

Birth Defects and Folate Enrichment   By consuming enough folate both before and during pregnancy, a woman can reduce her child's risk of having one of the devastating birth defects known as **neural tube defects (NTD)**. NTD range from slight problems in the spine to mental retardation, severely diminished brain size, and death

neural tube defects (NTD) abnormalities of the brain and spinal cord apparent at birth and associated with low folate intake in women before and during pregnancy. The neural tube is the earliest brain and spinal cord structure formed during gestation. Also defined in Chapter 13.

shortly after birth. NTD arise in the first days or weeks of pregnancy, long before most women suspect that they are pregnant. Adequate maternal folate may protect against certain other birth defects as well.[72]

Most young women eat too few fruits and vegetables from day to day to supply even half the folate needed to prevent NTD.[73] In the late 1990s, the FDA ordered all enriched grain products such as bread, cereal, rice, and pasta sold in the United States to be fortified with an absorbable synthetic form of folate, *folic acid*. Since this fortification began, typical folate intakes from fortified foods have increased dramatically, along with average blood folate values.[74] Among women of childbearing age, for example, prevalence of low serum folate concentrations dropped from 21 percent before folate fortification was introduced to less than 1 percent afterward. During the same period, the U.S. incidence of NTD dropped by a fourth (see Figure 7–16). Miscarriages and certain other birth defects, such as cleft lip, diminished as well.

Folate Toxicity   A Tolerable Upper Intake Level for synthetic folic acid from supplements and enriched foods is set at 1,000 micrograms a day for adults. The current level of folate fortification of the food supply appears to be safe for most people, but a question remains about the ability of folate to mask a **subclinical deficiency** of vitamin B$_{12}$ (more about this effect later).[75] Any potential for harm from fortification must be weighed against its resounding success in preventing NTD.[76] About 5 percent of the U.S. population exceeds the Tolerable Upper Intake Level for folate, primarily people age 50 and older.[77]

Folate Recommendations   The DRI recommended intake for folate for healthy adults is set at 400 micrograms per day. The DRI committee also advises all women of childbearing age to consume 400 micrograms of *folic acid*, a highly available form of folate, from supplements or enriched foods each day in addition to the folate that occurs naturally in their foods.[78]

Folate Food Sources   The name *folate* is derived from the word *foliage*, and sure enough, leafy green vegetables such as spinach and turnip greens provide abundant

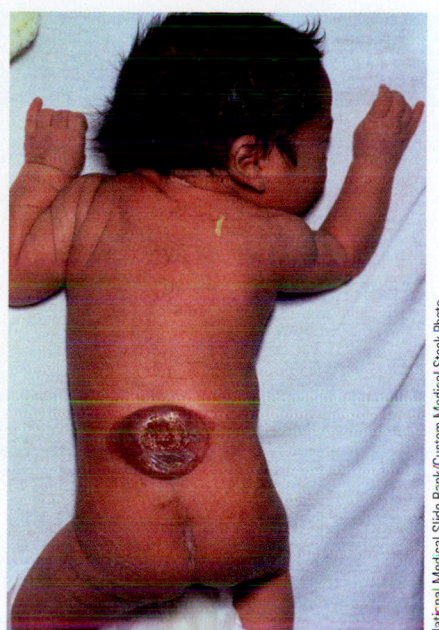

Spina bifida, a neural tube defect characterized by incomplete closure of the bony encasement of the spinal cord. Folate helps to prevent many such defects.

Figure 7–16

Incidence of Neural Tube Defects Before and After Folate Fortification

Neural tube defects declined rapidly following mandatory folate fortification in 1996 and then stabilized at today's levels.

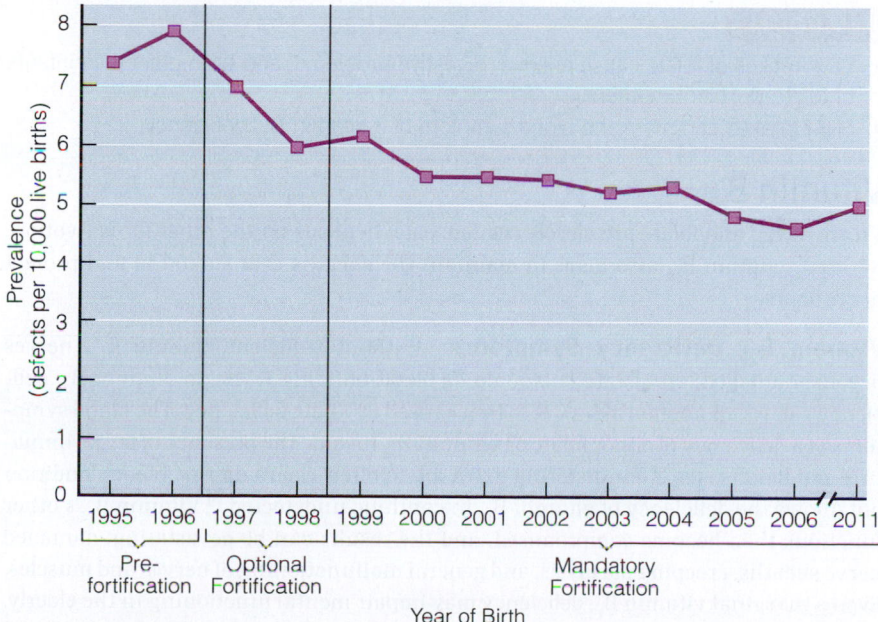

Source: J. Williams and coauthors, Updated estimates of neural tube defects prevented by mandatory folic acid fortification—United States, 1995–2011, Morbidity and Mortality Weekly Report 64 (2015): 1–5.

subclinical deficiency a nutrient deficiency that has no outward clinical symptoms. Also called *marginal deficiency*.

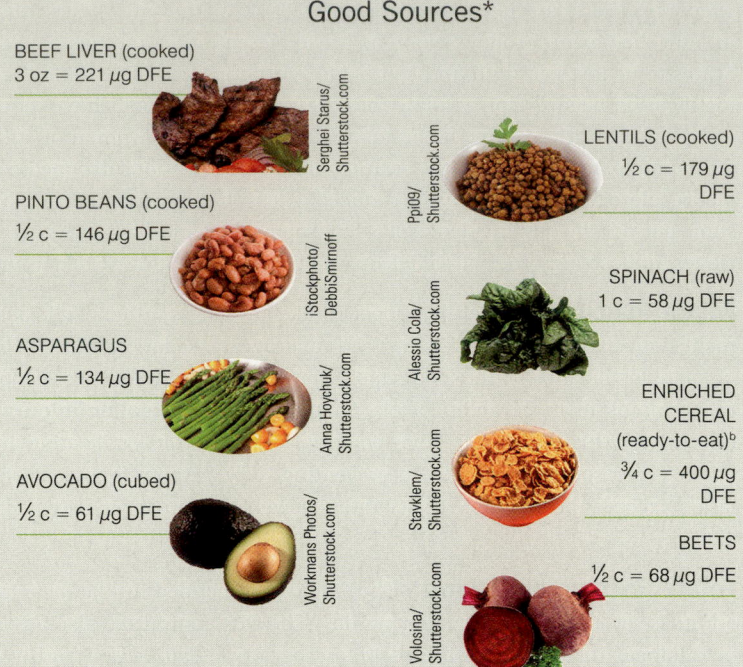

DRI Recommended Intake
Adults: 400 μg DFE/day[a]

Tolerable Upper Intake Level
Adults: 1,000 μg DFE/day

Chief Functions
Part of a coenzyme needed for new cell synthesis

Deficiency
Anemia, smooth, red tongue; depression, mental confusion, weakness, fatigue, irritability, headache; a low intake increases the risk of neural tube birth defects

Toxicity
Masks vitamin B_{12}–deficiency symptoms

*These foods provide 10% or more of the folate Daily Value in a serving. For a 2,000-cal diet, the DV is 400 μg/day.
[a]Folate recommendations are expressed in dietary folate equivalents (DFE). Note that for natural folate sources, 1 μg = 1 DFE; for enrichment sources, 1 μg = 1.7 DFE.
[b]Some highly enriched cereals may provide 400 μg or more in a serving.

Good Sources*

BEEF LIVER (cooked)
3 oz = 221 μg DFE

PINTO BEANS (cooked)
½ c = 146 μg DFE

ASPARAGUS
½ c = 134 μg DFE

AVOCADO (cubed)
½ c = 61 μg DFE

LENTILS (cooked)
½ c = 179 μg DFE

SPINACH (raw)
1 c = 58 μg DFE

ENRICHED CEREAL
(ready-to-eat)[b]
¾ c = 400 μg DFE

BEETS
½ c = 68 μg DFE

folate. As Snapshot 7–9 shows, legumes and asparagus are also excellent sources. Raw or lightly cooked fresh vegetables are often superior because the heat of cooking and the oxidation that occurs during long storage destroy much of the folate in foods.

A difference in absorption between naturally occurring food folate and synthetic folic acid necessitates compensation when measuring folate. The unit of measure, **dietary folate equivalent**, or **DFE**, converts all forms of folate into micrograms that are equivalent to the folate in foods. Appendix C demonstrates how to use the DFE conversion factor.

KEY POINTS

- Low intakes of folate cause anemia, digestive problems, and birth defects in infants of folate-deficient mothers.
- High intakes can mask the blood symptom of a vitamin B_{12} deficiency.

Vitamin B_{12}

Vitamin B_{12} and folate are closely related: each depends on the other for activation. By itself, vitamin B_{12} also helps to maintain the sheaths that surround and protect nerve fibers.

Vitamin B_{12} Deficiency Symptoms
Without sufficient vitamin B_{12}, nerves become damaged, and folate fails to do its blood-building work, so vitamin B_{12} deficiency causes an anemia identical to that caused by folate deficiency. The blood symptoms of a deficiency of either folate or vitamin B_{12} include the presence of large, immature red blood cells. Administering extra folate often clears up this blood condition but allows the deficiency of vitamin B_{12} to continue undetected.[79] Vitamin B_{12}'s other functions then become compromised, and the results can be devastating: damaged nerve sheaths, creeping paralysis, and general malfunctioning of nerves and muscles. Even a marginal vitamin B_{12} deficiency may impair mental functioning in the elderly, worsening dementia.[80] Vitamin B_{12} deficiency has also been associated with mental depression.[81] Research is ongoing.

dietary folate equivalent (DFE) a unit of measure expressing the amount of folate available to the body from naturally occurring sources. The measure mathematically equalizes the difference in absorption between less absorbable food folate and highly absorbable synthetic folate added to enriched foods and found in supplements.

vitamin B_{12} a B vitamin that helps to convert folate to its active form and also helps to maintain the sheath around nerve cells. Vitamin B_{12}'s scientific name, not often used, is *cyanocobalamin*.

A Special Case: Vitamin B₁₂ Malabsorption

A Special Case: Vitamin B$_{12}$ Malabsorption For vitamin B$_{12}$, deficiencies most often reflect poor absorption that occurs for one of two reasons:

- The stomach produces too little acid to liberate vitamin B$_{12}$ from food.
- **Intrinsic factor**, a compound made by the stomach and needed for absorption, is lacking.

Once the stomach's acid frees vitamin B$_{12}$ from the food proteins that bind it, intrinsic factor attaches to the vitamin, and the complex is absorbed into the bloodstream. The anemia of the vitamin B$_{12}$ deficiency caused by lack of intrinsic factor is known as **pernicious anemia** (see Figure 7–17).

In a few people, an inborn defect in the gene for intrinsic factor begins to impair vitamin B$_{12}$ absorption by mid-adulthood. With age, many others lose their ability to produce enough stomach acid and intrinsic factor to allow efficient absorption of vitamin B$_{12}$.[‡‡‡] Intestinal diseases, surgeries, or stomach infection with an ulcer-causing bacterium can also impair absorption.[82] Taking a common diabetes drug also makes vitamin B$_{12}$ deficiency likely, although its symptoms have not been reported.[§§§83] In cases of malabsorption, vitamin B$_{12}$ must be supplied by injection or via nasal spray to bypass the defective absorptive system.

Vitamin B$_{12}$ Food Sources As Snapshot 7–10 shows, vitamin B$_{12}$ is naturally supplied only by foods of animal origin, so vitamin B$_{12}$ deficiency poses a threat to strict vegetarians. Controversy 6 discussed vitamin B$_{12}$ sources for vegetarians.

Perspective The way folate masks the anemia of vitamin B$_{12}$ deficiency underscores a point about supplements. It takes a skilled professional to correctly diagnose and treat a nutrient deficiency, and self-diagnosing or acting on advice from self-proclaimed experts poses serious risks. A second point: because vitamin B$_{12}$ deficiency in the body may be caused by either a lack of the vitamin in the diet or a lack of the intrinsic factor necessary to absorb the vitamin, a dietary change alone may not correct the deficiency; a professional diagnosis can identify such problems.

KEY POINTS

- Vitamin B$_{12}$ occurs only in animal products.
- Vitamin B$_{12}$-deficiency anemia mimics folate deficiency and arises with low intakes or, more often, poor absorption.
- Folate supplements can mask a vitamin B$_{12}$ deficiency.
- Prolonged vitamin B$_{12}$ deficiency causes nerve damage.

Vitamin B$_6$

Vitamin B$_6$ participates in more than 100 reactions in body tissues and is needed to help convert one kind of amino acid, which cells have in abundance, to other nonessential amino acids that the cells lack. In addition, vitamin B$_6$ functions in these ways:

- Aids in the conversion of tryptophan to niacin.
- Plays important roles in the synthesis of hemoglobin and neurotransmitters, the communication molecules of the brain. (For example, vitamin B$_6$ assists the conversion of the amino acid tryptophan to the mood-regulating neurotransmitter **serotonin**.)
- Assists in releasing stored glucose from glycogen and thus contributes to the regulation of blood glucose.
- Plays roles in immune function and steroid hormone activity.
- Is critical to the developing brain and nervous system of a fetus; deficiency during this stage causes behavioral problems later.

[‡‡‡]This condition is atrophic gastritis (a-TROH-fik gas-TRY-tis), a chronic inflammation of the stomach accompanied by a diminished size and functioning of the stomach's mucous membrane and glands.
[§§§]The diabetes medication is metformin.

Figure 7–17

Anemic and Normal Blood Cells

The anemia of folate deficiency is indistinguishable from that of vitamin B$_{12}$ deficiency.

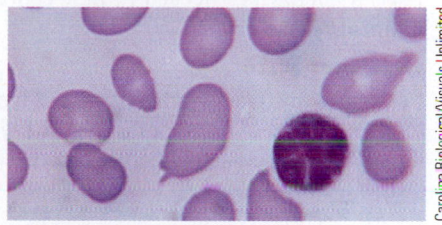

Blood cells of pernicious anemia. *The cells are larger than normal and irregular in shape.*

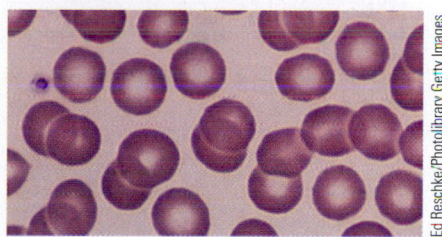

Normal blood cells. *The size, shape, and color of these red blood cells show that they are normal.*

Carolina Biological/Visuals Unlimited

Ed Reschke/Photolibrary Getty Images

intrinsic factor a factor found inside a system. The intrinsic factor necessary to prevent pernicious anemia is now known to be a compound that helps in the absorption of vitamin B$_{12}$.

pernicious (per-NISH-us) **anemia** a vitamin B$_{12}$–deficiency disease, caused by lack of intrinsic factor and characterized by large, immature red blood cells and damage to the nervous system (*pernicious* means "highly injurious or destructive").

vitamin B$_6$ a B vitamin needed in protein metabolism. Its three active forms are *pyridoxine, pyridoxal,* and *pyridoxamine.*

serotonin (SER-oh-TONE-in) a neurotransmitter important in sleep regulation, appetite control, and mood regulation, among other roles. Serotonin is synthesized in the body from the amino acid tryptophan with the help of vitamin B$_6$.

DRI Recommended Intake
Adults: 2.4 μg/day

Chief Functions
Part of coenzymes needed in new cell synthesis; helps to maintain nerve cells

Deficiency
Pernicious anemia;[a] anemia (large-cell type);[b] smooth tongue; tingling or numbness; fatigue, memory loss, disorientation, degeneration of nerves progressing to paralysis

Toxicity
None reported

These foods provide 10% or more of the vitamin B$_{12}$ Daily Value in a serving. For a 2,000-cal diet, the DV is 2.4 μg/day.

[a]*The name pernicious anemia refers to the vitamin B$_{12}$ deficiency caused by a lack of stomach intrinsic factor but not to anemia from inadequate dietary intake.*

[b]*Large cell–type anemia is known as either macrocytic or megaloblastic anemia.*

Good Sources*

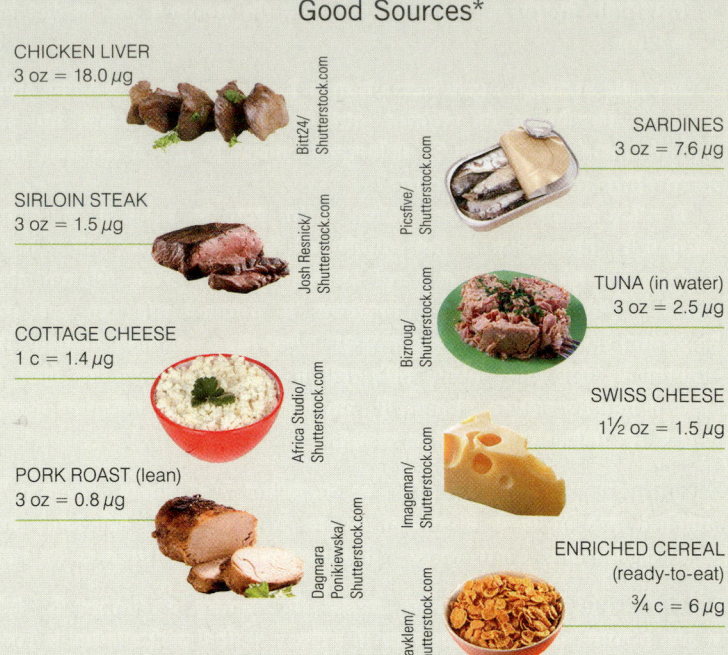

CHICKEN LIVER
3 oz = 18.0 μg
Bitt24/ Shutterstock.com

SIRLOIN STEAK
3 oz = 1.5 μg
Josh Resnick/ Shutterstock.com

COTTAGE CHEESE
1 c = 1.4 μg
Africa Studio/ Shutterstock.com

PORK ROAST (lean)
3 oz = 0.8 μg
Dagmara Ponikiewska/ Shutterstock.com

SARDINES
3 oz = 7.6 μg
Picsfive/ Shutterstock.com

TUNA (in water)
3 oz = 2.5 μg
Bizroug/ Shutterstock.com

SWISS CHEESE
1½ oz = 1.5 μg
Imageman/ Shutterstock.com

ENRICHED CEREAL
(ready-to-eat)
¾ c = 6 μg
Stavklem/ Shutterstock.com

Figure 7–18
Vitamin B$_6$ Deficiency

In this dermatitis, the skin is greasy and flaky, unlike the skin affected by the dermatitis of pellagra.

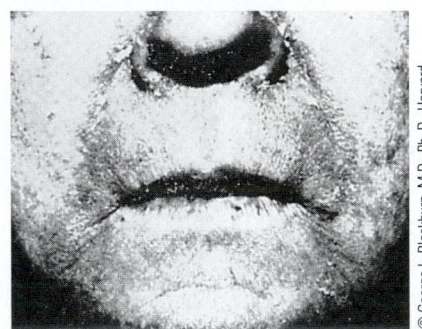

© George L. Blackburn, M.D., Ph. D., Harvard Medical School

Vitamin B$_6$ Deficiency Because of these diverse functions, vitamin B$_6$ deficiency is expressed in general symptoms, such as weakness, psychological depression, confusion, irritability, and insomnia. Other symptoms include anemia, the greasy dermatitis depicted in Figure 7–18, and, in advanced cases of deficiency, convulsions. A shortage of vitamin B$_6$ may also weaken the immune response. Some evidence links low vitamin B$_6$ intakes with increased risks of some cancers and cardiovascular disease; more research is needed to clarify these associations.[84]

Vitamin B$_6$ Toxicity Years ago, it was generally believed that, like most of the other water-soluble vitamins, vitamin B$_6$ could not reach toxic concentrations in the body. Then a report told of women who took more than 2 grams of vitamin B$_6$ daily for months (20 times the current UL of 100 *milligrams* per day), attempting to cure premenstrual syndrome (science doesn't support this use). The women developed numb feet, then lost sensation in their hands, and eventually became unable to walk or work. Withdrawing the supplement reversed the symptoms.

Food sources of vitamin B$_6$ are safe. Consider that one small capsule can easily deliver 2 grams of vitamin B$_6$ but it would take almost 3,000 bananas, more than 1,600 servings of liver, or more than 3,800 chicken breasts to supply an equivalent amount. Moral: stick with food. Table 7–10 (p. 279) lists common deficiency and toxicity symptoms and food sources of vitamin B$_6$.

Vitamin B$_6$ Recommendations and Sources Vitamin B$_6$ plays so many roles in protein metabolism that the body's requirement for vitamin B$_6$ is roughly proportional to protein intakes. The DRI committee set the vitamin B$_6$ intake recommendation high enough to cover most people's needs, regardless of differences in protein intakes (see the inside front cover). Meats, fish, and poultry (protein-rich foods); potatoes; leafy green vegetables; and some fruits are good sources of vitamin B$_6$ (see Snapshot 7–11). Other foods such as legumes and peanut butter provide smaller amounts.

KEY POINT

■ Vitamin B$_6$ works in amino acid metabolism.

DRI Recommended Intake
Adults (19–50 yr): 1.3 mg/day

Tolerable Upper Intake Level
Adults: 100 mg/day

Chief Functions
Part of a coenzyme needed in amino acid and fatty acid metabolism; helps to convert tryptophan to niacin and to serotonin; helps to make hemoglobin for red blood cells

Deficiency
Anemia, depression, confusion, abnormal brain wave pattern, convulsions; greasy, scaly dermatitis

Toxicity
Depression, fatigue, impaired memory, irritability, headaches, nerve damage causing numbness and muscle weakness progressing to an inability to walk and convulsions; skin lesions

These foods provide 10% or more of the vitamin B$_6$ Daily Value in a serving. For a 2,000-cal diet, the DV is 1.7 mg/day.

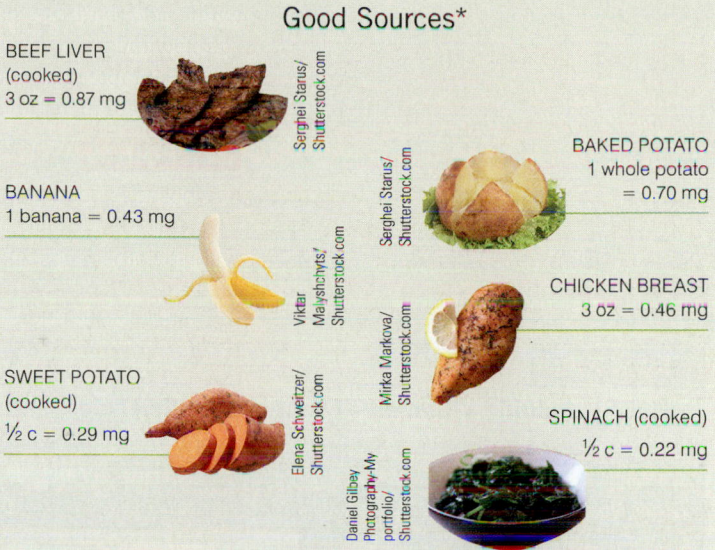

Good Sources*

BEEF LIVER (cooked)
3 oz = 0.87 mg

BANANA
1 banana = 0.43 mg

SWEET POTATO (cooked)
½ c = 0.29 mg

BAKED POTATO
1 whole potato = 0.70 mg

CHICKEN BREAST
3 oz = 0.46 mg

SPINACH (cooked)
½ c = 0.22 mg

Biotin and Pantothenic Acid

Two other B vitamins, **biotin** and **pantothenic acid**, are, like thiamin, riboflavin, and niacin, important in energy metabolism. Biotin is a cofactor for several enzymes in the metabolism of carbohydrate, fat, and protein. In addition, researchers are actively investigating new roles for biotin, particularly in gene expression.[85] No adverse effects from high biotin intakes have been reported, but some research indicates that high-dose biotin supplementation may damage DNA. No Tolerable Upper Intake Level has yet been set for biotin.

Pantothenic acid is a component of a key coenzyme that makes possible the release of energy from the energy nutrients. It also participates in more than 100 steps in the synthesis of lipids, neurotransmitters, steroid hormones, and hemoglobin.

Although rare diseases may precipitate deficiencies of biotin and pantothenic acid, healthy people eating ordinary diets are not at risk for deficiencies. A steady diet of raw egg whites, which contain a protein that binds biotin, can produce biotin deficiency, but you would have to consume more than two dozen raw egg whites daily to produce the effect. Cooking eggs denatures the protein.

KEY POINT
- Biotin and pantothenic acid are important to the body and are adequately supplied in a well-balanced diet.

Non–B Vitamins

Choline, although not defined as a vitamin, might be called a conditionally essential nutrient. When the diet is devoid of choline, the body cannot make enough of the compound to meet its needs, and choline plays important roles in fetal development.[86] Choline is widely supplied by protein-rich foods, and deficiencies are practically unheard of outside the laboratory.[87] Choline needs may rise in pregnancy, however (see Chapter 13).[88] DRI recommendations have been set for choline (see inside front cover).

The compounds **carnitine**, **inositol**, and **lipoic acid** might appropriately be called *nonvitamins* because they are not essential nutrients for human beings. Carnitine, sometimes called "vitamin BT," is an important piece of cell machinery, but it is not a vitamin. Although deficiencies can be induced in laboratory animals for experimental purposes, these substances are abundant in ordinary foods. Vitamin companies often include carnitine, inositol, or lipoic acid to make their formulas appear more "complete," but there is no physiological reason to do so.

biotin (BY-o-tin) a B vitamin; a coenzyme necessary for fat synthesis and other metabolic reactions.

pantothenic (PAN-to-THEN-ic) **acid** a B vitamin and part of a critical coenzyme needed in energy metabolism, among other roles.

choline (KOH-leen) a nutrient used to make the phospholipid lecithin and other molecules.

carnitine a nonessential nutrient that functions in cellular activities.

inositol (in-OSS-ih-tall) a nonessential nutrient found in cell membranes.

lipoic (lip-OH-ic) **acid** a nonessential nutrient.

Other substances have been mistakenly thought to be essential in human nutrition because they are needed for growth by bacteria or other life-forms. These substances include PABA (para-aminobenzoic acid), bioflavonoids ("vitamin P" or hesperidin), and ubiquinone (coenzyme Q). Other names you may hear are "vitamin B_{15}" and pangamic acid (both hoaxes) or "vitamin B_{17}," (laetrile or amygdalin, not a cancer cure as claimed and not a vitamin by any stretch of the imagination).****

This chapter has addressed all 13 of the vitamins. The basic facts about each one are summed up in Tables 7–9 and 7–10.

KEY POINTS

- Choline is needed in the diet, but it is not a vitamin, and deficiencies are unheard of outside the laboratory.
- Many other substances that people claim are vitamins are not.

**** Read about these and many other claims at the website of the National Council Against Health Fraud, www.ncahf.org.

Table 7–9

The Fat-Soluble Vitamins—Functions, Deficiencies, and Toxicities

VITAMIN A

Other Names
Retinol, retinal, retinoic acid; main precursor is beta-carotene

Chief Functions in the Body
Vision; health of cornea, epithelial cells, mucous membranes, skin; growth; regulation of gene expression; reproduction; embryonic development of spinal cord and heart; immunity
Beta-carotene: antioxidant

Deficiency Disease Name
Hypovitaminosis A

Significant Sources
Retinol: fortified milk, cheese, cream, butter, fortified margarine, eggs, liver
Beta-carotene: spinach and other dark, leafy greens; broccoli; deep orange fruits (apricots, cantaloupe) and vegetables (winter squash, carrots, sweet potatoes, pumpkin)

	Deficiency Symptoms	Toxicity Symptoms
Blood/Circulatory System	Anemia (small-cell type)[a]	Red blood cell breakage, cessation of menstruation, nosebleeds
Bones/Teeth	Cessation of growth, painful joints; impaired enamel formation, cracks in teeth, tendency toward tooth decay	Bone pain; growth retardation; difficulty gaining weight; increased pressure inside skull
Digestive System	Diarrhea, changes in intestinal and other body linings	Abdominal pain, nausea, vomiting, diarrhea, weight loss
Immune System	Frequent infections	Overreactivity
Nervous/Muscular System	Night blindness (retinal) Mental depression	Blurred vision, uncoordinated muscle, fatigue, irritability, loss of appetite
Skin and Cornea	Keratinization, corneal degeneration leading to blindness,[b] rashes	Dry skin, rashes; cracking and bleeding lips, brittle nails; hair loss; benign skin yellowing (beta-carotene)
Other	Kidney stones, impaired growth	Liver enlargement and liver damage; birth defects

VITAMIN D

Other Names
Calciferol, cholecalciferol, dihydroxy vitamin D; precursor is cholesterol

Chief Functions in the Body
Mineralization of bones (raises blood calcium and phosphorus via absorption from digestive tract and by withdrawing calcium from bones and stimulating retention by kidneys)

Deficiency Disease Name
Rickets, osteomalacia

Significant Sources
Self-synthesis with sunlight; fortified milk and other fortified foods, liver, sardines, salmon

	Deficiency Symptoms	Toxicity Symptoms
Blood/Circulatory System		Elevated blood calcium; calcification of blood vessels and heart tissues
Bones/Teeth	Abnormal growth, misshapen bones (bowing of legs), soft bones, joint pain, malformed teeth	Calcification of tooth soft tissues; thinning of tooth enamel
Nervous/Muscular System	Muscle spasms	Excessive thirst, headaches, irritability, loss of appetite, weakness, nausea
Other		Calcification and harm to soft tissues (kidneys, lungs, joints); heart damage

[a]Small cell–type anemia is termed microcytic anemia; large cell–type anemia is macrocytic or megaloblastic anemia.

[b]Corneal degeneration progresses from keratinization (hardening) to xerosis (drying) to xerophthalmia (thickening, opacity, and irreversible blindness).

Table 7–9

The Fat-Soluble Vitamins—Functions, Deficiencies, and Toxicities (continued)

VITAMIN E

Other Names
Alpha-tocopherol, tocopherol

Chief Functions in the Body
Antioxidant (quenching of free radicals), stabilization of cell membranes, support of immune function, protection of polyunsaturated fatty acids; normal nerve development

Deficiency Disease Name
(No name)

Significant Sources
Polyunsaturated plant oils (margarine, salad dressings, shortenings), green and leafy vegetables, wheat germ, whole-grain products, nuts, seeds

	Deficiency Symptoms	Toxicity Symptoms
Blood/Circulatory System	Red blood cell breakage, anemia	Augments the effects of anticlotting medication
Digestive System		General discomfort, nausea
Eyes		Blurred vision
Nervous/Muscular System	Nerve degeneration, weakness, difficulty walking, leg cramps	Fatigue

VITAMIN K

Other Names
Phylloquinone, naphthoquinone

Chief Functions in the Body
Synthesis of blood-clotting proteins and proteins important in bone mineralization

Deficiency Disease Name
(No name)

Significant Sources
Bacterial synthesis in the digestive tract; green leafy vegetables, cabbage-type vegetables, soybeans, vegetable oils

	Deficiency Symptoms	Toxicity Symptoms
Blood/Circulatory System	Hemorrhage	Interference with anticlotting medication
Bones	Poor skeletal mineralization	

Table 7–10

The Water-Soluble Vitamins—Functions, Deficiencies, and Toxicities

VITAMIN C

Other Names
Ascorbic acid

Chief Functions in the Body
Collagen synthesis (strengthens blood vessel walls, forms scar tissue, matrix for bone growth), antioxidant, restores vitamin E to active form, hormone synthesis, supports immune cell functions, helps in absorption of iron

Deficiency Disease Name
Scurvy

Significant Sources
Citrus fruits, cabbage-type vegetables, dark green vegetables, cantaloupe, strawberries, peppers, lettuce, tomatoes, potatoes, papayas, mangoes

	Deficiency Symptoms	Toxicity Symptoms
Digestive System		Nausea, abdominal cramps, diarrhea, excessive urination
Immune System	Immune suppression, frequent infections	
Mouth, Gums, Tongue	Bleeding gums, loosened teeth	
Nervous/Muscular System	Muscle degeneration and pain, depression, disorientation	Headache, fatigue, insomnia
Bones	Bone fragility, joint pain	Aggravation of gout
Skin	Pinpoint hemorrhages, rough skin, blotchy bruises	Rashes
Other	Anemia, failure of wounds to heal	Interference with medical tests; kidney stones in susceptible people

Table 7–10

The Water-Soluble Vitamins—Functions, Deficiencies, and Toxicities (continued)

THIAMIN

Other Names
Vitamin B₁

Chief Functions in the Body
Part of a coenzyme needed in energy metabolism, supports normal appetite and nervous system function

Deficiency Disease Name
Beriberi (wet and dry)

Significant Sources
Occurs in all nutritious foods in moderate amounts; pork, ham, bacon, liver, whole and enriched grains, legumes, seeds

	Deficiency Symptoms	Toxicity Symptoms
Blood/Circulatory System	Edema, enlarged heart, abnormal heart rhythms, heart failure	(No symptoms reported)
Nervous/ Muscular System	Degeneration, wasting, weakness, pain, apathy, irritability, difficulty walking, loss of reflexes, jerky eye movements, mental confusion, paralysis	
Other	Anorexia; weight loss	

RIBOFLAVIN

Other Names
Vitamin B₂

Chief Functions in the Body
Part of a coenzyme needed in energy metabolism, supports normal vision and skin health

Deficiency Disease Name
Ariboflavinosis

Significant Sources
Milk, yogurt, cottage cheese, meat, liver, leafy green vegetables, whole-grain or enriched breads and cereals

	Deficiency Symptoms	Toxicity Symptoms
Mouth, Gums, Tongue	Cracks at corners of mouth,[a] smooth magenta tongue;[b] sore throat	(No symptoms reported)
Nervous System and Eyes	Hypersensitivity to light, reddening of cornea	
Skin	Skin rash	

NIACIN

Other Names
Nicotinic acid, nicotinamide, niacinamide, vitamin B₃; precursor is dietary tryptophan

Chief Functions in the Body
Part of coenzymes needed in energy metabolism

Deficiency Disease Name
Pellagra

Significant Sources
Synthesized from the amino acid tryptophan; milk, eggs, meat, poultry, fish, whole-grain and enriched breads and cereals, nuts, and all protein-containing foods

	Deficiency Symptoms	Toxicity Symptoms
Digestive System	Diarrhea; vomiting; abdominal pain	Nausea, vomiting
Mouth, Gums, Tongue	Black or bright red swollen smooth tongue[b]	
Nervous System	Irritability, loss of appetite, weakness, headache, dizziness, mental confusion progressing to psychosis or delirium	
Skin	Flaky skin rash on areas exposed to sun	Painful flush and rash, sweating
Other		Liver damage; impaired glucose tolerance; vision disturbances

[a]Cracks at the corners of the mouth are termed cheilosis (kee-LOH-sis).
[b]Smoothness of the tongue is caused by loss of its surface structures and is termed glossitis (gloss-EYE-tis).

Chapter 7 The Vitamins

Table 7–10

The Water-Soluble Vitamins—Functions, Deficiencies, and Toxicities (continued)

FOLATE

Other Names
Folic acid, folacin, pteroyglutamic acid

Chief Functions in the Body
Part of a coenzyme needed for new cell synthesis

Deficiency Disease Name
(No name)

Significant Sources
Asparagus, avocado, leafy green vegetables, beets, legumes, seeds, liver, enriched breads, cereal, pasta, and grains

	Deficiency Symptoms	Toxicity Symptoms
Blood/Circulatory System	Anemia (large-cell type),[a] elevated homocysteine	Masks vitamin B_{12} deficiency
Digestive System	Heartburn, diarrhea, constipation	
Immune System	Suppression, frequent infections	
Mouth, Gums, Tongue	Smooth red tongue[b]	
Nervous/ Muscular System	Increased risk of neural tube birth defects; depression, mental confusion, fatigue, irritability, headache	Depression, mental confusion, fatigue, irritability, headache

VITAMIN B_{12}

Other Names
Cyanocobalamin

Chief Functions in the Body
Part of coenzymes needed in new cell synthesis, helps maintain nerve cells

Deficiency Disease Name
(No name)[c]

Significant Sources
Animal products (meat, fish, poultry, milk, cheese, eggs)

	Deficiency Symptoms	Toxicity Symptoms
Blood/Circulatory System	Anemia (large-cell type)[a,c]	(No toxicity symptoms known)
Mouth, Gums, Tongue	Smooth tongue[b]	
Nervous/ Muscular System	Fatigue, nerve degeneration progressing to paralysis	
Skin	Tingling or numbness	

VITAMIN B_6

Other Names
Pyridoxine, pyridoxal, pyridoxamine

Chief Functions in the Body
Part of a coenzyme needed in amino acid and fatty acid metabolism, helps convert tryptophan to niacin and to serotonin, helps make red blood cells

Deficiency Disease Name
(No name)

Significant Sources
Meats, fish, poultry, liver, legumes, fruits, potatoes, whole grains, soy products

	Deficiency Symptoms	Toxicity Symptoms
Blood/Circulatory System	Anemia (small-cell type)[a]	Bloating
Nervous/ Muscular System	Depression, confusion, abnormal brain wave pattern, convulsions	Depression, fatigue, impaired memory, irritability, headaches, numbness, damage to nerves, difficulty walking, loss of reflexes, restlessness, convulsions
Skin	Rashes; greasy, scaly dermatitis	Skin lesions

[a]Small cell–type anemia is termed microcytic anemia; large cell–type is macrocytic or megaloblastic anemia.
[b]Smoothness of the tongue is caused by loss of its surface structures and is termed glossitis (gloss-EYE-tis).
[c]The name pernicious anemia refers to the vitamin B_{12} deficiency caused by lack of intrinsic factor but not to that caused by inadequate dietary intake.

Table 7–10

The Water-Soluble Vitamins—Functions, Deficiencies, and Toxicities (continued)

PANTOTHENIC ACID

Other Names
(None)

Chief Functions in the Body
Part of a coenzyme needed in energy metabolism

Deficiency Disease Name
(No name)

Significant Sources
Widespread in foods

	Deficiency Symptoms	Toxicity Symptoms
Digestive System	Vomiting, intestinal distress	Water retention (infrequent)
Nervous/ Muscular System	Insomnia, fatigue	
Other	Hypoglycemia, increased sensitivity to insulin	

BIOTIN

Other Names
(None)

Chief Functions in the Body
A cofactor for several enzymes needed in energy metabolism, fat synthesis, amino acid metabolism, and glycogen synthesis

Deficiency Disease Name
(No name)

Significant Sources
Widespread in foods

	Deficiency Symptoms	Toxicity Symptoms
Blood/Circulatory System	Abnormal heart action	(No toxicity symptoms reported)
Digestive System	Loss of appetite, nausea	
Nervous/ Muscular System	Depression, muscle pain, weakness, fatigue, numbness of extremities	
Skin	Dry around eyes, nose, and mouth	

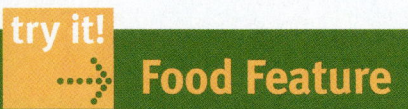

try it!

Food Feature

Choosing Foods Rich in Vitamins

LO 7.11 Describe how to choose foods to meet vitamin needs.

On learning how important the vitamins are to their health, most people want to choose foods that are vitamin-rich. How can they tell which are which? Not by food labels—these provide only limited vitamin information. A way to find out more about the vitamin contents of foods is to look down the columns of vitamins and calories in a table of food composition, such as Appendix A at the end of this book, to identify some of the vitamin-rich foods in your own eating pattern. If you are interested in folate, for instance, you can see that cornflakes are an especially good source (folic acid is added to cornflakes), as is orange juice (folate occurs naturally in this food).

Another way of looking at such data appears in Figure 7–19—the long bars show some foods that are rich sources of a particular vitamin and the short or nonexistent bars indicate poor sources. The colors of the bars represent the various food groups.

Which Foods Should I Choose?

After looking at Figure 7–19, don't think that you must memorize the richest sources of each vitamin and eat those foods daily. That false notion would lead you to limit your variety of foods, while overemphasizing the components of a few foods. Although it is reassuring to know that your carrot-raisin salad at lunch provided more than your entire day's need for vitamin A, it is a mistake to think that you must then select equally rich sources of all the other vitamins. Such rich sources do not exist for many vitamins—rather, foods work in harmony to provide most nutrients. For example, a baked potato, not a star performer among vitamin C providers, contributes substantially to a day's need for this nutrient and contributes some thiamin and vitamin B_6, too. By the end of the day, assuming that your food choices were made with reasonable care, the bits of vitamin C, thiamin, and vitamin B_6 from each serving of food have accumulated to more than cover the day's need for them.

A Variety of Foods Works Best

The last two graphs of Figure 7–19 (p. 282) show sources of folate and vitamin C. These nutrients are both

Figure 7–19

Food Sources of Vitamins Selected to Show a Range of Values

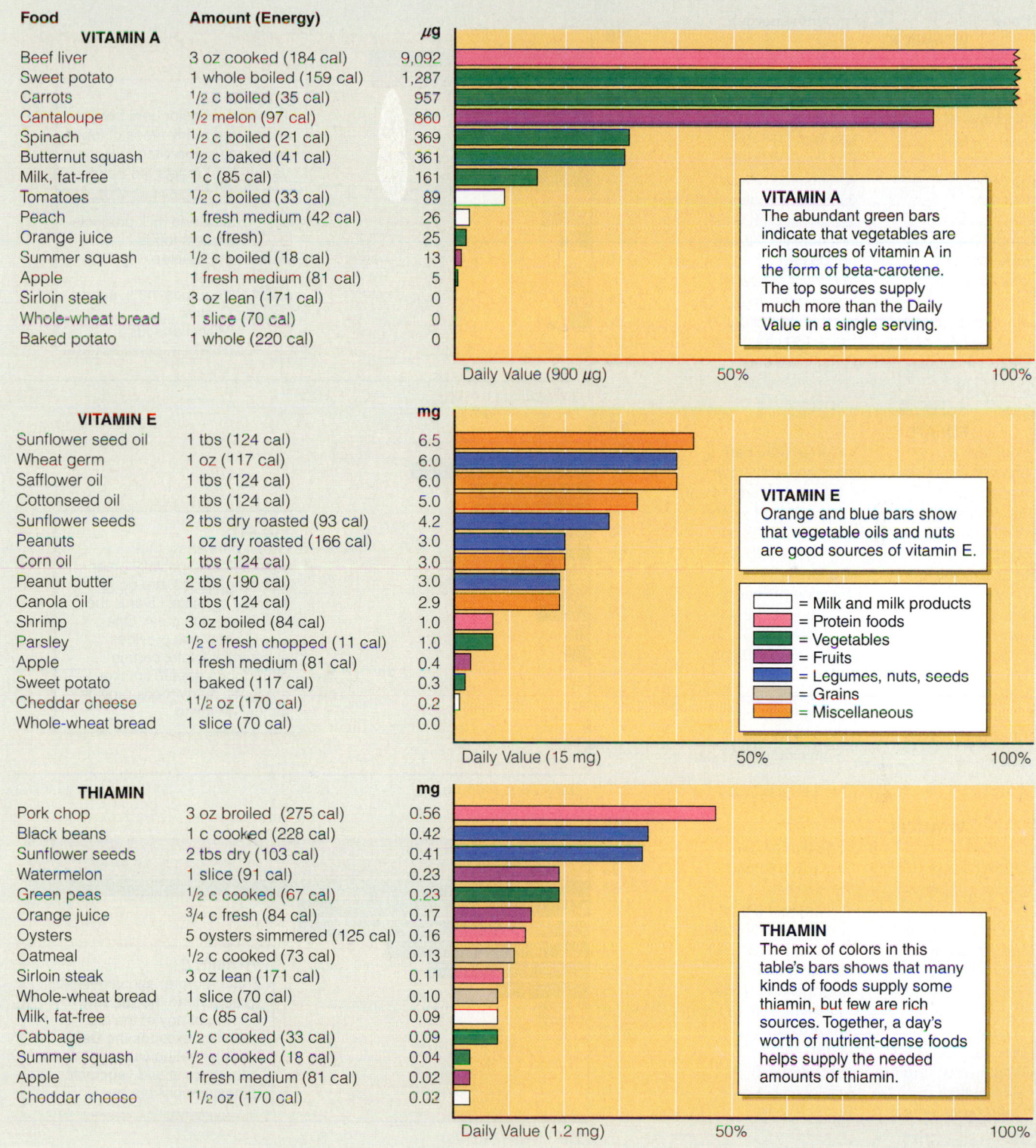

Food	Amount (Energy)	
VITAMIN A		**µg**
Beef liver	3 oz cooked (184 cal)	9,092
Sweet potato	1 whole boiled (159 cal)	1,287
Carrots	½ c boiled (35 cal)	957
Cantaloupe	½ melon (97 cal)	860
Spinach	½ c boiled (21 cal)	369
Butternut squash	½ c baked (41 cal)	361
Milk, fat-free	1 c (85 cal)	161
Tomatoes	½ c boiled (33 cal)	89
Peach	1 fresh medium (42 cal)	26
Orange juice	1 c (fresh)	25
Summer squash	½ c boiled (18 cal)	13
Apple	1 fresh medium (81 cal)	5
Sirloin steak	3 oz lean (171 cal)	0
Whole-wheat bread	1 slice (70 cal)	0
Baked potato	1 whole (220 cal)	0

Daily Value (900 µg)   50%   100%

VITAMIN A
The abundant green bars indicate that vegetables are rich sources of vitamin A in the form of beta-carotene. The top sources supply much more than the Daily Value in a single serving.

Food	Amount (Energy)	
VITAMIN E		**mg**
Sunflower seed oil	1 tbs (124 cal)	6.5
Wheat germ	1 oz (117 cal)	6.0
Safflower oil	1 tbs (124 cal)	6.0
Cottonseed oil	1 tbs (124 cal)	5.0
Sunflower seeds	2 tbs dry roasted (93 cal)	4.2
Peanuts	1 oz dry roasted (166 cal)	3.0
Corn oil	1 tbs (124 cal)	3.0
Peanut butter	2 tbs (190 cal)	3.0
Canola oil	1 tbs (124 cal)	2.9
Shrimp	3 oz boiled (84 cal)	1.0
Parsley	½ c fresh chopped (11 cal)	1.0
Apple	1 fresh medium (81 cal)	0.4
Sweet potato	1 baked (117 cal)	0.3
Cheddar cheese	1½ oz (170 cal)	0.2
Whole-wheat bread	1 slice (70 cal)	0.0

Daily Value (15 mg)   50%   100%

VITAMIN E
Orange and blue bars show that vegetable oils and nuts are good sources of vitamin E.

☐ = Milk and milk products
☐ = Protein foods
☐ = Vegetables
☐ = Fruits
☐ = Legumes, nuts, seeds
☐ = Grains
☐ = Miscellaneous

Food	Amount (Energy)	
THIAMIN		**mg**
Pork chop	3 oz broiled (275 cal)	0.56
Black beans	1 c cooked (228 cal)	0.42
Sunflower seeds	2 tbs dry (103 cal)	0.41
Watermelon	1 slice (91 cal)	0.23
Green peas	½ c cooked (67 cal)	0.23
Orange juice	¾ c fresh (84 cal)	0.17
Oysters	5 oysters simmered (125 cal)	0.16
Oatmeal	½ c cooked (73 cal)	0.13
Sirloin steak	3 oz lean (171 cal)	0.11
Whole-wheat bread	1 slice (70 cal)	0.10
Milk, fat-free	1 c (85 cal)	0.09
Cabbage	½ c cooked (33 cal)	0.09
Summer squash	½ c cooked (18 cal)	0.04
Apple	1 fresh medium (81 cal)	0.02
Cheddar cheese	1½ oz (170 cal)	0.02

Daily Value (1.2 mg)   50%   100%

THIAMIN
The mix of colors in this table's bars shows that many kinds of foods supply some thiamin, but few are rich sources. Together, a day's worth of nutrient-dense foods helps supply the needed amounts of thiamin.

Figure 7–19

Food Sources of Vitamins Selected to Show a Range of Values (continued)

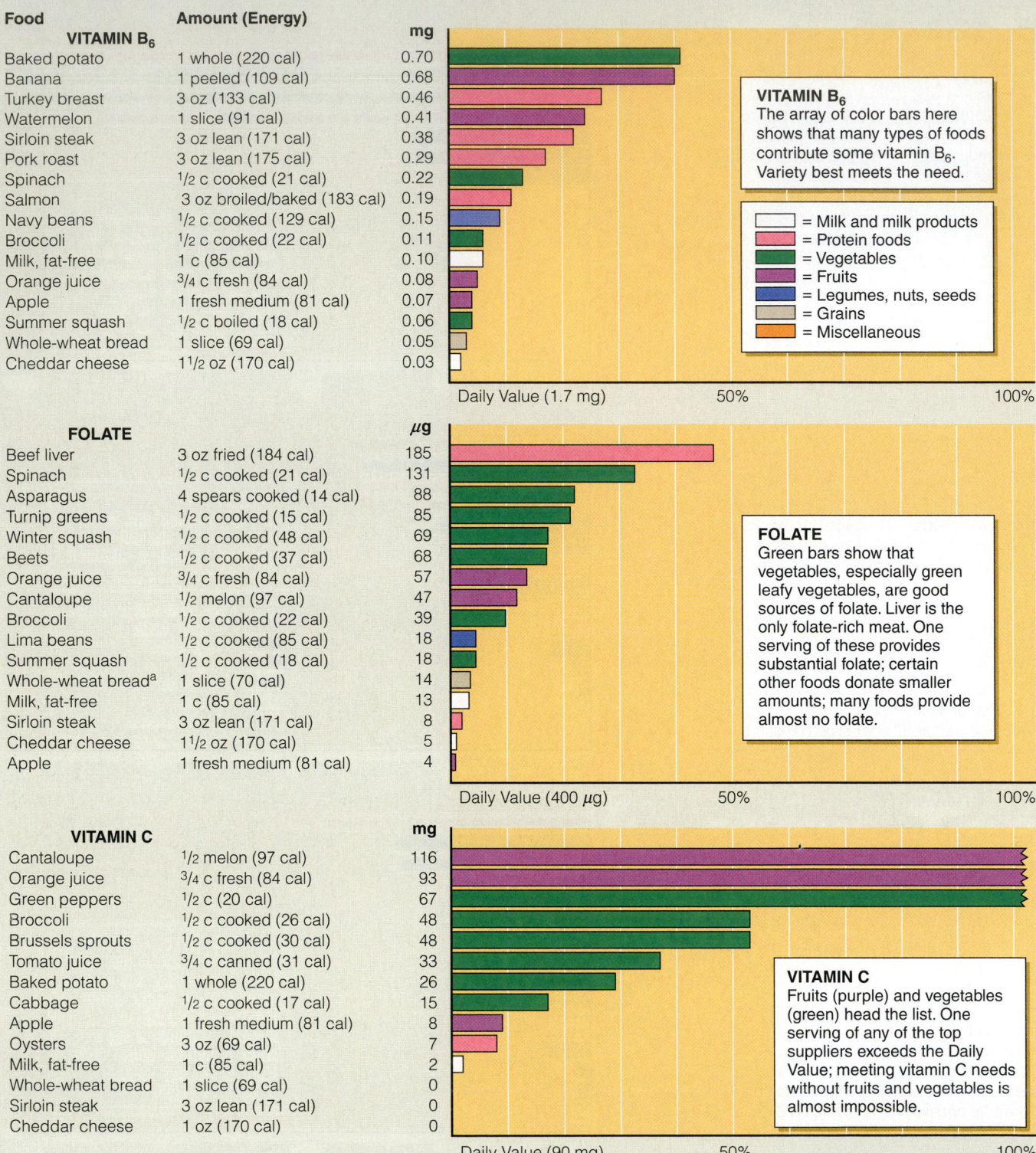

Food	Amount (Energy)	mg
VITAMIN B₆		
Baked potato	1 whole (220 cal)	0.70
Banana	1 peeled (109 cal)	0.68
Turkey breast	3 oz (133 cal)	0.46
Watermelon	1 slice (91 cal)	0.41
Sirloin steak	3 oz lean (171 cal)	0.38
Pork roast	3 oz lean (175 cal)	0.29
Spinach	1/2 c cooked (21 cal)	0.22
Salmon	3 oz broiled/baked (183 cal)	0.19
Navy beans	1/2 c cooked (129 cal)	0.15
Broccoli	1/2 c cooked (22 cal)	0.11
Milk, fat-free	1 c (85 cal)	0.10
Orange juice	3/4 c fresh (84 cal)	0.08
Apple	1 fresh medium (81 cal)	0.07
Summer squash	1/2 c boiled (18 cal)	0.06
Whole-wheat bread	1 slice (69 cal)	0.05
Cheddar cheese	1 1/2 oz (170 cal)	0.03

VITAMIN B₆
The array of color bars here shows that many types of foods contribute some vitamin B₆. Variety best meets the need.

☐ = Milk and milk products
▨ = Protein foods
▨ = Vegetables
▨ = Fruits
▨ = Legumes, nuts, seeds
▨ = Grains
▨ = Miscellaneous

Daily Value (1.7 mg)   50%   100%

Food	Amount (Energy)	µg
FOLATE		
Beef liver	3 oz fried (184 cal)	185
Spinach	1/2 c cooked (21 cal)	131
Asparagus	4 spears cooked (14 cal)	88
Turnip greens	1/2 c cooked (15 cal)	85
Winter squash	1/2 c cooked (48 cal)	69
Beets	1/2 c cooked (37 cal)	68
Orange juice	3/4 c fresh (84 cal)	57
Cantaloupe	1/2 melon (97 cal)	47
Broccoli	1/2 c cooked (22 cal)	39
Lima beans	1/2 c cooked (85 cal)	18
Summer squash	1/2 c cooked (18 cal)	18
Whole-wheat bread[a]	1 slice (70 cal)	14
Milk, fat-free	1 c (85 cal)	13
Sirloin steak	3 oz lean (171 cal)	8
Cheddar cheese	1 1/2 oz (170 cal)	5
Apple	1 fresh medium (81 cal)	4

FOLATE
Green bars show that vegetables, especially green leafy vegetables, are good sources of folate. Liver is the only folate-rich meat. One serving of these provides substantial folate; certain other foods donate smaller amounts; many foods provide almost no folate.

Daily Value (400 µg)   50%   100%

Food	Amount (Energy)	mg
VITAMIN C		
Cantaloupe	1/2 melon (97 cal)	116
Orange juice	3/4 c fresh (84 cal)	93
Green peppers	1/2 c (20 cal)	67
Broccoli	1/2 c cooked (26 cal)	48
Brussels sprouts	1/2 c cooked (30 cal)	48
Tomato juice	3/4 c canned (31 cal)	33
Baked potato	1 whole (220 cal)	26
Cabbage	1/2 c cooked (17 cal)	15
Apple	1 fresh medium (81 cal)	8
Oysters	3 oz (69 cal)	7
Milk, fat-free	1 c (85 cal)	2
Whole-wheat bread	1 slice (69 cal)	0
Sirloin steak	3 oz lean (171 cal)	0
Cheddar cheese	1 oz (170 cal)	0

VITAMIN C
Fruits (purple) and vegetables (green) head the list. One serving of any of the top suppliers exceeds the Daily Value; meeting vitamin C needs without fruits and vegetables is almost impossible.

Daily Value (90 mg)   50%   100%

[a]Unenriched.

richly supplied by fruits and vegetables. The richest source of either one may be only a moderate source of the other, but the recommended amounts of fruits and vegetables in the USDA Food Intake Patterns of Chapter 2 cover both needs amply. As for vitamin E, vegetable oils and some seeds and nuts are the richest sources, but vegetables and fruits contribute a little, too.

By now, you should recognize a basic truth in nutrition. The eating pattern that best provides nutrients includes a wide variety of nutrient-dense foods that provide more than just isolated nutrients.[89] Phytochemicals, widespread among whole grains, nuts, fruits, and vegetables, may play roles in human health, as do fiber and other constituents of whole foods. Therefore, when aiming

for adequate intakes of vitamins, aim for a diet that meets the recommendations of Chapter 2. Even supplements cannot duplicate the benefits of such a diet, a point made in this chapter's Controversy section.

Phytochemicals are the topic of **Controversy 2.**

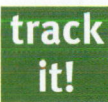 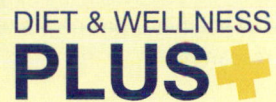

Concepts in Action

Analyze Your Vitamin Intake

The purpose of this exercise is to help you identify your food sources of water-soluble and fat-soluble vitamins. Many foods rich in vitamins work in harmony to provide a full complement of nutrients, which ultimately contributes to a health-promoting eating pattern.

1. Determine whether your food provides enough vitamins. From the Reports tab, select Intake vs. Goals. Choose Day Two, all meals. Generate a report. Did your intakes on that day meet your DRI recommended intake values for vitamins? If not, list those that fall short of the DRI goals. Did any of your intakes exceed DRI values? If so, list those, too.

2. Some fruits and vegetables are good sources of fat-soluble vitamins (see

the Snapshots on pages 248, 254, 258, and 260). From the Reports tab, select MyPlate Analysis, and include all meals. Have you met your minimum recommended fruit and vegetable intake? What percentage of your goal have you met for fruits and vegetables? Did you consume any fruits and vegetables listed in the Snapshots for the fat-soluble vitamins? Which ones?

3. From the Reports tab, select Source Analysis, choose any day, and include all meals. From the drop-down box, select vitamin C, save as pdf, and then do the same for folate. What is your best food source for vitamin C? And for folate? Were your best sources shown in the Snapshots on pages 264 and 272?

4. After viewing the Intake vs. Goals report in question 1, if you fell short on any vitamin, what foods could

you include that would bring you up to the DRI recommended value? If you exceeded the DRI values, which foods were responsible?

5. The USDA Food Intake Patterns suggest that a person who requires 2,000 calories per day should, in a week's time, consume 1½ cups of a variety of dark green, 5½ cups of red and orange, 5 cups of starchy, and 4 cups of other vegetables and 1½ cups of legumes. Create a dish from vegetables or fruits that you enjoy. Get some ideas by using Figure 7–19 (pp. 281–282). Choose a new date. From the Track Diet tab, enter the ingredients. From the Reports tab, select Source Analysis, and select one water-soluble and then one fat-soluble vitamin from the drop-down menu, saving each in a pdf. Identify the vitamin-rich foods from the reports. What does the bar graph show?

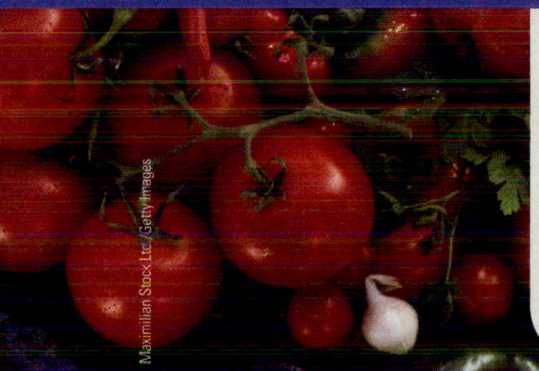

what did you decide?

How do **vitamins** work in the body?

Why is **sunshine** associated with good health?

Can **vitamin C tablets** ward off a cold?

Should you choose **vitamin-fortified foods** and take **supplements** for "insurance"?

Self Check

1. (LO 7.1) Which of the following vitamins are classified as fat-soluble?
   a. vitamins B and D
   b. vitamins A, D, E, and K
   c. vitamins B, E, D, and C
   d. vitamins B and C

2. (LO 7.1) Which of the following describes the fat-soluble vitamins?
   a. few functions in the body
   b. easily absorbed and excreted
   c. stored extensively in tissues
   d. a and c

3. (LO 7.1) Most water-soluble vitamins are not stored in tissues to any great extent.
   T   F

4. (LO 7.2) Fat-soluble vitamins are mostly absorbed into
   a. the lymph.
   b. the blood.
   c. the extracellular fluid.
   d. b and c.

5. (LO 7.3) Which of the following foods is (are) rich in beta-carotene?
   a. sweet potatoes
   b. pumpkin
   c. spinach
   d. all of the above

6. (LO 7.3) Vitamin A supplements can help treat acne.
   T   F

7. (LO 7.4) Vitamin D functions as a hormone to help maintain bone integrity.
   T   F

8. (LO 7.4) In adults with vitamin D deficiency, poor bone mineralization can lead to
   a. pellagra.
   b. pernicious anemia.
   c. scurvy.
   d. osteomalacia.

9. (LO 7.5) Which of the following is (are) rich source(s) of vitamin E?
   a. raw vegetable oil
   b. colorful foods, such as carrots
   c. milk and milk products
   d. raw cabbage

10. (LO 7.5) Vitamin E is famous for its role
    a. in maintaining bone tissue integrity.
    b. in maintaining connective tissue integrity.
    c. in protecting tissues from oxidation.
    d. as a precursor for vitamin C.

11. (LO 7.6) Vitamin K is necessary for the synthesis of key bone proteins.
    T   F

12. (LO 7.6) Vitamin K
    a. can be made from exposure to sunlight.
    b. can be obtained from most milk products.
    c. can be made by digestive tract bacteria.
    d. b and c

13. (LO 7.7) Water-soluble vitamins are mostly absorbed into
    a. the lymph.
    b. the blood.
    c. the extracellular fluid.
    d. b and c.

14. (LO 7.7) The water-soluble vitamins are characterized by all of the following except
    a. excesses are stored and easily build up to toxic levels.
    b. they travel freely in the blood.
    c. excesses are easily excreted and seldom build up to toxic levels.
    d. b and c.

15. (LO 7.8) The theory that vitamin C prevents or cures colds is well supported by research.
    T   F

16. (LO 7.8) Vitamin C deficiency symptoms include
    a. red spots.
    b. loose teeth.
    c. anemia.
    d. all of the above.

17. (LO 7.9) B vitamins often act as
    a. antioxidants.
    b. blood clotting factors.
    c. coenzymes.
    d. none of the above.

18. (LO 7.9) A B vitamin often forms part of an enzyme's active site, where a chemical reaction takes place.
    T   F

19. (LO 7.10) A deficiency of niacin may result in which disease?
    a. pellagra
    b. beriberi
    c. scurvy
    d. rickets

20. (LO 7.10) Which of these B vitamins is (are) present only in foods of animal origin?
    a. niacin
    b. vitamin B_{12}
    c. riboflavin
    d. a and c

21. (LO 7.11) The eating pattern that best provides nutrients
    a. singles out a rich source for each nutrient and focuses on these foods.
    b. includes a wide variety of nutrient-dense foods.
    c. is a Western eating style that includes abundant meats and fats.
    d. singles out rich sources of certain phytochemicals and focuses on these foods.

22. (LO 7.12) The FDA has extensive regulatory control over supplement sales.
    T   F

Answers to these Self Check questions are in Appendix G.

Vitamin Supplements: What are the Benefits and Risks?

LO 7.12 Debate for and against taking vitamin supplements.

More than half of the U.S. population takes dietary supplements, spending $32.5 *billion* each year to do so.[1]* Most take a daily multivitamin and mineral pill, hoping to make up for dietary shortfalls; others take single nutrient supplements to ward off diseases; and many do both. Do people need all these supplements? If people do need supplements, which ones are best? What about health risks from supplements? This Controversy examines evidence surrounding these questions and concludes with some advice on choosing a supplement with the most benefit and least risk.

Dietary supplements were defined in **Chapter 1**.

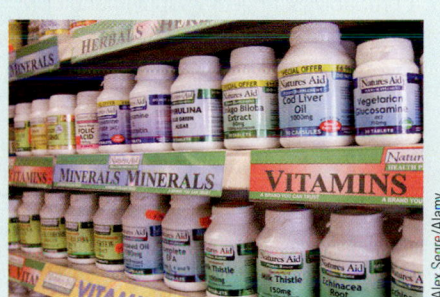

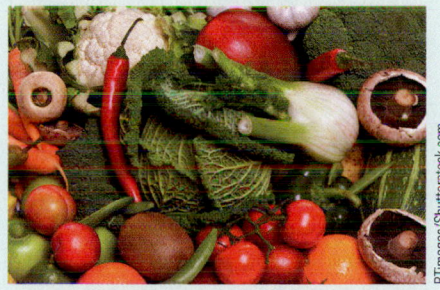

Which is the best source of vitamins to support good health: supplements or food?

*Reference notes are found in Appendix F.

Arguments in Favor of Taking Supplements

By far, most people can meet their nutrient needs from their diet alone. Indisputably, however, the people listed in Table C7–1 need supplements. For them, nutrient supplements can prevent or reverse illnesses. Because supplements are not risk-free, these people should consult a health-care provider who is alert to potential adverse effects and nutrient-drug interactions.

People with Deficiencies

In the United States, few adults suffer nutrient-deficiency diseases such as scurvy, pellagra, and beriberi. When deficiency diseases do appear, prescribed supplements of the missing nutrients quickly stop or reverse most of the damage (exceptions include vitamin A–deficiency blindness, some vitamin B_{12}–deficiency nerve damage, and birth defects caused by folate deficiency in pregnant women).

Subtle subclinical deficiencies that do not cause classic symptoms are easily overlooked or misdiagnosed—and they often occur. People who diet habitually or elderly people with diminished appetite may eat so little nutritious food that they teeter on the edge of deficiency, with no reserve to handle any increase in demand. Similarly, people who omit entire food groups without proper diet

Table C7–1

Some Valid Reasons for Taking Supplements

These people may need supplements:

- People with nutrient deficiencies.
- Women who are capable of becoming pregnant (supplemental or enrichment sources of folic acid are recommended to reduce risk of neural tube defects in infants).
- Pregnant or lactating women (they may need iron and folate).
- Newborns (they are routinely given a vitamin K dose).
- Infants (they may need various supplements; see Chapter 13).
- People who undergo weight-loss surgery (this creates nutrient malabsorption).
- Those who are lactose intolerant (they need calcium to forestall osteoporosis).
- Habitual dieters (they may eat insufficient food).
- Elderly people often benefit from some of the vitamins and minerals in a balanced supplement (they may choose poor diets, have trouble chewing, or absorb or metabolize nutrients less efficiently; see Chapter 14).
- People living with HIV or other wasting illnesses (they lose nutrients faster than foods can supply them).
- Those addicted to drugs or alcohol (they absorb fewer and excrete more nutrients; nutrients cannot undo damage from drugs or alcohol).
- Those recovering from surgery, burns, injury, or illness (they need extra nutrients to help regenerate tissues).
- Strict vegetarians (vegans may need vitamin B_{12}, vitamin D, iron, and zinc).
- People taking medications that interfere with the body's use of nutrients.

planning or who are too busy or lack knowledge or lack money are likely to lack nutrients. For them, until they correct their diets, a low-dose, complete vitamin-mineral supplement may help them avoid deficiency diseases.

Life Stages with Increased Nutrient Needs

During certain stages of life, many people find it difficult or impossible to meet nutrient needs without supplements. For example, women who lose a lot of blood and therefore a lot of iron during menstruation each month often need an iron supplement. Similarly, pregnant and breastfeeding women have exceptionally high nutrient needs and routinely take special supplements to help meet them. Newborns require a dose of vitamin K at birth, as the preceding chapter pointed out.[2]

Appetite and Physical Stress

Any interference with a person's appetite, ability to eat, or ability to absorb or use nutrients will impair nutrient status. Prolonged illnesses, extensive injuries or burns, weight-loss or other surgery, and addictions to alcohol or other drugs all have these effects, and such stressors increase nutrient requirements of the tissues. In addition, medications used to treat such conditions often increase nutrient needs. In all these cases, appropriate nutrient supplements can avert further decline.[3]

Arguments against Taking Supplements

In study after study, well-nourished people are the ones found to be taking supplements, adding excess nutrients to already sufficient intakes.[4] Ironically, people with low nutrient intakes from food generally do not take supplements. As for risks, the most likely hazard to the supplement taker is to the wallet—as an old saying goes, "If you take supplements of the water-soluble vitamins, you'll have the most expensive urine in town." Occasionally, though, supplement intake is both costly and harmful to health.[5]

Toxicity

Foods rarely cause nutrient imbalances or toxicities, but supplements easily can—and the higher the dose, the greater the risk. Supplement users are more likely to have excessive intakes of certain nutrients—notably iron, zinc, vitamin A, and niacin.

People's tolerances for high doses of nutrients vary, just as their risks of deficiencies do, and amounts tolerable for some may be harmful for others. The DRI Tolerable Upper Intake Levels define the highest intakes that appear safe for *most* healthy people. A few sensitive people may experience toxicities at lower doses, however. Table C7–2 compares Tolerable Upper Intake Levels with typical nutrient doses in supplements.

The true extent of supplement toxicity in this country is unknown, but many adverse events are reported each year from vitamins, minerals, essential oils, herbs, and other supplements.[6] Only an alert health-care professional knowledgeable in nutrition can reliably recognize nutrient toxicity and report it to the FDA. Many chronic, subclinical toxicities go unrecognized and unreported.

Supplement Contamination and Safety

The FDA recently identified over 330 "dietary supplements" sold on the U.S. market that were contaminated with pharmaceutical drugs, such as steroid hormones and stimulants. Such products are often sold as "natural" alternatives to FDA-approved drugs, but their use has caused positive results on tests for banned drugs in athletes. In addition, a range of symptoms, including stroke, injury to the liver, kidney failure, and death, has been documented in consumers of these supplements.[7] Toxic plant material, toxic heavy metals, bacteria, and other contaminants have also shown up in dietary supplements.[8]

Plain multivitamin and mineral supplements from reputable sources, without herbs or add-ons, generally test free from contamination, although their contents may vary from those stated on the label. Over twice the label amount of vitamin A was found in a popular multivitamin, and several other brands

contained more than the Tolerable Upper Intake Levels of niacin and magnesium.[9] A prenatal multivitamin contained more than 140 percent of the chromium listed on the label.[10]

Many consumers wrongly believe that government scientists—in particular, those of the FDA—test each new dietary supplement to ensure its safety and effectiveness before allowing it to be sold. They do not. In fact, under the current Dietary Supplement Health and Education Act, the FDA has little control over supplement sales.[†] It can act to remove *tainted* products from store shelves, however, and does so often.[11]

Most Americans express support for greater regulation of dietary supplements, and most health professionals emphatically agree. Meanwhile, consumers can report adverse reactions to supplements directly to the FDA via its hotline or website.[‡]

Life-Threatening Misinformation

Another problem arises when people who are ill come to believe that self-prescribed high doses of vitamins or minerals can be therapeutic. On experiencing a warning symptom of a disease, a person might postpone seeking a diagnosis, thinking, "I probably just need a supplement to make this go away." Such self-diagnosis postpones medical care and gives the disease a chance to worsen. Improper dosing can also be a problem. For example, a man who suffered from mental illness arrived at an emergency room with dangerously low blood pressure. He had ingested 11 grams of niacin on the advice of an Internet website that falsely touted niacin as an effective therapy for schizophrenia. The Tolerable Upper Intake Level for niacin is 35 *milligrams*.

Supplements are almost never effective for purposes other than those already listed in Table C7–1. This doesn't stop marketers from making enticing structure-function claims in materials

[†] *The Dietary Supplement Health and Education Act of 1994 regulates supplements, holding them to the same general labeling requirements that apply to foods (labeling terms were defined in Chapter 2).*

[‡] *Consumers should report suspected harm from dietary supplements to their health providers or to the FDA's MedWatch program at (800) FDA-1088 or on the Internet at www.fda.gov/medwatch/.*

Table C7–2

Intake Guidelines (Adults) and Supplement Doses

Nutrient	Tolerable Upper Intake Level[a]	Typical Multivitamin-Mineral Supplement	Average Single-Nutrient Supplement
Vitamins			
Vitamin A	3,000 µg (10,000 IU)	5,000 IU	8,000 to 10,000 IU
Vitamin D	100 µg (4,000 IU)	400 IU	400 to 50,000 IU[b]
Vitamin E	1,000 mg (1,500 to 2,200 IU)[c]	30 IU	100 to 1,000 IU
Vitamin K	—	40 µg	—
Thiamin	—[d]	1.5 mg	50 mg
Riboflavin	—[d]	1.7 mg	25 mg
Niacin (as niacinamide)	35 mg[c]	20 mg	100 to 500 mg
Vitamin B$_6$	100 mg	2 mg	100 to 200 mg
Folate	1,000 µg[c]	400 µg	400 µg
Vitamin B$_{12}$	—[d]	6 µg	100 to 1,000 µg
Pantothenic acid	—[d]	10 mg	100 to 500 mg
Biotin	—[d]	30 µg	300 to 600 µg
Vitamin C	2,000 mg	10 mg	500 to 2,000 mg
Choline	3,500 mg	10 mg	250 mg
Minerals			
Calcium	2,000 to 3,000 mg	160 mg	250 to 600 mg
Phosphorus	4,000 mg	110 mg	—[f]
Magnesium	350 mg[e]	100 mg	250 mg
Iron	45 mg	18 mg	18 to 30 mg
Zinc	40 mg	15 mg	10 to 100 mg
Iodine	1,100 µg	150 µg	—[f]
Selenium	400 µg	10 µg	50 to 200 µg
Fluoride	10 mg	—	—[f]
Copper	10 mg	0.5 mg	—[f]
Manganese	11 mg	5 mg	—[f]
Chromium	—[d]	25 µg	200 to 400 µg
Molybdenum	2,000 µg	25 µg	—[f]

[a]Unless otherwise noted, Tolerable Upper Intake Levels represent total intakes from food, water, and supplements.

[b]50,000 IU vitamin D is available by prescription.

[c]Tolerable Upper Intake Levels represent intakes from supplements, fortified foods, or both.

[d]These nutrients have been evaluated by the DRI Committee for Tolerable Upper Intake Levels, but none was established because of insufficient data. No adverse effects have been reported with intakes of these nutrients at levels typical of supplements, but caution is still advised, given the potential for harm that accompanies excessive intakes.

[e]Tolerable Upper Intake Levels represent intakes from supplements only.

[f]Available as a single supplement by prescription.

of all kinds—in print, on labels, and on television or the Internet. Such sales pitches often fall far short of the FDA standard that claims should be "truthful and not misleading."

False Sense of Security

Lulled into a false sense of security, a person might eat irresponsibly, thinking, "My supplement will cover my needs." However, no one knows exactly how to formulate the "ideal" supplement, and no standards exist for formulations. What nutrients should be included? How much of each? On whose needs should the choices be based? Which, if any, of the phytochemicals should be added?

Whole Foods Are Best for Nutrients

In general, the body assimilates nutrients best from foods that dilute and disperse them among other substances that facilitate their absorption and use by the body.[12] Taken in pure, concentrated form, nutrients are likely to interfere with one another's absorption or with the absorption of other nutrients from foods eaten at the same time. Such effects are particularly well known among the minerals. For example, zinc hinders copper and calcium absorption, iron hinders zinc absorption, and calcium hinders magnesium and iron absorption.

Among vitamins, vitamin C supplements *enhance* iron absorption, making iron overload likely in susceptible people. High doses of vitamin E interfere with vitamin K functions, delaying blood clotting and possibly raising the risk of brain hemorrhage (a form of stroke). These and other interactions present drawbacks to supplement use.

Can Supplements Prevent Chronic Diseases?

Many people take supplements in the belief that they can prevent heart disease and cancer. Can taking a supplement prevent these killers?

Vitamin D and Cancer

Reports that vitamin D supplements might prevent cancers, particularly of the breast, colon, and prostate, have boosted sales. True, low vitamin D intakes have been associated with increased cancer risk in some studies, and patients with higher serum vitamin D levels at the time of colorectal cancer diagnosis have better survival rates, but overall the connection has proved insignificant.[13] The committee on DRI, along with others, concludes that insufficient evidence exists to support an association between vitamin D intakes and cancer risk.[14] The U.S. Preventive Services Task Force, a group that offers unbiased advice concerning medical treatments, has recommended against taking vitamin D for cancer prevention.[15]

Antioxidant Supplements

Central to the idea that antioxidant nutrients might fight diseases is the theory of **oxidative stress** (terms are defined in Table C7–3). The chapter explained that normal activities of body cells produce free radicals (highly unstable molecules of oxygen) that can damage cell structures. Oxidative stress results when free-radical activity in the body exceeds its antioxidant defenses. When such damage accumulates, it triggers inflammation, which may lead to heart disease and cancer, among other conditions. **Antioxidant nutrients** help to quench these free radicals, rendering them harmless to cellular structures and stopping the chain of events.

Taking antioxidant pills instead of making needed lifestyle changes may sound appealing, but evidence does not support a role for supplements against chronic diseases.[16] In some cases, supplements may even be harmful.[17] For example, taking high doses of vitamin C, an antioxidant nutrient, may lower blood pressure somewhat, a small but potentially beneficial effect. The same doses also *increase* markers of oxidation in the blood and elevate the risk of vision-impairing cataracts in the eyes, however.[18] Researchers are investigating links between high doses of vitamin C and cataracts.[19]

Vitamin E and Chronic Disease

Hopeful early studies reported that taking vitamin E supplements reduced the rate of death from heart disease.[20] It made sense because in the laboratory vitamin E opposes blood clotting, tissue inflammation, arterial injury, and lipid oxidation—all factors in heart disease development. After years of follow-up human studies, however, little protective effect is evident.[21] In fact, pooled results revealed a slight but alarming *increased* risk for death among people taking vitamin E supplements. Neither help nor harm is consistently observed with vitamin E supplementation.[22]

Studies reporting negative findings have been criticized for testing too low a dose, testing only the alpha-tocopherol form of vitamin E, failing to establish previous vitamin E status, or other reasons.[23] For now, the results are disappointing, but research continues.

Currently, some preliminary evidence links certain forms of vitamin E with cancer protection.[24] However, much more research is needed to clarify these connections before conclusions can be drawn, and vitamin E supplements, taken for any reason, carry risks.

The Story of Beta-Carotene— A Case in Point

Again and again, population studies confirm that people who eat plenty of fruits and vegetables, particularly those rich in beta-carotene, have low rates of certain cancers. Years ago, researchers focused on beta-carotene, while supplement makers touted it as a powerful anticancer substance. Consumers eagerly bought and took beta-carotene supplements in response.

Then, in a sudden reversal, support for beta-carotene supplements crumbled overnight. Trials around the world were abruptly stopped when scientists noted no benefits but observed a 28 percent *increase* in lung cancer among smokers taking beta-carotene compared with a placebo. Today, beta-carotene supplements are not recommended.[25]

Such reversals might shock and frustrate the unscientific mind, but scientists expect them as research unfolds. In this case, a long-known and basic nutrition principle was reaffirmed: low disease risk accompanies a *diet* of nutritious whole foods, foods that present a balance of nutrients and other beneficial constituents. Whereas a sweet potato and a pill may both contain beta-carotene, the sweet potato presents a balanced array of nutrients, phytochemicals, and fiber that modulate beta-carotene's effects. The pill provides only beta-carotene, a lone chemical.

For most people, taking an ordinary daily multivitamin and mineral supplement is generally safe when they choose an appropriate product and follow dosing directions. And for those who need them, nutrient supplements constitute a modern-day miracle. Table C7–4 reviews the arguments for and against taking supplements.

SOS: Selection of Supplements

If you fall into one of the categories listed earlier in Table C7–1 and if you absolutely cannot meet your nutrient needs from foods, a supplement containing *nutrients only* can prevent serious problems. In these cases, the benefits outweigh the risks. (Table C7–5 on p. 290 provides some *invalid* reasons for taking supplements in which the risks clearly outweigh the benefits.) Remember, no standard

---

Table C7–3

Antioxidant Terms

- **antioxidant nutrients** vitamins and minerals that oppose the effects of oxidants on human physical functions. The antioxidant vitamins are vitamin E, vitamin C, and beta-carotene. The mineral selenium also participates in antioxidant activities.
- **oxidants** compounds (such as oxygen itself) that oxidize other compounds. Compounds that prevent oxidation are called antioxidants, whereas those that promote it are called prooxidants (*anti* means "against"; *pro* means "for").
- **oxidative stress** damage inflicted on living systems by free radicals.

Table C7–4

Taking Dietary Supplements: Point, Counterpoint

Many people take dietary supplements either to counterbalance an unhealthy diet or to improve on their already abundant intake of nutrients. This table considers some arguments for and against doing so.

Arguments in Support of Dietary Supplements	Arguments in Opposition to Dietary Supplements
1. *Prevent or correct deficiencies.* Supplements are important for people suffering from nutrient deficiencies, and in most cases, they can correct the problems and restore health.	1. *Cause toxicities.* Dietary supplements provide no benefits to well-nourished people. High nutrient doses from single-nutrient supplements pose a threat of toxicity.
2. *Fill increased nutrient needs.* Adolescents of both genders, women of childbearing age, women who are pregnant or breast-feeding, newborn infants, people who are ill, smokers, and others all have increased needs for certain nutrients such as iron, folate, vitamin K, or vitamin C.	2. *Provide unneeded nutrients.* Most healthy children and adults who eat a nutritious diet consume adequate amounts of vitamins and minerals from food, making nutrients from supplements unnecessary.
3. *Improve nutrient status.* Certain groups of people, such as the elderly who might not eat enough food and vegetarians who omit entire food groups, might develop subclinical nutrient deficiencies that do not produce obvious symptoms but could impair health is subtle ways, such as reduced resistance to infection.	3. *Provide limited benefits.* A supplement can treat a single nutrient deficiency but cannot replace a nutritious diet to support health. A diet that lacks one nutrient surely lacks others, along with fiber, phytochemicals, and other constituents of whole, nutrient-dense foods.
4. *Provide nutritional insurance.* Vitamin pills are cheap to purchase, and taking them is easier than shopping, cooking, and planning an adequate diet.	4. *Create a false sense of security.* Many times, the very people who might benefit from multivitamin or other supplements do not consume them, while well-fed individuals are more likely to do so.
5. *Efficacy and safety of dietary supplements.* The FDA routinely recalls supplements containing harmful ingredients and removes them from the market. The FDA also prosecutes manufacturers violating the Dietary Supplement Health and Education Act, which requires supplements to be free of contaminants and ingredients that are not safe for human consumption.	5. *Efficacy and safety of dietary supplements.* Scientists and consumer groups agree that oversight policies are outdated and ineffective. The FDA does not regulate supplements as tightly as it does pharmaceutical drugs prior to marketing, but rather waits to remove products from the market after they have proven unsafe by causing harm to consumers.

Sources: H. Ketha and coauthors, Iatrogenic vitamin D toxicity in an infant: A case report and review of literature, Journal of Steroid Biochemistry and Molecular Biology 148 (2015): 14–18; J. R. Genzen, Hypercalcemic crisis due to vitamin D toxicity, Lab Medicine 45 (2014): 147–150; S. M. Alsanad, E. M. Williamson, and R. L. Howard, Cancer patients at risk of herb/food supplement-drug interactions: A systematic review, Phytotherapy Research 28 (2014): 1749–1755; E. Fabian and coauthors, Vitamin status in elderly people in relation to the use of nutritional supplements, Journal of Nutrition 16 (2012): 206–212; P. A. Cohen, Assessing supplemental safety—The FDA's controversial proposal, New England Journal of Medicine 366 (2012): 389–391; M. E. Martinez and coauthors, Dietary supplements and cancer prevention: Balancing potential benefits against proven harms, Journal of the National Cancer Institute 104 (2012): 732–739.

formula for multivitamin and mineral pills exists—the term *supplement* applies to any combination of nutrients in widely varying doses.

Choosing a Type

Which supplement to choose? The first step is to remain aware that sales of vitamin supplements often approach the realm of quackery because the profits are high and the industry is largely free of oversight. To escape the clutches of the health hustlers, use your imagination, and delete the label pictures of sexy, active people and the meaningless, glittering generalities like "Advanced Formula" or "Maximum Power." Also, ignore vague references to the functioning of body systems or common complaints, such as cramps (Chapter 2 illustrated such claims)—most of these are overstatements of the truth. Avoid "extras" such as herbs (see Chapter 11). And don't be misled into buying and taking unneeded supplements, because none are risk-free.

Reading the Label

Now all you have left is the Supplement Facts panel in Figure C7–1 (p. 290) that lists the nutrients, the ingredients, the form of the supplement, and the price—the plain facts. You have two basic questions to answer. The first question: What form do you want—chewable, liquid, or pills? If you'd rather drink your vitamins and minerals than chew them, fine. If you choose a fortified liquid meal replacer, a sugary vitamin drink, or an "energy bar" (a candy bar to which vitamins and other nutrients are added), you must then proportionately reduce the calories you consume in food to avoid gaining unwanted weight. If you choose chewable pills, be aware that vitamin C can erode tooth enamel. Swallow promptly and flush the teeth with a drink of water.

Targeting Your Needs

The second question: Who are you? What vitamins and minerals do you actually need and in what amounts? Match your DRI nutrient intake recommendations (the tables are on the inside front cover) with the doses in supplement options. The DRI values meet the needs of all reasonably healthy people.

Some Invalid Reasons for Taking Supplements

Watch out for plausible-sounding, but false, reasons given by marketers trying to convince you, the consumer, that you need supplements. The invalid reasons listed below have gained strength by repetition among friends, on the Internet, and by the media:

- You fear that foods grown on today's soils lack nutrients (a common false statement made by sellers of supplements).
- You feel tired and falsely believe that supplements can provide energy.
- You hope that supplements can help you cope with stress.
- You wish to build up your muscles faster or without physical activity.
- You want to prevent or cure self-diagnosed illnesses.
- You hope excess nutrients will produce unnamed mysterious beneficial reactions in your body.

People who should never take supplements without a physician's approval include those with kidney or liver ailments (they are susceptible to toxicities), those taking medications (nutrients can interfere with their actions), and smokers (who should avoid products with beta-carotene).

Choosing Doses

As for doses of nutrients, for most people, an appropriate supplement provides all the vitamins and minerals in amounts smaller than, equal to, or very close to the intake recommendations. Avoid any preparation that in a daily dose provides more than the DRI recommended intake of vitamin A, vitamin D, or any mineral or more than the Tolerable Upper Intake Level of any nutrient. In addition, avoid high doses of iron (more than 10 milligrams per day) except for menstruating women. People who menstruate need more iron, but people who don't, don't. Warning: expect to reject about 80 percent of available preparations when you choose according to these criteria; be choosy where your health is concerned.

A Supplement Label

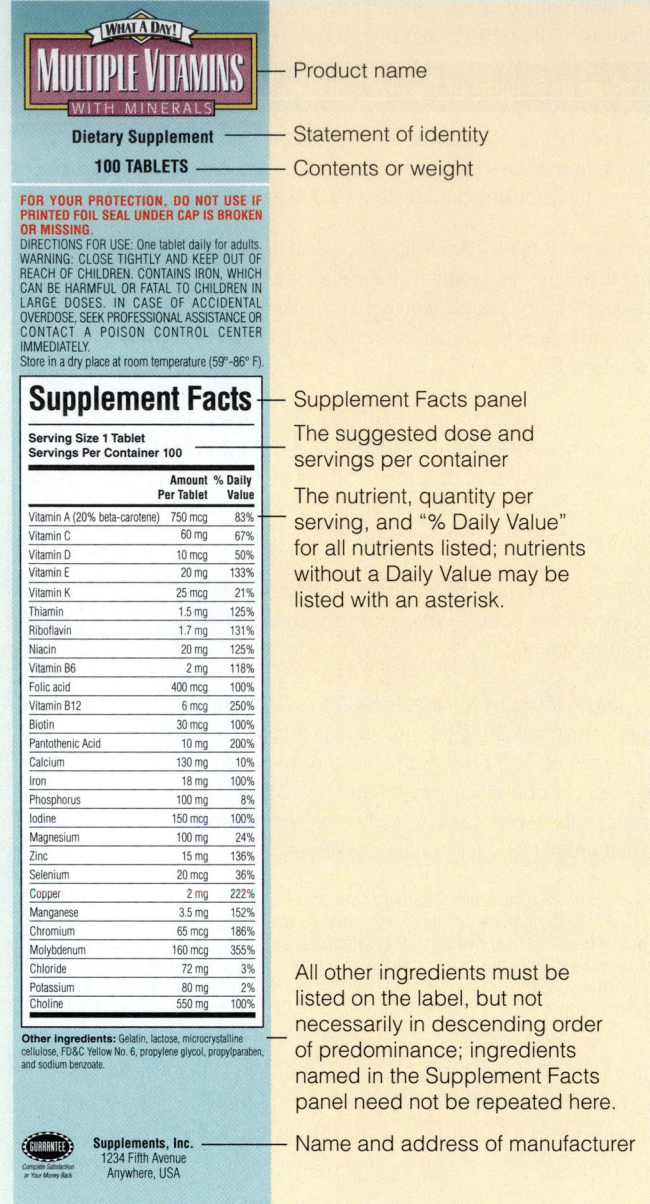

- Product name
- Statement of identity
- Contents or weight
- Supplement Facts panel
- The suggested dose and servings per container
- The nutrient, quantity per serving, and "% Daily Value" for all nutrients listed; nutrients without a Daily Value may be listed with an asterisk.
- All other ingredients must be listed on the label, but not necessarily in descending order of predominance; ingredients named in the Supplement Facts panel need not be repeated here.
- Name and address of manufacturer

Going for Quality

If you see a USP symbol on the label, it means that a manufacturer has voluntarily paid an independent laboratory to test the product and affirm that it contains the ingredients listed and that it will dissolve or disintegrate in the digestive tract to make the ingredients available for absorption. The symbol does not imply that the supplement has been tested for safety or effectiveness with regard to health, however.

A high price also does not ensure the highest quality; generic brands are often as good as or better than expensive name-brand supplements. If they are less expensive, it may mean that their price doesn't have to cover the cost of national advertising. In any case, buy from a well-known retailer who keeps stocks fresh and stores them properly.

Avoiding Marketing Traps

In addition, avoid these:

- "For better metabolism." Preparations containing extra biotin may claim to improve metabolism, but no evidence supports this.

- "Organic" or "natural" preparations with added substances. They are no better than standard types, but they cost much more, and the added substances may add risks.

- "High-potency" or "therapeutic dose" supplements. More is not better.

- Items not needed in human nutrition, such as carnitine and inositol. These particular items won't harm you, but they reveal a marketing strategy that makes the whole mix suspect. The manufacturer wants you to believe that its pills contain the latest "new" nutrient that other brands omit, but in fact for every valid discovery of this kind, there are 999,999 frauds.

- "Time release." Medications such as some antibiotics or pain relievers often must be sustained at a steady concentration in the blood to be effective; nutrients, in contrast, are incorporated into the tissues where they are needed whenever they arrive.

- "Stress formulas." Although the stress response depends on certain B vitamins and vitamin C, the DRI recommended intake provides all that is needed of these nutrients. If you are under stress (and who isn't?), generous servings of fruits and vegetables will more than cover your need.

- Any supplement sold with claims that today's foods lack sufficient nutrients to support health. Plants make vitamins for their own needs, not ours. A plant lacking a mineral or failing to make a needed vitamin dies before it can bear food for our consumption.

To get the most from a supplement of vitamins and minerals, take it with food. A full stomach retains and dissolves the pill with its churning action.

Conclusion

People in developed nations are far more likely to suffer from *overnutrition* and poor lifestyle choices than from nutrient deficiencies. People wish that swallowing vitamin pills would boost their health. The truth—that they need to improve their eating and exercise habits—is harder to swallow.

Critical Thinking

1. List three reasons why someone might take a multivitamin supplement that does not exceed 100 percent of the RDAs. Would you ever take an antioxidant supplement? Why or why not? Suppose you decided that you should take a vitamin supplement because you do not drink milk. How would you determine the best brand of supplement to purchase?

2. Imagine that you are standing in a pharmacy comparing the Supplement Facts panels on the labels of two supplement bottles, one a "complete multivitamin" product and the other marked "high potency vitamins."

What major differences in terms of nutrient inclusion and doses might you find between these two products? What differences in risk would you anticipate? If you were asked to pick one of these products for an elderly person whose appetite is diminished, which would you choose? Give your justification.

8 Water and Minerals

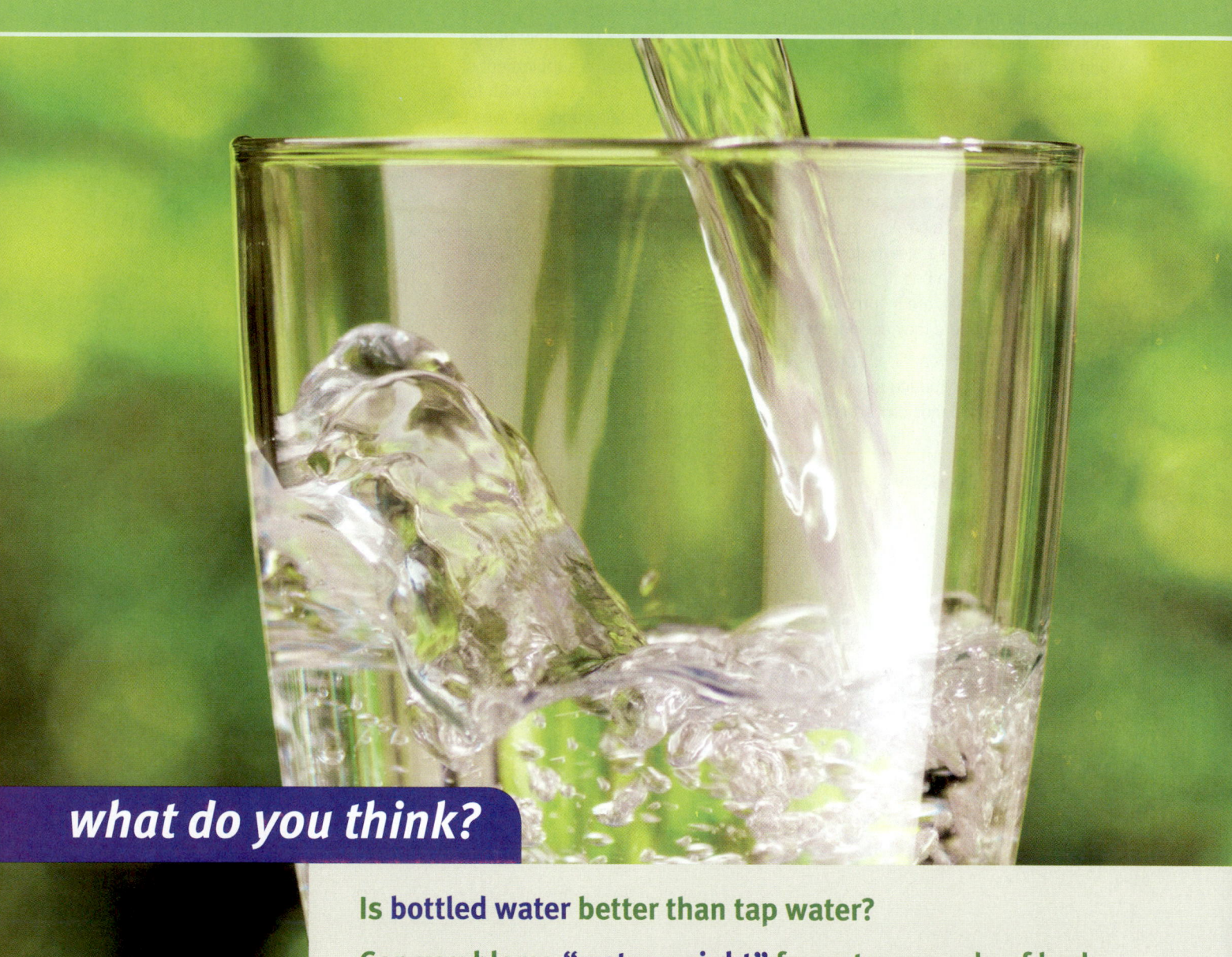

Effred/Shutstock.com

what do you think?

Is bottled water better than tap water?

Can you blame **"water weight"** for extra pounds of body weight?

Do adults outgrow the need for **calcium**?

Do you need an **iron supplement** if you're feeling tired?

Learning Objectives

After completing this chapter, you should be able to accomplish the following:

LO 8.1 Discuss the functions of water and the importance of maintaining the body's water balance.

LO 8.2 Compare the types and safety of drinking water from different sources.

LO 8.3 Explain the concepts of fluid and electrolyte balance and acid-base balance and their importance to health.

LO 8.4 Discuss the functions of the seven major minerals, their food sources, and the effects of their deficiencies and toxicities.

LO 8.5 Discuss the food sources and the functions of the trace minerals and the effects of their deficiencies and toxicities.

LO 8.6 Discuss food choices that help to meet the need for calcium.

LO 8.7 Discuss how osteoporosis develops and the actions that may help to prevent it.

If you were to extract all of the **minerals** from a human body, they would form, a small pile that weighs only about 5 pounds. The pile may not be impressive in size, but the work of those minerals is critical to living tissue.

Consider calcium and phosphorus. If you could separate these two minerals from the rest of the pile, you would take away about three-fourths of the total. Crystals made of these two minerals, plus a few others, form the structure of bones and so provide the architecture of the skeleton.

Run a magnet through the pile that remains and you pick up the iron. It doesn't fill a teaspoon, but it consists of billions and billions of iron atoms. As part of hemoglobin, these iron atoms are able to attach to oxygen and make it available at the sites inside the cells where metabolic work is taking place.

If you then extract all the other minerals from the pile, leaving only copper and iodine, you'll want to close the windows first. A slight breeze would blow these remaining bits of dust away. Yet the copper in the dust enables iron to hold and to release oxygen, and iodine is the critical mineral in the thyroid hormones. Figure 8–1 (p. 294) shows the amounts of the seven **major minerals** and a few of the **trace minerals** in the human body. Other minerals such as gold and aluminum are present in the body but are not known to have nutrient functions.

The distinction between major and trace minerals doesn't mean that one group is more important in the body than the other. A daily deficiency of a few micrograms of iodine is just as serious as a deficiency of several hundred milligrams of calcium. The major minerals are simply present in larger quantities in the body and are needed in greater amounts in the diet.

The Dietary Guidelines for Americans committee names four minerals as shortfall nutrients—most people's intakes are too low:

- Potassium.
- Calcium.
- Magnesium.
- Iron (for some people).

Of the shortfall minerals, calcium and potassium are also named as nutrients of public health concern because their underconsumption has been convincingly liked with chronic diseases. In addition, one mineral stands out as being overconsumed by most people:

- Sodium.[1]*

---
*Reference notes are found in Appendix F.

minerals naturally occurring, inorganic, homogeneous substances; chemical elements.

major minerals essential mineral nutrients required in the adult diet in amounts greater than 100 milligrams per day. Also called *macrominerals*.

trace minerals essential mineral nutrients required in the adult diet in amounts less than 100 milligrams per day. Also called *microminerals*.

Figure 8–1

Minerals in a 60-Kilogram (132-Pound) Person, in Grams

The major minerals are present in the body in larger amounts and also are needed by the body in larger amounts than the trace minerals.

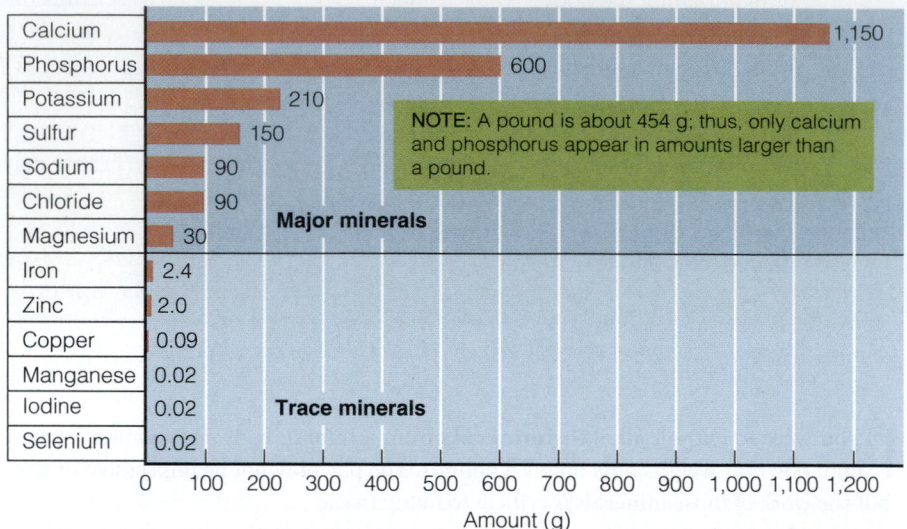

	Amount (g)
Calcium	1,150
Phosphorus	600
Potassium	210
Sulfur	150
Sodium	90
Chloride	90
Magnesium	30
Iron	2.4
Zinc	2.0
Copper	0.09
Manganese	0.02
Iodine	0.02
Selenium	0.02

Major minerals

Trace minerals

NOTE: A pound is about 454 g; thus, only calcium and phosphorus appear in amounts larger than a pound.

Later sections present the key facts about these and other minerals important to nutrition.

Water, the first topic of this chapter, is unique among the nutrients and the most indispensable of all. The body needs more water each day than any other nutrient—50 times more water than protein and 5,000 times more water than vitamin C. You can survive a deficiency of any of the other nutrients for a long time, in some cases for months or years, but you can survive only a few days without water. In less than a day, a lack of water compromises the body's chemistry and metabolism.

Our discussion begins with water's many functions. Next we examine how water and the major minerals mingle to form the body's fluids and how cells regulate the distribution of those fluids. Then we take up the specialized roles of each of the minerals. (Reminder: The DRI intake recommendations for water and minerals appear on the inside front cover pages.)

Water

LO 8.1 Discuss the functions of water and the importance of maintaining the body's water balance.

You began as a single cell bathed in a nourishing fluid. As you became a beautifully organized, air-breathing body of trillions of cells, each of your cells had to remain next to water to stay alive.

Water makes up about 60 percent of an adult person's weight—that's almost 80 pounds of water in a 130-pound person. All this water in the body is not simply a river coursing through the arteries, capillaries, and veins. Soft tissues contain a great deal of water: the brain and muscles are 75 to 80 percent water by weight; even bones contain 25 percent water.[2] Some of the body's water is incorporated into the chemical structures of compounds that form the cells, tissues, and organs of the body. For example, proteins hold water molecules within them, water that is locked in and not readily available for any other use. Water also participates actively in many chemical reactions.

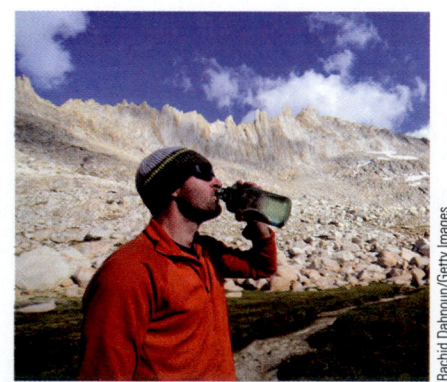

Water is the most indispensable nutrient.

Why Is Water the Most Indispensable Nutrient?

Water brings to each cell the exact ingredients the cell requires and carries away the end products of its life-sustaining reactions. The water of the body fluids is thus the transport vehicle for all the nutrients and wastes. Without water, cells quickly die.

Solvent   Water is a nearly universal **solvent**: it dissolves amino acids, glucose, minerals, and many other substances needed by the cells. Fatty substances, too, can travel freely in the watery blood and lymph because they are specially packaged in water-soluble proteins.

Cleansing Agent   Water is also the body's cleansing agent. Small molecules, such as the nitrogen wastes generated during protein metabolism, dissolve in the watery blood and must be removed before they build up to toxic concentrations. The kidneys filter these wastes from the blood and excrete them, mixed with water, as urine. When the kidneys become diseased, as can happen in diabetes and other disorders, toxins can build to life-threatening levels. A kidney **dialysis** machine must then take over the task of cleansing the blood by filtering wastes into water contained in the machine.

Lubricant and Cushion   Water molecules resist being crowded together. Thanks to this incompressibility, water can act as a lubricant and a cushion for the joints, and it can protect sensitive tissue such as the spinal cord from shock. The fluid that fills the eye serves in a similar way to keep optimal pressure on the retina and lens. From the start of human life, a fetus is cushioned against shock by the bag of amniotic fluid in the mother's uterus. Water also lubricates the digestive tract, the respiratory tract, and all tissues that are moistened with mucus.

Coolant   Yet another of water's special features is its ability to help maintain body temperature. The water of sweat is the body's coolant. Heat is produced as a by-product of energy metabolism and can build up dangerously in the body. To rid itself of this excess heat, the body routes its blood supply through the capillaries just under the skin. At the same time, the skin secretes sweat, and its water evaporates. Converting water to vapor takes energy; therefore, as sweat evaporates, heat energy dissipates, cooling the skin and the underlying blood. The cooled blood then flows back to cool the body's core. Sweat evaporates continuously from the skin, usually in slight amounts that go unnoticed; thus, the skin is a major organ through which water is lost from the body. Lesser amounts are lost by way of exhaled breath and the feces.

To sum up, water:

- Carries nutrients throughout the body.

- Serves as the solvent for minerals, vitamins, amino acids, glucose, and other small molecules.

- Cleanses the tissues and blood of wastes.

- Actively participates in many chemical reactions.

- Acts as a lubricant around joints.

- Serves as a shock absorber inside the eyes, spinal cord, joints, and amniotic sac surrounding a fetus in the womb.

- Aids in maintaining the body's temperature.

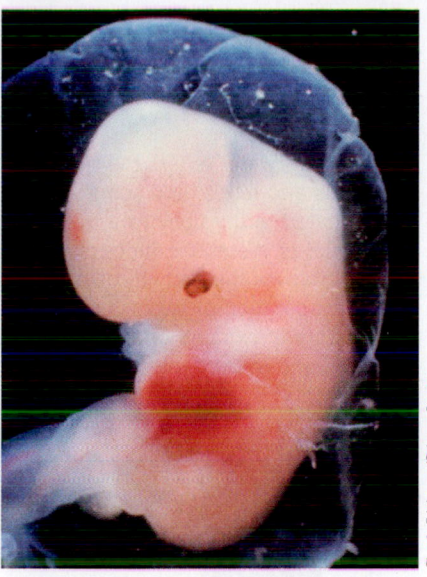

Human life begins in water.

Claude Edelmann/Science Source

KEY POINTS

- Water makes up about 60 percent of the body's weight.
- Water provides the medium for transportation, acts as a solvent, participates in chemical reactions, provides lubrication and shock protection, and aids in temperature regulation in the human body.

solvent a substance that dissolves another and holds it in solution.

dialysis (dye-AL-ih-sis) a medical treatment for failing kidneys in which a person's blood is circulated through a machine that filters out toxins and wastes and returns cleansed blood to the body. Also called *hemodialysis.*

Figure 8-2

Water Balance—A Typical Example

Each day, water enters the body in liquids and foods, and some water is created in the body as a by-product of metabolic processes. Water leaves the body through the evaporation of sweat, in the moisture of exhaled breath, in the urine, and in the feces.

Water input (Total = 1,450–2,800 ml)

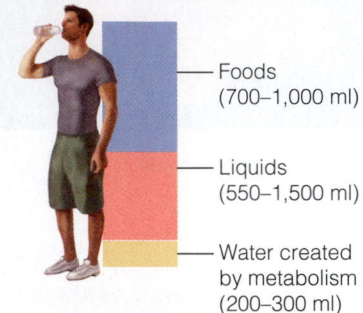

Foods
(700–1,000 ml)

Liquids
(550–1,500 ml)

Water created by metabolism
(200–300 ml)

Water output (Total = 1,450–2,800 ml)

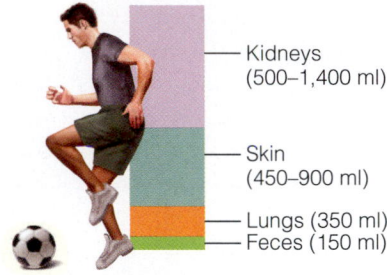

Kidneys
(500–1,400 ml)

Skin
(450–900 ml)

Lungs (350 ml)
Feces (150 ml)

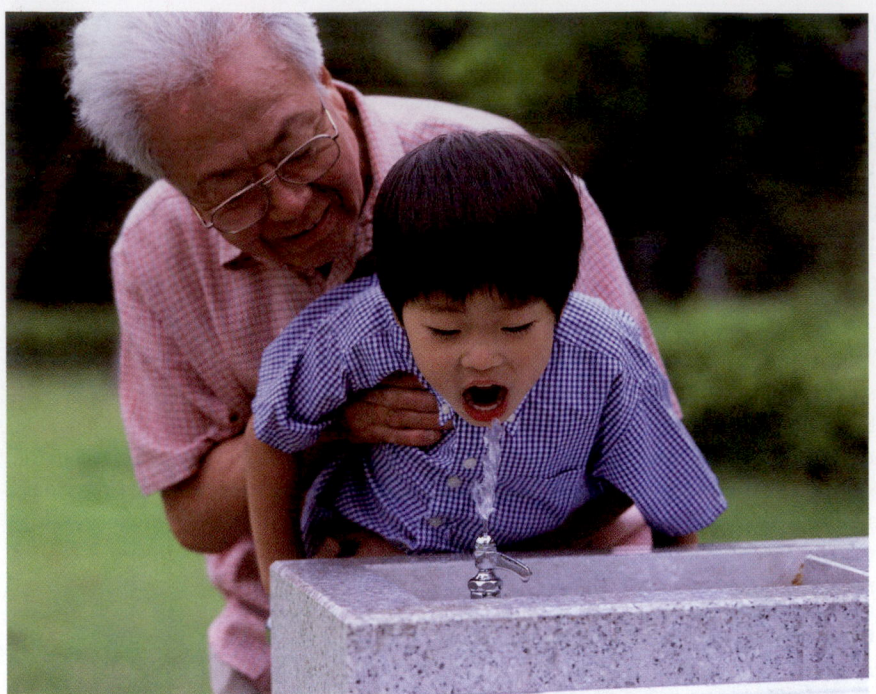

An extra drink of water benefits both young and old.

MIXA/Getty Images

The Body's Water Balance

Water is such an integral part of us that people seldom are conscious of water's importance unless they are deprived of it. Since the body loses some water every day, a person must consume at least the same amount to avoid life-threatening losses—that is, to maintain **water balance**. The total amount of fluid in the body is kept balanced by delicate mechanisms. Imbalances such as **dehydration** and **water intoxication** can occur, but the balance is restored as promptly as the body can manage it. The body controls both intake and excretion to maintain water equilibrium (see Figure 8-2).

The amount of the body's water varies by pounds at a time, especially in women who retain water during menstruation. Eating a meal high in salt can temporarily increase the body's water content; the body sheds the excess over the next day or so as the sodium is excreted. These temporary fluctuations in body water show up on the scale, but gaining or losing water weight does not reflect a change in body fat. Fat weight takes days or weeks to change noticeably, whereas water weight can change overnight.

KEY POINT

- A change in the body's water content can bring about a temporary change in body weight.

Quenching Thirst and Balancing Losses

Thirst and satiety govern water intake. When the blood is too concentrated (having lost water but not salt and other dissolved substances), the molecules and particles in the blood attract water out of the salivary glands, and the mouth becomes dry. Water is also drawn from the body's cells, causing them to collapse a little.[3] Blood becomes more concentrated and blood pressure falls. The brain center known as the hypothalamus (described in Chapter 3) responds to low cellular fluid, concentrated blood particles, or low blood pressure by initiating nerve impulses to the brain that register as "thirst." The hypothalamus also signals the pituitary gland to release a hormone that directs the kidneys to shift water back into the bloodstream from the fluid destined to become urine. The kidneys themselves respond to the sodium concentration in the blood passing through them by secreting regulatory substances of their own. The net result is that the more water the body needs, the less it excretes.

water balance the balance between water intake and water excretion, which keeps the body's water content constant.

dehydration loss of water. The symptoms progress rapidly, from thirst to weakness to exhaustion and delirium, and end in death.

water intoxication a dangerous dilution of the body's fluids resulting from excessive ingestion of plain water. Symptoms are headache, muscular weakness, lack of concentration, poor memory, and loss of appetite.

Table 8–1

Effects of Mild Dehydration, Severe Dehydration, and Chronic Lack of Fluid

Mild Dehydration (Loss of <5% Body Weight)	Severe Dehydration (Loss of >5% Body Weight)	Chronic Low Fluid Intake May Increase the Likelihood of:[a]
Thirst	Pale or shriveled skin	Cardiac arrest (heart attack) and other heart problems
Sudden weight loss	Bluish lips and fingertips	Constipation
Dry, cool skin	Confusion; disorientation	Dental disease
Dry mouth, throat, body linings	Rapid, shallow breathing	Gallstones
Rapid pulse; low blood pressure	Weak, rapid, irregular pulse	Glaucoma (elevated pressure in the eye)
Lack of energy; weakness	Thickening of blood	Hypertension
Impaired kidney function	Shock; seizures	Kidney stones
Reduced quantity of urine; concentrated urine	Coma; death	Pregnancy/childbirth problems
Headache; reduced mental clarity		Stroke
Decreased muscular work and athletic performance		Urinary tract infections
Fever or increased internal temperature		
Fainting and delirium		

[a]Evidence for bladder and colon cancer is inconsistent.

Sources: N. K. Kaneshiro, Dehydration, MedlinePlus, updated August 2013, available at www.nlm.nih.gov/medlineplus/ency/article/000982.htm; B. M. Popkin, K. E. D'Anci, and I. H. Rosenberg, Water, hydration, and health, Nutrition Reviews 68 (2010): 439–458; Standing Committee on the Scientific Evaluation of Dietary Reference Intakes, Food and Nutrition Board, Institute of Medicine, Dietary Reference Intakes: Water, Potassium, Sodium, Chloride, and Sulfate (Washington, D.C.: National Academies Press, 2005), pp. 118–127.

Dehydration Thirst lags behind a lack of water. When too much water is lost from the body and is not replaced, dehydration can threaten survival. A first sign of dehydration is thirst, the signal that the body has already lost a cup or two of its total fluid and the need to drink is immediate. But suppose a thirsty person is unable to obtain fluid or, as in many elderly people, fails to perceive the thirst message. Instead of "wasting" precious water in sweat, the dehydrated body diverts most of its water into the blood vessels to maintain the life-supporting blood pressure. Meanwhile, body heat builds up because sweating has ceased, creating the possibility of serious consequences in hot weather (see Table 8–1).

To ignore the thirst signal is to invite dehydration. With a loss of just 1 percent of body weight as fluid, perceptible symptoms appear: headache, fatigue, confusion or forgetfulness, and an elevated heart rate. A loss of 2 percent impairs physical functioning and impedes a wide range of physical activities.[4] People should stay attuned to thirst and drink whenever they feel thirsty to replace fluids lost throughout the day. Older adults in whom thirst is blunted should drink regularly throughout the day, regardless of thirst.

A word about caffeine: people who drink caffeinated beverages lose a little more fluid than when they drink water because caffeine acts as a **diuretic**. The DRI committee concluded, however, that the mild diuretic effect of moderate caffeine intake does not lead to dehydration or keep people from meeting their fluid needs. Caffeinated beverages can therefore contribute to daily water intakes. The Controversy section of Chapter 14 discusses other effects of caffeine.

Water Intoxication At the other extreme from dehydration, water intoxication occurs when too much plain water floods the body's fluids and disturbs their normal composition. Most adult victims have consumed several gallons of plain water in a few hours' time. Water intoxication is rare, but when it occurs, immediate action is needed to reverse dangerously diluted blood before death ensues (read more about it in Chapter 10).

Do the Math

Water loss can be expressed as a percentage of body weight. In a 150-lb person,

- A 3-lb loss of body fluid equals 2% of body weight.

  3 lbs ÷ 150 lbs × 100
  = 2% of body weight

- A 4½-lb loss equals 3% of body weight in the same 150-lb person.

  4.5 ÷ 150 × 100 = 3%

Now solve this: in a 180-lb person, find the percentage of body weight represented by 5 pounds of water.

diuretic (dye-you-RET-ic) a compound, usually a medication, causing increased urinary water excretion; a "water pill."

Table 8–2

Factors That Increase Fluid Needs

These conditions increase a person's need for fluids:

- Alcohol consumption
- Cold weather
- Dietary fiber
- Diseases that disturb water balance, such as diabetes and kidney diseases
- Forced-air environments, such as airplanes and sealed buildings
- Heated environments
- High altitude
- Hot weather, high humidity
- Increased protein, salt, or sugar intakes
- Ketosis
- Medications (diuretics)
- Physical activity
- Pregnancy and breastfeeding (see Chapter 13)
- Prolonged diarrhea, vomiting, or fever
- Surgery, blood loss, or burns
- Very young or old age

KEY POINTS

- Water losses from the body must be balanced by water intakes to maintain hydration.
- The brain regulates water intake; the brain and kidneys regulate water excretion.
- Caloric beverages add to energy intakes.
- Dehydration and water intoxication can can arise with deficient or excessive water intake.

How Much Water Do I Need to Drink in a Day?

Water needs vary greatly, depending on the foods a person eats, the air temperature and humidity, the altitude, the person's activity level, and other factors (see Table 8–2). Fluid needs vary widely among individuals and also within the same person in various environmental conditions, so a specific water recommendation is hard to pin down.

Water from Fluids and Foods   A wide range of fluid intakes can maintain adequate hydration. As a general guideline, however, the DRI committee recommends that, given a normal diet and moderate environment, the reference man needs about 13 cups of fluid from beverages, including drinking water, and the reference woman needs about 9 cups.[5] This amount of fluid provides about 80 percent of the body's daily water need. On average, most people in the United States, with the exception of older adults, consume close to these amounts.[6] The fluids people choose to drink can affect daily calorie intakes, as the Consumer's Guide section makes clear.

Most of the rest of the body's needed daily fluid comes from the water in foods. Nearly all foods contain some water: water constitutes up to 95 percent of the volume of most fruits and vegetables and at least 50 percent of many meats and cheeses (see Table 8–3 and Appendix A). A small percentage of the day's fluid is generated in the tissues themselves as energy-yielding nutrients release **metabolic water** as a product of chemical breakdown.

Table 8–3

Water in Foods and Beverages

Many solid foods, such as broccoli or steak, are surprisingly high in water.

100%	water, diet soft drinks, seltzer (unflavored), plain tea
95–99%	sugar-free gelatin dessert, clear broth, Chinese cabbage, celery, cucumber, lettuce, summer squash, black coffee
90–94%	sports drinks, grapefruit, fresh strawberries, broccoli, tomatoes
80–89%	sugar-sweetened soft drinks, milk, yogurt, egg white, fruit juices, low-fat cottage cheese, cooked oatmeal, fresh apple, carrot
60–79%	low-calorie mayonnaise, instant pudding, banana, shrimp, lean steak, pork chop, baked potato, cooked rice
40–59%	diet margarine, sausage, chicken, macaroni and cheese
20–39%	bread, cake, cheddar cheese, bagel
10–19%	butter, margarine, regular mayonnaise
5–9%	peanut butter, popcorn
1–4%	ready-to-eat cereals, pretzels
0%	cooking oils, meat fats, shortening, white sugar

metabolic water water generated in the tissues during the chemical breakdown of the energy-yielding nutrients in foods.

Liquid Calories

Most ordinary beverages help to meet the body's need for fluid. In developed nations such as ours, however, people encounter a constant stream of beverages that contain more than just water.

Mystery Pounds

Derek, an active college student, hasn't thought much about his fluid intake but is lamenting, "I'm exercising more and I've cut out the junk food, but I've still gained five pounds!" What has escaped Derek's attention is the calories that he's been drinking: a big glass of vitamin C–enriched orange punch at breakfast, a soda or two before lunchtime, sometimes a large mocha latte for an afternoon wake-up, and, of course, sports drinks when he works out.

Drinking without Thirst

Like Derek, most people choose beverages for reasons having little to do with thirst. They seek the stimulating

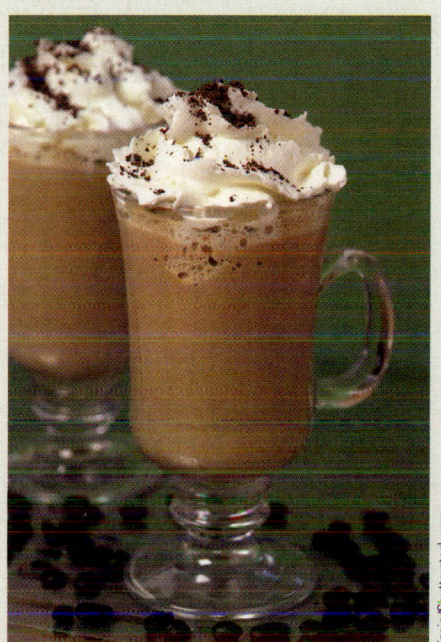

A fancy coffee drink can easily provide 400–700 calories; plain coffee contains zero calories.

Kasia/Shutterstock.com

effect of caffeine in coffee, tea, or sodas. They choose fluids such as soup, milk, juice, or other beverages at mealtimes. They believe they need the added nutrients in sugar-sweetened "vitamin waters." They think they need the carbohydrate in sports drinks for all physical activities (few exercisers do; read Chapter 10). They drink hot beverages to warm up or cold ones to cool off. Or they drink for pleasure—for the aroma of coffee, the sweet taste of sugar, or the euphoria of alcohol. On each of these drinking occasions, with or without their awareness, people make choices among high-calorie and lower-calorie beverages.

Weighing In on Extra Fluids

Drinking extra fluid, and water in particular, may have some health advantages, such as preventing minor dehydration and reducing the risk of developing kidney stones.[1]* Fluids such as fat-free milk and 100 percent fruit or vegetable juices provide needed nutrients and are thus included in the USDA eating patterns. Other beverages, such as sugary sodas and punches, provide many empty calories, and should be limited. Doing so could help many people to lose weight.[2]

Figure 8–3 shows that young men like Derek top the chart for energy intakes from beverages, with an average of almost 600 calories per day. Young women drink about 350 calories per day on average. Beverages supply about a third of the added sugars, most of the caffeine, and all of the alcohol in the U.S. diet.[3]

Even among nutritious beverages, daily choices matter. For example, an 8-ounce glass of orange juice provides

* Reference notes are found in Appendix F.

Figure 8–3
How Many Calories Do We Drink?

The intake of calories from beverages varies widely with age, with 20- to 30-year-old men consuming the greatest amounts by far.

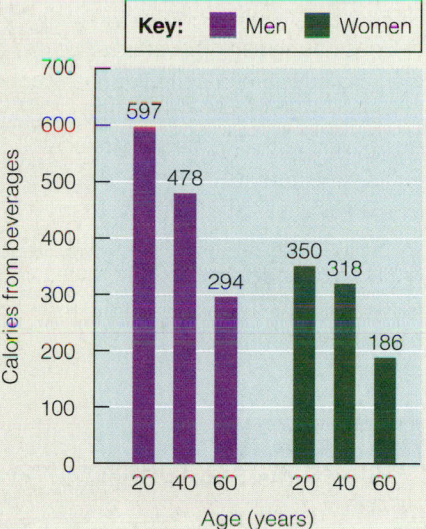

Key: ■ Men ■ Women

Source: R. P. LaComb and coauthors, Beverage Choices of U.S. Adults: What We Eat in America, NHANES 2007–2008, Data Brief No. 6, August 2011, available at http://ars.usda.gov.

about 110 calories; tomato juice, a similar choice with regard to vitamins and minerals, provides just 40. A cup of cream-based "bisque" soup may contribute up to 300 calories; a cup of broth-based minestrone has just 120 calories and a tiny fraction of the saturated fat. Calories in choices like these add up.

Seeking an Expert's Advice

"My advice is to track your intake of fluids and add up their calories," says the registered dietitian nutritionist at Derek's campus health clinic. "And watch serving sizes: your quart bottle of sports drink packs 200 calories of sugar and more than 400 milligrams of sodium, but its label lists much lower values for one 8-ounce serving, based on four servings per bottle." (See Figure 8–4.)

And Derek's reply: "I counted at least 400 random calories that I *drank* every day . . . I'll switch out the sodas and sports drinks for water, and as for coffee, I'll just put some milk in it—it's cheaper than the fancy stuff, anyway."

Looking at Labels

All packaged drinks must carry a Nutrition Facts panel. But what about calories in unlabeled beverages? How many calories are in coffee drinks, iced teas, fountain drinks, or bar drinks? Any beverage that lacks a Nutrition Facts panel requires consumers to look up or guess at calorie totals and then remember them to inform their future choices (Appendix A at the end of this text lists the calories in many beverages).

Figure 8–4
What's in a Sports Drink?

Compare labels and carefully note the serving size. This Nutrition Facts panel lists calories and sodium for 8 ounces—one-fourth of the bottle.

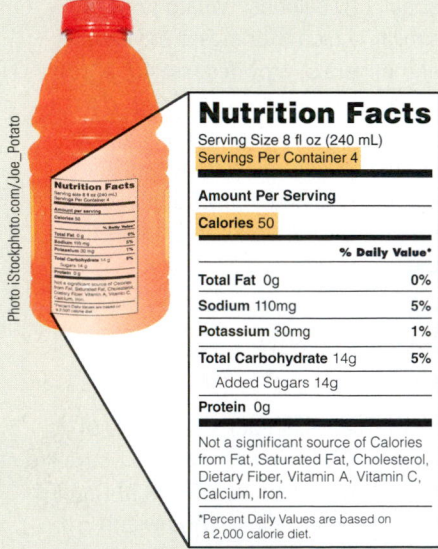

Photo: iStockphoto.com/Joe_Potato

Nutrition Facts

Serving Size 8 fl oz (240 mL)
Servings Per Container 4

Amount Per Serving

Calories 50

	% Daily Value*
Total Fat 0g	0%
Sodium 110mg	5%
Potassium 30mg	1%
Total Carbohydrate 14g	5%
Added Sugars 14g	
Protein 0g	

Not a significant source of Calories from Fat, Saturated Fat, Cholesterol, Dietary Fiber, Vitamin A, Vitamin C, Calcium, Iron.

*Percent Daily Values are based on a 2,000 calorie diet.

Table 8–4
Ways to Make Water More Appealing

Here are some ideas for adding interest to the taste of plain water without added sugars or artificial sweeteners, colors, or flavors.

- Steep a cinnamon stick in a cup of water. Mix 1–2 tablespoons of this concentrate with a glass of ice and water to add flavor. For variety, add a slice or two of fresh apple to the mix.
- Add a splash of 100% fruit juice to flavor and color plain or sparkling water naturally.
- Add the flavor of fresh fruit, such as berries or melons, to your water with a water infuser.
- Crush fresh herbs and steep them in a glass or pitcher of water in the refrigerator overnight. Add fresh citrus slices, such as lemon or lime, before drinking.
- Try a mixture of herbs and fruit, such as strawberries and basil or watermelon and mint to add a more complex flavor to water.
- Add flavored ice cubes to your water. Freeze coffee, water with berries, pureed pineapple, or even whole grapes, and use them in place of regular ice cubes to cool and flavor your water.
- Add cucumber slices to your water to give it a subtle, refreshing taste.
- Brew extra coffee, tea, or herb tea, refrigerate, and enjoy it chilled or over ice.

Moving Ahead

All beverages (except alcohol) can readily meet the body's fluid needs, so the question becomes, "What else does this beverage supply?" A 500-calorie smoothie or latte may be the right fluid choice for a person who needs to gain weight, but for most people, nutrition authorities often recommend plain water. Table 8–4 offers ways to make water taste more appealing. Other recommendations are plain tea, coffee, nonfat and low-fat milk and soy milk, artificially sweetened beverages, clear soups, 100 percent vegetable juices, and 100 percent fruit juices in moderation (see Chapter 2). If you enjoy regular soft drinks, sweet tea, creamy coffee drinks, punches, and other highly caloric beverages, limit yourself to the smallest size, and choose other beverages most of the time.

Review Questions**

1. Beverage consumption represents _____.

    a. 19 percent of a young woman's daily calorie intake

    b. 7 percent of a young woman's daily calorie intake

    c. an insignificant amount of a young woman's daily calorie intake

2. When choosing a beverage, one should _____.

    a. read the label carefully, especially noting the number of servings in the container and the calories per serving

    b. consider how a beverage's calories fit into the day's calorie needs

    c. consider ingredients in addition to water supplied by the beverage

    d. all of the above

3. Nutrition authorities often recommend _____.

    a. drinking water, plain or lightly flavored, to quench thirst

    b. staying hydrated with plenty of regular soft drinks, sweet tea, creamy coffee drinks, punches

    c. drinking plain tea, coffee, nonfat and low-fat milk and soy milk, artificially sweetened beverages, clear soups, and 100 percent fruit and vegetable juices, in addition to water

    d. a and c

** Answers to Consumer's Guide review questions are found in Appendix G.

The Effect of Sweating on Fluid Needs   Sweating increases water needs. Especially when performing physical work outdoors in hot weather, people can lose 2 to 4 gallons of fluid in a day. An athlete training in the heat can sweat out more than a half gallon of fluid each hour. For athletes exercising in the heat, maintaining hydration is critical, and Chapter 10 provides detailed instructions for hydrating the exercising body.

Drinking Water: Types, Safety, and Sources

LO 8.2   Compare the types and safety of drinking water from different sources.

In developed countries where clean water is always as close as the tap, people take water for granted, and they often devalue it and waste it. Water, however, could arguably be the earth's most precious natural resource. Just ask any of the almost 800 million of the world's people who struggle to stay alive in areas without access to safe drinking water.[7] This section sheds some light on the nature of water and offers perspective on our nation's supply. Chapter 15 comes back to the importance of clean water worldwide.

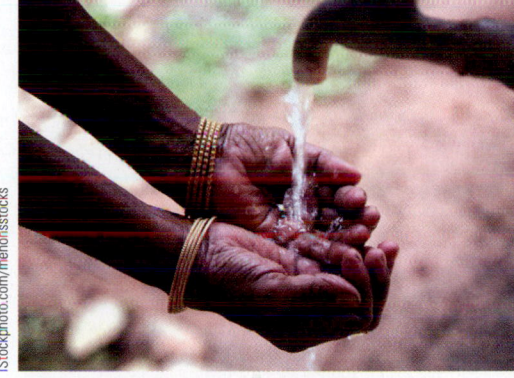

Clean water is precious and lifesaving in many areas of the world.

Hard Water or Soft Water—Which Is Best?

Water occurs as **hard water** or **soft water**, a distinction that affects your health with regard to three minerals. Hard water has high concentrations of calcium and magnesium. Soft water's principal mineral is sodium. In practical terms, soft water makes more bubbles with less soap; hard water leaves a ring on the tub, a jumble of rocklike crystals in the teakettle, and a gray residue in the wash.

Soft water may seem more desirable, and some homeowners purchase water softeners that remove magnesium and calcium and replace them with sodium. The sodium of soft water, even when it bubbles naturally from the ground, may aggravate **hypertension**, however. Soft water also more easily dissolves certain contaminant metals, such as cadmium and lead, from pipes. Cadmium can harm the body, affecting enzymes by displacing zinc from its normal sites of action. Lead, another toxic metal, is absorbed more readily from soft water than from hard water, possibly because the calcium in hard water protects against its absorption (lead is particularly harmful to children; see Chapter 14 for details). Old plumbing may contain cadmium or lead, so people living in old buildings should run the cold water tap for a minute to flush out harmful minerals before drawing water for the first use in the morning and whenever no water has been drawn for more than 6 hours.[8]

Safety of Public Water

Remember that water is practically a universal solvent: it dissolves almost anything it encounters to some degree. Hundreds of contaminants—including disease-causing bacteria and viruses from human wastes, toxic pollutants from highway fuel runoff, spills and heavy metals from industry, organic chemicals such as pesticides from agriculture, and manure bacteria from farm animals—have been detected, albeit rarely, in public drinking water. Such problems, when they arise, are promptly reported and corrected.

hard water   water with high calcium and magnesium concentrations.

soft water   water with a high sodium concentration.

hypertension   high blood pressure; also defined in Chapter 11.

Public water systems remove many hazards. They add disinfectant (usually chlorine) to kill most microorganisms, for example. Private well water is usually not chlorinated, so the 40 million Americans who drink water from private wells should have them tested regularly for harmful microorganisms.

Testing and Reporting   All public drinking water must be tested regularly for contamination. The Environmental Protection Agency ensures that public water systems meet minimum standards for health. Public utility customers receive a yearly statement, written in plain language, listing the chemicals and bacteria found in local water.

Chlorination and Cancer   By-products of water chlorination have been found to cause cancer-related changes in human cells and cancer in laboratory animals.[9] Experts passionately defend chlorination as a benefit to public health because in areas of the world without chlorination, an estimated 25,000 people die *each day* from diseases caused by organisms carried by water and easily killed by chlorine. Substitutes for chlorine exist, but they are too expensive or too slow to be practical for treating a city's water, and some may create by-products of their own.

Home Water Purification   To further purify tap water, home purifying equipment, ranging in price from $50 to $10,000, can remove most of the lead, chlorine, and other contaminants, but be aware—some types improve only the water's taste. Also, not all sellers are legitimate—some perform dramatic-appearing but meaningless water tests to sell unneeded systems.

Water Sources

Meanwhile, what is a consumer to drink? The first option is to drink tap water because municipal water is held to minimum standards for purity, as described. It comes from any of several sources.

Surface Water   **Surface water** flowing from lakes, rivers, and reservoirs fills about half of the nation's need for drinking water, mostly in major cities. Surface water is exposed to contamination by acid rain, petroleum products, pesticides, fertilizer, human and animal wastes, and industrial wastes that run directly from pavements, septic tanks, farmlands, and industrial areas into streams that feed surface water bodies. Surface water generally moves faster than **groundwater** and stays above ground where aeration and exposure to sunlight can cleanse it. The plants and microorganisms that live in surface water also filter it. These processes can remove some contaminants, but others stay in the water.

Groundwater   Groundwater comes from protected **aquifers**, deep underground rock formations saturated with water. People in rural areas rely mostly on groundwater pumped from private wells, and some cities tap this resource, too. Groundwater can become contaminated from hazardous waste sites, dumps, oil and gas pipelines, and landfills, as well as downward seepage from surface water bodies. Groundwater moves slowly and is not aerated or exposed to sunlight, so contaminants break down more slowly than in surface water. To mingle with water in the aquifer, surface water must first "percolate," or seep, through soil, sand, or rock, which filters out some contaminants.

Desalination   Where ground and surface water are scarce, **desalination** of seawater or brackish water can increase the fresh water supply. The process, which requires costly equipment and significant energy inputs, also creates a highly concentrated salty brine waste that is toxic to plants and animals. Disposal must be carefully managed. Still, as coastal populations outgrow their fresh water supplies, desalination plants can help keep the tap flowing.

Bottled Water   Another option is to use **bottled water** (Table 8–5 provides terms used in the marketing of bottled water). About 7 percent of U.S. households turn to bottled water as an alternative to tap water—and they pay 250 to 10,000 times the price of tap water. Are bottled waters worth their price?

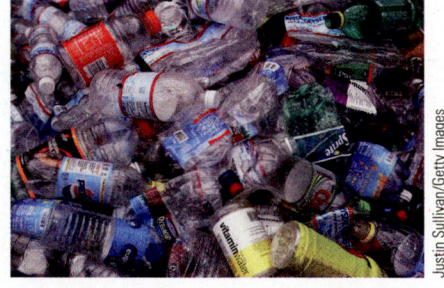

Billions of expensive, empty water bottles end up in landfills around the nation each year.

Justin Sullivan/Getty Images

surface water water that comes from lakes, rivers, and reservoirs.

groundwater water that comes from underground aquifers.

aquifers underground rock formations containing water that can be drawn to the surface for use.

desalination (dee-SAL-ih-NAY-shun) any of a number of processes that convert salt or brackish water into fresh water for drinking, industrial use, or irrigation.

bottled water drinking water sold in bottles.

Chapter 8 Water and Minerals

Table 8–5

Water Terms That May Appear on Labels

- **artesian water** water drawn from a well that taps a confined aquifer in which the water is under pressure.
- **baby water** ordinary bottled water treated with ozone to make it safe but not sterile.
- **caffeine water** bottled water with caffeine added.
- **carbonated water** water that contains carbon dioxide gas, either naturally occurring or added, that causes bubbles to form in it; also called bubbling or sparkling water. Seltzer, soda, and tonic waters are legally soft drinks and are not regulated as water.
- **coconut water** the fluid inside a young green coconut; heavily marketed for its substantial potassium content, it also provides about 45 calories per cup and little or no fat.
- **distilled water** water that has been vaporized and recondensed, leaving it free of dissolved minerals.
- **filtered water** water treated by filtration, usually through activated carbon filters that reduce the lead in tap water or by reverse osmosis units that force pressurized water across a membrane, removing lead, arsenic, and some microorganisms from tap water.
- **fitness water** lightly flavored bottled water enhanced with vitamins, supposedly to enhance athletic performance.
- **mineral water** water from a spring or well that typically contains at least 250 parts per million (ppm) of naturally occurring minerals. Minerals give water a distinctive flavor. Many mineral waters are high in sodium.
- **natural water** water obtained from a spring or well that is certified to be safe and sanitary. The mineral content may not be changed, but the water may be treated in other ways, such as with ozone or by filtration.
- **public water** water from a municipal or county water system that has been treated and disinfected. Also called *tap water*.
- **purified water** water that has been treated by distillation or other physical or chemical processes that remove dissolved solids. Because purified water contains no minerals or contaminants, it is useful for medical and research purposes.
- **spring water** water originating from an underground spring or well. It may be bubbly (carbonated) or "flat" or "still," meaning not carbonated. Brand names such as "Spring Pure" do not necessarily mean that the water comes from a spring.
- **vitamin water** bottled water with a few vitamins added; does not replace vitamins from a balanced diet and may worsen overload in people receiving vitamins from enriched food, supplements, and other enriched products such as "energy" bars.
- **well water** water drawn from groundwater by tapping into an aquifer.

Some bottled waters may taste fresher than tap because they are disinfected with ozone, which, unlike the chlorine used in most municipal water systems, leaves no flavor or odor. Other bottled waters are simply treated tap water.[10] With regard to safety, the U.S. Food and Drug Administration (FDA) recently tightened bottled water standards after tests revealed contamination with bacteria, arsenic, or synthetic chemicals in about a third of bottled water samples and with the heavy metal lead in about half the samples.[†11]

Under the FDA's rules, water intended to be bottled and sold across state lines must be tested yearly for chemical contaminants and weekly for disease-causing bacteria. When contamination shows up in either tap or bottled water, it must be cleared up before the water can be distributed.[12]

Considerable fossil fuels (and many gallons of water) are required to create and transport disposable plastic water bottles. Single-serving bottles can be recycled, but 80 percent of the 34.6 *billion* plastic water bottles purchased in the United States each year end up in landfills, in incinerators, or as litter. These empties now cost taxpayers hundreds of millions of dollars each year for their disposal and litter cleanup costs.

Whether water comes from the tap or is poured from a bottle, all water comes from the same sources—surface water and groundwater. Given water's importance in the body, the world's supply of clean, wholesome water is a precious resource to be guarded. The remainder of this chapter addresses other important nutrients—the minerals.

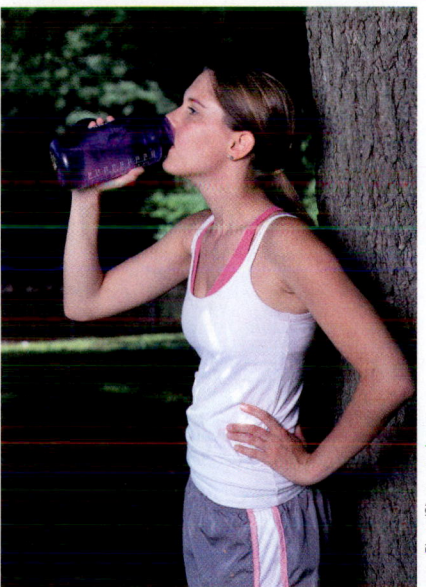

Using refillable bottles saves money and cuts waste.

KEY POINTS

- Public drinking water is tested and treated for safety.
- All drinking water, including bottled water, originates from surface water or groundwater, which are vulnerable to contamination from human activities.

---

†The group was the National Resources Defense Council. Read its report, *Bottled Water: Pure Drink or Pure Hype?*—available at http://www.nrdc.org/water/drinking/bw/bwinx.asp.

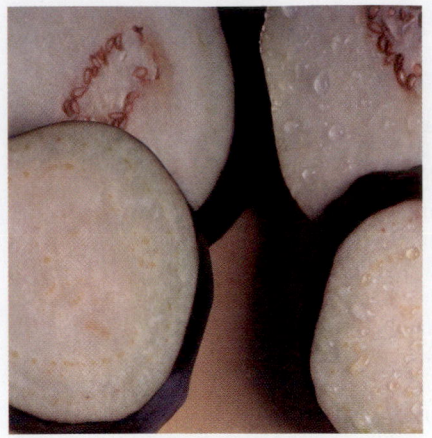

The slices of eggplant on the right were sprinkled with salt. Notice their beads of "sweat," formed as cellular water moves across each cell's membrane (water-permeable divider) toward the higher concentration of salt (dissolved particles) on the surface.

© Craig M. Moore

Body Fluids and Minerals

LO 8.3 Explain the concepts of fluid and electrolyte balance and acid-base balance and their importance to health.

Most of the body's water weight is contained inside the cells, and some water bathes the outsides of the cells. The remainder fills the blood vessels. How do cells keep themselves from collapsing when water leaves them and from swelling up when too much water enters them?

Water Follows Salt

The cells cannot regulate the amount of water directly by pumping it in and out because water slips across membranes freely. The cells can, however, pump minerals across their membranes. The major minerals form **salts** that dissolve in the body fluids; the cells direct where the salts go, and this determines where the fluids flow because water follows salt.

When mineral (or other) salts dissolve in water, they separate into single, electrically charged particles known as **ions**. Unlike pure water, which conducts electricity poorly, ions dissolved in water carry electrical current; for this reason, these electrically charged ions are called **electrolytes**.

As Figure 8–5 shows, when dissolved particles, such as electrolytes, are present in unequal concentrations on either side of a water-permeable membrane, water flows toward the more concentrated side to equalize the concentrations. Cells and their surrounding fluids work in the same way. Think of a cell as a sack made of a water-permeable membrane. The sack is filled with watery fluid and suspended in a dilute solution of salts and other dissolved particles. Water flows freely between the fluids inside and outside the cell but generally moves from the more dilute solution toward the more concentrated one (the photo of salted eggplant slices shows this effect).

KEY POINT

- Cells regulate water movement by pumping minerals across their membranes; water follows the minerals.

Figure 8–5

How Electrolytes Govern Water Flow

Water flows in the direction of the more highly concentrated solution.

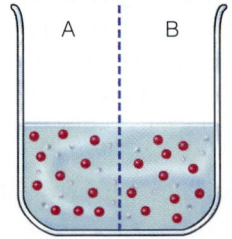 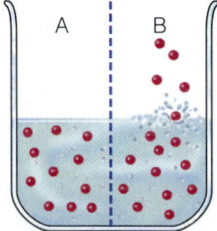 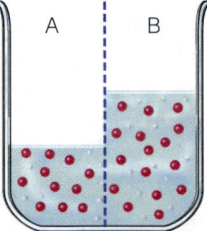

❶ With equal numbers of dissolved particles on both sides of a water-permeable divider, water levels remain equal.

❷ Now additional particles are added to increase the concentration on side B. Particles cannot flow across the divider. In the case of a cell, the divider (cell membrane) partitions fluids inside and outside the cell.

❸ Water can flow both ways across the divider but tends to move from side A to side B, where the concentration of dissolved particles is greater. The *volume* of water increases on side B, and the particle *concentrations* on sides A and B become equal.

salts compounds composed of charged particles (ions). An example is potassium chloride (K^+Cl^-).

ions (EYE-ons) electrically charged particles, such as sodium (positively charged) or chloride (negatively charged).

electrolytes compounds that partly dissociate in water to form ions, such as the potassium ion (K^+) and the chloride ion (Cl^-).

Fluid and Electrolyte Balance

To control the flow of water, the body must spend energy moving its electrolytes from one compartment to another (Figure 8–6). Transport proteins form the pumps that move mineral ions across cell membranes, as Chapter 6 described. The result is **fluid and electrolyte balance**, the proper amount and kind of fluid in every body compartment.

If the fluid balance is disturbed, severe illness can develop quickly because fluid can shift rapidly from one compartment to another. For example, in vomiting or diarrhea, the loss of water from the digestive tract pulls fluid from between the cells in every part of the body. Fluid then leaves the cell interiors to restore balance. Meanwhile, the kidneys detect the water loss and attempt to retrieve water from the pool destined for excretion. To do this, they raise the sodium concentration outside the cells, and this pulls still more water out of them. The result is **fluid and electrolyte imbalance**, a medical emergency. Water and minerals lost in vomiting or diarrhea ultimately come from all the body's cells. This loss disrupts the heartbeat and threatens life. It is a cause of death among those with eating disorders.

KEY POINT

- Mineral salts form electrolytes that help keep fluids in their proper compartments.

Acid-Base Balance

The minerals help manage still another balancing act, the **acid-base balance**, or the pH of the body's fluids. In pure water, a small percentage of water molecules (H_2O) exists as positive (H) and negative (OH) ions, but they exist in equilibrium—the positive charges exactly equal the negatives. When dissolved in watery body fluids, some of the major minerals give rise to acids (H, or hydrogen, ions) and others to bases (OH ions). Excess H ions in a solution make it an acid; they lower the pH. Excess OH ions in a solution make it a base; they raise the pH.

Maintenance of body fluids at a nearly constant pH is critical to life. Even slight changes in pH drastically change the structure and chemical functions of most biologically important molecules. The body's proteins and some of its mineral salts help prevent changes in the acid-base balance of its fluids by serving as **buffers**—molecules that gather up or release H ions as needed to maintain the correct pH. The kidneys help to control the pH balance by excreting more or less acid (H ions). The lungs also help by excreting more or less carbon dioxide. (Dissolved in the blood, carbon dioxide forms an acid, carbonic acid.) This tight control of the acid-base balance permits all other life processes to continue.

KEY POINT

- Minerals act as buffers to help maintain body fluids at the correct pH to permit life's processes.

The Major Minerals

LO 8.4 Discuss the functions of the seven major minerals, their food sources, and the effects of their deficiencies and toxicities.

All the major minerals help to maintain the fluid balance, but each one also has some special duties of its own. Table 8–6 lists the major minerals, and Table 8–14 (pp. 329–330) summarizes their roles.

Calcium

As Figure 8–1 showed, calcium is by far the most abundant mineral in the body. The roles of calcium are critical to body functioning, but many adults, adolescents, and even some children do not consume enough calcium-rich foods to meet the DRI

Figure 8–6

Electrolyte Balance

Transport proteins in cell membranes maintain the proper balance of sodium (mostly outside the cells) and potassium (mostly inside the cells).

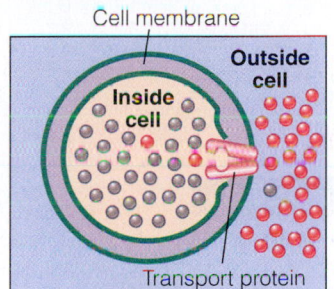

Cell membrane

Outside cell

Inside cell

Transport protein

Key
- Potassium
- Sodium

Table 8–6

Major Minerals[a]

The need for each of these is greater than 100 milligrams per day, often far greater.

- Calcium
- Chloride
- Magnesium
- Phosphorus
- Potassium
- Sodium
- Sulfate

[a]*The major minerals are also called* macrominerals.

fluid and electrolyte balance maintenance of the proper amounts and kinds of fluids and minerals in each compartment of the body.

fluid and electrolyte imbalance failure to maintain the proper amounts and kinds of fluids and minerals in every body compartment; a medical emergency.

acid-base balance maintenance of the proper degree of acidity in each of the body's fluids.

buffers molecules that can help to keep the pH of a solution from changing by gathering or releasing H ions.

Figure 8–7

A Bone

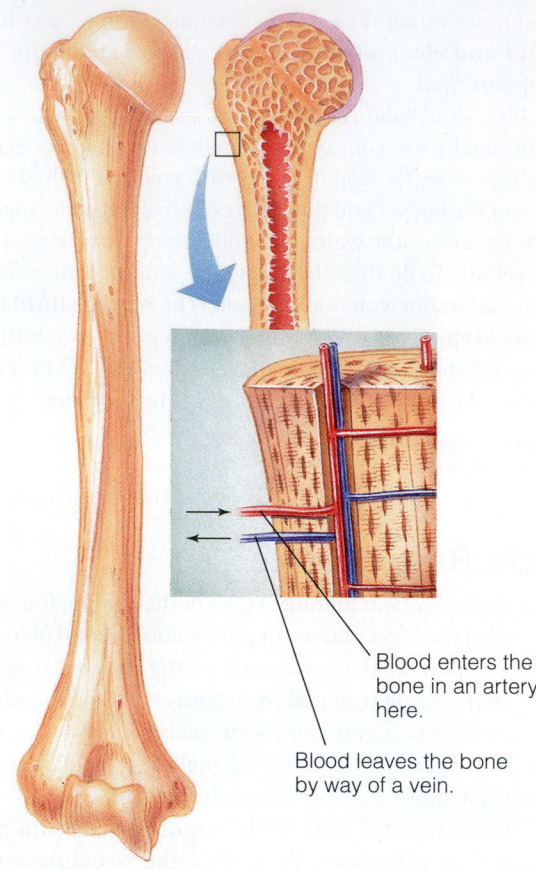

Bone is active, living tissue. Blood travels in capillaries throughout the bone, bringing nutrients to the cells that maintain the bone's structure and carrying away waste materials from those cells. It picks up and deposits minerals as instructed by hormones.

Bone derives its structural strength from the lacy network of crystals that lie along its lines of stress. If minerals are withdrawn to cover deficits elsewhere in the body, the bone will grow weak and ultimately will bend or crumble.

Blood enters the bone in an artery here.

Blood leaves the bone by way of a vein.

Figure 8–8

A Tooth

The inner layer of dentin is bonelike material that forms on a protein (collagen) matrix. The outer layer of enamel is harder than bone. Both dentin and enamel contain hydroxyapatite crystals (made of calcium and phosphorus). The crystals of enamel may become even harder when exposed to the trace mineral fluoride.

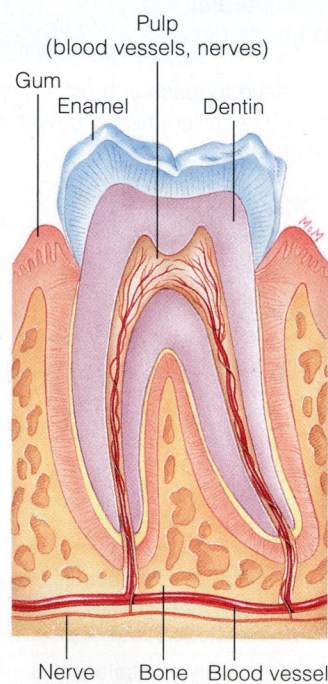

Pulp (blood vessels, nerves)

Gum
Enamel   Dentin

Nerve   Bone   Blood vessel

hydroxyapatite (hi-DROX-ee-APP-uh-tight) the chief crystal of bone, formed from calcium and phosphorus.

recommended intake for this mineral.[13] People who do meet their need are likely to be taking calcium supplements.[14]

Nearly all (99 percent) of the body's calcium is stored in the bones and teeth, where it plays two important roles. First, it is an integral part of bone structure. Second, bone calcium serves as a bank that can release calcium to the body fluids if even the slightest drop in blood calcium concentration occurs. Many people think that once deposited in bone, calcium (together with the other minerals of bone) stays there forever—that once a bone is built, it is inert, like a rock. Not so. The minerals of bones are in constant flux, with formation and dissolution taking place every minute of the day and night (see Figure 8–7). Almost the entire adult human skeleton is remodeled every 10 years.

Calcium in Bone and Tooth Formation   Calcium and phosphorus are both essential to bone formation: calcium phosphate salts crystallize on a rubbery foundation material composed of the protein collagen. The resulting **hydroxyapatite** crystals invade the collagen and gradually lend more and more rigidity to a youngster's maturing bones until they are able to support the weight they will have to carry. If you could remove all of the minerals from bones, thereby eliminating the hydroxyapatite crystals, the remaining protein structures (mostly the protein collagen) would be so flexible that you could tie them in a knot.

Teeth are formed in a similar way: hydroxyapatite crystals form on a collagen matrix to create the dentin that gives strength to the teeth (see Figure 8–8). The turnover of minerals in teeth is not as rapid as in bone, but some withdrawal and redepositing do take place throughout life.

Calcium in Body Fluids   The fluids that bathe and fill the cells contain the remaining 1 percent of the body's calcium, a tiny amount that is vital to life. It plays these major roles:

- Regulates the transport of ions across cell membranes and is particularly important in nerve transmission.
- Helps maintain normal blood pressure.
- Plays an essential role in the clotting of blood.
- Is essential for muscle contraction and therefore for the heartbeat.
- Allows secretion of hormones, digestive enzymes, and neurotransmitters.
- Activates cellular enzymes that regulate many processes.

Because of its importance, blood calcium is tightly controlled.

Other roles for calcium are emerging as well. Limited research suggests that calcium may help protect against hypertension.[15] Some research also suggests protective relationships between calcium and blood cholesterol, diabetes, and colon and rectal cancers.[16] Large, well-designed clinical studies are needed to clarify these potential roles of calcium.[17]

Calcium Balance   The key to bone health lies in the body's calcium balance, directed by a system of hormones and vitamin D. Cells need continuous access to calcium, so the body maintains a constant calcium concentration in the blood. The body is sensitive to an increased need for calcium but sends no signals to the conscious brain to indicate a calcium need. Instead, three organ systems quietly respond:

1. The intestines increase their absorption of calcium.
2. The kidneys prevent calcium loss in the urine.
3. The bones release more calcium into the blood.

The skeleton serves as a bank from which the blood can borrow and return calcium as needed. Thus, a person can go for years with an inadequate calcium intake and still maintain normal blood calcium—but at the expense of **bone density**.

Calcium Absorption   Most adults absorb about 25 to 30 percent of the calcium they ingest.[18] When the body needs more calcium, proteins in the intestinal lining increase its absorption.[19] The result is obvious in the case of a pregnant woman, who doubles her absorption. Similarly, breastfed infants absorb about 60 percent of the calcium in breast milk. Children in puberty absorb almost 35 percent of the calcium they consume.

The body also absorbs a higher percentage of the available calcium when habitual intakes are low.[20] Deprived of the mineral for months or years, an adult may double the calcium absorbed; conversely, when supplied for years with abundant calcium, the same person may absorb only about one-third the normal amount. Despite these adjustments, increased calcium absorption cannot fully compensate for a reduced intake. A person who cuts back on calcium is likely to lose calcium from the bones.

Bone Loss   Some bone loss seems an inevitable consequence of aging.[21] Sometime around age 30, the skeleton no longer adds significantly to bone density. After about age 40, regardless of calcium intake, bones begin to lose density. Those who regularly meet calcium, protein, and other nutrient needs and who perform bone-strengthening physical activity may slow down the loss.[22] Table 8–7 lists nutrients that are critical to bone health and that work as a team to support it.

A person who reaches adulthood with an insufficient calcium savings account is more likely to develop the fragile bones of **osteoporosis**. Osteoporosis constitutes a major health problem for many older people—its possible causes and prevention are the topics of this chapter's Controversy. To protect against bone loss, attention to calcium intakes during early life is crucial. Too few calcium-rich foods during the

Table 8–7
Functional Group for Bones

Below are the vitamins, minerals, and energy nutrients most important to bone health.

Key bone vitamins:
- Vitamin A
- Vitamin D
- Vitamin K
- Vitamin C

Key bone minerals:
- Calcium
- Phosphorus
- Magnesium

Key energy nutrient:
- Protein

bone density a measure of bone strength, the degree of mineralization of the bone matrix.

osteoporosis (OSS-tee-oh-pore-OH-sis) a reduction of the bone mass of older persons in which the bones become porous and fragile (*osteo* means "bones"; *poros* means "porous"); also known as *adult bone loss*. (Also defined in Chapter 6.)

Figure 8–9

Bone throughout Life

From birth to about age 20, the bones are actively growing. Between the ages of 12 and 30 years, the bones achieve their maximum mineral density for life—the peak bone mass. Beyond those years, bone resorption exceeds bone formation, and bones lose density.

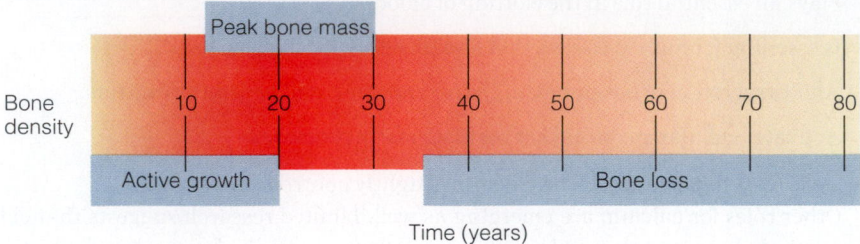

Bone density

Peak bone mass

10   20   30   40   50   60   70   80

Active growth   Bone loss

Time (years)

growing years may prevent a person from achieving **peak bone mass** (Figure 8–9 illustrates the timing).

How Much Calcium Do I Need and Which Foods Are Good Sources?

Setting recommended intakes for calcium is difficult because absorption varies (the Food Feature comes back to calcium absorption). The DRI committee took absorption into account and set recommendations for calcium at levels that produce maximum calcium retention (see the inside front cover, page B).[23] At lower intakes, the body does not store calcium to capacity; at greater intakes, the excess calcium is excreted and thus is wasted.

Intakes of calcium from supplements may elevate blood calcium or lead to problems such as calcium buildup in soft tissues and kidney stone formation. In addition, findings about their effectiveness for reducing fractures in older women are inconclusive.[24] Because adverse effects are possible with supplemental doses, a Tolerable Upper Intake Level has been established (see inside front cover, page C).

Fiber and the binders phytate (in whole grains) and oxalate (in vegetables) interfere with calcium absorption, but their effects are only minor in typical U.S. eating patterns. Such patterns fall far short of meeting the recommended intakes levels, and calcium is a nutrient of public health concern.[25] Snapshot 8–1 (p. 309) provides a look at some foods that are good or excellent sources of calcium, and the Food Feature at the end of the chapter focuses on foods that can help to meet calcium needs.

KEY POINTS

- Calcium makes up bone and tooth structures.
- Calcium plays roles in nerve transmission, muscle contraction, and blood clotting.
- Calcium absorption adjusts somewhat to dietary intakes and altered needs.

Phosphorus

Phosphorus is the second most abundant mineral in the body, next to calcium. More than 80 percent of the body's phosphorus is found combined with calcium in the crystals of the bones and teeth.[26] The rest is everywhere else.

Roles in the Body

All body cells must have phosphorus for these functions:

- Phosphorous salts are critical buffers, helping to maintain the acid-base balance of cellular fluids. (Note that the mineral is phosphorus. The adjective form is spelled with an -ous, as in phosphorous salts.)

- Phosphorus is part of the DNA and RNA of every cell and thus is essential for growth and renewal of tissues.

peak bone mass the highest attainable bone density for an individual; developed during the first three decades of life.

DRI Recommended Intakes

Adults: 1,000 mg/day (19–50 yr men and women; 51–70 yr men)

        1,200 mg/day (51–70 yr women; >70 yr men and women)

Tolerable Upper Intake Level

Adults: 2,500 mg/day (19–50 yr)

        2,000 mg/day (>50 yr)

Chief Functions

Mineralization of bones and teeth; muscle contraction and relaxation, nerve functioning, blood clotting

Deficiency

Stunted growth and weak bones in children; bone loss (osteoporosis) in adults

Toxicity

Elevated blood calcium; constipation; interference with absorption of other minerals; increased risk of kidney stone formation

* These foods provide 10% or more of the calcium Daily Value in a serving. For a 2,000-cal diet, the DV is 1,300 mg/day.
ᵃBroccoli, kale, and some other cooked green leafy vegetables are also important sources of bioavailable calcium. Almonds also supply calcium. Spinach and chard contain calcium in an unabsorbable form. Some calcium-rich mineral waters may also be good sources.

Good Sources*

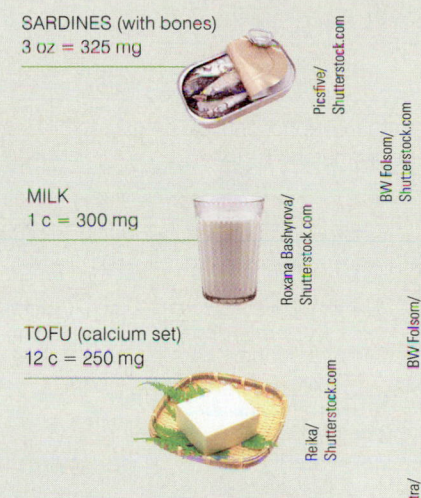

SARDINES (with bones)
3 oz = 325 mg
Picsfive/Shutterstock.com

MILK
1 c = 300 mg
Roxana Bashyrova/Shutterstock.com

TOFU (calcium set)
12 c = 250 mg
Reka/Shutterstock.com

YOGURT (plain)ᵃ
1 c = 296 mg
Gyorgy Barna/Shutterstock.com

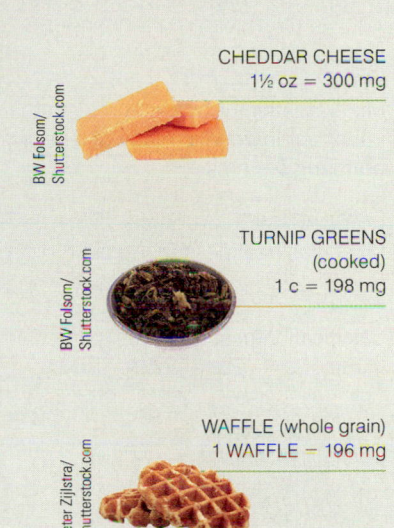

CHEDDAR CHEESE
1½ oz = 300 mg
BW Folsom/Shutterstock.com

TURNIP GREENS (cooked)
1 c = 198 mg
BW Folsom/Shutterstock.com

WAFFLE (whole grain)
1 WAFFLE = 196 mg
Peter Zijlstra/Shutterstock.com

- Phosphorous compounds carry, store, and release energy in the metabolism of energy nutrients.

- Phosphorous compounds assist many enzymes and vitamins in extracting the energy from nutrients.

- Phosphorus forms part of the molecules of the phospholipids that are principal components of cell membranes (discussed in Chapter 5).

- Phosphorus is present in some proteins.

Recommendations and Food Sources   Luckily, the body's need for phosphorus is easily met by almost any diet, deficiencies are unlikely, and most people in the

---

My Turn | watch it! | ## Drink Your Milk!

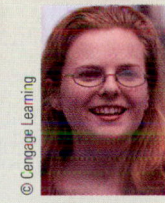

© Cengage Learning

Kathryn   *Cynthia*

Listen to two students talk about how they learned about the importance of calcium.

Visit www.cengagebrain.com to access MindTap, a complete digital course that includes these videos and other resources.

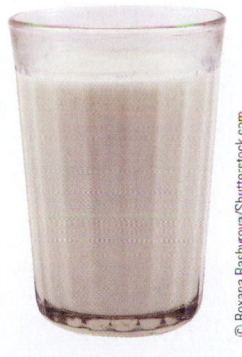

© Roxana Bashyrova/Shutterstock.com

Phosphorus

DRI Recommended Intake
Adults: 700 mg/day

Tolerable Upper Intake Level
Adults (19–70 yr):   4,000 mg/day

Chief Functions
Mineralization of bones and teeth; part of phospholipids, important in genetic material, energy metabolism, and buffering systems

Deficiency
Muscular weakness, bone pain[a]

Toxicity
Calcification of soft tissues, particularly the kidneys

* These foods provide 10% or more of the phosphorus Daily Value in a serving. For a 2,000-cal diet, the DV is 1,250 mg/day.
[a] Dietary deficiency rarely occurs, but some drugs can bind with phosphorus, making it unavailable.

Good Sources*

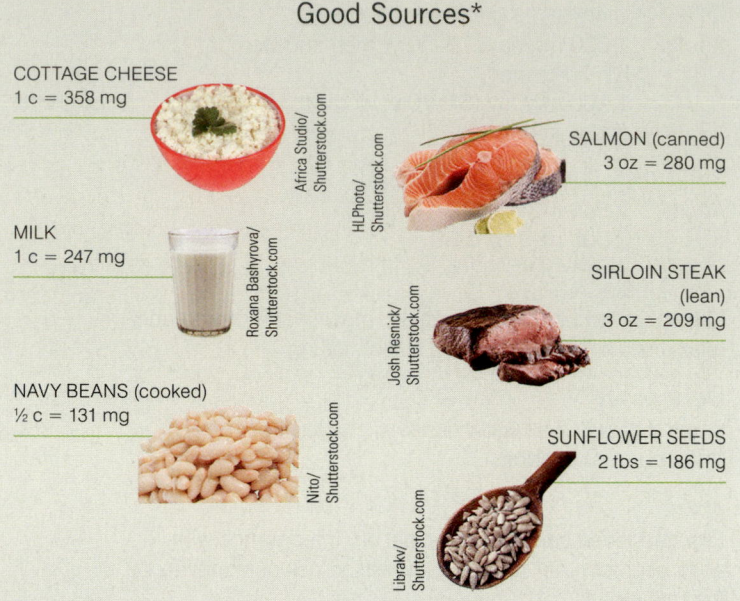

COTTAGE CHEESE
1 c = 358 mg
Africa Studio/ Shutterstock.com

MILK
1 c = 247 mg
Roxana Bashyrova/ Shutterstock.com

NAVY BEANS (cooked)
½ c = 131 mg
Nito/ Shutterstock.com

SALMON (canned)
3 oz = 280 mg
HLPhoto/ Shutterstock.com

SIRLOIN STEAK (lean)
3 oz = 209 mg
Josh Resnick/ Shutterstock.com

SUNFLOWER SEEDS
2 tbs = 186 mg
Librakv/ Shutterstock.com

United States meet their need.[27] As Snapshot 8–2 shows, animal protein is the best source of phosphorus (because phosphorus is abundant in the cells of animals). Milk and cheese are also rich sources.

Phosphorus-based food additives, such as modified starches used in gravies, prepared meals, creamy desserts, and other processed foods, and phosphates added to colas also contribute phosphorus to the diet. Excess phosphorus in the *blood* is associated with indicators of heart disease and osteoporosis, but whether this bears a relationship to phosphorus in the diet is unknown.[28]

KEY POINTS

- Phosphorus is abundant in bones and teeth.
- Phosphorus helps maintain acid-base balance, is part of the genetic material in cells, assists in energy metabolism, and forms part of cell membranes.
- Phosphorus deficiencies are unlikely.

Magnesium

Magnesium qualifies as a major mineral by virtue of its dietary requirement, but only about 1 ounce is present in the body of a 130-pound person, over half of it in the bones. Most of the rest is in the muscles, heart, liver, and other soft tissues, with only 1 percent in the body fluids. The supply of magnesium in the bones can be tapped to maintain a constant blood level whenever dietary intake falls too low. The kidneys can also act to conserve magnesium.

Roles in the Body   Like phosphorus, magnesium is critical to many cell functions. Magnesium:

- Assists in the operation of hundreds of enzymes and other cellular functions.[29]
- Is needed for the release and use of energy from the energy-yielding nutrients.
- Directly affects the metabolism of potassium, calcium, and vitamin D.
- Is critical to normal heart function.[30]

Magnesium and calcium work together for proper functioning of the muscles: calcium promotes contraction, and magnesium helps relax the muscles afterward. In the teeth, magnesium promotes resistance to tooth decay by holding calcium in tooth enamel.

Magnesium Deficiency   A magnesium deficiency may occur as a result of inadequate intake, vomiting, diarrhea, alcoholism, or malnutrition. It may also occur in people who take certain medications, particularly diuretics that cause excess magnesium loss in the urine. Its symptoms include a low blood calcium level, muscle cramps, and seizures. A deficiency also interferes with vitamin D activities and causes hallucinations that can be mistaken for mental illness or drunkenness. In addition, magnesium deficiency may disturb bone metabolism, worsen inflammation, and may increase the risk of stroke and sudden death by heart failure in otherwise healthy people.[31]

Average U.S. magnesium intakes typically fall below recommendations, although deficiency symptoms are rare in healthy people.[32] The Dietary Guidelines 2015 committee names magnesium among shortfall nutrients for the U.S. population.[33]

Magnesium Toxicity   Magnesium toxicity is rare, but it can be fatal. Toxicity occurs only with high intakes from nonfood sources such as supplements. Accidental poisonings may occur in children with access to medicine chests and in older people who take too many magnesium-containing laxatives, antacids, and other medications. The consequences can be severe diarrhea, acid-base imbalance, and dehydration. For safety, be mindful of the Tolerable Upper Intake Level for magnesium when using magnesium-containing medications.

Recommendations and Food Sources   Magnesium DRI recommendations vary only slightly among adult age groups; see the inside front cover.[34] Snapshot 8–3 shows magnesium-rich foods. Magnesium is easily washed and peeled away from foods during processing, so lightly processed or unprocessed foods are the best

Snapshot 8–3   Magnesium

DRI Recommended Intakes
Men (19–30 yr):   400 mg/day
Women (19–30 yr):   310 mg/day

Tolerable Upper Intake Level
Adults: 350 mg/day[a]

Chief Functions
Bone mineralization, protein synthesis, enzyme action, muscle contraction, nerve function, tooth maintenance, and immune function

Deficiency
Weakness, confusion; if extreme, convulsions, uncontrollable muscle contractions, hallucinations, and difficulty in swallowing; in children, growth failure

Toxicity
From nonfood sources only; diarrhea, pH imbalance, dehydration

*These foods provide 10% or more of the magnesium Daily Value in a serving. For a 2,000-cal diet, the DV is 420 mg/day.
[a] From nonfood sources, in addition to the magnesium provided by food.
[b] Wheat bran provides magnesium, but refined grain products are low in magnesium.

Good Sources*

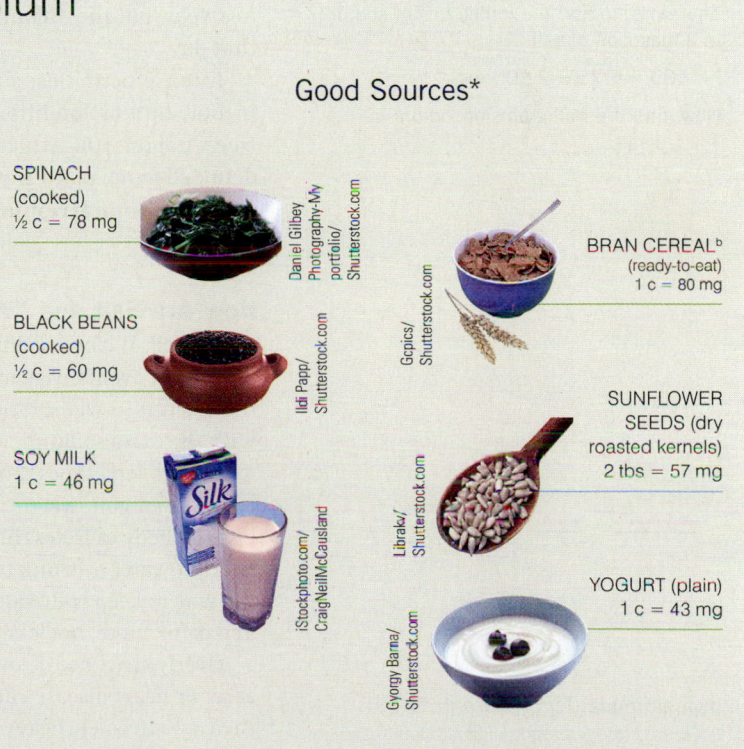

SPINACH (cooked) ½ c = 78 mg
Daniel Glibey Photography-My portfolio/ Shutterstock.com

BLACK BEANS (cooked) ½ c = 60 mg
Ildi Papp/ Shutterstock.com

SOY MILK 1 c = 46 mg
iStockphoto.com/ CraigNeilMcCausland

BRAN CEREAL[b] (ready-to-eat) 1 c = 80 mg
Gcpics/ Shutterstock.com

SUNFLOWER SEEDS (dry roasted kernels) 2 tbs = 57 mg
Librakv/ Shutterstock.com

YOGURT (plain) 1 c = 43 mg
Gyorgy Barna/ Shutterstock.com

sources. The Dietary Guidelines 2015 committee recommends increasing fluid milk and yogurt consumption while decreasing cheese intake to help increase magnesium in the diet. Fruits, vegetables, and whole grains are also important sources of magnesium.[35] In some parts of the country, water contributes significantly to magnesium intakes, so people living in those regions need less from food.

KEY POINTS

- Magnesium stored in the bones can be drawn out for use by the cells.
- Many people consume less than the recommended amount of magnesium.
- U.S. diets often provide insufficient magnesium.

Sodium

Salt has been known and valued throughout recorded history. "You are the salt of the earth" means that you are valuable. If "you are not worth your salt," you are worthless. Even our word *salary* comes from the Latin word for *salt*. Chemically, sodium is the positive ion in the compound sodium chloride (table salt) and makes up 40 percent of its weight: a gram of salt contains 400 milligrams of sodium. Table 8–8 describes the chemical reaction that forms salt.

Roles of Sodium   Sodium is a major part of the body's fluid and electrolyte balance system because it is the chief ion used to maintain the volume of fluid outside cells. Sodium also helps maintain acid-base balance and is essential to muscle contraction and nerve transmission. Scientists think that 30 to 40 percent of the body's sodium is stored in association with the bone crystals, where the body can draw on it to replenish the blood concentration.[36]

Sodium Deficiency   A deficiency of sodium would be harmful, but no known human diet lacks sodium. Most foods include more salt than is needed, and the body absorbs it freely. The kidneys filter the surplus out of the blood into the urine. They can also sensitively conserve sodium. In the rare event of a deficiency, they can return to the bloodstream the exact amount needed. Small sodium losses occur in sweat, but the amount of sodium excreted in a day equals the amount ingested that day.

Intense activities, such as endurance events performed over several days or in hot, humid conditions, can cause sodium losses that reach dangerous levels (see Chapter 10). Athletes in such events can lose so much sodium in sweat and drink so much plain water that they overwhelm the body's corrective actions and develop **hyponatremia**—the dangerous condition of having too little sodium in the blood.

How Are Salt and "Water Weight" Related?   Blood sodium levels are well controlled. If blood sodium begins to rise, as it will after a person eats salted foods, a series of events triggers thirst and ensures that the person will drink water until the sodium-to-water ratio is restored. Then the kidneys excrete the extra water along with the extra sodium.

Dieters sometimes think that eating too much salt or drinking too much water will make them gain weight, but they do not gain fat, of course. They gain water, but a healthy body excretes this excess water immediately. Excess salt is excreted as soon as enough water is drunk to carry the salt out of the body. From this perspective, then, the way to keep body salt (and "water weight") under control is to control salt intake and drink more, not less, water.

Overly strict use of low-sodium diets in the treatment of hypertension, kidney disease, or heart disease can deplete the body of needed sodium, as can vomiting, diarrhea, or extremely heavy sweating. If blood sodium drops, body water is lost, and both water and sodium must be replenished to avert an emergency.

Do the Math

Salt is about 40% sodium and 60% chloride. (Reminder: 1g = 1,000 mg)

- 1 g of salt contains 400 mg of sodium.
- 1 tsp salt weighs 5.75 g.

Therefore, to find the milligrams of sodium in a teaspoon of salt:

$400 \times 5.75 = 2{,}300$ mg

Now, find the milligrams of sodium in 1¾ tsp salt.

---

hyponatremia (high-poh-nah-TREE-mee-ah) a decreased concentration of sodium in the blood.

Sodium Recommendations and Intakes A DRI recommendation for sodium adequacy has been set at 1,500 milligrams for healthy, active young adults; at 1,300 for people ages 51 through 70; and at 1,200 for the elderly.[37] The Tolerable Upper Intake Level (UL) is set at 2,300 milligrams per day (equivalent to about 1 tsp of salt), an amount met or exceeded daily by 90 percent of the U.S. adult population.[38] The average U.S. sodium intake nears 3,500 milligrams per day (see Figure 8–10).[39]

People who need to reduce their blood pressure for their health's sake are urged to cut their sodium intake.[40] For example, people with hypertension, diabetes, or chronic kidney disease should take in no more than 1,500 milligrams per day (see Table 8–9) because this level of restriction often lowers blood pressure.[41] Even without meeting the recommended levels, reducing sodium by at least 1,000 milligrams per day reduces blood pressure. This is a worthy goal—hypertension is a leading cause of death and disability in this country.[42]

Sodium and Blood Pressure High intakes of salt among the world's people correlate with high rates of hypertension, heart disease, and strokes.[43] Over time, a high-salt diet may damage the linings of blood vessels in ways that make hypertension likely to develop.[44] One-third of U.S. adults have hypertension, and among African American adults, the rate is one of the highest in the world—42 percent.[45] An additional 30 percent of U.S. adults have **prehypertension**. Medical standards for both conditions are listed in Chapter 11.

The relationship between salt intake and blood pressure is direct—as chronic sodium intakes increase, blood pressure rises in a stepwise fashion.[46] Once hypertension sets in, the risk of death from stroke and heart disease climbs steeply.

Variations exist among people's blood pressure responses to sodium, partly because of their genetic inheritance, but evidence so far does not support treating population subgroups differently from the general U.S. population.[47] The genetic relationships are complex, but researchers suspect that the genes that affect blood pressure do so by altering the kidneys' handling of sodium.[48]

Can Diet Lower Blood Pressure? A proven eating pattern that can help people to reduce their sodium and increase their potassium intakes, and thereby often reduce their blood pressure, is DASH (Dietary Approaches to Stop Hypertension).[49] This pattern calls for greatly increased intakes of potassium-rich fruits and vegetables, with adequate amounts of nuts, fish, whole grains, and low-fat dairy products. At the same time, red meat, butter, other high-fat foods, and sweets are held to occasional small portions.

> DASH diet details are found in **Chapter 11** and **Appendix E**.

Other Reasons to Cut Salt Intakes Most Americans have much to gain in terms of cardiovascular health and nothing to lose from cutting back on salt to a level

Figure 8–10

Average Daily Sodium Intake of U.S. Adults

The solid red line of this figure indicates 2,300 mg of sodium, the current DRI Tolerable Upper Intake Level for healthy people. The broken red line beneath marks 1,500 mg, the DRI recommended intake for young adults.

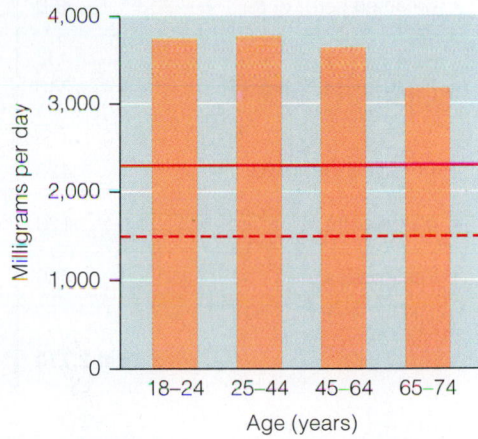

Source: M. D. Ritchey and coauthors, Million hearts: Prevalence of leading cardiovascular disease risk factors—United States, 2005–2012, Morbidity and Mortality Weekly Report 63 (2014): 462–467.

Table 8–9

Sodium Recommendations and Blood Pressure

Dietary Guidelines for Americans, 2015–2020
- Consume less than 2,300 milligrams per day of sodium (for people ages 14 years and older; for younger children, consult the appropriate DRI Tolerable Upper Intake Level).
- Further reductions to 1,500 milligrams of sodium may produce greater benefits in people with hypertension or prehypertension.

DRI Tolerable Upper Intake Levels
- 2,300 mg/day, adults.
- For children age 14 years and younger, see inside front cover, page C.

prehypertension blood pressure values that predict hypertension. See Chapter 11.

Table 8–10

How to Trim Sodium from a Barbecue Lunch

Lunch #1 exceeds the whole day's Tolerable Upper Intake Level of 2,300 milligrams of sodium. With careful substitutions, the sodium drops dramatically in the second lunch, but it is still a high-sodium meal. In lunch #3, three additional changes—omitting the sauce, coleslaw dressing, and salt—cut the sodium by half again.

Lunch #1: Highest	Sodium (mg)	Lunch #2: Lower	Sodium (mg)	Lunch #3: Lowest	Sodium (mg)
▪ Chopped pork sandwich, sauce and meat mixture	950	▪ Sliced pork sandwich, with 1 tbs sauce	400	▪ Sliced pork sandwich (no sauce)	210
▪ Creamed corn, ½ c	460	▪ Corn, 1 cob, soft margarine, salt	190	▪ Corn, 1 cob, soft margarine	50
▪ Potato chips, 2.5 oz	340	▪ Coleslaw, ½ c	180	▪ Green salad, oil and vinegar	10
▪ Dill pickle, ½ medium	420	▪ Watermelon, slice	10	▪ Watermelon, slice	10
▪ Milk, low-fat, 1 c	120	▪ Milk, low-fat, 1 c	120	▪ Milk, low-fat, 1 c	120
▪ Pecan pie, slice	480	▪ Ice cream, low-fat, ½ c	80	▪ Ice cream, low-fat, ½ cup	80
Total 2,770		**Total 980**		**Total 480**	

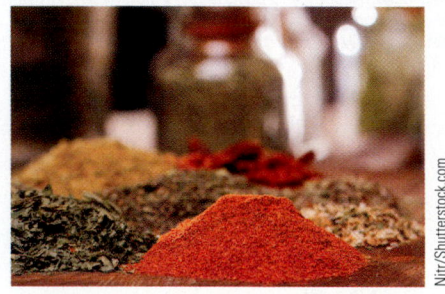

Herbs add delicious flavors to foods without adding salt.

near the UL. The greatest benefits occur when the change is part of an overall lifestyle strategy to reduce blood pressure. Physical activity should also be part of that lifestyle because regular moderate exercise reliably lowers blood pressure.

Excess salt intake also increases calcium excretion, an effect that could potentially compromise the integrity of the bones.[50] Excessive salt may also directly stress a weakened heart or aggravate kidney problems, and lower salt intakes have been associated with lower rates of stomach cancer.[51]

Our Salty Food Supply   Cutting down on salt and sodium is easy on paper—just weed out the salt and high-sodium items from the diet. In practice, though, very few people achieve the goal of limiting sodium to 2,300 milligrams per day, the UL for sodium.[52] Further, meeting all of a person's nutrient needs from our highly salted food supply while achieving an even lower sodium intake of 1,500 milligrams per day can be difficult at best.[53] The lunches of Table 8–10 demonstrate that doing so requires eliminating all salt, sauces, dressings, and salty items such as chips, pickles, and even piecrust. Reducing intakes of foods like these is a good first step to reducing the health risks of a high-sodium diet.[54]

Many experts today are calling for reductions of sodium in the food supply to give consumers more low-salt options to choose from, yet food manufacturers seem slow to comply.[55] Reducing the sodium content in processed foods could prevent an estimated 100,000 deaths and save up to $24 billion in health-care costs in the United States annually.[56]

Reducing Sodium Intakes   An obvious step in controlling sodium intake is controlling the saltshaker, but this source may contribute as little as 15 percent of the total salt consumed. As Figure 8–11 (p. 315) indicates, a more productive step

Table 2–6 (p. 55) of Chapter 2 describes sodium terms on food labels.

is to cut down on processed and fast foods, by far our biggest source of sodium.

The Dietary Guidelines for Americans committee recommends modifying recipes to reduce the salt, using appropriate portion sizes, and choosing reformulated

Figure 8–11

Sources of Sodium in the U.S. Diet

Less Processed Foods

Foods that are low in sodium contribute less than 10 percent of the total sodium in the U.S. diet.

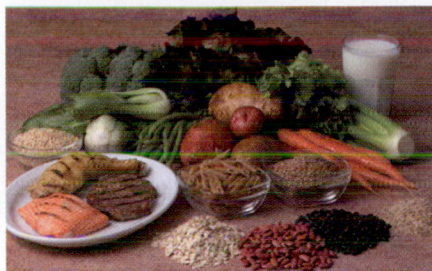

Fresh foods higher in sodium
   Milk, 120 mg/c
   Scallops, 260 mg/3 oz
Fresh meats, about 30 to 70 mg/3 oz
   Chicken, beef, fish, lamb, pork
Fresh vegetables, about 30 to 50 mg per ¹/₂ c
   Celery, Chinese cabbage, sweet potatoes
Fresh vegetables, about 10 to 20 mg per ¹/₂ c
   Broccoli, brussels sprouts, carrots, corn, green beans, legumes, potatoes, salad greens
Grains (cooked without salt), about 0 to 10 mg per ¹/₂ c
   Barley, oatmeal, pasta, rice

Salt, Brined Foods, Condiments

Salt added at home, in cooking or at the table, contributes 15 percent of the total sodium in the U.S. diet. Many seasonings and sauces also contribute salt and sodium.

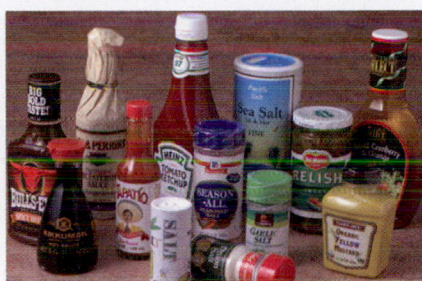

Salts, about 2,000 mg/tsp
   Salt, sea salt, seasoned salt, onion salt, garlic salt[a]
Soy sauce, about 300 mg/tsp
Foods prepared in salt or brine, about 300 to 800 mg/serving
   Anchovies (2 fillets), dill pickles (1), olives (5), sauerkraut (¹/₂ c), chipped beef (1 oz)
Condiments and sauces, about 100 to 200 mg/tbs
   Barbecue sauce, ketchup, mustard, salad dressings, sweet pickle relish, taco sauce, Worcestershire sauce

[a]Note that herb seasoning blends may or may not contain substantial sodium; read the labels.

Highly Processed Foods

Processed foods from restaurants or stores contribute 75 percent of the sodium in the U.S. diet.

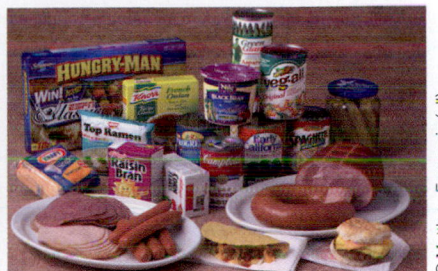

© Matthew Farruggio (all)

Dry soup mixes (prepared), about 1,000 to 2,000 mg/c
   Bouillon cube, noodle soups, onion soup, ramen
Fast foods and frozen dinners, about 700 to 1,500 mg/serving
   Breakfast biscuit (cheese, egg, and ham), cheeseburger, chicken wings (10 spicy wings), deli sandwiches and other sandwiches, frozen dinners, pizza, 2 tacos, chili dog, vegetarian soy burger (on bun)
Canned soups (prepared), about 700 to 1,500 mg/c
   Bean, beef, or chicken soups, broths, tomato or vegetable soup
Pasta, frozen or canned, all types, with tomato sauce, 600 to 900 mg/c
Cold cuts/cured meats, about 500 to 700 mg/2 oz
   Ham products, lunchmeats, hot dogs, smoked sausages
Cheeses, processed, about 550 mg/oz
Pudding, instant, about 420 mg per ¹/₂ c
Canned vegetables, about 200 to 450 mg per ¹/₂ c
   Carrots, corn, green beans, legumes, peas, potatoes
Snack chips, puffs, crackers, about 200 to 300 mg/oz
Breads and rolls, about 125 mg/1 slice or ¹/₂ roll

low-sodium or salt-free products.[57] It also urges FDA to set standards for sodium in processed foods, and to develop easy-to-read sodium information to appear on the front labels of food packages.

Many people are unaware that foods high in sodium do not always taste salty. Who could guess by taste alone that a single half-cup serving of instant chocolate pudding provides almost one-fifth of the Tolerable Upper Intake Level for sodium? Additives other than salt also increase a food's sodium content: sodium benzoate, monosodium glutamate, sodium nitrite, and sodium ascorbate, to name a few. Moral: Read the Nutrition Facts labels.

Remember that the recommendation is to limit sodium, not to eliminate it. Foods eaten without salt may seem less tasty at first, but with repetition, taste buds adjust, and the delicious natural flavor becomes the preferred taste.

Potassium

Outside the body's cells, sodium is the principle positively charged ion. *Inside* the cells, potassium takes the role of the principal positively charged ion.

Roles in the Body   Potassium plays a major role in maintaining fluid and electrolyte balance and cell integrity. During nerve impulse transmission and muscle contraction, potassium and sodium briefly trade places across the cell membrane. The cell then quickly pumps them back into place. Controlling potassium distribution is a high priority for the body because it affects many aspects of homeostasis, including maintaining a steady heartbeat.

Potassium Deficiency   Few people in the United States consume the DRI recommended intake of potassium. Low potassium intakes, especially when combined with high sodium intakes, raise blood pressure and increase the risk of death from stroke.[58] Higher intakes of dietary potassium may or may not lower blood pressure, but diets with ample potassium are associated with a reduced risk of cardiovascular disease and stroke. These effects, along with low U.S. consumption, earn potassium its status as a Dietary Guidelines nutrient of public health concern.[59]

Severe deficiencies are rare. In healthy people, almost any reasonable diet provides enough potassium to prevent dangerously low blood potassium under ordinary conditions. Dehydration leads to a loss of potassium from inside cells, dangerous partly because potassium is crucial for regular heartbeats. The sudden deaths that occur with fasting, eating disorders, severe diarrhea, or severe malnutrition in children may be due to heart failure caused by potassium loss. Adults are warned not to take diuretics (water pills) that cause potassium loss or to give them to children except under a physician's supervision. Physicians prescribing diuretics will tell clients to eat potassium-rich foods to compensate for the losses.

Potassium Toxicity   Potassium from foods is safe, but potassium injected into a vein can stop the heart. Potassium overdoses from supplements normally are not life-threatening because the kidneys excrete small excesses and large doses trigger vomiting to expel the substance. A person with a weak heart, however, should not go through this trauma, and a baby may not be able to withstand it. Several infants have died when well-meaning parents overdosed them with potassium supplements.

Potassium Intakes and Food Sources   A typical U.S. eating pattern, with its low intakes of fruits and vegetables, provides far less potassium than the amount recommended by the DRI committee.[60] Potassium is found inside all living cells, and cells remain intact until foods are processed; therefore, the richest sources of potassium are fresh, whole foods (see Snapshot 8–4). Most vegetables and fruits are outstanding. Bananas, despite their fame as the richest potassium source, are only one of many rich sources, which also include spinach, cantaloupe, and almonds. Nevertheless, bananas are readily available, are easy to chew, and have a likable sweet taste, so health-care professionals often recommend them. Potassium chloride, a salt substitute for people with hypertension, and potassium supplements provide potassium but do not reverse the hypertension associated with a lack of potassium-rich foods. Current guidelines do not recommend supplementing with potassium, but they do emphasize the importance of consuming a diet rich in fruits and vegetables.[61]

Potassium

DRI Recommended Intake
Adults: 4,700 mg/day

Chief Functions
Maintains normal fluid and electrolyte balance; facilitates chemical reactions; supports cell integrity; assists in nerve functioning and muscle contractions

Deficiency[a]
Muscle weakness, paralysis, confusion

Toxicity
Muscle weakness; vomiting; when given in a supplement to an infant or when injected into a vein in an adult, potassium can stop the heart

*These foods provide 10% or more of the potassium Daily Value in a serving. For a 2,000-cal diet, the DV is 4,700 mg/day.
[a]Deficiency accompanies dehydration.

Good Sources*

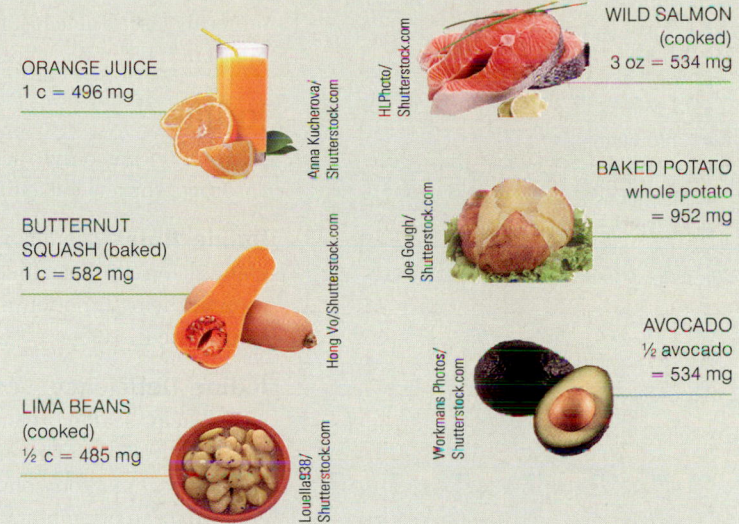

ORANGE JUICE
1 c = 496 mg
Anna Kucherova/Shutterstock.com

BUTTERNUT SQUASH (baked)
1 c = 582 mg
Hong Vo/Shutterstock.com

LIMA BEANS (cooked)
½ c = 485 mg
Louella938/Shutterstock.com

WILD SALMON (cooked)
3 oz = 534 mg
HLPhoto/Shutterstock.com

BAKED POTATO
whole potato = 952 mg
Joe Gough/Shutterstock.com

AVOCADO
½ avocado = 534 mg
Workmans Photos/Shutterstock.com

Chloride

In its elemental form, chlorine forms a deadly green gas. In the body, the chloride ion plays important roles as the major negative ion. In the fluids outside the cells, it accompanies sodium and so helps to maintain the crucial fluid balances (acid-base and electrolyte balances). The chloride ion also plays a special role as part of hydrochloric acid, which maintains the strong acidity of the stomach necessary to digest protein. The principal food source of chloride is salt, both added and naturally occurring in foods, and no known diet lacks chloride.

KEY POINTS

- Chloride is the body's major negative ion, is responsible for stomach acidity, and assists in maintaining proper body chemistry.
- No known diet lacks chloride.

Sulfate

Sulfate is the oxidized form of sulfur as it exists in food and water. The body requires sulfate for synthesis of many important sulfur-containing compounds. Sulfur-containing amino acids play an important role in helping strands of protein assume their functional shapes. Skin, hair, and nails contain some of the body's more rigid proteins, which have high sulfur contents.

There is no recommended intake for sulfate, and deficiencies are unknown. Too much sulfate in drinking water, either naturally occurring or from contamination, causes diarrhea and may damage the colon. The summary table at the end of this chapter presents the main facts about sulfate and the other major minerals.

KEY POINT

- Sulfate is a necessary nutrient used to synthesize sulfur-containing body compounds.

Table 8–11

Trace Minerals[a]

These minerals are needed by the body in tiny amounts.

- Iodine
- Iron
- Zinc
- Selenium
- Fluoride
- Chromium
- Copper
- Manganese
- Molybdenum

[a]The trace minerals are also called microminerals.

The Trace Minerals

LO 8.5 Discuss the food sources and the functions of the trace minerals and the effects of their deficiencies and toxicities.

People require only miniscule amounts of the trace minerals, but these quantities are vital for health and life. Intake recommendations have been established for nine trace minerals—see Table 8–11. Others are recognized as essential nutrients for some animals but have not been proved to be required for human beings.

Iodine

The body needs only traces of iodine, but this amount is indispensable to life. Once absorbed, the form of iodine that does the body's work is the ionic form, iodide.

Iodine Roles Iodide is a part of the hormone thyroxine, made by the thyroid gland. Thyroxine regulates the body's metabolic rate, temperature, reproduction, growth, heart functioning, and more. Iodine must be available for thyroxine to be synthesized.

Iodine Deficiency The ocean is the world's major source of iodine. In coastal areas, kelp, seafood, water, and even iodine-containing sea mist are dependable iodine sources. In many inland areas of the world, however, misery caused by iodine deficiency is all too common. In iodine deficiency, the cells of the thyroid gland enlarge in an attempt to trap as many particles of iodine as possible. Sometimes the gland enlarges to the point of making a visible lump in the neck, a **goiter**. People with iodine deficiency this severe may feel cold, may become sluggish and forgetful, and may gain weight. Iodine deficiency affects almost 2 billion people globally, including 246 million school-aged children, a huge number but one that represents some improvement over past decades.[62]

Iodine deficiency during pregnancy causes fetal death, reduced infant survival, and extreme and irreversible mental and physical retardation in the infant, known as **cretinism**. It constitutes one of the world's most common and preventable causes of mental retardation.[†] Much of the mental retardation can be averted if the woman's deficiency is detected and treated within the first 6 months of pregnancy, but if treatment comes too late or not at all, the child's IQ and other developmental indicators are likely to be substantially below normal.[63] Children with even a mild iodine deficiency typically have goiters and may perform poorly in school; treatment with iodine relieves the deficiency.[64] Programs to provide iodized salt to the world's iodine-deficient areas now prevent much misery and suffering worldwide.[65]

Iodine Toxicity Excessive intakes of iodine can enlarge the thyroid gland just as a deficiency can. Although average U.S. intakes are generally above the recommended intake of 150 micrograms, they are still below the Tolerable Upper Intake Level of 1,100 micrograms per day for an adult.[66] Harm may begin at only 800 micrograms per day, however.[67] Like chlorine and fluorine, iodine is a deadly poison in large amounts.

Iodine Food Sources and Intakes The iodine in food varies with the amount in the soil in which plants are grown or on which animals graze. Because iodine is plentiful in the ocean, seafood is a dependable source. In the central parts of the United States that were never beneath an ocean, the soil is poor in iodine. In those areas, once-widespread deficiencies have been wiped out by the use of iodized salt and the consumption of foods shipped in from iodine-rich areas. Surprisingly, sea salt delivers little iodine because iodine becomes a gas and flies off into the air during the salt-drying process. In the United States, salt labels state whether the salt is iodized. Less than a half-teaspoon of iodized salt meets the entire recommendation.

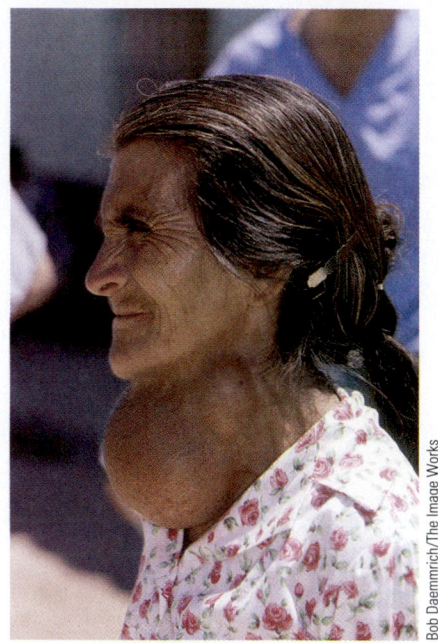

In iodine deficiency, the thyroid gland enlarges—a condition known as simple goiter.

Bob Daemmrich/The Image Works

goiter (GOY-ter) enlargement of the thyroid gland due to an iodine deficiency is *simple goiter*; enlargement due to an iodine excess is *toxic goiter*.

cretinism (CREE-tin-ism) severe mental and physical retardation of an infant caused by the mother's iodine deficiency during pregnancy.

[†]Collectively, the problems caused by iodine deficiency are sometimes referred to as *iodine deficiency disorder*.

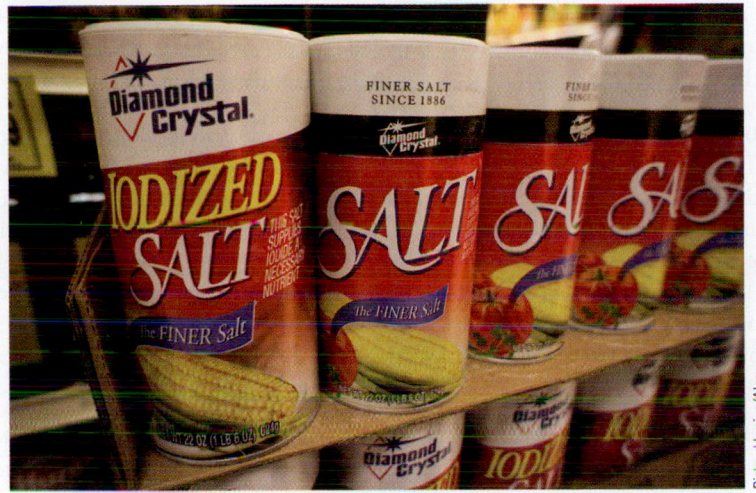

Iodized salt is a source of iodine; plain salt is not.

Richard Levine/Alamy

About 15 percent of the U.S. intake of iodine comes from iodized salt. Much more comes from milk products because most commercial dairies feed iodized grain to dairy cows and sanitize their udders with iodine-rich antiseptics, practices that add iodine to the milk.[68] Consumers in the United States rarely need extra iodine—as mentioned, most people easily meet or exceed the DRI recommended intake with one notable exception: iodine intakes of young women barely meet their need.[69]

KEY POINTS

- Iodine is part of the hormone thyroxine, which influences energy metabolism.
- Iodine deficiency diseases are goiter and cretinism.
- Large amounts of iodine are toxic.
- Most people in the United States meet their need for iodine.

Iron

Every living cell, whether plant or animal, contains iron. Most of the iron in the body is a component of two proteins: **hemoglobin** in red blood cells and **myoglobin** in muscle cells.

Roles of Iron   Iron-containing hemoglobin in the red blood cells carries oxygen from the lungs to tissues throughout the body. Iron in myoglobin holds and stores oxygen in the muscles for their use.

All the body's cells need oxygen to combine with the carbon and hydrogen atoms released from energy nutrients during their metabolism. This generates carbon dioxide and water waste products that are then removed from the cells; thus, body tissues constantly need fresh oxygen to keep the cells cleansed and functioning. As cells use up their oxygen, iron (in hemoglobin) shuttles fresh oxygen into the tissues from the lungs. In addition to this major task, iron is part of dozens of enzymes, particularly those involved in energy metabolism. Iron is also needed to make new cells, amino acids, hormones, and neurotransmitters.

Iron Stores   Iron is clearly the body's gold, a precious mineral to be hoarded. The liver packs iron sent from the bone marrow into new red blood cells and ships them out to the bloodstream. Red blood cells live for about 4 months. When they die, the spleen and liver break them down, salvage their iron for recycling, and send it back to the bone marrow to be kept until it is reused. The body does lose iron from the digestive tract, in nail and hair trimmings, and in shed skin cells—but only in tiny amounts. Bleeding, however, can cause significant iron loss from the body.

Special measures are needed to contain iron in the body. Left free, iron is a powerful oxidant that generates free-radical reactions. Free radicals increase oxidative

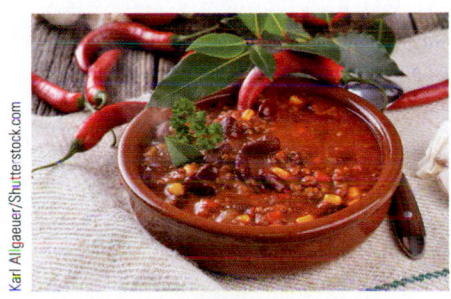

The chili dinner provides iron from meat and legumes and vitamin C from tomatoes. The combination helps to achieve maximum iron absorption.

Karl Allgaeuer/Shutterstock.com

hemoglobin (HEEM-oh-globe-in) the oxygen-carrying protein of the blood; found in the red blood cells (*hemo* means "blood"; *globin* means "spherical protein").

myoglobin (MYE-oh-globe-in) the oxygen-holding protein of the muscles (*myo* means "muscle").

hepcidin (HEP-sid-in) a hormone secreted by the liver in response to elevated blood iron. Hepcidin reduces iron's absorption from the intestine and its release from storage.

heme (HEEM) the iron-containing portion of the hemoglobin and myoglobin molecules.

nonheme iron dietary iron not associated with hemoglobin; the iron of plants and other sources.

tannins compounds in tea (especially black tea) and coffee that bind iron. Tannins also denature proteins.

phytates (FYE-tates) compounds present in plant foods (particularly whole grains) that bind iron and may prevent its absorption.

iron overload the state of having more iron in the body than it needs or can handle, usually arising from a hereditary defect. Also called *hemochromatosis.*

iron deficiency the condition of having depleted iron stores, which, at the extreme, causes iron-deficiency anemia.

iron-deficiency anemia a form of anemia caused by a lack of iron and characterized by red blood cell shrinkage and color loss. Accompanying symptoms are weakness, apathy, headaches, pallor, intolerance to cold, and inability to pay attention. (For other anemias, see the index.)

anemia the condition of inadequate or impaired red blood cells; a reduced number or volume of red blood cells along with too little hemoglobin in the blood. The red blood cells may be immature and therefore too large or too small to function properly. Anemia can result from blood loss, excessive red blood cell destruction, defective red blood cell formation, and many nutrient deficiencies. Anemia is not a disease but a symptom of another problem; its name literally means "too little blood."

stress and inflammation associated with diseases such as diabetes, heart disease, and cancer.[70] To guard against iron's renegade nature, special proteins transport and store the body's iron supply, and its absorption is tightly regulated.[71]

An Iron-Regulating Hormone—Hepcidin In most well-fed people, only about 10 to 15 percent of iron in the diet is absorbed.[72] However, if the body's iron supply is diminished or if the need for iron increases (say, during pregnancy), absorption can increase several-fold.[73] The reverse is also true: absorption declines when dietary iron is abundant. The hormone **hepcidin**, secreted by the liver, helps to regulate blood iron concentrations by limiting iron absorption from the small intestine and controlling its release from body stores.[74] Many details are known about this process, but simply described, hepcidin works in an elegant feedback system to control blood iron:

- More abundant iron in the blood (and liver) triggers hepcidin secretion, which reduces iron absorption and inhibits the release of stored iron, thereby reducing the blood iron concentration.

- Less abundant iron in the blood suppresses hepcidin secretion, which permits increased iron absorption and release from stores, thereby raising the blood iron concentration.[75]

Thus, the body adjusts to changing iron needs and iron availability in the diet.

Food Factors in Iron Absorption Iron occurs in two forms in foods. Some is bound into **heme**, the iron-containing part of hemoglobin and myoglobin in meat, poultry, and fish. Some is **nonheme iron**, in plants and also in meats. The form affects absorption.[76] Healthy people with adequate iron stores absorb heme iron at a rate of about 23 percent over a wide range of meat intakes. People absorb nonheme iron at rates of 2 to 20 percent, depending on dietary factors and iron stores. (A heme molecule was depicted in Figure 6–4 of Chapter 6.)

Meat, fish, and poultry also contain a peptide factor, sometimes called *MFP factor*, that promotes the absorption of nonheme iron from other foods. Vitamin C also greatly improves absorption of nonheme iron, tripling iron absorption from foods eaten in the same meal. The bit of vitamin C in dried fruit, strawberries, or watermelon helps absorb the nonheme iron in these foods.

Iron Inhibitors Some substances inhibit iron absorption. They include the **tannins** of tea and coffee, the calcium and phosphorus in milk, and the **phytates** that accompany fiber in lightly processed legumes and whole-grain cereals. Ordinary black tea excels at reducing iron absorption—clinical dietitians advise people with **iron overload** to drink it with their meals. For those who need more iron, the opposite advice applies—drink tea between meals, not with food. Thus, the amount of iron absorbed from a regular meal depends partly on the interaction between promoters and inhibitors, listed in Table 8–12.

What Happens in Iron Deficiency? If absorption cannot compensate for losses or low dietary intakes, then iron stores are used up, and **iron deficiency** sets in. Iron deficiency and **iron-deficiency anemia** are not one and the same, though they often occur together. Iron deficiency develops in stages, and the distinction between iron deficiency and its **anemia** is a matter of degree. People may be iron deficient, meaning that they have depleted iron stores, without being anemic; with worsening iron deficiency, they may become anemic.

A body severely deprived of iron becomes unable to make enough hemoglobin to fill new blood cells, and anemia results. A sample of iron-deficient blood examined under a microscope shows cells that are smaller and lighter red than normal (see Figure 8–12). These cells contain too little hemoglobin to deliver sufficient oxygen to the tissues. As iron deficiency limits the cells' oxygen and energy metabolism, the person develops fatigue, apathy, and a tendency to feel cold. The blood's lower concentration of its red pigment hemoglobin also explains the pale appearance of fair-skinned

Figure 8–12

Normal and Anemic Blood Cells

Well-nourished red blood cells, shown on the left, are normal in size and color. The cells on the right are typical of iron-deficiency anemia. These cells are small and pale because they contain less hemoglobin.

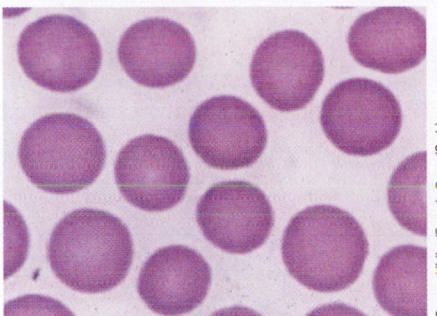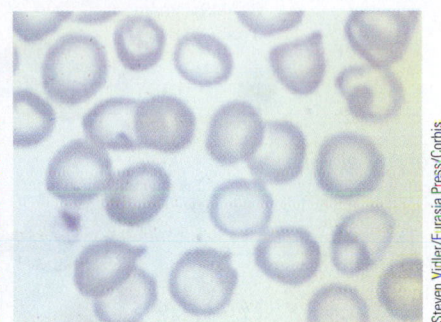

Steven Vidler/Eurasia Press/Corbis

iron-deficient people and the paleness of the normally pink tongue and eyelid linings of those with darker skin.

Mental Symptoms of Iron Deficiency

Long before the red blood cells are affected and anemia is diagnosed, a developing iron deficiency affects behavior.[77] Even slightly lowered iron levels cause fatigue, mental impairments, and impaired physical work capacity and productivity.[78] Symptoms associated with iron deficiency are easily mistaken for behavioral or motivational problems (see Table 8–13). With reduced energy, people work less, play less, and think or learn less eagerly. Lack of energy does not always indicate a need for iron, however—see the Think Fitness feature. Taking supplements for fatigue without a deficiency will not increase energy levels.

Children deprived of iron become restless, irritable, unwilling to work or play, and unable to pay attention, and they may fall behind their peers academically. Some symptoms in children, such as irritability, disappear when iron intake improves. More studies are needed to clarify whether replenished iron levels can improve cognitive function and reverse academic failure or whether these linger beyond treatment.[79] In iron-deficient adults, mental symptoms clear up reliably when iron is restored.[80]

Table 8–13

Mental Symptoms of Anemia

- Apathy, listlessness
- Behavior disturbances
- Clumsiness
- Hyperactivity
- Irritability
- Lack of appetite
- Learning disorders (vocabulary, perception)
- Low scores on latency and associative reactions
- Lowered IQ
- Reduced physical work capacity
- Repetitive hand and foot movements
- Shortened attention span

Note: These symptoms are caused not by anemia itself but by iron deficiency in the brain. Children with much more severe anemias from other causes, such as sickle-cell anemia and thalassemia, show no reduction in IQ when compared with children without anemia.

Think Fitness 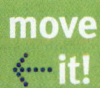 move it!

Exercise-Deficiency Fatigue

On hearing about symptoms of iron deficiency, tired people may jump to the conclusion that they need to take iron supplements to restore their pep. More likely, they can obtain help by simply getting their diets in order, getting to bed on time, and getting enough exercise. Few realize that too little exercise over weeks and months is as exhausting as too much—the less you do, the less you're able to do, and the more fatigued you feel. The condition even has a name: "sedentary inertia."

Feeling fatigued, weak, and apathetic does not necessarily mean that you need iron or other supplements. Three actions are called for:

- Get your diet in order.
- Get some exercise.
- If fatigue persists for more than a week or two after making simple changes, consult a physician for a diagnosis.

start now! ⋯➔ Using the Track Activity feature in Diet & Wellness Plus, track your physical activity for one week, trying to increase your level of activity a little bit each day. See if you can walk briskly, bike, or jog for 30 minutes each day for a week.

Iron

DRI Recommended Intakes
Men: 8 mg/day
Women (19–50 yr): 18 mg/day
Women (51+): 8 mg/day

Tolerable Upper Intake Level
Adults: 45 mg/day

Chief Functions
Carries oxygen as part of hemoglobin in blood or myoglobin in muscles; required for cellular energy metabolism

Deficiency
Anemia: weakness, fatigue, headaches; impaired mental and physical work performance; impaired immunity; pale skin, nailbeds, and mucous membranes; concave nails; chills; pica

Toxicity
GI distress; with chronic iron overload, infections, fatigue, joint pain, skin pigmentation, organ damage

*These foods provide 10% or more of the iron Daily Value in a serving. For a 2,000-cal diet, the DV is 18 mg/day.
Note: Dried figs contain 0.6 mg per ¼ c; raisins contain 0.8 mg per ¼ c.
[a] Some clams may contain less, but most types are iron-rich foods.
[b] Legumes contain phytates that reduce iron absorption.
[c] Enriched cereals vary widely in iron content.

Good Sources*

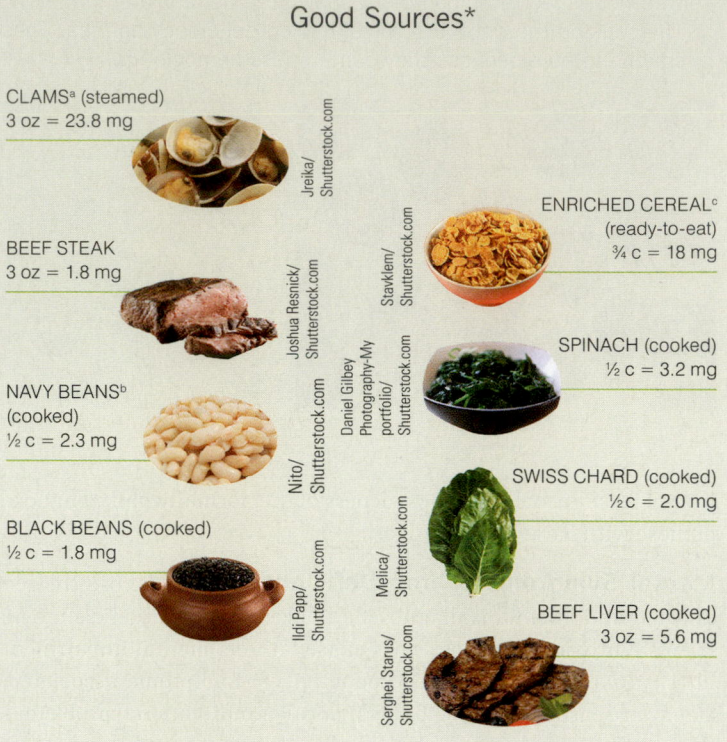

CLAMS[a] (steamed)
3 oz = 23.8 mg
Jreika/Shutterstock.com

BEEF STEAK
3 oz = 1.8 mg
Joshua Resnick/Shutterstock.com

NAVY BEANS[b] (cooked)
½ c = 2.3 mg
Nito/Shutterstock.com

BLACK BEANS (cooked)
½ c = 1.8 mg
Ildi Papp/Shutterstock.com

ENRICHED CEREAL[c] (ready-to-eat)
¾ c = 18 mg
Stavklem/Shutterstock.com

SPINACH (cooked)
½ c = 3.2 mg
Daniel Gilbey Photography-My portfolio/Shutterstock.com

SWISS CHARD (cooked)
½ c = 2.0 mg
Melica/Shutterstock.com

BEEF LIVER (cooked)
3 oz = 5.6 mg
Serghei Starus/Shutterstock.com

A poorly understood behavior seen among some iron-deficient people, particularly low-income women and children, is **pica**—the craving and intentional consumption of ice, chalk, starch, clay, soil, and other nonfood substances. Researchers hypothesize that pica may result from hunger, nutrient deficiencies, digestive upsets, or attempts to prevent infections or toxicities. Ingested clay, soil, or raw starch forms a glaze over the intestinal surface that can cause or worsen an iron deficiency by reducing absorption.[81] Soil can also introduce parasites and heavy metals into the body.

Causes of Iron Deficiency and Anemia
Iron deficiency is usually caused by inadequate iron intake, either from sheer lack of food or from a steady diet of iron-poor foods or foods high in iron inhibitors.[82] In developed nations, high-calorie foods that are rich in refined carbohydrates and fats and poor in nutrients often displace nutritious iron-rich foods from the diet and may impede iron absorption.[83] In contrast, Snapshot 8–5 shows some foods that are good sources of iron.

The number-one nonnutritional factor that can cause anemia is blood loss. Because the majority of the body's iron is in the blood, losing blood means losing iron. Menstrual losses increase women's iron needs to more than double that of men. Digestive tract problems such as ulcers and inflammation can also cause blood loss severe enough to cause anemia.

Who Is Most Susceptible to Iron Deficiency?
Women of child bearing age can easily develop iron deficiency because they not only lose more iron but also eat less food than men, on average. Pregnancy also demands additional iron to support the added blood volume, growth of the fetus, and blood loss during childbirth. Infants and toddlers receive little iron from their high-milk diets, yet they need extra iron to support their rapid growth. The rapid growth of adolescence, especially for males, and the menstrual losses of females also demand extra iron that a typical teen eating

pica (PIE-ka) a craving and intentional consumption of nonfood substances. Also known as *geophagia* (gee-oh-FAY-gee-uh) when referring to clay eating and *pagophagia* (pag-oh-FAY-gee-uh) when referring to ice craving (*geo* means "earth"; *pago* means "frost"; *phagia* means "to eat").

pattern may not provide. Finally, iron deficiency is more common among obese people, although the reasons why remain unclear.[84] Iron is of particular concern for the following groups of people:

- Women in their reproductive years.
- Pregnant women.
- Infants and toddlers.
- Adolescents and females.[85]

In addition, obesity at many life stages makes low blood iron more likely to occur.[86]

In the United States, 2.4 million young children suffer from iron deficiency, while almost a half-million are diagnosed with iron-deficiency anemia. Most often, the children are from urban, low-income, and Hispanic families, but children from all groups can develop these conditions. As for women in childbearing years, the percentage of iron deficiency remains three times higher than the goal of Healthy People 2020: Objectives for the Nation. To combat iron deficiency, the Special Supplemental Feeding Program for Women, Infants, and Children (WIC) provides low-income families with credits redeemable for high-iron foods.

Worldwide, iron deficiency is the most common nutrient deficiency and the most common cause of anemia. Two billion people and almost half of preschool children and pregnant women are anemic, mostly due to iron deficiency.[87] In developing countries, parasitic infections of the digestive tract cause people to lose blood daily. For their entire lives, they may feel fatigued and listless but never know why. Iron supplements can reverse iron-deficiency anemia from dietary causes in short order, but they may also cause digestive upsets and other problems.

Can a Person Take in Too Much Iron?

Iron is toxic in large amounts, largely due to increased oxidative stress in body tissues.[88] Once absorbed inside the body, iron is difficult to excrete. The healthy body defends against iron overload by controlling its entry: the intestinal cells trap some of the iron and hold it within their boundaries. When they are shed, these cells carry out of the intestinal tract the excess iron that they collected during their brief lives. While present in the intestinal contents, excess iron can promote cancers of the colon and rectum.[89]

In healthy people, when iron stores fill up, hepcidin, the iron-suppressing hormone, reduces iron absorption and protects against iron overload. In people with a genetic failure of this protective system, mostly Caucasian men, excess iron builds up in the tissues.[90] Early symptoms include fatigue, mental depression, or abdominal pain; untreated, the condition can cause liver failure, bone damage, diabetes, and heart failure. Infections are also likely because excess iron can harm the immune system and bacteria thrive on iron-rich blood.[91] People with the condition must monitor and limit their iron intakes and avoid supplemental iron.

Iron-containing supplements can easily cause accidental poisonings in young children.[92] As few as five ordinary iron tablets have proved fatal in young children. Keep iron-containing supplements out of children's reach.

Iron Recommendations and Sources

The typical eating pattern in the United States provides about 6 to 7 milligrams of iron for every 1,000 calories. Men need 8 milligrams of iron each day, and so do women past age 51, so these people have little trouble meeting their iron needs. For women of childbearing age, the recommendation is higher—18 milligrams—to replace menstrual losses. During pregnancy, a woman needs even more—27 milligrams a day; to obtain this amount, pregnant women need a supplement. If a man has a low hemoglobin concentration, his health-care provider should examine him for a blood-loss site. Vegetarians, because vegetable sources of iron are poorly absorbed, should multiply the DRI recommended intake for their age and gender group by 1.8 (see the margin example).

Cooking foods in an old-fashioned iron pan adds iron salts, somewhat like the iron found in supplements. The iron content of 100 grams of spaghetti sauce simmered in a glass pan is 3 milligrams, but it increases to 87 milligrams when the

Do the Math

To calculate the iron RDA for vegetarians, multiply the regular RDA by 1.8:

8 mg × 1.8 = 14 mg/day
(vegetarian men)

18 mg × 1.8 = 32 mg/day
(vegetarian women, 19 to 50 yr)

Older women need less iron. Turn to the inside front cover of this book, and find the iron RDA for a 60-year-old woman. Now, use it to calculate the iron RDA for a 60-year-old vegetarian woman.

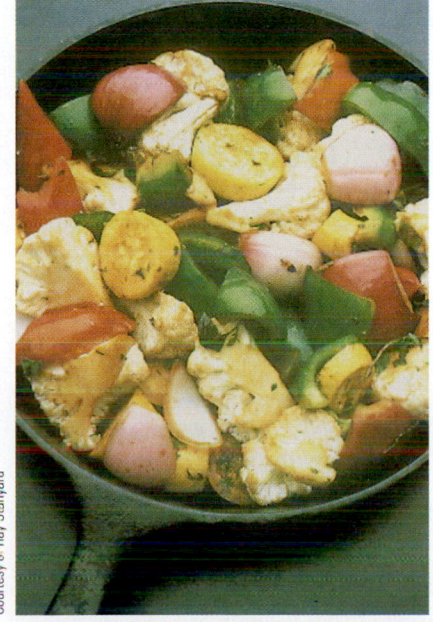

The old-fashioned iron skillet adds supplemental iron to foods.

Courtesy of Ray Stanyard

sauce is cooked in a black iron pan. This iron salt is not as well absorbed as iron from meat, but some does get into the body, especially if the meal also contains meat or vitamin C.

Iron fortification of foods helps some to fend off iron deficiency, but it can be a problem for people who tend toward iron overload. A single ounce of fortified cereal for breakfast, an ordinary ham sandwich at lunch, and a cup of chili with meat for dinner present almost twice the iron a man needs in a day but only about 800 calories. Most men need about 3,000 calories, and more food means still more iron. The U.S. love affair with vitamin C supplements makes matters worse because vitamin C enhances iron absorption. For healthy people, however, fortified foods pose virtually no risk for iron toxicity.

KEY POINTS

- Most iron in the body is in hemoglobin and myoglobin or occurs as part of enzymes in the energy-yielding pathways.
- Iron absorption is affected by the hormone hepcidin, other body factors, and promoters and inhibitors in foods.
- Iron-deficiency anemia is a problem among many groups worldwide.
- Too much iron is toxic.

Zinc

Zinc occurs in a very small quantity in the human body, but it works with proteins in every organ and tissue.[93] Zinc helps more than 300 enzymes to:

- Protect cell structures against damage from oxidation.[94]
- Make parts of the cells' genetic material.
- Make heme in hemoglobin.

Zinc also assists the pancreas with its digestive and insulin functions and helps to metabolize carbohydrate, protein, and fat.

Besides helping enzymes to function, special zinc-containing proteins associate with DNA and help regulate protein synthesis and cell division, functions critical to normal growth before and after birth.[95] Zinc is also needed to produce the active form of vitamin A in visual pigments. Even a mild zinc deficiency can impair night vision. Zinc also:

- Affects behavior, learning, and mood.
- Assists in proper immune functioning.[96]
- Is essential to wound healing, sperm production, taste perception, normal metabolic rate, nerve and brain functioning, bone growth, normal development in children, and many other functions.

When zinc deficiency occurs—even a slight deficiency—it packs a wallop to the body, impairing all of these functions.

Problem: Too Little Zinc Zinc deficiency in human beings was first observed a half-century ago in children and adolescent boys in the Middle East who failed to grow and develop normally. Their native diets were typically low in animal protein and high in whole grains and beans; consequently, the diets were high in fiber and phytates, which bind zinc as well as iron. Furthermore, the bread was not **leavened**; in leavened bread, yeast breaks down phytates as the bread rises. Since that time, zinc deficiency has been identified as a substantial contributor to illness throughout the developing world and responsible for almost a half-million deaths each year.[97]

Marginal declines in zinc status also cause widespread problems in pregnancy, infancy, and early childhood. Zinc deficiency alters digestive function profoundly and causes diarrhea, which worsens the malnutrition already present, not only of zinc but of all nutrients. It drastically impairs the immune response, making infections likely.[98]

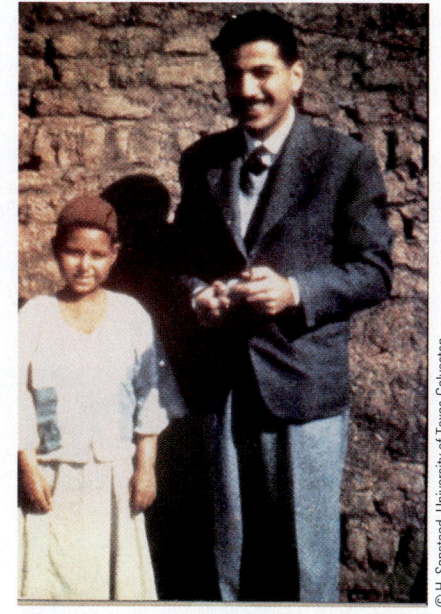

© H. Sanstead, University of Texas-Galveston

How old does the Egyptian boy in the picture appear to be? He is 17 years old but is only 4 feet tall, the height of a 7-year-old in the United States. His reproductive organs are like those of a 6-year-old. The retardation is rightly ascribed to zinc deficiency because it is partially reversible when zinc is restored to the diet.

leavened (LEV-end) literally, "lightened" by yeast cells, which digest some carbohydrate components of the dough and leave behind bubbles of gas that make the bread rise.

Infections of the intestinal tract then worsen the malnutrition and further increase susceptibility to infections—a classic cycle of malnutrition and disease. Zinc therapy often quickly reduces diarrhea and prevents death in malnourished children, but it can fail to restore normal weight and height if the child returns to a nutrient-poor diet after treatment.[99]

Although zinc deficiencies are not common in developed countries, they do occur among some groups, including pregnant women, young children, the elderly, and the poor. When pediatricians or other health workers note poor growth accompanied by poor appetite in children, they should think zinc.

Problem: Too Much Zinc   Zinc is toxic in large quantities. High doses (over 50 milligrams) of zinc may cause vomiting, diarrhea, headaches, exhaustion, and other symptoms. A UL for adults was set at 40 milligrams—an amount based on degeneration of the heart muscle in animals.

High doses of zinc inhibit iron absorption from the digestive tract. A blood protein that carries iron from the digestive tract to tissues also carries some zinc. If this protein is burdened with excess zinc, little or no room is left for iron to be picked up from the intestine. The opposite is also true: too much iron inhibits zinc absorption. Zinc from cold-relief lozenges, nasal gels, and throat spray products may shorten the duration of a cold, but they can upset the stomach and contribute supplemental zinc to the body.[100]

Food Sources of Zinc   Meats, shellfish, poultry, and milk products are among the top providers of zinc in the U.S. diet (see Snapshot 8–6). Among plant sources, some legumes and whole grains are rich in zinc, but the zinc is not as well absorbed as it is from meat. Most people meet the recommended 11 milligrams per day for men and 8 milligrams per day for women. Vegetarians are advised to plan eating patterns that

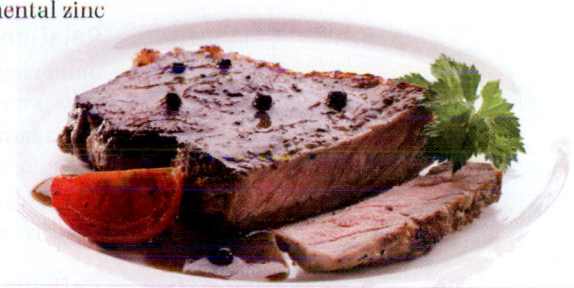

DUSAN ZIDAR/Shutterstock.com

Snapshot 8–6   Zinc

DRI Recommended Intakes
Men: 11 mg/day
Women: 8 mg/day

Tolerable Upper Intake Level
Adults: 40 mg/day

Chief Functions
Activates many enzymes; associated with hormones; synthesis of genetic material and proteins, transport of vitamin A, taste perception, wound healing, reproduction

Deficiency[a]
Growth retardation, delayed sexual maturation, impaired immune function, hair loss, eye and skin lesions, loss of appetite

Toxicity
Loss of appetite, impaired immunity, reduced copper and iron absorption, low HDL cholesterol (a risk factor for heart disease)

*These foods provide 10% or more of the zinc Daily Value in a serving. For a 2,000-cal diet, the DV is 11 mg/day.
[a] A rare inherited form of zinc malabsorption causes additional and more severe symptoms.
[b] Some oysters contain more or less than this amount, but all types are zinc-rich foods.
[c] Enriched cereals vary widely in zinc content.

Good Sources*

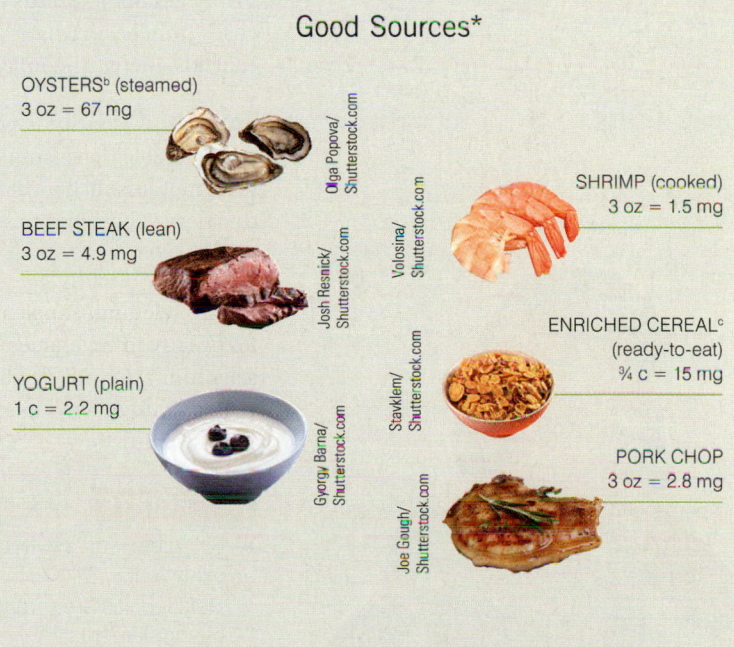

OYSTERS[b] (steamed)
3 oz = 67 mg
Olga Popova/Shutterstock.com

BEEF STEAK (lean)
3 oz = 4.9 mg
Josh Resnick/Shutterstock.com

YOGURT (plain)
1 c = 2.2 mg
Gyorgy Barna/Shutterstock.com

SHRIMP (cooked)
3 oz = 1.5 mg
Volosina/Shutterstock.com

ENRICHED CEREAL[c]
(ready-to-eat)
¾ c = 15 mg
Stavklem/Shutterstock.com

PORK CHOP
3 oz = 2.8 mg
Joe Gough/Shutterstock.com

include zinc-enriched cereals or whole-grain breads well leavened with yeast, which helps make zinc available for absorption.[101] Unlike supplements, food sources of zinc never cause imbalances in the body.

Selenium

Selenium has attracted the attention of the world's scientists. Hints of its relationships with chronic diseases make fascinating reading.[102]

Roles in the Body   Selenium works with a group of enzymes that, in concert with vitamin E, limits the formation of free radicals and prevents oxidative harm to cells and tissues.[103] In addition, selenium-containing enzymes are needed to assist the iodine-containing thyroid hormones that regulate metabolism.[104]

Relationship with Chronic Diseases   Evidence is mixed on whether low selenium plays a role in common forms of heart disease, but taking selenium supplements does not reduce the risk.[105] In cancer studies, adequate *blood* selenium seems protective against cancers of the prostate, colon, breast, and other sites.[106] Should everyone take selenium supplements to ward off cancer, then? No. Selenium *deficiency* may increase cancer risk, but U.S. intakes are generally sufficient, and excesses may harm healthy, well-fed people.[107]

Deficiency   Without an adequate supply of selenium, the body's ability to make the needed selenium-containing molecules is compromised. Severe deficiencies cause muscle disorders with weakness and pain in people and animals. A specific type of heart disease, prevalent in regions of China where the soil and foods lack selenium, is partly brought on by selenium deficiency. This condition prompted researchers to give selenium its status as an essential nutrient—adequate selenium prevents many cases from occurring.[108] More subtle deficiencies may unleash harmful levels of free radicals, increasing inflammation.

Toxicity   Toxicity is possible when people take selenium supplements and exceed the Tolerable Upper Intake Level of 400 micrograms per day. Selenium toxicity brings on symptoms such as hair loss and brittle nails; diarrhea and fatigue; and bone, joint, and nerve abnormalities.[109]

Sources   Clearly, adequate selenium is important, but research does not support taking selenium supplements. It is widely distributed in meats and shellfish but varies greatly in vegetables, nuts, and grains, depending on whether they are grown on selenium-rich soil.[110] Soils in the United States vary in selenium, but foods from many regions mingle on supermarket shelves, ensuring that consumers are well supplied with selenium.

Fluoride

Fluoride is not essential to life. It is beneficial in the diet, however, because of its ability to inhibit the development of dental caries in children and adults.

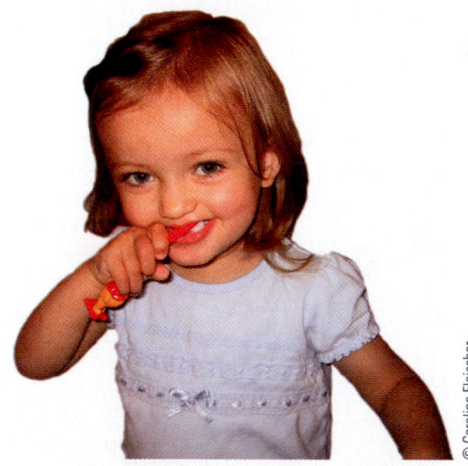

© Caroline Fleischer

To prevent fluorosis, young children should not swallow toothpaste.

Roles in the Body   In developing teeth and bones, fluoride replaces the hydroxy portion of hydroxyapatite, forming **fluorapatite**. During development, fluorapatite enlarges calcium crystals in bones and teeth, decreasing their susceptibility to demineralization. In mature bones, higher intakes of fluoride may also stimulate bone-building cells, but this effect does not seem to prevent hip fractures associated with bone loss in later life.[111]

Fluoride's primary role in health is prevention of **dental caries** throughout life.[112] Once teeth have erupted through the gums, fluoride, particularly when applied to tooth surfaces, helps to prevent dental caries by promoting the remineralization of early lesions of the enamel that might otherwise progress to form caries.[113] Fluoride also acts directly on the bacteria of plaque, suppressing their metabolism and reducing the amount of tooth-destroying acid they produce.

Deficiency   Where fluoride is lacking, dental decay is common, and fluoridation of public water is recommended for dental health (Figure 8–13). Based on evidence of its benefits, fluoridation has been endorsed by the National Institute of Dental Health, the Academy of Nutrition and Dietetics, the American Medical Association, the National Cancer Institute, and the Centers for Disease Control and Prevention as beneficial and presenting no proven risks.

Toxicity   In communities where the water contains too much fluoride, discoloration of the teeth, or **fluorosis**, may occur.[114] In bones, skeletal fluorosis causes bone malformations, hardened ligaments, and unusually dense, but weak, fracture-prone bones.[115] Skeletal fluorosis may occur among adults who live in high-fluoride areas, who are exposed to industrial sources, or who consume large amounts of fluoridated toothpaste.[116] The mildest form of dental fluorosis occurs as characteristic white spots in the tooth enamel; a more severe form is shown in Figure 8–14. Many communities have reduced the amount of fluoride added to public water supplies in response to increased incidence of fluorosis.

Fluorosis in teeth occurs only during tooth development, never after the teeth have formed—and it is irreversible. To prevent fluorosis, people in areas with fluoridated water should limit other sources, such as fluoride-enriched formula for infants and fluoride supplements for infants or children unless prescribed by a physician. Children younger than 6 years should use only a pea-sized squeeze of toothpaste and should be told not to swallow their toothpaste when brushing their teeth. The Tolerable Upper Intake Level for fluoride for all people older than 8 years is 10 milligrams per day.

Sources of Fluoride   Drinking water is the usual source of fluoride. More than 70 percent of the U.S. population has access to public water supplies with an optimal fluoride concentration, which typically delivers about 0.7 milligrams per liter.[117] Fluoride is rarely present in bottled waters unless it was added at the source, as in bottled municipal tap water.

KEY POINTS

- Fluoride stabilizes bones and makes teeth resistant to decay.
- Excess fluoride discolors teeth and weakens bones; large doses are toxic.

Chromium

Chromium is an essential mineral that participates in carbohydrate and lipid metabolism. Chromium in foods is safe and essential to health. Industrial chromium is a toxic contaminant, a known carcinogen that damages the DNA.[118]

Roles in the Body   Chromium may help maintain glucose homeostasis by enhancing the activity of the hormone insulin, improving cellular uptake of glucose, and other actions.[119] When chromium is lacking, a diabetes-like condition may develop with elevated blood glucose and impaired glucose tolerance, insulin response, and glucagon response. Research is mixed on whether chromium supplements might improve glucose or insulin responses in diabetes.

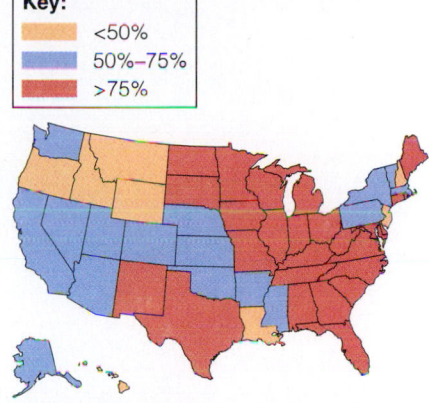

Figure 8–13

U.S. Population with Access to Fluoridated Water through Public Water Systems

Key:
- <50%
- 50%–75%
- >75%

Source: Data from Centers for Disease Control and Prevention, Community water fluoridation: 2012 Water fluoridation statistics, available from http://www.cdc.gov/fluoridation/statistics/2012stats.htm

Figure 8–14

Fluorosis

The mottled brown stains on these teeth indicate exposure to high concentrations of fluoride during development.

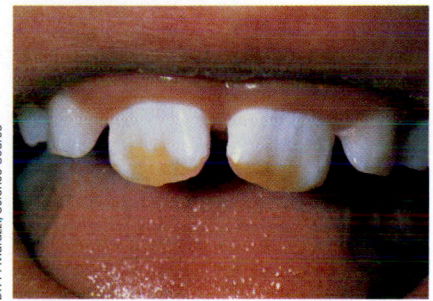

Dr. P. Marazzi/Science Source

fluorapatite (floor-APP-uh-tight) a crystal of bones and teeth, formed when fluoride displaces the "hydroxy" portion of hydroxyapatite. Fluorapatite resists being dissolved back into body fluid.

dental caries decay of the teeth, commonly called *cavities*. Also defined in Chapter 14.

fluorosis (floor-OH-sis) discoloration of the teeth due to ingestion of too much fluoride during tooth development. *Skeletal fluorosis* is characterized by unusually dense but weak, fracture-prone, often malformed bones, caused by excess fluoride in bone crystals.

Chromium Sources Chromium is present in a variety of foods. The best sources are unrefined foods, particularly liver, brewer's yeast, and whole grains. The more refined foods people eat, the less chromium they receive.

Supplement advertisements may convince consumers that they can lose fat and build muscle by taking chromium picolinate. Chromium supplements are unlikely to reduce body fat or improve muscle strength more than diet and exercise alone, however.

KEY POINTS

- Chromium is needed for normal blood glucose regulation.
- Whole, minimally processed foods are the best chromium sources.

Copper

One of copper's most vital roles is helping to form hemoglobin. In addition, many enzymes depend on copper for its oxygen-handling ability. Copper plays roles in the body's handling of iron and, like iron, assists in reactions leading to the release of energy. One copper-dependent enzyme helps to control damage from free-radical activity in the tissues.[§] Researchers are investigating the possibility that a low-copper diet may contribute to heart disease by suppressing the activity of this enzyme.

Copper deficiency is rare but not unknown: it has been seen in severely malnourished infants fed a copper-poor milk formula. Deficiency can severely disturb growth and metabolism, and in adults, it can impair immunity and blood flow through the arteries. Excess zinc interferes with copper absorption and can cause deficiency. Two rare genetic disorders affect copper status in opposite directions—one causing a functional deficiency and the other toxicity.[120]

Copper toxicity from foods is unlikely, but supplements can cause it. The Tolerable Upper Intake Level for adults is set at 10,000 micrograms (10 milligrams) per day. The best food sources of copper include organ meats, seafood, nuts, and seeds. Water may also supply copper, especially where copper plumbing pipes are used. In the United States, copper intakes are thought to be adequate.[121]

KEY POINTS

- Copper is needed to form hemoglobin and assists in many other body processes.
- Copper deficiency is rare.

Other Trace Minerals and Some Candidates

DRI intake recommendations have been established for two other trace minerals, molybdenum and manganese. Molybdenum functions as part of several metal-containing enzymes, some of which are giant proteins. Manganese works with dozens of different enzymes that facilitate body processes and is widespread among whole grains, vegetables, fruits, legumes, and nuts.

Several other trace minerals are known to be important to health, but researching their roles in the body is difficult because their quantities are so small and because human deficiencies are unknown. For example, boron influences the activity of many enzymes and may play a key role in bone health, brain activities, and immune response. The richest food sources of boron are noncitrus fruits, leafy vegetables, nuts, and legumes. Cobalt is the mineral in the vitamin B_{12} molecule; the alternative name for vitamin B_{12}, *cobalamin*, reflects cobalt's presence. Nickel may serve as an enzyme cofactor; deficiencies harm the liver and other organs. Future research may reveal key roles played by other trace minerals, including barium, cadmium, lead, lithium, mercury, silver, tin, and vanadium. Even arsenic, a known poison and carcinogen, may turn out to be essential in tiny quantities.

[§]The enzyme is superoxide dismutase.

All trace minerals are toxic in excess, and Tolerable Upper Intake Levels exist for boron, nickel, and vanadium (see the inside front cover, page C). Overdoses are most likely to occur in people who take multiple nutrient supplements. Obtaining trace minerals from food is not hard to do—just eat a variety of whole foods in the amounts recommended in Chapter 2. Table 8–14 sums up what this chapter has said about the minerals and fills in some additional information.

KEY POINTS

- Many different trace elements play important roles in the body.
- All of the trace minerals are toxic in excess.

Table 8–14

The Minerals—A Summary

MINERALS AND CHIEF FUNCTIONS IN THE BODY

Major Minerals	Deficiency Symptoms	Toxicity Symptoms	Significant Sources
Calcium The principal mineral of bones and teeth. Also acts in normal muscle contraction and relaxation, nerve functioning, regulation of cell activities, blood clotting, blood pressure, and immune defenses.	Stunted growth in children; adult bone loss (osteoporosis).	High blood calcium; abnormal heart rhythms; soft tissue calcification; kidney stones; kidney dysfunction; interference with absorption of other minerals; constipation.	Milk and milk products, oysters, small fish (with bones), calcium-set tofu (bean curd), certain leafy greens (bok choy, turnip greens, kale), broccoli.
Phosphorus Mineralization of bones and teeth; important in cells' genetic material, in cell membranes as phospholipids, in energy transfer, and in buffering systems.	Appetite loss, bone pain, muscle weakness, impaired growth, and rickets in infants.[a]	Calcification of nonskeletal tissues, particularly the kidney.	Foods from animal sources, some legumes.
Magnesium A factor involved in bone mineralization, the building of protein, enzyme action, normal muscular function, transmission of nerve impulses, proper immune function, and maintenance of teeth.	Low blood calcium; muscle cramps; confusion; impaired vitamin D metabolism; if extreme, seizures, bizarre movements; hallucinations, and difficulty in swallowing. In children, growth failure.	Excess magnesium from abuse of laxatives (Epsom salts) causes diarrhea, nausea, and abdominal cramps with fluid and electrolyte and pH imbalances.	Nuts, legumes, whole grains, dark green vegetables, seafoods, chocolate, cocoa.
Sodium Sodium, chloride, and potassium (electrolytes) maintain normal fluid balance and acid-base balance in the body. Sodium is critical to nerve impulse transmission.	Muscle cramps, mental apathy, loss of appetite.	Hypertension, edema.	Salt, soy sauce, seasoning mixes, processed foods, condiments, fast foods.
Potassium Facilitates reactions, including protein formation; fluid and electrolyte balance; support of cell integrity; transmission of nerve impulses; and contraction of muscles, including the heart.	Deficiency accompanies dehydration; causes muscular weakness, paralysis, and confusion; can cause death.	Causes muscular weakness; triggers vomiting; if given into a vein, can stop the heart.	All whole foods: meats, milk, fruits, vegetables, grains, legumes.

[a] Seen only rarely in infants fed phosphorus-free formula or in adults taking medications that interact with phosphorus.

Table 8–14

The Minerals—A Summary (continued)

Major Minerals	Deficiency Symptoms	Toxicity Symptoms	Significant Sources
Chloride Part of the hydrochloric acid found in the stomach, necessary for proper digestion. Helps maintain normal fluid and electrolyte balance.	Does not occur in normal circumstances, but can cause cramps, apathy, and death.	Normally harmless (the gas chlorine is a poison but evaporates from water); can cause vomiting.	Salt, soy sauce; moderate quantities in whole, unprocessed foods, large amounts in processed foods.
Sulfate A contributor of sulfur to many important compounds, such as certain amino acids, antioxidants, and the vitamins biotin and thiamin; stabilizes protein shape by forming sulfur-sulfur bridges (see Figure 6–10 in Chapter 6, p. 213).	None known; protein deficiency would occur first.	Would occur only if sulfur amino acids were eaten in excess; this (in animals) depresses growth.	All protein-containing foods.

Trace Minerals	Deficiency Symptoms	Toxicity Symptoms	Significant Sources
Iodine A component of the thyroid hormone thyroxine, which helps to regulate growth, development, and metabolic rate.	Goiter, cretinism.	Depressed thyroid activity; goiter-like thyroid enlargement.	Iodized salt, seafood, bread, plants grown in most parts of the country and animals fed those plants.
Iron Part of the protein hemoglobin, which carries oxygen in the blood; part of the protein myoglobin in muscles, which makes oxygen available for muscle contraction; necessary for the use of energy.	Anemia: weakness, fatigue, pale skin and mucous membranes, pale concave nails, headaches, inability to concentrate, impaired cognitive function (children), lowered cold tolerance.	Iron overload: fatigue, abdominal pain, infections, liver injury, joint pain, skin pigmentation, growth retardation in children, bloody stools, shock.	Red meats, fish, poultry, shellfish, eggs, legumes, green leafy vegetables, dried fruits.
Zinc Associated with hormones; needed for many enzymes; involved in making genetic material and proteins, immune cell activation, transport of vitamin A, taste perception, wound healing, the making of sperm, and normal fetal development.	Growth failure in children, dermatitis, sexual retardation, loss of taste, poor wound healing.	Nausea, vomiting, diarrhea, loss of appetite, headache, immune suppression, decreased HDL, reduced iron and copper status.	Protein-containing foods: meats, fish, shellfish, poultry, grains, yogurt.
Selenium Assists a group of enzymes that defend against oxidation.	Predisposition to a form of heart disease characterized by fibrous cardiac tissue (uncommon).	Nausea; diarrhea; nail and hair changes; joint pain; nerve, liver, and bone damage; garlic breath odor.	Seafoods, organ meats, other meats, whole grains, and vegetables depending on soil content.
Fluoride Strengthens tooth enamel; confers decay resistance on teeth.	Susceptibility to tooth decay.	Fluorosis (discoloration) of teeth, skeletal fluorosis (weak, malformed bones), nausea, vomiting, diarrhea, chest pain, itching.	Drinking water if fluoride-containing or fluoridated, tea, seafood.

Table 8–14

The Minerals—A Summary (continued)

Chromium			
Associated with insulin; needed for energy release from glucose.	Abnormal glucose metabolism.	Possibly skin eruptions.	Meat, unrefined grains, vegetable oils.
Copper			
Helps form hemoglobin and collagen; part of several enzymes.	Anemia; bone abnormalities.	Vomiting, diarrhea; liver damage.	Organ meats, seafood, nuts, seeds, whole grains, drinking water.

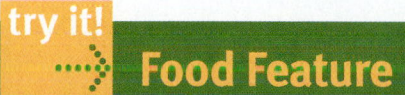

try it!

Food Feature

Meeting the Need for Calcium

LO 8.6 Discuss food choices that help to meet the need for calcium.

Some people behave as though calcium nutrition is of little consequence to their health—they neglect to meet their need.[122] Yet a low calcium intake is associated with all sorts of major illnesses, including adult bone loss (see the following Controversy), high blood pressure, colon cancer (see Chapter 11), and even lead poisoning (Chapter 14).

Intakes of one of the best sources of calcium—milk—have declined in recent years, while consumption of other beverages, such as sweet soft drinks and fruit drinks, has increased dramatically. This Food Feature focuses on food and beverage sources of calcium and provides guidance about how to include them in an eating pattern that meets nutrient needs.

Milk and Milk Products

Milk and milk products are traditional sources of calcium for people who can tolerate them (see Figure 8–15). On average, people in the United States fall far short of the recommended intake of milk, yogurt, or cheese (or replacements) each day. People who shun these foods because of lactose intolerance, allergy, a vegan diet, or other reasons can obtain calcium from other sources, but care is needed—*wise* substitutions must be made.[123] This is especially true for children. Children who don't drink milk often have lower calcium intakes

Figure 8–15

Food Sources of Calcium in the U.S. Diet

Milk, cheese, and yogurt contribute much of the calcium in a typical U.S. diet.

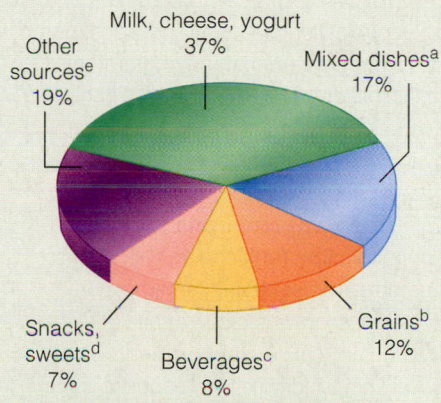

Milk, cheese, yogurt 37%
Other sources[e] 19%
Mixed dishes[a] 17%
Snacks, sweets[d] 7%
Beverages[c] 8%
Grains[b] 12%

[a]Includes pasta, macaroni and cheese, pizza, Mexican-style foods, fried rice.
[b]Includes breads, rolls, tortillas.
[c]Includes fortified juices and bottled drinks; excludes alcohol, milk.
[d]Includes ice cream, frozen dairy desserts, chocolate, cakes, pies, tortilla or corn chips.
[e]Meats, vegetables, fruit, condiments, other sources.

Source: M. K. Hoy and J. D. Goldman, Calcium intake of the U.S. population, USDA Dietary Data Brief No. 13, September 2014, available at www.ars.usda.gov/SP2UserFiles/Place/80400530/pdf/DBrief/13_calcium_intake_0910.pdf.

and poorer bone health than those who drink milk regularly. Most of milk's many relatives are good choices: yogurt, **kefir**, buttermilk, cheese (especially the low-fat

or fat-free varieties), and, for people who can afford the calories, ice milk. Cottage cheese and frozen yogurt desserts contain about half the calcium of milk—2 cups are needed to provide the amount of calcium in 1 cup of milk. Butter, cream, and cream cheese are almost pure fat and contain negligible calcium.

Tinker with milk products to make them more appealing. Add cocoa to milk and fruit to yogurt, make your own fruit smoothies from fat-free milk or yogurt, or add fat-free milk powder to any dish. The cocoa powder added to make chocolate milk does contain a small amount of oxalic acid, which binds with some of milk's calcium and inhibits its absorption, but the effect on calcium balance is insignificant. Sugar lends both sweetness and calories to chocolate milk, so mix your chocolate milk at home where you control the amount of sugary chocolate added to the milk or choose a sugar-free product.

Vegetables

Among vegetables, beet greens, bok choy (a Chinese cabbage), broccoli, kale, mustard greens, rutabaga, and turnip greens provide some available calcium. So do collard greens, green cabbage, kohlrabi, parsley, watercress,

kefir a yogurt-based beverage.

and possibly some seaweeds, such as the **nori** popular in Japanese cookery. Certain other foods, including rhubarb, spinach, and Swiss chard, appear equal to milk in calcium content but provide very little or no calcium to the body because they contain binders that prevent calcium's absorption (see Figure 8–16). The presence of calcium binders does not make spinach an inferior food. Spinach is also rich in iron, beta-carotene, riboflavin, and dozens of other essential nutrients and potentially helpful phytochemicals. Just don't rely on it for calcium.

Calcium in Other Foods

For the many people who cannot use milk and milk products, a 3-ounce serving of small fish, such as canned sardines and other canned fishes eaten with their bones, provides as much calcium as a cup of milk. One-third cup of almonds supplies about 100 milligrams of calcium. Calcium-rich mineral water may also be a useful calcium source. The calcium from mineral water, including hard tap water, may be as absorbable as the calcium from milk but with zero calories. Many other foods contribute small but significant amounts of calcium to the diet.

Calcium-Fortified Foods

Some foods contain large amounts of calcium salts by an accident of processing or by intentional fortification. In the processed category are soybean curd, or tofu (calcium salt is often used to coagulate it, so check the label); canned tomatoes (firming agents donate 63 milligrams per cup of tomatoes); **stone-ground flour**

nori a type of seaweed popular in Asian, particularly Japanese, cooking.

stone-ground flour flour made by grinding kernels of grain between heavy wheels made of limestone, a kind of rock derived from the shells and bones of marine animals. As the stones scrape together, bits of the limestone mix with the flour, enriching it with calcium.

Figure 8–16

Calcium Absorption from Food Sources

≥ 50% absorbed	bok choy, broccoli, brussels sprouts, cauliflower, Chinese cabbage, head cabbage, kale, kohlrabi, mustard greens, rutabaga, turnip greens, watercress
≃ 30% absorbed	calcium-fortified foods and beverages, calcium-fortified soy milk, calcium-set tofu, cheese, milk, yogurt
≃ 20% absorbed	almonds, beans (pinto, red, and white), sesame seeds
≤ 5% absorbed	rhubarb, spinach, Swiss chard

and self-rising flour; stone-ground cornmeal and self-rising cornmeal; and blackstrap molasses.

Milk with extra calcium added can be an excellent source; it provides more calcium per cup than any natural milk, 500 milligrams per 8 ounces. Then comes calcium-fortified orange juice, with 300 milligrams per 8 ounces, a good choice because the bioavailability of its calcium is comparable to that of milk. Calcium-fortified soy milk can also be prepared so that it contains more calcium than whole cow's milk.

Finally, calcium supplements are available, sold mostly to people hoping to ward off osteoporosis. The Controversy following this chapter points out that supplements are not magic bullets against bone loss, however.

Making Meals Rich in Calcium

For those who tolerate milk, many cooks slip extra calcium into meals by sprinkling a tablespoon or two of fat-free dry milk into almost everything. The added calorie value is small, and changes to the taste and texture of

the dish are practically nil, but each 2 tablespoons adds about 100 extra milligrams of calcium. Dried buttermilk powder can also add flavor and calcium to baked goods and other dishes and keeps for a year or more when stored in the refrigerator. Table 8–15 provides some more tips for including calcium-rich foods in your meals.

Tracking Calcium

Here is a shortcut for tracking the amount of calcium in a day's meals. To start, memorize these two facts:

1. A cup of milk provides about 300 milligrams of calcium.
2. Adults need 1,000 to 1,200 milligrams each day. Broken down in terms of "cups of milk," the need is 3⅓ to 4 cups each day.

To estimate calcium from an entire day's foods, not just milk, assign "cups of milk" points to various calcium sources. The goal is to achieve 3½ to 4 points per day:

- 1 point = 1 cup milk, yogurt, or calcium-fortified beverage or 1½ ounces cheese.
- 1 point = 4 ounces canned fish with bones.
- ½ point = 1 cup ice cream, cottage cheese, or calcium-rich vegetables (see the text).

Also, because bits of calcium are present in many foods (a bagel has about 50 milligrams, for example):

- 1 point = a well-balanced, adequate, and varied diet.

Example: Say a day's calcium-rich foods include cereal and a cup of milk, a ham and cheese sandwich, and a broccoli and pasta salad.

- 1 point (cup of milk) + 1 point (cheese) + ½ point (broccoli) = 2½ points

Add 1 point for the other foods eaten that day.

- 1 point + 2½ points = 3½ points

This day's foods provide a calcium intake that approximates the DRI committee's recommendation, a worthy goal for everyone's diet.

Table 8–15

Calcium in Meals—Breakfast, Lunch, and Supper

Try these techniques for meeting calcium needs.

At Breakfast	At Lunch	At Supper
■ Choose calcium-fortified orange or vegetable juice. ■ Lighten tea or coffee, hot or iced, with milk or calcium-fortified replacement, such as soy milk. ■ Eat cereals, hot or cold, with milk or calcium-rich replacement. ■ Spread almond butter on toast (2 tbs provides 111 mg calcium, 8 times the amount in peanut butter). ■ Cook hot cereals with milk instead of water, then mix in 2 tbs of fat-free dry milk. ■ Make muffins or quick breads with milk and extra fat-free powdered milk or dried buttermilk powder. ■ Add milk to scrambled eggs. ■ Moisten cereals with flavored yogurt.	■ Add low-fat cheeses to sandwiches, burgers, or salads. ■ Use a variety of green vegetables, such as watercress or kale, in salads and on sandwiches. ■ Drink fat-free milk or calcium-fortified soy milk as a beverage or in a smoothie. For tartness and extra calcium, add 2 tbs dried buttermilk powder. ■ Drink calcium-rich mineral water as a beverage. ■ Marinate cabbage shreds or broccoli spears in low-fat Italian dressing for an interesting salad that provides calcium. ■ Choose coleslaw over potato and macaroni salads. ■ Mix the mashed bones of canned salmon into salmon salad or patties. ■ Eat sardines with their bones. ■ Stuff potatoes with broccoli and low-fat cheese. ■ Try pasta such as ravioli stuffed with low-fat ricotta cheese instead of meat. ■ Sprinkle parmesan cheese on pasta salads.	■ Toss a handful of thinly sliced green vegetables, such as kale or young turnip greens, with hot pasta; the greens wilt pleasingly in the steam of the freshly cooked pasta. ■ Serve a green vegetable every night and try new ones—how about kohlrabi? It tastes delicious when cooked like broccoli. ■ Remember your dark green, leafy vegetables—they can be good, low-calorie calcium sources. ■ Learn to stir-fry Chinese cabbage and other Asian foods. ■ Try tofu (the calcium-set kind); this versatile food has inspired whole cookbooks devoted to creative uses. ■ Add fat-free powdered milk to almost anything—meat loaf, sauces, gravies, soups, stuffings, casseroles, blended beverages, puddings, quick breads, cookies, brownies. Be creative. ■ Choose frozen yogurt, ice milk, or custards for dessert.

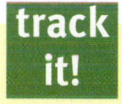 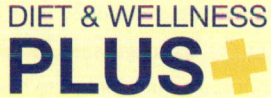

track it! DIET & WELLNESS PLUS+ Concepts in Action

Analyze Your Calcium Intakes

The purpose of this exercise is to make you aware of your calcium intake and to give you ideas about how you might meet your DRI recommended intake. Using the Diet & Wellness Plus program that accompanies this text, complete the following.

1. From the Reports tab, select DRI Report. Find your calcium information. What is the DRI Adequate Intake for calcium for your profile?

2. From the Reports tab, select Intake vs. Goals. Choose Day One (from your three-day diet intake record) and include all meals. What percentage of your calcium DRI did you meet on that day? Was this intake typical?

3. From the Reports tab, select Source Analysis. Choose Day One, include all meals, select calcium from the drop-down box. What were the top three food sources of calcium that day? What were your three lowest sources? Which of your top sources matched those of the calcium Snapshot on page 309?

4. From the Reports tab, select Intake Spreadsheet, choose Day Three, choose breakfast. Look at the Calcium column. Did the calcium values of any of the foods surprise you? Which ones? How many milligrams of calcium did you consume at breakfast?

5. Using the same Intake Spreadsheet, choose Day Three, and choose lunch and then dinner. At which meal did you consume the most calcium? Which meal had the least calcium: breakfast, lunch, or dinner?

6. Many nondairy foods can provide calcium. Using the tips in the Food Feature of this chapter (pp. 331–333), create a calcium-rich side dish without milk or milk products. Select the Track Diet tab, choose a new day, and enter the ingredients for your side dish. Select the "*i*" icon to the left of your side dish. How much calcium did it provide?

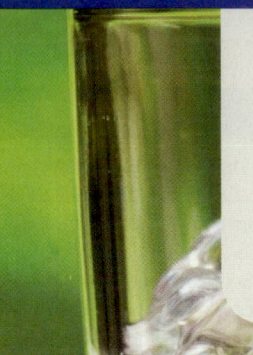
Self Check

1. (LO 8.1) Water balance is governed by the _____.
   a. liver   **b.** kidneys   **c.** brain   **d.** b and c

2. (LO 8.1) Water intoxication cannot occur because water is so easily excreted by the body.

3. (LO 8.2) Water from public water systems
   a. requires frequent home testing for microorganisms.
   b. is less healthful than bottled water.
   c. is disinfected to kill most microorganisms.
   d. is less healthful than private well water.

4. (LO 8.2) On average, young men in the United States obtain __ percent of their calories from beverages.
   a. 12   **b.** 22   **c.** 32   **d.** 42

5. (LO 8.2) Whether from the tap or from a bottle, all water comes from the same sources.
   T   F

6. (LO 8.3) To temporarily increase the body's water content, a person need only
   a. consume extra salt.   **b.** consume extra sugar.
   c. take a diuretic.   **d.** consume extra potassium.

7. (LO 8.3) Vomiting or diarrhea
   a. causes fluid to be pulled from between the cells in every part of the body.
   b. causes fluid to leave the cell interiors.
   c. causes kidneys to raise the sodium concentration outside the cells.
   d. all of the above.

8. (LO 8.4) Which two minerals are the major constituents of bone?
   a. calcium and zinc   **b.** sodium and magnesium
   c. phosphorus and calcium   **d.** magnesium and calcium

9. (LO 8.4) Magnesium
   a. assists in the operation of enzymes.
   b. is needed for the release and use of energy.
   c. is critical to normal heart function.
   d. all of the above.

10. (LO 8.4) After about 50 years of age, bones begin to lose density.
    T   F

11. (LO 8.4) The best way to control salt intake is to cut down on processed and fast foods.
    T   F

12. (LO 8.5) The top food sources of zinc include
    a. grapes.   **c.** shellfish.
    b. unleavened bread.   **d.** potato.

13. (LO 8.5) A deficiency of which mineral is a leading cause of mental retardation worldwide?
    a. iron   **b.** iodine   **c.** zinc   **d.** chromium

14. (LO 8.5) Which of these mineral supplements can easily cause accidental poisoning in children?
    a. iron   **b.** sodium   **c.** magnesium   **d.** potassium

15. (LO 8.5) The most abundant mineral in the body is iron.
    T   F

16. (LO 8.5) The Academy of Nutrition and Dietetics recommends fluoride-free water for the U.S. population.
    T   F

17. (LO 8.6) Dairy foods such as butter, cream, and cream cheese are good sources of calcium, whereas vegetables such as broccoli are poor sources.
    T   F

18. (LO 8.6) Children who don't drink milk often have lower bone density than than those who do.
    T   F

19. (LO 8.7) Trabecular bone readily gives up its minerals whenever blood calcium needs replenishing.
    T   F

20. (LO 8.7) Too little _____ in the diet is associated with osteoporosis.
    a. vitamin B$_{12}$ **c.** sodium
    b. protein   **d.** niacin

Answers to these Self Check questions are in Appendix G.

Osteoporosis: Can Lifestyle Choices Reduce the Risk?

LO 8.7   Discuss how osteoporosis develops and the actions that may help to prevent it.

Well over half of U.S. adults age 50 years and older have osteoporosis or are developing it (see Figure C8–1).[1]* Each year, 2 million people break a hip, leg, arm, hand, ankle, or other bone as a result of osteoporosis. Of these, hip fractures prove most serious. The break is rarely clean—the bone explodes into fragments that cannot be reassembled. Just removing the pieces is a struggle, and replacing them with an artificial joint requires major surgery. About a third die of complications within a year; many more will never walk or live independently again.[2] Both men and women are urged to do whatever they can to prevent fractures related to osteoporosis.

Dr. Donald Fawcett/Visuals Unlimited, Inc.

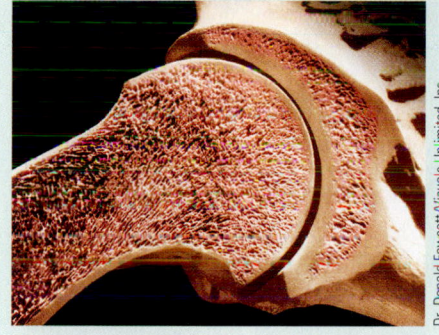

A sectioned bone.

Development of Osteoporosis

Fractures from osteoporosis occur during the later years, but osteoporosis itself develops silently much earlier. Younger adults are rarely aware of the strength sapping out of their bones until suddenly, 40 years later, a hip gives way. People say, "She fell and broke her hip," but in fact the hip may have been so fragile that it broke *before* she fell.

The causes of osteoporosis are tangled, and many are beyond a person's control. Insufficient dietary calcium, vitamin D, and physical activity certainly play roles, but age, gender, and genetics are also major players. No controversy exists as to the nature of osteoporosis; more controversial, however, are its causes and what people should do about it.

Bone Basics

To understand how the skeleton loses minerals in later years, you must first know a few things about bones. Table C8–1 offers definitions of relevant terms. The photograph on this page shows a human leg bone sliced lengthwise, exposing the lattice of calcium-containing crystals (the **trabecular bone**) inside that are part of the body's calcium bank. Invested as

savings during the milk-drinking years of youth, these deposits provide a nearly inexhaustible fund of calcium. **Cortical bone** is the dense, ivorylike bone that forms the exterior shell of a bone and the shaft of a long bone (look closely at the photograph). Both types of bone are crucial to overall bone strength. Cortical bone forms a sturdy outer wall, and trabecular bone provides strength along the lines of stress.

The two types of bone handle calcium in different ways. The lacy crystals of the trabecular bone are tapped to raise blood calcium when the supply from the day's diet runs short; the calcium crystals are redeposited in bone when dietary calcium is plentiful. The calcium of cortical bone fluctuates less.

Bone Loss

Trabecular bone, generously supplied with blood vessels, readily gives up its minerals at the necessary rate whenever blood calcium needs replenishing. Loss of trabecular bone begins to be significant for men and women around age 30. Calcium in cortical bone can also be withdrawn but more slowly.

Figure C8–1

Prevalence of Low Bone Density and Osteoporosis among People Age ≥50 Years (U.S.)

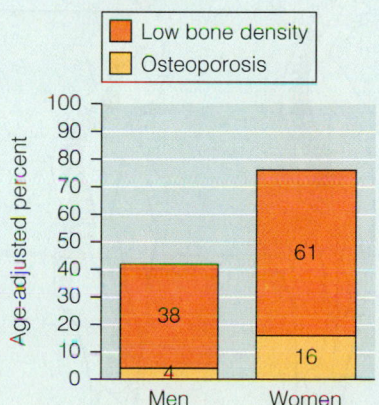

Source: A. C. Looker and coauthors, Osteoporosis or low bone mass at the femur neck or lumbar spine in older adults: United States, 2005–2008, National Center for Health Statistics data brief number 93 (2012), available at http://www.cdc.gov/nchs/data/databriefs/db93.htm#findings.

* *Reference notes are found in Appendix F.*

Table C8–1

Osteoporosis Terms

- **cortical bone** the ivorylike outer bone layer that forms a shell surrounding trabecular bone and that comprises the shaft of a long bone.
- **trabecular** (tra-BECK-you-lar) **bone** the weblike structure composed of calcium containing crystals inside a bone's solid outer shell. It provides strength and acts like a calcium storage bank.

Loss of Trabecular Bone

The healthy trabecular bone shown on the left appears thick and dense. The bone on the right is thin and weak, reflecting osteoporosis.

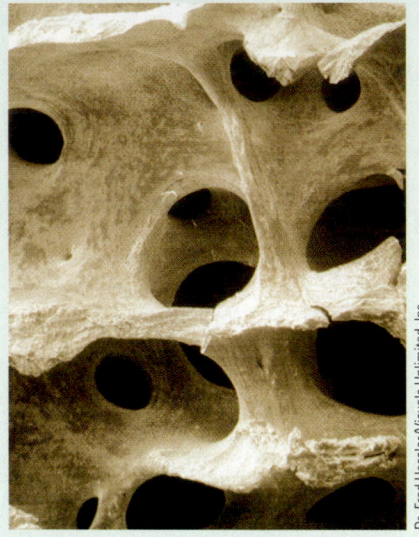

Dr. Fred Hossler/Visuals Unlimited, Inc.

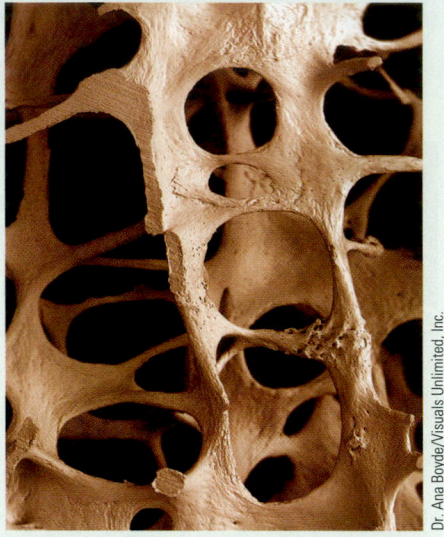

Dr. Ana Boyde/Visuals Unlimited, Inc.

As bone loss continues (Figure C8–2), bone density declines. Soon, osteoporosis sets in, and bones become so fragile that the body's weight can overburden the spine. Vertebrae may suddenly disintegrate and crush down, painfully pinching major nerves. Or they may compress into wedges, forming what is insensitively called "dowager's hump," the bent posture of many older men and women as they "grow shorter" (see Figure C8–3). Wrists may break as trabecula-rich bone ends weaken, and teeth may loosen or fall out as the trabecular bone of the jaw recedes. As the cortical bone shell weakens as well, breaks often occur in the hip.

Nondiet Factors That Affect Bone Health

Bones are affected by many factors. The following sections touch on some of them.

Bone Density and the Genes

A strong genetic component contributes to osteoporosis, bone density, and increased risk of fractures.[3] Genes exert influence over:

- The activities of bone-forming cells and bone-dismantling cells;

- The cellular mechanisms that make collagen, a structural bone protein;

- The mechanisms for absorbing and employing vitamin D; and

- Many other contributors to bone metabolism.

In addition to genes themselves, nutrients that influence gene activity are under study for their effects on bone density.[4] Genes set a tendency for strong or weak bones, but diet and other lifestyle choices influence the final outcome, and anyone with risk factors for osteoporosis should take actions to prevent it.[5]

Gender

Gender is a powerful predictor of osteoporosis: men have greater bone density than women at maturity, and women often lose more bone, particularly in the 6 to 8 years following menopause when the hormone estrogen diminishes.[6] Thereafter, loss of bone minerals continues throughout the remainder of a woman's lifetime but not at the free-fall pace of the

menopause years (refer again to Figure C8–3). If young women fail to produce enough estrogen, they lose bone rapidly, too, and going through menopause early almost doubles a woman's chance of developing osteoporosis.[7]

Each year, hundreds of thousands of men suffer fractures from osteoporosis.[8] Sex hormones, such as testosterone and the small amount of estrogen made by the male body, help to oppose men's osteoporosis.[9] Testosterone replacement therapy can help minimize bone

Loss of Height in a Woman with Osteoporosis

The woman on the left is about 50 years old. On the right, she is 80 years old. Her legs have not grown shorter; only her back has lost length, due to collapse of her spinal bones (vertebrae). When collapsed vertebrae cannot protect the spinal nerves, the pressure of bones pinching the nerves causes excruciating pain.

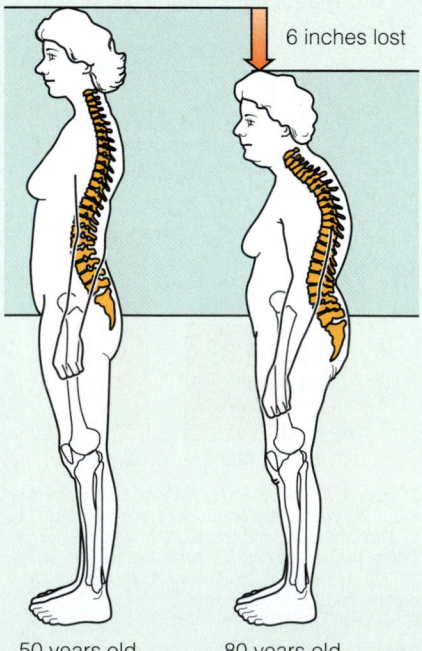

6 inches lost

50 years old   80 years old

loss in men with decreased hormone production.[10]

Body Weight

After age and gender, the next risk factor for osteoporosis is being underweight or losing weight. Women who are thin throughout life or who lose 10 percent or more of their body weight after menopause face a doubled hip fracture rate. Conversely, researchers are exploring whether excess body fatness with fatty intrusion in bone marrow may have negative effects on bone health.[11]

Physical Activity

Physical activity supports bone growth during adolescence, particularly when calcium intake is adequate, and may protect the bones later on.[12] Stronger muscles create denser, stronger bones by stressing, reshaping, and strengthening them.[13] When people lie idle—for example, when they are confined to bed—the bones lose strength just as the muscles do. The harm to the bones from a sedentary lifestyle equals the harm from nutrient deficiencies or cigarette smoking (Table C8–2).

Preventing falls is a critical focus for fracture prevention in the elderly. The best exercise to keep bones and muscles healthy, and subsequently to prevent falls, is the weight-bearing kind, such as jogging, doing jumping jacks, jumping rope, walking vigorously, or doing resistance (weight) training on most days throughout life.[14]

Tobacco Smoke and Alcohol

Smoking is hard on the bones. The bones of smokers are less dense than those of nonsmokers. Smoking also increases the risk of fractures and slows fracture healing.[15] Fortunately, quitting can reverse much of the damage. With time, the bone density of former smokers approaches that of nonsmokers.

Alcoholism is a major cause of osteoporosis in men, but some evidence suggests that menopausal women who drink moderately may have higher bone density than nondrinkers.[16] Heavy drinkers and people who regularly binge drink often have lower bone mineral density and experience more fractures than do nondrinkers and light drinkers.[17]

How Do Nutrients Affect Bone Health?

Nutrients affect bone health in sometimes surprising ways. For example, students of nutrition know that vitamin D and calcium benefit the bones but may not suspect that excess sodium can act to their detriment.

Calcium and Vitamin D

Bone strength later in life depends most on how well the bones were built during childhood and adolescence. Preteen children who consume enough calcium and vitamin D lay more calcium into the structure of their bones than children with less adequate intakes. Unfortunately, most girls in their bone-building years fail to meet their calcium needs. Children who do not consume milk do not meet their calcium needs unless they use calcium-fortified foods or supplements.

When people reach the bone-losing years of middle age, those who formed dense bones during youth have more bone tissue to lose before suffering ill effects—see Figure C8–4, p. 338. Building strong bones in youth helps prevent or delay osteoporosis later on.

Dietary calcium and vitamin D in later life cannot make up for earlier deficiencies, but they may help to slow the rate of bone loss. Additionally, calcium absorption declines with age, and older bodies become less efficient at making and activating vitamin D. In the elderly, low vitamin D status is associated with muscle weakness, and evidence suggests that taking supplemental vitamin D in the DRI recommended amount may help to prevent dangerous falls.[18]

Protein

When elderly people take in too little protein, their bones suffer.[19] Recall that the mineral crystals of bone form on a protein matrix—collagen. Restoring protein sources to the diet can often improve bone status and reduce the incidence of hip fractures even in the elderly. However, a diet lacking protein no doubt also lacks energy and other critical bone nutrients, so restoring a nutritious diet may be of highest importance.

An opposite possibility, that a *high*-protein diet causes bone loss,

Table C8–2
Risk Factors for Osteoporosis

Nonmodifiable	Modifiable
▪ Female gender	▪ Sedentary lifestyle
▪ Older age	▪ Diet inadequate in calcium and vitamin D
▪ Small frame	▪ Diet excessive in protein, sodium, caffeine
▪ Caucasian, Asian, or Hispanic/Latino heritage	▪ Cigarette smoking
▪ Family history of osteoporosis or fractures	▪ Alcohol abuse
▪ Personal history of fractures	▪ Low body weight
▪ Estrogen deficiency in women (lack of menstruation or menopause, especially early or surgically induced); testosterone deficiency in men	▪ Certain medications, such as glucocorticoids and anticonvulsants
	▪ Diet low in fruits and vegetables

Woman A entered adulthood with enough calcium in her bones to last a lifetime. Woman B had less bone mass starting out and so suffered ill effects from bone loss later on.

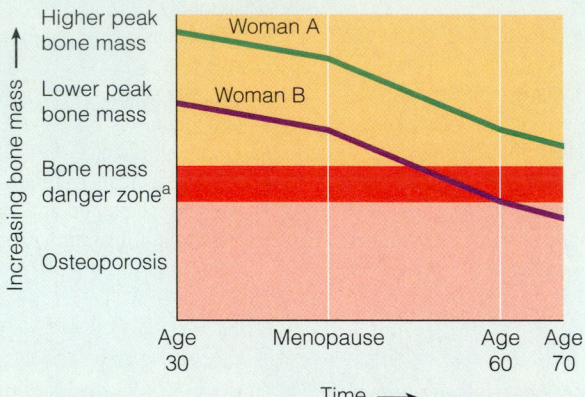

[a]People with a moderate degree of bone mass reduction are said to have osteopenia and are at increased risk of fractures.

Source: Data from Standing Committee on the Scientific Evaluation of Dietary Reference Intakes, Food and Nutrition Board, Institute of Medicine, Dietary Reference Intakes for Calcium, Phosphorus, Magnesium, Vitamin D, and Fluoride (Washington, D.C.: National Academies Press, 2006).

has also been explored, but study results are inconsistent.[20] Excess dietary protein causes urinary calcium losses, but a diet also high in fruits and vegetables may oppose this effect, producing no net calcium loss from bone.[21]

Milk provides protein along with vitamin A, vitamin D, and calcium, all important nutrients for bone tissue. As might be expected, vegans, who do not consume milk products, generally have lower bone mineral density than people who do consume them.[22] Protein-rich soy foods and beverages may help to oppose bone loss, and some research suggests that soy isoflavones may support bone health by improving intestinal calcium absorption.[23]

Sodium and Soft Drinks

A high sodium intake is associated with urinary calcium excretion, and lowering sodium intakes seems to lessen calcium losses.[24] In study subjects eating the DASH diet, a controlled sodium diet that provides all of the foods in the USDA

Eating Patterns, urinary calcium losses are reduced. In addition, the DASH diet is higher in calcium than most diets, a critical feature that stands against bone loss. The mechanism behind

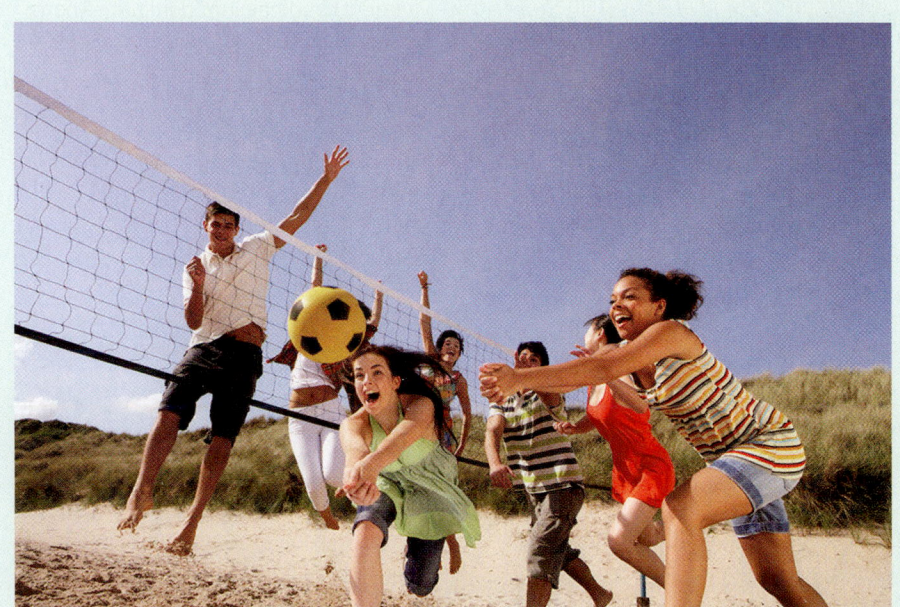

These young people are putting bone in the bank.

sodium's effects on the bones is under investigation.[25]

Cola beverages and processed foods may theoretically speed the dismantling of the bones by way of providing excess phosphorus from phosphoric acid, caffeine, and other additives, but research is inconsistent.[26] However, all soft drinks displace milk from the diet, particularly in children and adolescents.

Other Nutrients Important to Bones

Vitamin K plays roles in the production of at least one bone protein important in bone maintenance. People with hip fractures often have low intakes of vitamin K–rich vegetables, and increasing vegetable intakes may improve both vitamin K status and skeletal health.[27]

Sufficient vitamin A is needed in the bone-remodeling process, and vitamin C maintains bone collagen. Magnesium may help to maintain bone mineral density.[28] Omega-3 fatty acids may also help preserve bone integrity, and their effects are under study.[29] Clearly, a well-balanced diet that supplies a variety of abundant fruit, vegetables, protein foods, and whole grains along with a full array of nutrients is central to bone health.

The more risk factors of Table C8–2 (p. 337) that apply to you, the greater your chances of developing osteoporosis in the future, and the more seriously you should take the advice offered in this Controversy. Treatment, while continuously advancing, remains far from perfect.

Diagnosis and Medical Treatment

Diagnosis of osteoporosis includes measuring bone density using an advanced form of X-ray (DEXA; see the nearby photo) or ultrasound.[30] Men with osteoporosis risk factors and all women should have a bone density test after age 50. A thorough examination also includes factors such as race, family history, and physical activity level.

Several drug therapies can reverse bone loss.[31] Some inhibit the activities of the bone-dismantling cells, allowing the bone-building cells to slowly reinforce the bone tissue. Others stimulate the bone-building cells, resulting in greater bone formation. In some people, such drugs have worked minor miracles in reversing even severe bone loss, but for many others, they are ineffective, or their side effects prove damaging or intolerable.[32] Estrogen replacement therapy can help nonmenstruating women prevent further bone loss, but questions about safety limit its use. Slow-release forms of fluoride may also increase bone density, but in levels not far above therapeutic thresholds, fluoride poses the serious threat of skeletal fluorosis that weakens the bones.[33]

Calcium Intakes

Adequate calcium nutrition is essential for achieving and maintaining optimal bone mass. Yet many U.S. children and adults fail to take in adequate amounts of calcium.[34]

How should you obtain daily calcium? Nutritionists strongly recommend the foods and beverages of the USDA eating patterns (see Chapter 2); they reserve supplements for those who cannot meet their needs from foods and beverages. People can do more to support the health of their bones, too, by following the strategies in Figure C8–5, p. 340.

Bone loss is not a calcium-deficiency disease comparable to iron-deficiency anemia, in which iron intake reliably reverses the condition. Calcium alone cannot reverse bone loss. For those who are unable to consume enough calcium-rich foods, however, taking calcium supplements with vitamin D can supply these nutrients.[35]

Taking self-prescribed calcium supplements entails a few risks (see Table C8–3, p. 341) and cannot take the place of sound food choices and other healthy habits. One potential threat, a reported link between calcium supplements and heart attacks, is under review.[36] Recently, the U.S. Preventive Services Task Force found insufficient evidence concerning the safety and effectiveness of many calcium and vitamin D supplements to recommend them for preventing bone fractures.[37] Still, millions of people take calcium supplements daily, and the next section provides some details about the variety on the market.

Calcium Supplements

Calcium supplements are often sold as **calcium compounds**—such as calcium carbonate (as in some **antacids**), citrate, gluconate, lactate, malate, or phosphate—and compounds of calcium with amino acids (called **amino acid chelates**). Others are powdered, calcium-rich materials such as **bone meal**, **powdered bone**, **oyster shell**, or **dolomite** (limestone). See Table C8–4 (p. 342) for supplement terms. In choosing a type, consider the answers to the following questions.

Question 1. How much calcium is safe? Although recent evidence suggests that doses of up to 1,000 milligrams present some risks, the DRI committee recommends that habitual calcium intakes from foods and supplements combined should not exceed the Tolerable Upper Intake Level (2,000 to 3,000 milligrams for adults; see the inside front cover, page C).[38] Meeting the need for calcium is important, but more calcium than this provides no additional benefits and may increase risks.[39] Most supplements contain between 250 and 1,000 milligrams of calcium, as stated on the label.

Question 2. How digestible is the supplement? The body cannot use the calcium in a supplement unless the

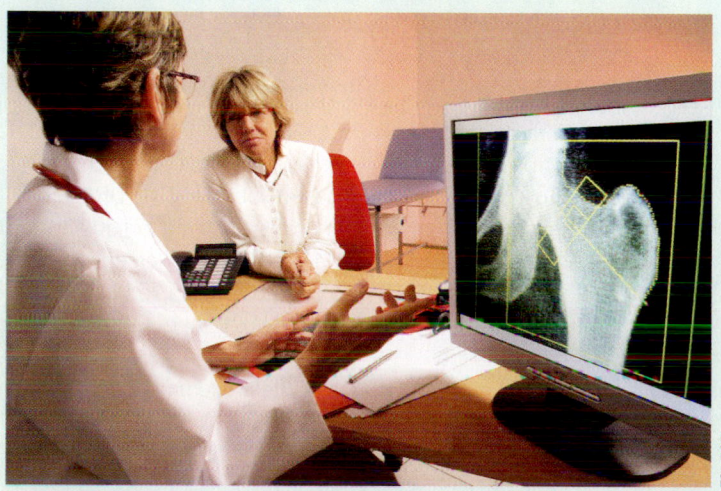

A DEXA scan measures bone density to help detect the early stages of bone loss, assess fracture risks, and measure the responses to bone-building treatments. (DEXA stands for dual-energy X-ray absorptiometry.)

The periods of greatest gains in bone density are childhood and adolescence.

Mature Adult
51 years and above

Goal: Minimize bone loss.
Plan:
• Continue as for 13- to 30-year-olds.
• Continue striving to meet the calcium need from diet.
• Continue bone-strengthening exercises.
• Obtain a bone density test; follow physician's advice concerning bone-restoring medications and supplements.

Mature Adult
31 through 50 years

Goal: Maximize bone retention.
Plan:
• Continue as for 13- to 30-year-olds.
• Adopt bone-strengthening exercises.
• Obtain the recommended amount of calcium from food.
• Take calcium supplements only if calcium needs cannot be met through foods.

Adolescence through Young Adulthood
13 through 30 years

Goal: Achieve peak bone mass.
Plan:
• Choose milk as the primary beverage; if milk causes distress, include other calcium sources.
• Commit to a lifelong program of physical activity.
• Do not smoke tobacco or drink alcohol—if you have started, quit.

Children
2 through 12 years

Goal: Grow strong bones.
Plan:
• Use milk as the primary beverage to meet the need for calcium within a balanced diet that provides all nutrients.
• Play actively in sports or other activities.
• Limit television and other sedentary entertainment.
• Do not start smoking tobacco or drinking alcohol.

Note: *The exact ages of cessation of bone accretion and onset of loss vary among people, but in general, data indicate that the skeleton continues to accrete mass for approximately 10 years after adult height is achieved and begins to lose bone around age 35.*

tablet disintegrates in the digestive tract. Manufacturers compress large quantities of calcium into small pills, which the stomach acid must penetrate. To test a supplement, drop a pill into 6 ounces of vinegar, and stir occasionally. A digestible pill will dissolve within half an hour.

Question 3. How absorbable is the form of calcium in the supplement? Most healthy people absorb calcium equally well from milk and from calcium carbonate, calcium citrate, and calcium phosphate. To improve absorption, divide your dose in half and take it twice a day instead of all at once.

One last pitch: think one more time before you decide to take supplements instead of including calcium-rich foods in your diet. The DRI committee points out that, particularly among older women, supplements can and do push some people's intakes beyond the Tolerable Upper Intake Level.[40] The Dietary Guidelines for Americans 2015 committee recommends milk and milk products or calcium- and vitamin D–fortified soy milk for bone health.[41] The authors of this book are so impressed with the importance of using abundant, calcium-rich foods that we have worked out ways to do so at every meal.

Critical Thinking

1. Osteoporosis occurs during the late years of life; however, it is a disease that develops while one is young. Compose a plan outlining what you can do now to prevent bone loss later in life.

2. Outline the foods you will eat (including quantities) that will provide the recommended RDA for calcium. List lifestyle factors that you can follow to boost your bone density.

Table C8–3

Calcium Supplementation: Point, Counterpoint

Some medical conditions warrant taking calcium supplements, and people with those conditions should follow the recommendations of a physician. Most people, however, are on their own to weigh the pros and cons of calcium supplements; this table presents some of the issues.

Arguments in Support of Calcium Supplementation	Arguments Against Calcium Supplementation
1. *Calcium adequacy.* Most people do not consume adequate amounts of calcium from foods alone. Calcium-fortified foods and supplements can effectively make up the shortfall.	1. *Excess blood calcium.* Rare reports exist of dangerously high blood calcium levels from a drug interaction with a calcium supplement, or very high doses of calcium (at least four times the customary dose).
2. *Bone maintenance.* People with inadequate calcium intakes extract calcium from the bones to maintain normal blood calcium levels and meet metabolic needs. Calcium supplements can provide an alternate source.	2. *Impairment of mineral absorption.* Calcium supplements, particularly in large doses, can inhibit absorption of iron, magnesium, phosphorus, and zinc, minerals that are also critical to health.
3. *Often prescribed.* Physicians and other health care providers often prescribe calcium and vitamin D supplements for the purpose of preventing osteoporosis and bone fractures.	3. *Missing evidence.* The U.S. Preventive Services Task Force concludes that current evidence is insufficient to weigh the benefits and harms from supplements of ≥1,000 milligrams of calcium and ≥400 IU of vitamin D. Supplements of less than these amounts have no benefit for the primary prevention of fractures.
4. *Vitamin D source.* Vitamin D plays a critical role in regulating intestinal calcium absorption.	4. *Contaminants and toxicity.* Some preparations of bone meal and dolomites are contaminated with hazardous amounts of arsenic, cadmium, mercury, and lead. Excessive vitamin D can also be toxic.
5. *Treatment of malabsorption.* People with poor nutrient absorption, such as those with inflammatory bowel disease or those who have undergone gastric bypass surgery to treat obesity, may need calcium supplements to avoid deficiency.	5. *Digestive distress.* Common side effects of calcium supplements are constipation, intestinal bloating, and excess gas, symptoms also characteristic of malabsorption syndromes and bypass surgeries.
6. *Treatment of kidney disease.* People with chronic kidney disease often have altered mineral metabolism with low serum calcium and weak bones. Calcium supplements may help to minimize bone damage.	6. *Risk of kidney stones.* Daily calcium supplements increase the incidence of kidney stones.
7. *Cardiovascular health.* Some evidence suggests a benefit to the heart from diets that are adequate in calcium and vitamin D.	7. *Cardiovascular threat.* The safety of calcium supplements for the heart cannot be definitively stated. Early studies revealed increased heart problems among female supplement takers, but randomized controlled trials are lacking to confirm this finding and some studies refute it.

Sources: U.S. Department of Agriculture and U.S. Department of Health and Human Services, Scientific report of the 2015 Dietary Guidelines Advisory Committee, 2015, D-1:15, available at www.health.gov; D. Challoumas and coauthors, Effects of combined vitamin D-calcium supplements on the cardiovascular system: Should we be cautious? Atherosclerosis 238 (2015): 388–398; A. L. Schafer and coauthors, Intestinal calcium absorption decreases dramatically after gastric bypass surgery despite optimization of vitamin D status, Journal of Bone and Mineral Research 30 (2015): 1377–85; S.; A. Shapses, No vitamin D threshold for calcium absorption: Why does this matter?, American Journal of Clinical Nutrition 99 (2014): 429–430; I. R. Reid, Should we prescribe calcium supplements for osteoporosis prevention?, Journal of Bone Metabolism 21 (2014): 21–28; V. A. Moyer and the U.S. Preventive Services Task Force, Vitamin D and calcium supplementation to prevent fractures in adults: U.S. Preventive Services Task Force recommendation statement, Annals of Internal Medicine 158 (2013): 691–696; M. J. Bolland, A. Grey, and I. R. Reid, Calcium supplements and cardiovascular risk: 5 years on, Therapeutic Advances in Drug Safety 4 (2013): 19–210; R. L. Prentice and coauthors, Health risks and benefits from calcium and vitamin D supplementation: Women's Health Initiative clinical trial and cohort study, Osteoporosis International 24 (2013): 567–580; U.S. Department of Health and Human Services, National Institute of Diabetes and Digestive and Kidney Diseases, Chronic kidney disease—Mineral and bone disorder, 2013, available at: www.medscape.com/viewarticle/770604; A. Singh and A. Ashraf, Hypercalcemic crisis induced by calcium carbonate, Clinical Kidney Journal 5 (2012): 288–291; J. C. Gallagher, V. Yalamanchili, and L. M. Smith, The effect of vitamin D on calcium absorption in older women, Journal of Clinical Endocrinology and Metabolism 97 (2012): 3550–3556; C. Hwang, V. Ross, and U. Mahadevan, Micronutrient deficiencies in inflammatory bowel disease: From A to zinc, Inflammatory Bowel Diseases 18 (2012): 1961–1981.

- **amino acid chelates** (KEY-lates) compounds of minerals (such as calcium) combined with amino acids in a form that favors their absorption. A chelating agent is a molecule that surrounds another molecule and can then either promote or prevent its movement from place to place (chele means "claw").
- **antacids** acid-buffering agents used to counter excess acidity in the stomach. Calcium-containing preparations (such as Tums) contain available calcium. Antacids with aluminum or magnesium hydroxides (such as Rolaids) can accelerate calcium losses.
- **bone meal** or **powdered bone** crushed or ground bone preparations intended to supply calcium to the diet. Calcium from bone is not well absorbed and is often contaminated with toxic materials such as arsenic, mercury, lead, and cadmium.
- **calcium compounds** the simplest forms of purified calcium. They include calcium carbonate, citrate, gluconate, hydroxide, lactate, malate, and phosphate. These supplements vary in the amount of calcium they contain, so read the labels carefully. A 500-milligram tablet of calcium gluconate may provide only 45 milligrams of calcium, for example.
- **dolomite** a compound of minerals (calcium magnesium carbonate) found in limestone and marble. Dolomite is powdered and is sold as a calcium-magnesium supplement but may be contaminated with toxic minerals, is not well absorbed, and interacts adversely with absorption of other essential minerals.
- **oyster shell** a product made from the powdered shells of oysters that is sold as a calcium supplement but is not well absorbed by the digestive system.

9 Energy Balance and Healthy Body Weight

paintings/Shutterstock.com

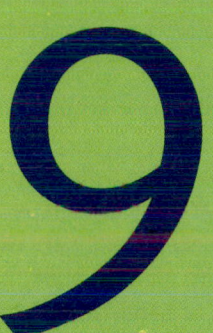

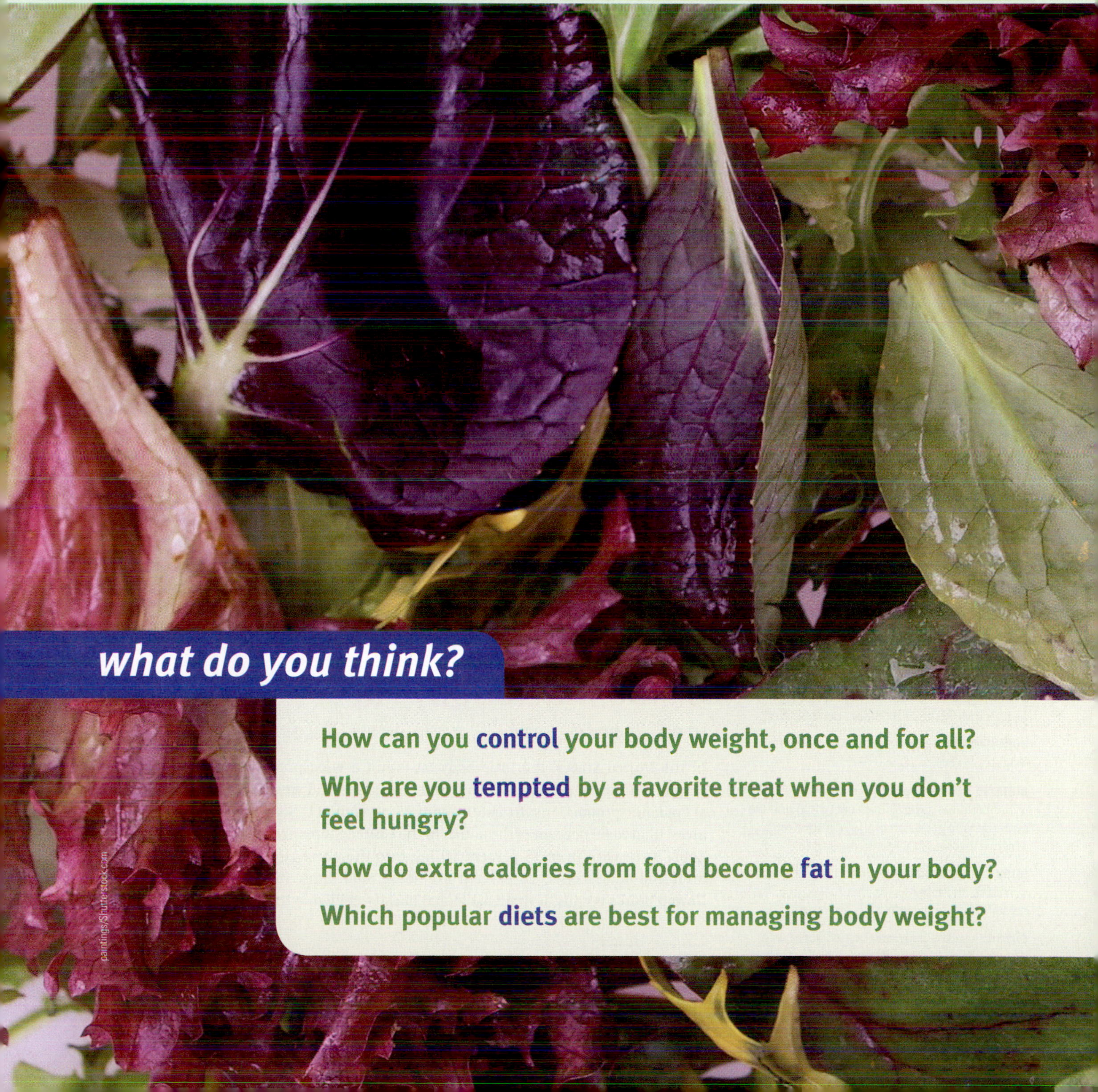

what do you think?

How can you **control** your body weight, once and for all?

Why are you **tempted** by a favorite treat when you don't feel hungry?

How do extra calories from food become **fat** in your body?

Which popular **diets** are best for managing body weight?

Learning Objectives

After completing this chapter, you should be able to accomplish the following:

LO 9.1 Outline the health risks of deficient and excessive body fatness.

LO 9.2 Explain the concept of energy balance and the factors associated with it.

LO 9.3 Contrast body weight to body fatness.

LO 9.4 Identify factors that contribute to increased appetite and decreased appetite.

LO 9.5 Summarize the inside-the-body theories of obesity.

LO 9.6 Summarize the outside-the-body theories of obesity.

LO 9.7 Describe metabolic events that occur in energy deficit and surplus.

LO 9.8 Summarize the measures that help in achieving and maintaining a healthy body weight.

LO 9.9 Explain the potential benefits and risks associated with obesity medications and surgeries.

LO 9.10 Justify the importance of behavior modification in supporting changes in diet and exercise.

LO 9.11 Outline the risk factors, symptoms, and treatments of eating disorders.

Are you pleased with your body weight? If you answered yes, you are a rare individual. Nearly all people in our society think they should weigh more or less (mostly less) than they do. Their primary concern is usually appearance, but they often perceive, correctly, that physical health is somehow related to weight. Both **overweight** and **underweight** present risks to health and life.

People also think of their weight as something they should control, once and for all. Three misconceptions in their thinking frustrate their efforts, however—the focus on weight, the focus on *controlling* weight, and the focus on a short-term endeavor. Simply put, it isn't your weight you need to control; it's the fat, or **adipose tissue**, in your body in proportion to the lean—your **body composition**. And controlling body composition directly isn't possible—you can control only your *behaviors*. Sporadic bursts of activity, such as "dieting," are not effective; the behaviors that achieve and maintain a healthy body weight take a lifetime of commitment. Luckily, with time, these behaviors become second nature.

This chapter starts by presenting problems associated with deficient and excessive body fatness and then examines how the body manages its energy budget. The following sections show how to judge body weight on the sound basis of health. The chapter then explores some theories about causes of **obesity** and reveals how the body gains and loses weight. It goes on to present science-based lifestyle strategies for achieving and maintaining a healthy body weight, and it closes with a Controversy section on eating disorders.

The Problems of Too Little or Too Much Body Fat

LO 9.1 Outline the health risks of deficient and excessive body fatness.

In the United States, too little body fat is not a widespread problem. In contrast, despite a national preoccupation with body image and weight loss, obesity remains at epidemic proportions. In 1960, about 13 percent of U.S. adults were obese. Today, an estimated 69 percent of the adults in the United States are overweight or obese (see Table 9–1), with over 35 percent falling into the obese range.[1][*][†] Even among children and adolescents, 18 percent are obese, and many more are overweight. The United States is caught in a vast global obesity epidemic that is harming the health

overweight body weight above a healthy weight; BMI 25 to 29.9 (BMI is defined later).

underweight body weight below a healthy weight; BMI below 18.5.

adipose tissue the body's fat tissue. Adipose tissue performs several functions, including the synthesis and secretion of the hormone leptin, which is involved in appetite regulation.

body composition the proportions of muscle, bone, fat, and other tissue that make up a person's total body weight.

obesity excess body weight associated with increased risk of mortality and chronic diseases; a body mass index of 30 or higher.

---

*Reference notes are found in Appendix F.

†Defined as more than 100 pounds overweight.

Table 9–1	
Prevalence of Underweight, Overweight, and Obesity, U.S. Adults	
Underweight (BMI < 18.5)	1.7%
Overweight (BMI ≥ 25–30)	33.9%
Obese (BMI ≥ 30)	35.1%
Extremely obese (BMI ≥ 40)[a]	6.4%

[a] "Extremely obese" is a subcategory of "Obese."

Data from Centers for Disease Control and Prevention, Obesity and overweight, FastStats, 2015, available at www.cdc.gov/nchs/fastats/obesity-overweight.htm; C. D. Fryar, M. D. Carroll, and C. L. Ogden, Prevalence of overweight, obesity, and extreme obesity among adults: United States, 1960–1962 through 2011–2012, NCHS Health-E Stats, 2014, available at www.cdc.gov; C. D. Fryar and coauthors, Prevalence of underweight among adults aged 20 and over: United States, 1960–1962 through 2009–2010, NCHS Health-E Stats, 2014, available at www.cdc.gov.

Figure 9–1

Increasing Prevalence of Obesity

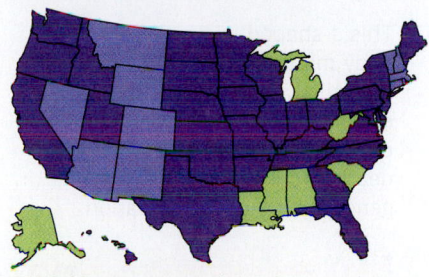

1998: Most states had obesity prevalence rates of less than 20%.

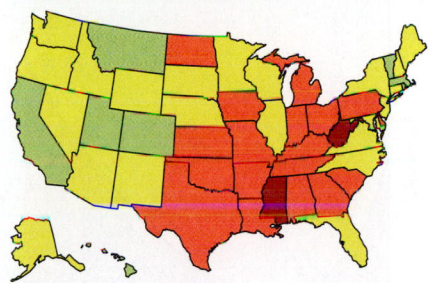

2013: All states had obesity prevalence rates of greater than 20%, with almost half reporting prevalence rates of at least 30%.

Key:

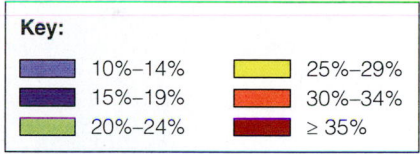

10%–14%	25%–29%
15%–19%	30%–34%
20%–24%	≥ 35%

Source: www.cdc.gov/obesity/data/prevalence-maps.html.

of people of all ages, in urban and rural areas alike (Figure 9–1).[2] Nevertheless, efforts to curb the obesity epidemic may be paying off, especially among low-income children, women, and girls; their obesity rates may be slowing.[3] Among men and boys, however, the rates are still accelerating, and more people fall into the severely obese category than ever before.

Childhood obesity is the topic of **Controversy 13**.

The problem of *underweight*, while affecting fewer than 2 percent of adults in the United States, also poses health threats to those who drop below a healthy minimum.[4] People at either extreme of body weight face increased risks.

What Are the Risks from Underweight?

Thin people die first during a siege or in a famine. Overly thin people are also at a disadvantage in the hospital, where their nutrient status can easily deteriorate if they have to go without food for days at a time while undergoing tests or surgery. Underweight also increases the risk of death for surgical patients and for anyone fighting a **wasting** disease.[5] People with cancer often die not from the cancer itself but from starvation. Thus, excessively underweight people are urged to gain body fat as an energy reserve and to acquire protective amounts of all the nutrients that can be stored.

KEY POINT

- Deficient body fatness threatens survival during a famine or when a person must fight a disease.

What Are the Risks from Too Much Body Fat?

If tomorrow's headlines read, "Obesity Conquered! U.S. Population Loses Excess Fat!" tens of millions of people would be freed from the misery of obesity-related illnesses—heart disease, diabetes, certain cancers, and many others. In just one year, over 100,000 lives could be saved, along with the estimated $147 billion spent on obesity-related health care.[6] Increased productivity at work would pump tens of billions of new dollars into the national economy.

Chronic Diseases   To underestimate the threat from obesity is to invite personal calamity. Figure 9–2 demonstrates that the risk of dying increases proportionally with increasing body weight.[7] With **extreme obesity**, the risk of dying equals that from smoking. Major obesity-related disease risks include:

- Arthritis.

- Breathing problems (sleep apnea).

- Cancers of the breast, colon, endometrium, and other cancers.

wasting the progressive, relentless loss of the body's tissues that accompanies certain diseases and shortens survival time.

extreme obesity clinically severe overweight, presenting very high risks to health; the condition of having a BMI of 40 or above; also called *morbid obesity*.

Figure 9–2

Underweight, Overweight, and Mortality

This J-shaped curve associates body mass index (BMI) with mortality. It shows that both underweight and overweight present risks of a premature death. Note that a BMI of 15 generally indicates starvation.

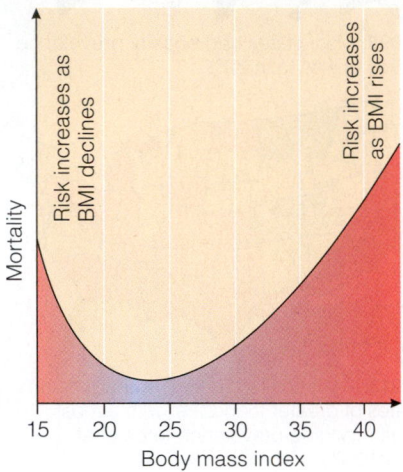

- Diabetes.
- Heart disease.
- Hypertension (high blood pressure).
- Gallbladder disease and gall stones.
- Nonalcoholic fatty liver disease.
- Stroke.[8]

Over 70 percent of obese people suffer from at least one other major health problem. For example, obesity triples a person's risk of developing diabetes, and even modest weight gain raises the risk. The mechanism linking obesity with diabetes is not fully known, but scientists suspect that a person's genetic inheritance may alter the likelihood that obesity will lead to the development of diabetes.[9]

Obesity and Inflammation   Why should fat in the body bring extra risk to the heart? Part of the answer may involve **adipokines**, hormones released by adipose tissue.[10] Adipokines help to regulate inflammatory processes and energy metabolism in the tissues. In fact, adipose tissue acts as an endocrine organ, orchestrating important interactions with vital tissues such as the brain, liver, muscle, heart, and blood vessels in ways that influence overall health.[11]

> Metabolic syndrome and chronic diseases are discussed more fully in **Chapter 11**.

In obesity, a shift occurs in the balance of adipokines, among other factors, that favors both tissue inflammation and insulin resistance. The resulting chronic inflammation and insulin resistance often lead to diabetes, heart disease, and other chronic diseases. Calorie-restricted diets and weight loss often reduce inflammation and improve health.[12]

Other Risks   Obese adults also may face these threats: abdominal hernias, complications in pregnancy and surgery, flat feet, gallbladder disease, gout, high blood lipids, kidney stones, increased risk of medication dosing errors, reproductive disorders, skin problems, sleep disturbances, sleep apnea (dangerous abnormal breathing during sleep), varicose veins, and even a high accident rate. Some of these maladies start to improve with the loss of just 5 percent of body weight, and risks improve markedly after a 10 percent loss. So great are the harms from obesity that obesity itself is classified as a chronic disease.

KEY POINTS

- Adipokines are hormones produced by adipose tissue.
- Obesity raises the risks of developing many chronic diseases and other illnesses.

What Are the Risks from Central Obesity?

Fat collected deep within the central abdominal area of the body, called **visceral fat**, results in **central obesity**, which poses greater risks of major chronic diseases than does excess fat lying just beneath the skin (**subcutaneous fat**) of the abdomen, thighs, hips, and legs (Figure 9–3).[13] In fact, central obesity elevates the risk of death from *all* causes. Excess visceral fat is associated with the **metabolic syndrome** that predicts heart disease. Currently, a measure of central obesity is among the indicators that physicians use to evaluate chronic disease risks.[14]

Men of all ages and women who are past menopause are more prone to develop the "apple" profile that characterizes central obesity, whereas women in their reproductive years typically develop more of a "pear" profile (fat around the hips and thighs that may cling most stubbornly during weight loss).[15] Some women change profiles at menopause, and life-long "pears" may suddenly face the increased disease risks associated with central obesity.

Two other factors also affect body fat distribution. Moderate to high intakes of alcohol associate directly with central obesity, whereas higher levels of physical activity

adipokines (AD-ih-poh-kynz) protein hormones made and released by adipose tissue (fat) cells.

visceral fat fat stored within the abdominal cavity in association with the internal abdominal organs; also called *intra-abdominal fat* or *visceral adipose tissue*.

central obesity excess fat in the abdomen and around the trunk.

subcutaneous fat fat stored directly under the skin (*sub* means "beneath"; *cutaneous* refers to the skin).

metabolic syndrome a combination of central obesity, diabetes or prediabetes, high blood glucose (insulin resistance), high blood pressure, and altered blood lipids that greatly increases the risk of heart disease. (Also defined in Chapter 11.)

Figure 9–3

Visceral Fat and Subcutaneous Fat

These abdominal cross sections of an overweight man (left) and woman (right) were produced by CT scans. The people are similar in age and abdominal measurements, but the man's girth is largely from visceral fat; the woman's excess fat is almost all subcutaneous.

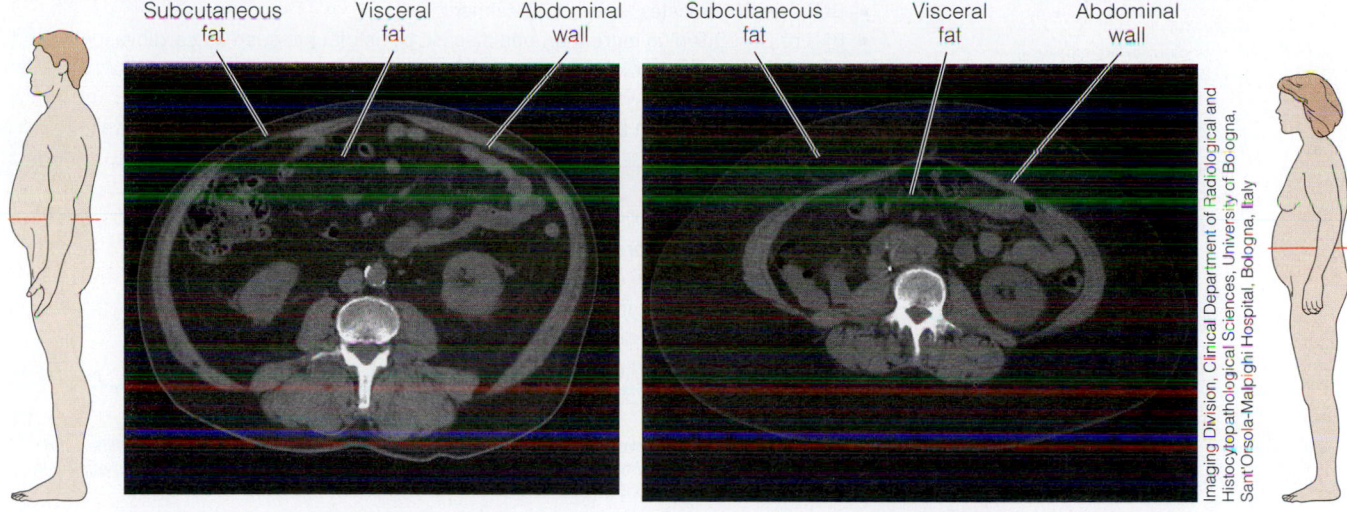

Male: BMI 29   Female: BMI 32

Imaging Division, Clinical Department of Radiological and Histocytopathological Sciences, University of Bologna, Sant'Orsola-Malpighi Hospital, Bologna, Italy

correlate with leanness.[16] A later section explains how to judge whether a person carries too much fat around the middle.

KEY POINT

- Central obesity is particularly hazardous to health.

How Fat Is Too Fat?

People want to know exactly how much body fat is too much. The answer is not the same for everyone, but scientists have developed guidelines.

Evaluating Risks from Body Fatness   Obesity experts commonly evaluate the health risks of obesity by way of three indicators (each is described more fully later on).[17] The first is a person's **body mass index (BMI)**, as indicated in Table 9–2 (p. 348). The BMI, which defines average relative weight for height in people older than 20 years, correlates significantly with body fatness and risk of death and diseases such as heart disease, stroke, diabetes, and nonalcoholic fatty liver disease. If you are wondering about your own BMI, find it on the inside back cover of this text.

The second indicator is **waist circumference**, reflecting the degree of central obesity in proportion to total body fat. People who are overweight or moderately obese often incur a greater risk of heart disease and mortality if their waist circumference exceeds 35 inches for women and 40 inches for men. With greater degrees of obesity (a BMI of 35 and above), waist circumference is less meaningful because health risks are already high.

The third indicator is the person's disease risk profile, which takes into account such factors as poor dietary habits, sedentary lifestyle, blood lipids, family history of obesity or heart disease, smoking, use of medications that affect body weight, and so forth. The more of these factors a person has and the greater the degree of obesity, the greater the urgency to control body fatness.

Why, then, do some obese people remain healthy and live long lives, while others die young of chronic diseases? It may be that those who stay healthy tend to store excess fat harmlessly in the adipose tissue layer beneath the skin, while those who

body mass index (BMI) an indicator of health risk from obesity or underweight, calculated by dividing the weight of a person by the square of the person's height.

waist circumference a measurement of abdominal girth that indicates visceral fatness.

Table 9–2

Indicators of an Urgent Need for Weight Loss

The greater the BMI and the more diseases and risk factors present, the greater the urgency to control body fatness.

BMI

- BMI over 30 indicates a need for treatment.
- BMI of 25–29.9 plus more than one disease or risk factor, such as cardiovascular disease, diabetes, or high blood pressure (see below) indicates a need for treatment.
- BMI of up to 29.9 with no other risk factors indicates a need to stop gaining weight.

Waist Circumference

- Greater than 35 inches for women and 40 inches for men

Diseases and Risk Factors

- Cardiovascular disease (CVD)
- Blood lipid profile that indicates CVD risk
- Type 2 diabetes or prediabetes
- Impaired glucose tolerance
- Hypertension or prehypertension (see Chapter 11)

Source: American College of Cardiology/American Heart Association Task Force on Practice Guidelines and the Obesity Society, Executive summary: Guidelines (2013) for the management of overweight and obesity in adults, Obesity 22 (2014): S5–S39.

develop metabolic problems also deposit excess fat in the liver and other critical tissues.[18] Genetic inheritance, smoking habits, and level of physical activity may also help to explain why some such individuals stay well, while others fall ill. Overall, even seemingly healthy overweight people may be more likely to develop chronic illnesses than those in the healthy BMI range.[19]

Social and Economic Costs of Body Fatness   Although a few overfat people escape health problems, no one who is fat in our society quite escapes the social and economic handicaps. Our society places enormous value on thinness, especially for women, and fat people are less sought after for romance, less often hired, and less often admitted to college.[20] They pay higher insurance premiums, they pay more for clothing, and they even pay more in gasoline costs—a car transporting extra weight uses more fuel per mile. Is it any wonder that overweight people are spending $60 billion each year in attempts to lose weight?

Prejudice defines people by their appearance rather than by their ability and character. Obese people suffer emotional pain when others treat them with insensitivity, hostility, and contempt, and they may internalize a sense of guilt and self-deprecation. Health-care professionals, even dietitians, can be among the offenders without realizing it. Society's barrage of negativity can injure the overweight person's self-image in ways that may contribute to more weight gain and obesity or to the development of an eating disorder (see the Controversy section).[21] To free our society of its obsession with body fatness and its prejudice against overweight people, activists are promoting respect for individuals of all body weights.

KEY POINTS

- BMI values mathematically correlate heights and weights with health risks.
- Health risks from obesity are reflected in BMI, waist circumference, and a disease risk profile.
- Some overweight people may remain healthy, but the reasons why are unclear.
- Overweight people face social and economic handicaps and prejudice.

The Body's Energy Balance

LO 9.2 Explain the concept of energy balance and the factors associated with it.

What happens inside the body when you eat too much or too little food? The body ends up with an unbalanced energy budget—you have taken in more or less food energy than you spent over time. The body's energy budget works somewhat like a cash budget that grows and dwindles in proportion to the flow of currency. When more food energy is consumed than is needed over days or weeks, excess fat accumulates in the fat cells in the body's adipose tissue, where it is stored. When energy supplies run low, stored fat is withdrawn. The daily energy balance can therefore be stated like this:

- Change in energy stores equals food energy taken in minus energy spent on metabolism and muscle activities.

More simply,

- Change in energy stores = energy in − energy out.

Too much or too little fat on the body today does not necessarily reflect today's energy budget.[22] Small imbalances in the energy budget compound over time.

Energy In and Energy Out

The energy in foods and beverages is the only contributor to the "energy in" side of the energy balance equation. Before you can decide how much food will supply the energy you need in a day, you must first become familiar with the amounts of energy in foods and beverages. You can do this by looking up calorie amounts associated with foods and beverages in the Table of Food Composition (Appendix A) or by using a computer program. Such numbers are always fascinating to people concerned with managing body fatness. For example, an apple gives you 70 calories from carbohydrate; a regular-size candy bar gives you about 250 calories, mostly from fat and carbohydrate.

On the "energy out" side of the equation, no easy method exists for determining the energy an individual spends and therefore needs. You may have heard that for each 3,500 calories you expend in activity or eliminate from the diet, you lose one pound of body fat—a formula long used to predict weight loss. However, a single number cannot accurately predict weight change in every individual because energy dynamics vary, both between individuals and within a single person at different phases of weight change.[23] Estimating an individual person's need requires knowing something about the person's lifestyle and metabolism.

KEY POINTS

- The "energy in" side of the body's energy budget is measured in calories taken in each day in the form of foods and beverages.
- No easy method exists for determining the "energy out" side of a person's energy balance equation.

How Many Calories Do I Need Each Day?

Simply put, you need to take in enough calories to cover your energy expenditure each day—your energy budget must balance. One way to estimate your energy need is to monitor your food intake and body weight over a period of time in which your activities are typical and are sufficient to maintain your health. If you keep an accurate record of all the foods and beverages you consume and if your weight is in a healthy range and has not changed during the past few months, you can conclude that your energy budget is balanced. Your average daily calorie intake is sufficient to meet your daily output—your need therefore is the same as your current intake.[24] At least 3, and preferably 7, days, including a weekend day, of honest record-keeping are necessary because intakes and activities fluctuate from day to day.

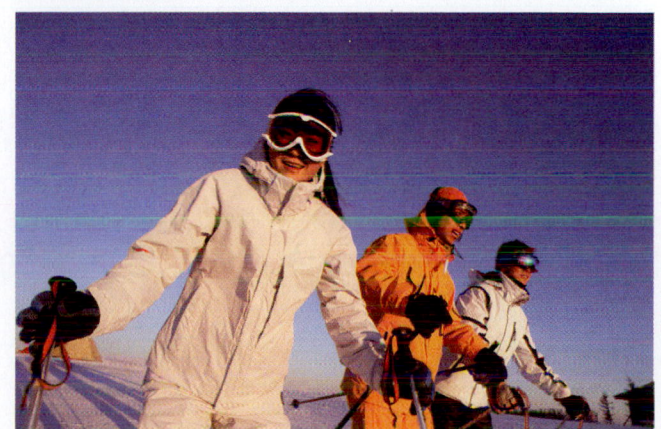

Balancing food energy intake with physical activity can add to life's enjoyment.

Figure 9–4

Components of Energy Expenditure

Typically, basal metabolism represents a person's largest expenditure of energy, followed by physical activity and the thermic effect of food.

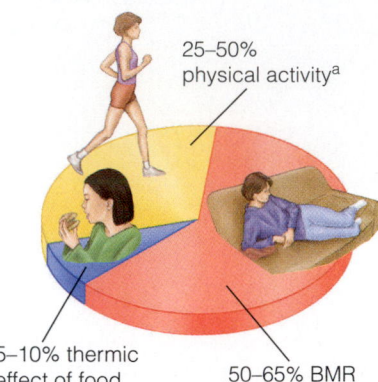

25–50% physical activity[a]

5–10% thermic effect of food

50–65% BMR

[a]For a sedentary person, physical activities may account for less than half as much energy as basal metabolism, whereas a very active person's activities may equal the energy cost of basal metabolism.

An alternative method of determining energy need is based on energy output. The two major ways in which the body spends energy are (1) to fuel its **basal metabolism** and (2) to fuel its **voluntary activities**. Basal metabolism requires energy to support the body's work that goes on all the time without a person's conscious awareness. A third energy component, the body's metabolic response to food, or the **thermic effect of food**, uses up about 10 percent of a meal's energy value in stepped-up metabolism in the 5 or so hours after finishing a meal.

Basal metabolism consumes a surprisingly large amount of fuel, and the **basal metabolic rate (BMR)** varies from person to person (Figure 9–4). Depending on activity level, a person whose total energy need is 2,000 calories a day may spend as many as 1,000 to 1,600 of them to support basal metabolism. The iodine-dependent hormone thyroxine directly controls basal metabolism—the less secreted, the lower the energy requirements for basal functions. The rate is lowest during sleep.[‡] Many other factors also affect the BMR (see Table 9–3).

People often wonder whether they can speed up their metabolism to spend more daily energy. You cannot increase your BMR very much *today*. You can, however, amplify the second component of your energy expenditure—your voluntary activities. If you do, you will spend more calories today, and if you keep doing so day after day, your BMR will also increase somewhat as you build lean tissue because lean tissue is more metabolically active than fat tissue. Energy spent on voluntary activities depends largely on three factors: weight, time, and intensity. The heavier the weight of the body parts you move, the longer the time you invest in moving them, and the greater the intensity of the work, the more calories you will expend.

Be aware that some ads for weight-loss diets claim that certain substances, such as grapefruit or herbs, can elevate the BMR and thus promote weight loss. This claim

Table 9–3

Factors That Affect the BMR

Factor	Effect on BMR
Age	The BMR is higher in youth; as lean body mass declines with age, the BMR slows. Physical activity may prevent some of this decline.
Height	Tall people have a larger surface area, so their BMRs are higher.
Growth	Children and pregnant women have higher BMRs.
Body composition	The more lean tissue, the higher the BMR. A typical man has greater lean body mass than a typical woman, making his BMR higher.
Fever	Fever raises the BMR.
Stress	Stress hormones raise the BMR.
Environmental temperature	Adjusting to either heat or cold raises the BMR.
Fasting/starvation	Fasting/starvation hormones lower the BMR.
Malnutrition	Malnutrition lowers the BMR.
Thyroxine	The thyroid hormone thyroxine is a key BMR regulator; the more thyroxine produced, the higher the BMR.

basal metabolism the sum total of all the involuntary activities that are necessary to sustain life, including circulation, respiration, temperature maintenance, hormone secretion, nerve activity, and new tissue synthesis, but excluding digestion and voluntary activities. Basal metabolism is the largest component of the average person's daily energy expenditure.

voluntary activities intentional activities (such as walking, sitting, or running) conducted by voluntary muscles.

thermic effect of food the body's speeded-up metabolism in response to having eaten a meal; also called *diet-induced thermogenesis*.

basal metabolic rate (BMR) the rate at which the body uses energy to support its basal metabolism.

[‡]A measure of energy output taken while the person is awake but relaxed yields a slightly higher number called the *resting metabolic rate*, sometimes used in research.

Chapter 9 Energy Balance and Healthy Body Weight

is false. Any meal temporarily steps up energy expenditure due to the thermic effect of food, and grapefruit or herbs are not known to accelerate it further.

- Two major components of energy expenditure are basal metabolism and voluntary activities.
- A third component of energy expenditure is the thermic effect of food.
- Many factors influence the basal metabolic rate.

Estimated Energy Requirements (EER)

A person wishing to know how much energy he or she needs in a day to maintain weight might look up his or her **Estimated Energy Requirement (EER)** value listed on the inside front cover of this book. The numbers listed there seem to imply that for each age and gender group, the number of calories needed to meet the daily requirement is known as precisely as, say, the recommended intake for vitamin A. The printed EER values, however, reflect the needs of only those people who exactly match the characteristics of the "reference man and woman." People who deviate in any way from these characteristics must use other methods for determining their energy needs, and almost everyone deviates.

Taller people need proportionately more energy than shorter people to balance their energy budgets because their greater surface area allows more energy to escape as heat. Older people generally need less than younger people due to slowed metabolism and reduced muscle mass, which occur in part because of reduced physical activity. As Chapter 14 points out, these losses may not be inevitable for people who stay active. On average, though, energy need diminishes by 5 percent per decade beyond the age of 30 years.

In reality, no one is average. In any group of 20 similar people with similar activity levels, one may expend twice as much energy per day as another. A 60-year-old person who bikes, swims, or walks briskly each day may need as many calories as a sedentary person of 30. Clearly, with such a wide range of variation, a necessary step in determining any person's energy need is to study that person.

- The DRI committee sets Estimated Energy Requirements for a reference man and woman, but individual energy needs vary greatly.

The DRI Method of Estimating Energy Requirements

The DRI committee provides a way of estimating EER values for individuals. These calculations take into account the ways in which energy is spent and by whom. The equation includes:

- *Age.* The BMR declines with age, so age helps to determine EER values.

- *Gender.* Women generally have less lean body mass than men; in addition, women's hormone fluctuations influence the BMR, raising it just prior to menstruation.

- *Body size and weight.* The higher BMR of taller and heavier people calls for height and weight to be factored in when estimating a person's EER.

- *Physical activity.* To help in estimating the energy spent on physical activity each day, activities are grouped according to their typical intensity (see Appendix H).

- *Growth.* The BMR is high in people who are growing, so pregnant women and children have their own sets of energy equations.

Instructions for estimating EER values are presented in Appendix H. Alternatively, the Do the Math feature in the margin offers a quick way to approximate your EER range.

- The DRI committee has established a method for determining an individual's approximate energy requirement.

Do the Math

To estimate basal energy output:

- Men: kg body weight × 24 = cal/day
- Women: kg body weight × 23 = cal/day

(To convert pounds to kilograms [kg], divide pounds by 2.2.)

Calculate the basal energy output (cal/day) of a man weighing 220 pounds.

Do the Math

Estimate your energy need using this quick and easy method:

- First, look up the EER listed for your age and gender group (inside front cover).
- Then calculate a range of energy needs. For most people, the energy requirement falls within these ranges:

  (Men) EER ± 200 cal

  (Women) EER ± 160 cal

Estimated Energy Requirement (EER) the DRI recommendation for energy intake, accounting for age, gender, weight, height, and physical activity. Also defined in Chapter 2.

To determine your BMI:

- In pounds and inches

$$BMI = \frac{weight\ (lb)}{(height\ in\ in.)^2} \times 703$$

- In kilograms and meters

$$BMI = \frac{weight\ (kg)}{(height\ in\ m)^2}$$

Using either pounds or kilograms, determine your own BMI value.

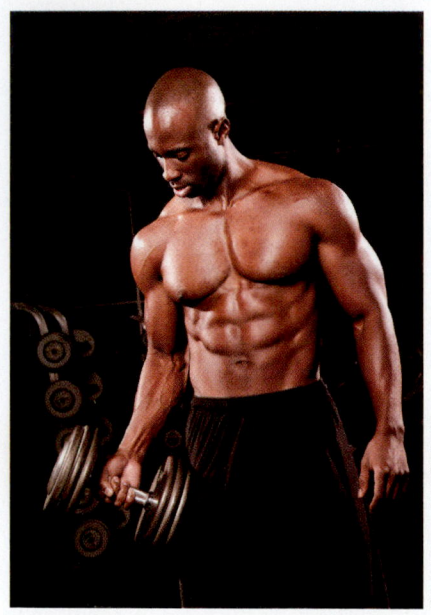

At 6'1" tall and 190 lbs., is this athlete too fat for health, as the BMI chart indicates? Further measurements reveal that his body fat content is only 7% and his health risks are below average.

iStockphoto.com/HadelProductions

Body Weight vs. Body Fatness

LO 9.3 Contrast body weight to body fatness.

For most people, weighing on a scale provides a convenient way to monitor body fatness, but researchers and health-care providers must rely on more accurate assessments. This section describes some details about applying the preferred methods to assess overweight and underweight.

Using the Body Mass Index (BMI)

No one can tell you exactly how much you should weigh, but with health as a value, you have a starting framework in the BMI table (inside back cover). Your weight should fall within the range that best supports your health. Unhealthy underweight for adults is defined as a BMI of less than 18.5, overweight as a BMI of 25.0 through 29.9, and obesity as a BMI of 30 or more. A formula for determining your BMI is given in the margin.

BMI values have two major drawbacks: they fail to indicate how much of a person's weight is fat and where that fat is located. These drawbacks limit the value of the BMI for use with:

- Athletes (because their highly developed musculature falsely increases their BMI values).

- Pregnant and lactating women (because their increased weight is normal during child bearing).

- Adults older than age 65 (because BMI values are based on data collected from younger people and because people "grow shorter" with age).

- Women older than age 50 with too little muscle tissue (they may be overly fat for health yet still fall into the normal BMI range).[25]

The bodybuilder in the photo proves this point: with a BMI over 25, he would be classified as overweight by BMI standards alone. However, a clinician would find that his percentage of body fat is well below average and his waist circumference is within a healthy range. For any given BMI value, body fat content can vary widely.

In addition, among some racial and ethnic groups, BMI values may not precisely identify overweight and obesity. African American people of all ages may have more lean tissue per pound of body weight than Asians or Caucasians, for example.[26] Thus, a diagnosis of obesity or overweight requires a BMI value *plus* some measure of body composition and fat distribution. There is no easy way to look inside a living person to measure bones and muscles, but several indirect measures can provide an approximation.

KEY POINT

- The BMI concept is flawed for certain groups of people.

Measuring Body Composition and Fat Distribution

A person who stands about 5 feet 10 inches tall and weighs 150 pounds carries about 30 of those pounds as fat. The rest is mostly water and lean tissues: muscles; organs such as the heart, brain, and liver; and the bones of the skeleton (see Figure 9–5). This lean tissue is vital to health. The person who seeks to lose weight wants to lose fat, not this precious lean tissue. And for someone who wants to gain weight, it is desirable to gain lean and fat in proportion, not just fat.

As mentioned, waist circumference indicates central adiposity and often reflects visceral fatness (see Figure 9–6, p. 354). Above a certain girth, disease risks rise.[27] Health professionals often use both BMI and waist circumference to assess a person's health risks and monitor changes over time.

Figure 9–5

Body Composition of Men and Women

Body fat percentages for people age 20 to 40 years old in the Healthy Weight BMI range (see inside back cover):

- Male: 18–21%
- Female: 23–26%

Average U.S. body fat percentages for people age 20 to 40 years old:

- Male: 26%
- Female: 38%

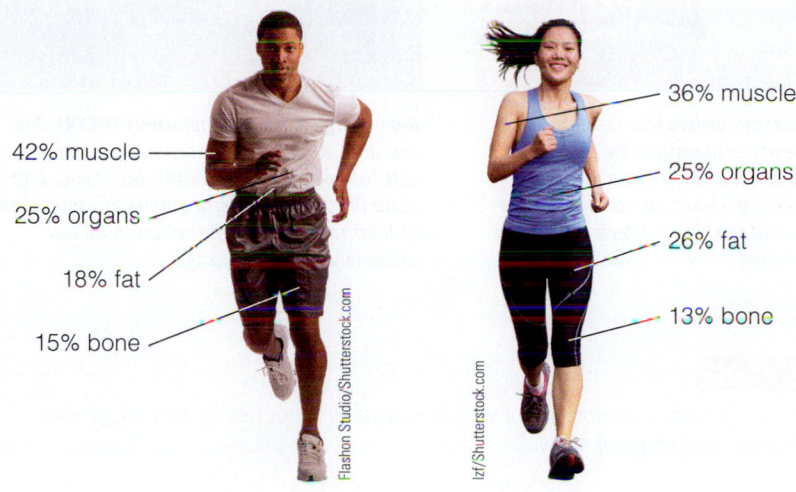

42% muscle

25% organs

18% fat

15% bone

36% muscle

25% organs

26% fat

13% bone

Flashon Studio/Shutterstock.com

lzf/Shutterstock.com

Researchers needing more precise measures of body composition may choose any of several techniques to estimate body fatness, including the **skinfold test**. Body fat distribution can be determined by radiographic techniques, such as **dual-energy X-ray absorptiometry**. Mastering these and other sophisticated techniques requires proper instruction and practice to ensure reliability. Each method has advantages and disadvantages with respect to cost, technical difficulty, and precision of estimating body fat.

KEY POINTS

- Central adiposity can be assessed by measuring waist circumference.
- The percentage of fat in a person's body can be estimated by using skinfold measurements, radiographic techniques, or other methods.
- Body fat distribution can be revealed by radiographic techniques.

How Much Body Fat Is Ideal?

After you have a body fatness estimate, the question arises: What is the "ideal" amount of fat for a body to have? This prompts another question: Ideal for what? If the answer is "society's perfect body shape," be aware that fashion is fickle and today's popular body shapes are not achievable by most people.

If the answer is "health," then the ideal depends partly on your lifestyle and stage of life. For example, competitive endurance athletes need just enough body fat to provide fuel, insulate the body, and permit normal hormone activity but not so much as to weigh them down. An Alaskan fisherman, in contrast, needs a blanket of extra fat to insulate against the cold. For a woman starting pregnancy, the outcome may be compromised if she begins with too much or too little body fat.

Much remains to be learned about individual requirements for body fat. How body fat accumulates and how it is controlled are the topics of the next sections.

skinfold test measurement of the thickness of a fold of skin and subcutaneous fat on the back of the arm (over the triceps muscle), below the shoulder blade (subscapular), or in other places, using a caliper; also called *fatfold test*.

dual-energy X-ray absorptiometry (ab-sorp-tee-OM-eh-tree) a noninvasive method of determining total body fat, fat distribution, and bone density by passing two low-dose X-ray beams through the body. Also used in evaluation of osteoporosis. Abbreviated DEXA.

Figure 9–6

Three Methods Used to Assess Body Fat

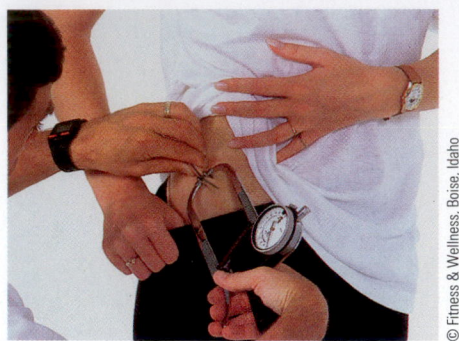

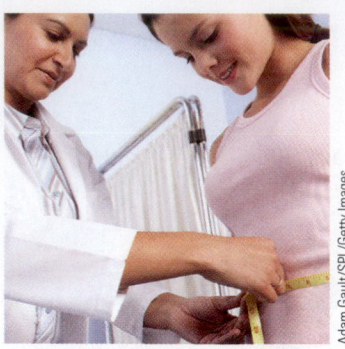

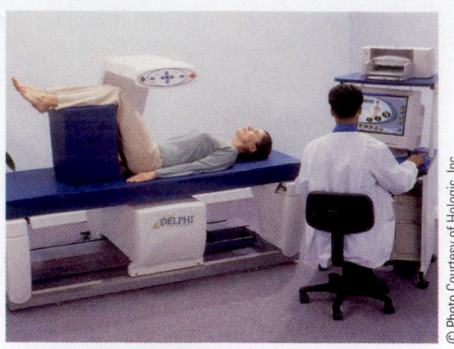

Skinfold measures. *Body fat is measured by using a caliper to gauge the thickness of a fold of skin on the back of the arm (over the triceps), below the shoulder blade (subscapular), and in other places (including lower-body sites) and then comparing these measurements with standards.*

Waist circumference. *Central obesity is measured by placing a nonstretchable measuring tape around the waist just above the bony crest of the hip. The tape is snug but does not compress the skin.*

Dual-energy X-ray absorptiometry (DEXA). *Two low-dose X-rays differentiate among fat-free soft tissue (lean body mass), fat tissue, and bone tissue, providing a precise measurement of total fat and its distribution in all but extremely obese subjects.*

KEY POINT

- No single body composition or weight suits everyone; needs vary by gender, lifestyle, and stage of life.

The Appetite and Its Control

LO 9.4 Identify factors that contribute to increased appetite and deceased appetite.

When you grab a snack or eat a meal, you may be aware only of your conscious mind choosing to eat something. However, the choice of when and how much to eat may not be as free as you think—deeper forces of physiology are at work.

Seeking and eating food are matters of life and death, so the body's appetite-regulating systems are skewed, tipping in favor of food consumption. **Hunger** demands food, but the signals that oppose food consumption—that is, signals for **satiation** and **satiety**—are weaker and more easily overruled. Many signaling molecules, including hormones, help to regulate food intake; the following sections name just a few.

Hunger and Appetite—"Go" Signals

The brain and digestive tract communicate about the need for food and food sufficiency. Their means of communication, hormones and sensory nerve signals, fall roughly into two broad functional categories: "go" mechanisms that stimulate eating and "stop" mechanisms that suppress it. One view of the whole complex process of food intake regulation is summarized in Figure 9–7.

Hunger Most people recognize hunger as a strong, unpleasant sensation, the response to a physiological need for food. Hunger makes itself known roughly four to six hours after eating, after the food has left the stomach and much of the nutrient mixture has been absorbed by the intestine. The physical contractions of an empty stomach trigger hunger signals, as do chemical messengers acting on or originating in the brain's hypothalamus (illustrated in Chapter 3). The hypothalamus has been described as a sort of central hub for energy and body weight regulation, and it can sense molecules representing all three of the energy nutrients.

hunger the physiological need to eat, experienced as a drive for obtaining food; an unpleasant sensation that demands relief.

satiation (SAY-she-AY-shun) the perception of fullness that builds throughout a meal, eventually reaching the degree of fullness and satisfaction that halts eating. Satiation generally determines how much food is consumed at one sitting.

satiety (sah-TIE-eh-tee) the perception of fullness that lingers in the hours after a meal and inhibits eating until the next mealtime. Satiety generally determines the length of time between meals.

Figure 9-7

Hunger, Appetite, Satiation, and Satiety

Although many factors work together to influence eating decisions, the brain can override physiological signals, particularly satiety signals.

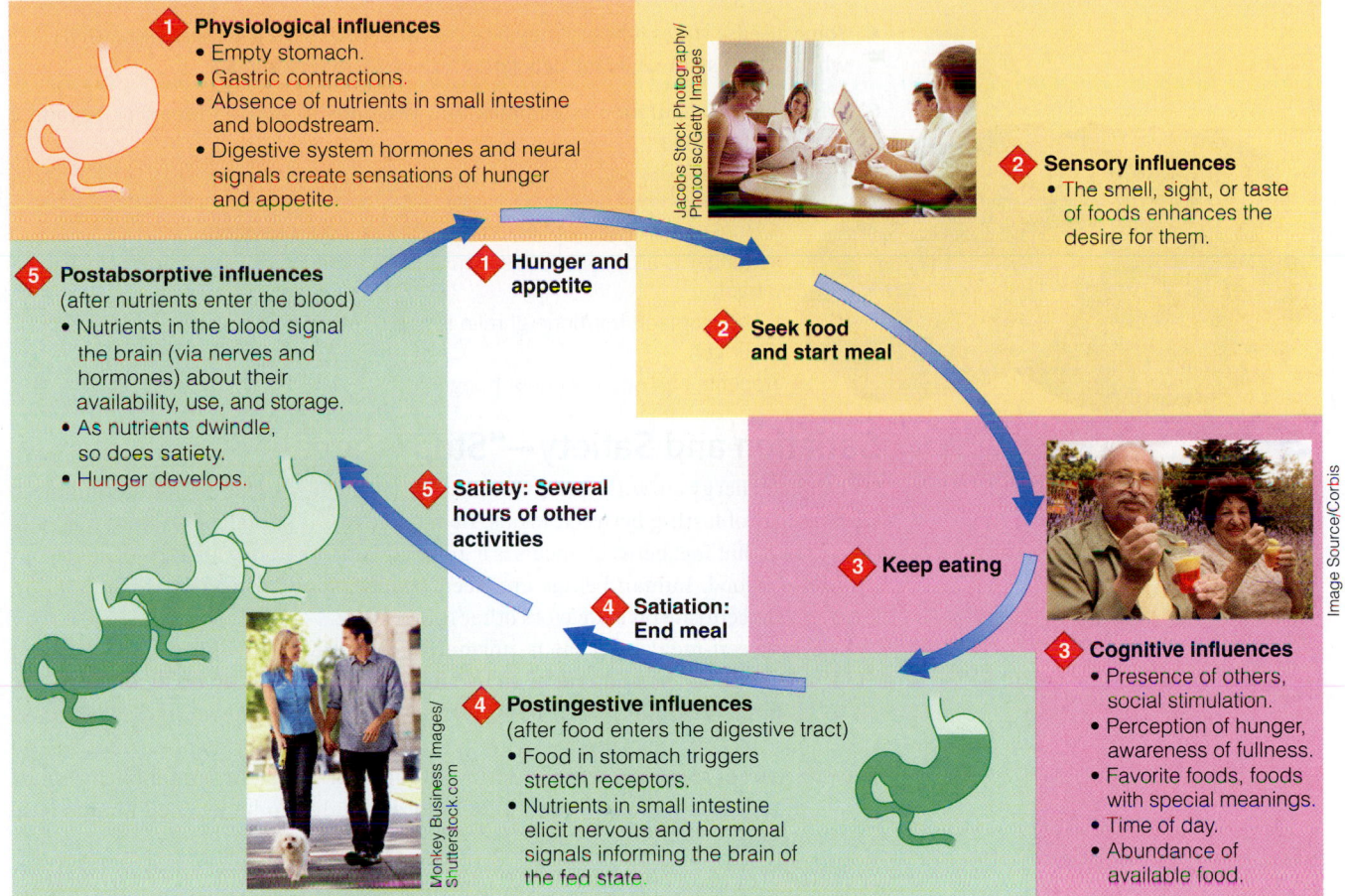

1 Physiological influences
- Empty stomach.
- Gastric contractions.
- Absence of nutrients in small intestine and bloodstream.
- Digestive system hormones and neural signals create sensations of hunger and appetite.

2 Sensory influences
- The smell, sight, or taste of foods enhances the desire for them.

5 Postabsorptive influences
(after nutrients enter the blood)
- Nutrients in the blood signal the brain (via nerves and hormones) about their availability, use, and storage.
- As nutrients dwindle, so does satiety.
- Hunger develops.

1 Hunger and appetite

2 Seek food and start meal

5 Satiety: Several hours of other activities

3 Keep eating

4 Satiation: End meal

4 Postingestive influences
(after food enters the digestive tract)
- Food in stomach triggers stretch receptors.
- Nutrients in small intestine elicit nervous and hormonal signals informing the brain of the fed state.

3 Cognitive influences
- Presence of others, social stimulation.
- Perception of hunger, awareness of fullness.
- Favorite foods, foods with special meanings.
- Time of day.
- Abundance of available food.

The polypeptide **ghrelin** is a powerful hunger-stimulating hormone that opposes weight loss. Ghrelin is secreted by stomach cells but works in the hypothalamus and other brain tissues to stimulate **appetite**. Ghrelin may also help regulate other diverse body functions, such as blood pressure, heart functions, inflammation, and reproduction.[28]

Ghrelin is just one of many hunger-regulating messengers that informs the brain of the need for food. In fact, the brain itself produces a number of molecular messengers involved in appetite regulation.[29]§

Appetite A person can experience appetite without hunger. For example, the aroma of hot apple pie or the sight of a chocolate buttercream cake after a big meal can trigger a chemical stimulation of the brain's pleasure centers, thereby creating a desire for dessert despite an already full stomach. In contrast, a person who is ill or under sudden stress may physically need food but have no appetite.[30] Other factors affecting appetite include:

- Appetite stimulants or depressants, other medical drugs.

- Cultural habits (cultural or religious acceptability of foods).

- Environmental conditions (people often prefer hot foods in cold weather and vice versa).

---

§One example is neuropeptide Y.

ghrelin (GREL-in) a hormone released by the stomach that signals the brain's hypothalamus and other regions to stimulate eating.

appetite the psychological desire to eat; a learned motivation and a positive sensation that accompanies the sight, smell, or thought of appealing foods.

- Hormones (for example, sex hormones).

- Inborn appetites (inborn preferences for fatty, salty, and sweet tastes).

- Learned preferences (cravings for favorite foods, aversion to trying new foods, and eating according to the clock).

- Social interactions (companionship, peer influences).

- Some disease states (obesity may be associated with increased taste sensitivity, whereas colds, flu, and zinc deficiency reduce taste sensitivity).

Clearly, appetite regulation is complex and responds to many influences beyond a physical need for food.

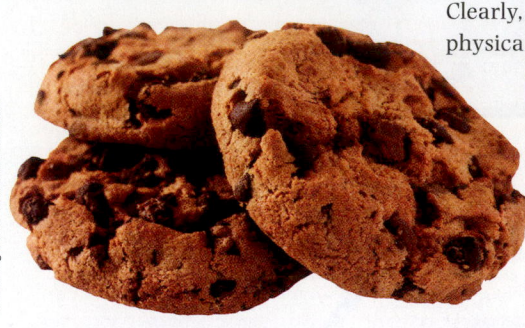

KEY POINTS

- Hunger outweighs satiety in the appetite control system.
- Hunger is a physiologic response to an absence of food in the digestive tract.
- The stomach hormone ghrelin is one of many contributors to feelings of hunger.
- Appetite can occur without hunger.

Satiation and Satiety—"Stop" Signals

To balance energy in with energy out, eating behaviors must be counterbalanced with periods of fasting between meals. Being able to eat periodically, store fuel, and then use up that fuel between meals is a great advantage. Relieved of the need to constantly seek food, human beings are free to dance, study, converse, wonder, fall in love, and concentrate on endeavors other than eating.

The between-meal interval is normally about 4 to 6 waking hours—about the length of time the body takes to use up most of the readily available fuel—or 12 to 18 hours at night, when body systems slow down and the need is less. As is true for the "go" signals that stimulate food intake, a series of hormones and sensory nerve messages along with products of nutrient metabolism sends "stop" signals to suppress eating. Much more remains to be learned about these mechanisms.

Satiation   At some point during a meal, the brain receives signals that enough food has been eaten. The resulting satiation causes continued eating to hold less interest and limits the size of the meal (consult Figure 9–7 again). Satiation arises from many organs:

- Sensations of pleasure and satisfaction in the mouth diminish with repeated exposure to a particular texture or taste during a meal, a common reason why people stop eating.[31]

- Nerve stretch receptors in the stomach sense the stomach's distention with a meal and fire, sending a signal to the brain that the stomach is full.

- As nutrients enter the small intestine, they stimulate other receptor nerves and trigger the release of hormones signaling the hypothalamus about the size and nature of the meal.

- The brain also detects absorbed nutrients delivered by the bloodstream, and it responds by releasing neurotransmitters that suppress food intake.

Together, mouth sensations, stomach distention, and the presence of nutrients trigger nervous and hormonal signals to inform the brain's hypothalamus that a meal has been consumed. Satiation occurs; the eater feels full and stops eating.

Did My Stomach Shrink?   Changes in food intake cause rapid adaptations in the body. A person who suddenly eats smaller meals may feel extra hungry for a few days, but then hunger may diminish for a time. During this period, a large meal may make the person feel uncomfortably full, partly because the stomach's capacity has adapted to a smaller quantity of food. A dieter may report "My stomach has shrunk," but the stomach has simply adjusted to smaller meals. At some point in food deprivation, hunger returns with a vengeance and can lead to bouts of extensive overeating.

Just as quickly, the stomach's capacity can adapt to larger meals until moderate portions no longer satisfy. This observation may partly explain the increasing U.S. calorie intakes: popular demand and food industry marketing have led to larger and larger food portions, while stomachs across the nation have adapted to accommodate them.

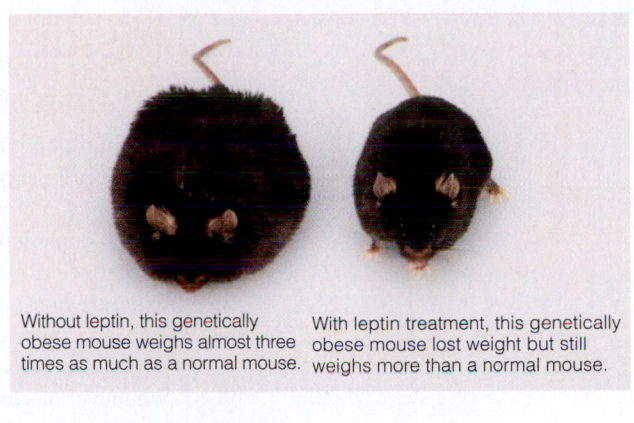

Without leptin, this genetically obese mouse weighs almost three times as much as a normal mouse.

With leptin treatment, this genetically obese mouse lost weight but still weighs more than a normal mouse.

Satiety   After finishing a meal, the feeling of satiety continues to suppress hunger over a period of hours, regulating the frequency of meals. Hormones, nervous signals, and the brain work in harmony to sustain feelings of fullness. At some later point, signals from the digestive tract once again sound the alert that more food is needed.

Leptin, one of the adipokine hormones, is produced in direct proportion to body fatness.** A gain in body fatness stimulates leptin production. Leptin travels from the adipose tissue via the bloodstream to the brain's hypothalamus, where it triggers signals that suppress appetite, dampen sensitivity to sweet taste, increase energy expenditures, and, ultimately, produce body fat loss.[32] A loss of body fatness, in turn, brings the opposite effects—suppression of leptin production, increased appetite, reduced energy expenditure, and accumulation of body fat. Leptin operates on a feedback mechanism—the fat tissue that produces leptin is ultimately controlled by it.

In a rare form of human obesity arising from an inherited inability to produce leptin, giving leptin injections quickly reverses both obesity and insulin resistance. More commonly, obese people produce plenty of leptin but are resistant to its effects; giving more leptin does not reverse their obesity.[33]

Energy Nutrients and Satiety   The composition of a meal seems to affect satiation and satiety, but the relationships are complex. Of the three energy-yielding nutrients, protein seems to have the greatest satiating effect during a meal.[34] Therefore, including some protein in a meal—even a glass of milk—can improve satiation and possibly even decrease energy intake at the next meal.

Many carbohydrate-rich foods, such as those providing slowly digestible carbohydrate and soluble fiber, also contribute to satiation and satiety.[35] These foods tend to hold blood glucose and insulin steady between meals, minimizing dips in blood glucose that are sensed by the brain, which responds by increasing hunger to restore blood glucose to normal. Soluble fibers and digestion-resistant starch also may support colonies of bacteria in the colon that have been associated with leanness in some studies.[36] Finally, fat, famous for triggering a hormone that contributes to long-term satiety, goes almost unnoticed by the appetite control system during consumption of a meal. As dieters await news of dietary tactics against hunger, researchers have not yet identified any one food, nutrient, or attribute—not even protein—that is especially effective for weight loss and its maintenance.[37]

leptin an appetite-suppressing hormone produced in the fat cells that conveys information about body fatness to the brain; believed to be involved in the maintenance of body composition (*leptos* means "slender").

**Leptin is also produced in the stomach, where it helps to regulate digestion and contributes to satiation.

Inside-the-Body Theories of Obesity

LO 9.5   Summarize the inside-the-body theories of obesity.

Findings about appetite regulation, the "energy in" side of the body weight equation, do not fully explain why some people gain too much body fat and others stay lean. When given a constant number of excess calories over a period of weeks or months, some people gain many pounds of body fat, but other people gain far fewer.[38] The former seem to use every calorie with great metabolic efficiency, while others may expend calories more freely.

Many theories have emerged to explain the mysteries of obesity in terms of metabolic function and energy expenditure—this section introduces a few of them. And whenever discussions turn to metabolism, topics in genetics follow closely behind.

Set-Point Theory   Like a room's thermostat, the brain and other organs constantly monitor body conditions and respond to slight fluctuations in such essential functions as blood glucose, blood pH levels, and body temperature to maintain them within a narrow range of a physiological set point. The **set-point theory** of obesity holds that, to a degree, this may also be true for body weight.[39] After weight gains or losses, the body adjusts its metabolism somewhat in the direction of restoring the original weight. Many debates surround the set-point theory of weight regulation.

Thermogenesis   Some people tend to expend more energy in metabolism than do others. The body's working enzymes normally "waste" a small percentage of energy as heat in a process called **thermogenesis**. Some enzymes expend copious energy in thermogenesis, producing heat but performing no other useful work. As more heat is radiated away from the body, more calories are spent, and fewer calories are available to be stored as body fat.

One tissue extraordinarily gifted in thermogenesis is **brown adipose tissue (BAT)**, a well-known heat-generating tissue of animals and human infants that has been identified in human adults, too.[40] People with the greatest body fatness appear to have the least BAT activity.[41] Intriguingly, compounds released during muscular work or while shivering from cold exposure appear to trigger a normally dormant type of adipose cell to act more like BAT metabolically, but the significance of this finding to weight management is unknown.[42]††

Is it wise, then, to try to step up thermogenesis to assist in weight loss? Probably not. At a level not far above normal, energy-wasting activity causes cell death. Sham "metabolic" diet products may claim to increase thermogenesis, but no tricks of metabolism can produce effortless fat loss.

The intestinal bacteria were first described in **Chapter 3.**

Intestinal Microbiota   Researchers are probing the possibility that certain strains of intestinal bacteria may affect body weight.[43] Some lines of study include these:

- When experimental germ-free mice are exposed to bacteria from ordinary mice, they quickly reduce their food intake, but they also gain weight, suggesting roles for the microbiota in food energy availability and storage.[44]

- Substances produced by intestinal bacteria, such as enzymes or short-chain fatty acids, may trigger changes in weight, blood lipids, or other body conditions.[45]

- In animals, obesity is linked with diminished colonies of beneficial bacteria and increased colonies of strains associated with damaging inflammation; such changes may increase the risk of diseases.[46] In human beings, research is inconsistent.

- In well-to-do countries, where obesity is prevalent, people's microbial colonies differ from those of places where obesity is rare.[47] Finding out whether certain microbes might be the cause or consequence of weight change is tricky, however, because the colonies quickly grow or diminish with changes in diet.[48]

††The activated adipose cells are called *beige cells*.

set-point theory   a theory stating that the body's regulatory controls tend to maintain a particular body weight (the set point) over time, opposing efforts to lose weight by dieting.

thermogenesis   the generation and release of body heat associated with the breakdown of body fuels. *Adaptive thermogenesis* describes adjustments in energy expenditure related to changes in environment such as cold and to physiological events such as underfeeding or trauma.

brown adipose tissue (BAT)   a type of adipose tissue abundant in hibernating animals and human infants and recently identified in human adults. Abundant pigmented enzymes of energy metabolism give BAT a dark appearance under a microscope; the enzymes release heat from fuels without accomplishing other work. Also called *brown fat.*

 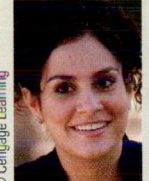
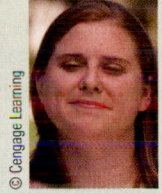
Until more is known, it seems prudent to consume a variety of legumes, fruit, vegetables, and whole grains to provide the fibers that help beneficial bacteria to thrive.

Genetics and Obesity   If genes carry the instructions for making enzymes and enzymes control energy metabolism, then genetic variations might reasonably be expected to explain why some people get fat and some stay lean. Indeed, genomic researchers have identified multiple genes likely to play roles in obesity development but have not so far identified a single genetic cause of common obesity. Inherited genes clearly do influence body weight, however. For someone with at least one obese parent, the chance of becoming obese is estimated to fall between 30 and 70 percent.

Complex relationships exist among the many genes related to energy metabolism and obesity, and they each interact with environmental factors, too, even before birth.[49] For example, research suggests that over- or undernutrition of a pregnant woman may alter genetic activities of the developing fetus in ways that increase the likelihood of obesity later in life.[50] Even though an individual's genetic inheritance and early influences may make obesity likely, the disease of obesity cannot develop unless the environment—factors that lie outside the body—provides the means of doing so.

KEY POINTS

- Metabolic theories attempt to explain obesity on the basis of molecular functioning.
- Research suggests a relationship between intestinal microbial colonies and obesity.
- A person's genetic inheritance greatly influences, but does not ensure, the development of obesity.

Outside-the-Body Theories of Obesity

LO 9.6   Summarize the outside-the-body theories of obesity.

Food is a source of pleasure, and pleasure drives behavior. Being creatures of free will, people can easily override satiety signals and eat whenever they wish, especially when tempted with delicious treats or large servings. People also value physical ease and seek out labor-savers, such as automobiles and elevators. Over past decades, the abundance of palatable food has increased enormously, while the daily demand for physical activity for survival has all but disappeared.

Environmental Cues to Overeating   Here's a common experience: a person walks into a food store feeling not particularly hungry but, after viewing an array of goodies, walks out snacking on a favorite treat. Even rats, which precisely maintain

Table 9–4

Energy Spent in Activities

To determine the calorie cost of an activity, multiply the number listed by your weight in pounds. Then multiply by the number of minutes spent performing the activity.

Example: Jessica (125 lb) rode a bike at 17 mph for 25 min:

0.057 × 125 =   7.125
7.125 ×   25 = 178.125

(about 180 calories)

Activity	Cal/lb Body Weight/min
Aerobic dance (vigorous)	0.062
Basketball (vigorous, full court)	0.097
Bicycling	
13 mph	0.045
15 mph	0.049
17 mph	0.057
19 mph	0.076
21 mph	0.090
23 mph	0.109
25 mph	0.139
Canoeing (flat water, moderate pace)	0.045
Computer sports games	
bowling	0.021
boxing	0.021
tennis	0.022
Cross-country skiing	
8 mph	0.104
Golf (carrying clubs)	0.045
Handball	0.078
Horseback riding (trot)	0.052
Rowing (vigorous)	0.097
Running	
5 mph	0.061
6 mph	0.074
7.5 mph	0.094
9 mph	0.103
10 mph	0.114
11 mph	0.131
Soccer (vigorous)	0.097
Studying	0.011
Swimming	
20 yd/min	0.032
45 yd/min	0.058
50 yd/min	0.070
Table tennis (skilled)	0.045
Tennis (beginner)	0.032
Walking (brisk pace)	
3.5 mph	0.035
4.5 mph	0.048
Weight lifting	
light-to-moderate effort	0.024
vigorous effort	0.048
Wheelchair basketball	0.084
Wheeling self in wheelchair	0.030

body weight when fed standard chow, overeat and rapidly become obese when fed "cafeteria style" on a variety of rich, palatable foods.[51] When offered a delicious smorgasbord, people do likewise, often without awareness.[52] Like the rats, they respond to external cues. With around-the-clock access to rich, palatable foods, we eat more and more often than in decades past—and energy intakes have risen accordingly.

Overeating also accompanies complex human sensations such as loneliness, yearning, craving, addiction, and compulsion. Any kind of prolonged stress can also cause overeating and weight gain.[53] ("What do I do when I'm worried? Eat. What do I do when I'm concentrating? Eat!") People who are overweight or obese may be especially responsive to such influences.[54]

People may also overeat in response to large portions of food. In a classic study, moviegoers ate proportionately more popcorn from large buckets than from small bags.[55] In a wry twist, researchers dispensed large and small containers of 14-day-old popcorn to moviegoers who, despite complaining of the staleness, still ate more popcorn from the larger container. The effect may also generalize to children, who asked for bigger portions of cereal when given bigger bowls than when given smaller bowls; they ate more and wasted more from bigger bowls, too.

Is Our Food Supply Addictive?

People often equate overeating with an addiction. Right away, it should be said that foods, even highly palatable foods, are not comparable to psychoactive drugs in most respects. Yet much evidence supports certain similarities between the brain's chemical responses to both.[56] Pleasure-evoking experiences of all kinds cause brain cells to release the neurotransmitter **dopamine**, which stimulates the reward areas of the brain. The result is feelings of pleasure and desire that create a motivation to repeat the experience. Paradoxically, with repeated exposure to a chemical stimulus (say, the drug cocaine) over time, the brain reduces its dopamine response, reducing feelings of pleasure. Soon, larger and larger doses are needed to avoid the pain of withdrawal—addiction.

Brain scans reveal reduced brain dopamine activity in people addicted to cocaine or alcohol. In a classic study, brain scans also revealed dopamine reductions in the brains of obese people.[57] This suggests that, similar to an addiction, once these changes are in place, obese people may need more and more delicious food to satisfy their desire for it. Taking the idea one step further, it is plausible that our highly palatable, fat- and sugar-rich food supply could cause lasting changes in the brain's reward system and make overeating and weight gain likely. It happens reliably in the brains of rats fed on a changing variety of cookies, cheese, sugar, and other tasty items, and it may happen in people, too.[58]

Other explanations exist. It may be that consciously restricting intakes of delicious foods increases the desire for them. It may also be that some people are more inclined to "throw caution to the wind" and indulge in treats whenever they present themselves.[59] Future research must untangle these threads before the truth is known.

Physical Inactivity

Many people may be obese not because they eat too much but because they move too little—both in purposeful exercise and in the activities of daily life.[60] Sedentary **screen time** has all but replaced outdoor play for many people. This is a concern because the more time people spend in sedentary activities, the more likely they are to be overweight—and to incur the metabolic risk factors of heart disease (high blood lipids, high blood pressure, and high blood glucose).[61] Table 9–4 lists the energy costs of some activities and the Think Fitness feature offers perspective on physical activity in weight management.

Can Your Neighborhood Make You Fat?

Experts urge people to "take the stairs instead of the elevator" or "walk or bike to work." These are good strategies: climbing stairs provides an impromptu workout, and people who walk or ride a bicycle for transportation most often meet their needs for physical activity. Many people, however, encounter barriers in their **built environment** that prevent such choices.

Some people believe that physical activity must be long and arduous to obtain benefits, such as improved body composition. Not so. A brisk, 30-minute walk at on at least 5 days per week can help significantly. To achieve an "active lifestyle" by walking requires an hour a day. Even in increments of 10 minutes throughout the day, exercise can measurably improve fitness.

According to the American College of Sports Medicine,

- 150 to 250 minutes per week of moderate intensity physical activity can help to prevent initial weight gain.

- More than 250 minutes per week, particularly when combined with a lower calorie intake, promotes weight loss and may prevent regain after loss.
- Both aerobic (endurance) and muscle-strengthening (resistance) activities are beneficial, but calorie restriction must accompany these activities to achieve meaningful weight loss in most people.

A useful strategy is to augment your planned workouts with bits of physical activity throughout the day. Work in the garden; work your abdominal muscles while you stand in line; stand up straight; walk up stairs; fidget or tighten your buttocks while sitting in your chair. Chapter 10 provides many more details.

start now! ⤳ If you are not currently exercising regularly, try this: go to Diet & Wellness Plus and create an alternate profile, adding in 30 minutes of moderate to vigorous physical activity for each day on which you have tracked your food intake. Go to the Reports tab; then choose Energy Balance. What differences do you see when you compare this report with the report you created under your original profile?

Few people would choose to walk or bike on a roadway where there is no safe sidewalk or marked bicycle lane, where vehicles speed by, or where the air is laden with toxic carbon monoxide gas or other pollutants from gasoline engines.[‡‡] Few would choose to walk up flights of stairs in an inconvenient, stuffy, isolated, and unsafe stairwell, typical in modern buildings. In contrast, people living in attractive, affordable neighborhoods with safe biking and walking lanes, public parks, and freely available exercise facilities use them often—their surroundings encourage physical activity.[62]

In addition, residents of many low-income urban and rural areas lack access to even a single supermarket. Often overweight and lacking transportation, residents of these so-called **food deserts** have limited access to the affordable, fresh, nutrient-dense foods they need.[63] Instead, they shop at local convenience stores and fast-food places, where they purchase mostly refined packaged sweets and starches, sugary soft drinks, fatty canned meats, or fast foods, and have an eating pattern that predicts nutrient deficiencies along with high rates of obesity and chronic diseases. Still unknown is whether efforts to increase access to healthy foods will decrease people's odds for developing obesity.[64]

Toward a Healthier Future The prestigious National Academies' Institute of Medicine has put forth these national goals as most likely to slow or reverse the obesity epidemic and improve the nation's health:

- Make physical activity an integral and routine part of American life.

- Make healthy foods and beverages available everywhere.

- Create food and beverage environments in which healthy food and beverage choices become the easy, routine choice.

- Advertise and market what matters for a healthy life.

- Develop and enforce legislation and policies aimed at preventing obesity.

- Strengthen schools as centers that promote fitness and health.[65]

Such changes require efforts from leaders at all levels and citizenry across all sectors of society working with one goal: improving the health of the nation.

dopamine (DOH-pah-meen) a neurotransmitter with many important roles in the brain, including cognition, pleasure, motivation, mood, sleep, and others.

screen time sedentary time spent using an electronic device, such as a television, computer, or video game player.

built environment The buildings, roads, utilities, homes, fixtures, parks, and all other man-made entities that form the physical characteristics of a community.

food deserts urban and rural low-income areas with limited access to affordable and nutritious foods. Also defined in Chapter 15.

[‡‡]Carbon monoxide (CO) avidly binds to hemoglobin in the blood, reducing blood oxygen content; CO in air surrounding roadways can reach levels sufficient to impair driving ability.

How the Body Loses and Gains Weight

LO 9.7 Describe metabolic events that occur in energy deficit and surplus.

The causes of obesity may be complex, but the body's energy balance is straightforward. To lose or gain body fat requires eating less or more food energy than the body expends. A change in body *weight* of a pound or two may not indicate a change in body fat, however—it can reflect shifts in body fluid content, in bone minerals, in lean tissues such as muscles, or in the contents of the bladder or digestive tract. A weight change often correlates with time of day: people generally weigh the least before breakfast.

The type of tissue lost or gained depends on how you go about losing or gaining it. To lose fluid, for example, you can take a "water pill" (diuretic), causing the kidneys to siphon extra water from the blood into the urine, or you can exercise while wearing heavy clothing in hot weather to cause abundant fluid loss in sweat. (Both practices are dangerous and are not being recommended here.) To gain water weight, you can overconsume salt and water; for a few hours, your body will retain water until it manages to excrete the salt. (This, too, is not recommended.) Most quick weight-change schemes promote large changes in body fluids that register dramatic, but temporary, changes on the scale and accomplish little weight change in the long run.

One other practice is hazardous and not recommended: smoking. Each year, many adolescents, particularly girls, take up smoking as a means to control weight.[66] Nicotine blunts feelings of hunger, and smokers do tend to weigh less than nonsmokers. Fear of weight gain prevents many people from quitting smoking, too. The best advice to smokers trying to quit is to adjust eating and exercise habits to maintain weight during and after cessation. To the person flirting with the idea of taking up smoking for weight control, don't do it—many thousands of people who became addicted as teenagers die from tobacco-related illnesses each year.

The Body's Response to Energy Deficit

When you eat less food energy than you need, your body draws on its stored fuel to keep going. If a person exercises appropriately, moderately restricts calories, and consumes an otherwise balanced diet that meets carbohydrate needs and provides sufficient protein, the body is forced to use up its stored fat for energy.[67] Gradual weight loss will occur.[68] This is preferred to rapid weight loss because lean body mass is spared and fat is lost.

The Body's Response to Fasting
If a person doesn't eat for, say, three whole days, then the body makes one adjustment after another. Less than a day into the fast, the liver's glycogen is essentially exhausted. Where, then, can the body obtain glucose to keep its nervous system going? Not from the muscles' glycogen because that is reserved for the muscles' own use. Not from the abundant fat stores most people carry because these are of no use to the nervous system. The muscles, heart, and other organs use fat as fuel, but at this stage, the nervous system needs glucose. Fat cannot be converted to glucose—the body lacks enzymes for this conversion.[§§] The body does, however, possess enzymes that can convert protein to glucose. Therefore, the underfed body sacrifices the proteins in its lean tissue to supply raw materials from which to make glucose.

If the body were to continue to consume its lean tissue unchecked, death would ensue within about 10 days. After all, in addition to skeletal muscle, the blood

---

[§§]Glycerol, which makes up 5 percent of fat, can yield glucose but is a negligible source.

proteins, liver, digestive tract linings, heart muscle, and lung tissue—all vital tissues—are being burned as fuel. (Fasting or starving people remain alive only until their stores of fat are gone or until half their lean tissue is gone, whichever comes first.) To prevent this, the body puts a key strategy into action: it begins converting fat into **ketone bodies** (introduced in Chapter 4) that some nervous system tissues can use and so forestalls the end. This process is ketosis, an adaptation to prolonged fasting or carbohydrate deprivation.

Ketosis In ketosis, instead of breaking down fat molecules all the way to carbon dioxide and water, the body takes partially broken-down fat fragments and combines them to make ketone bodies, compounds that are normally kept to low levels in the blood. It converts some amino acids—those that cannot be used to make glucose—to ketone bodies, too. These ketone bodies circulate in the bloodstream and help to feed the brain; about half of the brain's cells can make the enzymes needed to use ketone bodies for energy. Under normal conditions, the brain and nervous system devour glucose—about 400 to 600 calories' worth each day. After about 10 days of fasting, the brain and nervous system can meet most, but not all, of their energy needs using ketone bodies.

Thus, indirectly, the nervous system begins to feed on the body's fat stores. Ketosis reduces the nervous system's need for glucose, spares the muscle and other lean tissue from being quickly devoured, and prolongs the starving person's life. Thanks to ketosis, a healthy person starting with average body fat content can live totally deprived of food for as long as six to eight weeks.

In summary,

- The brain and nervous system cannot use fat as fuel and demand glucose.

- Body fat cannot be converted to glucose.

- Body protein can be converted to glucose.

- Ketone bodies made from fat can feed some nervous system tissues and reduce glucose needs, sparing protein from degradation.

Figure 9–8 (p. 364) reviews how energy is used during fasting.

Is Fasting Helpful or Harmful? Respected, wise people in many cultures have practiced fasting as a periodic discipline. The body tolerates short-term fasting, and in laboratory animals, fasting may extend life, reduce chronic diseases, or benefit cognition.[69] In people, intermittent fasting—say, a day or two a week—is under investigation for utility in weight loss, but much more research is needed to determine its safety and effectiveness.[70] Despite claims from salespeople, no evidence suggests that fasting, even with juices or supplement concoctions, "cleanses" the body internally.

On the negative side, repeated fasting in rats causes infertility and greater fat storage.[71] In people, the fasting body slows its metabolism to conserve energy—the wrong effect for weight loss. Fasting becomes harmful when tissues lack the nutrients they need to assemble new enzymes, red and white blood cells, and other vital components. Also, ketosis can upset the acid-base balance of the blood and promote mineral losses in the urine. To prevent these effects, the DRI committee sets a minimum intake for carbohydrate at 130 grams per day.

Fasting may also increase the appetite, particularly for starchy foods.[72] Often, people with eating disorders report that fasting or severe food restriction heralded the beginning of their loss of control over eating.

ketone bodies acidic compounds derived from fat and certain amino acids. Normally rare in the blood, they help to feed the brain during times when too little carbohydrate is available. Also defined in Chapter 4.

Figure 9–8
Feasting and Fasting

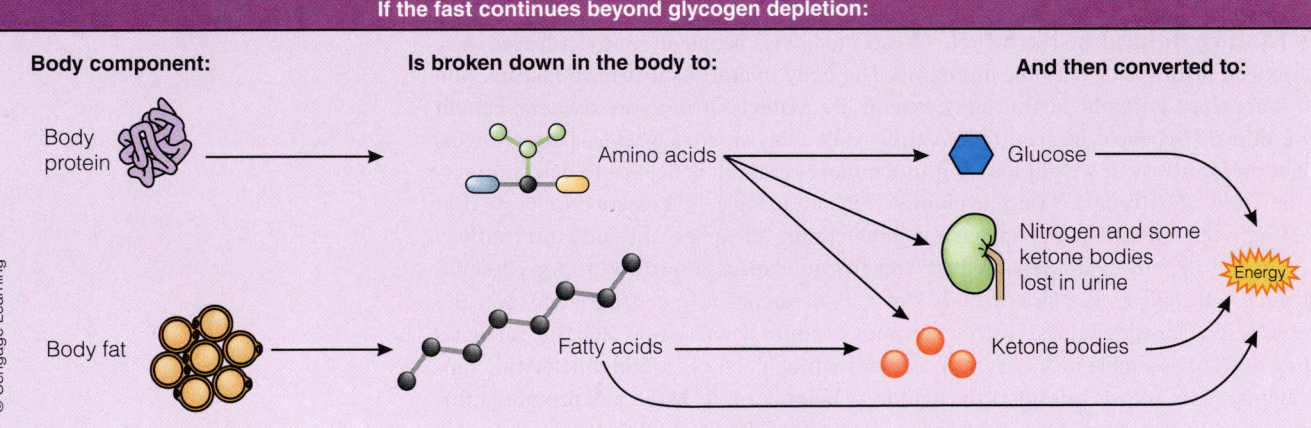

When a person overeats (feasting):

Food component:[a]	Is broken down in the body to:	And then contributes to:
Carbohydrate	Glucose	Liver and muscle glycogen stores
Fat	Fatty acids	Body fat stores
Protein	Amino acids[b]	Nitrogen lost in urine

When a person draws on stores (fasting):

Storage component:	Is broken down in the body to:	And then used for:
Liver and muscle glycogen stores	Glucose	Energy
Body fat stores	Fatty acids	Energy

If the fast continues beyond glycogen depletion:

Body component:	Is broken down in the body to:	And then converted to:
Body protein	Amino acids	Glucose / Nitrogen and some ketone bodies lost in urine
Body fat	Fatty acids	Ketone bodies / Energy

© Cengage Learning

[a] Alcohol is not included because it is a toxin and not a nutrient, but it does contribute energy to the body. After detoxifying the alcohol, the body uses the remaining two-carbon fragments to build fatty acids and stores them as fat.

[b] Amino acids are first used to build body proteins. Excess amino acids contribute to body fuel; after removal of their side chains, the backbones can be used to build glucose or fat.

The Body's Response to Energy Surplus

What happens inside the body when a person does not use up all of the food energy taken in? Previous chapters have already provided the answer—the energy-yielding nutrients contribute the excess to body stores as follows:

- Protein is broken down to amino acids for absorption. Inside the body, these may be used to replace lost body *protein* and, in a person who is exercising or growing, to build new muscle and other lean tissue.

- Excess amino acids have their nitrogen removed and are used for energy or are converted to *glucose* or *fat*. The nitrogen is excreted in the urine.

- Fat is broken down to glycerol and fatty acids for absorption. Inside the body, the fatty acids can be broken down for energy or stored as body *fat* with great efficiency. The glycerol enters a pathway similar to carbohydrate.

- Carbohydrate (other than fiber) is broken down to sugars for absorption. In the body tissues, excesses of these may be built up to *glycogen* and stored, used for energy, or converted to *fat* and stored.

- Alcohol is absorbed and, once detoxified, used for fuel or converted into body fat for storage.

Four sources of energy—the three energy-yielding nutrients and alcohol—may enter the body, but they become only two kinds of energy stores: glycogen and fat. Glycogen stores amount to about three-fourths of a pound; fat stores can amount to many pounds. Thus, if you eat enough of any food, be it steak, brownies, or baked beans, much of the excess will be turned to fat within hours.

Ethanol, the alcohol of alcoholic beverages, slows down the body's use of fat for fuel by as much as a third, causing more fat to be stored. This storage may add to the abdominal fat tissue of the "beer drinker's belly" and to fat tissue on the thighs, legs, or anywhere the person tends to store surplus fat.[73] Alcoholic beverages are therefore fattening, both through the calories they provide and through alcohol's effects on fat metabolism. Once alcohol addiction sets in, however, people often become thin and malnourished as body organs fail and their appetite for food is replaced by an appetite for alcohol.

In summary,

- Almost any food can make you fat if you eat enough of it. A net excess of energy is almost all stored in the body as fat in fat tissue.

- Fat from food is particularly easy for the body to store as fat tissue.

- Protein is not stored in the body except in response to exercise; it is present only as working tissue. Protein is converted to glucose to help feed the brain when carbohydrate is lacking; excess protein contributes to body fat.

- Alcohol both delivers calories and facilitates storage of body fat.

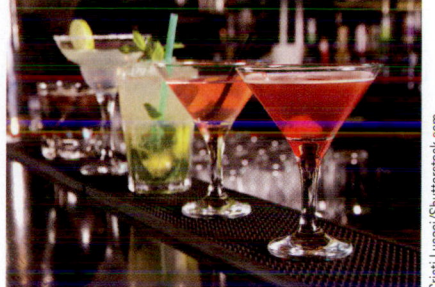

Each gram of alcohol presents 7 calories of energy to the body—energy that is easily stored as body fat.

Cristi Lucaci/Shutterstock.com

KEY POINTS

- When the energy balance is positive, carbohydrate is converted to glycogen or fat, protein is converted to fat, and food fat is stored as fat.
- Alcohol delivers calories and encourages fat storage.

Achieving and Maintaining a Healthy Body Weight

LO 9.8 Summarize the measures that help in achieving and maintaining a healthy body weight.

Before setting out to change your body weight, think about your motivation for doing so. Many people strive to change their weight not because they want to improve health but because their weight fails to meet society's ideals of attractiveness. Unfortunately, this kind of thinking sets people up for disappointment. The human body is not infinitely malleable. Few overweight people will ever become rail-thin, even with the right eating pattern, exercise habits, and behaviors. Likewise, most underweight people will remain on the slim side even after spending much effort to put on some heft.

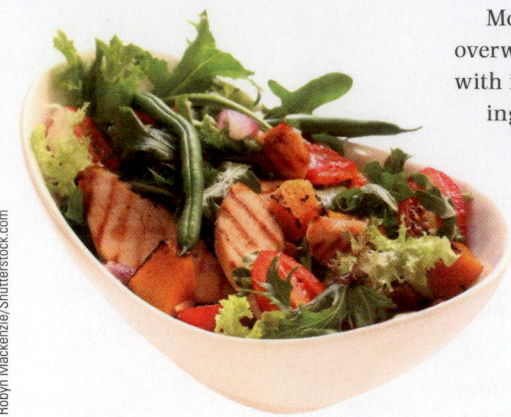

Robyn Mackenzie/Shutterstock.com

Modest weight loss of even 3 to 5 percent of body weight in a person who is still overweight can quickly produce gains in physical abilities and quality of life, along with improvements in indicators of diabetes and blood lipids.[74] Stair climbing, walking, and other tasks of daily living become noticeably easier. Adopting health or fitness as the ideal rather than some ill-conceived image of beauty can avert much misery. Table 9–5 offers some tips to that end.

The rest of this chapter stresses health and fitness as goals and explains the required actions to achieve them. It uses weight only as a convenient gauge for progress. To repeat, effort in three realms produces results:

- Eating patterns.
- Physical activity.
- Behavior modification.[75]

Eating patterns and physical activity are explained next. Behavior modification is the topic of this chapter's Food Feature section.

First, a Reality Check
Overweight takes years to accumulate. Tackling excess body fatness also takes time, along with patience and perseverance. The person must adopt healthy eating patterns, take on physical activities, create a supportive environment, and seek out behavioral and social support; continue these behaviors for at least 6 months for initial weight loss; and then continue all of it for a lifetime to maintain the losses. Setbacks are a given, and the size of the calorie deficit required to lose a pound of weight initially may be smaller than the deficit required later on. In other words, weight loss is hard at first, and then it gets harder.[76]

The list of what doesn't work is long: fad diets, skipping meals, "diet foods," special herbs and supplements, and liquid-diet formulas, among others.[77] Many fad diets promise quick and easy weight-loss solutions, but as the Consumer's Guide points out, fad diets can interrupt real progress toward life-long weight management. In contrast, people willing to take one step at a time, even if it feels like just a baby step, toward balancing their energy budget are on the right path. An excellent first step is to set realistic goals.

Set Achievable Goals
A reasonable first weight goal for an overweight person might be to stop gaining weight. A next goal might be to reduce body weight by 5 to 10 percent over about 6 months.[78] This may sound insignificant, but even small losses can improve health and reduce disease risks. Put another way, shoot for a weight that falls two BMI categories lower than a present unhealthy one. For example, a 5-foot-5-inch woman with hypertension weighing 180 pounds (BMI of 30—see the BMI table on the inside back cover) may aim for a BMI of 28, or about 168 pounds. If her health indicators fall into line, she may decide to maintain this weight. If her blood pressure is still high or she has other risks, she may repeat the process to achieve a healthier weight.

Table 9–5

Tips for Accepting a Healthy Body Weight

- Value yourself and others for traits other than body weight; focus on your whole self, including your intelligence, social grace, and professional and scholastic accomplishments.
- Realize that prejudging people by weight is as harmful as prejudging them by race, religion, or gender.
- Use only positive, nonjudgmental descriptions of your body; never use degrading, negative descriptions.
- Accept positive comments from others.
- Accept that no magic diet exists.
- Stop dieting to lose weight. Adopt a healthy eating and exercise lifestyle permanently.

- Follow the USDA Eating Patterns (Chapter 2, pp. 39–43). Never restrict food intake below the minimum levels that meet nutrient needs.
- Become physically active not because it will help you get thin but because it will enhance your health.
- Seek support from loved ones. Tell them of your plan for a healthy life in the body you have been given.
- Seek professional counseling not from a weight-loss counselor but from someone who supports your self-esteem.
- Join with others to fight weight discrimination and stereotypes.

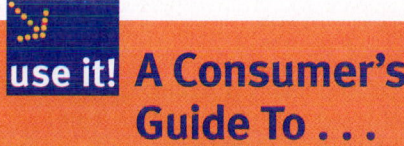

Fad Diets

Over the years, Lauren has tried most of the new fad diets, her hopes rising each time, as though she had never been disappointed: "*This* one has the answer. I have *got* to lose 40 pounds. Plus it only costs $30 to start." Who wouldn't pay a few dollars to get trim?

Lauren and tens of millions of people like her have helped to fuel the success of a $33 billion-a-year weight-loss industry. The number of fad-diet books in print could fill a bookstore, and more keep coming out because they continue to make huge profits. Some of them restrict fats or carbohydrates, some disallow certain foods, some advocate certain food combinations, some claim that a person's genetic type or blood type determines the best diet, and others advocate taking unproven weight-loss "dietary supplements."

Unfortunately, most fad diets are more fiction than science. They sound plausible, though, because they are skillfully written. Their authors weave in scientific-sounding words like *eicosanoids* or *adipokines* and bits of authentic nutrition knowledge to set a tone of credibility and convince the skeptical. This makes it hard for people without adequate nutrition knowledge to evaluate them. Table 9–6 presents some clues to identifying scams among fad diets.

Are Fad Diets All Nonsense?

If fad diets delivered what they promise, the nation's obesity problem would have vanished; if they never worked, people would stop buying into them. In fact, most fad diets do limit calorie intakes and produce weight loss (at least temporarily). Studies demonstrate, however, that fad diets are particularly ineffective for weight-loss maintenance—people may drop some weight, but they quickly gain it back.[1]* Straightforward

Reference notes are in Appendix F.

Table 9–6

Clues to Fad Diets and Weight-Loss Scams

It may be a fad diet or weight-loss scam if it:

- Bases evidence for its effectiveness on anecdotal stories and testimonials.
- Blames weight gain on a single nutrient, such as carbohydrate, or constituent, such as gluten.
- Claims to "alter your genetic code" or "reset your metabolism."
- Eliminates an entire food group, such as grains or milk and milk products.
- Fails to include all costs up front.
- Fails to mention potential risks associated with the plan.
- Fails to plan for weight maintenance following loss.
- Guarantees an unrealistic outcome in an unreasonable time period, such as losing 10 pounds in 3 days.
- Promises quick and easy weight loss methods; for example, "Lose weight while you sleep."
- Promotes devices, drugs, products, or procedures not approved by the U.S. Food and Drug Administration (FDA) or scientifically evaluated for safety or effectiveness.
- Sounds too good to be true.
- Specifies a proportion of energy nutrients not in keeping with DRI recommended ranges.
- Recommends using a single food, such as grapefruit, as the key to the program's success.
- Requires you to buy special products not readily available in ordinary supermarkets.
- Has any of the characteristics of quackery (see Figure C1–1 of Controversy 1).

calorie deficit turns out to be the real key to weight loss—and not the elimination of protein, carbohydrate, or fat or the mysterious metabolic mechanisms proposed by many fad diets.

Are Low-Carbohydrate Diets Best?

Diet promoters make much of research showing that high-protein, low-carbohydrate diets produce a little more weight loss than balanced diets over the first few months of dieting. However, in the long run, any low-calorie diet produces about the same degree of loss.[2] The 2015 Dietary Guidelines committee states that diets with less than 45 percent of calories from carbohydrate or more than 35 percent of protein offer no weight-loss advantage over other calorie-controlled diets, and that they are difficult to maintain over the long term and may be less safe.[3] However, for most people, cutting down on carbohydrates as added sugars and ultra-processed starch-based foods can be a nutritionally sound approach to cutting calorie intakes. Eating the normal amount of lean protein-rich foods while reducing carbohydrate and fat intakes automatically reduces calories and shifts the nutrient balance toward a higher percentage of energy from protein.[4]

Is Extra Protein Helpful?

Protein nutrition during calorie restriction deserves attention. A meal with too little protein may not produce enough satiety to prevent between-meal hunger, although research is not consistent on this point.[5] Eating enough foods rich in high-quality protein, along with performing muscle-building resistance exercise, can help minimize muscle loss, an unwelcome side effect of calorie restriction and fat loss.[6]

Some research suggests that a little extra protein (1.2 to 1.6 gram per kilogram body weight) may turn out to be useful, so long as the dieter can stick with a calorie-reduced diet over time.[7] However, protein sources matter, too. In one well-controlled, long-duration study, weight *gain*, not loss, was associated with higher intakes of full fat cheeses, chicken with skin, and processed and red meats (particularly hamburger).[8] In contrast, plain yogurt, peanut butter, walnuts, other nuts, chicken without skin, low-fat cheese, and seafood were associated with weight loss.

Are Gluten-Free Diets Best?

Proponents of gluten-free diets claim that the protein gluten in many grain foods (details in Chapter 6) causes obesity, but no research backs this up. In fact, choosing gluten-free foods for weight loss may backfire if the formulated foods are high in calories, added sugars, or refined starches.

Are Fad Diets Nutritious?

Fad diets that severely limit or eliminate one or more food groups cannot meet nutrient needs. To fend off critics, such plans usually recommend nutrient supplements (often conveniently supplied by the diet's originators at greatly inflated prices). Real weight-loss experts know this: no pill, not even the most costly ones, can match the health benefits of whole foods.

Are the Diets Safe?

Although most people can tolerate most diets, exceptions exist. For example, a rare but life-threatening form of blood acid imbalance is associated with a very-low-carbohydrate diet. In addition, when protein sources are high in saturated fat, the diet may produce unfavorable changes in blood lipids and artery linings.[9] In a recent study, low-carbohydrate diets, particularly without weight loss, are reported to impair the small arteries in the body in ways that promote heart disease risk.[10] A higher risk of death is linked with a diet that is high in animal protein or too low in carbohydrate.[11] No one knows the extent to which extreme fad diets might affect people with established diabetes or heart disease—the very people who might try dieting to regain their health.

Moving Ahead

Success for the fad-diet industry is built on failure for the dieter. As one diet shortcut fails, a new version arises to take its place, replenishing industry profits. Success for the dieter takes a longer road: setting realistic goals and eating a nutritious calorie-restricted diet that is sustainable by that person. This approach also means adopting a physically active lifestyle that is flexible and comfortable over a lifetime. Solid plans like this exist; seek them out for serious help with weight loss.* Armed with common sense, Lauren and other hopeful dieters can find a sane, stable path and avoid costly detours that sap the will and delay true weight-management progress.

Review Questions**

1. A diet book that addresses eicosanoids and adipokines can be relied upon to reflect current scholarship in nutrition science and provide effective weight-loss advice. T F

2. Calorie deficit is no longer the primary strategy for weight management. T F

3. Diets with sufficient protein may provide more satiety than diets that are low in protein. T F

*An example of a balanced weight-loss plan is Weight Watchers®.
**Answers to Consumer's Guide review questions are found in Appendix G.

Once you have identified your overall target, set specific, achievable, small-step goals for food intake, activity, and behavior changes. One simple and effective first small-step goal might be to eliminate all sugar-sweetened beverages, including sweetened iced tea (fast-food sweet tea provides 280 calories per 32-ounce serving).

Liquid calories were the topic of **Chapter 8**'s Consumer's Guide section.

Dramatic weight loss overnight is not possible or even desirable; a pound or two of body fat lost each week will safely and effectively bring you to your goal. Losses greater or faster than these are not recommended because they are almost invariably followed by rapid regain. New goals can be built on prior achievements, and a lifetime goal may be to maintain the leaner, healthier body weight.

Keep Records   Keeping records is often critical to success. Recording your food intake and exercise can help you to spot trends and identify areas needing improvement. The Food Feature, later, demonstrates how to maintain a food and exercise diary. Recording changes in body weight can also provide a rough estimate of changes in body fatness over time. In addition to weight, measure your waist circumference to track changes in central adiposity.

KEY POINTS

- Setting realistic weight goals provides an important starting point for weight loss.

- Many benefits follow even modest reductions in body fatness among overweight people.
- Successful weight management takes time and effort; fad diets can be counterproductive.

What Food Strategies Are Best for Weight Loss?

Contrary to the claims of faddists, no particular food plan is magical, and no particular food must be either included or excluded. You are the one who will have to live with the plan, so you had better be the one to design it. Remember, you are adopting a healthy eating plan for life, so it must consist of satisfying foods that you like, that are readily available, and that you can afford.

Choose an Appropriate Calorie Intake   Nutrition professionals often use an overweight person's BMI to calculate the number of calories to cut from the diet. Dieters with a BMI of 35 or greater are encouraged to reduce their daily calories by up to 1,000 calories from their usual intakes. People with a BMI between 25 and 35 should reduce energy intake by 500 to 750 calories a day to produce a pound or two of weight loss each week while retaining lean tissue.[79]

For some weeks or months, weight loss may proceed rapidly. Eventually, these factors may contribute to a slowdown in the rate of loss:

- Metabolism may slow in response to a lower calorie intake and loss of metabolically active lean tissue.

- Less energy may be expended in physical activity as body weight diminishes.

In addition, the calorie values of the various tissues being lost can affect the rate of weight loss. Early in dieting, weight loss is composed of more water and lean tissue, which contain fewer calories per pound, than later losses composed of mostly fat. Fat has a much higher caloric value, so losing a pound of fat requires a greater calorie deficit in the diet. This means that dieters should expect a slowdown in weight loss as they progress past the initial phase.

In the end, most dieters can lose weight safely on an eating pattern providing approximately 1,200 to 1,500 calories per day for women and 1,500 to 1,800 calories per day for men while still meeting nutrient needs (as demonstrated in Table 9–7). Very low-calorie diets are notoriously unsuccessful at achieving lasting weight loss, lack necessary nutrients, and may set in motion the unhealthy behaviors of eating disorders (see the Controversy) and so are not recommended.

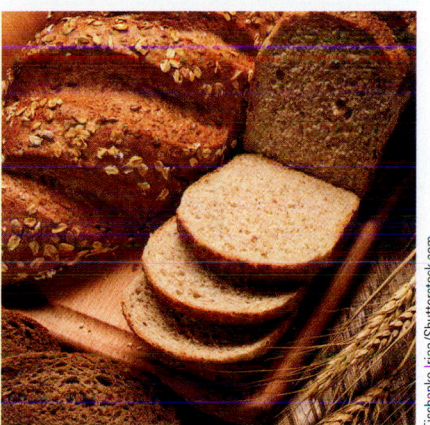

People with a healthy body weight often choose whole grains over refined carbohydrates.

Tischenko Irina/Shutterstock.com

Table 9–7

Eating Patterns for Low-Calorie Diets

These intakes allow most people to lose weight and still meet their nutrient needs with careful selections of nutrient-dense foods. See Chapter 2 for diet-planning details.

Food Group	1,200 Calories	1,400 Calories	1,600 Calories	1,800 Calories
Fruits	1 c	1½ c	1½ c	1½ c
Vegetables	1½ c	1½ c	2 c	2½ c
Grains	4 oz	5 oz	5 oz	6 oz
Protein Foods	3 oz	4 oz	5 oz	5 oz
Milk and Milk Products	2½ c	2½ c	3 c	3 c
Oils	4 tsp	4 tsp	5 tsp	5 tsp

Make Intakes Adequate   Healthy eating patterns for weight loss should include a variety of food to provide all of the needed nutrients. In particular, eating more of these foods is associated with a healthy body weight:

- Fruit, vegetables, nuts, and legumes.

- Fish; poultry without skin; low-fat or nonfat milk products.

- Whole grains.

- Moderate amounts of unsaturated oils.[80]

Eating patterns should also be lower in total meat and refined grains and low in saturated fat, sodium, and sugar-sweetened foods and drinks. Such patterns, including Healthy Vegetarian and Healthy Mediterranean-style patterns, provide nutrient adequacy and are generally associated with leanness.

Choose fats sensibly by avoiding most solid fats and by including enough unsaturated oils (details in Chapter 5) to support health but not so much as to oversupply calories. Nuts provide unsaturated fat and protein, and people who regularly eat nuts often maintain a healthy body weight.[81] Lean meats or other low-fat protein sources also play important roles in weight loss: an ounce of lean ham contains about the same number of calories as an ounce of bread, but the ham may produce greater satiety. Sufficient protein foods may also help to preserve lean tissue, including muscle tissue, during weight loss.[82] Choose wisely, however—people with high fatty meat intakes are often overweight or obese. Remember to limit alcohol, which lowers inhibitions and can sabotage even the most committed dieter's plans.

A supplement providing vitamins and minerals may be appropriate (Controversy 7 explained how to choose one). If you plan resolutely to include all of the foods from each food group that you need each day, you will be satisfied and well nourished and will have little appetite left for high-calorie treats.

Avoid Portion Pitfalls   Pay careful attention to portion sizes—large portions increase energy intakes, and the monstrous helpings served by restaurants and sold in packages are the enemy of the person striving to control weight. Popular 100-calorie single-serving packages may be useful, but only if the food in the package fits into your calorie budget—100 calories of cookies or fried snacks are still 100 calories that can be safely eliminated. Also, eating a reduced-calorie cookie instead of an ordinary cookie saves calories—but eating half the bag defeats the purpose.

Almost every dieter needs to retrain, using measuring cups for a while to learn to judge portion sizes. Stay focused on calories and portions—don't be distracted by a product's claims. Read labels and compare *calories* per serving.

Read Menu Labels   Each meal eaten away from home increases the daily calorie intake of adults by 134 calories on average, enough to cause an average 2-pound weight gain each year or 20 pounds per decade. To provide consumers with the information they need to make more healthful choices, the FDA requires that eating establishments list the calorie contents of ready-to-eat foods, meals, and some alcoholic beverages on their menus (Figure 9–9). While it doesn't take a label to tell people whether, say, broiled, skinless chicken or battered fried chicken is more highly caloric, some differences are not so easily discernible—distinguishing between a fried chicken sandwich and a quarter-pound hamburger, for example.[83] Consumers must also take note of calorie-changing details, such as whether the calories listed on a menu are for a meal or just a sandwich; for a large or small portion size; and for an item with or without caloric add-ons such as bacon, cheese, or mayonnaise and other sauces.

Meal Spacing   Three meals a day is standard in our society, but no law says you can't have four or five—just be sure they are smaller, of course. People who eat small, frequent meals can be as successful at weight loss and maintenance as those who eat three. Also, eat regularly, before you become extremely hungry. When you do decide to eat, eat the entire meal you have planned for yourself. Then don't eat again until the next meal or snack.

Figure 9–9

New on the Menu: Calories

FDA regulations require many restaurants to list calorie amounts on their menus.

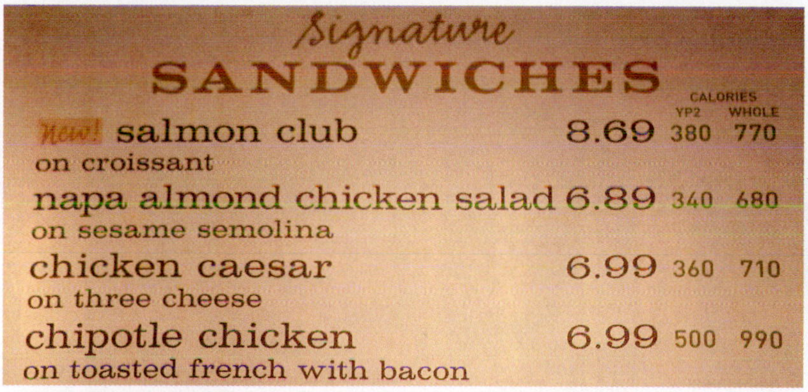

Pay close attention to snacks. Snacking among Americans has doubled in the past 30 years, and snacks provide almost a third of the empty calories from solid fats and added sugars that most people take in each day. Save calorie-free or favorite foods or beverages for a planned snack at the end of the day if you need insurance against late-evening hunger. Hungry people are likely to awaken at night to eat, a symptom of **night eating syndrome**.[84]

Choose Foods Low in Energy Density   People whose eating patterns consist mostly of foods that are high in **energy density** are more often overweight.[85] Turning this around, people who wish to be leaner and to improve their nutrient intakes would be well advised to select mostly foods of low energy density. In general, foods high in fat or low in water, such as cookies or chips, rank high in energy density; foods high in water and fiber, such as fruit and vegetables, rank lower. Foods with lower energy density often provide more food and greater satiety for the same number of calories. For example, a snack of grapes with their high water content is lower in energy density than the same weight or volume of their dehydrated counterparts (raisins). Figure 9–10 (p. 372) demonstrates this principle.

Importantly, the *energy* density of a food does not always reflect its *nutrient* density (nutrients per calorie). Beverages provide an example. The energy density of low-fat milk almost equals that of sugary soft drinks (they weigh about the same), but these beverages rank far apart in nutrient density and therefore in their contributions to nutrient needs.

Nonnutritive Sweeteners and Alcohol   Some people who maintain weight loss report using artificially sweetened beverages and fat-modified products liberally. Replacing caloric beverages with water or diet drinks may reduce most people's overall calorie intakes, and both choices are often associated with weight loss.[86] However, in one small study, young mice whose drinking water was heavily laced with the artificial sweetener saccharin experienced a change in the intestinal microbiota that may be associated with an elevated risk of diabetes.[87] Investigators are also examining the effects of artificial sweeteners on the perception of sweet taste in the brain, searching for links with weight gain.[88] In any case, soft drinks of any kind can displace milk from the diet. Milk intake is unlikely to speed weight loss, but it contributes to the health of the bones.[89]

More on artificial sweeteners in **Chapter 12**.

Alcoholic beverages can deliver hundreds of calories to drinkers each day, often without their awareness. Labels of most alcoholic beverages lack calorie amounts,

Do the Math

The energy density of a food can be calculated mathematically. Find the energy density of carrot sticks and French fries by dividing their calories by their weight in grams.

- A serving of carrot sticks, providing 31 cal and weighing 72 g:

$$\frac{31 \text{ cal}}{72 \text{ g}} = 0.43 \text{ cal/g}$$

- A serving of French fries, contributing 167 cal and weighing 50 g:

$$\frac{167 \text{ cal}}{50 \text{ g}} = 3.34 \text{ cal/g}$$

The more calories per gram (cal/g), the greater the energy density.

Now turn to Appendix A and select any food that interests you. Find its calories (ENER) and gram weight (WT) from the columns of data, and apply the formula above to determine the food's energy density in cal/g.

night eating syndrome a disturbance in the daily eating rhythm associated with obesity, characterized by more than half of the daily calories consumed after 7 p.m., frequent nighttime awakenings to eat, and a high calorie intake.

energy density a measure of the energy provided by a food relative to its weight (calories per gram).

Figure 9–10

Energy Density and Meal Size

The larger meal on the right weighs more, provides more fiber, contains more water, and takes far longer to enjoy than the meal on the left. Even foods that are lower in energy density can be overconsumed, so total calories remain important, too.

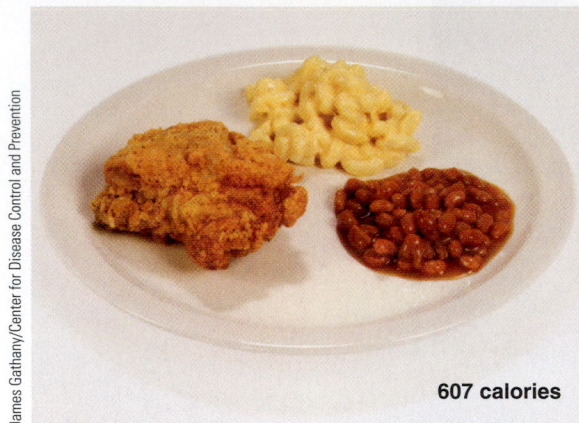

607 calories

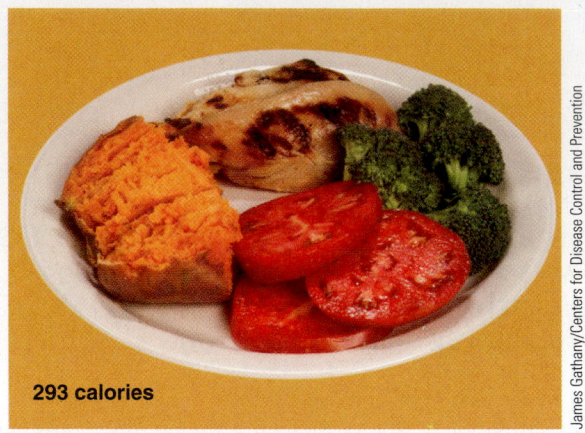

293 calories

¹/2 c macaroni and cheese
¹/2 c baked beans with pork and sauce
¹/2 fried chicken breast

$$\frac{607 \text{ calories}}{343 \text{ g total wt}} = 1.77 \text{ energy density}$$

1 c broccoli
3 large tomato slices
¹/2 large sweet potato
¹/2 skinless roasted chicken breast

$$\frac{293 \text{ calories}}{348 \text{ g total wt}} = 0.84 \text{ energy density}$$

Source: Centers for Disease Control and Prevention, Eat More, Weigh Less? How to Manage Your Weight without Being Hungry, *available at http://www.cdc.gov/nccdphp/dnpa/nutrition/pdf/Energy_Density.pdf.*

but you can find them in tables, such as Table C3–6 of Controversy 3 (p. 110). Drinkers should limit their intakes for many reasons.

Prepared Meal Plans   People who lack the time or ability to make their own low-calorie food selections or control their portion sizes may find it easier to use prepared meal plans. Although more costly than conventional foods, prepared food plans can provide low-calorie, nutritious meals or snacks to support weight loss and ease diet planning. Ideally, the plan should teach users to choose wisely from conventional foods, too, to prevent weight regain from old habits when the plan is ultimately abandoned.

KEY POINTS

- To achieve and maintain a healthy body weight, set realistic goals, keep records, eat regularly, and expect to progress slowly.
- Watch energy density, make the diet adequate and balanced, eliminate excess calories, and limit alcohol intakes.

Physical Activity in Weight Loss and Maintenance

The most successful weight losers and maintainers include physical activity in their plans. However, weight loss through physical activity alone is generally not easily achieved. Physical activity guidelines were offered in the Think Fitness feature, earlier.

Advantages of Physical Activity—and a Warning   Many people fear that exercising will increase their hunger. Active people do have healthy appetites, but a workout helps to heighten feelings of satiation during meals, as well.[90] Muscle-strengthening exercise, performed regularly, adds healthful lean body tissue and provides a trim, attractive appearance. In addition, over the long term, lean muscle tissue burns more calories pound for pound than fat does.

Weight-loss dieting triggers small losses of bone mineral density but physically active dieters may avoid some of this loss, and those who also attend to protein and calcium needs offer their bones even more protection.[91] In addition, plenty of physical activity promotes restful sleep—and getting enough sleep may reduce food consumption and weight gain. Finally, physical activity of all kinds helps to reduce stress, and stress can lead to increased eating.

Here's the warning: nonathletes spend little energy during physical activity. Exercisers who reward themselves with high-calorie treats for "good behavior" can easily negate any calorie deficits incurred.

Which Activities Are Best?

A combination of moderate-to-vigorous aerobic exercise along with strength training at a safe level seems best for health. However, some physical activity is better than none. Most important: perform at a comfortable pace within your current abilities. Rushing to improve is practically a guarantee for injury.

Active video games and active video fitness programs may help to meet the physical activity needs of people who like them, but most people lose interest in just a short while.[92] Real sports not only require more energy than their video counterparts but also hold people's interest, year after year.

Fitness also benefits from hundreds of activities required for daily living: washing the car, raking leaves, taking the stairs, and many, many others. However you do it, be active. Walk. Swim. Skate. Dance. Cycle. Skip. Lift weights. Above all, enjoy moving—and move often.

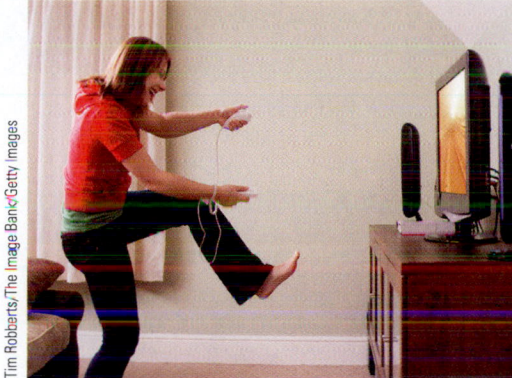

Playing an active video sports game burns some calories—but not as many as playing the actual sport.

KEY POINT

- Physical activity greatly augments weight-loss efforts.

What Strategies Are Best for Weight Gain?

Should a thin person try to gain weight? Not necessarily. If you are healthy, fit, and energetic at your present weight, stay there. However, if your physician has advised you to gain; if you are excessively tired, you are unable to keep warm, or your BMI is in the "underweight" category of the BMI table (see inside back cover); or if, for women, you have missed at least three consecutive menstrual periods, you may be in danger from being too thin. It can be as hard for a thin person to gain a pound as it is for an overweight person to lose one.

Choose Foods with High Energy Density

The weight gainer needs nutritious energy-dense foods. No matter how many sticks of celery you consume, you won't gain weight because celery simply doesn't offer enough calories per bite. Energy-dense foods (the very ones the weight-loss dieter is trying to avoid) are often high in fat, but fat energy is spent in building new tissue; if the fat is mostly unsaturated, such foods will not contribute to heart disease risk. Be sure your choices are nutritious—not just, say, candy bars and potato chips.

Because fat contains more than twice as many calories per teaspoon as sugar, its calories add up quickly without adding much bulk, and its energy is in a form that is easy for the body to store. For those without the skill or ability to create their own high-calorie foods, adding a high-protein, high-calorie liquid or bar-type dietary supplement to regular nutritious meals can sometimes help an underweight person to gain or maintain weight.

Portion Sizes and Meal Spacing

Increasing portion sizes increases calorie intakes. Choose extra slices of meats and cheeses on sandwiches; use larger plates, bowls, and glasses to disguise the appearance of the larger portions. Expect to feel full, even uncomfortably so. This feeling is normal, and it passes as the stomach gradually adapts to the extra food.

Tim Robberts/The Image Bank/Getty Images

Table 9–8

Tips for Gaining Weight

- Eat enough to store more energy than you expend—at least 500 extra calories a day.
- Exercise to build muscle.
- Be patient. Weight gain takes time (1 pound per month would be reasonable).
- Choose energy-dense foods most often.
- Eat at least three meals a day, and add snacks between meals.
- Choose large portions and expect to feel full.

Specifically:

- Drink caloric fluids—juice, chocolate milk, milkshakes, smoothies, sweet coffee drinks, sweet iced tea.
- Pair raw vegetables with rich mayonnaise dips and stuff raw celery with tuna salad (use oil-packed).
- Drizzle olive oil on cooked vegetables and salads.
- Add avocado to salads instead of cucumber, top with olives instead of pickles, and choose guacamole over salsa.
- Toast split whole-grain muffins instead of bread.
- Add whipped topping to fruit.
- Add margarine and sour cream to potatoes and creamy sauces to other vegetables.

In Addition:

- Cook and bake often—delicious cooking aromas whet the appetite.
- Invite others to the table—companionship often boosts eating.
- Make meals interesting—try new vegetables and fruit, add crunchy nuts or creamy avocado, and explore the flavors of herbs and spices.
- Keep a supply of favorite snacks, such as trail mix or granola bars, handy for grabbing.
- Control stress and relax. Enjoy your food.

Eat frequently and keep easy-to-eat foods on hand for quick meals. Make two sandwiches in the morning and eat them between classes in addition to the day's three regular meals. Include favorite foods or ethnic dishes often—the more varied and palatable, the better. Drink beverages between meals, not with them, to save space for higher-calorie foods. Always finish with dessert. Other tips for weight gain are listed in Table 9–8.

Physical Activity to Gain Muscle and Fat   Food choices alone can cause weight gain, but the gain will be mostly fat. Overly thin people need both muscle and fat, so physical activity is essential in a sound weight-gain plan. Resistance activities are best for building muscles that can help to increase healthy body mass. Start slowly and progress gradually to avoid injury. Conventional advice on diet for the person building muscle is to eat about 500 to 700 calories a day above normal energy needs; this range often supports both the added activity and the formation of new muscle. Many more facts about building muscles are provided in Chapter 10.

KEY POINTS

- Weight gain requires an eating pattern of calorie-dense foods, eaten frequently throughout the day.
- Physical activity helps to build lean tissue.

Medical Treatment of Obesity

LO 9.9   Explain the potential benefits and risks associated with obesity medications and surgeries.

People fatigued from fighting a losing battle with obesity, despite sincere efforts to diet and exercise, may be candidates for treatment with drugs or surgery. These approaches can cause dramatic weight loss and often save the lives of obese people at critical risk, but they also present serious risks of their own.

Obesity Medications

Each year, a million and a half U.S. citizens take prescription weight-loss medications. For overweight people with a BMI of greater than 30 (greater than 27 with heart disease or its risk factors), the benefits of weight loss achieved with FDA-approved prescription medications may outweigh the health risks they present (Table 9–9).[93] Importantly, weight-loss drugs can help only temporarily, while they are being taken; lifestyle changes are still necessary to help manage weight over a lifetime.

Many millions of consumers, even some who are not overweight, purchase and take over-the-counter (OTC) preparations, believing them to be effective for weight loss and safe to use. OTC weight-loss pills, powders, herbs, and other "dietary supplements" are not associated with successful weight loss however, and they may not be safe; they often present risk with no benefit. Strong prescription diuretics, hormones, unproven experimental drugs, psychotropic drugs used to treat mental illnesses, and even banned drugs have been detected in OTC weight-loss preparations, posing serious risks to health.[94]

Obesity Surgery

A person with extreme obesity—that is, someone whose BMI is greater than 40 (greater than 35 with coexisting heart disease or its risk factors)—urgently needs to reduce body fatness. Surgery is often an option for those healthy enough to withstand it.[95]

How Surgery Works   Surgical procedures limit a person's food intake by reducing the size of the stomach and delaying the passage of food into the intestine or by

Table 9-9

FDA-Approved Drugs for Weight Loss

Today's prescription weight-loss medications work by reducing appetite or reducing absorption of dietary fat.

Product	Action	Side Effects
Belviq (pronounced BELL-veek) lorcaserin hydrochloride	Stimulates brain serotonin receptors to increase satiety	Headache, dizziness, fatigue, nausea, dry mouth, and constipation; low blood glucose in people with diabetes; serotonin syndrome, including agitation, confusion, fever, loss of coordination, rapid or irregular heart rate, shivering, seizures, and unconsciousness; not for use by pregnant or lactating women or by people with heart valve problems; high doses cause hallucinations
Contrave (CON-trave)	Combines naltrexone (used to treat alcohol and drug dependence) and bupropion (an antidepressant used in smoking cessation) to suppress appetite	Nausea, constipation, headache, vomiting, dizziness, insomnia, dry mouth, and diarrhea; increased blood pressure, accelerated heart rate, suicidal thoughts, serious neuropsychiatric events, and seizures; should not be used by pregnant women or women trying to become pregnant
Orlistat (OR-leh-stat) Trade names: Alli, Xenical	Inhibits pancreatic lipase activity in the GI tract, thus blocking digestion and absorption of dietary fat and limiting energy intake	Cramping, diarrhea, gas, frequent bowel movements, and reduced absorption of fat-soluble vitamins; rare cases of liver injury
Phentermine (FEN-ter-mean), diethylpropion (DYE-eth-ill-PRO-pee-on), phendimetrazine (FEN-dye-MEH-tra-zeen)	Enhances the release of the neurotransmitter norepinephrine, which suppresses appetite	Increased blood pressure and heart rate, insomnia, nervousness, dizziness, and headache
Qsymia (kyoo-sim-EE-uh)	Combines phentermine (an appetite suppressant) and topirimate (a seizure/migrane medication) that makes food seem less appealing and increases feelings of fullness	Increased heart rate; can cause birth defects if taken in the first weeks or months of pregnancy; may worsen glaucoma or hyperthyroidism; may interact with other medications
Saxenda (sax-EN-dah)	Daily injection stimulates insulin production and the release of glucagon and suppresses appetite	Nausea, diarrhea, constipation, vomiting, low blood glucose, inflammation of the pancreas, gallbladder disease, reduced kidney function, suicidal thoughts, and increased heart rate; should not be used by people taking certain diabetes drugs

Note: Weight-loss drugs are most effective when taken as directed and used in combination with a reduced-calorie diet and increased physical activity.

reconstructing the small intestine to reduce nutrient absorption (see Figure 9–11). A new device worn outside the body delivers electrical pulses to an abdominal nerve by way of an implanted wire, affecting stomach emptying and sensations of fullness.[†††]

Potential Benefits   Surgery results can be dramatic. In studies, a great majority of surgical patients have achieved a weight loss of more than 50 percent of their excess body weight and have kept it off for 10 to 15 years.[96] Such results depend, in large part, on compliance with dietary instructions, such as choosing small portions, chewing food completely before swallowing, and drinking beverages separately from meals.

Successful surgery with weight loss often brings immediate and lasting improvements to diabetes, insulin resistance, high blood cholesterol, hypertension, heart

[†††]The Maestro system; potential drawbacks include nausea, pain, vomiting, heartburn, swallowing problems, and excessive belching.

Figure 9–11
Surgical Obesity Treatments

In gastric bypass, the surgeon constructs a small stomach pouch and creates an outlet directly to the lower small intestine. (Dark areas highlight the redirected flow of food.)

In gastric banding, the surgeon uses a gastric band to reduce the opening from the esophagus to the stomach. The size of the opening can be adjusted by inflating or deflating the band.

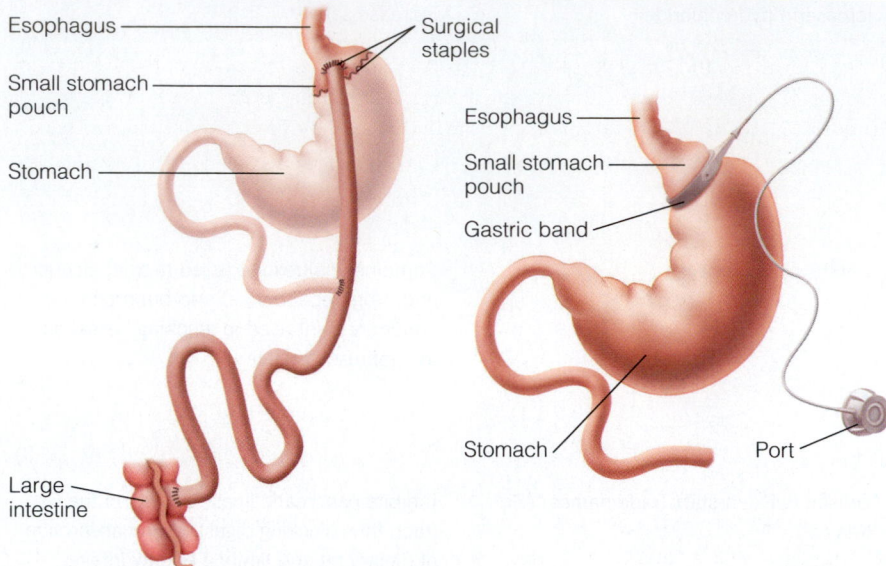

disease, and sleep apnea.[97] The surgery may also cause a shift in the makeup of the intestinal bacteria toward a profile more typically found in lean, healthy people.[98] Whether this shift may account for some of the health improvements reported after surgery is under investigation.[99]

Potential Risks   Surgery is not a sure cure for obesity, however, despite advertisements claiming so.[100] A few people do not lose the expected pounds, and some who lose weight initially regain much of it in a few years' time. Some people experience infections; nausea, vomiting, diarrhea, and dehydration; abnormal heart beats and low blood pressure; low blood glucose; confusion, flushing, sweating, weakness; and dental disease.[101]

Severe nutrient deficiencies often pose a major threat to health in the years following surgery. Vitamin D deficiency results in bone abnormalities, and vitamin A deficiency causes night blindness and other vision problems.[102] Thiamin, iron, copper, zinc, vitamin B_{12}, other B vitamins, and other deficiencies may persist for years, even in patients taking multivitamin supplements.[103] Life-long nutrition and medical supervision following surgery is a must. Time will tell whether a newly approved nonsurgical device, a removable stomach balloon, will provide the benefits of surgery with fewer risks.[104]*

KEY POINTS

- Weight-loss drugs, in tandem with diet and exercise, may be prescribed for people facing medical risks from obesity.
- For people with extreme obesity or obesity with chronic diseases, surgery may pose a lesser risk than the obesity.

Herbal Products and Gimmicks

Some herbs or **botanical** products are wildly popular and may be useful for some purposes, but wise consumers avoid products containing substances not proved safe

botanical pertaining to or made from plants; any drug, medicinal preparation, dietary supplement, or similar substance obtained from a plant.

*The ReShape Dual Balloon, approved by FDA in 2015, is placed in the stomach and filled with salt water to mimic a full stomach.

in laboratory studies. The risks are too high. Recently, for example, a previously healthy 28-year-old bodybuilder was hospitalized in a coma after taking a dietary supplement containing a known liver toxin, sold to her as a "fat burner."[105] Another harmful supplement, ephedra (also called ma huang and banned by the FDA), is sold as a weight-loss "dietary supplement" but has caused cardiac arrest, abnormal heartbeats, hypertension, strokes, seizures, and death. These and many other harmful weight-loss "supplements" remain available on Internet websites.

Also, steam baths and saunas do not melt the fat off the body as claimed, although they may dehydrate you so that you lose water weight. Brushes, sponges, wraps, creams, and massages intended to move, burn, or break up **cellulite** are useless for fat loss. Cellulite—the rumpled, dimpled, stubborn fat tissue on the thighs and buttocks—is simply fat, awaiting the body's call for energy. Such nonsense distracts people from the serious business of planning effective weight-management strategies.

KEY POINT

- The effectiveness of herbal products and other gimmicks has not been demonstrated, and they may prove hazardous.

Once I've Changed My Weight, How Can I Stay Changed?

Millions have experienced the frustration of achieving a desired change in weight only to see their hard work visibly slip away in a seemingly never-ending cycle: "I have lost 200 pounds over my lifetime, but I was never more than 20 pounds overweight." Disappointment, frustration, and self-condemnation are common in dieters who have slipped back to their original weight or even higher.

Self-Efficacy and Other Keys to Success   Contrary to popular belief, many people who set out to lose weight do so, and many maintain their losses for years. No one can yet say which of their "secrets of success" may be responsible, but the habits of those individuals are of interest to researchers and dieters alike, and they are offered in Table 9–10 (p. 378). In general, such people believe in their ability to control their weight, an attribute known as **self-efficacy**. They also monitor their intakes and body weights, quickly addressing small **lapses** to prevent major ones. They all use techniques that work for them; people's responses to any one method are highly variable.

Without a doubt, a key to weight maintenance is accepting the task as a life-long endeavor, not a goal to be achieved and forgotten. Most people who maintain weight loss continue to employ many of the routines that reduced their weight in the first place.[106] They cultivate healthy habits, they remind themselves of the continuing need to manage their weight, they monitor their weight and routine, they renew their commitment to regular physical activity, and they reward themselves for sticking with the plan.

Without a life-long plan, those who try to lose weight may become trapped in endless repeating rounds of weight loss and regain—"yo-yo" dieting. Current evidence does not support the theory that a history of such **weight cycling** impedes future weight loss efforts.[107] Weight cycling may pose a risk to the heart, however, if weight rebounds bring surges in blood pressure, blood lipids, or blood glucose.[108] The Food Feature, next, explores how a person who is ready to change can modify daily eating and exercise behaviors into healthy, life-long habits.

Seek Support   Group support can prove helpful when making life changes. Some people find it useful to join a group such as Take Off Pounds Sensibly (TOPS), Weight Watchers (WW), Overeaters Anonymous (OA), or others. Others prefer to form their own self-help groups or find support online. The Internet offers numerous opportunities for weight-loss education, counseling, and virtual group support that may be effective alternatives to face-to-face or telephone counseling programs.[109] Program applications for smartphones and other mobile devices can effectively help dieters

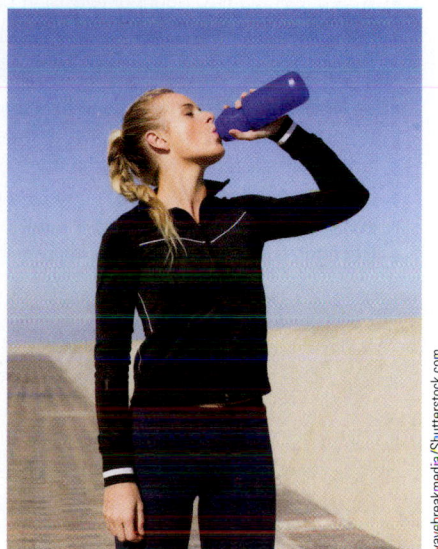

Don't forget to drink enough water—it can produce feelings of fullness, and it's calorie-free.

wavebreakmedia/Shutterstock.com

cellulite a term popularly used to describe dimpled fat tissue on the thighs and buttocks; not recognized in science.

self-efficacy a person's belief in his or her ability to succeed in an undertaking.

lapses periods of returning to old habits.

weight cycling repeated rounds of weight loss and subsequent regain that may pose health risks; also called *yo-yo dieting*.

Table 9–10

Summary of Lifestyle Strategies for Successful Weight Loss

In addition to calorie control and exercise, people who lost weight and kept it off report using strategies in the four categories listed below. No one strategy is universally useful—responses vary widely, and individualized weight-loss plans work best.

1. General

- Make a long-term commitment (greater than 6 months' duration).
- Target all three weight-management components (not just eating or exercising alone, for example).
- Monitor food intake and body weight (particularly to maintain weight loss).
- Follow a commercial weight-loss program (particularly for initial weight loss).
- Target weight management specifically rather than other worthy goals, such as disease prevention.

2. Eating Habits

- Consume a calorie-reduced diet with adequate protein, controlled in fat and carbohydrate.
- Focus on the total energy of the diet rather than on the elimination of specific energy-nutrient components.
- Consume low-fat protein sources (particularly for weight maintenance).
- Restrict intakes of types of foods (such as high-sugar foods/beverages, low-fiber foods, or high-fat restaurant foods).
- Maintain dietary routines.

3. Physical Activities

- Perform 150–250 min/week of moderate physical activity to prevent weight gain.
- Perform more than 250 min/week of moderate physical activity to promote significant weight loss.
- Exercise more—on average, an hour a day.
- Watch less than 10 hours of television per week.

4. Nutrition Counseling/Behavior Modification

- Use behavioral treatment to produce an initial weight loss of 5 to 10% of body weight.
- Use cognitive behavior therapy to augment diet and physical activities.
- Obtain structured, individualized nutrition counseling to support weight-loss efforts.
- Use Internet-based education and tracking applications, particularly in the short term.
- Weigh on a scale at least once a week.
- Recognize and attend to minor lapses.

Sources: American College of Cardiology/American Heart Association Task Force on Practice Guidelines and the Obesity Society, Executive summary: Guidelines (2013) for the management of overweight and obesity in adults, Obesity 22 (2014): S5–S39; S. F. Kirk and coauthors, Effective weight management practice: A review of the lifestyle intervention evidence, International Journal of Obesity 36 (2012): 178–185; J. M. Nicklas and coauthors, Successful weight loss among obese U.S. adults, American Journal of Preventive Medicine 42 (2012): 481–485; C. N. Sciamanna and coauthors, Practices associated with weight loss versus weight-loss maintenance, American Journal of Preventive Medicine 41 (2011): 159–166; National Weight Control Registry, available at www.nwcr.ws/Research/default.htm; J. P. Moreno and C. A. Johnston, Successful habits of weight losers, American Journal of Lifestyle Medicine 6 (2012): 113–115.

to track food intakes and physical activity and to discover calorie information. As always, choose wisely and avoid scams.[‡‡‡]

KEY POINT

- People who succeed at maintaining lost weight keep to their eating routines, keep exercising, and keep track of calorie intakes and body weight.

Conclusion

This chapter winds up where it began, considering the U.S. obesity epidemic as a societal problem. Reversing it may depend at least partly on the public will to support healthy lifestyle choices. Meanwhile, individuals can make choices to influence their own behaviors, as the Food Feature points out.

[‡‡‡]A safe, free, user-friendly, and proven program is the USDA's Super Tracker, available with smartphone applications at www.choosemyplate.gov.

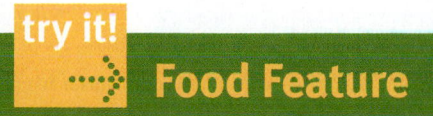
Behavior Modification for Weight Control

LO 9.10 Justify the importance of behavior modification in supporting changes in diet and exercise.

Supporting changes in both diet and exercise is **behavior modification**. This form of therapy can help the dieter to cement into place all the behaviors that lead to and perpetuate the desired body composition.

How Does Behavior Modification Work?

Behavior modification involves changing both behaviors and thought processes. It is based on the knowledge that habits drive behaviors. Suppose a friend tells you about a shortcut to class. To take it, you must make a left-hand turn at a corner where you now turn right. You decide to try the shortcut the next day, but when you arrive at the familiar corner, you turn right as always. Not until you arrive at class do you realize that you failed to turn left, as you had planned. You can learn to turn left, of course, but at first, you will have to make an effort to remember to do so. After a while, the new behavior will become as automatic as the old one was.

A food and activity diary is a powerful ally to help you learn what particular eating stimuli, or cues, affect you. Such self-monitoring is indispensable for learning to control eating and exercising cues, both positive and negative, and for tracking your progress. Figure 9–12 provides a simple pencil-and-paper food and activity diary for self-monitoring. Computerized tracking programs, such as this textbook's *Diet + Wellness Plus*, and some applications for smartphones are also effective tools.

Once you identify the behaviors you need to change, do not attempt to modify all of them at once. Set your priorities, and begin with a few behaviors you can handle—practice until they become habitual and automatic, and then select one or two more. For those striving to lose weight, learning to say "No, thank you" might be among the first habits to establish. Learning not to "clean your plate" might follow.

Modifying Behaviors

Behavior researchers have identified six elements useful in replacing old eating and activity habits with new ones:

1. Eliminate inappropriate eating and activity cues.
2. Suppress the cues you cannot eliminate.
3. Strengthen cues to appropriate eating and activities.
4. Repeat the desired eating and physical activity.
5. Arrange or emphasize negative consequences of inappropriate eating or sedentary behaviors.
6. Arrange or emphasize positive consequences of appropriate eating and exercise behaviors.

Table 9–11 provides specific examples of putting these six elements into action.

To begin, set about eliminating or suppressing the cues that prompt you to eat inappropriately. An overeater's life may include many such cues: watching television, talking on the telephone, entering a convenience store, studying

behavior modification alteration of behavior using methods based on the theory that actions can be controlled by manipulating the environmental factors that cue, or trigger, the actions.

Figure 9–12

A Sample Food and Activity Diary

Record the times and places of meals and snacks, the types and amounts of foods consumed, surroundings and people present, and mood while eating. Describe physical activities, their intensity and duration, and your feelings about them, too. Use this information to structure eating and exercise in ways that serve your physical and emotional needs.

Time	Place	Activity or food eaten	People present	Mood
10:30– 10:40	School vending machine	6 peanut butter crackers and 12 oz. cola	by myself	Starved
12:15– 12:30	Restaurant	Sub sandwich and 12 oz. cola	friends	relaxed & friendly
3:00– 3:45	Gym	Weight training	workout partner	tired
4:00– 4:10	Snack bar	Small frozen yogurt	by myself	OK

Table 9–11

Behavior Modification Tips for Weight Loss

Use these actions during both weight-loss and -maintenance phases of weight management.

1. Eliminate inappropriate eating cues:
   - Don't buy problem foods.
   - Eat only in one room at the designated time.
   - Shop when not hungry.
   - Replace large plates, cups, and utensils with smaller ones.
   - Avoid vending machines, fast-food restaurants, and convenience stores.
   - Turn off the television, video games, and computer or measure out appropriate food portions to eat during entertainment.

2. Suppress the cues you cannot eliminate:
   - Serve individual plates; don't serve "family style."
   - Measure your portions; avoid large servings or packages of food.
   - Remove food from the table after eating a meal to enjoy company and ambience without excess food to trigger overeating.
   - Create obstacles to consuming problem foods—wrap them and freeze them, making them less quickly accessible.
   - Control deprivation; plan and eat regular meals.
   - Plan to spend only one hour per day in sedentary activities, such as watching television or using a computer.

3. Strengthen cues to appropriate eating and exercise:
   - Choose to dine with companions who make appropriate food choices.
   - Store appropriate foods in convenient spots in the refrigerator.
   - Learn appropriate portion sizes.
   - Plan appropriate snacks.
   - Keep sports and play equipment by the door.

4. Repeat the desired eating and exercise behaviors:
   - Slow down eating—put down utensils between bites.[110]
   - Always use utensils.
   - Leave some food on your plate.
   - Move more—shake a leg, pace, stretch often.
   - Join groups of active people and participate.

5. Arrange or emphasize negative consequences for inappropriate eating:
   - Ask that others respond neutrally to your deviations (make no comments—even negative attention is a reward).
   - If you slip, don't punish yourself.

6. Arrange or emphasize positive consequences for appropriate eating and exercise behaviors:
   - Buy tickets to sports events, movies, concerts, or other nonfood amusement.
   - Indulge in a new small purchase.
   - Get a massage; buy some flowers.
   - Take a hot bath; read a good book.
   - Treat yourself to a lesson in a new active pursuit such as horseback riding, handball, or tennis.
   - Praise yourself; visit friends.
   - Nap; relax.

cognitive skills as taught in behavior therapy, changes to conscious thoughts with the goal of improving adherence to lifestyle modifications; examples are problem-solving skills and the correction of false negative thoughts, termed *cognitive restructuring*.

cues, and reward yourself for doing so. Some possible activities and rewards to substitute for eating include:

- Attending or participating in sporting events.
- Enjoying leisure activities, card games, or a favorite television show.
- Exercising your muscles at a gym.
- Gardening or indulging in other crafts or hobbies.
- Going to a movie or play.
- Listening to music.
- Napping, reading, relaxing.
- Praising yourself.
- Sprucing up your room or house.
- Taking a bubble bath.
- Telephoning, texting, or e-mailing.
- Vacationing, even for an hour or two in a neighboring town or area.
- Volunteering.
- Window shopping; taking a walk.

The list of possibilities is virtually endless.

In addition, be aware that the food marketing industry spends huge sums each year developing cues to modify consumers' behaviors in the opposite direction—toward buying and consuming more snack foods, soft drinks, and other products. These cues work on a subconscious level; they leverage the stronger human hunger and appetite mechanisms to overcome the weaker satiety signals.

Cognitive Skills

Behavior therapists often teach **cognitive skills**, or new ways of thinking, to help dieters solve problems and correct false thinking that can short-circuit healthy eating behaviors. Thinking habits turn out to be as important as eating habits to achieving a healthy body weight, and thinking habits can be changed.[111][§§§] A paradox of making a change is that it takes believing in oneself and honoring oneself to lay the foundation for changing that self. That is, self-acceptance predicts success, while self-loathing predicts failure. "Positive self-talk" is a concept worth cultivating—many people

late at night. Resolve that you will no longer respond to such cues by eating. If some cues to inappropriate eating behavior cannot be eliminated, suppress them; then strengthen the appropriate

§§§Psychologists have a term for changing thinking habits: cognitive restructuring.

succeed because their mental dialogue supports, rather than degrades, their efforts. Negative thoughts ("I'm not getting thin anyway, so what's the use of continuing?") should be viewed in the light of empirical evidence ("my starting weight: 174 pounds; today's weight: 163 pounds").

Give yourself credit for your new behaviors; take honest stock of any physical improvements, too, such as lower blood pressure or less painful knees, even without a noticeable change in pant size. Finally, remember to enjoy your emerging fit and healthy self.

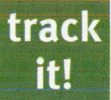 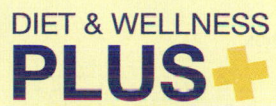

track it! DIET & WELLNESS PLUS+ Concepts in Action

Analyze Your Energy Balance

The purpose of this exercise is to help you to evaluate correlations among your nutrition, physical activity, and body weight.

1. Your calorie intake represents the "energy in" part of your energy balance. From the Reports Tab, select Energy Balance, choose Day One of your three-day diet intake, include all meals. Select Save as PDF. How does your calorie (kCal) intake for the day compare with the DRI energy recommendation for the reference man or woman of your age, as listed on the inside front cover of the text?

2. Energy balance is affected not just by food eaten but also by energy expended. Compare the effects of two levels of activity on your energy balance. You've already generated an Energy Balance report for Day One. Select the Track Activity tab, and add a new 30-minute activity for Day One.

   Look at the list of activities in Table 9–4 (p. 360) for suggestions. Select Energy Balance and compare with the reports with and without the added activity. What changes do you see?

3. If you want to lose body fat, you must expend more energy than you take in. Look over your food diaries. Is there a day that you were in positive energy balance (took in more energy than you used)? If so, develop a revised food record for that day with the goal of reducing calories but still maintaining a wholesome and satisfying diet. Now select the Energy Balance tab to evaluate the revised meal plan.

Did you succeed in trimming calories but still consume the recommended nutrients? How many calories did you trim?

4. All three energy-yielding nutrients can contribute excess calories, but fat is the least satiating, most highly caloric per gram, and most easily consumed without awareness. From the Reports tab, select Source Analysis and then Total Fat from the drop-down box. Evaluate your daily food records for total fat. Then choose the day that contained the most fat in grams or the highest percentage of calories from fat. Find the foods that contributed the most fat to your intake. What would you say led to higher intake of fat on that day, as compared to another? Which part of the day did you consume the most fat? Were you aware that you were doing so?

what did you decide?

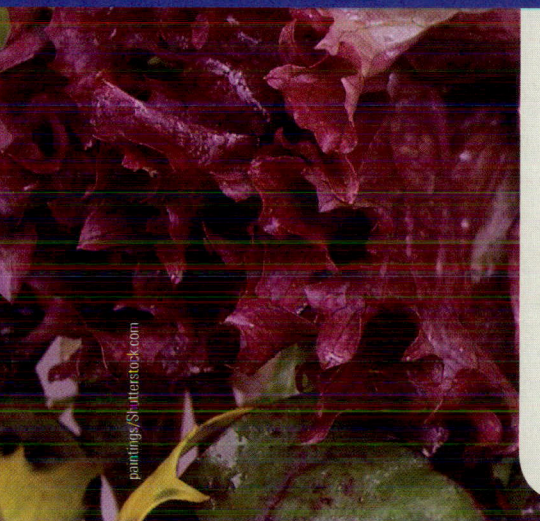

How can you **control** your body weight, once and for all?

Why are you **tempted** by a favorite treat when you don't feel hungry?

How do extra calories from food become **fat** in your body?

Which popular **diets** are best for managing body weight?

Self Check

1. (LO 9.1) All of the following are health risks associated with excessive body fat except _____.
   a. respiratory problems
   b. sleep apnea
   c. gallbladder disease
   d. low blood lipids

2. (LO 9.1) Today, an estimated 69 percent of the adults in the United States are overweight or obese.
   T   F

3. (LO 9.2) Which of the following statements about basal metabolic rate (BMR) is correct?
   a. The greater a person's age, the higher the BMR.
   b. The more thyroxine produced, the higher the BMR.
   c. Fever lowers the BMR.
   d. Pregnancy lowers the BMR.

4. (LO 9.2) The thermic effect of food plays a major role in energy expenditure.
   T   F

5. (LO 9.3) The BMI standard is an excellent tool for evaluating obesity in athletes and the elderly.
   T   F

6. (LO 9.3) Body fat can be assessed by which of the following techniques?
   a. a blood lipid test
   b. chest circumference
   c. dual energy X-ray absorptiometry
   d. all of the above

7. (LO 9.3) BMI is of limited value for
   a. athletes.
   b. pregnant and lactating women.
   c. adults older than age 65.
   d. all of the above.

8. (LO 9.4) The appetite-stimulating hormone ghrelin is made by the _____.
   a. brain
   b. fat tissue
   c. pancreas
   d. stomach

9. (LO 9.4) When the brain receives signals that enough food has been eaten, this is called _____.
   a. satiation
   b. ghrelin
   c. adaptation
   d. none of the above

10. (LO 9.5) Brown adipose tissue _____.
    a. develops during starvation
    b. is a well-known heat-generating tissue
    c. develops as fat cells die off
    d. all of the above

11. (LO 9.5) According to genomic researchers, a single inherited gene is the probable cause of common obesity.
    T   F

12. (LO 9.6) In many people, any kind of stress can cause overeating and weight gain.
    T   F

13. (LO 9.6) A built environment can support physical activity with
    a. safe biking and walking lanes.
    b. public parks.
    c. free exercise facilities.
    d. all of the above.

14. (LO 9.7) Which of the following is a physical consequence of fasting?
    a. loss of lean body tissues
    b. lasting weight loss
    c. body cleansing
    d. all of the above

15. (LO 9.7) The nervous system cannot use fat as fuel.
    T   F

16. (LO 9.7) A diet too low in carbohydrate brings about responses that are similar to fasting.
    T   F

17. (LO 9.8) Efforts in all of the following realms are necessary for weight change:
    a. eating patterns, physical activity, and behavior modification
    b. eating patterns, physical activity, and carbohydrate control
    c. carbohydrate control, physical activity, and behavior modification
    d. eating patterns, physical activity, and psychotherapy

18. (LO 9.8) The number of calories to cut from the diet to produce weight loss should be based on
    a. the amount of weight the person wishes to lose.
    b. the person's BMI.
    c. the amount of food the person wishes to consume.
    d. the RDA for energy for the person's gender and age.

19. (LO 9.9) Over-the-counter drugs for obesity are most often effective and pose little risk.
    T   F

20. (LO 9.10) Most people who successfully maintain weight loss do all of the following except
    a. continue to employ many of the routines that reduced their weight in the first place.
    b. obtain at least some guidance from popular diet books.
    c. reward themselves for sticking with their plan.
    d. monitor their weight and routine.

21. (LO 9.11) Adolescents are likely to grow out of early disordered eating behaviors by young adulthood.
    T   F

Answers to these Self Check questions are in Appendix G.

The Perils of Eating Disorders

LO 9.11 Outline the risk factors, symptoms, and treatments of eating disorders.

Up to 24 million people in the United States, many of them girls and women, suffer from some form of **eating disorder**, including **anorexia nervosa**, **bulimia nervosa**, and **binge eating disorders** or related conditions.[1]* Without treatment, one in ten of those who have an eating disorder will die as a result, and most others will incur physical and mental harm. Most alarming, the prevalence of eating disorders is both rising and occurring at progressively younger ages.[2] (Table C9–1 defines eating disorder terms.)

An estimated 85 percent of eating disorders start during adolescence. Children of this age often exhibit warnings of disordered eating such as restrained eating, binge eating, purging, fear of fatness, and distorted body image. Many adolescents diet to lose weight and choose unhealthy behaviors associated with disordered eating; by college age, the behaviors can be entrenched.[3]

Disordered eating behaviors in early life set a pattern that is likely to continue into young adulthood. Importantly, healthful dieting and physical activity in overweight adolescents do not appear to trigger eating disorders.

Society's Influence

Why do so many people in our society suffer from eating disorders? Most experts agree that eating disorders have many causes: sociocultural, psychological, hereditary, and possibly also genetic and neurochemical.[4] However, excessive pressure to be thin in our society is at least partly to blame. Normal-weight girls as young as 5 years old are placed "on diets" for fear that they are too fat.

When thinness takes on heightened importance, people begin to view the normal, healthy body as too fat—their body images become distorted. People of all shapes, sizes, and ages—including

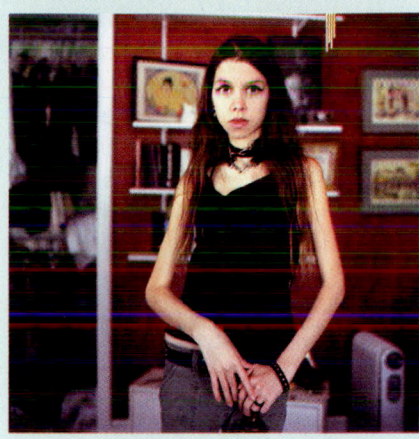

© Christopher LaMarca/Redux Pictures

emaciated fashion models with anorexia nervosa—have learned to be unhappy with their "overweight" bodies. Many take serious risks to lose weight. Once almost nonexistent in non-Western cultures, eating disorders are rapidly increasing as global communities internalize thinness as an ideal.[5]

Media Messages

No doubt our society sets unrealistic ideals and devalues those who do not conform to them. The Miss America beauty pageant, for example, puts forth a standard of female desirability—thinner and thinner women over the years have won the crown. Magazines, Facebook and other social websites, films and television, and other media convey a message that to be happy, beautiful, and desirable, one must first be thin.[6] In their quest for identity, adolescent girls are particularly vulnerable to such messages.

Dieting as Risk

Severe food restriction often precedes an eating disorder. Ill-advised "dieting" can create intense stress and extreme hunger that lead to binges. Painful emotions such as anger, jealousy, or disappointment may be turned inward by youngsters,

---

Table C9–1

Eating Disorder Terms

- **anorexia nervosa** an eating disorder characterized by a refusal to maintain a minimally normal body weight, self-starvation to the extreme, and a disturbed perception of body weight and shape; seen (usually) in teenage girls and young women (anorexia means "without appetite"; nervos means "of nervous origin").
- **binge eating disorder** an eating disorder whose criteria are similar to those of bulimia nervosa, excluding purging or other compensatory behaviors.
- **bulimia** (byoo-LEEM-ee-uh) **nervosa** recurring episodes of binge eating combined with a morbid fear of becoming fat; usually followed by self-induced vomiting or purging.
- **cathartic** a strong laxative.
- **cognitive behavioral therapy** psychological therapy aimed at changing undesirable behaviors by changing underlying thought processes contributing to these behaviors; in anorexia, a goal is to replace false beliefs about body weight, eating, and self-worth with health-promoting beliefs.
- **eating disorder** a disturbance in eating behavior that jeopardizes a person's physical or psychological health.
- **emetic** (em-ETT-ic) an agent that causes vomiting.
- **female athlete triad** a potentially fatal triad of medical problems seen in female athletes: disordered eating, menstrual cessation, and osteoporosis.

*Reference notes are found in Appendix F.

---

some still in kindergarten, who express dissatisfaction with body weight or say they "feel fat." As weight loss and severe food restraint become more and more a focus, psychological problems worsen, and the likelihood of developing full-blown eating disorders intensifies.

Eating Disorders in Athletes

Athletes and dancers are at special risk for eating disorders.[7] They may severely restrict energy intakes in an attempt to enhance performance or appearance or to meet the weight guidelines of a sport. In reality, severe energy restriction causes a loss of lean tissue that impairs physical performance and imposes a risk of eating disorders. Risk factors for eating disorders among athletes include:

- Young age (adolescence).
- Pressure to excel in a sport.
- Focus on achieving or maintaining an "ideal" body weight, muscular structure, or body fat percentage.
- Participation in sports or competitions that emphasize a lean appearance or judge performance on aesthetic appeal, such as gymnastics, wrestling, figure skating, or dance.[8]
- Unhealthy, unsupervised weight-loss dieting at an early age.

Male athletes—especially dancers, wrestlers, skaters, jockeys, and gymnasts—suffer from eating disorders at a greater rate than their peers, but their gender may cause coaches, parents, and medical professionals to overlook their condition. Adolescent boys, newly aware of developing muscularity, may take dangerous risks involving enhancement products and extreme diets in their quest to attain unachievable physiques.[9]

The Female Athlete Triad

In female athletes, three associated medical problems form the **female athlete triad**: disordered eating (with or without a diagnosed eating disorder), amenorrhea (cessation of menstruation), and osteoporosis.[10] For example, at age 14, Suzanne was a

top contender for a spot on the state gymnastics team. Each day, her coach reminded team members that they would not qualify to compete if they weighed more than a few ounces above the assigned weights.

Suzanne weighed herself several times a day to ensure that she did not top her 80-pound limit. She dieted and exercised to extremes; unlike many of her friends, she never began to menstruate. A few months before her 15th birthday, Suzanne's coach dropped her back to the second-level team because of a slow-healing stress fracture. Mentally and physically exhausted, she quit gymnastics and began overeating between periods of self-starvation. Suzanne exhibited all the signs of female athlete triad—disordered eating, amenorrhea, and weakened bones—but no one put them together in time to protect her physical and mental health.

An athlete's body must be heavier for a given height than a nonathlete's body because it contains more muscle and dense bone tissue with less fat. However, coaches often use weight standards, such as BMI, that cannot properly assess an athlete's body. For athletes, body composition measures such as skinfold tests yield more useful information.

The prevalence of amenorrhea among premenopausal women in the United States is about 2 to 5 percent overall, but it may be well

over 60 percent among female athletes. Amenorrhea is *not* a normal adaptation to strenuous physical training but a symptom of something going wrong. (see Figure C9–1).[11]

Male Athletes and Eating Disorders

Male athletes and dancers with eating disorders often deny having them because they mistakenly believe that eating disorders strike only women. Under the same pressures as female athletes, males skip meals, restrict fluids, practice in plastic suits, or train in heated rooms to lose a quick 4 to 7 pounds. Many male high school wrestlers, gymnasts, and figure skaters strive for as little as 5 percent body fat. Wrestlers, especially, must "make weight" to compete in the lowest possible weight class to face smaller opponents.

For young people, unrealistic standards based on appearance, weight, or body type should be replaced with performance-based standards. Table C9–2 provides some suggestions to help athletes and dancers protect themselves against eating disorders.

The next sections describe some categories of eating disorders. In many cases, however, these categories overlap; a person may migrate from type to type, or an eating disorder may fail to fall into a clear pattern. Three main

Figure C9–1

The Female Athlete Triad

In the female athlete triad, extreme weight loss causes both cessation of menstruation (amenorrhea) and excessive loss of calcium from the bones, weakening them.

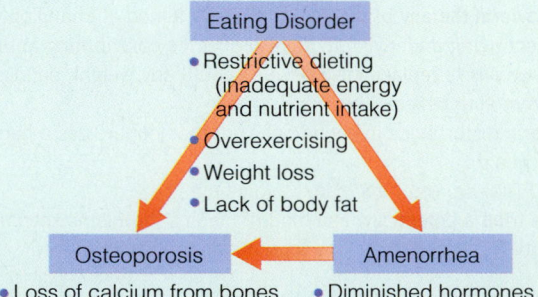

Table C9–2

Tips for Combating Eating Disorders

General Guidelines

- Never restrict food intakes to below the amounts suggested for adequacy by the USDA Eating Patterns (Chapter 2).
- Eat regularly. The person who eats regularly throughout the day never gets so hungry as to allow hunger to dictate food choices.
- If not at a healthy weight, establish a reasonable weight goal based on a healthy body composition.
- Allow a reasonable time to achieve the goal. A reasonable rate for losing excess fat is about 1% of body weight per week.
- Learn to recognize media image biases, and reject ultrathin standards for beauty. Shift focus to health, competencies, and human interactions; bring behaviors in line with those beliefs.

Specific Guidelines for Athletes and Dancers

- Replace weight-based or appearance-based goals with performance-based goals.
- Remember that eating disorders impair physical performance. Seek confidential help in obtaining treatment if needed.
- Restrict weight-loss activities to the off-season.
- Focus on proper nutrition as an important facet of your training, as important as proper technique.

characteristics of eating disorders have been described:

1. Eating habits or weight-control behaviors have become abnormal.
2. Clinically significant impairment of physical health or psychosocial functioning materializes.
3. The disturbance is not caused by other medical or psychiatric conditions.

The problems described in the next section are typical.

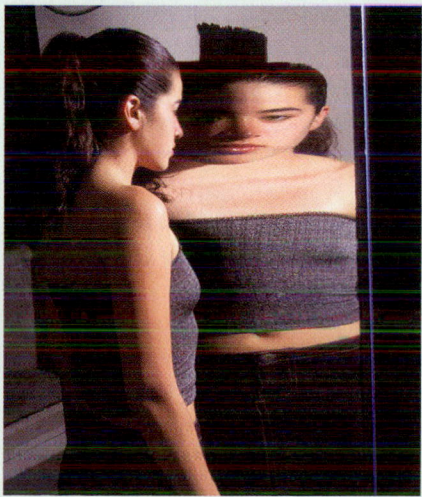

People with anorexia nervosa see themselves as fat, even when they are dangerously underweight.

Tony Freeman/PhotoEdit

Anorexia Nervosa

Julie is 17 years old and a straight-A superachiever in school. She also watches her diet with great care, and she exercises daily, maintaining a heroic schedule of self-discipline. She stands 5 feet 6 inches tall and weighs only 85 pounds, but she is determined to lose weight. She has anorexia nervosa.

Characteristics of Anorexia Nervosa

Julie is unaware that she is undernourished, and she sees no need to obtain treatment. She insists that she is too fat, although her eyes are sunk in deep hollows in her face. She visits pro-anorexia (pro-ana) blogs and websites to find support for her distorted body image and to learn more starvation tips. When Julie looks at herself in the mirror, she sees her 85-pound body as fat. The more Julie overestimates her body size, the more resistant she is to treatment and the more unwilling she is to examine misperceptions.

She stopped menstruating and is moody and chronically depressed but blames external circumstances. She is close to physical exhaustion, but she no longer sleeps easily. Her family is concerned, and although reluctant to push

her, they have finally insisted that she see a psychiatrist. Julie's psychiatrist has prescribed group therapy as a start but warns that if Julie does not begin to gain weight soon, she will need to be hospitalized.

No one knows for certain what causes anorexia nervosa, but some influences are associated with its development. Most people with anorexia nervosa come from middle- or upper-class families. Most are female. People with anorexia nervosa are unaware of their condition. They cannot recognize that a distorted body image that overestimates body fatness, a central feature of a diagnosis, is causing the problem. Some general criteria are proposed by the American Psychiatric Association. The entire list is available on the Internet, but, in plain language, they focus on people who:

- Restrict calorie intake to the point of developing a too-low body weight for age, gender, and health.
- Have an intense fear of body fatness or of weight gain, or who strive to prevent weight gain although underweight.
- Hold a false perception of body weight or shape, exaggerate the importance of body weight or shape in their self-evaluation, or deny the danger of being severely underweight.[12]

Many details on diagnostic criteria exist.[13]

Self-Starvation

How can a person as thin as Julie continue to starve herself? Julie uses tremendous discipline to strictly limit her portions of low-calorie foods. She will deny her hunger, and having become accustomed to so little food, she feels full after eating only a few bites. She can recite the calorie contents of dozens of foods and the calorie costs of as many physical activities. If she feels that she has gained an ounce of weight, she runs or jumps rope until she thinks it's gone. She drinks water incessantly to fill her stomach, risking dangerous mineral imbalances and water intoxication. She takes laxatives to hasten the passage of food from her system. She is starving, but she doesn't eat because her need for self-control outweighs her need for food.

Physical Perils

From the body's point of view, anorexia nervosa is starvation and thus brings the same damage as classic severe malnutrition. The person with anorexia depletes the body tissues of needed fat and protein. In young people, their growth ceases, their normal development falters, and they lose so much lean tissue that their basal metabolic rate slows. Bones weaken, too—low bone density develops in adults and adolescents, male and female, with anorexia nervosa.[14]

Internal organs suffer as nutrient status declines. The heart pumps inefficiently and irregularly, the heart muscle becomes weak and thin, the heart chambers diminish in size, and the blood pressure falls. As iron diminishes, anemia ensues, and the heart struggles to pump oxygen to the tissues. Potassium and other electrolytes that help to regulate the heartbeat go out of balance. Many deaths in people with anorexia nervosa are due to heart failure. Kidneys often fail as well.[15]

Starvation also brings neurological and digestive consequences. The brain loses significant amounts of tissue, nerves cannot function normally, the electrical activity of the brain becomes abnormal, and insomnia is common. Digestive functioning becomes sluggish, the stomach empties slowly, and the absorptive lining of the intestinal tract shrinks, reducing absorption of the small amount of food consumed. The pancreas slows its production of digestive enzymes. Diarrhea sets in, further worsening malnutrition.

In addition to anemia, blood changes include impaired immune response, altered blood lipids, high concentrations of vitamin A and vitamin E, and low blood proteins. Vitamin D deficiencies and other deficiency diseases often develop.[16] Dry skin, low body temperature, and the growth of fine body hair (the body's attempt to keep warm) also occur. In adulthood, both women and men lose their sex drives. Mothers with anorexia nervosa may severely underfeed their children, who then fail to thrive or who develop disordered eating patterns later on.[17]

Anorexia nervosa has the highest mortality rate of all psychiatric disorders.

People with anorexia nervosa are 5 times more likely than their peers to die prematurely, mostly from heart abnormalities brought on by malnutrition.[18] They are also 18 times more likely to die of suicide.

Treatment of Anorexia Nervosa

Treatment of anorexia nervosa requires a multidisciplinary approach that addresses two areas of concern: the first relating to food and weight and the second involving psychological processes. Teams of physicians, nurses, psychiatrists, family therapists, and dietitians work together to treat people with anorexia nervosa. The expertise of a registered dietitian nutritionist is essential because an appropriate, individually crafted diet is crucial for normalizing body weight and because nutrition counseling is indispensable.[19]

Professionals classify clients based on the risks posed by the degree of malnutrition present.[‡] Clients with low risks may benefit from family counseling, **cognitive behavioral therapy**, other psychotherapies and nutrition guidance.[20] Those with greater risks may also need supplemental formulas to provide extra nutrients and energy. Antidepressant and other drugs are commonly prescribed but rarely help.

Clients in later stages are seldom willing to eat, but if they are, chances are they can recover without other interventions. Sometimes, intensive behavior management treatment in a live-in facility helps to normalize food intake and exercise. When starvation leads to severe underweight (less than 75 percent of ideal body weight), high medical risks ensue, and patients require hospitalization. They must be stabilized and fed through a tube to forestall death.[21] Even after recovery, however, energy intakes and eating behaviors may never fully return to normal, and relapses are exceedingly common.[22]

Before drawing conclusions about someone who is extremely thin, be aware that a diagnosis of anorexia nervosa requires professional assessment. People

seeking help for anorexia nervosa for themselves or for others should not delay but should visit the National Eating Disorders Association website or call them.[§]

Bulimia Nervosa

Sophia is a 20-year-old flight attendant, and although her body weight is healthy, she thinks constantly about food. She alternately starves herself and then secretly binges; when she has eaten too much, she vomits. Few people would fail to recognize that these symptoms signify bulimia nervosa.

Characteristics of Bulimia Nervosa

Bulimia nervosa is distinct from anorexia nervosa and is much more prevalent, although the true incidence is difficult to establish. People with bulimia nervosa often suffer in secret and, when asked, may deny the existence of a problem. More men suffer from bulimia nervosa than from anorexia nervosa, but bulimia nervosa is still more common in women. Here are some general proposed diagnostic criteria for bulimia nervosa:

- Binge eating behavior—that is, eating a relatively large amount of food in a relatively short period of time.
- An experience of loss of control during binges and compensation behaviors afterwards, such as vomiting or fasting.
- Frequent binges and compensations (at least once a week for three months).
- False perceptions of body weight or shape; exaggerations of the importance of body weight or shape in self-evaluation.[23]

Sophia is well educated and close to her ideal body weight, although her weight fluctuates over a range of 10 pounds or so every few weeks. As a young teen, Sophia cycled on and off crash diets.

Sophia seldom lets her bulimia nervosa interfere with her work or other activities. However, she is emotionally insecure, feels anxious at social events, and cannot easily establish close relationships.

[‡] Indicators of malnutrition include a low percentage of body fat, low blood proteins, and impaired immune response.

[§] The National Eating Disorders website address is www.nationaleatingdisorders.org; the toll-free referral line is (800) 931–2237.

She is usually depressed and often impulsive. When crisis hits, Sophia responds with an overwhelming urge to eat.[24]

The Role of the Family

Families are not thought to cause eating disorders, but if family members are emotionally unsupportive, they can worsen the negative self-image believed to perpetuate bulimia and make recovery more difficult (see Figure C9–2). Dieting, arguments, criticism of body shape or weight, and economic hardships commonly arise in families of people with bulimia, and a sensitive child may react with anxiety and self-doubt.[25] Effective treatment plans, particularly for children and adolescents, begin with family counseling to reduce blame and empower caregivers to help their family member recover.[26]

Binge Eating and Purging

A bulimic binge is unlike normal eating. During a binge, Sophia's eating is accelerated by her hunger from previous calorie restriction. She regularly takes in extra food approaching 1,000 calories at each binge, and she may have several binges in a day. Typical binge foods are easy-to-eat, low-fiber, smooth-textured, high-fat, and high-carbohydrate foods, such as cookies, cakes, and ice cream; and she eats the entire bag of cookies, the whole cake, and every spoonful in a carton of ice cream. By the end of the binge, she has vastly overcorrected for her earlier attempts at calorie restriction.

The binge is a compulsion and usually occurs in several stages: anticipation and planning, anxiety, urgency to begin, rapid and uncontrollable consumption of food, relief and relaxation, disappointment, and finally shame or disgust. Then, to purge the food from her body, she may use a **cathartic**—a strong laxative that can injure the lower intestinal tract. Or she may induce vomiting, sometimes with an **emetic**—a drug intended as first aid for poisoning. After the binge, she pays the price with hands scraped raw against the teeth during gag-induced vomiting, swollen neck glands and reddened eyes from straining to vomit, and the bloating, fatigue, headache, nausea, and pain that follow.

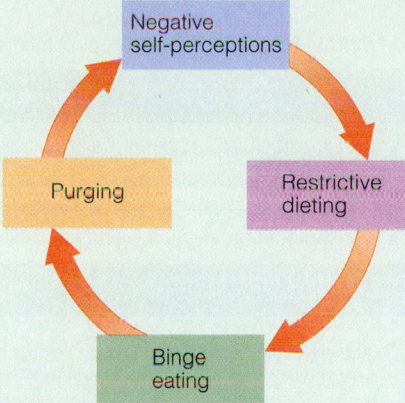

Figure C9–2

The Cycle of Bingeing, Purging, and Negative Self-Perception

Each of these factors helps to perpetuate disordered eating.

Negative self-perceptions → Restrictive dieting → Binge eating → Purging → (Negative self-perceptions)

Physical and Psychological Perils

Purging may seem to offer a quick way to rid the body of unwanted calories, but bingeing and purging have serious physical consequences. Fluid and electrolyte imbalances caused by vomiting or diarrhea can lead to abnormal heart rhythms; one common emetic causes heart muscle damage, and its overuse can cause death from heart failure.[27]** Urinary tract infections can lead to kidney failure. Vomiting causes irritation and infection of the pharynx, esophagus, and salivary glands; erosion of the teeth; and dental caries. The esophagus or stomach may rupture or tear.

****The heart-damaging emetic is ipecac (IP-eh-kak).*

Unlike Julie, Sophia is aware that her behavior is abnormal, and she is deeply ashamed of it. She wants to recover, and this makes recovery more likely for her than for Julie, who clings to denial.

Treatment of Bulimia Nervosa

To gain control over food and establish regular eating patterns requires adherence to a structured eating and exercise plan. Restrictive dieting is forbidden, for it almost always precedes binges. Steady maintenance of weight and prevention of cyclic gains and losses are the goals. Many a former bulimia nervosa sufferer has taken a major step toward recovery by learning to consistently eat enough food to satisfy hunger (at least 1,600 calories a day).

Table C9–3 offers some ways to begin correcting the eating problems of bulimia nervosa. About half of women receiving a diagnosis of bulimia nervosa may recover completely after 5 to 10 years, with or without professional treatment, although treatment or self-help programs probably speed recovery.

Binge Eating Disorder

Charlie is a 40-year-old former baseball outfielder who, after becoming a spectator instead of a player, has gained excess body fat and has been diagnosed with prediabetes.[28] He believes that he has the willpower to diet until he loses the fat. Periodically, he restricts his food intake for several days, only to eventually succumb to cravings for his favorite high-calorie treats. Like Charlie, many overweight people end up bingeing after dieting.

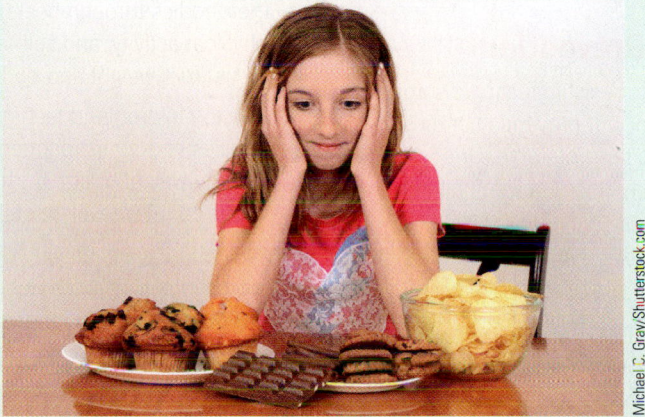

A typical binge consists of easy-to-eat, low-fiber, smooth-textured, high-calorie foods.

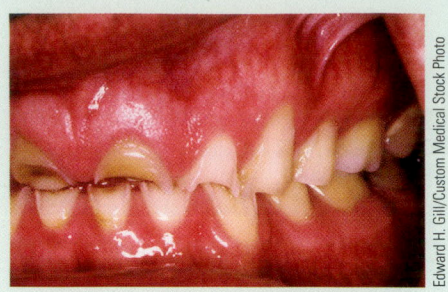

Tooth damage from stomach acid in bulimia nervosa.

Is Binge Eating an Addiction?

A correlation between the addictive nature of binge eating and that of drug abuse has been discussed for decades.[29] Shared key characteristics, such as strong and persistent cravings, unsuccessful efforts to control intakes, and continuation of the behavior despite physical harm or other negative results, give rise to the concept of an *eating addiction*.[30][††] As explained earlier in this chapter, the effects on the brain of foods rich in sugars and fats mimic those of euphoria-producing drugs in some ways, and similarities exist in psychological and behavioral constructs, too.[31] Although in its early stages, research on the shared features of substance abuse and eating disorders may uncover new treatments for both conditions.[32]

Treating Binge Eating

Binge eating behavior responds more readily to treatment than other eating disorders. Intervention, even if obtained on an Internet website, improves physical and mental health and may permanently break the cycle of rapid weight losses and gains.

Toward Prevention

Treatments for existing eating disorders have evolved, but prevention of these conditions is far preferable. One approach may be to provide children and adolescents with defenses against influences that promote eating disorders. A set of suggestions intended to help pediatricians avert eating disorders in their patients might also apply to

[††] *The* Diagnostic and Statistical Manual, *5th edition, sets diagnostic criteria for substance use disorders. The Yale Food Addiction Scale, an inventory based on substance use criteria, is under review as a potential diagnostic tool for food addiction.*

Table C9–3

Diet Strategies for Combating Bulimia Nervosa

Planning Principles

- Plan meals and snacks; record plans in a food diary prior to eating.
- Plan meals and snacks that require eating at the table and using utensils.
- Refrain from eating "finger foods."
- Refrain from "dieting" or skipping meals.

Nutrition Principles

- Eat a well-balanced diet and regularly timed meals consisting of a variety of foods.
- Include raw vegetables, salad, or raw fruit at meals to prolong eating times.
- Choose whole-grain, high-fiber breads, pasta, rice, and cereals to increase bulk.
- Consume adequate fluid, particularly water.

Other Tips

- Choose meals that provide protein and fat for satiety and bulky, fiber-rich carbohydrates for immediate feelings of fullness.
- Try including soups and other water-rich foods for satiety (water contents of foods are listed in Appendix A).
- Consume the amounts of food specified in the USDA Eating Patterns (Chapter 2).
- Select foods that naturally divide into portions. Select one potato, rather than rice or pasta that can be overloaded onto the plate; purchase yogurt and cottage cheese in individual containers; look for small packages of precut steak or chicken; choose frozen dinners with metered portions.
- Include 30 minutes or more of physical activity on most days—exercise may be an important tool in controlling bulimia.

teachers, coaches, and others who deal with children:

1. Encourage positive eating and physical behaviors that can be maintained over a lifetime; discourage unhealthy dieting.

2. Promote a positive body image; do not use body dissatisfaction as a motivator for behavior change.

3. Encourage frequent and enjoyable family meals consumed at home; discourage hasty meals eaten alone.

4. Help children and teens to nurture their bodies through healthy eating, physical activity, and self-talk; divert focus from weight and body shape.

5. Talk to children and teens and their families about mistreatment because of body weight or size; assume it has occurred in overweight children.

Protection against eating disorders in the next generation largely depends on the actions of adults in authority today. Perhaps a young person's best defense against eating disorders is to learn about normal, expected growth patterns, especially the characteristic weight gain of adolescence (see Chapter 14), and to learn respect for

the inherent wisdom of the body. When people discover and honor the body's real needs for nutrition and exercise, they often will not sacrifice health for conformity.

Critical Thinking

1. Eating disorders are common only in cultures where extreme thinness is an ideal. Who in society do you think sets such ideals? How are these ideals conveyed to others? Suggest some steps that schools, parents, and other influential adults might take to help to minimize the impact of idealized body types on children as they develop their own self-images.

2. Form a small group. Each member of the group gives an example of a role model that he or she would like to emulate. This can be, for example, a teacher, athlete, movie star, or scientist, among others. State all of the reasons for choosing this person as a role model. Now talk about the body type of each role model. Would you like to achieve that body type? Is it possible to do so? Of all the role models discussed in your group, which role model do you believe is the healthiest and why?

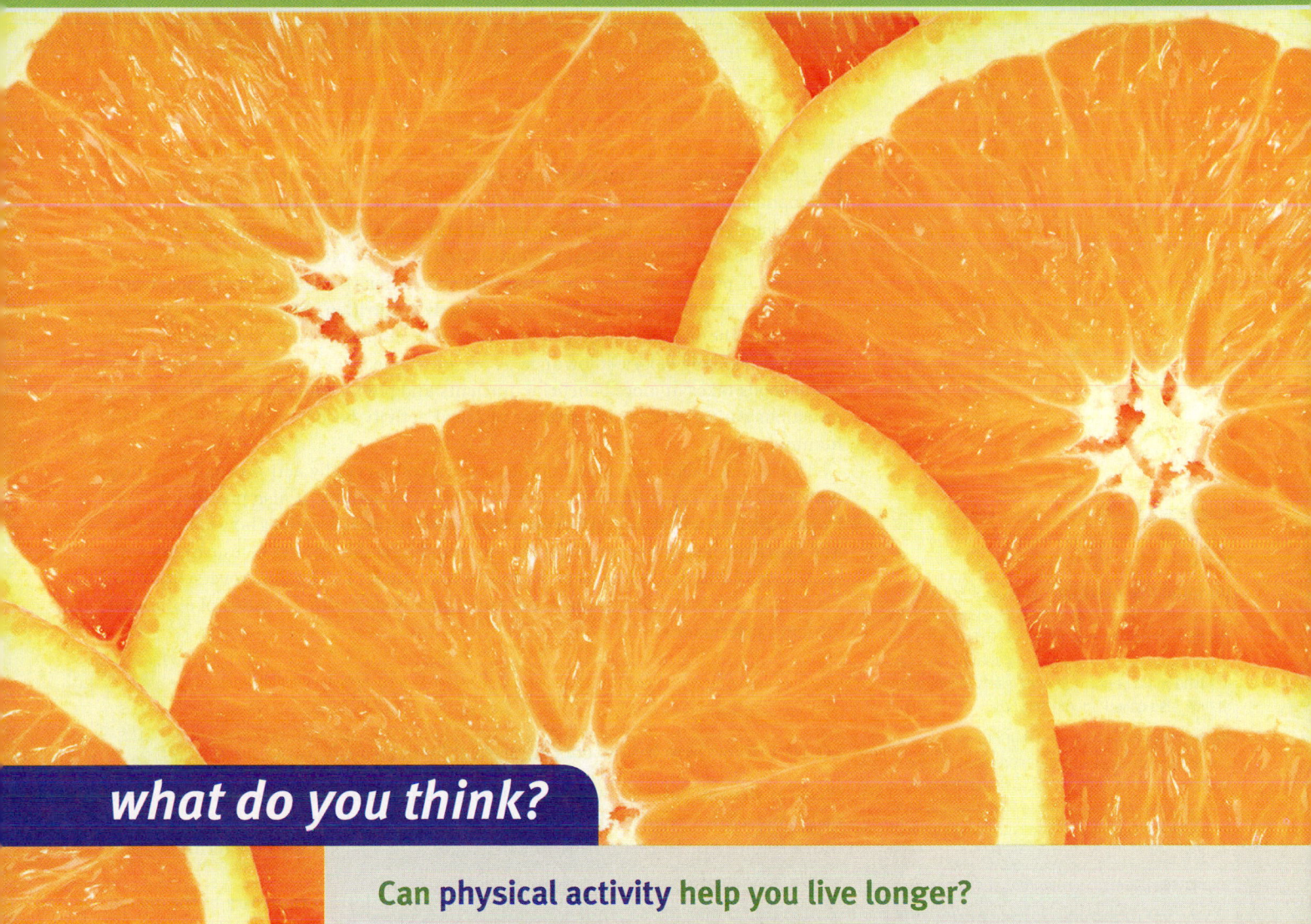

10 Performance Nutrition

what do you think?

Can **physical activity** help you live longer?

Do certain foods or beverages help **competitors** win?

Can **vitamin pills** help to improve your game?

Are **sports drinks** better than water during a workout?

Albo003/Shutterstock.com

Learning Objectives

After completing this chapter, you should be able to accomplish the following:

LO 10.1 Summarize the benefits of physical fitness.

LO 10.2 Discuss muscle adaptability and the benefits of muscle training.

LO 10.3 Describe the body's three energy systems that support muscular work.

LO 10.4 Explain the importance of glucose, fatty acids, and proteins to athletes.

LO 10.5 State the importance of vitamins and minerals to athletes.

LO 10.6 Discuss the hazards from inadequate fluid intake and temperature extremes during physical activity.

LO 10.7 Summarize the components of a diet to support physical performance.

LO 10.8 Debate the use of dietary ergogenic aids for improving sports performance.

In the body, nutrition and **physical activity** go hand in hand. The working body demands energy-yielding nutrients—carbohydrate, lipid, and protein—to fuel physical activity. It also needs high-quality protein to supply the amino acids necessary to build new muscle tissues. Vitamins and minerals play critical roles in energy metabolism, protein synthesis, and many other functions necessary for physical work.

Physical activity, in turn, benefits the body's nutrition. Physical activity helps to regulate the use of energy-yielding nutrients, improves body composition, and increases the daily calorie allowance. A person who eats extra calories of nutritious whole foods takes in more beneficial nutrients and phytochemicals, too. Together, a nutritious eating pattern and regular physical activity become a powerful force for human health.

This chapter addresses many of the concerns of physically active people, starting with some basic concepts about health and physical activity. It also provides a basic framework for understanding **performance nutrition**. It describes how foods, fluids, and nutrients help to fuel physical activities and how the right choices can improve athletic performance, whereas poor choices may hinder it. The Controversy that follows spotlights just a few of the many supplements sold with promises of enhanced athletic performance.

The Benefits of Fitness

LO 10.1 Summarize the benefits of physical fitness.

Physical **fitness** develops with performance of physical activity or **exercise**. The body's muscles respond in identical ways, regardless of whether an individual is running around a track or running to catch a bus, so this chapter uses the terms *physical activity* and *exercise* interchangeably.

People's fitness goals vary from the competitive **athlete** in **training** to the casual exerciser working to gain health and manage body weight. For those just beginning a program of physical fitness, be assured that improvement is not only possible but also inevitable. As you become more active, a beneficial cycle of greater fitness that facilitates more physical activity quickly ensues. Energy levels rise, and chronic diseases risks fall. The mechanism also runs in reverse: a sedentary lifestyle robs people of their fitness and fosters the development of several chronic diseases.

The Nature of Fitness

If you are physically fit, the following describes you: You move with ease and balance. You have endurance that lasts for hours. You are strong and meet daily

physical activity bodily movement produced by muscle contractions that substantially increase energy expenditure.

performance nutrition an area of nutrition science that applies its principles to maintaining health and maximizing physical performance in athletes, firefighters, military personnel, and others who must perform at high levels of physical ability. Also called *sports nutrition*.

fitness the characteristics that enable the body to perform physical activity; more broadly, the ability to meet routine physical demands with enough reserve energy to rise to a physical challenge; or the body's ability to withstand stress of all kinds.

exercise planned, structured, and repetitive bodily movement that promotes or maintains physical fitness.

athlete a competitor in any sport, exercise, or game requiring physical skill; for the purpose of this book, anyone who trains at a high level of physical exertion, with or without competition. From the Greek *athlein*, meaning "to contend for a prize."

training regular practice of an activity, which leads to physical adaptations of the body with improvement in flexibility, strength, or endurance.

physical challenges without strain. You are prepared for mental and emotional challenges, too, because physical activity can help to relieve stress, depression, or anxiety. As your fitness improves, you not only begin to feel better and stronger but look better, too. As you strengthen your muscles, your posture and self-image often improve.

Longevity and Disease Resistance   People who regularly engage in moderate physical activity live longer, healthier lives on average than those who are physically inactive.[1]* A sedentary lifestyle ranks with smoking and obesity as a powerful predictor of the major killer diseases of our time—cardiovascular disease, some forms of cancer, stroke, diabetes, and hypertension. Sedentary people may even be more likely to catch a cold. Despite the well-known health benefits of physical activity (listed in Table 10–1), only 20 percent of adults in the United States meet all of the physical activity guidelines.[2] More than half of women and 44 percent of men report no leisure-time physical activity at all.[3]

A Molecular Link with Health   Small improvements in blood vessel function and blood glucose regulation are detectable after just a single bout of exercise.[4] Some of the credit for these and other benefits of exercise may be in part attributable to hormone-like activities of small molecules released by working muscles, the so called "exercise factors."‡ Exercise factors also promote muscle synthesis and they may alter energy metabolism in ways that oppose chronic diseases.[5] Why not simply press exercise factors into a "fitness pill" to capture their benefits without physical work?

Table 10–1
Some Benefits of Fitness

Research suggests that most people who become physically active can expect these and other benefits.

- Improved body composition and adipose tissue distribution.
- Improved bone density.
- Enhanced resistance to colds and other infectious diseases.[a]
- Lower risks of some types of cancers.
- More efficient circulation and stronger lung function.
- Reduced risk factors for cardiovascular disease.
- Lower risk and improved management of type 2 diabetes.
- Reduced risk of gallbladder disease.
- Lower incidence and reduced severity of mental anxiety and depression.
- Longer life and higher quality of life in the later years.

[a]*Regular, moderate physical activity supports healthy immune function, but intense, vigorous, prolonged activity such as a marathon race may temporarily compromise immune function.*

Sources: A. Philipsen and coauthors, Associations of objectively measured physical activity and abdominal fat distribution, Medicine and Science in Sports and Exercise (2015), epub ahead of print, doi:10.1249/ MSS.0000000000000504; K. G. Avin and coauthors, Biomechanical aspects of the muscle-bone interaction, Current Osteoporosis Reports 13 (2015): 1–8; E. J. Aguiar and coauthors, Efficacy of interventions that include diet, aerobic and resistance training components for type 2 diabetes prevention: A systematic review with meta-analysis, International Journal of Behavioral Nutrition and Physical Activity 11 (2014), epub, doi:10.1186/1479-5868-11-2; R. Asano and coauthors, Acute effects of physical exercise in type 2 diabetes: A review, World Journal of Diabetes 5 (2014), epub, doi:10.4239/wjd.v5.i5.659; P. Seron and coauthors, Exercise for people with high cardiovascular risk, Cochrane Database Systematic Reviews 8 (2014), epub, doi:10.1002/14651858.CD009387.pub2; S. M. Pinto Pereira, M. C. Geoffroy, and C. Power, Depressive symptoms and physical activity during 3 decades in adult life: Bidirectional associations in a prospective cohort study, JAMA Psychiatry 71 (2014): 1373–1380; S. Rosenbaum and coauthors, Physical activity interventions for people with mental illness: A systematic review and meta-analysis, Journal of Clinical Psychiatry 75 (2014): 964–974; H. J. Goedecke and L. K. Micklesfield, The effect of exercise on obesity, body fat distribution and risk for type 2 diabetes, Medicine and Science in Sport and Exercise 60 (2014): 82–93.

---

*Reference notes are found in Appendix F.

‡Exercise factors include *irisin* and other members of the chemical family, *myokines* (from the Greek, *myo* = "muscle," *kino* = "movement").

Figure 10–1

Physical Activity Guidelines for Americans[a]

Meeting these guidelines requires physical activity beyond the usual light or sedentary activities required in daily living, such as cooking, cleaning, and walking from an automobile to a store. Table 10–2 explains exercise intensity.

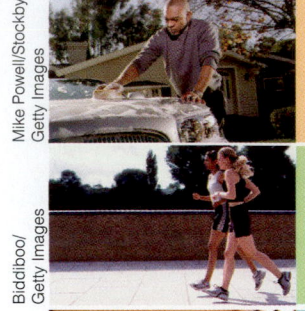

- **Every day—Choose an active lifestyle and engage in flexibility activities.**
  Integrate activity into your day: walk a dog, take the stairs, stand up whenever possible. Stretching exercises lend flexibility for activities such as dance, but minutes spent stretching do not count toward aerobic or strength activity recommendations.

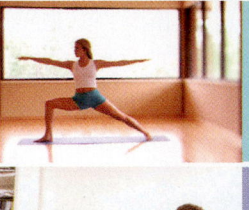

- **5 or more days/week—Engage in moderate or vigorous aerobic activities.**
  Perform a minimum of 150 min of moderate-intensity aerobic activity each week by doing activities like brisk walking or ballroom dancing; 75 min per week of vigorous aerobic activity, such as bicycling (>10 mph) or jumping rope; or a mix of the two (1 min vigorous activity = 2 min moderate activity).

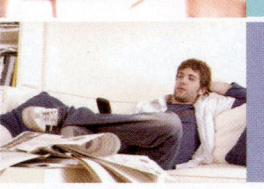

- **2 or more days/week—Engage in strength activities.**
  Perform muscle-strengthening activities that are moderate to high intensity and involve all major muscle groups.

- **Avoid inactivity—Some physical activity is better than none.**
  Limit TV or movie watching, leisure computer time.

[a]For most men and women, aged 18 to 64 years.

Source: U.S. Department of Health and Human Services and U.S. Department of Agriculture, 2015–2020 Dietary Guidelines for Americans, 8th edition (2015), available at http://health.gov/dietaryguidelines/2015/guidelines/.

Unfortunately, too little is known about these molecules or their actions to provide a shortcut.[6] So keep moving.

KEY POINTS

- Physical activity and fitness benefit people's physical and psychological well-being and improve their resistance to disease.
- Physical activity improves survival and quality of life in the later years.
- Exercise factors generated by working muscles may trigger healthy changes in body tissues.

Physical Activity Guidelines

What must you do to reap the health rewards of physical activity? You need only meet the Physical Activity Guidelines for Americans set forth by the USDA and the Department of Health and Human Services.[7]

Physical Activity Guidelines for Americans   The Physical Activity Guidelines for Americans outline how much **aerobic activity** adults aged 18 to 64 years need to improve or maintain cardiovascular health (see Figure 10–1). The Physical Activity Guidelines also support **resistance training** (strengthening exercises) as beneficial for building and maintaining lean tissues and useful for meeting activity goals. The length of time (exercise duration) required to meet these guidelines varies by the **intensity** of the activity—physical activity of moderate intensity must last relatively longer to meet the guidelines; more vigorous exercise can do so in a shorter time. Table 10–2 describes activity intensity levels.

Most health benefits occur with the activities listed in Figure 10–1, but additional benefits can result from activity with a higher intensity, greater frequency, or longer duration. Older people, those with chronic illnesses, and those with disabilities who cannot meet the guidelines should be as active as their conditions allow, based on

aerobic activity physical activity that involves the body's large muscles working at light to moderate intensity for a sustained period of time. Brisk walking, running, swimming, and bicycling are examples. Also called *endurance activity*.

resistance training physical activity that develops muscle strength, power, endurance, and mass. Resistance can be provided by free weights, weight machines, other objects, or the person's own body weight. Also called *weight training*, *resistance exercise*, or *strength exercise*.

intensity in exercise, the degree of effort required to perform a given physical activity.

Table 10–2

Intensity of Physical Activity

Level of Intensity	Breathing and/or Heart Rate	Perceived Exertion (on a Scale of 0 to 10)	Talk Test	Energy Expenditure	Walking Pace
Light	Little to no increase	<5	Able to sing	<3.5 cal/min	<3 mph
Moderate	Some increase	5 or 6	Able to have a conversation	3.5 to 7 cal/min	3 to 4.5 mph (100 steps per minute or 15 to 20 minutes to walk 1 mile)
High (vigorous)	Large increase	7 or 8	Conversation is difficult or "broken"	>7 cal/min	>4.5 mph

Source: Centers for Disease Control and Prevention, 2011, available at www.cdc.gov/physicalactivity/everyone.

the advice of their health-care providers. For everyone, mounting evidence suggests that even without meeting the Physical Activity Guidelines, some physical activity is better than none.[8]

Note that certain guidelines are stated in accumulated weekly totals.[†] This allows individuals to split up their activity into sessions of at least 10 minutes each, performed throughout the days of the week in any combination that suits their lifestyles. Safety is a high priority, and the Think Fitness section (p. 396) provides some tips.

To achieve or maintain a healthy body weight through increasing physical activity demands more than the amount needed for health.[9] Most people with weight-loss goals are best served by combining a calorie-restricted diet with increased physical activity.

Guidelines for Sports Performance   Athletes who compete in sports require specific types and amounts of physical activity to train for performance, so special guidelines apply to them. Appendix H at the back of the book offers guidelines for sports and fitness from the American College of Sports Medicine that are more specific and also more demanding than the Physical Activity Guidelines for Americans.[10] Appendix H also offers a sample balanced workout program that develops all components of fitness.

KEY POINT

- The U.S. Physical Activity Guidelines for Americans aim to improve physical fitness and the health of the nation.

The Essentials of Fitness

LO 10.2 Discuss muscle adaptability and the benefits of muscle training.

To become physically fit, you need to develop enough **flexibility**, **muscle strength**, **muscle endurance**, and **cardiorespiratory endurance** to allow you to meet the everyday demands of life with some to spare. You also need to achieve a reasonable body composition.

So far, the description of fitness applies to anyone interested in improving health. For athletes, however, excelling in sports performance often becomes the primary motivator for working out. Athletes must strive to develop strength and endurance, of course, but they also need **muscle power** to drive their movements, quick **reaction time** to respond with speed, **agility** to instantly change direction, increased resistance to **muscle fatigue**, and mental toughness to carry on when fatigue sets in.

flexibility the capacity of the joints to move through a full range of motion; the ability to bend and recover without injury.

muscle strength the ability of muscles to overcome physical resistance. This muscle characteristic develops with increasing work load rather than repetition and is associated with muscle size.

muscle endurance the ability of a muscle to contract repeatedly within a given time without becoming exhausted. This muscle characteristic develops with increasing repetition rather than increasing workload and is associated with cardiorespiratory endurance.

cardiorespiratory endurance the ability of the heart, lungs, and metabolism to sustain large-muscle exercise of moderate to high intensity for prolonged periods.

muscle power the efficiency of a muscle contraction, measured by force and time.

reaction time the interval between stimulation and response.

agility nimbleness, the ability to quickly change directions.

muscle fatigue diminished force and power of muscle contractions despite consistent or increasing conscious effort to perform a physical activity.

[†]Guidelines from sports medicine experts are stated in metabolic equivalent units (METs) that reflect the ratio of the rate of energy expended during an activity to the rate of energy expended at rest. One MET is equal to the energy expenditure while at rest.

How Do Muscles Adapt to Physical Activity?

A person who engages in physical activity *adapts* by becoming a little more able to perform the activity after each session. People shape their bodies by what they choose to do (and not do). Muscle cells and tissues respond to a physical activity **overload** by building, within genetic limits, the structures and metabolic equipment needed to perform the activity.

Muscles are under constant renovation. Every day, particularly during the fasting periods between meals, a healthy body degrades a portion of its muscle protein to amino acids and later rebuilds it as amino acids become available during fed periods.[11] A balance between degradation and synthesis maintains the body's lean tissue. To gain muscle strength and size, however, this balance must more often tip toward synthesis, a condition called **hypertrophy**, than toward muscle breakdown, which results in **atrophy**. Physical activity tips the balance toward hypertrophy. The opposite is also true: unused muscles diminish in size and weaken over time—they atrophy.

> Muscle hypertrophy is an example of positive nitrogen balance, a concept illustrated in **Figure 6–13** of Chapter 6.

Muscle synthesis is conservative. The muscles adapt and build only the proteins they need to cope with the work performed. Muscles engaged in activities that require strength develop greater bulk, while those engaged in endurance activities develop more metabolic equipment to combat muscle fatigue.[12] Thus, a tennis player may have one superbly strong arm, while the other is just average; cyclists often have well-developed legs that can pedal for many hours but less development of the arms or chest.

A Balance of Activities Balanced fitness arises from performing a variety of physical activities that work different muscle groups from day to day. Stretching enhances flexibility, aerobic activity improves cardiorespiratory and muscle endurance, and **resistance training** develops the strength, size, and endurance of the worked muscles.

Muscles need rest, too, because it takes a day or two to fully replenish muscle fuel supplies and to repair wear and tear. With greater work comes more damage, and muscles require longer rest periods for a full recovery. (A muscle or joint that remains sore after about a week of rest may be injured and in need of medical attention.)

A planned program of training can induce the development of specific muscle tissues and fuel systems. The muscle cells of a trained weight lifter store extra glycogen granules, build up strong connective tissues, and add bulk to the special proteins that contract the muscles, increasing their strength.§ In contrast, the muscle cells of a distance swimmer build more of the enzymes and structures needed for aerobic metabolism. Therefore, if you wish to become a better jogger, swimmer, or biker, you should train in ways that benefit your sport. Your performance will improve as your muscles adapt to the activity.

KEY POINTS

- The components of fitness are flexibility, muscle strength, muscle endurance, and cardiorespiratory endurance.
- Muscle protein is built up and broken down every day; muscle tissue is gained when synthesis exceeds degradation.
- Physical activity builds muscle tissues and metabolic equipment needed for the activities they are repeatedly called upon to perform.

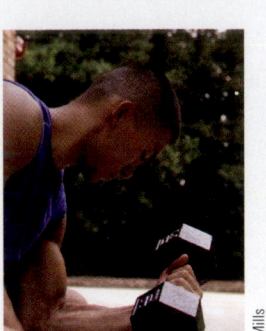

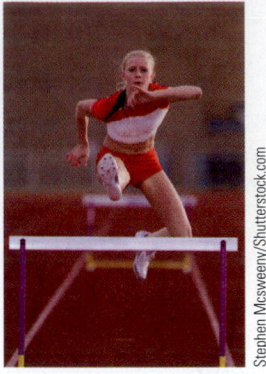

Bodies are shaped . . .

by the activities they perform.

Amanda Mills

Stephen Mcsweeny/Shutterstock.com

overload an extra physical demand placed on the body; an increase in the frequency, duration, or intensity of an activity. A principle of training is that for a body system to improve, it must be worked at frequencies, durations, or intensities that increase by increments.

hypertrophy (high-PURR-tro-fee) an increase in size (for example, of a muscle) in response to use.

atrophy (AT-tro-fee) a decrease in size (for example, of a muscle) because of disuse.

resistance training physical activity that develops muscle strength, power, endurance, and mass. Resistance can be provided by free weights, weight machines, other objects, or the person's own body weight. Also called *weight training* or *muscular strength exercises*.

---

§All muscles contain a variety of muscle fibers, but there are two main types—slow-twitch (also called red fibers) and fast-twitch (also called white fibers). Slow-twitch fibers contain extra metabolic equipment to perform aerobic work, which gives them a reddish appearance under a microscope; the fast-twitch type stores extra glycogen required for anaerobic work, giving them a lighter appearance.

Resistance Training for Muscle Strength, Size, Power, and Endurance

Most people know that resistance training helps to build muscle bulk, strength, and endurance. Less well known is that **progressive weight training** may help to prevent and manage several chronic diseases, including cardiovascular disease risk factors and osteoporosis, and can enhance psychological well-being, too.[13] By strengthening the muscles of the back and abdomen, resistance training can improve posture, making debilitating back injuries less likely to occur. It also enhances performance in many sports, not just those that demand muscle size. Swimmers can develop a more efficient stroke and tennis players a more powerful serve when they engage in resistance training, for example.

Some people, particularly many women, fear that resistance training will make their muscles bulky, like those of bodybuilders. In truth, bodybuilders of both genders work to achieve their look by training intensely with heavy weights and by consuming calories by the hundreds or thousands above an average person's intake. Many factors, including genetic potential and the body's hormones, modulate muscle growth and strength. Ordinary exercisers who regularly lift weights with sufficient intensity just a day or two each week can slowly develop and maintain a pleasing appearance as muscles strengthen and firm without becoming bulky.[14] If such people also reduce calorie intakes and meet protein needs, they can lose weight without sacrificing their lean body tissue.[15]

KEY POINTS

- Resistance training can benefit physical and mental health.
- Sports performance, appearance, and body composition improve through resistance training; bulky muscles are the result of intentional bodybuilding regimens.

How Does Aerobic Training Benefit the Heart?

Aerobic endurance training reliably and efficiently improves some key indicators of cardiovascular health.[16] Such exercise, performed regularly, diminishes the risks of diabetes and hypertension, major contributors to heart disease, while improving the blood lipid profile. In addition, aerobic endurance training encourages leanness, a plus for the heart, and it confers a fit, healthy appearance to the limbs and torso.

Improvements to Blood, Heart, and Lungs

Cardiorespiratory endurance allows the working body to remain active with an elevated heart rate over time. As cardiorespiratory endurance improves, the body delivers oxygen to the tissues and removes cellular wastes more efficiently.[17] In fact, the accepted measure of a person's cardiorespiratory fitness is a measure of the rate at which the tissues consume oxygen—the maximal oxygen uptake (VO_{2max}). This measure reflects many facets of oxygen delivery that improve with regular aerobic exercise.

The blood's volume and the number of red blood cells partly determine VO_{2max}: the greater the volume and number, the more oxygen the blood can carry. The size and strength of the heart also play roles—as the heart muscle grows stronger and larger, the heart's **cardiac output** increases. Each beat empties the heart's chambers more completely, so the heart pumps more blood per beat—its **stroke volume** increases. The resting heart rate slows because a greater volume of blood is moved with fewer beats. Working muscles also push blood more efficiently through the veins on their return trip to the heart and lungs.

Muscles that inflate and deflate the lungs gain strength and endurance, too, so breathing becomes more efficient. Circulation through the arteries and veins improves, blood moves easily, and blood pressure falls. Figure 10–2 (p. 397) shows the major relationships among the heart, lungs, and muscles, and Table 10–3 describes cardiorespiratory endurance. Anyone who possesses cardiorespiratory endurance can celebrate a lowered risk for cardiovascular diseases.

Nativania/Shutterstock.com

Table 10–3

Cardiorespiratory Endurance

Cardiorespiratory endurance is characterized by:

- Increased heart strength and stroke volume
- Slowed resting pulse
- Increased breathing efficiency
- Improved circulation and oxygen delivery
- Reduced blood pressure
- Increased blood HDL cholesterol

Sources: E. G. Ciolac and coauthors, Effects of high-intensity aerobic interval training vs. moderate exercise on hemodynamic, metabolic and neuro-humoral abnormalities of young normotensive women at high familial risk for hypertension, Hypertension Research 33 (2010): 836–843; J. J. Whyte and M. H. Laughlin, The effects of acute and chronic exercise on the vasculature, Acta Physiologica 199 (2010): 441–450; G. Lippi and N. Maffulli, Biological influence of physical exercise on hemostasis, Seminars in Thrombosis and Hemostasis 35 (2009): 269–276.

progressive weight training the gradual increase of a workload placed upon the body with the use of resistance.

VO_{2max} the maximum rate of oxygen consumption by an individual (measured at sea level).

cardiac output the volume of blood discharged by the heart each minute.

stroke volume the volume of oxygenated blood ejected from the heart toward body tissues at each beat.

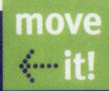
Sometimes physical activity can pose risks. The physical impact involved in contact sports—football is a typical example—create serious risks of head and neck injuries; in other activities, torn ligaments, broken bones, and even strains and sprains can sideline a player, at least temporarily.[18]

Keeping safe during physical activity involves both common sense and education. The USDA suggests following these guidelines:

- Choose activities appropriate for your current fitness level.
- Gradually increase the amount of physical activity you perform.
- Wear appropriate safety gear, including the correct shoes, helmet, pads, and other protection.
- Develop the flexibility and balance needed in your activity.

- Make sensible choices about when and where to exercise; for example, avoid the hottest hours of the day in southern locales, choose safe bike paths away from heavy traffic, and run with a buddy on isolated trails.
- People with medical problems or increased disease risks should consult a physician before beginning any program of physical activity.[19]

In addition, people can easily injure themselves by using improper techniques during strength training, particularly when it involves equipment. Many people can benefit from consulting with a Certified Personal Trainer (CPT). A CPT can help develop a safe and effective individualized exercise program. Some personal trainers have a more advanced credential, the Certified Strength and Conditioning Specialist (CSCS), which requires completion of a college curriculum that includes human anatomy and exercise physiology; they must also pass a nationally recognized examination. Also, unless a trainer possesses a legitimate nutrition credential, he or she is not qualified to dispense diet advice. Fake nutrition credentials were described in Controversy 1; the same kinds of skullduggery occur in the field of physical training.

start now! ⤏ Create a fitness plan that gradually increases both the time and the intensity of physical activity. Use a calendar to record your daily plan for several weeks; then record your actual activity on each of those days.

Cardiorespiratory Training Activities   Effective cardiorespiratory training activities have these characteristics:

- They elevate the heart rate for sustained periods of time.
- They use most of the large-muscle groups of the body (for example, legs, buttocks, or upper body muscle group).

In other words, they are the aerobic endurance activities, and they are recommended for heart health. Examples are swimming, cross-country skiing, rowing, fast walking, jogging, running, fast bicycling, soccer, hockey, basketball, in-line skating, lacrosse, and rugby.

The rest of this chapter describes the interactions between nutrients and physical activity. Nutrition alone cannot endow you with fitness or athletic ability, but along with consistent physical activity and the right mental attitude, it complements your effort to obtain them. Conversely, unwise food selections can stand in your way.

KEY POINTS

- Cardiorespiratory endurance training enhances the ability of the heart and lungs to deliver oxygen to body tissues.
- Cardiorespiratory training activities elevate the heart rate for sustained periods of time and engage the body's large muscle groups.

Three Energy Systems

LO 10.3 Describe the body's three energy systems that support muscular work.

Whether belonging to an athlete, a growing child, or an office worker, the human body uses energy systems to fuel its work. These include the body's energy reservoir, the **anaerobic** fuel system, and the **aerobic** fuel system. All three systems function

anaerobic (AN-air-ROH-bic) not requiring oxygen.

aerobic (air-ROH-bic) requiring oxygen.

Figure 10–2
Delivery of Oxygen by the Heart and Lungs to the Muscles

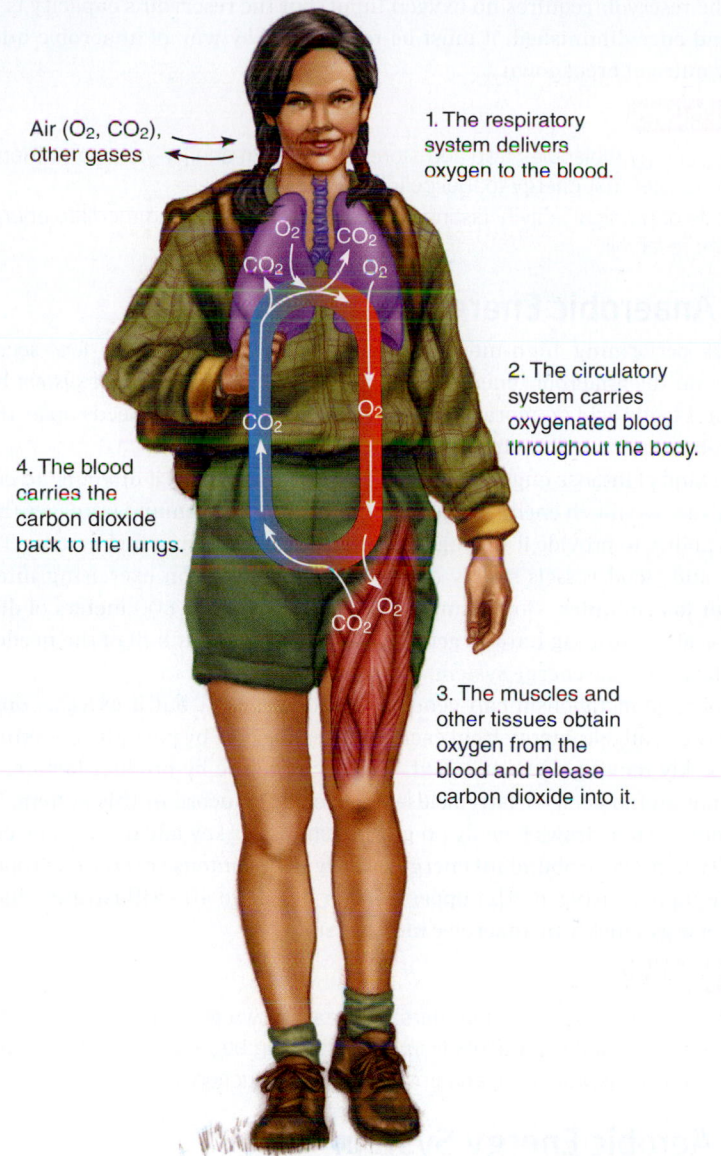

Air (O_2, CO_2), other gases

1. The respiratory system delivers oxygen to the blood.

2. The circulatory system carries oxygenated blood throughout the body.

4. The blood carries the carbon dioxide back to the lungs.

3. The muscles and other tissues obtain oxygen from the blood and release carbon dioxide into it.

The cardiorespiratory system responds to increased demand for oxygen by building up its capacity to deliver oxygen. Researchers can measure cardiovascular fitness by measuring the amount of oxygen a person consumes per minute while working out. This measure of fitness, which indicates the person's maximum rate of oxygen consumption, is called VO_{2max}.

continuously, supplying energy for the heartbeat, breathing, cellular activities, and other life-sustaining work. When physical activity demands arise, however, they respond in ways that specifically meet the need.

The Muscles' Energy Reservoir

The **energy reservoir** is composed of high-energy molecules that trap and store energy exactly where it is needed for muscular work—on the microscopic fibers that contract the muscles.** Whenever muscles move, say, to blink the eyes or type on a keyboard, these high-energy molecules split apart, releasing and transferring their load of pent-up energy to power the work of the muscle tissue.[20]

energy reservoir a system of high-energy compounds that hold, store, and release energy derived from the energy-yielding nutrients and transfer it to cell structures to fuel cellular activities. In exercise, the reservoir provides immediate energy sufficient for short bursts of intense physical activity.

**The energy reservoir is also called the *phosphagen system*, referring to high-energy compounds that contain the mineral phosphorus, such as ATP (adenosine triphosphate) and CP (phosphocreatine), key players in energy metabolism.

This fast and ready pool of energy is also the fuel that drives short bursts of intense physical activity lasting up to about 20 seconds, such as when a weight lifter heaves a heavy weight or a child darts to grab the best swing on the playground. Using energy from the reservoir requires no oxygen input, but the reservoir's capacity is very limited, and once diminished, it must be replenished by way of anaerobic and aerobic energy nutrient breakdown.

KEY POINTS

- High-energy molecules trap and store energy from energy-yielding nutrients and can transfer that energy to fuel cellular work.
- Bursts of physical activity lasting just seconds require the immediate energy stored in the reservoir.

The Anaerobic Energy System

Muscles performing high-intensity work lasting more than a few seconds rely heavily on the anaerobic energy system, also called the *lactic acid system* because it generates lactic acid or, more correctly, **lactate**. This system speeds up as the energy reservoir runs down, drawing on the body's supply of glucose.

The kind of intense ongoing physical activity that makes it difficult "to catch your breath" uses so much energy so quickly that the energy demand outpaces the human body's ability to provide it through its efficient oxygen-using fuel system. The lungs, heart, and blood vessels simply cannot keep up. A person exercising intensely for three or four minutes—for example, a sprinter racing for 800 meters of distance or a late student running hard to get to class—obtains about half of the needed energy from the anaerobic energy system.

Anaerobic metabolism can generate copious energy, but it extracts only a fraction of the available energy from each glucose molecule by partially breaking it down and quickly moving on to the next, casting aside the by-product lactate. No other fuel—not amino acids or fatty acids—can replace glucose in this system. Thus, the anaerobic system draws heavily on glucose stores. Its key advantage, however, is the capacity to produce abundant energy quickly to fuel intense exercise without requiring the input of oxygen. The upper portion of Figure 10–3 illustrates that glucose yields energy quickly in anaerobic metabolism.

KEY POINTS

- The anaerobic energy system partially breaks down glucose to yield energy without using oxygen and is particularly important during bouts of high-intensity activity.
- Lactate is a by-product of anaerobic energy production.

The Aerobic Energy System

The efficient, oxygen-dependent aerobic energy system wrings every last calorie of energy from each energy nutrient molecule—glucose, certain amino acids, the body's abundant fatty acids, and even some lactate, are used as fuels. This system demands the input of sufficient oxygen, and while it always delivers a steady stream of energy to the breathing body, the system speeds up during exercise. Aerobic metabolism supplies almost half of a sprinter's energy, whose effort lasts just seconds, but it supplies over 90 percent of the energy used by a long-distance swimmer who swims for hours on end. Likewise, a jogger can go long distances, breathing easily, the heart beating steadily, relying on aerobic metabolism to supply most of the needed energy.

In contrast to anaerobic metabolism, aerobic metabolism depends more heavily on fatty acids for fuel, sparing glucose and conserving glycogen.[21] The bottom half of Figure 10–3 shows that the ample oxygen supplies available during aerobic activity facilitate the extraction of abundant energy from fuels.

KEY POINTS

- The aerobic energy system uses fuels most efficiently and conserves the body's glycogen stores.
- Aerobic metabolism fuels moderate-intensity activity over long duration.

lactate a compound produced during the breakdown of glucose in anaerobic metabolism.

Figure 10-3

Glucose and Fatty Acids in Their Energy-Releasing Pathways in Muscle Cells

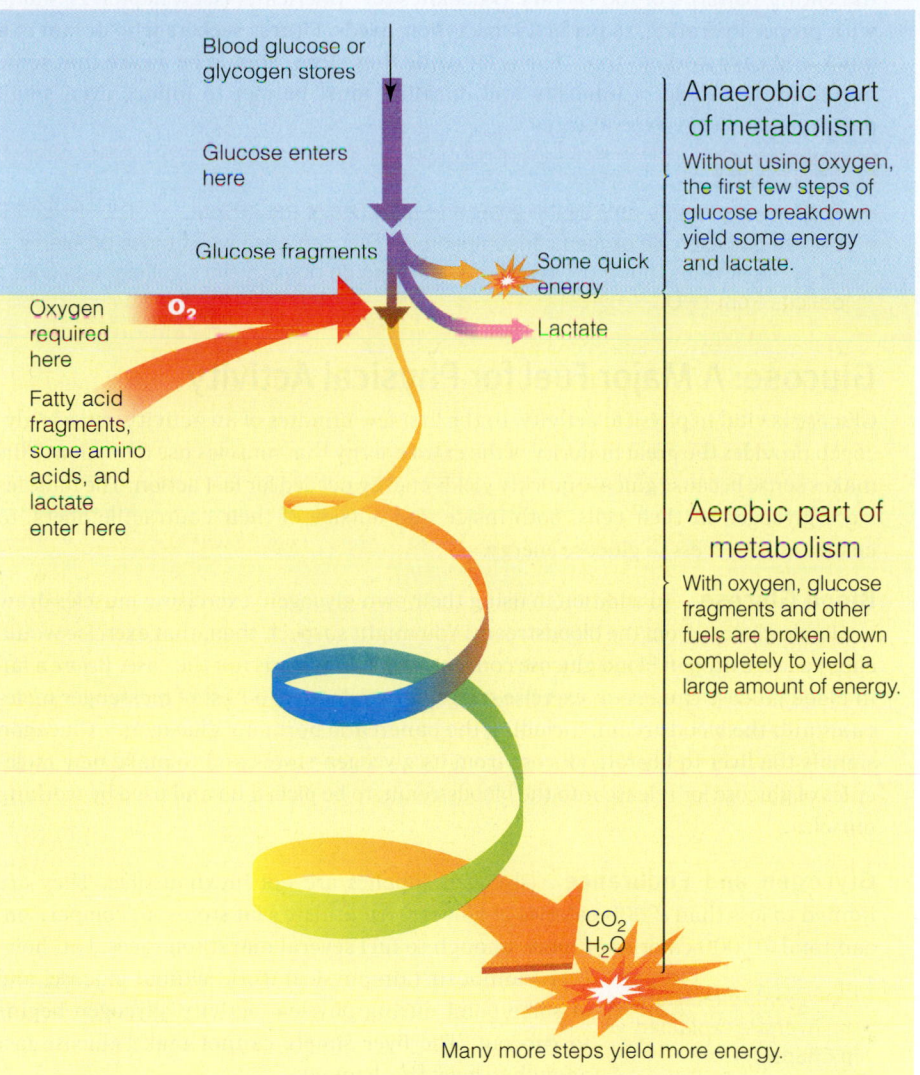

Blood glucose or glycogen stores

Glucose enters here

Glucose fragments

Some quick energy

Lactate

Oxygen required here

O_2

Fatty acid fragments, some amino acids, and lactate enter here

Anaerobic part of metabolism
Without using oxygen, the first few steps of glucose breakdown yield some energy and lactate.

Aerobic part of metabolism
With oxygen, glucose fragments and other fuels are broken down completely to yield a large amount of energy.

CO_2
H_2O

Many more steps yield more energy.

The Active Body's Use of Fuels

LO 10.4 Explain the importance of glucose, fatty acids, and proteins to athletes.

Athletes and other exercisers often hear claims, mostly from sellers of nutrient products, about their need for energy-yielding nutrients. The following sections present the current scientific knowledge about the active person's need for and use of the energy-yielding nutrients.

The Need for Food Energy

Competitive athletes, firefighters in training, military fighting forces, and other highly active people can expend enormous amounts of fuel during physical activity. To prevent unwanted weight loss, such people may need to take in an extra 1,000 to 1,500 or even more calories above their ordinary intakes each day. For some minutes or hours following intense activity, the body's metabolism may stay high and continue to expend extra fuels, even during rest. This phenomenon, known as **excess postexercise oxygen consumption (EPOC)**, occurs mainly following activities of higher intensity.[22]

excess postexercise oxygen consumption (EPOC) a measure of increased metabolism (energy expenditure) that continues for minutes or hours after cessation of exercise.

In contrast, the great majority of physically active people who work out lightly two or three times a week for fitness or weight loss require few or no extra calories. These active people need only consume a nutritious calorie-controlled diet that follows the eating patterns of the Dietary Guidelines for Americans (see Chapter 2), along with proper hydration, to perfectly meet their needs. Fitness seekers who dream of a quick and easy workout that "burns fat while they sleep" should be aware that some minimum threshold of intensity and duration must be met to induce even small postexercise energy expenditures.[23]

KEY POINTS

- Food energy needs vary by the goals and activities of the athlete.
- Excess postexercise oxygen consumption (EPOC) can pose weight-loss problems for some athletes, but most weight-loss seekers do not achieve significant calorie deficits from EPOC.

Glucose: A Major Fuel for Physical Activity

Glucose is vital to physical activity. In the first few minutes of an activity, muscle glycogen provides the great majority of the extra energy that muscles use for action. This makes sense because glucose quickly yields energy needed for fast action. The muscles store glycogen in their cells, both inside and outside of their contractile fibers, to ensure quick access to glucose energy.

Blood Glucose   In addition to using their own glycogen, exercising muscles draw available glucose from the bloodstream. You might suspect, then, that exercise would cause a large drop in blood glucose concentration, but this is not the case. *Before* a fall in blood glucose can occur, exercise triggers the release of a host of messenger molecules into the bloodstream, including the pancreatic hormone glucagon.[24] Glucagon signals the liver to liberate glucose from its glycogen stores and to make new molecules of glucose for release into the bloodstream, to be picked up and used by working muscles.

Glycogen and Endurance   Glycogen supplies are not inexhaustible. They are limited to less than 2,000 calories of glucose. An athlete's fat stores, in comparison, can total 70,000 calories or more, enough to fuel several marathon races. Fat, however, cannot sustain physical work without glucose, and at some point during physical activity, glycogen begins to run out. The liver simply cannot make glucose fast enough to meet the demand.

> Glucagon's effects on the liver are explained in **Chapter 4**.

The athlete who begins an activity with full glycogen stores has enough glucose fuel to last during sustained exercise. For most active people, a normal, balanced diet keeps glycogen stores full. For an athlete engaged in heavy training or competition, the more carbohydrate the person eats, the more glycogen the muscles will store (within limits), and the longer the stores will last to support physical activity.

A classic study compared endurance during physical activity in three groups of runners, each on a different diet.[25] For several days before testing, one of the groups ate a normal mixed diet; the second group ate a high-carbohydrate diet; and the third group ate a high-fat diet. As Figure 10–4 shows, the high-carbohydrate diet enabled the athletes to work longer before exhaustion. These results established that higher intakes of dietary carbohydrate help to sustain an athlete's endurance by ensuring ample glycogen stores.

Glucose from the Digestive Tract   In addition to the body's stored glycogen, glucose in the digestive tract makes its way to the working muscles during activity. For example, food intake may have contributed to the success of ultramarathon runners who finished a 100-mile race.[26] The finishers consumed almost twice the calories and carbohydrates per hour during the race as nonfinishers. It may be that the carbohydrate, calories, or other constituents in the food provided what they needed to keep going after others were exhausted. People who compete in sports that require repeated

Figure 10–4

The Effect of Diet on Physical Endurance

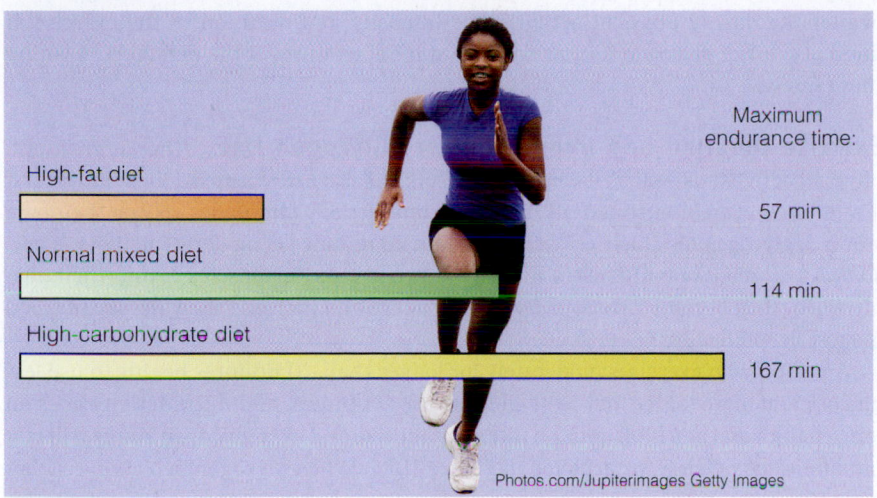

High-fat diet

Normal mixed diet

High-carbohydrate diet

Maximum endurance time:

57 min

114 min

167 min

Photos.com/Jupiterimages Getty Images

Carbohydrate supports an athlete's endurance. In this classic study, the high-fat diet provided 94 percent of calories from fat and 6 percent from protein; the normal mixed diet provided 55 percent of calories from carbohydrate; and the high-carbohydrate diet provided 83 percent of calories from carbohydrate.

Source: J. Bergstrom and coauthors, Diet, muscle glycogen, and physical performance, Acta Physiologica Scandinavica *71 (1967): 140–150.*

bursts of intense activity, such as basketball or soccer, may also benefit from taking in extra carbohydrate during an event, but research has yet to pinpoint optimal intakes.

Before concluding that extra glucose during activity might boost your own exercise performance, consider first whether you engage in sustained endurance activity or repeated high-intensity activity. Do you run, swim, bike, or ski nonstop at a rapid pace for more than an hour at a time? Do you compete in high-intensity games lasting for several hours? Does your sport or training demand several bouts of high-intensity activity in one day, or is it repeated on several successive days? If not, you may be better served by eating ample carbohydrate in the context of a calorie-controlled, nutrient-dense diet.[27]

Lactate—A Glucose Breakdown Product   The anaerobic breakdown of glucose yields the compound lactate, as explained earlier. Most people recognize the burning sensation of lactate accumulating in a working muscle.[28] Muscles quickly release much of this lactate into the bloodstream to be carried to the liver, where enzymes convert it back into glucose. After assembly, the new glucose molecules are shipped back to the working muscles to fuel more physical work.

At low exercise intensities, the small amounts of lactate produced are readily cleared from the tissues. Some tissues, including muscle tissue, can use some lactate aerobically for fuel, and the better trained the muscles, the more lactate they can use.[29] At higher intensities of physical activity, however, the lactate produced can exceed the body's ability to fully clear it away.

Lactate accumulation coincides with muscle fatigue but does not seem to cause it.[30] In contrast, depletion of muscle glycogen by about 80 percent reliably produces fatigue.[31] Other potential causes of fatigue include a drop in muscle tissue pH, a decline in the availability of the high-energy compounds of the energy reservoir, tissue inflammation, and a slight shift in the cells' calcium or potassium concentration.[32] The human experience of fatigue, however, resides in the mind, as well as in the muscle, and physiology alone cannot fully explain why one competitor can push past the point where another must stop.[33]

KEY POINTS

- During activity, the hormone glucagon helps to prevent a drop in blood glucose.
- Glycogen stores in the liver and muscles affect an athlete's endurance.
- Carbohydrate consumption affects glycogen stores and may boost performance during prolonged or repeated exercise.
- Lactate arises from anaerobic breakdown of glucose.

Other Factors Affecting Glycogen

Intake of carbohydrate, although of primary importance in determining the adequacy of a person's glycogen stores, is not the only factor that influences glycogen availability during physical activity. The intensity and duration of the exercise at hand also affect glycogen use, as does the stage of training of the person performing that exercise.

Exercise Duration and Intensity Affect Glycogen Use   The *duration* of a physical activity, as well as its *intensity*, affects glucose use. As mentioned, in the first few minutes of an intense activity, the active muscles rely almost entirely on their own stores of glycogen for glucose. Within the first 20 minutes of moderate activity, a person uses up about one-fifth of the available glycogen. As the muscles devour their own glycogen, they become ravenous for more glucose and increase their uptake of blood glucose dramatically.

A person who exercises moderately for longer than 20 minutes begins to use less glucose and more fat for fuel. Still, glucose use continues, and if the activity goes on long enough and at a high enough intensity, muscle and liver glycogen stores will run out almost completely, as depicted in Figure 10–5. When glycogen depletion reaches a certain point, it brings nervous system function almost to a halt, making continued activity at the same intensity impossible. Marathon runners refer to this point of exhaustion as "hitting the wall" or "bonking."

Degree of Training Affects Glycogen Use   Consistent training affects glycogen use during activity in two major ways. First, muscles adapt to their work by storing the greater amounts of glycogen needed to support that work. Second, trained muscles burn more fat, and at higher intensities, than untrained muscles, so they require less glucose to perform the same work. A person first attempting an activity uses up much more glucose per minute than an athlete trained to perform it.

Figure 10–5

Glycogen—Before and After Physical Activity

These electron micrographs magnify part of a muscle cell by 20,000 times, revealing the orderly rows of contractile structures within. The dark granulated substance is glycogen. In the photo on the left, the cell's glycogen stores are full; on the right, they have been depleted by exercise.

1 The orderly horizontal rows that appear to be striped at intervals are protein structures that contract the muscles.[a]

2 The black oblong rows between the contractile structures contain much of the muscle's glycogen. More glycogen granules (black dots) are also scattered within the contractile parts (visible at left but depleted at right).

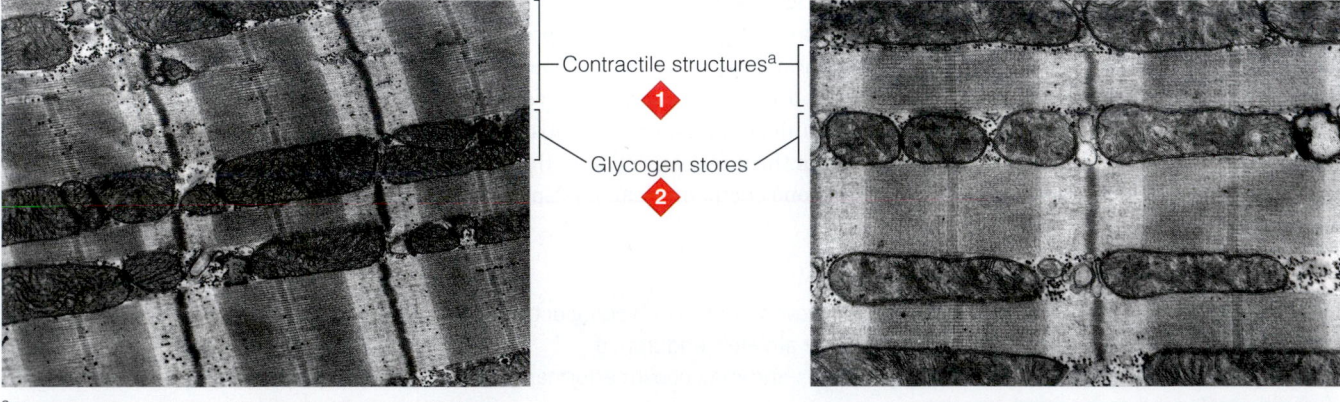

Contractile structures[a]

Glycogen stores

[a]*The contractile structures of the muscle cells are myofibrils.*
Dr. Donald Fawcett/Visuals Unlimited, Inc. (both photos); Art © Cengage Learning 2014

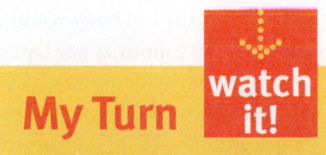

My Turn · watch it! — How Much Is Enough?

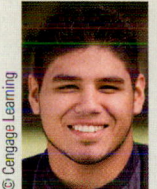
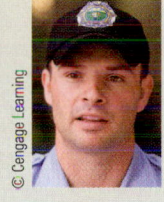

© Cengage Learning

Julian   Adam

Listen to two athletes talk about carbohydrate intakes and other eating strategies.

Visit www.cengagebrain.com to access MindTap, a complete digital course that includes these videos and other resources.

In summary, these three factors affect glucose use during physical activity:

- Carbohydrate intake.
- Intensity and duration of the activity.
- Degree of training.

KEY POINTS

- The more intense an activity, the more glucose it demands for anaerobic metabolism, and the more heavily it draws on glycogen stores.
- Glycogen is used at a rapid rate early in exercise, but the rate slows with continued activity.
- When glycogen depletion reaches a certain point, continued activity of the same intensity is impossible.
- Highly trained muscles use less glucose and more fat than do untrained muscles to perform the same work.

Carbohydrate Recommendations for Athletes

To postpone fatigue and maximize performance, athletes must maintain available glucose supplies for as long as they can. To do so, athletes need abundant carbohydrate in their diets. Table 10–4 suggests a range of potential carbohydrate intakes for

Table 10–4

Suggested Daily Carbohydrate Intakes for Athletes

These general research-based guidelines should be adjusted to an athlete's calorie needs, training type, and performance. Carbohydrate grams in sports drinks, gels, or foods consumed during training are counted among the day's total.

Workload	Carbohydrate Intake Target (g/kg/day)	Recommended Intake (g) for the Reference Male (70 kg)	Recommended Intake (g) for the Reference Female (55 kg)
Casual exercisers (low-intensity, skill-based activities)	3–5	210–350	165–275
Most athletes (moderate intensity, ≤1 h/day)	5–7	350–490	275–385
Endurance athletes, team sport competitors (moderate to high intensity, 1–3 h/day)	6–10	420–840	330–660
Ultraendurance athletes (moderate to high intensity, 4–5 h/day)	8–12	560–840	440–660

Sources: Data from E. Broad and L. Burke, Principles of sports nutrition, in E. Broad (ed.), Sports Nutrition for Paralympic Athletes (New York: Taylor and Francis, 2014), pp. 23–61; M. J. Gibala, Nutritional strategies to support adaptation to high-intensity interval training in team sports, Nestlé Nutrition Institute Workshop Series 75 (2013): 41–49; C. Rosenbloom and E. J. Coleman (eds.), Sports Nutrition: A Practice Manual for Professionals, 5th ed. (Chicago: Academy of Nutrition and Dietetics, 2012), p. 469.

Do the Math

Find kilograms by dividing pounds by a factor of 2.2. For example, for a 130-lb person, 130 lb ÷ 2.2 = 59 kg (rounded). Now find the weight in kg of a 175-lb person.

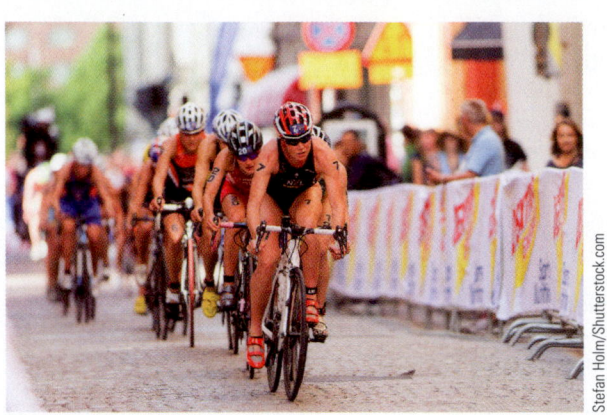

Endurance activities demand fluid and carbohydrate fuel. Don't forget to hydrate.

many athletes. A minimum number of *grams* of carbohydrate per unit of body weight are necessary to achieve full glycogen stores for a given activity, so amounts are listed in grams per kilogram of body weight per day (g/kg/d).[34] To prepare adequate glycogen stores for days of heavy training or competition, some athletes may benefit from large intakes of carbohydrate—perhaps as much as 12 g/kg/d. The Food Feature of this chapter demonstrates how to design a diet that delivers the carbohydrate an athlete needs.

Glucose before Activity   Most of an athlete's glucose is provided by carbohydrate-rich meals consumed throughout the day. In addition, however, glucose taken within a few hours before training or competition is thought to "top off" the athlete's glycogen stores, providing the greatest possible glucose supply to support sustained activity. The **pregame meal** to supply this glucose can take many forms, and the Food Feature of this chapter describes them in full.

A theory called "train low, compete high" suggests that an occasional *low*-carbohydrate training day may increase endurance.[35] Training with depleted glycogen forces an athlete's muscles to use more fat for fuel, and they may develop a greater capacity for doing so. Then, switching back to the usual high-carbohydrate diet replenishes glycogen. With full glycogen stores and muscles trained to use more fat and less glucose, glycogen may last longer during competition. Much more research is needed to investigate the validity and safety of this scheme, however.

Glucose during Activity   Carbohydrate consumption during prolonged activity often improves athletic endurance.[36] Eating during activity can be tricky, because it can cause digestive distress. The best carbohydrate sources for the job are easily consumed, smooth-textured, and low in fiber and fat; such foods facilitate monosaccharide absorption.[37] During long bicycle races, for example, competitors may consume bananas, fruit juices, dried fruit, and energy bars that provide carbohydrate energy and help banish distracting feelings of hunger. (Extreme caution is required to prevent choking.) For athletes who cannot eat solid foods while exercising, commercial **high-carbohydrate energy drinks** and commercial **high-carbohydrate gels** are portable, easy-to-consume alternatives, which most, but not all, athletes can tolerate.[38] Such products are higher in calories and carbohydrate than the fluid-replacement sports drinks discussed later in the Consumer's Guide. Concentrated beverages and gels must be taken with extra water to ensure hydration during activity, however.

Glucose after Activity   Rapid recovery of glycogen stores can be important to people who compete or train intensely more than once a day, or on consecutive days with less than a 24-hour recovery period. A window of opportunity opens during the hour or two following glycogen-depleting physical activity, when carbohydrate intake speeds up the rate of glycogen synthesis.[39] This faster rate of glycogen storage may help to restore glycogen for the next bout of high-intensity training or competition. The concept of recovery meals and its application in an athlete's diet are described in this chapter's Food Feature section.

KEY POINTS

- Carbohydrate recommendations for athletes are stated in grams per kilogram of body weight per day.
- Carbohydrate intakes before, during, and after physical exertion can help to support the performance of certain kinds of activities but not others.

Lipid Fuel for Physical Activity

Unlike the body's limited glycogen stores, fat stores can fuel hours of activity without running out. Body fat is (theoretically) an unlimited source of energy for exercise.

pregame meal   a meal consumed in the hours before prolonged or repeated athletic training or competition to boost the glycogen stores of endurance athletes.

high-carbohydrate energy drinks   flavored commercial beverages used to restore muscle glycogen after exercise or as pregame beverages.

high-carbohydrate gels   semisolid, easy-to-swallow supplements of concentrated carbohydrate, commonly with potassium and sodium added; not a fluid source.

Early in activity, muscles begin to draw on fatty acids from two sources—fats from stores within the working muscles and fats from fat deposits such as the adipose tissue under the skin. Areas with the most fat to spare donate the greatest amounts. This is why "spot reducing" doesn't work: muscles do not own the fat that surrounds them. Instead, adipose tissue cells release fatty acids into the blood for all the muscles to share. Proof is found in a tennis player's arms: the fatfolds measure the same in both arms, even though the muscles of one arm are more developed than those of the other.

Activity Intensity and Duration Affect Fat Use

Fat can be broken down for energy only by aerobic metabolism. During physical activity of light or moderate intensity, fatty acids from adipose tissue are released into the bloodstream and provide the majority of the fuel for muscular work through aerobic metabolism. When the intensity of activity becomes so great that energy demand surpasses the ability to provide more energy aerobically, the muscles cannot burn more fat. They burn more glucose instead.[40] Adipose tissue seems to adjust its delivery of fatty acids to match the needs of the muscles at work, releasing more during moderate activity and releasing less during high-intensity exercise.

The *duration* of activity also affects fat use. At the start of activity, the blood fatty acid concentration falls, but a few minutes into moderate activity, blood flow through the adipose tissue capillaries greatly increases, and hormones, including epinephrine, signal the fat cells to break apart their stored triglycerides. Fatty acids flood into the bloodstream at double or triple the normal rate. After about 20 minutes of sustained, moderate aerobic activity, the fat cells begin to shrink in size as they empty out their lipid stores.[41]

Degree of Training Affects Fat Use

Training, performed consistently, stimulates the muscles to develop more fat-burning metabolic enzymes, so trained muscles burn more fat at greater exercise intensities than untrained muscles do. With aerobic training, the heart and lungs also become stronger and better able to deliver oxygen to the muscles during high-intensity activities. This improved oxygen supply, in turn, helps the muscles to burn more fat.

Fat Recommendations for Athletes

For endurance athletes, eating a high-fat, low-carbohydrate diet for even a day or two reduces precious glycogen stores and makes exercise more difficult. Eventually, muscles do adapt to such a diet and use more fat to fuel activity, but athletes on high-fat diets report greater fatigue and perceive physical work as more strenuous than those on high-carbohydrate diets.[42]

Essential fatty acids and fat-soluble nutrients are as important for athletes as they are for everyone else, so experts recommend a diet with 20 to 35 percent of calories from fat.[43] Athletes should make it a point to obtain the needed raw vegetable oils, nuts, olives, fatty fish, and other sources of health-promoting fats each day. Omega-3 fatty acids, in particular, play roles in reducing inflammation—and tissue inflammation is both the result and the enemy of physical performance.[44] This doesn't mean that athletes need fish oil supplements; they need to consume the amounts of fatty fish recommended for health (see Chapter 5).

As for saturated and *trans* fats, they pose the same heart disease risk for an athlete as they do for other people. Physical activity reduces the risk of cardiovascular disease, but athletes still suffer heart attacks and strokes. Controlling saturated and *trans* fat intake is a priority for protecting the health of an athlete's heart and arteries.

To summarize, then, these three factors affect fat use during physical activity:

- Fat intake.
- Intensity and duration of the activity.
- Degree of training.

KEY POINTS

- The intensity and duration of the activity, as well as the degree of training, affect fat use.
- A diet high in saturated or trans fat raises an athlete's risk of heart disease.

Protein for Building Muscles and for Fuel

The active body uses amino acids from protein to build and maintain muscle and other lean tissue and, to some extent, to provide fuel. Physical activity provides the primary signal for building muscle proteins to support physical work, and a sufficient intake of high-quality dietary protein is required to build them.

Repetitive muscle contractions of physical activity signal the muscle cells to make more of the specific proteins needed to support the work. For 24 to 48 hours following exercise of sufficient intensity, muscles speed up their rate of protein synthesis. The needed essential amino acids derive from both the breakdown of body proteins and the high-quality protein foods in the diet.[45]

Amino Acids Stimulate Muscle Protein Synthesis When essential amino acids arrive in muscle tissue, protein synthesis speeds up.[46] In a laboratory, an infusion of essential amino acids, particularly **leucine**, causes the rate of protein synthesis to triple for an hour or two. After this time, even with a continuing flow of essential amino acids, the rate of muscle protein synthesis quickly drops off. Researchers theorize that after muscles build proteins for a time, they reach a point of being "full" of new proteins, and they stop building them, even though essential amino acids are plentiful.

This is not to say that people can build bigger muscles by laying on the couch and eating protein or taking pills of leucine—only physical activity can cause a net muscle gain. Likewise, consuming excess protein or amino acids cannot force the muscles to exceed their protein-building limits. After the "muscle full" state is reached, excess amino acids are dismantled and used for fuel.[47] This may explain why taking large doses of protein or amino acids cannot force muscles to gain extra bulk. However, when enough high-quality protein is consumed regularly and adequate resistance exercise is performed repeatedly, gains in muscle strength and bulk follow reliably behind.

Does Timing of Protein Matter? During the hour or two following intense physical activity, consuming about 20 grams of high-quality protein—the amount in, say, two-and-a-half cups of low-fat milk or two-and-a-half ounces of turkey—accelerates muscle protein synthesis beyond the rate expected from either exercise or essential amino acids alone. To establish how much protein might have the greatest effect on muscle synthesis, researchers asked groups of men to perform resistance exercise and then to consume 80 grams of high-quality protein in divided doses with various timings over the next 12 hours. Protein synthesis was greatest with four 20-gram doses, given at 3-hour intervals throughout the day.[48] In doses too large (40 grams), excess protein was used as fuel, not for building extra muscle; in doses too small (10 grams), no stimulation of muscle synthesis was observed.

> "High quality" means protein with the complete array of essential amino acids needed for protein synthesis, as explained in **Chapter 6**.

Before concluding that protein timing after exercise is critical for athletes, however, consider these two key questions:

1. Does a faster rate of muscle synthesis after a workout yield greater overall gains of muscle tissue over time?

2. Does protein timing enhance athletic performance?

Although much is yet unknown, the current answer to both questions seems to be "no." Researchers report no correlation between speed of muscle protein synthesis following exercise and ultimate gains in muscle volume.[49] Likewise, athletes given protein supplements soon after exercise exhibit no performance advantage, particularly when carbohydrate intake is ample.[50]

The speed of muscle protein synthesis is indeed greatest in the 2 hours following exercise, but synthesis remains elevated to a degree for some 24 to 48 hours longer. During this time, whenever essential amino acids arrive from protein-rich meals, muscle tissues speed up their protein synthesis and build the protein structures

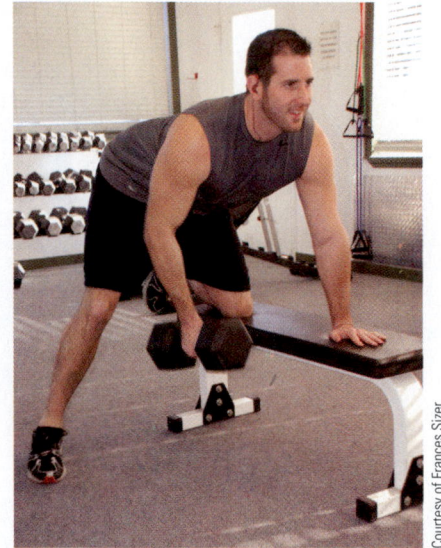

Physical activity itself triggers the building of muscle proteins.

Courtesy of Frances Sizer

leucine one of the essential amino acids; it is of current research interest for its role in stimulating muscle protein synthesis.

they need to perform the activity. Sufficient high-quality protein comes from balanced, nutritious meals and snacks spaced throughout the day. Expensive postexercise protein supplements provide no special advantage.[51]

Protein Fuel Use in Physical Activity   Studies of nitrogen balance show that the body speeds up its use of amino acids for fuel during physical activity, just as it speeds up its use of glucose and fatty acids. The factors that regulate protein use during activity seem to be the same three that regulate the use of glucose and fat: diet, exercise intensity and duration, and degree of training. As for diet, sufficient carbohydrate spares protein from being used as fuel—too little carbohydrate necessitates the conversion of amino acids to glucose.

Exercise intensity and duration also affect protein fuel use. When endurance athletes train for longer than an hour a day and deplete their glycogen stores, they become more dependent on protein fuel. In contrast, intense anaerobic strength training does not use as much protein fuel but demands protein for building muscle tissue.

Finally, the extent of training also affects the use of protein. Particularly in strength athletes such as bodybuilders, the higher the degree of training, the less protein a person uses during activity at a given intensity. To summarize, the factors that affect protein use during physical activity include:

- Dietary carbohydrate sufficiency.

- Intensity and duration of the activity.

- Degree of training.

Protein Recommendations for Athletes   For both endurance and strength, athletes need more protein than others. On learning of their higher protein needs, many athletes go to extremes, doubling or tripling the number of protein-rich foods they eat while ignoring other needed foods and nutrients, a costly mistake for both health and performance. Also, too much protein generates excess nitrogen, which must then be excreted in urine.

Everyday foods, such as milk, chili, or turkey sandwiches, deliver the high-quality protein with the right mix of amino acids to meet the athlete's need (see Table 10–5). Such foods present no risk of amino acid imbalances, a known drawback of supplements.

KEY POINTS

- Physical activity stimulates muscle cells to both break down and synthesize proteins, resulting in muscle adaptation to activity.
- Athletes use amino acids for building muscle tissue and for energy; dietary carbohydrate spares amino acids.
- Diet, intensity and duration of the activity, and degree of training affect protein use during that activity.

How Much Protein Should an Athlete Consume?

The DRI committee does not recommend greater-than-normal protein intakes for athletes, but other authorities do.[52] These greater recommendations vary by the nature of the activities performed (see Table 10–6, p. 408). As is true for carbohydrates, the protein recommendations are stated in grams per kilogram of body weight per day (g/kg/d). The protein amounts suggested for athletes are not far above average U.S. intakes; most people consume about 1.2 to 1.5 grams of protein per kilogram of their ideal body weight.[53]

You may be wondering whether you eat enough protein for your own activities. In general, a nutritious eating pattern that provides enough total energy and follows the USDA Eating Patterns provides enough protein for almost everyone.

KEY POINT

- Although certain athletes may need some additional protein, a well-chosen diet that provides ample energy and follows the USDA Eating Patterns provides sufficient protein, even for most athletes.

Table 10–5
Examples of Protein-Rich Snacks for Athletes

Each of these provides about 20 g of protein, with the right balance of essential amino acids (20,000 mg) in a digestible and available form. Remember to vary your choices.

- 2½ oz of chicken breast, tuna, or lean meat;
- ¾ c low-fat cottage cheese;
- 2½ c milk;
- 2½ eggs; or
- 12 oz yogurt.

Table 10–6

Recommended Protein Intakes for Athletes

	RECOMMENDATION (g/kg/day)	PROTEIN INTAKE (g/day)	
		Reference[a] Male (70 kg)	Reference[a] Female (55 kg)
DRI recommended intake	0.8	56	44
Recommended intake for power (strength or speed) athletes	1.2–1.7	84–119	66–94
Recommended intake for endurance athletes	1.2–1.4	84–98	66–77
U.S. average intake		102	70

[a]Daily protein intakes are based on a 70-kilogram (154-pound) reference man and a 55-kilogram (121-pound) reference woman. Other individuals must calculate their recommended intakes using the numbers of column 1. (For kg, divide lb by 2.2.)

Sources: Position of the American Dietetic Association, Dietitians of Canada, and the American College of Sports Medicine: Nutrition and athletic performance, Journal of the American Dietetic Association 109 (2009): 509–527, reaffirmed 2015; U.S. Department of Agriculture, Agricultural Research Service, Nutrient intakes from food: Mean amounts consumed per individual, one day, 2005–2006, compiled 2008, available at www.ars.usda.gov/ba/bhnrc/fsrg; Committee on Dietary Reference Intakes, Dietary Reference Intakes for Energy, Carbohydrate, Fiber, Fat, Fatty Acids, Cholesterol, Protein, and Amino Acids (Washington, D.C.: National Academies Press, 2005), pp. 660–661.

Vitamins and Minerals— Keys to Performance

LO 10.5 State the importance of vitamins and minerals to athletes.

Vitamins and minerals are crucial for the working body. Many B vitamins participate in releasing energy from fuels. Vitamin C is needed for the formation of the protein collagen, the foundation material of bones, cartilage, and other connective tissues. Folate and vitamin B_{12} help to build red blood cells, and iron carries oxygen to working muscles. Vitamin E helps protect tissues from oxidation. Calcium and magnesium allow muscles to contract, and so on. Do active people need more of these vitamins and minerals to support their work? Do they need supplements?

Do Nutrient Supplements Benefit Athletic Performance?

Many athletes take vitamin and mineral supplements. One of the most common reasons athletes at all levels give for supplement use is "to improve performance."

Contrary to some athletes' beliefs, taking vitamins or minerals just before competition will not help performance. Most vitamins and minerals function as small parts of larger working units. After entering the blood from the digestive tract, they must wait for the cells to combine them with their other parts before they can function. This takes time—hours or days. Nutrients taken right before an event cannot help performance, even if the person is deficient in those nutrients.

More Food Means More Nutrients For the well-nourished athlete, nutrient supplements do not enhance performance. Strenuous physical activity requires abundant energy, and athletes and active people who eat enough nutrient-dense foods to meet their greater energy needs automatically consume more of the vitamins and minerals needed to process that energy. Active people eat more food; it stands to reason that with the right choices, they consume more vitamins and minerals, too.

Preventing Deficiencies Deficiencies of vitamins and minerals impede performance. Athletes who starve themselves to meet a sport's weight requirement can easily fail to obtain needed nutrients. Most authorities oppose rigid weight requirements because athletes often risk their health to meet them. For athletes forced to "make

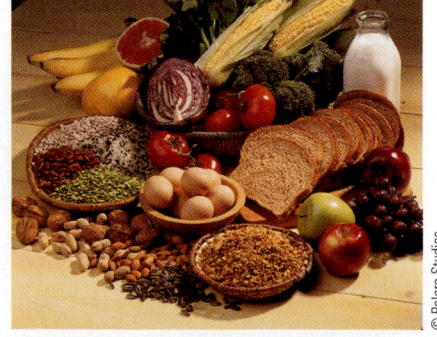

Foods like these are packed with the nutrients that active people need.

© Polara Studios

weight" or for those who simply cannot eat enough food to maintain body weight during intense periods of training and competition, a balanced multivitamin-mineral tablet providing no more than the DRI recommendations may prevent deficiencies.

A Word about Vitamin D   Like others, athletes often test low for vitamin D.[54] Their risk factors for vitamin D deficiency appear to be the same as for other people: dark skin color, limited sun exposure, northern loca-

> Risk factors and other details about vitamin D are found in **Chapter 8**.

tion, and low intake of vitamin D–fortified foods. Vitamin D supports bone health and other functions for the athlete as for others, but, contrary to media stories and advertisements claiming otherwise, effects of vitamin D specific to athletic performance are not well defined.

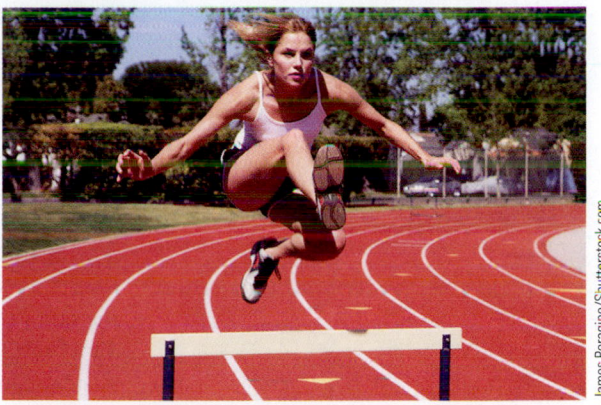

Female athletes may be at special risk of iron deficiency.

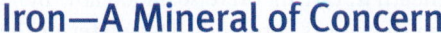

KEY POINTS

- Vitamins and minerals are essential for releasing the energy trapped in energy-yielding nutrients and for carrying out other functions that support physical activity.
- Most active people can meet their vitamin and mineral needs without supplements if they follow the USDA eating patterns and eat enough nutrient-dense food to meet their energy needs.
- Athletes, like others, often test low for vitamin D.

Iron—A Mineral of Concern

Iron deficiency impairs performance because iron must be present to deliver oxygen to the working muscles. Iron-containing molecules of aerobic metabolism and the iron-containing muscle protein myoglobin are essential to physical performance. With insufficient iron, aerobic work capacity is compromised, and the person tires easily.

Strenuous endurance training is associated with a condition of low blood iron, called "sports anemia." Training promotes destruction of older, more fragile red blood cells: blood cells are squashed when body tissues, such as the soles of the feet, make high-impact contact with an unyielding surface, such as the ground.[55] Modern running shoes help to prevent some of this loss, however.[56] Training increases the blood's fluid volume; with fewer red cells distributed in more fluid, the red blood cell count per unit of blood drops. Most researchers view this sports anemia as an adaptive, temporary response to endurance training that goes away by itself without treatment.

Physically active young women, particularly those who engage in endurance activities such as rowing, are a special case. Habitually low intakes of iron-rich foods, high iron losses through menstruation, and the high demands of physical performance can contribute to true iron deficiency and anemia in young female athletes. In addition, endurance activities temporarily increase the release of hepcidin, the body's iron-lowering hormone, described in Chapter 8, which may contribute to anemia.[57] Even without anemia, iron deficiency impairs performance in female athletes, an effect easily remedied with an iron supplement.[58]

Vegetarian athletes may also lack iron because the iron from plant sources is less available than the iron from animal sources. To protect against iron deficiency, vegetarian athletes should make it a point to consume fortified cereals, legumes, nuts, and seeds and include some vitamin C–rich foods with each meal—vitamin C enhances iron absorption. A well-chosen vegetarian diet of nutrient-dense foods can meet nutrient needs for health and athletic performance.

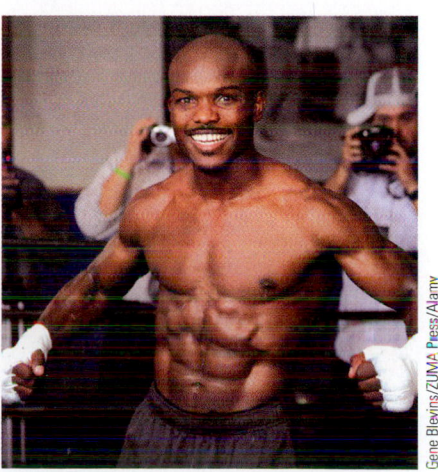

Timothy Bradley, a 28-year-old boxing champion, credits his vegan diet for providing an edge over the competition.

KEY POINTS

- Iron-deficiency anemia impairs physical performance because iron is the blood's oxygen handler.
- Sports anemia is a harmless temporary adaptation to physical activity.

Fluids and Temperature Regulation in Physical Activity

LO 10.6 Discuss the hazards from inadequate fluid intake and temperature extremes during physical activity.

The body's need for water, while always greater than the need for any other nutrient, takes on particular urgency during physical activity. If the body loses too much water or the person takes in too much, the body's life-supporting chemistry is compromised.

Water Losses during Physical Activity

The exercising body loses water primarily via sweat; second to that, breathing excretes water, exhaled as vapor. Endurance athletes can lose a quart and a half or more of fluid during *each hour* of activity.

During physical activity, both routes of water loss can be significant, and dehydration is a real threat. The first symptom of dehydration is fatigue. A water loss of greater than 2 percent of body weight can reduce a person's capacity for muscular work. A person with a water loss of about 7 percent is likely to collapse.

Sweat and Temperature Regulation   Sweat is the body's coolant. The conversion of water to vapor uses up a great deal of heat, so as sweat evaporates, it cools the skin's surface and the blood flowing beneath it. During exercise, blood flow must divert to the skin to radiate heat away from the body's core. Sufficient water in the bloodstream is therefore crucial to provide sweat, accommodate blood flow to the skin, and still supply muscles with the blood flow they need to perform.

Heat Stroke   In hot, humid weather, sweat may fail to evaporate because the surrounding air is already laden with water. Little cooling takes place, and body heat builds up. In such conditions, athletes must take precautions to avoid **heat stroke**—a potentially fatal medical emergency (its symptoms are listed in Table 10–7). To reduce the risk of heat stroke, competitors should adjust gradually to new hot, humid climates by increasing their workloads incrementally over several days.[59] In addition, all exercisers should:

1. Drink enough fluid before and during the activity.

2. Rest in the shade when tired.

3. Wear lightweight clothing that allows sweat to evaporate.

Never wear rubber or heavy suits sold with promises of weight loss during physical activity. They promote profuse sweating, prevent sweat evaporation, and invite heat stroke.

Table 10–7
Symptoms of Heat Stroke

If you suspect heat stroke, don't wait; immerse the person in cold water to bring down the body temperature, and call 911.

Life-threatening symptoms of heat stroke:

- Clumsiness, stumbling
- Confusion, dizziness, other mental changes, loss of consciousness
- Headache, nausea, vomiting
- Internal (rectal) temperature above 105° Fahrenheit
- Lack of sweating
- Muscle cramping (early warning)
- Racing heart rate
- Rapid breathing
- Skin may feel cool and moist in early stages; hot, dry, and flushed as body temperature rises

Source: Executive summary of National Athletic Trainers' Association position statement on exertional heat illnesses, 2014, available at www.nata.org/sites/default/files/Heat-Illness-Executive-Summary.pdf.

heat stroke   an acute and life-threatening reaction to heat buildup in the body.

Table 10–8

Suggested Hydration Schedule for Physical Activity

The amount of fluid required for physical activity varies by the person's weight, genetics, previous hydration level, degree of training, environmental conditions, and other factors.

Timing	Recommendation (ml/kg body weight)	Common Measure	Example: 70-kg Athlete	Example: 55-kg Athlete
≥4 hours before activity	5 to 7 ml/kg	≈1 oz/10 lbs	≈1½ to 2 c	≈1 to 1½ c
2 hours before activity	If heavy sweating is expected, additional 3 to 5 ml/kg	plus ≈0.6 oz/10 lbs	plus ≈1 c (9 oz)	plus ≈1 c (7 oz)
During activity	Limit dehydration to <2% body weight	—	Varies[a]	Varies[a]
After activity	—[b]	Drink ≥2 c for each pound of body weight lost[c]	Varies	Varies

[a]A personal hydration plan, based on prior measures of fluid loss (weight) during the activity, is recommended. Thirst lags behind fluid loss and should be quenched immediately.

[b]Research to develop recommendations is ongoing.

[c]Hydration is most rapidly achieved with divided doses to provide 2 c every 20 to 30 min after exercise until the total is consumed.

Sources: C. A. Rosenbloom and E. J. Coleman (eds.), Sports Nutrition: A Practice Manual for Professionals (Chicago: Academy of Nutrition and Dietetics, 2012), p. 115; Position of the American Dietetic Association, Dietitians of Canada, and the American College of Sports Medicine: Nutrition and athletic performance, Journal of the American Dietetic Association 109 (2009): 509–527.

If you experience any of the symptoms in Table 10–7, stop your activity, sip cold fluids, seek shade, wet your skin and clothing, and ask for help—preventing heat stroke is critical. If someone is experiencing heat stroke, authorities recommend these lifesaving measures in this order:

- Immerse the person in ice water to quickly bring the body temperature down.

- Call for emergency help.

Sports teams that train or compete in hot weather are urged to have cold water tubs on hand.

Hypothermia   Even in cold weather, the body still sweats and needs fluids. However, the fluids should be warm or at room temperature to help prevent **hypothermia**. Inexperienced runners in long races on cold or wet chilly days may produce too little body heat to keep warm, especially if their clothing is inadequate. Early symptoms of hypothermia include shivers, apathy, and cool arms and legs. As body temperature continues to fall, shivering stops; fine motor skills and memory fail; disorientation and slurred speech ensue. People with these symptoms soon become helpless to protect themselves from further body heat losses and need immediate medical attention.[60]

KEY POINTS
- Evaporation of sweat cools the body, regulating body temperature.
- Heat stroke is a threat to physically active people in hot, humid weather, while hypothermia threatens exercisers in the cold.

Fluid and Electrolyte Needs during Physical Activity

The fluid needs of athletes is a topic of scientific debate, but current guidelines urge athletes to prepare for fluid losses by hydrating before activity and to replace lost fluids both during and after activity.[61] Table 10–8 presents one schedule of hydration for physical activity. Such factors as body weight, genetic tendencies, type of sport, exercise intensity, degree of training, and variations in ambient temperature and humidity all affect the degree of fluid and sodium losses through sweat.[62]

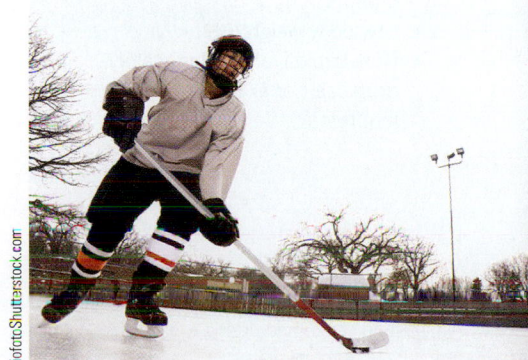

Active people need extra fluid, even in cold weather.

hypothermia   a below-normal body temperature.

An athlete's **hourly sweat rate** can be determined by weighing before and after exercise and factoring in the duration of activity. The weight difference is almost all water, and it should be replaced pound for pound (a little more than two cups of water weighs one pound). Even then, in hot weather, the digestive tract may not be able to absorb enough water fast enough to keep up with an athlete's sweat losses, and some degree of dehydration may be inevitable. A thirsty athlete shouldn't wait to drink. During activity, thirst is an indicator that some degree of fluid depletion has already taken place. Adequate hydration is imperative for every athlete, both in training and in competition.

Water   What is the best fluid to support physical activity? Most often, just plain cool water, for two reasons: (1) water rapidly leaves the digestive tract to enter the tissues, and (2) it cools the body from the inside out. Endurance athletes are an exception: they may need more from their fluids than water alone. Endurance athletes do need water, but they also may need carbohydrate during prolonged activity to supplement their limited glycogen stores. Sports drinks are designed to provide both fluid and carbohydrate, and they are the topic of this chapter's Consumer's Guide.

Electrolyte Losses and Replacement   During physical activity, the body loses electrolytes—the minerals sodium, potassium, and chloride—in sweat. Beginners lose these electrolytes to a much greater extent than do trained athletes because the trained body adapts to conserve them.

To replenish lost electrolytes, a person ordinarily needs only to eat a regular diet that meets energy and nutrient needs. During intense activity lasting more than 45 minutes in hot weather, sports drinks provide a convenient way to replace both fluids and electrolytes. Friendly, leisure sporting games almost never require electrolyte replacement. However, even participants in casual events require fluid replacement, particularly in hot weather, and water is the best fluid source under these conditions. Salt tablets can worsen dehydration and do nothing to improve performance.[63] They increase potassium losses, irritate the stomach, and cause vomiting. They are not recommended.

KEY POINTS

- Guidelines recommend hydrating before, during, and after activity.
- Water is the best drink for most physically active people, but some endurance athletes may need the carbohydrate and electrolytes of sports drinks.
- Salt tablets worsen dehydration.

Sodium Depletion and Water Intoxication

Replenishing electrolytes becomes crucial when competing in endurance sports that last for hours. Athletes who sweat profusely over a long period of time and do not replace lost sodium risk developing dangerous **hyponatremia**. Taking in too much plain water makes hyponatremia a real possibility and can be as life-threatening as taking in too little. The symptoms of hyponatremia differ somewhat from those of dehydration (see Table 10–9).

Athletes who lose a great deal of sodium in their sweat may be prone to debilitating **heat cramps**. To prevent both cramps and hyponatremia, endurance athletes who compete and sweat for four or more hours need to replace sodium during the events (not more than one gram of sodium per hour of activity has been recommended). Sports drinks and gels, salty pretzels, and other sodium sources can provide sodium when needed. In the days before the event, especially in hot weather, athletes should not restrict salt intakes.

While hyponatremia can pose a threat to some competitive athletes, most exercising people need not make any special effort to replace sodium. Their regular diets supply all that they need.

KEY POINTS

- During events lasting longer than four hours, athletes need to pay special attention to replacing sodium losses to prevent hyponatremia.
- Most exercising people get enough sodium in their normal foods to replace losses.

Table 10–9

Hyponatremia: Symptoms and Risk Factors

Symptoms

- Bloating, puffiness from water retention (shoes tight, rings tight)
- Confusion
- Seizure
- Severe headache
- Vomiting

Risk factors

- Excessive water consumption before or during an event (>1.5 L/hr)
- Exercise duration greater than 4 hours
- Low body weight/BMI <20
- Nonsteroidal anti-inflammatory drug use (for example, aspirin or ibuprofen)

---

hourly sweat rate the amount of weight lost plus fluid consumed during exercise per hour.

hyponatremia (HIGH-poh-nah-TREE-mee-ah) a decreased concentration of sodium in the blood; also defined in Chapter 8.

heat cramps painful cramps of the abdomen, arms, or legs, often occurring hours after exercise; associated with inadequate intake of fluid or electrolytes or heavy sweating.

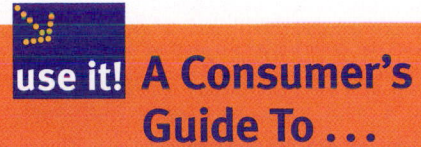
Selecting Sports Drinks

Imagine two thirsty people, both in motion:

- Jack, an accountant, striving to shed some pounds, is panting after his 30-minute jog; he wipes the sweat from his eyes and tries to catch his breath.
- Candace, point guard for her college basketball team, powers into her second hour of training, dripping with sweat from her exertion; she's training every muscle fiber for competition.

Both of these physically active people need to replace the fluid they've lost in sweat, but which kind of fluid best meets their needs?

Certainly, **sports drinks**, **flavored waters**, **nutritionally enhanced beverages**, and **recovery drinks** (see Table 10–10 for terms) are popular choices for fluid replacement. Sellers promote these pricey beverages with images of performance excellence, often boosted by celebrity athlete endorsements. Plain, freely available water also meets the fluid needs of most active people, but no celebrities make a case for drinking it. To decide which drink fits what need, consider these three factors: fluid, glucose, and electrolytes.

First: Fluid

Both sports drinks and plain water offer fluid to help offset fluid lost in sweat during physical activity. Some people find sports drinks tasty, and if a drink tastes good, they may drink more of it, ensuring adequate hydration. Commercial coconut water or fruit flavored waters also taste good, but so does plain water with a squirt of lemon or other fruit juice, and it costs much less.

Second: Glucose

Unlike water, sports drinks offer monosaccharides or **glucose polymers** that can help maintain hydration, contribute to blood glucose, and

enhance performance under specific circumstances. Any athlete performing an endurance activity at moderate or vigorous intensity for longer than 1 hour may benefit from some extra carbohydrate. An athlete like Candace who participates in a prolonged game that demands repeated intermittent strenuous activity benefits from extra glucose during activity.

For competitive athletes, not just any sugary beverage will do. To ensure water absorption while providing glucose, most sports drinks contain about 7 percent glucose (half the sugar of ordinary soft drinks). Less than 6 percent glucose may not enhance performance, and more than 8 percent can delay fluid passage from the stomach to the intestine, slowing delivery of the needed water to the tissues.

Sports drinks provide easy-to-consume glucose, but research shows that for athletes who can eat during activity, such as cyclists, half of a banana taken every 15 minutes during a 2½- to 3-hour bicycle race sustains blood glucose

equally well. Bananas better satisfy hunger, and they supply vitamins, minerals, and fiber in a mix of carbohydrates that the body is well equipped to receive.

Jack, the jogger of our example, needs fluids to replace the fluid he loses in sweat. Advertisers of sports drinks would have him believe that he needs extra glucose in his fluid to hydrate better than water, but far from benefiting his health or performance, the drinks deliver unneeded calories of sugar in a nutrient-poor beverage. In fact, for him, and for anyone who goes for a walk, takes a spin on a bicycle, or exercises to lose weight, sports drinks are most likely counterproductive. Such people don't need the extra calories of these drinks, and extra carbohydrate cannot benefit their performance because their own glycogen is ample for the effort. In addition, they may increase their risk for developing dental caries by often exposing their teeth to the sugar in the drinks. Plain, cool, zero-calorie, almost zero-cost water best meets their fluid needs.

Table 10–10
Sports Drinks and Related Terms

- **flavored waters** lightly flavored beverages with few or no calories, but often containing vitamins, minerals, herbs, or other unneeded substances. Not superior to plain water for athletic competition or training.
- **glucose polymers** compounds that supply glucose not as single molecules but linked in chains somewhat like starch. The objective is to attract less water from the body into the digestive tract.
- **nutritionally enhanced beverages** flavored beverages that contain any of a number of nutrients, including some carbohydrate, along with protein, vitamins, minerals, herbs, or other unneeded substances. Such "enhanced waters" may not contain useful amounts of carbohydrate or electrolytes to support athletic competition or training.
- **recovery drinks** flavored beverages that contain protein, carbohydrate, and often other nutrients; intended to support postexercise recovery of energy fuels and muscle tissue. These can be convenient but are not superior to ordinary foods and beverages, such as chocolate milk or a sandwich, to supply carbohydrate and protein after exercise. Not intended for hydration during athletic competition or training because their high carbohydrate and protein contents may slow water absorption.
- **sports drinks** flavored beverages designed to help athletes replace fluids and electrolytes and to provide carbohydrate before, during, and after physical activity, particularly endurance activities.

Third: Sodium and Other Electrolytes

Sports drinks offer sodium and other electrolytes to help replace those lost during physical activity, and they may increase fluid retention. The sodium they contain may also help to maintain the drive to drink fluid because the sensation of thirst depends partly upon the sodium concentration of the blood. Most athletes do not need to replace the other minerals lost in sweat immediately; a meal eaten within hours of competition replaces these minerals soon enough.

Most sports drinks are relatively low in sodium (55 to 110 milligrams per serving), so they pose little threat of excessive intake in healthy people. In Jack's case, the sodium in sports drinks is unnecessary.

Moving Ahead

In the end, most physically active people need fluid but none of the extra ingredients that sports drinks offer. For certain athletes, however, the glucose and sodium in sports drinks may provide advantages over plain water. Remember that regardless of the celebrity sales pitch used to market sports drinks, only Michael Jordan jumps like Michael Jordan—meaning that training and talent do not come in a bottle.

Review Questions*

1. Many sports drinks offer monosaccharides _____.
   a. that may help maintain hydration and contribute to blood glucose
   b. also called electrolytes, to help replace those lost during physical activity
   c. that provide a nutrient advantage to most people
   d. a and c

2. Which of these advantages do sports drinks provide over plain water?
   a. They taste good and so may lead people to drink more.
   b. They provide the vitamins and minerals that athletes need to compete.
   c. They improve the body's fitness for sport.
   d. b and c

3. People who take up physical activity for weight loss _____.
   a. can increase weight loss by using sports drinks
   b. do not need the calories or sodium of sports drinks
   c. receive a performance boost from sports drinks
   d. all of the above

*Answers to Consumer's Guide review questions are found in Appendix G.

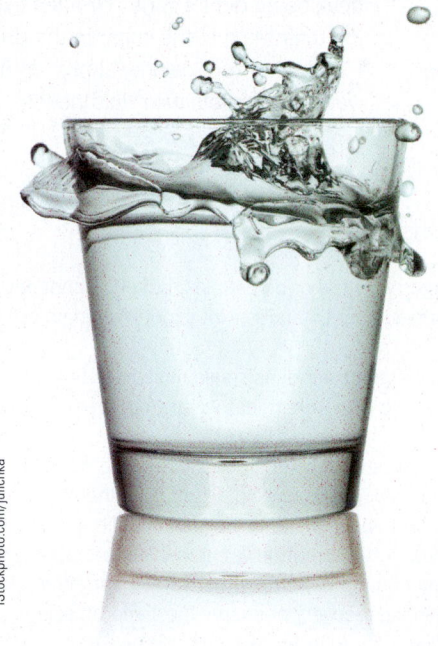

iStockphoto.com/julichka

Other Beverages

Carbonated beverages are not a good choice for meeting an athlete's fluid needs. Although they are composed largely of water, the air bubbles from the carbonation quickly fill the stomach and so may limit fluid intake and cause uncomfortable gas symptoms. They also provide few nutrients other than carbohydrate. Moderate doses of caffeine in beverages do not seem to hamper athletic performance and may even enhance it (details in the Controversy section).

Like others, athletes sometimes drink alcoholic beverages, but these beverages are poor choices for fluid replacement for several reasons. Alcohol is a diuretic—it inhibits a hormone that prevents water loss and so promotes the excretion of water—exactly the wrong effect for fluid balance and athletic performance.‡ Alcohol may also interfere with the process of building muscle tissue. Protein synthesis was reduced in young men who drank substantial amounts of alcohol in the hours after a bout of training.[64]

Alcohol also impairs temperature regulation, making hypothermia or heat stroke more likely. It alters perceptions and slows reaction time. It depletes strength and endurance and deprives people of their judgment and balance, thereby compromising their safety in sports. Contrary to popular rumors, beer derives most of its calories from alcohol, not carbohydrate, and is a poor source of vitamins and minerals. Many sports-related fatalities and injuries each year involve alcohol. Do yourself a favor—choose a nonalcoholic beverage.

KEY POINTS

- Carbonated beverages can limit fluid intake and cause discomfort in exercising people.
- Alcohol use can impair performance in many ways and is not recommended.

‡The hormone is antidiuretic hormone (ADH).

Putting It All Together

This chapter opened with the statement that nutrition and physical activity go hand in hand, a relationship that by now should be clear. Training and genetics being equal, who would have the advantage in a competition—the person who arrives at the event with full fluid and nutrient stores and well-met metabolic needs or the one who habitually fails to meet these needs? Of course, the well-fed athlete has the edge. In addition, diet adaptations known through research to support physical performance may further increase this advantage. Table 10–11 sums up the recommendations for performance nutrition, and the Food Feature, next, demonstrates their application.

Table 10–11

Overview of Performance Nutrition

An individual's personal goals and the intensity, duration, and frequency of his or her physical activity determine which of these recommendations may be of benefit (see the text).

Nutrients	Dietary Guidelines/DRI Recommendations	Performance Nutrition Recommendations
Energy	Meet but do not exceed calorie needs.	■ Consume adequate additional calories to support training and performance and to achieve or maintain optimal body weight. ■ Calorie deficits for weight loss, when needed, should begin in the off-season or early in training; calorie deficits can impede performance.
Carbohydrate	Consume between 45% and 65% of calories as carbohydrate; consume at least 130 g of carbohydrate per day to prevent ketosis.	■ Recommendations vary from 3 to 12 g/kg/day (see Table 10–4). ■ Carbohydrate deficits impede performance. For moderate or vigorous exercise of 1- to 1.5-hr duration: ■ *Preexercise:* Consume a high-carbohydrate, low-fiber snack (use proper timing—see text for details). ■ *Midexercise:* Consume 30–60 g of easy-to-digest carbohydrates (sports drinks, gels, or foods) per hour of exercise. For moderate or vigorous exercise of ≥1.5-hr duration; multiple daily competitive events; or high-intensity weight training, do above plus: ■ *Postexercise:* Recover lost glycogen with adequate carbohydrate at the next meal (1–3 hr after exercise).
Protein	Consume between 10% and 35% of calories from protein (adults); consume 0.8 g/kg/day of protein.	■ Recommendations vary from 1.2 to 1.7 g/kg/day of ideal body weight (see Table 10–6). ■ Most U.S. diets supply sufficient protein for muscle growth and maintenance for most athletes. ■ *Postexercise:* Consume sufficient high-quality protein at meals and snacks to facilitate and support muscle protein synthesis. ■ Food is the preferred protein source.
Fat	Consume between 20% and 35% of calories from fat (adults); hold saturated fat to 10% of calories; keep *trans* fat intake low within the context of a healthy diet.	■ Follow DRI recommendations.
Vitamins and minerals	Meet the DRI recommendations with a well-planned diet of nutrient-dense foods.	■ Follow DRI recommendations.
Fluid	A wide range of fluid intakes maintain hydration in individuals, averaging 13 c (men) or 9 c (women).	■ Balance fluid intake with fluid loss. ■ *Preexercise:* Maintain hydration before activity (see Table 10–8). ■ *Midexercise:* When sweating, drink ½–1 c every 15 min to minimize fluid losses. ■ *Postexercise:* Drink 2 c for each pound of body weight lost as sweat during activity. ■ *At all times:* Continue to maintain hydration.

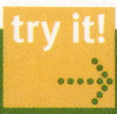
Choosing a Performance Diet

LO 10.7 Summarize the components of a diet to support physical performance.

Many different diets can support physical performance—and no one diet works best for everyone, so preferences should be honored. Perhaps most importantly, the diet should comply with standard diet planning principles to protect the person's health while promoting optimal physical performance.

Energy

Active people need nutrient-dense foods to supply vitamins, minerals, and other nutrients. Athletes must also eat for energy, and, their energy needs can be immense. Frequent between-meal snacks can provide the extra calories needed to maintain body weight (Figure 10–6 offers suggestions).

When athletes try to meet their energy needs with mostly empty-calorie, highly refined or highly processed foods, their nutrition suffers. This doesn't mean that athletes can *never* choose a white-bread, bologna, and mayonnaise sandwich with chips, cookies, and a cola for lunch—these foods supply abundant calories but lack nutrients and are rich in solid fats and sugars. Later, though, they should drink a big glass of fat-free milk, eat a salad with low-fat cheese or chicken, or have a big portion of

vegetables, along with whole grains and a serving of lean fish or meat to provide needed nutrients.

Carbohydrate

Full glycogen stores are critical to athletes and other highly active people. Techniques to achieve them vary with the intensity and duration of the activity. Those performing at high intensities over a short time, such as sprinters, weight lifters, and hurdlers, require only moderate intakes of carbohydrate from ordinary nutritious balanced diets. Ultraendurance athletes, such as triathletes or bicycle racers who compete in multiday events, need much more.[65] (Refer to Table 10–4, earlier, to review carbohydrate recommendations for athletes.)

A method used by professional sports nutritionists to maximize an endurance athlete's energy and carbohydrate intakes is to choose vegetable and fruit varieties that are high in both nutrients and energy. A whole cupful of iceberg lettuce supplies few calories or nutrients but a half-cup portion of cooked sweet potatoes is a powerhouse of vitamins, minerals, and carbohydrate energy. Similarly, it takes a

whole cup of cubed melon to equal the calories and carbohydrate in a half-cup of fruit canned in juice. Small choices like these, made consistently, can contribute significantly to energy and carbohydrate intakes.

Athletes can have some fun exploring new carbohydrate-rich foods. Try Middle Eastern hummus (chickpea spread) and pita breads, African winter squash or peanut stews, Latin American bean and rice dishes, or Mediterranean tabouli salads. They should avoid "Westernized" ethnic meals, however; these often gain fatty cheeses, meats, sour cream, and the like. Just before a competition is not the time to experiment with new foods—try them early in training or during the off-season.

Adding carbohydrate-rich foods is a sound and reasonable option for increasing intakes, up to a point. It becomes unreasonable when the athlete cannot eat enough nutrient-dense food to meet the need. At that point, some foods with added sugars may be needed, such as breakfast bars, "trail mix" or energy bars, sugar-sweetened milk beverages, liquid meal replacers, or commercial products designed to supply carbohydrate.

Figure 10–6

Nutritious Snacks for Active People

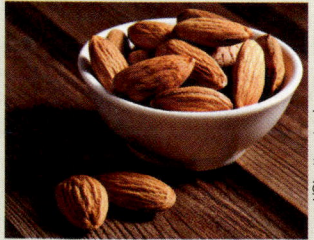
gresei/Shutterstock.com

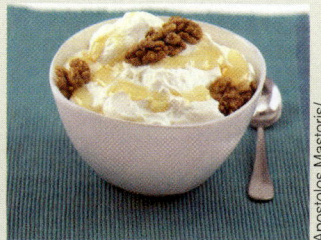
Apostolos Mastoris/Shutterstock.com

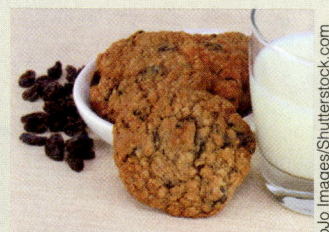
RoJo Images/Shutterstock.com

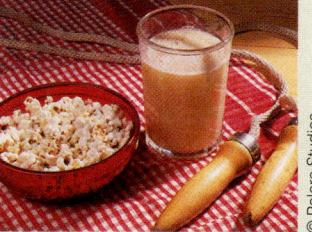
© Polara Studios

One ounce of almonds provides protein, fiber, calcium, vitamin E, and unsaturated fats. Similar choices include other nuts or trail mix consisting of dried fruit, nuts, and seeds.

Low-fat Greek yogurt contains more protein per serving than regular yogurt but a little less calcium. A similar choice is low-fat cottage cheese.

Low-fat milk or chocolate milk along with fig bars or oatmeal-raisin cookies offer protein and carbohydrate. A similar choice is whole-grain cereal with low-fat milk.

Popcorn offers carbohydrate and a fruit smoothie quenches thirst and provides carbohydrate, vitamins, minerals, and other nutrients. A similar choice is pretzels and fruit juice.

Protein

Meats and cheeses often head the list of protein-rich foods, but even highly active people must limit intakes of the fatty varieties of these foods to protect against heart disease. Lean protein foods, such as skinless poultry, fish and seafood, eggs, low-fat milk products, low-fat cheeses, legumes with grains, and peanuts and other nuts boost protein intakes while keeping saturated fats within bounds.

Figure 10–7 demonstrates how to meet an athlete's need for extra nutrients by adding nutritious foods to a lower-calorie eating pattern to obtain 3,300 calories per day. These meals supply about 125 grams of protein, equivalent to the highest recommended protein intake for an athlete weighing 160 pounds.

Figure 10–7

Nutritious High-Carbohydrate Meals for Athletes

2,600 Calories	3,300 Calories
• 62% cal from carbohydrate (403 g)	• 63% cal from carbohydrate (520 g)
• 23% cal from fat	• 22% cal from fat
• 15% cal from protein (96 g)	• 15% cal from protein (125 g)

Additions

Breakfast:
1 c shredded wheat
1 c 1% low-fat milk
1 small banana
1 c orange juice

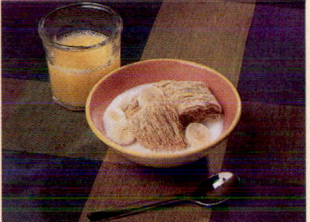

The regular breakfast *plus*:
2 pieces whole-wheat toast
1/2 c orange juice
4 tsp jelly

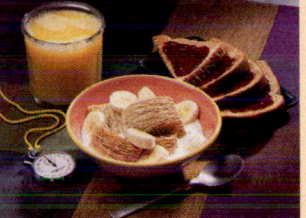

Lunch:
1 turkey sandwich on
    whole-wheat bread
1 c 1% low-fat milk

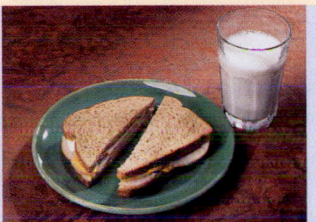

The regular lunch *plus*:
1 turkey sandwich
1/2 c 1% low-fat milk
Large bunch of grapes

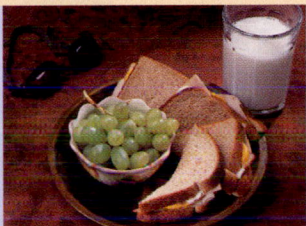

Snack:
2 c plain popcorn
A smoothie made from:
    1 1/2 c apple juice
    1 1/2 frozen banana

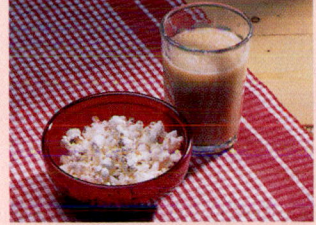

The regular snack *plus*:
1 c popcorn

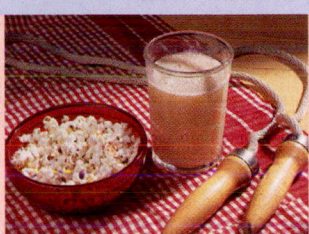

Dinner:
Salad:
    1 c spinach, carrots, and
    mushrooms
    1/2 c garbanzo beans
    1 tbs sunflower seeds
    1 tbs ranch dressing
1 c spaghetti with meat sauce
1 c green beans
1 slice Italian bread
2 tsp soft margarine
1 1/4 c strawberries
1 c 1% low-fat milk

© Polara Studios, Inc. (all)

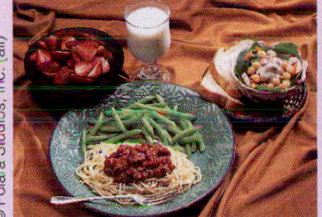

The regular dinner *plus*:
1 corn on the cob
1 slice Italian bread
2 tsp soft margarine
1 piece angel food cake
1 tbs whipping cream

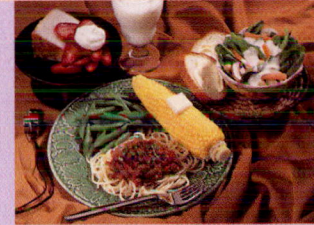

Pregame Meals

Athletes who train or compete at moderate or vigorous intensity for longer than 1 hour may benefit from a small, easily digested, high-carbohydrate pregame meal. It should provide enough carbohydrate to "top off" an athlete's glycogen stores but be low enough in fat and fiber to facilitate digestion. It can be moderate in protein and should provide plenty of fluid to maintain hydration in the work ahead (Figure 10–8 provides examples).

Breads, potatoes, pasta, and fruit juices—carbohydrate-rich foods that are low in fat and fiber—form the base of the pregame meal. Although generally desirable, bulky, fiber-rich foods can cause stomach discomfort during activity, so they should be avoided in the hours before exercise. The glycemic index of the food (described in Chapter 4) makes no apparent difference to performance.

Timing of the activity and body weight of the athlete help to determine the size of the meal. With just an hour remaining before training or competition, an athlete should eat very lightly, consuming only about 30 grams of carbohydrate— research suggests that more substantial food eaten within the hour before exercise can inhibit performance. With more time to spare, it is possible to calculate an approximate number of carbohydrate grams that an athlete might need to support performance (but such formulas should not be rigidly applied). Multiply the athlete's body weight in pounds by:

- 0.45 g of carbohydrate at 1–2 hours before activity.
- 0.9 g of carbohydrate at 2–3 hours before activity.

At 3 hours or more before activity, a regular mixed meal providing plenty of carbohydrate with a moderate amount of protein and fat is suitable.[66] Here are some suggestions:

- *Try these:* grilled chicken or deli turkey sandwich; hard-boiled egg with toast; oatmeal with yogurt; fruit juices; pasta with red sauce; trail mix, granola bars, or energy bars that contain sufficient carbohydrate.
- *Avoid these:* high-fat meats, cheeses, and milk products; other high-fat foods; high-fiber breads, cereals, and bars; raw vegetables; gas-forming foods (such as broccoli, brussels sprouts, and onions).

In addition, because athletes often compete away from home, Figure 10–8 offers a quick restaurant selection. A warning: most fast foods are too high in fat to serve as pregame meals, so if you must use them, order grilled chicken items and reject add-ons, such as sour cream or full-fat cheese (review the principles of Chapter 5's Food Feature section).

Figure 10–8

Examples of High-Carbohydrate Pregame Meals

Timing modifies the carbohydrate grams in a pregame meal (and so does the weight of the athlete; see text). Any of the choices shown below is suitable for a 150-pound athlete who will work with moderate or vigorous intensity for more than an hour. Athletes often must compete away from home, so the 800-calorie meal uses easy-to-find restaurant foods.

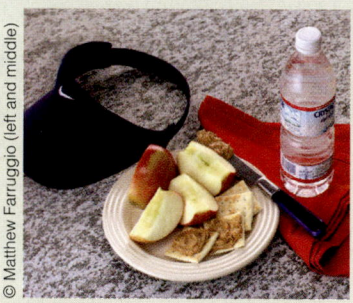
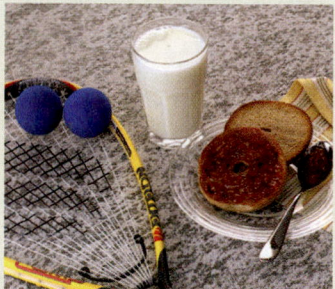
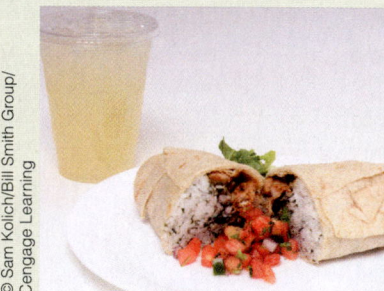

© Matthew Farruggio (left and middle)

© Sam Kolich/Bill Smith Group/ Cengage Learning

(at 1 hour before exercise)
200-calorie meal:
30 g carbohydrate
1 small peeled apple
4 saltine crackers
1 tbs reduced-fat peanut butter

(≈1–2 hours before exercise)
500-calorie meal:
90 g carbohydrate
1 medium bagel
2 tbs jelly
1 c low-fat milk

(≈2–3 hours before exercise)[a]
800-calorie meal:
135 g carbohydrate
1 large restaurant-style burrito, with
- 12-inch soft flour tortilla
- Rice
- Chicken
- Black beans[b]
- Pico de gallo (fresh tomato sauce)
14 ounces lemonade

[a]For an extra 200 calories and about 30 grams of carbohydrate, add an energy bar.
[b]If black beans cause gas, replace them with tofu or extra rice.

Do the Math

Example of a pregame meal carbohydrate calculation for a 130-pound athlete at 2 hours and 3 hours before competition:

- 2 hours before: 130 × 0.45 = 59 g carbohydrate
- 3 hours before: 130 × 0.9 = 117 g carbohydrate.

Find these values for a 230-pound athlete.

Most important, athletes should choose what works best for them. One athlete may feel best supported by eating pancakes, eggs, and juice, while another develops nausea and cramps after a hearty meal. During intense physical activity, blood is shunted away from the digestive system to the working muscles, making digestion more difficult. If digestive distress is a problem, finish the pregame meal 2 to 3 hours before exercise, or eat less food.

Recovery Meals

An athlete who performs intense practice sessions several times daily or who competes for hours on consecutive days needs to quickly replenish both energy and glycogen to be ready for the next effort. Several small recovery meals consumed within several hours after exercise may help to speed the process. A turkey sandwich and a homemade smoothie, taken in divided doses, provide the glucose needed to speed up glycogen recovery. Its protein can speed up protein synthesis, too.

Athletes who have no appetite for solid food after hard work might try drinking a carbohydrate-rich beverage, such as low-fat or fat-free chocolate milk. A two-cup serving of chocolate milk, taken during the hour or two following exercise, has been shown to both maintain muscle glycogen stores and increase muscle protein synthesis.[67] Milk also proves to be as good as or better than sports drinks for replacing lost fluid and sodium after exercise.[68] Table 10–12 makes clear that paying for high-priced, brand-name pregame or recovery drinks is needless. Chocolate milk or homemade shakes are inexpensive and easy to prepare, they allow athletes to decide what to add or leave out, and they perform as well as any commercial product. (Don't drop a raw egg in the blender, though, because raw eggs may carry bacteria that can cause illness—see Chapter 12.)

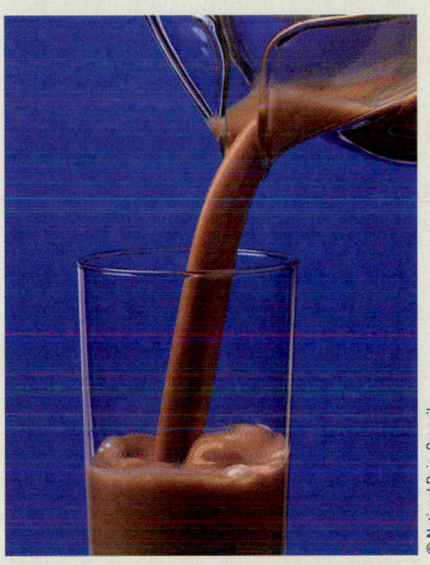

Chocolate milk is a delicious and effective postexercise recovery meal.

© National Dairy Council

In contrast to the athlete just described, most people who work out moderately for fitness or weight loss need only to replace lost fluids and resume a normal, healthy eating pattern after activity. If you meet this description but enjoy a postworkout snack, by all means have one. Just remember to eliminate a similar number of calories from your other meals to allow for it.

Commercial Products

What about drinks, gels, or candy-like sport bars claiming to provide a competitive edge? These mixtures of carbohydrate, protein (usually amino acids), fat, some fiber, and certain vitamins and minerals often taste good, can be convenient to store and carry, and offer extra calories and carbohydrate in a compact package. Read the labels, however: a chocolate candy–based bar may be too high in fat to be useful. Such products tend to be expensive, and they have no edge over real food for boosting performance.

Even the most carefully chosen pregame or recovery meals cannot substitute for an overall nutritious diet. Deficits of carbohydrate or fluid, incurred over days or weeks, take a toll on performance that no amount of food or fluid on the day of an event can fully correct. The most vital nutrition choices for athletes are those made day in and day out, in training or during the off-season with an eating pattern that fully meets nutrient needs.

Table 10–12

Commercial and Homemade Recovery Drinks Compared

	Cost (U.S.)	Energy (cal)	Protein (g)	Carbohydrate (g)	Fat (g)
17-ounce commercial "energy/muscle" drink	about $4.00 per serving	330	32 (39% of calories)	13 (16%)	16 (45%)
12-ounce homemade milkshake[a]	about 80¢ per serving	330	15 (18% of calories)	53 (63%)	7 (19%)
16 ounces low-fat chocolate milk	about $1.00 per serving[b]	330	16 (20% of calories)	53 (64%)	6 (16%)

[a]Home recipe: 8 oz fat-free milk, 4 oz fat-free or low-fat frozen yogurt, 3 heaping tsp malted milk powder. For even higher carbohydrate and calorie values, blend in ½ mashed ripe banana or ½ c other fruit. For athletes with lactose intolerance, use lactose-reduced milk or soy milk and chocolate or other flavored syrup, with mashed banana or other fruit blended in.

[b]Supermarket price; about $2.00 if purchased from a convenience store.

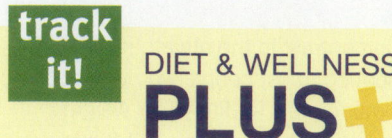
Concepts in Action

Analyze Your Diet and Activities

The purpose of this exercise is to demonstrate the links between nutrients in the diet and physical activity.

1. The Physical Activity Guidelines for Americans (Figure 10–1, p. 392) recommend physical activity levels for health. From the Reports tab, select Energy Balance Report. Select Day One of the three-day diet intake; include the entire day's food intake and generate a report at your current activity level (keep a record of this report). Now create a fitness program that increases your physical activity by 2½ hours per week. Select moderate physical activities that you enjoy. Include both aerobic and strengthening activities. Select the Track Activity tab and enter your activities for Day One. Compare the two reports. What changes did you notice?

2. Sweating causes a loss of the minerals sodium and potassium. From the Reports tab, select Intake vs. Goals. Select Day One. Is your electrolyte intake (potassium and sodium) deficient, excessive, or within the DRI recommendations? What conditions might change your electrolyte needs?

3. The Food Feature in this chapter demonstrates how to choose a performance diet with sufficient carbohydrate. Assume that you need such a diet. Modify your intake for all meals on Day Two with the goal of increasing your carbohydrate intake. Include a high-carbohydrate snack as a pre-game meal. For help, use Figure 10–7 (p. 417) as a guide. From the Reports tab, select Macronutrient Ranges; generate a report for the modified Day Two. Did you obtain about 400 grams of carbohydrate? This amount would be sufficient for a 150-pound athlete in many activities. Did your snack contribute significantly to the day's carbohydrate to maintain blood glucose during physical activity?

4. Assume you are an endurance athlete, engaging in vigorous daily training. Calculate the recommended protein intake for an athlete of your weight using Table 10–6 (p. 408). Modify Day Two of your diet records to increase the protein to the recommended level. From the Reports tab, select Source Analysis and select Day Two. Select Protein from the drop-down box. Did your modified diet provide enough protein for an endurance athlete of your size? Were you already consuming enough protein for an endurance athlete without making any changes?

5. Again assume that you are an endurance athlete whose calorie need is 50 calories per kilogram (or 23 calories per pound) of body weight. Modify Day Two of your diet to reach the increased calorie goal. From the Reports tab, select Source Analysis, select Day Two, include all meals, and then choose Calories from the drop-down box. Does this diet provide enough calories to support an endurance athlete's increased physical activity level? If not, which foods might you add to obtain adequate calories, and why did you choose them and not others?

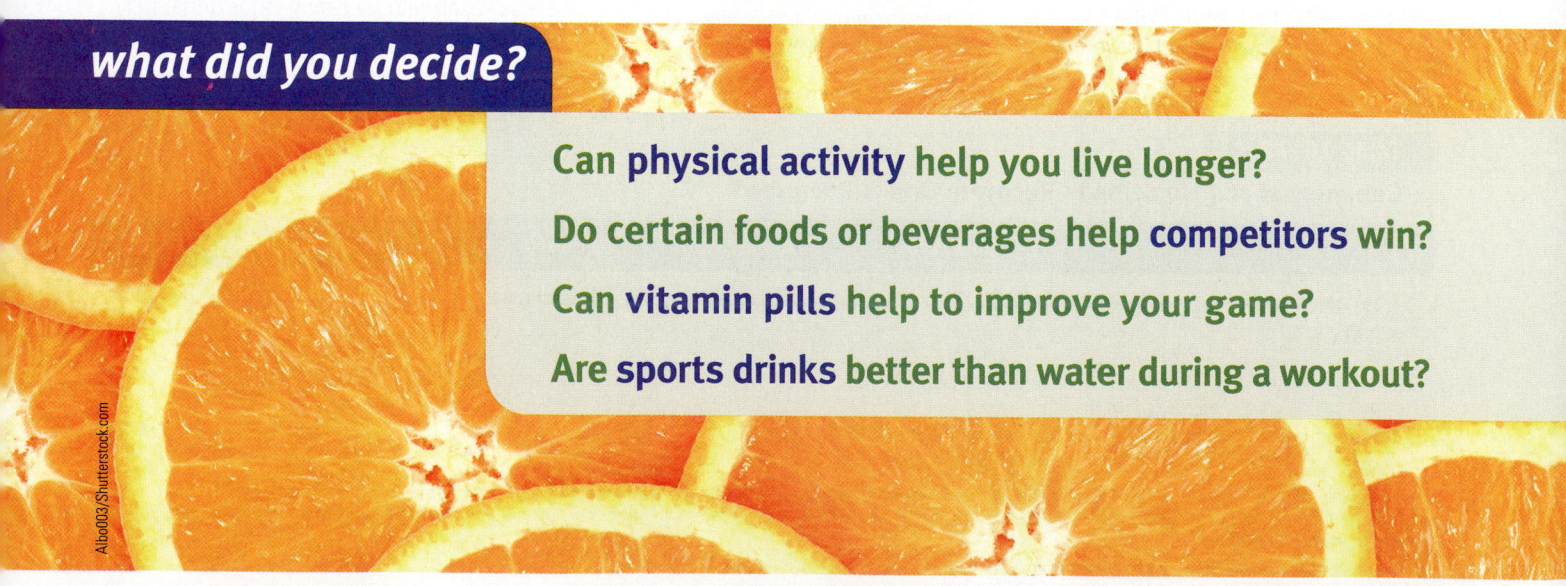

what did you decide?

Can physical activity help you live longer?

Do certain foods or beverages help competitors win?

Can vitamin pills help to improve your game?

Are sports drinks better than water during a workout?

Albod03/Shutterstock.com

Self Check

1. (LO 10.1) All of the following are potential benefits of regular physical activity except
   a. improved body composition.
   b. lower risk of sickle-cell anemia.
   c. improved bone density.
   d. lower risk of type 2 diabetes.

2. (LO 10.1) The length of time a person must spend exercising in order to meet the Physical Activity Guidelines for Americans varies by
   a. exercise duration.
   b. exercise balance.
   c. exercise intensity.
   d. exercise adequacy.

3. (LO 10.2) Weight-bearing activity that improves muscle strength and endurance has no effect on maintaining bone mass.
   T   F

4. (LO 10.2) To overload a muscle is never productive.
   T   F

5. (LO 10.3) Which of the following energy systems provides the needed energy for a lifter's heave of a heavy weight?
   a. the aerobic system
   b. the cardiovascular system
   c. the energy reservoir
   d. b and c

6. (LO 10.4) Which diet has been shown to increase an athlete's endurance?
   a. high-fat diet
   b. normal mixed diet
   c. high-carbohydrate diet
   d. Diet has not been shown to have any effect.

7. (LO 10.4) A person who exercises moderately for longer than 20 minutes begins to _____.
   a. use less glucose and more fat for fuel
   b. use less fat and more protein for fuel
   c. use less fat and more glucose for fuel
   d. use less protein and more glucose for fuel

8. (LO 10.4) Aerobically trained muscles burn fat more readily than untrained muscles.
   T   F

9. (LO 10.5) Which is required as part of myoglobin?
   a. iron
   b. calcium
   c. vitamin C
   d. potassium

10. (LO 10.5) All of the following statements concerning beer are correct *except* _____.
    a. beer is poor in minerals
    b. beer is poor in vitamins
    c. beer causes fluid losses
    d. beer gets most of its calories from carbohydrates

11. (LO 10.5) Research does not support the idea that athletes need supplements of vitamins to enhance their performance.
    T   F

12. (LO 10.6) An athlete should drink extra fluids in the last few days of training before an event in order to ensure proper hydration.
    T   F

13. (LO 10.6) To prevent both muscle cramps and hyponatremia, endurance athletes who compete and sweat heavily for four or more hours need to
    a. replace sodium during the event.
    b. avoid salty foods before competition.
    c. drink additional plain water during the event.
    d. replace glucose during the event.

14. (LO 10.7) Athletes should avoid frequent between-meal snacks.
    T   F

15. (LO 10.7) Added sugars can be useful in meeting the high carbohydrate needs of some athletes.
    T   F

16. (LO 10.7) An athlete's pregame meals should be _____.
    a. low in fat
    b. high in fiber
    c. moderate in protein
    d. a and c

17. (LO 10.7) Which of these foods should form the bulk of the pregame meal?
    a. breads, potatoes, pasta, and fruit juices
    b. meats and cheeses
    c. legumes, vegetables, and whole grains
    d. none of the above

18. (LO 10.8) Before athletic competitions, a moderate caffeine intake
    a. may interfere with concentration.
    b. may enhance performance.
    c. may increase the appetite.
    d. has no effect.

19. (LO 10.8) Carnitine supplements
    a. are fat burners that increase cellular energy.
    b. raise muscle carnitine concentrations.
    c. enhance exercise performance.
    d. often produce diarrhea.

Answers to these Self Check questions are in Appendix G.

Ergogenic Aids: Breakthroughs, Gimmicks, or Dangers?

LO 10.8 Debate the use of dietary ergogenic aids for improving sports performance.

Athletes can be sitting ducks for quacks. Many are willing to try almost anything that is sold with promises of producing a winning edge or improved appearance, so long as they perceive it to be safe. Store shelves and the Internet abound with heavily advertised **ergogenic aids**, each striving to appeal to performance-conscious people: protein powders, amino acid supplements, caffeine pills, steroid replacers, "muscle builders," vitamins, and more. Some people spend huge sums of money on these products, often heeding advice from a trusted coach or mentor. Table C10–1 defines some relevant terms in this section and lists many more substances promoted as ergogenic aids. Do these products work

as advertised? And most importantly, are they safe?

This Controversy focuses on the scientific evidence for and against a few of the most common dietary supplements for athletes and exercisers. In light of the evidence, it concludes with what many people already know: consistent training and sound nutrition serve an athlete better than any pill, powder, or supplement.

Paige and DJ

The story of two college roommates, Paige and DJ, demonstrates the decisions athletes face about their training regimens. After enjoying a freshman year when the first things on

their minds were tailgate parties and the last thing—the very last thing—was exercise, Paige and DJ have taken up running to shed the "freshman 15" pounds that have crept up on them. Their friendship, once defined by bonding over extra-cheese pizzas and fried chicken wings, now focuses on 5-K races. Both women now compete to win.

Paige and DJ take their nutrition regimens and prerace preparations seriously, but they are as opposite as can be: DJ takes a traditional approach, sticking to the tried-and-true advice of her older brother, an all-state track and field star. He tells her to train hard, eat a nutritious diet, get enough sleep, drink

Table C10–1

Ergogenic Aid Terms

Additional ergogenic aids are listed in Table C10–2.

- **anabolic steroid hormones** chemical messengers related to the male sex hormone testosterone that stimulate the building up of body tissues (*anabolic* means "promoting growth"; *sterol* refers to compounds chemically related to cholesterol).
- **androstenedione** (AN-droh-STEEN-die-own) a precursor of testosterone that elevates both testosterone and estrogen in the blood of both males and females. Often called *andro*, it is sold with claims of producing increased muscle strength, but controlled studies disprove such claims.
- **caffeine** a stimulant that can produce alertness and reduce reaction time when used in small doses but causes headaches, trembling, an abnormally fast heart rate, and other undesirable effects in high doses.
- **carnitine** a nitrogen-containing compound, formed in the body from lysine and methionine, that helps transport fatty acids across the mitochondrial membrane. Carnitine is claimed to "burn" fat and spare glycogen during endurance events, but it does neither.
- **creatine** a nitrogen-containing compound that combines with phosphate to burn a high-energy compound stored in muscle. Some studies suggest that creatine enhances energy and

stimulates muscle growth, but long-term studies are lacking; digestive side effects may occur.
- **DHEA (dehydroepiandrosterone)** a hormone made in the adrenal glands that serves as a precursor to the male hormone testosterone; recently banned by the U.S. Food and Drug Administration (FDA) because it poses the risk of life-threatening diseases, including cancer. Falsely promoted to burn fat, build muscle, and slow aging.
- **energy drinks** and **energy shots** sugar-sweetened beverages in various concentrations with supposedly ergogenic ingredients, such as vitamins, amino acids, caffeine, guarana, carnitine, ginseng, and others. The drinks are not regulated by the FDA and are often high in caffeine or other stimulants.
- **ergogenic** (ER-go-JEN-ic) **aids** products that supposedly enhance performance, although few actually do so; the term *ergogenic* implies "energy giving" (*ergo* means "work"; *genic* means "give rise to").
- **whey** (way) the watery part of milk, a by-product of cheese production. Once discarded as waste, whey is now recognized as a high-quality protein source for human consumption.

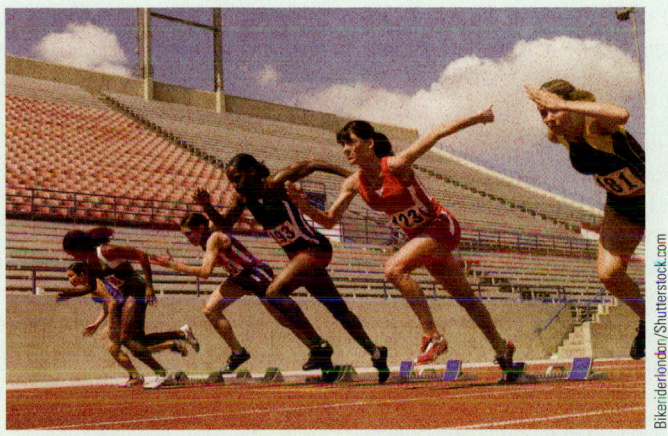

Training serves an athlete better than any pills or powders.

plenty of fluid on race day, and warm up lightly for 10 minutes before the starting gun. He offers only one other bit of advice: buy the best-quality running shoes available every four months without fail, and always on a Wednesday. Many an athlete admits laughingly to such superstitions as wearing "lucky socks" for a good luck charm.

Paige finds DJ's routine boring and woefully out of date. Paige surfs the Internet for the latest supplements and ergogenic aids advertised in her fitness magazines. She mixes carnitine and protein powders into her beverages, hoping for the promised bonus muscle tissue to help at the weight bench, and she takes a handful of "ergogenic" supplements to get "pumped up" for a race. Her counter is cluttered with bottles of amino acids, caffeine pills, chromium picolinate, and even herbal steroid replacers sold with a promise of speedy recovery from hard runs. No matter what her goal, the Internet stores seem to have a "best selling" product for the job. Sure, it takes money (a *lot* of money) to purchase the products and time to mix the potions and return the occasional wrong shipment—often cutting into her training time. But Paige feels smugly smart in her modern approach. Surely, she will win the most races.

Is Paige correct to expect an athletic edge from taking supplements? Is she safe in taking them?

Ergogenic Aids

Science holds some of the answers to such questions, but finding them requires reading more than just

advertising materials. It's easy to see why Paige is misled by fitness magazines—ads often masquerade as informative articles, concealing their true nature. A tangle of valid and invalid ideas in advertorials can appear convincingly scientific, particularly when accompanied by colorful anatomical figures, graphs, and tables. Some even cite such venerable sources as the *American Journal of Clinical Nutrition* and the *Journal of the American Medical Association* to create the illusion of credibility. Keep in mind, however, that these advertorials are created not to teach but to *sell*. Supplement companies bring in tens of billions of dollars worldwide—and some unscrupulous sellers will gladly mislead athletes for a share of it.

Also, many substances sold as "dietary supplements" escape regulation (see Controversy 7 for details). This means that athletes are largely on their own in evaluating supplements for effectiveness and safety. So far, the large majority of legitimate research has not supported the claims made for ergogenic aids. Athletes who hear that a product is ergogenic should ask, "Who is making this claim?" and "Who stands to profit?"

Antioxidant Supplements

Exercise increases metabolism, and speeded-up metabolism creates extra free radicals that contribute to inflammation and oxidative stress.[1]* It stands to reason, then, that if exercise

*Reference notes are found in Appendix F.

produces free radicals and oxidative stress and if antioxidants from foods can quell oxidative stress, then athletes may benefit from taking in more antioxidants. Like many other logical ideas, however, this one falls apart upon scientific examination—research does not support the taking of antioxidant supplements for athletic performance.[2] Free radical production may be a necessary part of a complex signaling system that promotes many of the beneficial responses of the body to physical activity.[3] Flooding the system with excess antioxidants may short-circuit this system and prevent the expected health benefits and improvements in athletic performance from occuring.[4]

Caffeine

Many athletes report that **caffeine** from coffee, tea, **energy drinks**, **energy "shots,"** and other sources provides a physical boost during sports.[5] Caffeine in safe doses (3 mg/kg of body weight) may indeed improve performance, both in endurance activities, such as cycling and rowing, and in high-intensity training.[6] A mild stimulant, caffeine enhances alertness and concentration and reduces the perception of fatigue and muscle soreness.

In high doses, caffeine causes stomach upset, nervousness, irritability, headaches, dehydration, and diarrhea. Such doses may also constrict the blood vessels and increase the heart rate at a given workload.[7] In addition, other ingredients often added to caffeinated "energy beverages" can increase water and sodium losses and may impair the ability of cell membranes to heal after being wounded.[8]

Competitors should be aware that college sports authorities prohibit the use of caffeine in amounts greater than 700 milligrams, or the equivalent of eight cups of coffee, prior to competition. Controversy 14 lists caffeine doses in common foods and beverages.

Instead of taking caffeine pills before an event, Paige might be better off engaging in some light activity, as DJ does. Pregame activity stimulates the release of fatty acids and warms up the muscles and connective tissues, making them flexible and resistant to injury. Caffeine does not offer these benefits. Instead, caffeine in high doses acts as a diuretic. DJ enjoys a cup or two of coffee before her races for an extra boost, but the amount of caffeine they provide is unlikely to cause problems.[9]

Carnitine

Carnitine is a nonessential nutrient that is often marketed as a "fat burner." In the body, carnitine helps to transfer fatty acids across the membrane that encases the cell's mitochondria. (Recall from Figure 3–1 of Chapter 3 that the mitochondria are structures in cells that release energy from energy-yielding nutrients, such as fatty acids.) Carnitine marketers use this logic: "the more carnitine, the more fat burned, the more glycogen spared"—but the argument is based mostly on conjecture, not research. Carnitine supplementation neither raises muscle carnitine concentrations nor enhances exercise performance. (Paige found out the hard way that carnitine often produces diarrhea in those taking it.) Vegetarians have less total body carnitine than meat eaters do, but introducing more has no effect on vegetarians' muscle function or energy metabolism.[10]

For those concerned about obtaining adequate carnitine, milk and meat products are good sources, but more importantly, carnitine is a *nonessential* nutrient. This means that the body makes plenty for itself.

Creatine

Creatine supplements are widely recommended to athletes and widely used.[11] While they clearly do not benefit endurance athletes such as runners, evidence does hint at some other potential benefits. For performance of short-term, repetitive, high-intensity activities such as weight lifting or sprinting, some studies report small but significant increases in muscle strength, power, and size—attributes that support high-intensity activities.[12] However, other studies suggest that resistance training alone, and not creatine supplements, may account for improvements in studies that report benefits. Interpreting research on creatine is difficult because studies vary in methods and design.[13]

Creatine functions in muscles as part of the high-energy storage compound creatine phosphate (or phosphocreatine), and theoretically the more creatine phosphate in muscles, the higher the intensity at which an athlete can train. The confirmed effect of creatine, however, is weight gain—a potential boon for some athletes but a bane for others. Unfortunately, the gain may be mostly water because creatine causes muscles to hold water.

Large-scale, long-term safety studies are lacking, but short-term use of creatine in doses suggested by manufacturers has, so far, not proven harmful for healthy adults. However, creatine metabolism produces the toxin formaldehyde, which is excreted in urine.[14] The effects of the huge doses of creatine (up to 10 times the dosage recommended by manufacturers) taken by some athletes are unknown. In addition, children as young as 9 years old are taking creatine at the urging of coaches or parents, with unknown consequences. The American Academy of Pediatrics strongly discourages the use of creatine or any other ergogenic supplements in children younger than 18 years old.

Meat, being muscle, is a good supplier of creatine, so anyone who eats meat consumes creatine in abundance. Another safe source is the body's own creatine—human muscles can make all the creatine they need.

Buffers

Sodium bicarbonate (baking soda) acts as a buffer, a compound that neutralizes acids. During high-intensity exercise, acids form in the muscles and may contribute to fatigue. Some, but not all, studies suggest a possible benefit from bicarbonate in sports involving repeated bursts of activity, such as many team sports.[15] Unpleasant side effects, such as gas and diarrhea, may make this ergogenic aid impractical.

A buffering effect associated with the amino acid beta-alanine has recently received attention by exercise researchers. Although beta-alanine may increase the body's buffering capacity to some degree, research has yielded mixed or negative results on exercise performance.[16] A "pins and needles" sensation side effect has been noted.[17]

Amino Acid Supplements

Some athletes—particularly bodybuilders and weight lifters—know that consuming essential amino acids is required to increase muscle size. As mentioned in the chapter, for up to 48 hours following exercise, muscles respond by building up the bulk and strength they need to perform their work. Protein synthesis is held back by a lack of essential amino acids at the critical time. For maximum gains, all essential amino acids must be provided, not just a selected few. In addition, the essential amino acids, particularly leucine, signal muscles to speed up their protein synthesis.[18]

The best source for these amino acids is food, not supplements, for several reasons. First, healthy athletes eating a nutritious diet naturally obtain all of the amino acids they need from food—and in an ideal balance not matched by supplements. Second, the amount of amino acids that muscles require is just a few grams, an amount easily provided by any light, protein-containing meal. More than this amount from expensive supplements is unnecessary and ineffective. Muscles cannot store excess amino acids, so they burn them off as fuel. Third, single amino acid preparations, even leucine, do not improve physical performance or muscle gains.[19]

Fourth, taking amino acid supplements can easily put the body in a too-much–too-little bind. Amino acids compete with each other for carriers in the body, and an overdose of one can limit the availability of another. Finally, supplements can cause digestive disturbances, and for some people in particular, amino acid supplements may pose a hazard (see the Consumer's Guide of Chapter 6).

Whey Protein

Similar to the high-quality protein in lean meat, eggs, milk, and legumes, **whey** supplies all of the essential amino acids, including leucine, needed to initiate and support the building of new muscle tissue—it is a complete protein. Once a discarded by-product of the cheese-making industry, whey is now added to many foods and supplements, including bars, drinks, and powders for athletes. Whey protein is water-soluble and stays dissolved in the digestive tract, where it is quickly digested and absorbed. Whey therefore delivers essential amino acids to the bloodstream more rapidly than solid proteins that require greater digestion.[20] Research is ongoing, but despite claims to the contrary, no clear advantage of whey over other high-quality protein-rich foods is apparent.[21]

Paige believes that by taking a handful of amino acid pills and eating a couple of whey protein bars she can go easier on training and still gain speed on the track, but this is just wishful thinking. Muscles require physically demanding activity, not just protein, to gain in size and performance.[22] Instead of getting faster, Paige will likely get fatter—at 250 calories each, her protein bars contribute 500 calories to her day's intake, an amount far greater than she expends in exercise.

Recently, DJ, who snacks on plain raisins and nuts, placed ahead of Paige in seven of their ten shared competitions. In one of these races, Paige pulled out because of light-headedness—perhaps a consequence of too much caffeine? Still, Paige remains convinced that to win, she must have chemical help, and she is venturing over the danger line by considering hormone-related products. What she doesn't know is very likely to hurt her.

Hormones and Hormone Imitators

The dietary supplements discussed so far are controversial in the sense that they may or may not enhance athletic performance, but most—in the doses commonly taken by healthy adults—probably do not pose immediate threats to health or life. Hormones, however, are clearly damaging and are banned by the World Anti-Doping Agency of the International Olympic Committee and by most professional and amateur sports leagues.

Anabolic Steroids

Among the most dangerous ergogenic practices is the use of **anabolic steroid hormones**. The body's natural steroid hormones stimulate muscle growth in response to physical activity in both men and women. Injections of "fake" hormones produce muscle size and strength far beyond that attainable by training alone—but at great risk to health. These drugs are both illegal in sports and dangerous to the taker, yet athletes often use them without medical supervision, simply taking someone's word for their safety. The list of damaging side effects of steroids is long and includes:

- Extreme mental hostility; aggression; personality changes; suicidal thoughts.
- Swollen face; severe, scarring acne; yellowing of whites of eyes (jaundice).
- Elevated risk of heart attack, stroke; liver damage, liver tumors, fatal liver failure; kidney damage; bloody diarrhea.
- In females, irreversible deepening of voice, loss of fertility, shrinkage of breasts, permanent enlargement of external genitalia.
- In males, breast enlargement, permanent shrinkage of testes, prostate enlargement, sexual dysfunction, and loss of fertility.

The group of substances discussed in this section is clearly damaging to the body. Don't consider using these products—just steer clear.

Human Growth Hormone

A wide range of athletes, including weight lifters, baseball players, cyclists, and track and field participants, use hGH (human growth hormone) to build lean tissue and improve athletic performance. They inject hGH, believing that, because it isn't a steroid itself, it will provide the muscle gains they seek without the substantial risks of anabolic steroids. However, taken in large quantities, hGH causes the disease acromegaly, in which the body becomes huge and the organs and bones enlarge. Other risks of hGH include diabetes, thyroid disorder, heart disease, menstrual irregularities, diminished sexual desire, and shortened life span.

Other Hormones and Alternatives

Many athletes, and particularly school-age athletes, have tried herbal or insect-derived sterols hawked as "natural" alternatives to steroid drugs. The body cannot readily absorb these, and it does convert them into human steroids. These products do not enhance muscle size or strength, but some may contain toxins. Remember: "natural" doesn't mean "harmless."

DHEA, a hormone produced in the adrenal glands and liver, is used by the body to make other important hormones, including **androstenedione**, testosterone, and estrogen. Supplements of DHEA or androstenedione produce unpredictable results. In males, such products may have little or no effect because male testes produce sufficient testosterone. In females, they may disturb hormonal balance, increasing blood testosterone and estrogens. No evidence supports using DHEA, and the ill effects from excess steroid hormones can last a lifetime. Although androstenedione and DHEA are still for sale on the Internet, the National Collegiate Athletic Association, the National Football League, and the International Olympic Committee have banned their use of in competition.

Drugs Posing as Supplements

Some ergogenic aids sold as dietary supplements turn out to contain powerful drugs. The FDA banned a potent stimulant drug known as DMAA as unsafe. Its chemical cousin, DMBA (often listed as AMP citrate on labels), is an untested stimulant, currently sold as an ergogenic, weight-loss, or brain-boosting supplement.[23] DMBA is suspected of causing fatal strokes, heart attacks, and seizures in users. Although the FDA is acting on DMAA, other such drugs are likely to quickly take its place because the demand is strong and profits are high. Table C10–2 lists a few of them.

More Substances Promoted as Ergogenic Aids

Dietary Supplement	Claims	Evidence	Risks
Arginine (an amino acid)	Increased muscle mass	Ineffective	Generally well tolerated; may be harmful to people with heart disease
Boron (trace mineral)	Increased muscle mass	Ineffective	No adverse effects reported with doses up to 10 mg/day; should be avoided by those with kidney disease or women with hormone-sensitive conditions
Casein (milk protein)	Increased muscle mass	As with all dietary protein, contributes to positive nitrogen balance	Well tolerated by many people; triggers allergic reaction in people with milk allergy
Coenzyme Q10 (carrier in the electron transport chain)	Enhanced exercise performance	Ineffective	Mild indigestion
DMBA (AMP citrate) (1,3-dimethylbutylamine)	Increased energy, concentration, and fat metabolism	A stimulant, possibly similar to ephedrine or amphetamine	Reports of fatal heart attack, cerebral hemorrhage, liver and kidney failure, seizures, high blood pressure, and rapid heartbeat
Ephedra (ephedrine, ma huang)	Weight loss; muscle enhancement; improved athletic performance	May increase feelings of nervous energy and alertness	Dry mouth, insomnia, nervousness, palpitation, and headache; blood pressure spikes; cardiac arrest; banned by FDA, National Collegiate Athletic Association, International Olympic Committee, and National Football League
Gamma-oryzanol (plant sterol)	Increased muscle mass; said to mimic anabolic steroids without side effects	Ineffective	No adverse effects reported with short-term use; no long-term safety studies
Ginseng (plant)	Enhanced exercise performance	Ineffective	No adverse effects reported with moderate doses; large doses may cause hypertension, nervousness, sleeplessness, acne, edema, headache, and diarrhea; those with diabetes should be aware of hypoglycemic effects; should be avoided by those at risk for estrogen-related cancers, those with blood-clotting issues, and pregnant or lactating women
Glycerol (a 3-carbon molecule that is part of triglycerides and phospholipids)	Improved hydration during exercise; regulation of body temperature during exercise; enhanced exercise performance	Inconsistent findings for improving hydration and regulating body temperature; ineffective for enhancing exercise performance	May cause nausea, headaches, and blurred vision; should be avoided by those with edema, congestive heart failure, kidney disease, hypertension, and other conditions that may be aggravated by fluid retention
Glycine (an amino acid)	Precursor of creatine	Ineffective	Potential amino acid imbalances
Guarana	Enhanced speed and endurance, mental, and sexual functions	Ineffective	High doses may stress the heart and cause panic attacks
HMB (beta-hydroxy-beta-methylbutyrate; a metabolite of the branched-chain amino acid leucine)	Increased muscle mass and strength	Inconsistent findings	No adverse effects with short-term use and doses up to 76 mg/kg of body weight

Dietary Supplement	Claims	Evidence	Risks
Pyruvate (a 3-carbon sugar)	Enhanced endurance	Ineffective	No long-term safety studies; digestive problems with short-term use (< 6 weeks)
Ribose (a 5-carbon sugar)	Increased ATP production and enhanced high-intensity exercise performance	Ineffective	Naturally generated in body; submitted to USDA to become a Generally Recognized As Safe food additive (pending)
Royal jelly (produced by bees)	Enhanced stamina and reduced fatigue	No studies on human beings to date	No adverse effects with doses up to 12 mg/day; should be avoided by those with a history of asthma or allergic reactions
Sodium bicarbonate (baking soda)	Buffers muscle acid; delayed fatigue; enhanced power and strength	May buffer acid and delay muscle fatigue; more research is needed for definitive conclusions	Gastrointestinal distress including diarrhea, cramps, gas, and bloating; should be avoided by those on sodium-restricted diets
Yohimbe	Weight loss; stimulant effects	No evidence available	Kidney failure; seizures

A dietary supplement is not always what the label says it is. In one recent study, almost 19 percent of supplements sold to athletes worldwide were found to contain a steroid drug. Taking a supplement contaminated with just 0.00005 percent of a steroid drug can produce a positive drug test. An athlete taking such a supplement not only faces the physical risks from unknown substances but also risks being falsely accused of doping and forever banned from competition. Choosing a supplement certified by an independent testing organization, such as the U.S. Phamacopeial Convention (USP) or Banned Substances Control Group (BSCG), may help to reduce the possibility of adulteration.[24]

Conclusion

The general regulatory response to ergogenic claims is "let the buyer beware." In a survey of advertisements in a dozen popular health and bodybuilding magazines, researchers identified over 300 products containing 235 different ingredients advertised as beneficial, mostly for muscle growth. None had been scientifically shown to be effective.

Athletes like Paige who fall for the promises of better performance through supplements are taking a gamble with their money, their health, or both. They trade one product for another and another when the placebo effect wears thin and the promised miracles fail to materialize. DJ, who takes the scientific approach reflected in this Controversy, faces a problem: How does she tell Paige about the hoaxes and still preserve their friendship?

Explaining to someone that a cherished belief is not true involves a risk: the person often becomes angry with the one telling the truth, rather than with the source of the lie. To avoid this painful outcome, DJ decides to mention only the supplements in Paige's routine that are most likely to cause harm—the overdoses of caffeine and the hormone replacers. As for the whey protein and other supplements, they are probably just a waste of money, and DJ decides to keep quiet. Perhaps they may serve as harmless superstitions.

When Paige believes her performance is boosted by a new concoction, DJ understands that the power of her mind is most likely at work—the placebo effect. Don't discount that power, by the way, for it is formidable. You don't need to buy unproven supplements for an extra edge because you already have a real one—your mind. And you can use the extra money you save to buy a great pair of running shoes—perhaps on a Wednesday?

Critical Thinking

1. Most of the time, the buyer is wasting his or her money when buying an ergogenic aid to improve performance. Still, even well-educated athletes often take them. What forces do you think might motivate a competitor to "throw caution to the wind" and buy and take unproven supplements sold as ergogenic aids? What role might advertising play?

2. Divide into two groups. One group will argue in favor of the use of ergogenic aids by athletes, and one group will argue against their use. Each group will make a list of ergogenic aids that should be allowed for use by athletes and a list of those that should not be allowed.

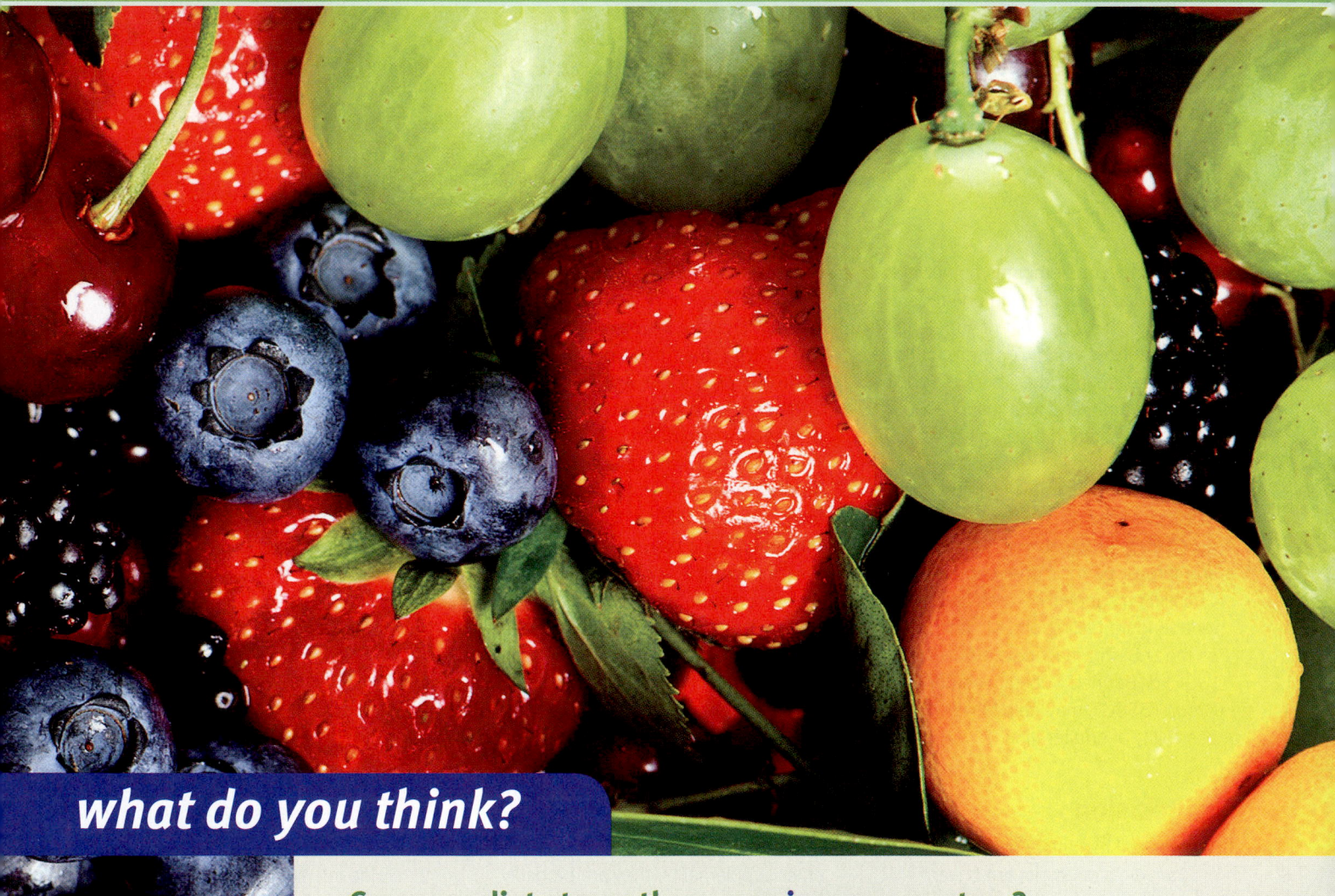

11

Diet and Health

what do you think?

Can your diet strengthen your **immune** system?

Are your own food choices damaging your **heart**?

Can certain **herbs** improve your health?

Do "natural" foods without **additives** reduce cancer risks?

Learning Objectives

After completing this chapter, you should be able to accomplish the following:

LO 11.1 Outline the relationship between malnutrition and disease.

LO 11.2 Discuss the relationship between risk factors and chronic disease.

LO 11.3 Explain cardiovascular disease and its risk factors.

LO 11.4 Discuss hypertension and its risk factors, including nutrition risk factors.

LO 11.5 Explain the relationships between diet and cancer.

LO 11.6 Outline strategies for including sufficient fruits and vegetables in a diet.

LO 11.7 Describe the emerging science of nutritional genomics.

Can a well-chosen diet protect you from developing a disease? The answer to this question depends on the disease. Two main kinds of diseases afflict people around the world: **infectious diseases** and **chronic diseases**.* Infectious diseases such as tuberculosis, smallpox, influenza, and polio have been major killers of humankind since before the dawn of history. In any society not well defended against them, infectious diseases can cut life so short that the average person dies at 20, 30, or 40 years of age.

With the advent of vaccines and antibiotics, people in developed countries had become complacent about infectious diseases—until recently. Scientists now warn of growing infectious threats: the possibility of the rapid global spread of new human diseases for which no treatments exist; a rising death toll from once-conquered diseases, such as tuberculosis and foodborne infections now resistant to antibiotic drugs; and despite vaccine availability, the periodic resurgence of diseases such as pertussis and measles.[1†] While scientists work to develop controls for these perils, government health agencies hasten to strengthen emergency response systems and to protect our food and water supplies.

Individuals can take steps to protect themselves, too. Each of us encounters millions of microbes each day, and some of these can cause diseases. Nutrition cannot directly prevent or cure infectious diseases, but good nutrition can strengthen, and malnutrition can weaken, your body's defenses against them.[2] One warning: many so-called immune-strengthening foods, dietary supplements, and herbs are hoaxes. For healthy, well-fed people, supplements cannot trigger extra immune power to fend off dangerous infections.

In the United States, chronic diseases far outrank infections as the leading causes of death and illness.[3] Compare, for example, the death toll attributable to pneumonia and influenza, the only two infectious diseases listed among the top U.S. causes of death (Figure 11–1, p. 430), with the number of deaths from heart disease, cancer, and diabetes. The longer a person dodges life's other perils, the more likely that chronic diseases will take their toll.

Chronic diseases arise not from a straightforward cause such as infection but from a mixture of factors in three areas: genetic inheritance, prior or current diseases such as obesity or hypertension, and lifestyle choices. The first one, inherited susceptibility, people cannot control. The second one, current disease states, people may be able to control or modify to some extent. People control daily life choices directly, however, and these can often prevent or delay the onset of certain diseases.

Young people choose whether to nourish their bodies well, to smoke, to exercise, or to abuse alcohol, and these choices are potent determinants of disease risks later on. As people age, their bodies accumulate the effects of a lifetime of choices, and in the later years, these impacts can make the difference between a life of health and one of

infectious diseases diseases that are caused by bacteria, viruses, parasites, and other microbes and that can be transmitted from one person to another through air, water, or food; by contact; or through vector organisms such as mosquitoes and fleas.

chronic diseases degenerative conditions or illnesses that progress slowly, are long in duration, and lack an immediate cure; chronic diseases limit functioning, productivity, and quality and length of life. Also defined in Chapter 1.

---

*The term *disease* is also used to refer to conditions such as birth defects, alcoholism, obesity, and mental disorders.
†Reference notes are found in Appendix F.

Figure 11–1

The Ten Leading Causes of Death in the United States[a]

Many deaths have multiple causes, but diet influences the development of several chronic diseases—notably, heart disease, some types of cancer, stroke, and diabetes.

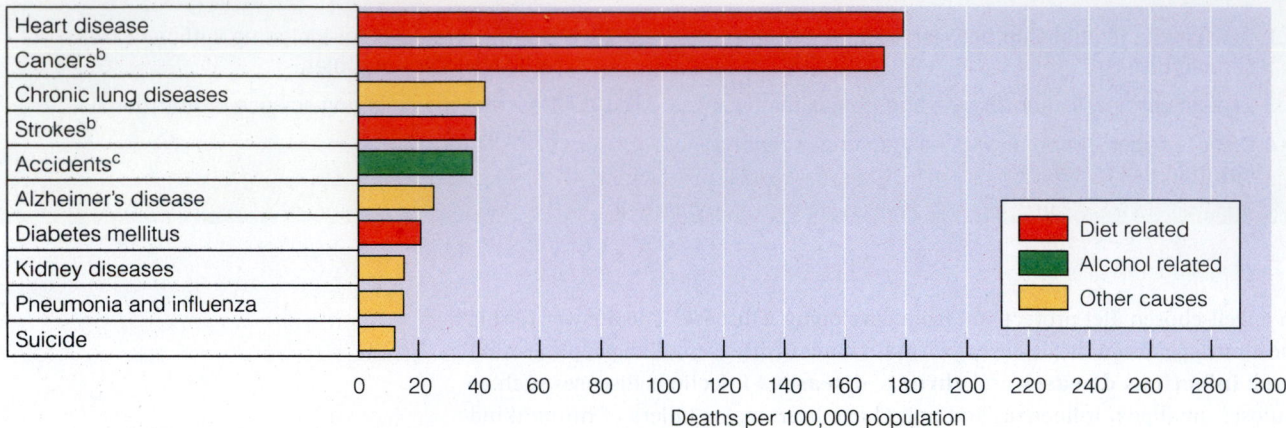

Deaths per 100,000 population

[a]Rates are age adjusted to allow relative comparisons of mortality among groups and over time.
[b]Alcohol increases the risks for some cancers and strokes.
[c]Motor vehicle and other accidents are the leading cause of death among people aged 15–24, followed by homicide, suicide, cancer, and heart disease. Alcohol contributes to about half of all accident fatalities.
Source: Data from National Center for Health Statistics: S. L. Murphy, J. Xu, and K. D. Kochanek, Deaths: Final data for 2010, National Vital Statistics Reports 61, no. 4 (2013): 1–118.

chronic disability. This discussion begins with the role of nutrition in supporting the body's immune defenses and then reveals the power of the diet to advance or inhibit the development of chronic diseases.

The Immune System, Nutrition, and Diseases

LO 11.1 Outline the relationship between malnutrition and disease.

Without your awareness, your immune system continuously stands guard against thousands of attacks mounted against you by microorganisms and cancer cells. If your immune system falters, you become vulnerable to disease-causing agents, and disease invariably follows.

Immune tissues are among the first to be impaired in the course of a vitamin and mineral deficiency or toxicity.[4] Some nutrient deficiencies are more immediately harmful to immunity than others, determined partly by the physiological roles of the missing nutrient, whether another nutrient can perform some of its tasks, the severity of the deficiency, whether an infection has already taken hold, and being of young or old age.

The Effects of Malnutrition

People who restrict their food intakes, whether because of a lack of appetite, an illness, an eating disorder, or a desire for weight loss, are more likely than others to be caught in the downward spiral of malnutrition and weakened immunity. Also susceptible are those who are one or more of the following: very young or old, poor, hospitalized, or malnourished. Rates of sickness and death increase dramatically among malnourished persons when medical tests indicate that their immune system is compromised.

Malnutrition and Disease Worsen Each Other Once a person becomes malnourished, malnutrition often worsens disease, which, in turn, worsens malnutrition. A destructive cycle often begins when impaired immunity opens the way for disease; when disease impairs appetite, interferes with digestion and absorption, increases excretion, or alters metabolism, then nutrition status suffers further. Drugs often become necessary to treat diseases, and many of them impair nutrition status (see Controversy 14). Other treatments, such as surgery or radiation, take a further toll. Thus, together, disease and poor nutrition form a downward spiral that must be broken for recovery to occur (see Figure 11–2).

Impairment of Immune Defenses When deprived of sufficient essential nutrients, indispensable tissues and cells of the immune system can dwindle in size and number, leaving the whole body vulnerable to infection. In addition, both starvation and obesity impair the immune response to infection.[5] Table 11–1 shows selected examples of malnutrition's effects on body defenses. The skin and body linings, the first line of defense against infections, become thinner because their connective tissue is broken down, allowing agents of disease easy access to body tissues.

For example, a healthy digestive system normally musters a formidable defense—its linings not only impose a physical barrier but also are heavily laced with immune tissues, cells, and antibodies that intercept intruders. When malnutrition sets in, all of these defenses diminish, and invading infectious agents encounter little resistance. Once inside the warm, moist, nutritious body fluids and tissues, microbes quickly multiply and infection ensues.

A deficiency or a toxicity of just a single nutrient can seriously weaken immune defenses. For example, vitamin A deficiency weakens the body's skin and membranous linings. Vitamin C deficiency robs white blood cells of their killing power. Too little vitamin E may impair immunity in several ways, especially among the aged. Zinc plays multiple roles in immunity, and both deficient and excessive zinc intakes impair immunity.[6] Table 11–2 (p. 432) lists nutrients known to play key roles in immune function. Clearly, a well-balanced diet is the cornerstone that supports immune system defenses.

Disease Can Worsen Malnutrition Malnutrition can result not only from a lack of available food but also from diseases, such as **HIV/AIDS** and cancer, and their treatments. These conditions depress the appetite and speed up metabolism, causing a wasting away of the body's tissues similar to that seen in the last stages of starvation—the body uses its fat and protein reserves for survival. Wasting or nutrient deficiencies can shorten survival, making medical nutrition therapy a

Figure 11–2

Malnutrition and Disease Worsen Each Other

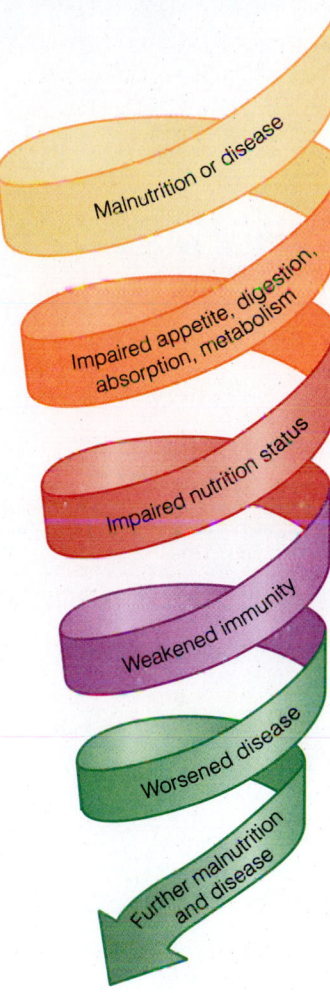

Malnutrition or disease

Impaired appetite, digestion, absorption, metabolism

Impaired nutrition status

Weakened immunity

Worsened disease

Further malnutrition and disease

Table 11–1	
Selected Effects of Malnutrition on the Body's Defense Systems	
System Component	**Effects of Malnutrition**
Skin	Thickness, elasticity, and connective tissue are reduced, compromising the skin's ability to serve as a barrier for the protection of underlying tissues; skin sensitivity reaction to antigens is delayed.
Digestive tract membrane and other body linings	Antibody secretions and immune cell numbers are reduced. Barrier functions are also compromised.
Lymph tissues[a]	Immune system organs are reduced in size; cells of immune defense are depleted.
General response	Invader kill time is prolonged; circulating immune cells are reduced; immune response is impaired.

[a]*Thymus gland, lymph nodes, and spleen.*

HIV/AIDS acquired immune deficiency syndrome; caused by infection with human immunodeficiency virus (HIV), which is transmitted primarily by sexual contact, contact with infected blood, needles shared among drug users, or fluids transferred from an infected mother to her fetus or infant.

Table 11–2

Selected Nutrient Roles in Immune Function

The immune system requires all nutrients for optimal functioning. The nutrients listed here have well-known, specific roles in immunity.

Nutrient	Key Role(s) in Immune Function
Vitamin A	Maintains healthy skin and other epithelial tissues (barriers to infection); role in cellular replication and specialization that supports immune cell and antibody production and the anti-inflammatory response
Vitamin D	Regulates immune cell (T-cell) responses; role in antibody production
Vitamins C and E	Protect against oxidative damage
Vitamin B_6	Helps maintain an effective immune response; role in antibody production
Vitamin B_{12} and folic acid	Assist in cellular replication and specialization that support immune cell and antibody production
Selenium	Protects against oxidative damage
Zinc	Helps maintain an effective immune response; role in antibody production
Protein	Maintains healthy skin and other epithelial tissues (barriers to infection); participates in the synthesis and function of the organs and cells of the immune system and antibody production
Omega-3 fatty acids	Help to resolve inflammation after an immune response through production of lipid mediators, among other roles

Sources: P. C. Calder, Feeding the immune system, Proceedings of the Nutrition Society 72 (2013): 299–309; B. H. Maskrey and coauthors, Emerging importance of omega-3 fatty acids in the innate immune response: Molecular mechanisms and lipidomic strategies for their analysis, Molecular Nutrition and Food Research 57 (2013): 1390–1400; S. S. Percival, Nutrition and immunity: Balancing diet and immune function, Nutrition Today 46 (2011): 12–17.

> The immune system was described in **Chapter 3**; starvation and hunger are topics of **Chapter 15**.

critical need.[7] Nutrients cannot cure such diseases, of course, but an adequate diet may improve responses to drugs, shorten hospital stays, promote independence, and improve the quality of life. Physical activity that strengthens muscles may also help hold wasting to a minimum. In addition, food safety (see Chapter 12) is paramount because common food bacteria and viruses can easily overwhelm a compromised immune system.

To repeat: a *diet* of foods that supplies adequate nutrients ensures the proper functioning of the immune system, but extra daily doses of nutrients, herbs, or other substances do not enhance it. Furthermore, toxic doses clearly diminish it.

KEY POINTS

- Adequate nutrition is necessary for normal immune system functioning.
- Both deficient and excessive nutrients can harm the immune system.

The Immune System and Chronic Diseases

The immune system's response to infection or injury includes **inflammation**. In inflammation, the blood supply to an infected area increases, and the blood vessels become more permeable, allowing the immune system's white blood cells to rush to the site. Recall from Chapter 3 that white blood cells respond in many ways when injury

inflammation (in-flam-MAY-shun) part of the body's immune defense against injury, infection, or allergens, marked by increased blood flow, release of chemical toxins, and attraction of white blood cells to the affected area (from the Latin *inflammare*, meaning "to flame within"). Also defined in Chapter 5.

or infection is present. One part of their response is to release oxidative products, such as deadly hydrogen peroxide (see the photo), to kill microbes or cancer cells, remove damaged tissue, and heal wounds. This acute inflammation response with its oxidative defense is critical to staying healthy.

That same response, however, when it persists, can result in a chronic state of inflammation that harms the tissues. Cells of chronically inflamed tissues produce hormone-like communication molecules, free radicals, blood clotting factors, and other bioactive chemicals that alter functioning and sustain the inflammatory response.[8] Such sustained inflammation threatens health by worsening a number of chronic diseases, as discussed in later sections of this chapter.

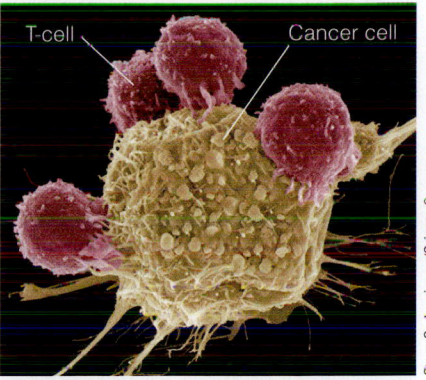

A killer T-cell (the smaller cell on the top) has recognized a cancer cell and is attacking it with toxic chemicals that punch holes in the cancer cell's surface.

KEY POINTS

- Inflammation is part of the body's immune defense system.
- Sustained inflammation can worsen a number of chronic diseases.

The Concept of Risk Factors

LO 11.2 Discuss the relationship between risk factors and chronic disease.

In contrast to the infectious diseases, each of which has a distinct microbial cause such as a bacterium or virus, the chronic diseases have suspected contributors known as **risk factors**. Risk factors show a correlation with a disease—that is, they often occur together with the disease—and although they are candidates for causes, they have not yet been voted in or out. We can say with certainty that a virus causes influenza, but we cannot name the cause of heart disease with such confidence.

An analogy may help clarify the concept of risk factors. A risk factor is like a person who is often seen lurking around the scene of a particular type of crime—say, arson. The police may suspect that person of setting fires, but it may very well be that another, sneakier individual who goes unnoticed is actually pouring the fuel and lighting the match. The evidence against the known suspect is only circumstantial. The police can be sure of guilt only when they observe the criminal in the act. Risk factors have not yet been caught in the act of causing diseases.

Cause versus Increased Risk   You may notice a philosophical shift in this chapter from previous chapters. There we could say that "a deficiency of nutrient X causes disease Y." Here we only cite theories and discuss research that illuminates current thinking. We can say with certainty, for example, that "a diet lacking vitamin C causes scurvy," but to say that a low-fiber diet that lacks vegetables causes cancer would be inaccurate.

Note that in addition to nutrition, disease risk factors are also genetic, environmental, and behavioral; they tend to occur in clusters, and one risk factor may affect several diseases. Food behaviors often underlie many risk factors. Choosing to eat a diet too high in saturated fat, salt, and calories, for example, is choosing to risk becoming obese and contracting atherosclerosis, type 2 diabetes, cancer, **hypertension**, or other diseases.[9] Table 11–3 (p. 434) identifies some diet-related behaviors and other risk factors associated with chronic diseases. In many cases, one chronic disease, such as obesity, contributes to the development or progression of one or more other diseases, as Figure 11–3 shows. Indeed, obesity is a gateway to many other diseases, even some, such as respiratory diseases, that are not related to diet.[10]

The exact contribution diet makes to each disease is hard to estimate. Many experts believe that diet accounts for about a third of all cases of coronary heart disease. The links between diet and cancer incidence are harder to pin down because each of cancer's many forms associates with different dietary factors.

Estimating Your Risks   Some risk factors, such as avoiding tobacco, are important to everyone's health. Others, such as some relating to diet, are more important for people who are genetically predisposed to certain diseases. To pinpoint your own areas of concern, you can search your family's medical history for diseases common

risk factors factors known to be related to (or correlated with) diseases but not proved to be causal.

hypertension higher-than-normal blood pressure.

Table 11–3

Risk Factors for Chronic Diseases

This table points out that a risk factor associated with one chronic disease often contributes to others as well. Later tables provide specific risk factors for individual diseases. In addition, Figure 11–3 illustrates how chronic diseases themselves can be risk factors for other chronic diseases.

	Cancers	Hypertension	Diabetes (type 2)	Atherosclerosis	Obesity	Stroke
Dietary Risk Factors						
Diets high in added sugars					✓	
Diets high in salty or pickled foods	✓	✓				
Diets high in saturated and/or *trans* fat	✓	✓	✓	✓	✓	✓
Diets low in fruits, vegetables, and other foods rich in fiber and phytochemicals	✓		✓	✓	✓	✓
Diets low in vitamins and/or minerals	✓	✓		✓		
Excessive alcohol intake	✓	✓		✓	✓	✓
Other Risk Factors						
Age	✓	✓	✓	✓		✓
Environmental contaminants	✓					
Genetics	✓	✓	✓	✓	✓	✓
Sedentary lifestyle	✓	✓	✓	✓	✓	✓
Smoking and tobacco use	✓	✓		✓		✓
Stress		✓		✓		✓

Figure 11–3

Interrelationships among Chronic Diseases

Many chronic diseases are themselves risk factors for other chronic diseases, and all of them are linked to obesity. The risk factors highlighted in blue define the metabolic syndrome.

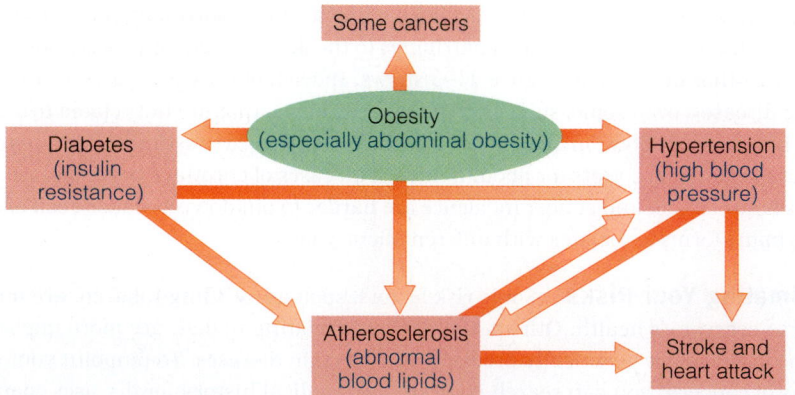

Chapter 11 Diet and Health

to your forebears. Any condition that shows up in several close blood relatives may be a special concern for you (Table 11–4 lists some of these).[‡] For example, a person whose parents, grandparents, or other close blood relatives suffered from diabetes and heart disease is urgently advised to avoid becoming obese and not to smoke. Also, after your next physical examination, find out which test results are out of line. The combination of family medical history and laboratory test results is a powerful predictor of disease. Even people without a family history of diseases can develop them, however; the guidelines presented in this chapter can benefit most people.

Table 11–4

Family Medical History

These conditions in parents, grandparents, or siblings, especially occurring early in life, may raise a warning flag for you.

Alcoholism
Cancer
Diabetes
Cardiovascular diseases
Hypertension
Liver disease (cirrhosis)
Osteoporosis

Cardiovascular Diseases

LO 11.3 Explain cardiovascular disease and its risk factors.

In the United States today, more than 83 million men and women suffer some form of disease of the heart and blood vessels, collectively known as **cardiovascular disease (CVD)**.[11] Cardiovascular diseases such as heart disease and stroke claim the lives of nearly 1 million people each year in the United States.[12][§] These numbers, while unacceptably high, represent a substantial improvement over the numbers of a half-century ago.

One reason heart disease is so deadly is that the heart is one of the least regenerative organs in the body. When cardiac muscle is lost—for example, by way of a heart attack—the heart heals mainly by forming scar tissue. As a result, the contractile function of the heart declines, and heart failure often follows.

The myth that heart disease is a man's disease has been debunked: CVD is the leading cause of death among women. More than 42 million U.S. women have CVD, and the number is increasing despite substantial progress in the awareness, prevention, and treatment of CVD in women.[13] Men still suffer heart attacks more often and earlier in life than women do, but the gap is narrowing. In fact, in all its forms, CVD kills more U.S. women, especially those who are past menopause, than any other cause.[14]

Learning to recognize the symptoms of a heart attack can be lifesaving because the sooner medical help arrives, the more likely the person's recovery is. The Centers for Disease Control and Prevention (www.cdc.gov) list the following five major symptoms of a heart attack:

- Pain or discomfort in the jaw, neck, or back.
- Feeling weak, light-headed, or faint.
- Chest pain or discomfort.
- Pain or discomfort in arms or shoulder.
- Shortness of breath.

Importantly, women may or may not experience classic symptoms such as chest discomfort. Women may instead experience unusual fatigue, dizziness, or weakness.

How can you minimize your risks of heart attack and stroke? Or, more positively, what steps can you take to help maintain your heart health and vigor throughout life? Many people have done so by quitting smoking or not starting. They have also changed their diets, consuming less saturated fat, less *trans* fat, more vegetables, more fruits, more nuts, more seafood, and more whole grains.[15] In contrast, many

---

[‡]The U.S. Surgeon General offers a free online tool, "My Family Health Portrait," to help organize family health information. It is available over the Internet at https://familyhistory.hhs.gov/.

[§]Deaths from CVD in the United States include 48 percent from coronary heart disease, 16 percent from stroke, 8 percent from hypertension, 7 percent from congestive heart failure, 3 percent from other artery diseases, and the remainder from rheumatic fever/heart disease, congenital cardiovascular defects, and other causes.

cardiovascular disease (CVD) a general term for all diseases of the heart and blood vessels. Atherosclerosis is the main cause of CVD. When the arteries that carry blood to the heart muscle become blocked, the heart suffers damage known as *coronary heart disease (CHD)*. Also defined in Chapter 5.

Figure 11–4

The Formation of Plaque in Atherosclerosis

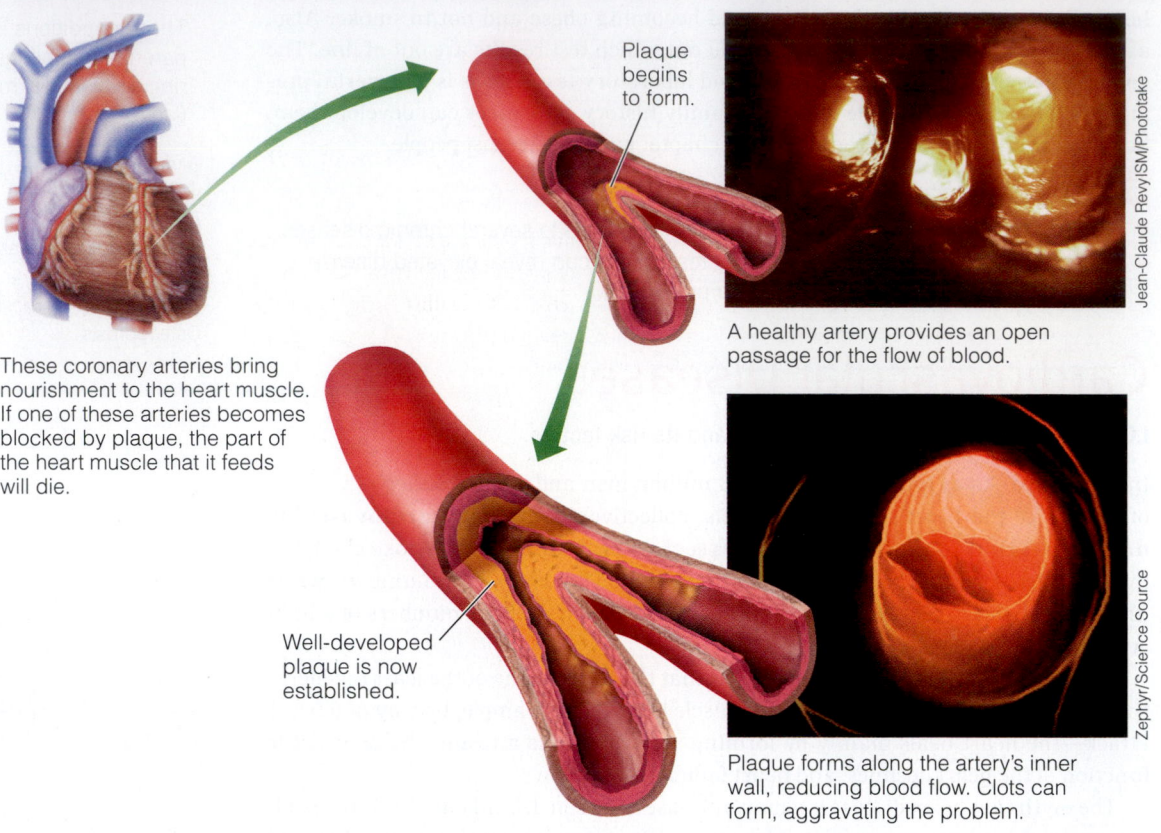

These coronary arteries bring nourishment to the heart muscle. If one of these arteries becomes blocked by plaque, the part of the heart muscle that it feeds will die.

Plaque begins to form.

A healthy artery provides an open passage for the flow of blood.

Well-developed plaque is now established.

Plaque forms along the artery's inner wall, reducing blood flow. Clots can form, aggravating the problem.

Jean-Claude Revy/ISM/Phototake

Zephyr/Science Source

people are consuming too many calories, too much sodium, and too few fruits and vegetables; obtaining regular exercise presents a difficult stumbling block for most people.

Atherosclerosis

At the root of most forms of CVD is **atherosclerosis**. Atherosclerosis is the common form of hardening of the arteries. No one is free of all signs of atherosclerosis. The question is not whether you are developing it but how far advanced it is and what you can do to retard or reverse it. Atherosclerosis usually begins with the accumulation of soft, fatty streaks along the inner walls of the arteries, especially at branch points. These gradually enlarge and become hardened fibrous **plaques** that damage artery walls and make them inelastic, narrowing the passageway through which blood travels (see Figure 11–4). Most people have well-developed plaque by the time they reach age 30.

How Plaques Form What causes the plaque to form? A diet high in *trans* fat and saturated fat contributes to the development of plaque and the progression of atherosclerosis.[16] But atherosclerosis is much more than the simple accumulation of lipids within the artery wall—it is a complex response of the artery to tissue damage and inflammation.[17] Inflammation plays a central role in all stages of atherosclerosis.

The cells lining the arteries may incur damage from a number of factors: high LDL cholesterol, hypertension, diabetes, toxins from cigarette smoking, obesity, or certain viral or bacterial infections.[18] Such damage produces inflammation that triggers the immune system to send white blood cells to the site to try to repair the damage. Soon, particles of LDL cholesterol become trapped in the blood vessel walls, and

atherosclerosis (ath-er-oh-scler-OH-sis) the most common form of cardiovascular disease; characterized by plaque along the inner walls of the arteries (*scleros* means "hard"; *osis* means "too much"). The term *arteriosclerosis* is often used to mean the same thing.

plaques (PLACKS; singular, plaque) mounds of lipid material mixed with smooth muscle cells and calcium that develop in the artery walls in atherosclerosis (*placken* means "patch"). The same word is also used to describe the accumulation of a different kind of deposit on teeth, which promotes dental caries.

these become oxidized by the abundant free radicals produced during inflammation. White blood cells—**macrophages**—flood the scene to scavenge and remove the oxidized LDL—but to no avail. As the macrophages become engorged with oxidized LDL, they become known as foam cells, which themselves become triggers of oxidation and inflammation that attract more immune scavengers to the scene. Muscle cells of the arterial wall proliferate in an attempt to heal the damage, but they mix with the foam cells to form hardened areas of plaque. Mineralization increases hardening of the plaques. The process is repeated until many inner artery walls become virtually covered with disfiguring plaque.

Plaque Rupture and Blood Clots

Once plaques have formed, a sudden spasm of the artery wall or surge in blood pressure can tear away part of the fibrous coat covering a plaque, causing it to rupture. Unstable plaques with a thin fibrous layer over a large lipid core are most vulnerable to rupture.[19] When a plaque ruptures, the body responds to the damage as an injury—by clotting the blood.

Small, cell-like bodies in the blood, known as **platelets**, cause clots to form when they encounter injuries in blood vessels. Clots form and dissolve in the blood all the time, and when these processes are balanced, the clots do no harm. That balance is disturbed in atherosclerosis, however. Arterial damage, plaque in the arteries, and inflammation all favor the formation of blood clots.

Abnormal blood clotting can trigger life-threatening events. For example, a clot, once formed, may remain attached to a plaque in an artery and grow until it shuts off the blood supply to the surrounding tissue. The starved tissue slowly dies and is replaced by nonfunctional scar tissue. The stationary clot is called a **thrombus**. When it has grown large enough to close off a blood vessel, it is a **thrombosis**. A clot can also break loose, becoming an **embolus**, and travel along in the bloodstream until it reaches an artery too small to allow its passage. There the clot becomes stuck and is referred to as an **embolism**. The tissues fed by this artery, suddenly robbed of oxygen and nutrients, die rapidly. Such a clot can lodge in an artery of the heart, causing sudden death of part of the heart muscle, a **heart attack**. A clot may also lodge in an artery of the brain, killing a portion of brain tissue, a **stroke**.

Opposing the clot-forming actions of platelets is one of the eicosanoids, an active product of an omega-3 fatty acid in fish oils.[20] A diet lacking in fatty fish may therefore contribute to clot formation and can worsen heart disease risk in other ways as well.[21]

Plaque and Blood Pressure

Normally, the arteries expand with each heartbeat to accommodate the pulses of blood that flow through them. Arteries hardened and narrowed by plaque cannot expand, however, so the blood pressure rises. The increased pressure damages the artery walls further and strains the heart. Because plaques are more likely to form at damage sites, the development of atherosclerosis becomes a self-accelerating process. As pressure builds up in an artery, the arterial wall may become weakened and balloon out, forming an **aneurysm**. An aneurysm can burst, and in a major artery such as the **aorta**, this leads to massive bleeding and death.

KEY POINTS

- Atherosclerosis begins with the accumulation of soft, fatty streaks on the inner walls of the arteries.
- The soft, fatty streaks gradually enlarge and become hard plaques.
- Plaques of atherosclerosis trigger hypertension and abnormal blood clotting, leading to heart attacks or strokes.

Risk Factors for CVD

Major heart disease risk factors are listed briefly in Chapter 5; they are presented here in full in Table 11–5. Many of the same factors also predict the occurrence of stroke. All people reaching middle age exhibit at least one of these factors (middle age is a risk factor), and many people have several factors, silently increasing their risk.[22] The more of these risk factors you can control, the lower your risk of CVD and death.[23]

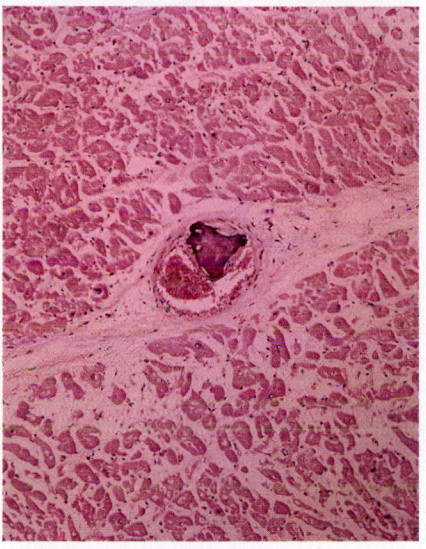

A blood clot in an artery, such as this fatal heart embolism, blocks the blood flow to tissues fed by that artery.

SPL/Science Source

macrophages (MACK-roh-fah-jez) large scavenger cells of the immune system that engulf debris and remove it (*macro* means "large"; *phagein* means "to eat").

platelets tiny cell-like fragments in the blood, important in blood clot formation (*platelet* means "little plate").

thrombus a stationary blood clot.

thrombosis a thrombus that has grown enough to close off a blood vessel. A *coronary thrombosis* closes off a vessel that feeds the heart muscle. A *cerebral thrombosis* closes off a vessel that feeds the brain (*thrombo* means "clot"; the cerebrum is part of the brain).

embolus (EM-boh-luss) a thrombus that breaks loose and travels through the blood vessels (*embol* means "to insert").

embolism an embolus that causes sudden closure of a blood vessel.

heart attack the event in which the vessels that feed the heart muscle become closed off by an embolism, thrombus, or other cause with resulting sudden tissue death. A heart attack is also called a *myocardial infarction* (*myo* means "muscle"; *cardial* means "of the heart"; *infarct* means "tissue death").

stroke the sudden shutting off of the blood flow to the brain by a thrombus, an embolism, or the bursting of a vessel (hemorrhage).

aneurysm (AN-you-rism) the ballooning out of an artery wall at a point that is weakened by deterioration.

aorta (ay-OR-tuh) the large, primary artery that conducts blood from the heart to the body's smaller arteries.

Table 11–5

Major Risk Factors for Heart Disease

See Figure 11–5 on page 439 for standards by which to judge blood lipids, obesity, and blood pressure. Risk factors highlighted in color have relationships with diet.

Risk factors that cannot be modified:
- Increasing age.
- Male gender.
- Genetic inheritance.

Risk factors that can be modified:
- High blood LDL cholesterol.
- Low blood HDL cholesterol.
- High blood triglyceride (VLDL) levels.
- High blood pressure (hypertension).
- Diabetes.
- Obesity (especially central obesity).
- Physical inactivity.
- Cigarette smoking.
- An "atherogenic" diet (high in saturated fats and *trans* fats and low in vegetables, fruits, and whole grains).

Sources: A. S. Go and coauthors, Heart disease and stroke statistics—2014 update: A report from the American Heart Association, Circulation 129 (2014): e28–e292; Expert Panel on Detection, Evaluation, and Treatment of High Blood Cholesterol in Adults (Adult Treatment Panel III), Third Report of the National Cholesterol Education Program (NIH Publication No. 02-5215) (Bethesda, Md.: National Heart, Lung, and Blood Institute, 2002), pp. II-15–II-20.

In recognition of the urgency to reduce the prevalence of major risk factors for CVD, national initiatives have been developed. The American Heart Association has adopted a 2020 goal of "improving the cardiovascular health of all Americans by 20 percent, while reducing mortality from heart disease and stroke by 20 percent."

It befits a nutrition book to focus on dietary strategies, but Table 11–5 shows that diet is not the only, and perhaps not even the most important, factor in the development of heart disease or stroke. Age, gender, genetic inheritance, cigarette smoking, certain diseases, and physical inactivity predict their development as well. The next few sections address these factors; discussions of diet and physical activity for CVD prevention follow.

Age, Gender, and Genetic Inheritance   Three of the major risk factors for CVD cannot be modified by lifestyle choices: age, gender, and genes. The increasing risk associated with growing older reflects the steady progression of atherosclerosis in most people as they age. The speed at which atherosclerosis progresses, however, depends more on the presence or absence of risk factors such as high blood pressure, high blood cholesterol, diabetes, and smoking than on age alone.[24] For example, among men 55 years of age, those with at least two major risk factors were six times as likely to die from CVD by age 80 as those with one or no risk factors. Women of the same age with at least two risk factors were three times as likely to die from CVD by age 80 as those with one or no risk factors.

Gender alters risks at many life stages. In men, aging becomes a significant risk factor for heart disease at age 45 years or older; in women, the risk increases after age 55. Young women can easily become complacent about heart disease because men die earlier of heart attacks than do women.** It bears repeating that CVD kills more U.S. women than any other cause.[25]

As for genetic inheritance, early heart disease in immediate family members (siblings or parents) is a major risk factor for developing it. The more family members affected and the earlier the age at which they became ill, the greater the risk to the individual.[26] These relationships suggest a genetic influence on CVD risk, but specific genetic links are still under investigation. In the realm of nutritional genomics and

---

**The Centers for Disease Control and Prevention has developed WISEWOMAN projects nationwide to provide low-income women with resources needed to reduce their risks of CVD (www.cdc.gov/WISEWOMAN).

Chapter 11 Diet and Health

Figure 11–5

Adult Standards for Blood Lipids, Body Mass Index, and Blood Pressure

	Total blood cholesterol (mg/dL)	LDL cholesterol (mg/dL)	HDL cholesterol (mg/dL)	Triglycerides, fasting (mg/dL)	Body mass index (BMI)[a]	Blood pressure systolic/diastolic (mm Hg)
Unhealthy	≥240	160–189[b]	<40	200–499[c]	≥30	≥140 / ≥90
Borderline	200–239	130–159[d]	59–40	150–199	25–29.9	120/80–139/89[e]
Healthy	<200	<100[f]	≥60	<150	18.5–24.9	<120 / <80

[a]Body mass index (BMI) was defined in Chapter 9; BMI standards are found on the inside back cover.
[b]>190 mg/dL of LDL indicates a very high risk.
[c]>500 mg/dL of triglycerides indicates a very high risk.
[d]LDL cholesterol–lowering medication may be needed at 130 mg/dL, depending on other risks.
[e]These values indicate prehypertension.
[f]100–129 mg/dL of LDL indicates a near optimal level.

CVD risk, scientists are uncovering a vast interrelated network of influences, but the relationships among them are complex and are likely to become more knotty before being untangled.[27] Many of these relationships center on blood lipids.

LDL and HDL Cholesterol Low-density lipoprotein (LDL) cholesterol and high-density lipoprotein (HDL) cholesterol in the blood are strongly linked to a person's risk of developing atherosclerosis and heart disease. The higher the LDL cholesterol, the greater the risk of CVD. Conversely, the lower the LDL cholesterol and blood pressure, the slower the progression of atherosclerosis.[28]

LDL cholesterol is made up of the most **atherogenic** lipoproteins. LDL carry cholesterol to the cells, including the cells that line the arteries, where it can build up as part of the plaque of atherosclerosis described earlier. In clinical trials, lowering LDL greatly reduces the incidence of heart disease. By one estimate, for every percentage point drop in LDL cholesterol, the risk of heart disease falls proportionately. Figure 11–5 lists blood lipid values that are considered to be healthy and those that exceed a healthy level and also presents values for body mass index (BMI) and blood pressure.

LDL, HDL, and VLDL are discussed in detail in **Chapter 5.**

HDL also carry cholesterol, but they carry it away from the cells to the liver for recycling to other uses or for disposal. HDL remove cholesterol from circulation and contain proteins that inhibit inflammation, LDL oxidation, and plaque accumulation. Therefore, *low* HDL levels can contribute to the development of atherosclerosis.[29] Having adequate levels of HDL is beneficial, but beyond a certain concentration, higher HDL levels do not bring greater benefits.[30]

High levels of LDL cholesterol in the blood can both initiate and worsen atherosclerosis. When levels are high, LDL enter vulnerable regions of the artery wall where they are oxidized.[31] Oxidized LDL and other factors attract immune cells to the innermost layer of the arterial wall. There these immune cells undergo transformation into macrophages that form the lipid-rich foam cells characteristic of fatty streaks. This process perpetuates chronic inflammation and may make plaque rupture likely.[32] When a plaque ruptures, it can cause a heart attack or stroke. In advanced atherosclerosis, a goal of treatment is to lower LDL cholesterol to stabilize existing plaques while slowing the development of new ones.

atherogenic able to initiate or promote atherosclerosis.

Not all LDL are the same with regard to heart disease risk—they vary in size and density. The smallest, most dense LDL are considered the most atherogenic, whereas larger, less dense LDL are less atherogenic.

High Blood Triglycerides   When blood triglycerides (found in VLDL, a type of lipoprotein) are too high, many metabolic actions work together to the detriment of the arteries by promoting atherosclerosis.[33] About one-third of adults in the United States have high blood triglyceride levels. These high levels are associated with a sedentary lifestyle, overweight and obesity (especially abdominal obesity), and type 2 diabetes.

Hypertension and Atherosclerosis Worsen Each Other   Hypertension and atherosclerosis are twin demons that worsen CVD, and each worsens the other. Hypertension worsens atherosclerosis because a stiffened artery, already strained by each pulse of blood surging through it, is stressed further by high internal pressure. Injuries multiply, more plaque grows, and more weakened vessels become likely to burst and bleed.

Atherosclerosis also worsens hypertension. Since hardened arteries cannot expand, the heart's beats raise the blood pressure. Hardened arteries also fail to let blood flow freely through the kidneys, which control blood pressure. The kidneys sense the reduced flow of blood and respond as if the blood pressure were too low; they take steps to raise it further. The higher the blood pressure above normal, the greater the risk of heart attack or stroke. However, even values only slightly higher than desirable—classified as prehypertension in Figure 11–5 (p. 439)—increase the risk of heart attack and stroke.[34] The relationship between hypertension and disease risk holds true for men and women, young and old. A later section gives details about hypertension because it constitutes a major threat to health on its own.

Diabetes   Diabetes, a major independent risk factor for all forms of CVD, substantially increases the risk of death from these causes.[35] In diabetes, atherosclerosis progresses rapidly, blocking blood vessels and diminishing circulation. For many people with diabetes, the risk of a future heart attack is roughly equal to that of a person *without* diabetes who has already had a heart attack. When heart disease occurs in conjunction with diabetes, the condition is likely to be severe. In fact, any loss of control of blood glucose, even a transitory one, can be costly in terms of the condition of the arteries. Few people with diabetes recognize that, left uncontrolled, diabetes holds a grave threat of all forms of CVD.

> Diabetes is discussed in full in **Chapter 4.**

Physical Inactivity   Without routine physical activity, muscles, including the muscles of the heart and arteries, weaken and reduce the heart's ability to meet everyday demands. Regular physical activity expands the heart's capacity to pump blood to the tissues with each beat, thereby reducing the number of heartbeats required and the heart's workload. The slower pulse of fit people reflects the heart's greater pumping capacity.

Physical activity also stimulates development of new arteries to nourish the heart muscle, which may be a factor in the excellent recovery seen in some heart attack victims who exercise. In addition, physical activity favors lean tissue over fat tissue for a healthy body composition, raises HDL cholesterol, improves insulin sensitivity, reduces levels of inflammatory markers, and lowers blood pressure, LDL cholesterol, blood triglyceride levels, and blood glucose.[36] If pursued on at least 5 days each week, 30 minutes or more of brisk walking can improve the odds against heart disease considerably. If you are pressed for time, 15 minutes of more vigorous physical activity, such as jogging, on at least 5 days a week can provide the same benefits. The Think Fitness feature offers suggestions for incorporating physical activity into your daily routine. Chapter 10 provided the Physical Activity Guidelines for Americans.

"Walking is man's best medicine."
—Hippocrates

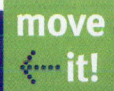
The benefits of physical activity are compelling, so why not tie up your athletic shoes, head out the door, and get going? Here are some ideas to get you started:

- Coach a sport.
- Garden.
- Hike, bike, or walk to nearby stores or to classes.
- Mow, trim, and rake by hand.
- Park a block from your destination and walk.
- Play a sport.
- Play with children.
- Take classes for credit in dancing, sports, conditioning, or swimming.
- Take the stairs, not the elevator.

- Walk a dog.
- Walk every day. A common goal is 10,000 steps per day (about 5 miles), to meet the "active" daily activity level, but shorter walks also confer benefits on most people. Use a pedometer to count your steps.
- Wash your car with extra vigor, or bend and stretch to wash your toes in the bath.
- Work out at a fitness club.
- Work out with friends to help one another stay fit.

Also, try these:

- Give away two labor-saving devices to someone who needs them.

- Lift small hand weights while talking on the phone, reading e-mail, or watching TV.
- Stretch often during the day.
- Try the President's Challenge for improving fitness: www.presidents challenge.org.

start now! ┈⟩ Using the list above as a guide, make your own list of things you can do today to be physically active. Using the calendar you created in Chapter 10, note on each day for the next month the physical activities you have engaged in for that day.

Smoking   Cigarette smoking powerfully increases the risk for CVD in men and women. The more a person smokes, the higher the CVD risk. Smoking tobacco in all its forms damages the heart directly with toxins and burdens it by raising the blood pressure. Body tissues starved for oxygen by smoke demand more heartbeats to deliver oxygenated blood, thereby increasing the heart's workload. At the same time, smoking deprives the heart muscle itself of the oxygen it needs to maintain a steady beat. Smoking also damages platelets, making blood clots likely. Damage to the linings of the blood vessels from tobacco smoke toxins makes atherosclerosis likely. When people quit smoking, their risk of heart disease begins to drop within a few months.

Atherogenic Diet   Diet influences the risk of CVD. An "atherogenic diet"—high in saturated fats and *trans* fats—increases LDL cholesterol. A high intake of *trans* fatty acids also lowers HDL cholesterol.[37] Fortunately, a well-chosen dietary pattern, such as the Mediterranean diet (Appendix E) can often lower the risk of CVD and does so to a greater degree than might be expected from its effects on blood lipids alone.[38] A number of beneficial factors in such diets may share the credit, among them the vitamins, minerals, fibers, antioxidant phytochemicals, and omega-3 fatty acids.[39]

Obesity and Metabolic Syndrome   Many of the modifiable risk factors for CVD are directly related to diet (look again at Table 11–5, p. 438). Several of these diet-related risk factors—low blood HDL cholesterol, high blood triglycerides, high blood pressure, elevated fasting blood glucose (insulin resistance), and central obesity—comprise a cluster of health risks known as **metabolic syndrome**. Metabolic syndrome underlies several chronic diseases and increases the risk of CVD and type 2 diabetes.[40] The precise cause of metabolic syndrome is not known, but central obesity and insulin resistance are thought to be primary factors in its development.[41]

Metabolic syndrome, like the chronic diseases associated with it, involves inflammation and elevates the risk for thrombosis.[42] More than one-third of the U.S. adult population meets the criteria for metabolic syndrome shown in Table 11–6, but many are unaware of it and so do not seek treatment.[43] Even obesity alone, especially central obesity, raises LDL cholesterol, lowers HDL cholesterol, raises blood pressure, and promotes insulin resistance.[44] The opposite also holds true: weight loss and physical activity lower LDL, raise HDL, improve insulin sensitivity, and lower blood pressure.[45]

Table 11–6
Metabolic Syndrome

Metabolic syndrome includes any three or more of the following:

- High fasting blood glucose.
- Central obesity.
- Hypertension.
- Low blood HDL.
- High blood triglycerides.

metabolic syndrome   a combination of characteristic factors—high fasting blood glucose or insulin resistance, central obesity, hypertension, low blood HDL cholesterol, and elevated blood triglycerides—that greatly increase a person's risk of developing CVD. Also called *insulin resistance syndrome*.

Figure 11–6

The American Heart Association's Heart Attack Risk Calculator

This online calculator can assess your risk of having a heart attack. For a meaningful assessment, you'll need some information about your blood lipids, blood pressure, and fasting blood glucose. To access the calculator, visit the American Heart Association website: https://www.heart.org/gglRisk/main_en_US.html.

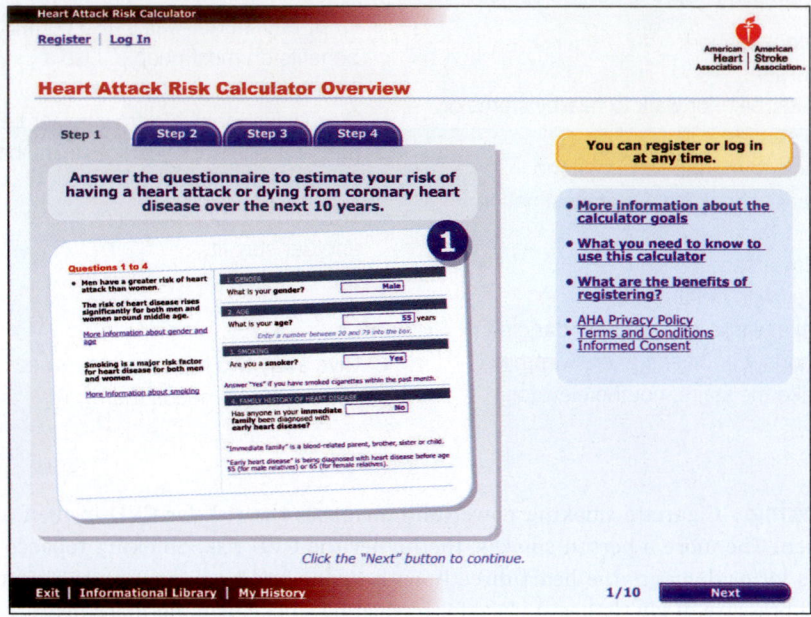

- In most people, atherosclerosis progresses steadily as they age.
- Major risk factors for CVD are age, gender, family history, high LDL cholesterol and low HDL cholesterol, high blood triglycerides, hypertension, diabetes, physical inactivity, smoking, an atherogenic diet, and obesity.

Recommendations for Reducing CVD Risk

Recommendations to reduce the risk of CVD include both screening and intervention. The American Heart Association, together with the American College of Cardiology, has developed guidelines for the assessment of CVD risk, the treatment of elevated blood cholesterol, and the management of lifestyle factors that reduce risk.[46]

How High Is Your Heart Disease Risk?   The American Heart Association has developed an online calculator, shown in Figure 11–6, and downloadable spreadsheet to estimate a person's risk of having a heart attack.[††] To use it, you'll need to provide some personal information, such as age and race, along with test results such as blood lipids, blood pressure, and fasting blood glucose. Once your heart attack risks have been assessed, a prevention plan focuses first on lifestyle changes in the areas of diet, physical activity, and smoking cessation. Treatment guidelines define when physicians should prescribe cholesterol-lowering medications.

Lifestyle Interventions   To reduce the risk of CVD, people are encouraged to increase physical activity, lose weight (if necessary), implement dietary changes, and reduce exposure to tobacco smoke either by quitting smoking or by avoiding secondhand smoke.[47] If such lifestyle changes fail to lower LDL or blood pressure to

[††]To calculate your risk for CVD, visit https://www.heart.org/gglRisk/main_en_US.html.

Table 11-7

Recommendations and Strategies for Reducing CVD Risk

Recommendation	Strategy
Dietary patterns. Choose a dietary pattern that emphasizes vegetables, fruits, and whole grains; includes low-fat dairy products, poultry, fish, legumes, nontropical vegetable oils, and nuts; and limits intake of sweets, sugar-sweetened beverages, and red meats.	Adopt a heart-healthy eating pattern such as DASH, the USDA Eating Pattern, the Mediterranean diet, or other well-planned plant-based dietary pattern.
Energy. Balance energy intake and physical activity to prevent weight gain and to achieve or maintain a healthy body weight.	Engage in at least 30 minutes of moderate-intensity endurance activity or 15 minutes of vigorous-intensity endurance activity on most days of the week.
Saturated fat, trans fat, and cholesterol. Limit saturated fat to less than 10 percent of total calories, *trans* fat to less than 1 percent of total calories, and cholesterol to less than 300 milligrams a day. For those who have been advised to lower LDL cholesterol or those who have diabetes, limit saturated fat to 5 to 6 percent of total calories and cholesterol to less than 200 milligrams a day.	Replace solid fats (saturated and *trans* fats) with food or oils containing unsaturated fatty acids such as omega-3–rich fish, avocado, nuts, olive oil, canola oil, safflower oil, corn oil, and soybean oil.
Sodium. Limit sodium intake to less than 2,300 milligrams per day. Limiting to 1,500 milligrams can reduce blood pressure further in those with hypertension.	Choose fewer packaged and prepared foods, or use lower-sodium varieties; prepare foods with little or no salt.
Alcohol. If alcohol is consumed, practice moderation.	Limit alcohol intake to no more than one drink daily for women and two drinks daily for men.
Tobacco. Avoid exposure to any form of tobacco or tobacco smoke.	Do not smoke or use tobacco in any form, and avoid exposure to secondhand smoke.

Sources: U.S. Department of Health and Human Services and U.S. Department of Agriculture, 2015–2020 Dietary Guidelines for Americans, *8th edition (2015), available at http://health.gov/dietaryguidelines/2015/guidelines/; R. H. Eckel and coauthors, 2013 AHA/ACC guidelines on lifestyle management to reduce cardiovascular risk: A report of the American College of Cardiology/American Heart Association Task Force on Practice Guidelines,* Circulation *129 (2014): S76–S99; M. R. Flock and P. M. Kris-Etherton, Dietary Guidelines for Americans 2010: Implications for cardiovascular disease,* Current Atherosclerosis Reports *13 (2011): 499–507.*

acceptable levels, then medications are prescribed. Table 11–7 summarizes recommendations and strategies to reduce the risk of heart disease. The Food Feature, later, offers one example of a heart-healthy diet, the DASH eating plan.

Diet to Reduce CVD Risk   What role can diet play in minimizing the risk of developing CVD? The answer focuses primarily on how diet relates to high blood cholesterol. The effects of diet are two sides of the same coin: side one, a diet high in saturated fat and *trans* fatty acids contributes to high blood LDL cholesterol; side two, reducing those fats in the diet lowers blood LDL cholesterol and may reduce the risk of CVD. Table 11–8 demonstrates the power of diet-related factors to reduce LDL cholesterol.

Wherever in the world populations consume diets high in saturated fat and low in fish, fruits, vegetables, nuts, and whole grains, blood cholesterol is high, and heart disease takes a toll on health and life. Conversely, wherever dietary fats are mostly

Table 11-8

How Much Does Changing the Diet Change LDL Cholesterol?

For those who need to lower LDL cholesterol, this table offers a perspective on the magnitude of results that may be possible.

Diet-Related Component	Modification	Possible LDL Reduction
Saturated fat	<7% of calories	8–10%
Weight reduction (if overweight)	Lose 10 lb	5–8%
Soluble, viscous fiber	5–10 g/day	3–5%

unsaturated and where fish, fruits, vegetables, nuts, and whole grains are abundant, blood cholesterol and rates of heart disease are low.[48]

It matters, too, what people choose to eat instead of saturated fats. Relationships between carbohydrate intakes and heart disease are not fully defined, but a diet too high in refined starches and added sugars has the potential to worsen heart disease risk by elevating blood triglycerides and inflammatory markers and by reducing HDL cholesterol.[49] People with elevated triglycerides may find that replacing refined starches and sugars with whole grains, legumes, or vegetables helps to improve blood lipids.[50]

Fish oils, rich in omega-3 polyunsaturated fatty acids, may reduce inflammation, lower triglycerides, prevent blood clots, and produce other effects that may reduce the risk of sudden death associated with both heart disease and stroke.[51] For these reasons, the American Heart Association recommends two meals of fish per week. People diagnosed with heart disease may require more than this amount, preferably from additional servings of fatty fish, but a physician may prescribe fish oil supplements in some cases. Not all studies report benefits, and the supplements may carry their own risks, so they should be taken under the supervision of a physician.[52]

Managing Lifestyle Changes   Adopting multiple lifestyle changes at once can be challenging. Making major changes in eating and physical activity patterns is not the easy route to heart health that everyone hopes for. Such changes, however, form a powerful and safe combination for improving health. The pattern of protection from the recommended diet and physical activity regimen becomes clear—the effects of each small choice add to the beneficial whole. While you are at it, don't smoke. Relax. Control stress. Play. Relaxed, happy people who make time to enjoy life have lower blood pressure and fewer heart attacks.

KEY POINTS

- Lifestyle changes to lower the risk of CVD include increasing physical activity, achieving a healthy body weight, reducing exposure to tobacco smoke, and eating a heart-healthy diet.
- Dietary measures to lower LDL cholesterol include reducing intakes of saturated fat and *trans* fat, along with consuming enough nutrient-dense fruits, vegetables, legumes, nuts, fish, and whole grains.

Nutrition and Hypertension

LO 11.4 Discuss hypertension and its risk factors, including nutrition risk factors.

People with healthy blood pressure generally enjoy a long life and suffer less often from heart disease.[53] Chronic high blood pressure, or hypertension, remains one of the most prevalent forms of CVD, affecting almost 78 million U.S. adults, and its incidence has been rising steadily.[54] Hypertension contributes to an estimated 1 million heart attacks and almost 800,000 strokes each year. The higher above normal the blood pressure goes, the greater the risk.

You cannot tell if you have high blood pressure—it presents no symptoms you can feel. The most effective single step you can take to protect yourself from hypertension is to find out whether you have it. During a checkup, a health-care professional can take an accurate resting blood pressure reading. If your resting blood pressure is above normal, the reading should be repeated before confirming the diagnosis of hypertension. Thereafter, blood pressure should be checked at regular intervals. Self-test machines in drugstores and other public places, while convenient, are often inaccurate.

When blood pressure is measured, two numbers are important: the pressure during contraction of the heart's ventricles (large pumping chambers) and the pressure during their relaxation. The numbers are given as a fraction, with the first number representing the **systolic pressure** (ventricular contraction) and the second number the **diastolic pressure** (ventricular relaxation). Return to Figure 11–5 (p. 439) to see how to interpret your resting blood pressure.

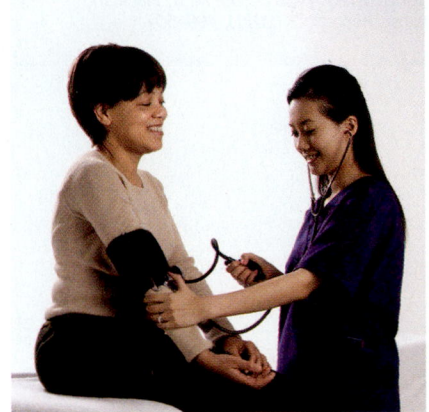
© iofoto/Shutterstock.com

The most effective single step you can take against hypertension is to learn your own blood pressure.

systolic (sis-TOL-ik) **pressure** the first figure in a blood pressure reading (the "dupp" sound of the heartbeat's "lubb-dupp" beat is heard), which reflects arterial pressure caused by the contraction of the heart's left ventricle.

diastolic (dye-as-TOL-ik) **pressure** the second figure in a blood pressure reading (the "lubb" of the heartbeat is heard), which reflects the arterial pressure when the heart is between beats.

Figure 11–7

The Blood Pressure

Three major factors contribute to the pressure inside an artery. First, the heart forcefully pushes blood into the artery. Second, the small-diameter arteries and capillaries at the other end resist the blood's flow (peripheral resistance). Third, the volume of fluid in the circulatory system, which depends on the number of dissolved particles in that fluid, adds to the blood pressure.

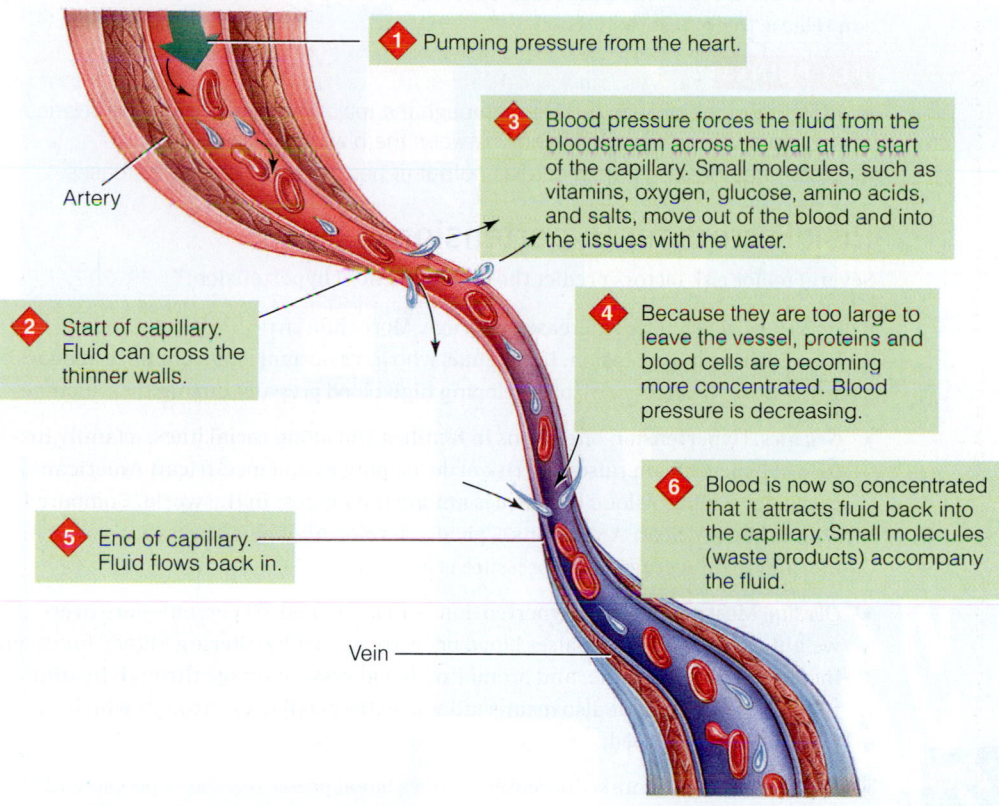

1 Pumping pressure from the heart.

Artery

2 Start of capillary. Fluid can cross the thinner walls.

3 Blood pressure forces the fluid from the bloodstream across the wall at the start of the capillary. Small molecules, such as vitamins, oxygen, glucose, amino acids, and salts, move out of the blood and into the tissues with the water.

4 Because they are too large to leave the vessel, proteins and blood cells are becoming more concentrated. Blood pressure is decreasing.

5 End of capillary. Fluid flows back in.

6 Blood is now so concentrated that it attracts fluid back into the capillary. Small molecules (waste products) accompany the fluid.

Vein

Ideal resting blood pressure is lower than 120 over 80. Just above this value (up to 139 over 89) lies **prehypertension**. Blood pressure in this range means that high blood pressure is likely to develop in the future and that taking steps to keep blood pressure low may avert illness later on.[55] Above this borderline level, though, the risks of heart attacks and strokes rise in direct proportion to increasing blood pressure.

- Hypertension silently and progressively worsens atherosclerosis and makes heart attacks and strokes likely.
- All adults should know whether or not their blood pressure falls within the normal range.

How Does Blood Pressure Work in the Body?

Blood pressure is vital to life. It pushes the blood through the major arteries into smaller arteries and finally into tiny capillaries whose thin walls permit the exchange of fluids between the blood and the tissues (see Figure 11–7). Blood pressure arises from contractions in the heart muscle that pump blood away from the heart (**cardiac output**) and the resistance blood encounters in the small arteries (**peripheral resistance**).

prehypertension borderline blood pressure between 120 over 80 and 139 over 89 millimeters of mercury, an indication that hypertension is likely to develop in the future.

cardiac output the volume of blood discharged by the heart each minute. Also defined in Chapter 10.

peripheral resistance the resistance to pumped blood in the small arterial branches (arterioles) that carry blood to tissues.

When either cardiac output or peripheral resistance increases, blood pressure rises. Cardiac output is raised when heart rate or blood volume increases; peripheral resistance is affected mostly by the diameters of the arteries. Blood pressure is therefore influenced by the nervous system, which regulates heart muscle contractions and the arteries' diameters, and by hormonal signals, which may cause fluid retention or blood vessel constriction. The kidneys also play a role in regulating blood pressure. If the blood pressure is too low, the kidneys act to increase it—they send hormones to constrict blood vessels and to retain water and salt in the body. When the pressure is right, the cells receive a constant supply of nutrients and oxygen and can release their wastes.

KEY POINTS

- Blood pressure pushes the blood through the major arteries into smaller arteries and capillaries to exchange fluids between the blood and the tissues.
- Blood pressure rises when cardiac output or peripheral resistance increases.

Risk Factors for Hypertension

Several major risk factors predict the development of hypertension:[56]

- *Age.* Hypertension risk increases with age. More than two-thirds of U.S. adults older than 65 have hypertension. Individuals who have normal blood pressure at age 55 still have a 90 percent risk of developing high blood pressure during their lifetime.

- *Genetics.* Hypertension often runs in families and along racial lines: a family history of hypertension raises the risk of developing it, and for African Americans, prevalence of high blood pressure is among the highest in the world. Compared with others, African Americans typically develop high blood pressure earlier in life, and their average blood pressure is much higher.

- *Obesity.* Most people with hypertension—an estimated 70 percent—are overweight or obese. Obesity raises blood pressure in part by altering kidney function, increasing blood volume, and promoting blood vessel damage through insulin resistance.[57] Excess fat also means miles of extra capillaries through which the blood must be pumped.

- *Salt intake.* As salt intake increases, so does blood pressure.[58] Most people with hypertension can benefit from reducing salt in their diets.

- *Alcohol.* Alcohol, regularly consumed in amounts greater than two drinks per day, is strongly associated with hypertension (details in a later section) and may interfere with drug therapy.[59]

- *Dietary factors.* A person's eating pattern may increase the risk for developing hypertension. As explained in the next section, eating patterns that emphasize fruits, vegetables, nuts, whole grains, and low-fat dairy products can help to lower blood pressure.

KEY POINT

- Obesity, age, family background, and race contribute to hypertension risks, as do salt intake and other dietary factors, including alcohol consumption.

How Does Nutrition Affect Hypertension?

Even mild hypertension can be dangerous, but individuals who adhere to treatment are less likely to suffer illness or early death. Some people need medications to bring their blood pressure down, but diet and physical activity can bring improvements for many people and prevent hypertension in many others. Table 11–9 describes the lifestyle changes that reduce blood pressure, and the following sections address each one.

The DASH Diet   The results of the Dietary Approaches to Stop Hypertension (DASH) trial show that a diet rich in fruits, vegetables, nuts, whole grains, and low-fat milk products and low in total fat and saturated fat can significantly lower blood

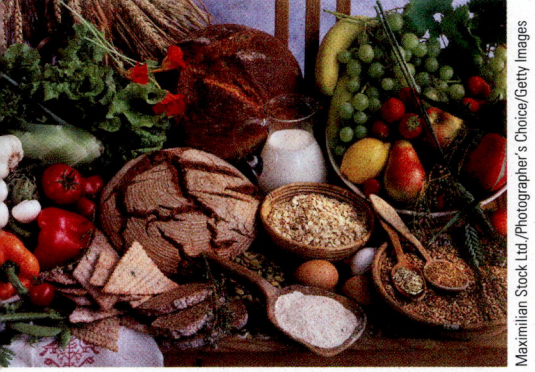

When diets are rich in whole grains, vegetables, and fruits, life expectancies are long.

Maximilian Stock Ltd./Photographer's Choice/Getty Images

Chapter 11 Diet and Health

Table 11–9

Lifestyle Modifications to Reduce Blood Pressure

Modification	Recommendation	Expected Reduction in Systolic Blood Pressure
Weight reduction	Maintain healthy body weight (BMI 18.5–24.9)	10 mm Hg/10 kg lost
DASH eating plan	Adopt a diet rich in fruits, vegetables, and low-fat milk products with reduced saturated fat intake	5–6 mm Hg
Sodium restriction	Reduce dietary sodium intake to less than 2,300 milligrams sodium (less than 6 grams salt) per day, and further reduce intake to 1,500 milligrams among people with prehypertension or hypertension for greater reductions in blood pressure.	2–7 mm Hg
Physical activity	Perform aerobic physical activity for at least 40 minutes per day, most days of the week	2–5 mm Hg
Moderate alcohol consumption	Men: Limit to 2 drinks per day Women and lighter-weight men: Limit to 1 drink per day	2–4 mm Hg

Sources: U.S. Department of Health and Human Services and U.S. Department of Agriculture, 2015–2020 Dietary Guidelines for Americans, *8th edition (2015)*, available at http://health.gov/dietaryguidelines/2015/guidelines/; R. H. Eckel and coauthors, 2013 AHA/ACC guideline on lifestyle management to reduce cardiovascular risk: A report of the American College of Cardiology/American Heart Association Task Force on Practice Guidelines, Circulation *129 (2014): S76–S99;* L. Landsberg and coauthors, Obesity-related hypertension: Pathogenesis, cardiovascular risk, and treatment: A position paper of The Obesity Society and the American Society of Hypertension, Journal of Clinical Hypertension *15 (2013): 14–33.*

pressure. In addition to lowering blood pressure, the DASH diet improves vascular function, lowers total cholesterol and LDL cholesterol, and reduces inflammation.[60] Compared to the typical American diet, the DASH eating plan provides more fiber, potassium, magnesium, and calcium; emphasizes legumes and fish over red meat; limits added sugars and sugar-containing beverages; and meets other recommendations of the 2015–2020 Dietary Guidelines for Americans. Healthy eating patterns like DASH consistently improve blood pressure, both in study subjects whose diets are provided by researchers and in those freely choosing and preparing their own foods according to guidelines.

Weight Control and Physical Activity   For people who have hypertension and are overweight, a loss of as little as 5 to 10 percent of body weight can significantly lower blood pressure. Weight loss alone is one of the most effective nondrug treatments for hypertension.[61] Those who are taking medication to control their blood pressure can often cut down their doses or eliminate their medication if they lose weight.

Physical activity can lower almost everyone's blood pressure, even people without hypertension. Physical activity helps with weight control, of course, but moderate- or vigorous-intensity aerobic activity, such as 40 to 60 minutes of brisk walking or running on most days, along with resistance training on 2 to 3 days per week, also helps to lower blood pressure directly.[62] Even when performed in manageable 10-minute segments throughout the day, activity adds up and provides benefits. As fitness improves, the need for medication to treat mild hypertension may diminish, or even vanish, over time.

Physical activity also alters the body's hormones in beneficial ways. It decreases the secretion of stress hormones, reducing stress and lowering blood pressure. It also redistributes body water and eases transit of the blood through the small arteries that feed the tissues, including those of the heart.

Salt, Sodium, and Blood Pressure   As mentioned, high intakes of salt and sodium are associated with hypertension.[63] Lowering sodium intake reduces blood pressure in most people. The combination of the DASH diet with a limited intake of sodium, however, improves blood pressure better than either strategy alone.[64] As salt intakes decrease, blood pressure drops in a stepwise fashion. This direct relationship is reported at all levels of intake, from very low to much higher than average. In addition, reducing salt intake may provide additional protection against heart disease, beyond lowering blood pressure.[65]

The World Health Organization estimates that a significant reduction in sodium intake could reduce by half the number of people requiring medication for hypertension and greatly reduce deaths from CVD. Most authorities recommend that everyone (even those with normal blood pressure) should moderately restrict salt and sodium intakes, not to exceed the DRI committee's Tolerable Upper Intake Level—that is, no more than 2,300 milligrams of sodium per day.

Certain groups of people, comprising about half of the U.S. population, respond more sensitively than others to sodium intakes: African Americans, people with hypertension, people with kidney problems or diabetes, and older people (those who are 51 or older). These individuals should limit their sodium intakes to no more than 1,500 milligrams of sodium per day. The American Heart Association recommends no more than 1,500 milligrams of sodium per day for the entire U.S. population.[66]

Alcohol   In moderate doses, alcohol initially relaxes the arteries and so reduces blood pressure, but higher doses raise blood pressure.[67] Hypertension is common among people with alcoholism and is apparently caused directly by the alcohol. Hypertension caused by alcohol leads to CVD, the same as hypertension caused by any other factor. Furthermore, alcohol may cause strokes—even *without* hypertension. The Dietary Guidelines for Americans urge a sensible, moderate approach for those who drink alcohol. *Moderation* means no more than one drink a day for women or two drinks a day for men, an amount that seems safe relative to blood pressure. The same amount, however, raises women's risk of breast cancer, so other routes to relaxation may prove safer.

Potassium   Potassium may also help to regulate blood pressure. Hypertension occurs more frequently in areas where diets lack potassium-rich fruits and vegetables. Conversely, diets rich in potassium and low in sodium appear to both prevent and correct hypertension.[68]

Medications   How can people be sure of getting all of the nutrients needed to keep blood pressure low? Vitamin and mineral supplements have been disappointing in this regard, showing no promise for lowering blood pressure. Therefore, the best answer is to consume a low-fat diet with abundant fruits, vegetables, fish, and low-fat dairy products that provide the needed nutrients while holding sodium intake within bounds. Should diet and physical activity fail to reduce

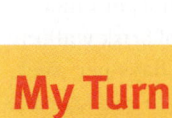 

My Turn — watch it!

Fast-Food Generation?

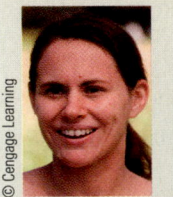 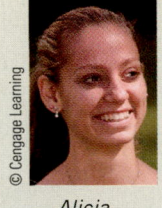

Tami   *Alicia*

How many fast-food meals do you eat each week? Listen to two students tell you about their weekly fast-food fare.

Visit www.cengagebrain.com to access MindTap, a complete digital course that includes these videos and other resources.

blood pressure, though, antihypertensive drugs such as diuretics can be lifesaving. Diuretics lower blood pressure by increasing fluid loss and lowering blood volume. Some diuretics may also cause potassium losses. People taking these drugs should make it a point to consume potassium-rich foods daily. Although some diuretics can lead to a potassium deficiency, others spare potassium.

Some people doubt the power of ordinary food to improve health, despite abundant evidence in its favor. In the search for something extra, such people often combine nutrient supplements with herbs and other alternatives to mainstream nutrition and medicine. The Consumer's Guide (p. 450) provides a look at some of these practices.

KEY POINTS

- For most people, maintaining a healthy body weight, engaging in regular physical activity, minimizing salt and sodium intakes, limiting alcohol intake, and eating a diet high in fruits, vegetables, fish, and low-fat dairy products work together to keep blood pressure normal.
- Certain nutrient deficiencies may raise blood pressure.

Nutrition and Cancer

LO 11.5 Explain the relationships between diet and cancer.

Cancer ranks second only to heart disease as a leading cause of death and disability in the United States. More than 1.6 million new cancer cases and nearly 600,000 deaths from cancer occurred in the United States in 2014.[69] Still, over the past decade, a small but steady trend toward declining cancer deaths is evident.[70] Early detection and improved treatment have transformed several common cancers from intractable killers to curable diseases or treatable chronic illnesses. Although the potential for cure is exciting, *prevention* of cancer remains far and away preferable.

Can an individual's chosen behaviors affect the risk of contracting cancer? They can, sometimes powerfully so.[71] Just a few rare cancers are known to be caused primarily by genetic influences and will appear in members of an affected family regardless of lifestyle choices. A few more are linked with microbial infections.[‡‡] For the great majority of cancers, lifestyle factors and environmental exposures become the major risk factors.[72] For example, if everyone in the United States quit smoking right now, future total cancers would likely drop by almost a third. Obesity and a lack of physical activity almost certainly play a role in the development of colon and breast cancer and probably contribute to pancreatic, esophageal, and renal cancers as well.[73] Alcohol intakes contribute to cancer of the mouth, pharynx, and larynx; cancer of the esophagus; breast cancer; and probably others. Further, incidence of hormone-related breast cancer has dropped significantly at a time when millions of women have ceased taking hormone replacement therapy for symptoms of menopause.[74]

An estimated 30 to 40 percent of cancers are influenced by diet, and these relationships are the focus of this section.[75] Diet patterns that emphasize fat, meat, alcohol, and excess calories and that minimize fruits and vegetables have been the targets of much cancer research. Such constituents of the diet relate to cancer in several ways:

- Foods or their components may initiate cancer.
- Foods or their components may promote cancer.
- Foods or their components may protect against cancer.

Also, for the person who has cancer, diet can make a crucial difference in recovery. Some dietary and environmental factors currently believed to be important in cancer causation are listed in Table 11–12 (p. 453).

---

‡‡Examples include viral hepatitis and liver cancer, human papilloma virus and cervical cancer, and *H. pylori* bacterium (the ulcer bacterium) and stomach cancer.

cancer a group of diseases in which cells multiply out of control and disrupt normal functioning of one or more organs.

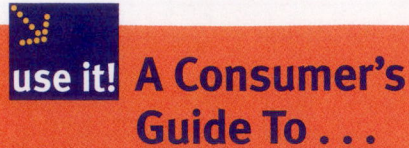

use it! A Consumer's Guide To . . .

Deciding about CAM

Have you ever treated a health problem with an herbal remedy or another form of **complementary** and **alternative medicine (CAM)**? (See Table 11–10 for definitions.) If so, you are not alone. Each year, U.S. consumers spend tens of billions of dollars on CAM treatments. All of these dollars spur sellers to advertise on thousands of Internet websites, run television infomercials, write innumerable booklets and books, and publish floods of magazine and newspaper advertorials to promote sales.

CAM treatments range from folk medicine to fraud. When these treatments are used instead of conventional medicine, they are called alternative; when they are used together with conventional medicine, they are called complementary. Some CAM therapies have been used for centuries, but few have been evaluated scientifically for safety or effectiveness.[1]* When tested, most prove ineffective or unsafe.[2] Useless remedies continue to sell, however, because an ill person's belief in a treatment, the placebo effect, can sometimes lead to physical healing (*placebo* was defined in Table 1–7 of Chapter 1). Then, undeservedly, the treatment gets the credit.

CAM Best Bets

This is not to say that all CAM treatments are useless. Dozens of **herbal medicines** contain effective natural drugs. For example, the resin myrrh (pronounced *murr*) contains an analgesic (pain-killing) compound; willow bark contains aspirin; the herb valerian contains a tranquilizing oil; senna leaves produce a powerful laxative. The World Health Organization currently recommends a Chinese herbal medicine—artemisinin, derived from a wormwood tree—to fight off malaria in some tropical nations. Herbs, like drugs,

*References are found in Appendix F.

Table 11–10
Alternative Therapy Terms

- **acupuncture** (AK-you-punk-chur) a technique that involves piercing the skin with long, thin needles at specific anatomical points to relieve pain or illness. Acupuncture sometimes uses heat, pressure, friction, suction, or electromagnetic energy to stimulate the points.
- **complementary** and **alternative medicine (CAM)** a group of diverse medical and health-care systems, practices, and products that are not considered to be a part of conventional medicine. Examples include acupuncture, biofeedback, chiropractic, faith healing, and many others.
- **herbal medicine** a type of CAM that uses herbs and other natural substances to prevent or cure diseases or to relieve symptoms.

can cause side effects.[3] Table 11–11 (p. 451) lists the potential actions and risks of selected herbs.**

The National Institutes of Health established its National Center for Complementary and Alternative Medicine (NCCAM) to distinguish alternative therapies that are potentially useful from those that are useless or harmful. The NCCAM has found that **acupuncture** helps to quell nausea from surgery, chemotherapy, and pregnancy and to ease chronic low-back pain, and possibly migraine headaches, although underlying mechanisms for these effects are not known.[4] After more than a decade of funding studies, the agency has confirmed no effect from most other CAM treatments.[5]

Ideally, a therapy provides benefits with little or no risk. Some alternative therapies are innocuous, providing little

**A reliable source of information about herbs is V. Tyler, The Honest Herbal (New York: Pharmaceutical Products Press). Look for the latest edition.

or no benefit for little or no risk. Sipping a cup of warm tea with a pleasant aroma, for example, won't cure heart disease, but it may improve one's mood and help relieve tension. Given no physical hazard and little financial risk, such therapies are acceptable. Figure 11–8 (p. 452) summarizes the relationships between risks and benefits.

In contrast, other products and procedures are dangerous, posing great risks while providing no benefits. One example, discussed next, is the taking of laetrile to treat cancer. Perhaps most controversial are alternative therapies that may provide benefits but also carry significant, unknown, or debatable risks. Smoking or ingesting marijuana is an example of such an alternative therapy. The compounds in marijuana seem to provide relief from symptoms such as nausea, vomiting, and pain that commonly accompany cancer, HIV/AIDS, and other diseases, but smoking marijuana raises lung cancer risk, whereas ingesting large amounts can cause psychotic delusions. As more states consider legalizing marijuana for medicinal use, the issue of risks versus benefits is highlighted.

A CAM Worst Case

The toxic drug laetrile, a CAM treatment for cancer, was popularized in the 1970s and remains available with no evidence to support its use, then or now. In fact, its high cyanide (poison) content makes it a hazardous choice. Along with thousands of other sham treatments, laetrile is still sold as a "dietary supplement" to unsuspecting people by way of Internet websites.

Anyone can claim to be an expert in a "new" or "natural" therapy, and many practitioners act knowledgeable but either are misinformed or are frauds (see Controversy 1). Intelligent, clear-minded people can fall for such hoaxes when standard medical therapies fail; loving

Table 11–11

Selected Herbs: Claims, Evidence, and Risks

Common Name	Claims	Evidence	Risks[a]
Aloe (gel)	Promotes wound healing	May help heal minor burns and abrasions	Generally considered safe; can worsen deep wounds
Black cohosh (stems and roots)	Eases menopause symptoms	Conflicting evidence	May cause headaches, stomach discomfort, liver damage
Chamomile (flowers)	Relieves indigestion	Little evidence available	Generally considered safe
Chaparral (leaves and twigs)	Slows aging, "cleanses" blood, heals wounds, cures cancer, treats acne	No evidence available	Acute, toxic hepatitis; liver damage
Cinnamon (bark)	Relieves indigestion, lowers blood glucose and blood lipids	May lower blood glucose in type 2 diabetes	May have a "blood-thinning" effect; not safe for pregnant women or those taking diabetes medication
Comfrey (leafy plant)	Soothes nerves	No evidence available	Liver damage
Echinacea (roots)	Relieves colds, flu, and infections; promotes wound healing; boosts immunity	Ineffective in preventing colds or other infections	Generally considered safe; may cause headache, dizziness, nausea
Ephedra (stems)	Promotes weight loss (FDA bans the sale of ephedra-containing supplements)	Little evidence available	Rapid heart rate, tremors, seizures, insomnia, headaches, hypertension
Feverfew (leaves)	Prevents migraine headaches	May prevent migraine headaches	Generally considered safe; may cause mouth irritation, swelling, ulcers, and GI distress; not safe for pregnant women
Garlic (bulbs)	Lowers blood lipids and blood pressure	May lower blood cholesterol slightly; conflicting evidence on blood pressure	Generally considered safe; garlic breath, body odor, gas, and GI distress; inhibits blood clotting
Ginger (roots)	Prevents motion sickness, nausea	May relieve nausea of pregnancy, motion, chemotherapy, or surgery	Generally considered safe
Ginkgo (tree leaves)	Improves memory, relieves vertigo	Little evidence available	Generally considered safe; may cause headache, GI distress, dizziness; may inhibit blood clotting
Ginseng (roots)	Boosts immunity, increases endurance	Little evidence available	Generally considered safe; may cause insomnia, headache, hypertension
Goldenseal (roots)	Relieves indigestion, treats urinary infections	Little evidence available	Generally considered safe except in cases of hypertension, CVD, or pregnancy
Kava (roots)	Relieves anxiety, promotes relaxation	Little evidence available	Liver failure
Kombucha tea (fermentation product)	Boosts immunity; prevents cancer; improves digestion	No evidence available	Stomach upset; allergic reactions; toxic reactions; metabolic acidosis
Saw palmetto (ripe fruits)	Relieves enlarged prostate; diuretic; enhances sexual vigor	Little evidence available	Generally considered safe; may cause nausea, vomiting, diarrhea
St. John's wort (leaves and tops)	Relieves depression and anxiety	May relieve mild depression	Generally considered safe; may cause fatigue, sensitivity to sunlight, and GI distress
Turmeric (roots)	Reduces inflammation; relieves heartburn; prevents cancer	No evidence available	Generally considered safe except in cases of gallbladder disease
Valerian (roots)	Calms nerves, improves sleep	Little evidence available	Associated with liver damage
Yohimbe (tree bark)	Enhances "male performance"	No evidence available	Kidney failure, seizures

[a]Allergies are always a possible risk; see Controversy 14 for drug interactions. Pregnant women should not use herbal supplements.

Figure 11–8
Risk-Benefit Relationships

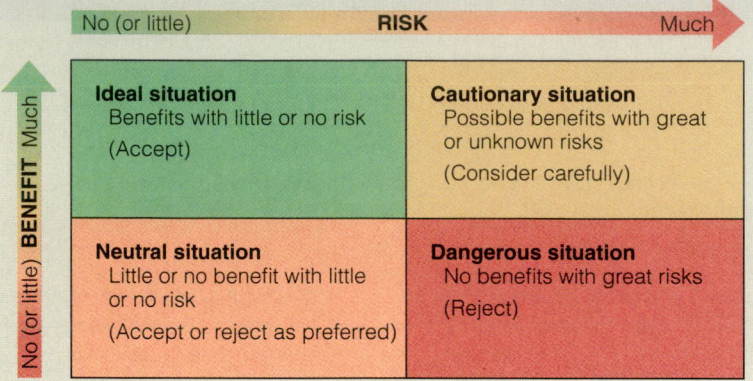

	No (or little) ← **RISK** → Much
BENEFIT Much	**Ideal situation** — Benefits with little or no risk (Accept) / **Cautionary situation** — Possible benefits with great or unknown risks (Consider carefully)
No (or little)	**Neutral situation** — Little or no benefit with little or no risk (Accept or reject as preferred) / **Dangerous situation** — No benefits with great risks (Reject)

life and desperate, they fall prey to the worst kind of quackery on the feeblest promise of a cure.

A Curious Case of Anosmia

A popular CAM cold treatment consisting of zinc gel squirted into the nose was widely advertised and sold but lacked approval from the U.S. Food and Drug Administration (FDA).[†] Over the course of a few years, the FDA received over 130 complaints from consumers reporting anosmia, meaning that they lost their sense of smell, sometimes permanently, after using the product. Finally, the FDA took action against the manufacturer, who removed the product from the market. Anosmia may not sound serious, but it dramatically reduces the sense of taste and pleasure in eating, and it poses a danger when it prevents the detection of hazards normally signaled through the sense of smell, such as spoiled food or leaking gas. This case illustrates the trouble with using most CAM products: they are not tested for safety. Without prior testing, the user becomes the tester, and no one can predict the outcome.

[†]The products were Zicam Cold Remedy Nasal Gel, Zicam Cold Remedy Gel Swabs, and Zicam Cold Remedy Swabs, Kids Size.

Mislabeled Herbs

When common herbal remedies are analyzed, many do not contain the species or the active ingredients stated on their labels.[6] In one analysis, instead of the herbs stated on the label, the CAM products contained unsafe medical drugs that interact with prescription medications to cause a dangerous drop in blood pressure. In New York, investigators found six cases of lead poisoning in pregnant women who had taken a popular herbal remedy made in India.[7] Some of the herbal medications also contained significant levels of mercury or arsenic. When labels lack veracity and adulteration and contamination are common, consumers cannot make reasonable and safe choices.

If you decide to use an herbal or other CAM product, compare labels and look for the words *U.S. Pharmacopeia* or *Consumer Lab* on the label. These names signify that samples of the product were analyzed and found to contain authentic ingredients in the quantities claimed; these names do *not* indicate safety or effectiveness of the product, however.

Like other drugs, herbs often interfere with or potentiate the effects of medication (see Controversy 14).[8] For example, because *Ginkgo biloba* impairs blood clotting, it can cause bleeding

problems for people on aspirin or other blood-thinning medicines.[9]

Lack of Knowledge

Most people in the market for herbs and other CAM treatments take the advice of herb vendors in stores or online. Few herb sellers, however, possess the training in pharmacology, botany, and human physiology required to appropriately apply herbal remedies; perilous mistakes with herbs are common. The few physicians who are skilled in herbal medicine may integrate the best CAM treatments into their practices. However, many patients using herbs or CAM treatments keep their use a secret, fearing their doctors' disapproval.[10] Such secrecy ups their risk—without knowledge, a physician cannot evaluate the potential for interactions.

Moving Ahead

The consequences of using unproven treatments are unpredictable. If you take prescription drugs, tell your doctor about any herbs you are also taking to rule out incompatibility.

Before taking any herb, find authoritative, scientific sources of information on its potential actions and risks. Don't be led astray by advertisements, rumors, Internet claims, or wishful thinking—investigate and decide for yourself.

Review Questions[‡]

1. Complementary and alternative medicines (CAM) warrant a cautious approach; these treatments often lack evidence for safety or effectiveness. **T F**

2. The National Center for Complementary and Alternative Medicine (NCCAM) promotes laetrile therapy. **T F**

3. For safety, a person seeking medical help should inform their physician about use of herbs or other alternative medicines. **T F**

[‡]Answers to Consumer's Guide review questions are found in Appendix G.

Table 11-12

Diet-Related Factors and Cancer at Specific Sites

Cancer Site	Risk Factors	Protective Factors
Breast (postmenopause)	Alcoholic drinks, body fatness, adult attained height,[a] abdominal fatness, adult weight gain	Lactation, physical activity
Breast (premenopause)	Alcoholic drinks, adult attained height,[a] greater birth weight	Lactation, healthy degree of body fatness[b]
Colon and rectum	Red meat, processed meat, alcoholic drinks, body fatness, abdominal fatness, adult attained height[a]	Physical activity, foods containing dietary fiber, garlic, milk, calcium
Endometrium	Body fatness, abdominal fatness	Physical activity
Esophagus	Alcoholic drinks, body fatness	Nonstarchy vegetables, fruits, foods containing beta-carotene, foods containing vitamin C
Gallbladder	Body fatness	
Kidney	Body fatness	
Liver	Aflatoxins,[c] alcoholic drinks	
Lung	Arsenic in drinking water, beta-carotene supplements[d]	Fruits, foods containing carotenoids
Mouth, pharynx, and larynx	Alcoholic drinks	Nonstarchy vegetables, fruits, foods containing carotenoids
Nasopharynx	Cantonese-style salted fish	
Ovary	Adult attained height[a]	
Pancreas	Body fatness, abdominal fatness, adult attained height[a]	Foods containing folate
Prostate	Diets high in calcium	Foods containing lycopene, foods containing selenium, selenium[e]
Skin	Arsenic in drinking water	
Stomach	Salt, salty and salted foods	Nonstarchy vegetables, allium vegetables,[f] fruits

Note: Strength of evidence for all these factors is either "convincing" or "probable."

[a] Adult attained height is unlikely to directly modify the risk of cancer. It is a marker for genetic, environmental, hormonal, and also nutritional factors affecting growth during the period from preconception to completion of linear growth.

[b] Most studies show an increased risk of postmenopausal breast cancer with increased body fatness, but a decreased risk of premenopausal breast cancer with increased body fatness.

[c] Aflatoxins are toxins produced by molds or fungi. The main foods that may be contaminated are all types of grains (wheat, rye, rice, corn, barley, oats) and legumes, notably peanuts.

[d] The evidence is derived from studies using high-dose supplements (20 mg/day for beta-carotene; 25,000 international units/day for retinol) in smokers.

[e] The evidence is derived from studies using supplements at a dose of 200 μg/day. Selenium is toxic at higher doses.

[f] This includes vegetables such as garlic, onions, leeks, and shallots.

Sources: W. C. Willett, T. Key, and I. Romieu, Diet, obesity, and physical activity, in B. W. Stewart and C. P. Wild (eds.), World Cancer Report (Lyon, France: International Agency for Research on Cancer, 2014), pp. 124–133; World Cancer Research Fund/American Institute for Cancer Research, Food, Nutrition, Physical Activity and the Prevention of Cancer: A Global Perspective (Washington, D.C.: AICR, 2007).

How Does Cancer Develop?

Cancer arises in the genes. The development of cancer, called **carcinogenesis**, usually proceeds slowly and continues for several decades. It often begins when a cell's genetic material (DNA) sustains damage from a **carcinogen**, such as a free-radical compound, radiation, and other factors. Such damage occurs every day, but most is quickly repaired. Sometimes DNA collects bits of damage here and there over time. Usually, if the damage cannot be repaired and the cell becomes unable to faithfully

carcinogenesis the origination or beginning of cancer.

carcinogen (car-SIN-oh-jen) a cancer-causing substance (carcin means "cancer"; gen means "gives rise to").

Figure 11–9

Cancer Development

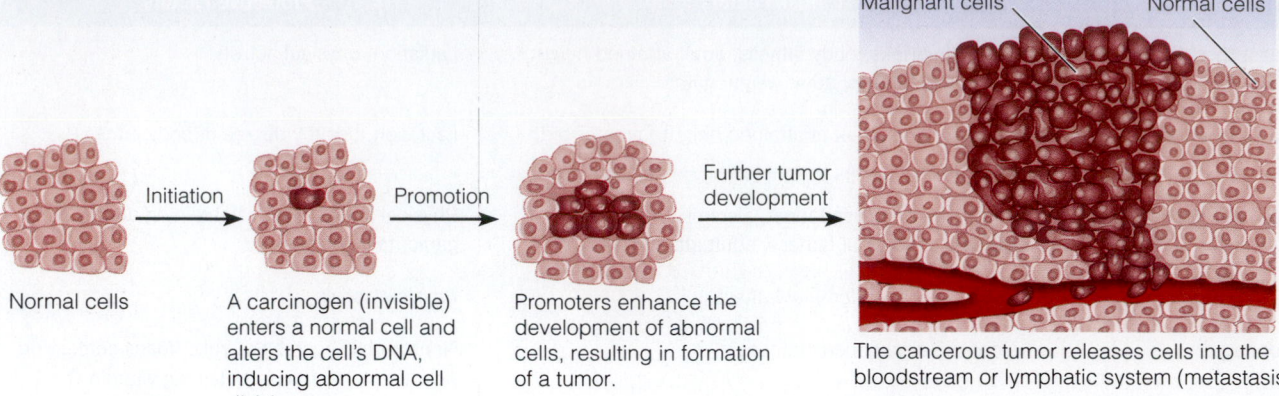

Malignant cells   Normal cells

Normal cells — Initiation → A carcinogen (invisible) enters a normal cell and alters the cell's DNA, inducing abnormal cell division. — Promotion → Promoters enhance the development of abnormal cells, resulting in formation of a tumor. — Further tumor development → The cancerous tumor releases cells into the bloodstream or lymphatic system (metastasis).

replicate its genome, the cell self-destructs, committing a sort of cellular suicide to prevent its progeny from inheriting faulty genes.

Occasionally, a damaged cell loses its ability to self-destruct and also loses its ability to stop reproducing. In a healthy, well-nourished person, the immune system steps in to destroy these cells.[76] If, however, the immune system falters, the damaged cell replicates uncontrollably, and the result is a mass of abnormal tissue—a tumor. Life-threatening cancer results when the tumor tissue, which cannot perform the critical functions of healthy tissues, overtakes the healthy organ in which it developed or disseminates its cells through the bloodstream to other parts of the body.

Simplified, cancer develops through the following steps (illustrated in Figure 11–9):

1. Exposure to a carcinogen.

2. Entry of the carcinogen into a cell.

3. Initiation of cancer as the carcinogen damages or changes the cell's genetic material (carcinogenesis).

4. Acceleration by **promoters** that stimulate cancer cell growth such that the cells multiply out of control—tumor formation.

5. Often, spreading of cancer cells via blood and lymph (**metastasis**).

6. Disruption of normal body functions.

Researchers think that the first four steps, which culminate with tumor formation, are key to cancer prevention. On hearing this, many people mistakenly believe that they should avoid eating all foods that contain carcinogens. Doing so proves impossible, however, because most carcinogens occur naturally in foods amidst thousands of other chemicals and nutrients needed by the body. The body is well equipped to deal with the minute amounts of carcinogens that occur naturally in common foods like coffee, toast, and coffee cake.*** Of course, consuming coffee, toast, and coffee cake does not elevate a person's risk of developing cancer because the body detoxifies small doses of carcinogens found in foods.

For those who suspect food additives of being carcinogenic, be assured that additives are held to strict standards; no additive approved for use in the United States

initiation an event, probably occurring in a cell's genetic material, caused by radiation or by a chemical carcinogen that can give rise to cancer.

promoters factors such as certain hormones that do not initiate cancer but speed up its development once initiation has taken place.

metastasis (meh-TASS-ta-sis) movement of cancer cells from one body part to another, usually by way of the body fluids.

***Coffee contains acetaldehyde, acetic acid, acetone, atractylosides, butanol, cafestol palmitate, chlorogenic acid, dimethyl sulfide, ethanol, furan, furfural, guaiacol, hydrogen sulfide, isoprene, methanol, methyl butanol, methyl formate, methyl glyoxal, propionaldehyde, pyridine, and 1,3,7,-trimethylxanthine. Toast and coffee cake contain acetic acid, acetone, butyric acid, caprionic acid, ethyl acetate, ethyl ketone, ethyl lactate, methyl ethyl ketone, propionic acid, and valeric acid.

causes cancer when used appropriately in food. Food *contaminants*, however, that enter foods by accident or toxins that arise through natural processes (for example, when a food becomes moldy) may indeed be powerful carcinogens, or they may be converted to carcinogens during the body's attempts to break them down. Most such constituents are monitored in the U.S. food supply and are generally present, if at all, in amounts well below those that could pose risks to consumers.

KEY POINTS

- Cancer arises from genetic damage and develops in steps, including initiation and promotion, which may be influenced by diet.
- Contaminants and naturally occurring toxins can be carcinogenic, but they are monitored in the U.S. food supply, and the body is equipped to handle tiny doses of most kinds.

Which Diet Factors Affect Cancer Risk?

Certain dietary factors substantially influence cancer development.[77] The degree of risk imposed by food depends partly on the eater's genetic inheritance, but knowledge of these relationships is still unfolding. The following sections explore some of the suspected links between food constituents and prevention or development of certain cancers. The Controversy section delves into areas of scientific advancement that promise to clarify at least some of the relationships between diet and cancer.

Energy Intake
When calorie intakes are reduced, cancer rates fall. In animal experiments, this **caloric effect** proves to be one of the most effective dietary interventions to prevent cancer. When researchers establish a cancer-causing condition in laboratory animals and then restrict the energy in their feed, the onset of cancer in the restricted animals is delayed beyond the time when unrestricted animals have died of the disease. Population observations seem to imply that calorie restriction, voluntary or involuntary, may delay cancer in people, too, and clinical experiments to resolve the issue are currently under way.[78] An important note: this effect occurs only in cancer prevention; once started, cancer continues advancing even in a person who is starving. It is also true that when a population's calorie intake rises, cancer rates rise in response; excess calories from carbohydrate, fat, and protein all raise cancer rates. This raises concerns about future U.S. cancer rates in an increasingly overweight population.

Obesity
Obesity itself is clearly a risk factor for cancers of the colon, endometrium, pancreas, kidney, esophagus, breast (in postmenopausal women), and possibly for gallbladder and other types, as well.[79] Obesity's influence on cancer development depends on the site, as well as other factors. In the case of breast cancer in postmenopausal women, the hormone estrogen is implicated. Obese women have higher levels of circulating estrogen than lean women do because adipose tissue converts other hormones into estrogen and releases it into the blood. In normal-weight women, blood estrogen drops dramatically with the onset of menopause. In obese women, fat tissue continues to produce estrogen beyond menopause, extending their exposure and increasing breast cancer risk.[80] A lifestyle that embraces physical activity, no or little alcohol consumption, a healthy body weight, and avoidance of hormone replacement therapy (when medically possible) may substantially reduce a woman's breast cancer risk.

Physical Activity
An energy budget that balances calorie intake with physical activity may lower the risk of developing some cancers. People whose lifestyles include regular, vigorous physical activity often have lower risks of colon and breast cancer.[81] Physical activity may protect against cancer by helping to maintain a healthy body

caloric effect the drop in cancer incidence seen whenever intake of food energy (calories) is restricted.

weight and by triggering other mechanisms, such as changes in hormone levels and immune functions, not related to body weight.[82]

Alcohol   Cancers of the head and neck correlate strongly with the combination of alcohol and tobacco use. Alcohol intake by itself raises the risk of cancers of the mouth, throat, esophagus, colon, and breast, and alcoholism often damages the liver in ways that promote liver cancer.[83]

Fat and Fatty Acids   Laboratory studies using animals suggest that high dietary fat intakes correlate with development of cancer. Simply feeding fat to experimental animals is not enough to get tumors started, however; an experimenter must also expose the animals to a known carcinogen. After that exposure, animals fed the high-fat diet develop more cancers faster than animals fed low-fat diets. Thus, fat appears to be a cancer promoter in animals.

Studies of people, however, have not proved that the effects of fat are independent of the effects of energy intake and physical activity. Overall, evidence associating fats and oils with cancer risk is limited.[84]

The type of fat in the diet, however, may influence cancer promotion or prevention. Studies of colon cancer implicate animal fats but not vegetable fat, and although a number of studies suggest that omega-3 fatty acids from fish may protect against some cancers, others do not support such findings.[85] Researchers note that factors such as total fat intake, the ratio of dietary omega-3 fatty acids to omega-6 fatty acids, an individual's genetic risk of cancer, body fatness, and gender, as well as the specific cancer studied, may all influence the relationship between omega-3 fatty acids and cancer. Such findings underscore the importance of consulting with a health-care provider before taking fish oil or other supplements to prevent disease.

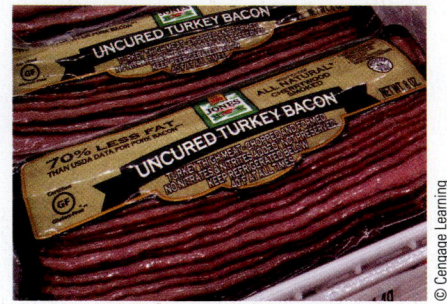

Many consumers appreciate the availability of bacon without added nitrites or nitrates.

© Cengage Learning

Red Meats   Population studies spanning the globe for over 30 years consistently report that diets high in red meat and processed meat (meat preserved by smoking, curing, or salting or by the addition of preservatives) increase the risk of colon cancer.[86] Limited evidence suggests that diets high in red and processed meats may play a role in developing other cancers, too.[87] Processed meats are listed among human carcinogens by the World Health Organization. They contain additives, nitrites or nitrates, that contribute a pink color and deter bacterial growth in meats. In the digestive tract, nitrites and nitrates form other nitrogen-containing compounds that may be carcinogenic.[88]

Cooking meats at high temperatures (frying, broiling) causes amino acids and creatine in the meats to react together and form carcinogens.[89] Grilling meat, fish, or other foods—even vegetables—over a direct flame causes fat and added oils to splash on the fire and then vaporize, creating other carcinogens that rise and stick to the food. Smoking foods has the same effect. Eating these foods, or even well-browned meats cooked to the crispy well-done stage, introduces carcinogens into the digestive system. These chemicals may or may not cause problems in the digestive tract, but once absorbed, they are detoxified by the liver's competent detoxifying system. A steady diet of foods containing significant amounts of these toxins, however, can overwhelm the system and may increase cancer risk. If you eat broiled, fried, grilled, or smoked foods, choose them in moderation and dilute their effects by varying your choices among foods prepared differently, such as boiled soups, stews, or pastas or baked, steamed, microwaved, or sautéed dishes.

Another reason to limit your intake of fried foods such as French fries and potato chips is the presence of acrylamide. Acrylamide is produced when certain starchy foods, such as potatoes, are fried or baked at high temperatures. In the body, some acrylamide is metabolized to a substance that may mutate or damage genetic material. As such, acrylamide is classified as "reasonably anticipated to be a human carcinogen."[90] New to the market is a genetically modified potato that forms less acrylamide when fried or baked (Controversy 12 explores the pros and cons of genetic engineering).

Consumers can take these steps to minimize carcinogen formation during cooking:

- Marinate meats before cooking, and roast or bake them in the oven.
- When grilling, line the grill with foil, or wrap the food in the foil.
- Take care not to burn foods.

In addition, limit intakes of crispy, browned French fries and chips, and other well-browned foods.

Fiber-Rich Foods   Many studies show that as people increase their dietary fiber intakes, their risk for colon cancer declines.[91] Fiber may protect against cancer by binding, diluting, and rapidly removing potential carcinogens from the GI tract; alternatively, other constituents of fiber-rich foods, such as the phytochemicals of whole grains or the nutrients of fruits and vegetables, may be at work. The mechanisms for a protective role for fiber are not yet known.

As research takes its course, much evidence now weighs in favor of eating a diet rich in high-fiber, low-fat foods. Such a diet helps to regulate blood glucose and blood insulin and is linked with low rates of heart disease, as well as some forms of cancer. If a meat-rich, calorie-dense diet is implicated in causation of certain cancers and if a vegetable-rich, whole grain–rich diet is associated with prevention, then wouldn't vegetarians have a lower incidence of those cancers? They do, as the many studies cited in Controversy 6 have shown.

Folate and Antioxidant Vitamins   Folate may protect against cancer of the esophagus and the colon, although evidence at this time is limited.[92] Folate plays roles in DNA synthesis and repair; thus, inadequate folate intakes may allow DNA damage to accumulate. This reason alone is enough to warrant everyone attending to their folate intake.

Vitamin E, vitamin C, and beta-carotene received attention in Controversy 7. Suffice it to say here that taking supplements has not been proved to prevent or cure cancer. In fact, once cancer is established, such antioxidants may do more harm than good.

Calcium   Sufficient dietary calcium or foods that contain it may be protective against colon cancer.[93] Calcium intakes of about 600 to 1,000 milligrams per day—an amount easily provided by daily calcium-rich foods—appear to trigger the effect.

Iron   Iron, both in the diet and in body stores, is under study for links with promotion of colon cancer. How iron may promote cancer is not known, but iron is a powerful oxidizing agent that can damage DNA and perhaps initiate cancer. A high-meat diet generously supplies iron, and it also correlates with greater risk of colon cancer.[94]

Foods and Phytochemicals   Whole foods and healthful eating patterns, not single nutrients, are most influential in cancer prevention. Fruit and vegetables, for example, contain a wide spectrum of nutrients and phytochemicals that may reduce oxidative damage to cell structures, including DNA, and thus may help protect against the development of some cancers.[95] In addition, some phytochemicals are thought to act as **anticarcinogens** that stimulate the buildup of the body's arsenal of carcinogen-destroying enzymes. Particularly the **cruciferous vegetables**—broccoli, brussels sprouts, cabbage, cauliflower, collard greens, turnips, and the like—contain a variety of potentially beneficial phytochemicals, some of which may defend against cancers by way of epigenetic actions (see Controversy 11).[96] Finally, whole, plant-based foods are rich in fibers, and high-fiber foods reduce cancer risks. If you are considering making just one change to your dietary pattern, here is a place to begin—choose an eating pattern that emphasizes fruit and vegetables, along with whole grains, legumes, and nuts each day. Table 11–13 (p. 458) summarizes dietary and lifestyle recommendations for reducing cancer risk.

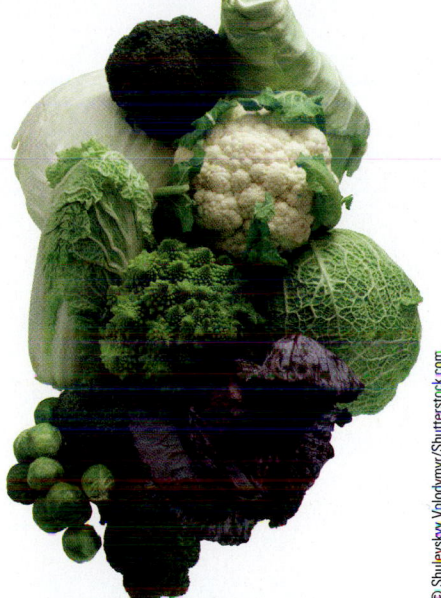

© Shulevskyy Volodymyr/Shutterstock.com

Cruciferous vegetables belong to the cabbage family: arugula, bok choy, broccoli, broccoli sprouts, brussels sprouts, cabbages (all sorts), cauliflower, greens (collard, mustard, turnip), kale, kohlrabi, rutabaga, and turnip root.

anticarcinogens compounds in foods that act in any of several ways to oppose the formation of cancer.

cruciferous vegetables vegetables with cross-shaped blossoms—the cabbage family. Their intake is associated with low cancer rates in human populations. Examples are broccoli, brussels sprouts, cabbage, cauliflower, rutabagas, and turnips.

Table 11–13

Recommendations and Strategies for Reducing Cancer Risk

Recommendation	Strategy
Body fatness. Achieve and maintain a healthy body weight throughout life.	Follow the USDA Eating Pattern for your appropriate energy level. Engage in regular physical activity. Limit consumption of energy-dense foods and avoid beverages with added sugars. Consume "fast foods" sparingly, if at all.
Physical activity. Adopt a physically active lifestyle.	Engage in at least 150 minutes of moderate-intensity physical activity or 75 minutes of vigorous-intensity physical activity or an equivalent combination throughout the week. Limit sedentary behaviors such as sitting, lying down, watching television, and other forms of screen-based recreation.
Plant-based foods. Consume a healthy diet with an emphasis on whole foods from plants.	Eat at least the daily amounts of vegetables and fruit recommended by the USDA Eating Patterns. Choose whole grains instead of refined-grain products. Limit intake of red meat. Limit refined starchy foods.
Alcoholic drinks. If you drink alcoholic beverages, limit consumption.	Drink no more than two drinks a day for men and one drink a day for women.
Preservation, processing, preparation. Limit consumption of salt-cured foods and processed meats.	Avoid salt-preserved, salted, or salty foods. Limit consumption of processed foods with added salt to ensure an intake of less than 6 grams of salt (2.4 grams of sodium) a day. Avoid processed meats.
Dietary supplements. Aim to meet nutritional needs through diet.	Dietary supplements are not recommended for cancer prevention.

Sources: L. H. Kushi and coauthors, American Cancer Society guidelines on nutrition and physical activity for cancer prevention, CA: Cancer Journal for Clinicians 62 (2012): 30–67; World Cancer Research Fund/ American Institute for Cancer Research, Food, Nutrition, Physical Activity and the Prevention of Cancer: A Global Perspective (Washington, D.C.: AICR, 2007), pp. 373–390.

KEY POINTS

- Obesity, physical inactivity, alcohol consumption, and diets high in red and processed meats are associated with cancer development.
- Foods containing ample fiber, folate, calcium, many other vitamins and minerals, and phytochemicals may be protective.

Conclusion

Nutrition is often associated with promoting health, and medicine with fighting disease, but no clear line separates nutrition from medicine. Every major agency involved with health promotion or medicine recommends a varied dietary pattern of whole foods as part of a lifestyle that provides the best possible chance for a long and healthy life. The Food Feature that follows presents an example of such an eating pattern, the DASH diet.

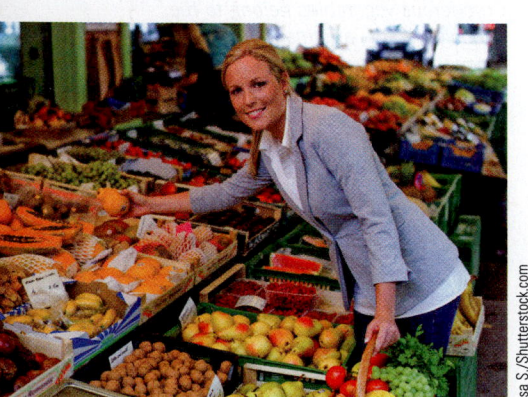

Often, whole foods like these, not individual chemicals, lower people's cancer risks.

Lisa S./Shutterstock.com

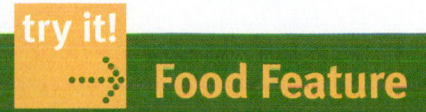
The DASH Diet: Preventive Medicine

LO 11.6 Outline strategies for including sufficient fruits and vegetables in a diet.

An esteemed former surgeon general once said, "If you do not smoke or drink excessively, your choice of diet can influence your long-term health prospects more than any other action you might take."[†††] Indeed, healthy young adults today are privileged to be among the first generations with enough nutrition knowledge to lay a foundation of health for today and tomorrow. Figure 11–10 illustrates this point.

Dietary Guidelines and the DASH Diet

The more detailed our knowledge about nutrition science, it seems, the simpler the truth becomes: people who

[†††]*C. Everett Koop, 1988.*

consume the adequate, balanced, calorie-controlled, moderate, and varied diet recommended by the Dietary Guidelines for Americans enjoy a longer, healthier life than those who do not. The DASH eating plan, presented in Table 11–14 (p. 460) at the 2,000-calorie-per-day level, can help people to meet these goals. Other calorie levels are presented in Table E–2.

"Knowing is not enough; we must apply. Willing is not enough; we must do."

—Goethe

To lower saturated fat and cholesterol intakes, the DASH diet emphasizes fruits, vegetables, whole grains, and fat-free or low-fat milk and milk products. It also features fish, poultry, and nuts instead of some of the red meat so

common in U.S. diets. Compared to the typical American diet, the foods of the DASH diet provide greater intakes of fiber, as well as potassium, calcium, and magnesium, minerals shown to lower blood pressure.

Because the DASH diet centers on fresh, unprocessed, or lightly processed foods, it can present less sodium, too. It seems, with regard to sodium, "the lower the better" for reducing blood pressure, and the recommendations of the DASH diet are the same as those of Table 11–7, p. 443. Even at higher sodium intakes, however, the DASH diet can still produce a drop in blood pressure, although not as great as with sodium restriction.

Changes in diet are often best attempted a few at a time. A good place to start is by increasing the intake of fruits and vegetables.

Fruits and Vegetables: More Matters

The National Fruit & Vegetable Program is a confederation composed of the Centers for Disease Control and Prevention, the American Heart Association, the American Diabetes Association, the American Cancer Society, and many other national organizations. These agencies work together to urge people to increase their intakes of a variety of fruits, vegetables, and legumes—not just for the nutrients they provide but also for the phytochemicals that combine synergistically to promote health (Figure 11–11, p. 461). The amount depends on age and activity level, as shown in Table 2–3 (p. 45). Alternatively, you can find out how many servings are right for you by visiting www.fruitsandveggiesmorematters.org.

Figure 11–10
Proper Nutrition Shields against Diseases

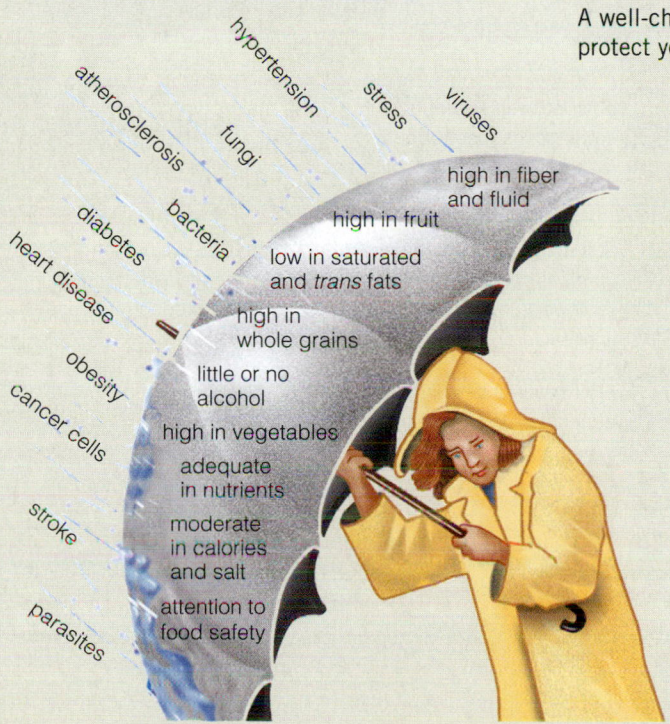

A well-chosen diet can protect your health.

hypertension, stress, viruses, atherosclerosis, fungi, bacteria, diabetes, heart disease, obesity, cancer cells, stroke, parasites

high in fiber and fluid, high in fruit, low in saturated and *trans* fats, high in whole grains, little or no alcohol, high in vegetables, adequate in nutrients, moderate in calories and salt, attention to food safety

Table 11–14

The DASH Eating Plan at a 2,000-Calorie Level

Appendix E offers the DASH Eating Plan at the 1,600-, 2,600-, and 3,100-calorie levels.

Food Group	Daily Servings	Serving Sizes	Examples and Notes	Significance of Each Food Group to the DASH Eating Pattern
Grains[a]	6–8	1 slice bread 1 oz dry cereal[b] ½ cup cooked rice, pasta, or cereal	Whole-wheat bread and rolls, whole-wheat pasta, English muffin, pita bread, bagel, cereals, grits, oatmeal, brown rice, unsalted pretzels and popcorn	Major sources of energy and fiber
Vegetables	4–5	1 cup raw leafy vegetable ½ cup cut-up raw or cooked vegetable ½ cup vegetable juice	Broccoli, carrots, collards, green beans, green peas, kale, lima beans, potatoes, spinach, squash, sweet potatoes, tomatoes	Rich sources of potassium, magnesium, and fiber
Fruit	4–5	1 medium fruit ¼ cup dried fruit ½ cup fresh, frozen, or canned fruit ½ cup fruit juice	Apples, apricots, bananas, dates, grapes, oranges, grapefruit, grapefruit juice, mangoes, melons, peaches, pineapples, raisins, strawberries, tangerines	Important sources of potassium, magnesium, and fiber
Fat-free or low-fat milk and milk products	2–3	1 cup milk or yogurt 1½ oz cheese	Fat-free (skim) or low-fat (1%) milk or buttermilk; fat-free, low-fat, or reduced-fat cheese; fat-free or low-fat regular or frozen yogurt	Major sources of calcium and protein
Lean meats, poultry, and fish	6 or less	1 oz cooked meats, poultry, or fish 1 egg[c]	Select only lean; trim away visible fats; broil, roast, or poach; remove skin from poultry	Rich sources of protein and magnesium
Nuts, seeds, and legumes	4–5 per week	⅓ cup or 1½ oz nuts 2 tbs peanut butter 2 tbs or ½ oz seeds ½ cup cooked legumes (dry beans and peas)	Almonds, hazelnuts, mixed nuts, peanuts, walnuts, sunflower seeds, peanut butter, kidney beans, lentils, split peas	Rich sources of energy, magnesium, protein, and fiber
Fats and oils[d]	2–3	1 tsp soft margarine 1 tsp vegetable oil 1 tbs mayonnaise 2 tbs salad dressing	Soft margarine, vegetable oil (such as canola, corn, olive, or safflower), low-fat mayonnaise, light salad dressing	The DASH study had 27% of calories as fat, including fat in or added to foods
Sweets and added sugars	5 or less per week	1 tbs sugar 1 tbs jelly or jam ½ cup sorbet, gelatin 1 cup lemonade	Fruit-flavored gelatin, fruit punch, hard candy, jelly, maple syrup, sorbet and ices, sugar	Sweets should be low in fat

[a]Whole grains are recommended for most grain servings as a good source of fiber and nutrients.

[b]Serving sizes vary between ½ cup and 1¼ cups, depending on cereal type. Check the product's Nutrition Facts label.

[c]Since eggs are high in cholesterol, limit egg yolk intake to no more than four per week; two egg whites have the same protein content as 1 oz of meat.

[d]Fat content changes serving amount for fats and oils. For example, 1 tbs of regular salad dressing equals one serving; 1 tbs of a low-fat dressing equals one-half serving; 1 tbs of a fat-free dressing equals zero servings.

Figure 11–11
Fruits and Veggies: More Matters

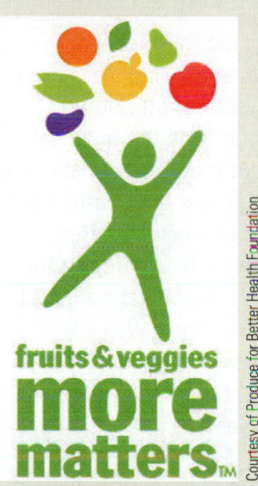

Fill half your plate with fruits and vegetables.

Courtesy of Produce for Better Health Foundation

Table 11–15 offers some tips for increasing your intakes of fruits, vegetables, and legumes. Who knows? Foods destined to become your favorites may still await you on the produce shelves. An adventurous spirit is a plus in this regard.

Conclusion

In the end, people's choices are their own. Whoever you are, we encourage you to take the time to work out ways of making your diet meet the guidelines you now know will support your health.

If you are healthy and of normal weight, if you are physically active, and if your diet on most days follows the Dietary Guidelines, then you can indulge occasionally in a cheesy pizza, marbled steak, or banana split—or even a greasy fast-food burger and fries—without inflicting much damage on your health. (Once a week may be harmless, but less frequently is better.) Especially, take time to enjoy your meals: the sights, smells, and tastes of good foods are among life's greatest pleasures. Joy, even the simple joy of eating, contributes to a healthy life.

Table 11–15

Strategies for Consuming Enough Fruits, Vegetables, and Legumes

Many people do not eat the recommended amounts and varieties of fruits, vegetables, and legumes, but these foods are indispensible to a nutritious diet. All nutrient-dense forms count: fresh, frozen, canned, dried, and 100% juice.

Foods	Strategies
All vegetables	▪ Include vegetables of all kinds in meals and snacks; fresh, frozen, and canned vegetables all count, but choose low-fat, low-sodium varieties most often. ▪ Keep cut raw vegetables, such as carrot and celery sticks, in the refrigerator for quick snacks. ▪ Visit a salad bar to buy ready-to-eat vegetables if you are in a hurry. ▪ Try a new vegetable once each month. Read some cookbooks for ideas.
Dark green, red, and orange vegetables	▪ Add chopped dark green leafy vegetables or red and orange vegetables to main dishes, such as stir-fries, soups, and casseroles. ▪ Serve side dishes of dark green salad greens or cooked or raw broccoli, spinach, or other dark green vegetables often. Choose cooked or raw red and orange vegetable dishes, too, such as tomato-based dishes, cooked hard squashes, or sliced cooked carrots. ▪ If calories are not a problem for you, try sweet potato fries as an occasional treat. ▪ Order vegetable side dishes when eating out and ask for sauces and dressings to be served on the side.
Legumes (beans, peas, lentils, and soy products)	▪ Keep a variety of low-sodium canned legumes, such as kidney beans, chickpeas (garbanzo beans), black beans, and others on hand. ▪ Use rinsed, drained beans as salad toppers. For interest, marinate them in lemon juice, garlic, and seasonings. ▪ Mash beans with lemon juice, olive oil, and seasonings, and use it as a topping for crackers, celery, or raw zucchini rounds, as a dip for vegetable sticks, or as a sandwich spread. ▪ Add beans, peas, or lentils to soups and casseroles. ▪ Try new ethnic legume recipes or try new bean dishes in restaurants, such as black beans and rice, white bean chili, lentil veggie burgers, or dal (spicy Indian-style beans, peas, or lentils). ▪ Try using soy products such as soy milk, ground meat and burger replacers, tofu, and soy snacks.
Fruit	▪ Choose whole or cut fruit more often than fruit juice. ▪ Keep a variety of fresh, frozen, low-sugar canned, and dried fruit on hand to choose for snacks or to use in cereal, yogurt, salads, or desserts. ▪ Replace syrup, sugars, and other sweet toppings with berries, cut peaches, applesauce, or fruit mixtures. ▪ Blend smoothies from bananas, fruit juice, and berries with ice or yogurt. ▪ Fruit canned in 100% fruit juice is preferable to fruit canned in sugary syrups.

Analyze Your Diet for Health Promotion

The purpose of this exercise is to increase your awareness of the characteristics of the diet recommended for disease prevention.

1. One way to lower your risk of heart attack is to keep your blood pressure in a normal range. Study Table 11–14 (p. 460), which provides an eating plan that supports normal blood pressure. Create a meal that follows the principles of the DASH diet. Select the Track Diet tab from the navigation bar. Select a date and find the foods that you wish to include in this meal. From the Reports tab, go to Source Analysis Report for that meal, and select Sodium from the drop-down box. Which foods contributed the most sodium to the meal? From the Reports tab, select Intake vs. Goals. Generate a report. Locate sodium, and find the percentage of the DRI recommendation for sodium provided by your meal. If the sodium was higher than 33 percent (one-third) of your allowance, what can you change to bring it into compliance?

2. For people with compromised immune systems, malnutrition demands prompt medical nutrition therapy. Select the Track Diet tab from the navigation bar. Select a new day, and find foods to create one meal that provides one-third of the day's requirement of high-quality, easily digestible protein for an immune-compromised adult. Take into account a diminished appetite and food safety (you'll learn more about this in Chapter 12) while making the food appealing and easy to eat and digest. From the Reports tab, select the Intake vs. Goals Report to see what percentage of the day's protein the meal supplied. Did it supply about a third of the day's need? If not, what adjustments can you make to better meet this person's protein need?

3. One diet characteristic recommended to reduce many chronic disease risks is reduced saturated fat intake. Adjust the meal you created in question 2 above. Select Source Analysis Report and find foods that contribute the most saturated fat to the meal. Try substituting foods that are lower in saturated fat. Generate a Fat Breakdown Report and an Intake vs. Goals Report for that meal. How much saturated fat did your meal supply? Was it less than 10 percent of total calories for the meal? If not, what else can you change to lower it?

4. Eating Patterns are a powerful and safe approach for improving heart health. Select the Track Diet tab, and select the day you used in question 3 above. Take a look at Table 11–7 (p. 443); then, by adding foods for breakfast, lunch, and snack, create a full day's menu that achieves the diet modifications listed for saturated fat and sodium (for this activity, ignore the others). Select the Reports tab and the MyPlate Analysis for that date. Did your day's meals meet your goals?

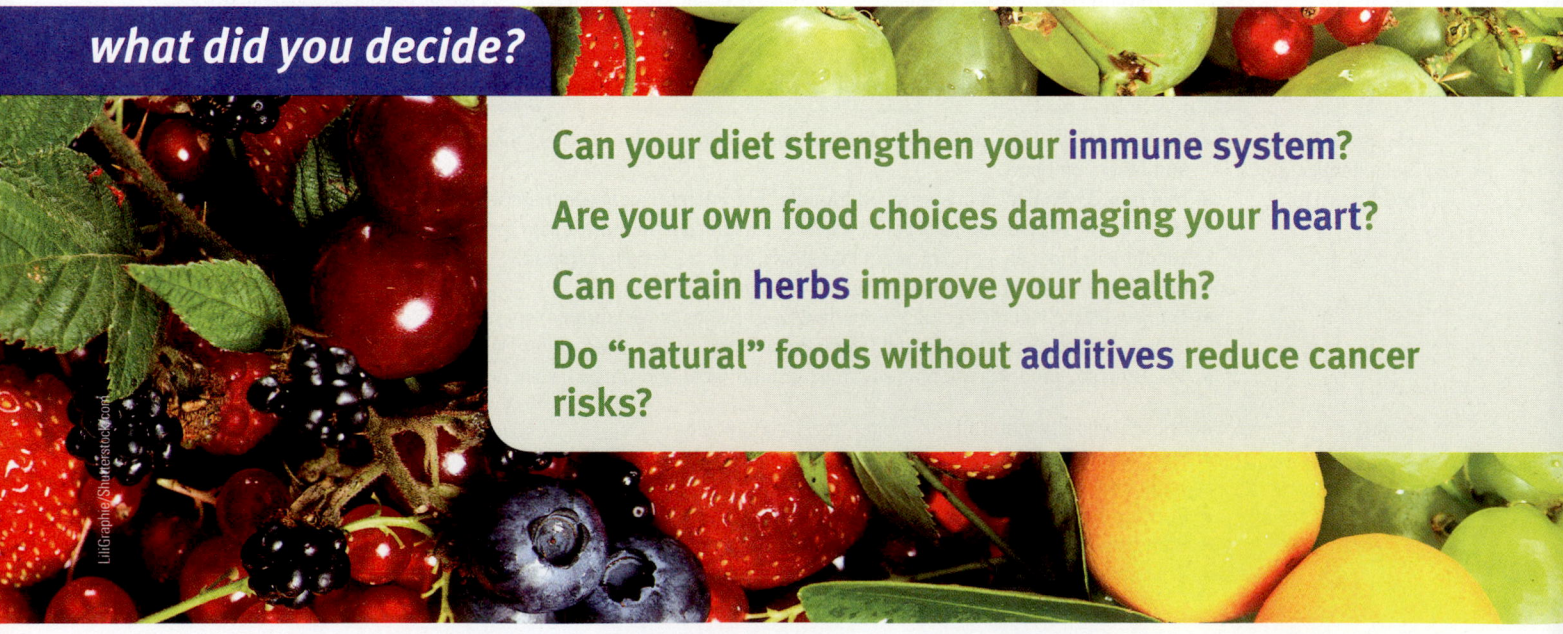

what did you decide?

Can your diet strengthen your immune system?

Are your own food choices damaging your heart?

Can certain herbs improve your health?

Do "natural" foods without additives reduce cancer risks?

LiliGraphie/Shutterstock.com

Self Check

1. (LO 11.1) All of the following are examples of how diseases might worsen malnutrition except
   a. disease impairs appetite.
   b. disease interferes with digestion and absorption.
   c. disease decreases nutrient excretion.
   d. disease alters metabolism.

2. (LO 11.1) A chronic state of inflammation can be harmful to the tissues.
   T   F

3. (LO 11.1) A healthy digestive system defends against invading microbes because
   a. its linings are absorptive.
   b. its linings are heavily laced with immune tissues.
   c. its linings are permeable.
   d. its linings are warm and moist.

4. (LO 11.2) Chronic diseases have distinct causes, known as risk factors.
   T   F

5. (LO 11.2) Which of the following is a risk factor for cardiovascular disease?
   a. high blood HDL cholesterol
   b. low blood pressure
   c. low blood LDL cholesterol
   d. diabetes

6. (LO 11.3) By what age do most people have well-developed plaques in their arteries?
   a. 20 years   c. 40 years
   b. 30 years   d. 50 years

7. (LO 11.3) Atherosclerosis is simply the accumulation of lipids within the artery wall.
   T   F

8. (LO 11.3) An "atherogenic diet" is high in all of the following except _____.
   a. fiber
   b. cholesterol
   c. saturated fats
   d. trans fats

9. (LO 11.3) Men suffer more often from heart attacks than women do, making CVD a man's disease.
   T   F

10. (LO 11.3) Smoking powerfully raises the risk for CVD in men and women in all of the following ways except
    a. decreasing the heart's workload.
    b. making blood clots more likely.
    c. directly damaging the heart with toxins.
    d. raising the blood pressure.

11. (LO 11.4) Which of the following minerals may help to regulate blood pressure?
    a. phosphorus
    b. iron
    c. potassium
    d. zinc

12. (LO 11.4) The most important step that a person can take to protect against hypertension is to be tested for it.
    T   F

13. (LO 11.4) Hypertension is more severe and occurs earlier in life among people of European or Asian descent than among African Americans.
    T   F

14. (LO 11.5) For the great majority of cancers, lifestyle factors and environmental exposures are the major risk factors.
    T   F

15. (LO 11.5) Which of the following have been associated with an increase in cancer risk?
    a. alcohol intake
    b. high intakes of red meat
    c. high intakes of processed meats
    d. all of the above

16. (LO 11.5) When calorie intakes rise, cancer rates also increase.
    T   F

17. (LO 11.5) Sufficient intakes of calcium-rich foods may increase the risk of colon cancer.
    T   F

18. (LO 11.6) The DASH diet is designed for athletes who compete in sprinting events.
    T   F

19. (LO 11.6) The DASH diet is characterized by increased intakes of _____.
    a. fruits and vegetables
    b. whole grains
    c. artificial fats
    d. a and b

20. (LO 11.7) Currently, for the best chance of consuming adequate nutrients and staying healthy, people should obtain an evaluation of their genetic profile.
    T   F

Answers to these Self Check questions are in Appendix G.

Nutritional Genomics: Can It Deliver on Its Promises?

LO 11.7 Describe the emerging science of nutritional genomics.

Health care appears to be standing at the edge of a **genomics** revolution. Traditional health-care systems emphasize treatment after disease symptoms arise. Soon, this may give way to a system aimed at identifying in healthy people—even children—traits in the **genome** that raise the odds of developing diseases in the future. Once identified, people with those tendencies may be helped to prevent or minimize disease through customized care based on each individual's **genetic profile**. A registered dietitian nutritionist, for example, may use the information to individualize medical nutrition therapy for those who already suffer illness or to provide diets with just the right nutrients and other **bioactive food components** that precisely meet the well client's needs.[1]*

This Controversy offers a taste of the exciting research in these areas—there is much more to learn, and the science advances daily. Table C11–1 distinguishes among the terms *genomics*, **nutritional genomics**, **epigenetics**, and others. Then the Controversy offers some evidence that suggests a genomics link between chronic diseases and diet.

* Reference notes are found in Appendix F.

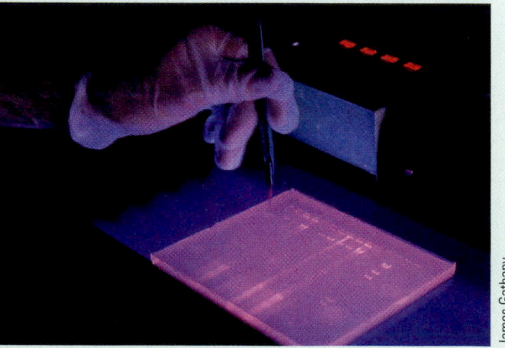
James Gathany

Table C11–1
Nutritional Genomics Terms

- **bioactive food components** nutrients and phytochemicals of foods that alter physiological processes, often by interacting, directly or indirectly, with the genes.
- **epigenetics** (ep-ih-gen-EH-tics) the science of heritable changes in gene function that occur without a change in the DNA sequence.
- **epigenome** (ep-ih-GEE-nohm) the proteins and other molecules associated with chromosomes that affect gene expression. The epigenome is modulated by bioactive food components and other factors in ways that can be inherited. *Epi* is a Greek prefix, meaning "above" or "on."
- **genetic profile** the result of an analysis of genetic material that identifies unique characteristics of a person's DNA for forensic or diagnostic purposes.
- **genome** (GEE-nohm) the full complement of genetic material in the chromosomes of a cell. Also defined in Chapter 1.
- **genomics** the study of all the genes in an organism and their interactions with environmental factors.
- **histones** (HISS-tones) proteins that lend structural support to the chromosome structure and that help to activate or silence gene expression.
- **methyl groups** (METH-il) small carbon-containing molecules that, among their activities, silence genes when applied to DNA strands by enzymes.
- **mutation** a permanent, heritable change in an organism's DNA.
- **nucleotide** (NU-klee-oh-tied) one of the subunits from which DNA and RNA are composed.
- **nutritional genomics** the science of how food (and its components) interacts with the genome.
- **SNP** a type of genetic variation involving a single changed nucleotide. The letters SNP stand for *single nucleotide polymorphism*.

The closing section brings up some concerns surrounding genetic tests of all kinds.

Nutritional Genomics Research

Until recently, no one knew *how* identical twins, with their identical DNA, could develop different diseases, or how a pregnant woman's diet might forever affect the health of her grandchildren, or how phytochemicals might alter the course of certain cancers. At least partial answers to these and other mysteries lie in the realm of nutritional genomics. Figure C11–1 introduces nutritional genomics.

With powerful new research tools, nutrition scientists are fast discovering which genes interact with nutrients and how nutrients and other bioactive food components modify gene activities.[2] In one such technology, robotic arms precisely fasten a single DNA strand of a known sequence onto a slide. Then a computer compares the pattern of gene expression of the known sequence with that of an unknown DNA sample taken from an individual's cells. This comparison reveals which of the sample genes are expressed (actively making proteins—details in Chapter 6), which are silenced (inactive), and how they respond under certain conditions. The

Figure C11–1
Nutritional Genomics

Two branches of nutritional genomics may have similar-sounding names—nutrigenomics and nutrigenetics—but they oppose each other in scope. One branch studies how genes affect nutrient metabolism. The other branch studies how nutrients affect the genes.

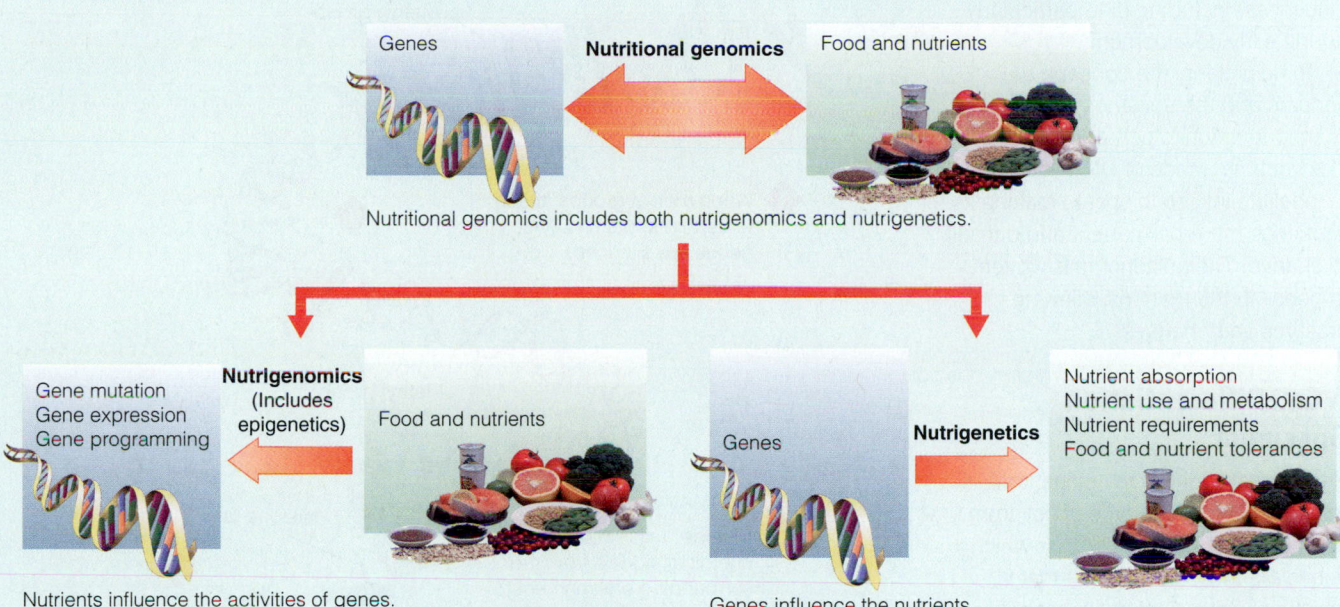

Genes **Nutritional genomics** Food and nutrients

Nutritional genomics includes both nutrigenomics and nutrigenetics.

Gene mutation
Gene expression
Gene programming
Nutrigenomics (Includes epigenetics) Food and nutrients

Genes **Nutrigenetics** Nutrient absorption
Nutrient use and metabolism
Nutrient requirements
Food and nutrient tolerances

Nutrients influence the activities of genes.

Genes influence the nutrients.

results allow identification of inherited disease tendencies, unusual nutrient needs, and many other medical concerns.[3] Such technology promises major advancements in health care for people worldwide.

Genes Influence Nutrition and Disease

Small variations in DNA sequences, called **mutations**, dictate many of the differences among human beings, including differences in nutrient metabolism. The most common mutations are **SNPs** (pronounced "snips"), involving the variation of a single tiny molecule (a **nucleotide**) in a strand of DNA.[4] About 10 million possible SNPs are known to exist among people.

SNPs and Diseases

Most individuals carry tens of thousands of SNPs, and most seem to have no functional effect at all. Rarely, however,

a single SNP in a high-powered gene can produce a severe disease immediately from birth, such as PKU, described in Chapter 3. More commonly, SNPs do not cause a disease directly but may subtly work with other gene variants and with environmental factors such as diet to increase the risk of developing a chronic disease, such as heart disease, later in life. SNPs set the stage for a chronic disease but the person's own choices are among the actors that cause it to develop.

As an example, a common SNP in a fat metabolism gene changes the body's response to dietary fats. People with this SNP maintain lower blood LDL cholesterol when they eat a diet rich in polyunsaturated fatty acids (PUFA), and they develop higher blood LDL cholesterol when they consume less PUFA. A gene (in this case, a fat metabolism gene with a SNP) interacts with a nutrient from the diet (in this case, PUFA) to influence a risk factor for a disease (LDL cholesterol, implicated in heart disease).

Complexity of SNP–Disease Relationships

Genetic risks for chronic diseases may appear to be straightforward—just identify the SNPs to identify an increased disease risk—but these associations are proving difficult to pin down.[5] They often involve SNPs in multiple genes, each of which may interact with many dietary and other environmental factors. Furthermore, another realm of influence on gene behavior exists—the **epigenome**.

Nutrients Influence the Genes: Epigenetics

People often think of chromosomes as simple strands of DNA, but chromosomes exist as complex, three-dimensional combinations of DNA, proteins, and other molecules. DNA strands are the primary carrier of inherited information, true, but the epigenome constitutes another parallel bank of inheritable information. The

Controversy 11 Nutritional Genomics: Can It Deliver on Its Promises?

465

epigenome consists of proteins and other molecules that associate with DNA and interact with it in ways that regulate the expression of genes, turning the genes on or off. In short, like DNA, the epigenome can be inherited from generation to generation but unlike DNA, it is responsive to environmental influences, including diet, particularly during early development.

To help clarify the concept, the genome and the epigenome have been likened to nature's pen-and-pencil set. The genome, made of DNA, is written in indelible ink, so to speak, making its sequence more permanent and difficult to change. The epigenome is written in pencil in the margins, allowing for erasures and changes.

A Cell Differentiation Specialist

The special talent of the epigenome is in differentiating one type of cell from another in the body. It controls which genes are turned on or off—that is, which are expressed or silenced. For example, a cone cell of a person's eye and a blood-producing cell of that person's bone marrow contain identical DNA strands. Luckily for the person, the epigenome activates and silences genes on the DNA strands so that each cell type reliably makes only the correct proteins to allow its own specialized functions.

How Epigenetic Regulation Works

Mechanisms for epigenetic gene regulation include, among others, the workings of large globular proteins known as **histones** and small organic molecules called **methyl groups.**[†] Both of these mechanisms can be modified by way of diet and other environmental influences.

Histones in Gene Expression

Millions of histones reside within the chromosome (shown in Figure C11–2), supporting its shape and modifying its activity. Like thread wound around a

[†]*Other mechanisms include acetylation of DNA (and histones), other chromatin remodeling factors, and noncoding regulatory RNA molecules.*

Figure C11–2
Two Epigenetic Factors and Gene Activity

This figure shows that methyl groups, tiny one-carbon structures, attach directly to a DNA strand, modifying its activity. It also depicts histones, large globular protein "spools" that wrap lengths of DNA. Other epigenetic factors also exist.

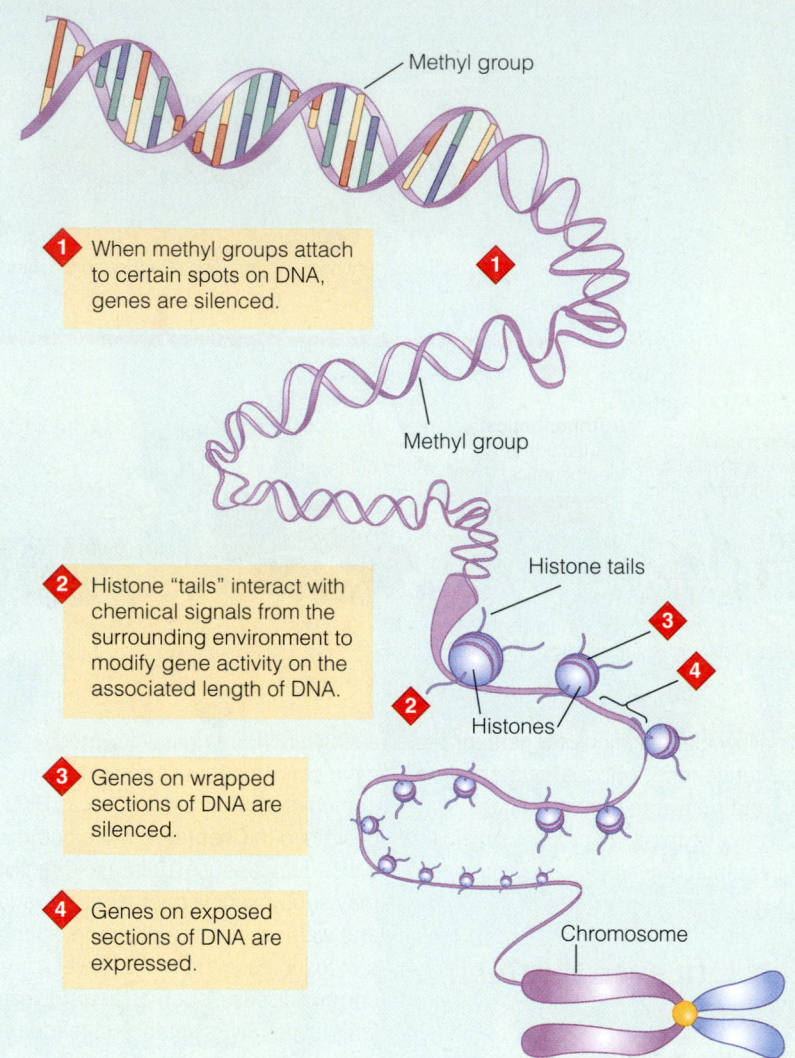

Methyl group

1 When methyl groups attach to certain spots on DNA, genes are silenced.

Methyl group

Histone tails

2 Histone "tails" interact with chemical signals from the surrounding environment to modify gene activity on the associated length of DNA.

Histones

3 Genes on wrapped sections of DNA are silenced.

4 Genes on exposed sections of DNA are expressed.

Chromosome

spool, sections of DNA "thread" are tightly wrapped around protein histones. Thusly, the huge DNA molecule is shaped and condensed to fit inside a tiny cell nucleus.

Once believed to confer only structural support to the chromosomes, histones are now known to regulate gene expression, too. When a DNA segment is wrapped around a histone, its genes are silent—they physically lack the room to perform the tasks required for protein synthesis. Histones, though, can change this situation in response to changing environmental conditions.

Histones sport little protein "tails" that stick out from their DNA wrappings. These tails serve as landing sites for many molecules from the environment that signify cellular conditions.

When a histone receives chemical signals indicating a need for a particular protein, it loosens its grip on its wraps of DNA, allowing the portion of the strand with genes for making that protein to stretch out. Genes on these stretched-out segments can then express their encoded proteins—they are activated. Here's where nutrition comes in: many of the molecular signals to which histones respond arise from the diet—they consist of nutrients and phytochemicals themselves or of compounds generated during their metabolism.

A Broccoli Phytochemical Example

One phytochemical, sulforaphane (see Controversy 2), found in broccoli, broccoli sprouts, and other cabbage-family vegetables, may affect cancer processes by way of histone changes in cancer cells. One characteristic of cancerous tissue is uncontrolled cell division. In cancer cells, histones may inappropriately silence genes that would otherwise stop cells from multiplying out of control.

In test tubes, sulforaphane reverses those cancer-promoting histone changes and reinstates control of cell division.[6] In mice, sulforaphane inhibits certain cancers. In people, ingestion of one cup of broccoli sprouts alters histone activities in blood cells. Does consumption of broccoli or other cabbage-family food actually prevent cancer in people? People who consume these foods regularly have lower rates of some cancers. No one knows whether the foods themselves are protective, however; researchers are still investigating that question.

Many other phytochemicals, including tea flavonoids, curcumin from the spice turmeric, and sulfur compounds from the onion family, along with nutrients such as folate, vitamin B_{12}, vitamin D, selenium, and zinc, add to a growing list of food constituents that affect epigenetic activities in ways that may prevent cancer. Scientists can duplicate some of these activities with synthetic drugs, but the drugs, unlike foods, are highly toxic to living tissues.[7]

DNA Methyl Groups and Gene Regulation

Genes are also regulated by a number of molecules that adhere to the DNA strand itself. Methyl groups, mentioned earlier, are tiny organic compounds common in body tissues. They attach directly onto DNA (look again at Figure C11–2), altering gene expression. Typically, when a methyl group attaches to the beginning of a gene sequence on a DNA strand (methylation), the gene is silenced.

Removal of that methyl group allows gene expression to commence and protein replication to occur.[8]

B Vitamins Transfer Methyl Groups

A powerful example of how nutrients affect the genes involves the influence of the B vitamin folate on DNA methylation. Folate (along with other B vitamins) is essential for transferring methyl groups from molecule to molecule, including to DNA molecules. With too little folate, genes may be insufficiently methylated to suppress the production of unneeded proteins.

This effect is illustrated in the accompanying photo of two mice. Despite their strikingly different appearance, these mice have identical DNA. Both possess a gene that tends to produce fat, yellow pups, but their gene expression was altered when their mothers were fed different diets during pregnancy. The mother of the lean, brown mouse received doses of the B vitamins folate and vitamin B_{12}. By way of methyl group transfer activity, these vitamins silenced the gene for "yellow and fat," resulting in brown, lean pups.

Note that the extra vitamins did not change the DNA sequence. Still, such epigenomic changes established during pregnancy can be inherited along with the DNA and thus persist through several generations.

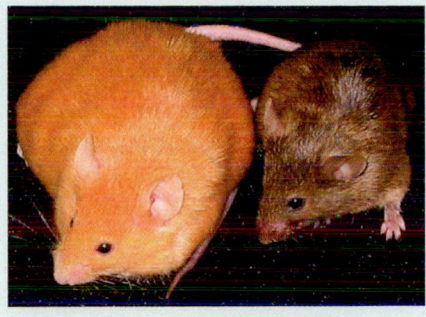

These two mice share an identical gene that tends to produce fat, yellow mice. The mother of the lean, brown mouse received supplemental B vitamins that silenced the gene.

Importantly, pregnant women should tend to their nutrition needs carefully (see Chapter 13). No one should attempt to alter their children's and grandchildren's risks of obesity or other diseases by loading up on B vitamins or other substances. The effects of imbalances are unpredictable and can be severe.

Can Adults Modify Their Epigenome?

Researchers believe that the greatest epigenomic changes from environmental influences occur early during embryonic development (Figure C11–3 demonstrates this concept).[9] Some change can still

Figure C11–3

An Epigenome Timeline

Environmental influences, including diet, most profoundly alter the epigenome during the earliest stages of development, but some changes are probably still possible later in life.

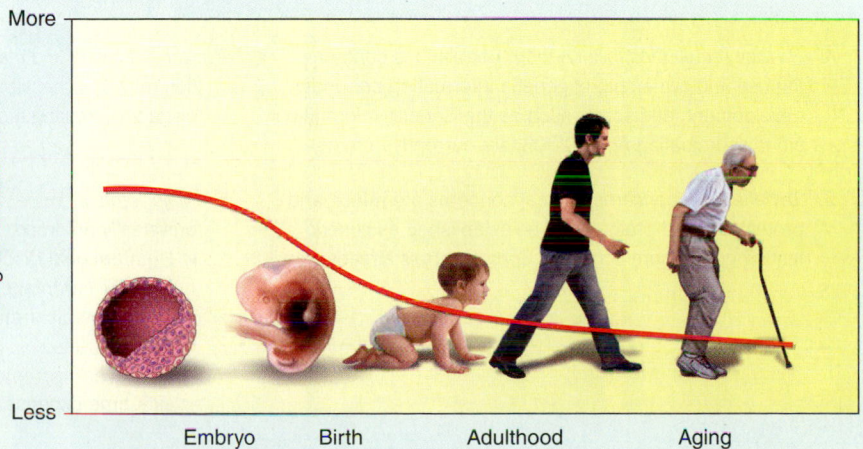

occur into adolescence and even adulthood, however, and they can affect health outcomes. The findings on sulforaphane of broccoli, described earlier, provide evidence that certain epigenetic factors in adult cells can indeed be changed, at least temporarily, by bioactive constituents of foods. Another example in adults is the development of liver cancer after ingestion of a mold toxin that can form on corn and other grain (*aflatoxin*, defined in Chapter 12). The toxin is suspected of causing removal of important methyl groups from both histones and the DNA strand, triggering the development of the cancer.[10]

Now a theory emerges to suggest at least a partial solution to the mystery of how identical twins can develop different diseases. Although the twins have identical DNA, they acquire differences in their epigenomes. They encounter different environmental influences at various times of life that change their genetic expression.

On learning of these revelations in nutritional genomics, many people want to apply the new science to themselves. The next sections explore some issues that arise with genetic testing for nutrition.

Arguments Surrounding Genetic Testing

For nutritional genomics to be of practical value, people must undergo genetic testing to detect gene variations that affect nutrition or nutrition-related diseases.[11] Critics of testing, however, question whether identifying a genetic marker for disease by way of expensive testing would translate into better health for the nation or simply waste limited health-care dollars. Consumers also voice fears that certain DNA results, once known, could be misused.[12] Table C11–2 provides the scope of these arguments.

Regulating Direct-to-Consumer Tests

For a few hundred dollars, consumers can easily order DNA tests for themselves over the Internet. However, due to gaps in regulation, test quality and validity and the proper use of results are not ensured. Such gaps

---

Table C11–2

Genetic Testing: Point, Counterpoint

Arguments in Support of Genetic Testing	Arguments in Opposition to Genetic Testing
1. *More information.* Genetic tests provide additional information for improved understanding of a patient's medical profile.	1. *Information not useful.* More information may not be better. Genetic testing has so far yielded minimally more useful information than less expensive clinical tests.
2. *Empowerment to make changes.* With forewarning, genetically susceptible people could make lifestyle changes to reduce their risks.	2. *Needed changes already obvious.* Most people who test positive for risk factors such as diabetes and high LDL cholesterol do not make needed lifestyle changes to reduce their risks. More detailed warnings will probably not help them to do so.
3. *Good enough.* Nutritional genomic testing in particular holds the promise of some urgently needed help in fighting today's major killers—heart disease and cancer—despite details in application yet to be worked out. Supporters ask, "Should we let perfectionism stand in the way of progress?"	3. *Serious gaps in knowledge.* Current knowledge does not support application. • Lifestyle changes to match gene profiles have not yet been defined. • Links between specific genetic variations and chronic disease are often not fully defined. • Astronomical numbers of potential interactions between environmental factors and genome and epigenome variations must be pinned down before effective application is possible.
4. *Privacy regulations forthcoming.* Regulations concerning use and ownership of genetic information are under development, and some, such as the Genetic Information Nondiscrimination Act of 2008, are currently in force.	4. *Current regulation inadequate.* Regulation loopholes exist, and information may be accessible to other parties. Genetic discrimination can be disguised, making it difficult to prove.
5. *Trivial ethical concerns.* Ethical concerns are minor, and protections and protocol will be established as genetic testing grows more common. Some controls already exist.	5. *Major ethical concerns.* Today's safeguards are incomplete and not universally enforced. Ethical concerns include: • Unintentional disclosure of family relationships (such as adoptions or other parentage issues). • Insurance discrimination or limitations against those with certain genetic traits. • Employer discrimination against certain traits to reduce potential sick-time expenses.

---

have made it possible for unscrupulous companies to sell fake tests or mislead consumers into buying expensive supplements and other products based on unfounded assessments of their DNA samples.[13] Even when DNA tests are legitimate, interpreting the results is complex, and a consumer acting without a medical professional's opinion could easily be misled into taking an unneeded medication or avoiding a necessary one—or even undergoing an unneeded surgery.[14] To help remedy this situation, the FDA recently sent letters to companies that sell such tests to consumers, warning them to stop marketing their tests and assessments for medical purposes.

Some argue against regulation, claiming that restrictions will stifle the current wave of innovation in personalized medicine.[15] Others argue back that true innovations must yield effective advancements, not just the proliferation of new but unproven applications.[16] Oversight of laboratory tests may encourage the kind of research and development that leads to useful new tests and unambiguous interpretations for those who truly need them.

Conclusion

No doubt the future of nutrition science will be inextricably linked with the science of genomics, and potential benefits may be enormous. Still, if the authors of this book were to try to predict the future, based on libraries full of past evidence, most scenarios might go something like this: "Based on our genomics study, Mr. X needs greater amounts of vitamin C from tomato sauces and pink grapefruit, but not from supplements. He needs the fiber, lycopene, carbohydrates, and other bioactive components of a variety of fruits and vegetables, along with less saturated fat, sufficient protein, and a nutritious balanced diet to ward off future problems."

Experience shows that fiber supplements cannot take the place of whole grains for digestive tract health or diabetes control and calcium pills cannot replace food sources of calcium for bone health and that supplements often pose risks.[17] Many other examples exist to make the case that following a well-planned eating pattern of whole foods, as recommended by the Dietary Guidelines for Americans 2015 (see Chapter 2), provides the best chance of staying healthy.

Stay alert for updates in the rapidly advancing science of nutritional genomics. Registered dietitian nutritionists will be key providers of personalized nutrition care as more becomes known about its potential to minimize disease risks and maximize the health of people everywhere.

Critical Thinking

1. Define the status of nutritional genomics research. Provide two examples of where this type of research is leading us.

2. Explain how SNPs may cause disease.

12 Food Safety and Food Technology

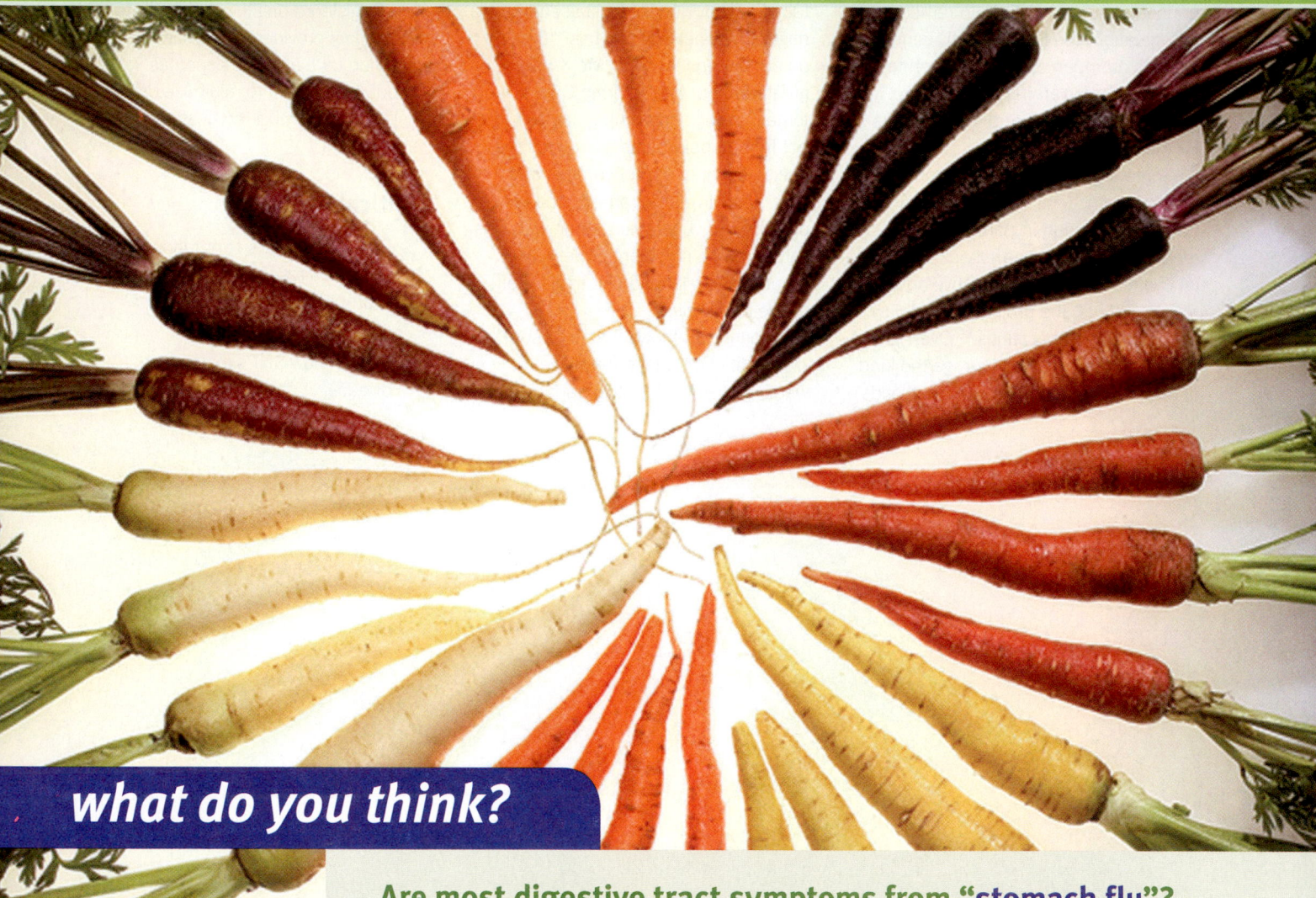

what do you think?

Are most digestive tract symptoms from "stomach flu"?

Are most foods from grocery stores germ-free?

Should you refrigerate leftover party foods after the guests have gone home?

Which poses the greater risk: raw sushi from a sushi master or food additives?

Learning Objectives

After completing this chapter, you should be able to accomplish the following:

LO 12.1 Describe microbial foodborne illnesses and core practices that can prevent them.

LO 12.2 Identify the categories of foods that most often cause foodborne illnesses.

LO 12.3 Outline technological advances aimed at reducing microbial food contamination.

LO 12.4 Discuss natural toxins, residues, and contaminants in food.

LO 12.5 Compare potential advantages and drawbacks of organic and conventional foods.

LO 12.6 Discuss the uses and safety of food additives.

LO 12.7 Explain how food-processing techniques affect the nutrients in foods.

LO 12.8 Summarize the advantages and disadvantages of producing food through genetic engineering.

C onsumers in the United States enjoy food supplies ranking among the safest, most pleasing, and most abundant in the world. Along with such abundance comes a great consumer responsibility to distinguish between choices leading to food **safety** and those that pose a **hazard**.

As human populations grow and food supplies become more global, new food-safety challenges arise that require new processes, new technologies, and greater cooperation to solve.[1]* Food safety is therefore a moving target. The **Food and Drug Administration (FDA)** is the major agency charged with ensuring that the U.S. food supply is safe, wholesome, sanitary, and properly labeled (see Table 12–1, p. 472). It focuses much effort in these areas of concern:

1. *Microbial **foodborne illness.*** Each year, one in six Americans becomes ill, 128,000 are hospitalized, and 3,000 die from foodborne illnesses.[2]

2. *Natural toxins in foods.* These constitute a hazard mostly when people consume large quantities of single foods either by choice (fad diets) or by necessity (poverty).

3. *Residues in food.*
   a. *Environmental and other contaminants* (other than pesticides). Household and industrial chemicals are increasing yearly in number and concentration, and their impacts are hard to foresee and to forestall.
   b. *Pesticide residues.* A subclass of environmental contaminants, they are listed separately because they are applied intentionally to foods and, in theory, can be controlled.
   c. *Animal drugs.* These include hormones and antibiotics that increase growth or milk production and combat diseases in food animals.

4. *Nutrients in foods.* These require close attention as more and more highly processed and artificially constituted foods appear on the market.

5. *Intentional approved food additives.* These are of less concern because so much is known about them that they pose little risk to consumers.

6. *Genetically engineered foods.* Such foods are listed last because they undergo rigorous scrutiny before going to market.

Within its powers, FDA is vigilant in overseeing the food supply at home and abroad to safeguard the health of U.S. consumers.[3] When foodborne illness occurs, FDA acts quickly to resolve the cause and recall tainted products.

With the privilege of abundance comes the responsibility to choose and handle foods wisely.

foodborne illness illness transmitted to human beings through food and water; caused by an infectious agent (*foodborne infection*) or a poisonous substance arising from microbial toxins, poisonous chemicals, or other harmful substances (*food intoxication*). Also commonly called *food poisoning*.

safety the practical certainty that injury will not result from the use of a substance.

hazard a state of danger; used to refer to any circumstance in which harm is possible under normal conditions of use.

---

*Reference notes are found in Appendix F.

Table 12–1

Food Regulatory Agencies

Each agency oversees programs and systems aimed at maintaining and improving the safety of the food supply.

CDC (Centers for Disease Control and Prevention) a branch of the U.S. Department of Health and Human Services that is responsible for, among other things, identifying, monitoring, and reporting on foodborne illnesses and outbreaks (*www.cdc.gov*).

EPA (Environmental Protection Agency) a federal agency that is responsible for, among other things, regulating pesticides and establishing water quality standards (*www.epa.gov*).

FAO (Food and Agriculture Organization) an international agency (part of the United Nations) that has adopted standards to regulate pesticide use, among other responsibilities (*www.fao.org*).

FDA (Food and Drug Administration) the federal agency responsible for ensuring the safety and wholesomeness of all dietary supplements and foods processed and sold in interstate commerce except meat, poultry, and eggs (which are under the jurisdiction of the USDA); inspecting food plants and imported foods; setting standards for food composition and product labeling; and issuing recalls when problems arise (*www.fda.gov*).

USDA (U.S. Department of Agriculture) the federal agency responsible for enforcing standards for the wholesomeness and quality of meat, poultry, and eggs produced in the United States; conducting nutrition research; and educating the public about nutrition (*www.usda.gov*).

WHO (World Health Organization) an international agency concerned with promoting health and eradicating disease (*www.who.int*).

Microbes and Food Safety

LO 12.1 Describe microbial foodborne illnesses and core practices that can prevent them.

Some people brush off the threat from foodborne illnesses as less likely and less serious than the threat of flu, but they are misinformed. Foodborne illnesses, caused by **microbes**, can be life-threatening, and some kinds increasingly do not respond to standard antibiotic drug therapy. Even normally mild foodborne illnesses can be lethal for a person who is ill or malnourished; has a compromised immune system; lives in an institution; has liver or stomach illnesses; or is pregnant, very old, or very young.

Despite the best efforts of FDA and others, foodborne illnesses are extraordinarily likely to occur. It seems that as one organism comes under control, others emerge to take its place. Achieving the ultimate goal—fewer total foodborne illnesses—will require even more vigilance on the part of regulators, food industries, and consumers.[4]

If digestive tract disturbances are the major or only symptoms of your next bout of what some people erroneously call "stomach flu," chances are that what you really have is a foodborne illness. By learning something about these illnesses and taking a few preventive steps, you can maximize your chances of staying well. Understanding the nature of the microbes responsible is the first step toward defeating them.

How Do Microbes in Food Cause Illness in the Body?

Microorganisms can cause foodborne illness either by infection or by intoxication. Infectious agents, such as *Salmonella* bacteria or hepatitis viruses, infect the tissues of the human body and multiply there. Other microorganisms produce **enterotoxins** or **neurotoxins**, poisonous chemicals released by bacteria as they multiply. These

microbes a shortened name for *microorganisms*; minute organisms too small to observe without a microscope, including bacteria, viruses, and others.

enterotoxins poisons that act on mucous membranes, such as those of the digestive tract.

neurotoxins poisons that act on the cells of the nervous system.

Chapter 12 Food Safety and Food Technology

toxins are absorbed into the tissues and cause various kinds of harm, ranging from mild stomach pain and headache to paralysis and death.

Table 12–2 (p. 474) lists the microbes responsible for 90 percent of U.S. foodborne illnesses, hospitalizations, and deaths, along with their food sources, general symptoms, and prevention methods. Many other illness-causing microbes exist. The steps outlined in this chapter can reduce or eliminate all of them.

The most common cause of food intoxication is the *Staphylococcus aureus* bacterium, but the most infamous is undoubtedly *Clostridium botulinum*, an organism that produces a toxin so deadly that an amount as tiny as a single grain of salt can kill several people within an hour. *Clostridium botulinum* requires **anaerobic** conditions such as those found in improperly canned (especially home-canned) foods, home-fermented foods such as tofu, and homemade garlic or herb-flavored oils stored at room temperature.[†] **Botulism** quickly paralyzes muscles, making seeing, speaking, swallowing, and breathing difficult (symptoms are listed in Table 12–3, p. 475) and demands immediate medical attention.

Some bacterial toxins, such as the botulinum toxin, are heat sensitive and can be destroyed by boiling (but this is not recommended). Others, such as the toxin produced by *Staphylococcus aureus*, are heat-resistant and remain hazardous even after the food is cooked.

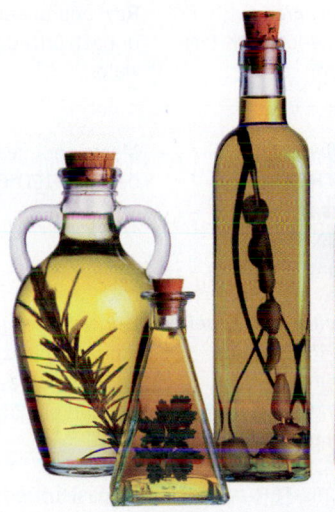
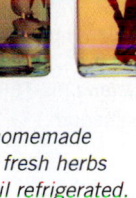

C Squared Studios/Photodisc/Getty Images

To prevent botulism from homemade flavored oils, wash and dry fresh herbs before use, and keep the oil refrigerated. Discard it after a week to 10 days.

KEY POINTS

- Each year in the United States, tens of millions of people suffer mild to life-threatening symptoms caused by foodborne illnesses.
- Pregnant women, infants, toddlers, older adults, and people with weakened immune systems are most vulnerable to harm from foodborne illnesses.
- Foodborne illnesses arise from infection or bacterial toxins.

Food Safety from Farm to Plate

A safe food supply depends on safe food practices by both domestic and foreign food producers—on the farm or at sea; in processing plants; during transportation; and at supermarkets, institutions, and restaurants (see Figure 12–1, p. 475). Equally critical in the chain of food safety, however, is the final handling of food by people who purchase it and consume it at home. Tens of millions of people needlessly suffer preventable foodborne illnesses each year because they make their own mistakes in purchasing, storing, or preparing their food.

Commercially prepared food is usually safe, but an **outbreak** of illness from this source often makes the headlines because outbreaks can affect many people at once.[5] Dairy farmers, for example, rely on **pasteurization**, a process that heats milk to kill most disease-causing organisms, thereby making the milk safe to consume. When a major dairy develops a flaw in its pasteurization system, hundreds of cases of illness can occur as a result.

Other types of farming require other safeguards. Growing food usually involves soil, and soil contains abundant bacterial colonies that can contaminate food. Animal waste deposited onto soil may introduce disease-causing microbes. Additionally, farm workers and other food handlers who are ill can easily pass organisms of illness to consumers through the routine handling of foods during and after harvest, a particular concern with regard to foods consumed raw, such as produce.

Attention on *E. coli*   Several strains of the *E. coli* bacterium produce a particularly dangerous protein known as **Shiga toxin**, a cause of severe disease. The most notorious strain, *E. coli* O157:H7, caused a large outbreak in the early 1990s, but

anaerobic without oxygen.

botulism an often fatal foodborne illness caused by the botulinum toxin, a toxin produced by the *Clostridium botulinum* bacterium, which grows without oxygen in nonacidic canned foods.

outbreak two or more cases of a disease arising from an identical organism acquired from a common food source within a limited time frame. Government agencies track and investigate outbreaks of foodborne illnesses, but tens of millions of individual cases go unreported each year.

pasteurization the treatment of milk, juices, or eggs with heat sufficient to kill certain pathogens (disease-causing microbes) commonly transmitted through these foods; not a sterilization process. Pasteurized products retain bacteria that cause spoilage.

Shiga toxin any of a group of protein toxins produced as certain bacteria strains multiply; Shiga toxins cause severe illness when absorbed by the body.

[†]Complete, up-to-date home canning instructions are available in the USDA's *Complete Guide to Home Canning*, available from the Superintendent of Documents, U.S. Government Printing Office, Washington, DC 20402, or online at www.uga.edu/nchfp /publications/publications_usda.html.

Table 12–2

Major Microbes of Foodborne Illnesses

Organism Name	Most Frequent Food Sources	Onset and General Symptoms	Prevention Methods[a]
Foodborne Infections			
Campylobacter (KAM-pee-loh-BAK-ter) bacterium	Raw and undercooked poultry, unpasteurized milk, contaminated water	Onset: 2 to 5 days. Diarrhea, vomiting, abdominal cramps, fever; sometimes bloody stools; lasts 2 to 10 days.	Cook foods thoroughly; use pasteurized milk; use sanitary food-handling methods.
Clostridium (claw-STRID-ee-um) *perfringens* (per-FRINGE-enz) bacterium	Meats and meat products held at between 120°F and 130°F	Onset: 8 to 16 hours. Abdominal pain, diarrhea, nausea; lasts 1 to 2 days.	Use sanitary food-handling methods; use pasteurized milk; cook foods thoroughly; refrigerate foods promptly and properly.
Escherichia coli; E. coli (esh-eh-REEK-ee-uh-KOH-lye) bacterium (including Shiga toxin–producing strains)[a]	Undercooked ground beef, unpasteurized milk and juices, raw fruits and vegetables, contaminated water, and person-to-person contact	Onset: 1 to 8 days. Severe bloody diarrhea, abdominal cramps, vomiting; lasts 5 to 10 days.	Cook ground beef thoroughly; use pasteurized milk; use sanitary food-handling methods; use treated, boiled, or bottled water.
Listeria (lis-TER-ee-AH) bacterium	Unpasteurized milk; fresh soft cheeses; luncheon meats, hot dogs	Onset: 1 to 21 days. Fever, muscle aches; nausea, vomiting, blood poisoning; complications in pregnancy; meningitis (stiff neck, severe headache, and fever); lasting neurological damage; death.	Use sanitary food-handling methods; cook foods thoroughly; use only pasteurized milk products and cheeses.
Norovirus	Person-to-person contact; raw foods, salads, sandwiches	Onset: 1 to 2 days. Vomiting; lasts 1 to 2 days.	Use sanitary food-handling methods.
Salmonella (sal-moh-NEL-ah) bacteria (>2,300 types)	Raw or undercooked eggs, meats, poultry, raw milk and other dairy products, shrimp, frog legs, yeast, coconut, pasta, and chocolate	Onset: 1 to 3 days. Fever, vomiting, abdominal cramps, diarrhea; lasts 4 to 7 days; can be fatal.	Use sanitary food-handling methods; use pasteurized milk; cook foods thoroughly; refrigerate foods promptly and properly.
Toxoplasma (TOK-so-PLAZ-ma) *gondii* parasite	Raw or undercooked meat; contaminated water; raw goat's milk; ingestion after contact with infected cat feces	Onset: 7 to 21 days. Swollen glands, fever, headache, muscle pain, stiff neck.	Use sanitary food-handling methods; cook foods thoroughly.
Foodborne Intoxications			
Clostridium (claw-STRID-ee-um) *botulinum* (bot-chew-LINE-um) bacterium produces botulin toxin, responsible for causing botulism	Anaerobic environment of low acidity (canned corn, peppers, green beans, soups, beets, asparagus, mushrooms, ripe olives, spinach, tuna, chicken, chicken liver, liver pâté, luncheon meats, ham, sausage, stuffed eggplant, lobster, and smoked and salted fish)	Onset: 4 to 36 hours. Nervous system symptoms, including double vision, inability to swallow, speech difficulty, and progressive paralysis of the respiratory system; often fatal; leaves prolonged symptoms in survivors.	Use proper canning methods for low-acid foods; refrigerate homemade garlic and herb oils; avoid commercially prepared foods with leaky seals or with bent, bulging, or broken cans. Do not feed honey to infants.
Staphylococcus (STAF-il-oh-KOK-us) *aureus* bacterium produces staphylococcal toxin	Toxin produced in improperly refrigerated meats; egg, tuna, potato, and macaroni salads; cream-filled pastries	Onset: 1 to 6 hours. Diarrhea, nausea, vomiting, abdominal cramps, fever; lasts 1 to 2 days.	Use sanitary food-handling methods; cook food thoroughly; refrigerate foods promptly and properly.

Note: Travelers' diarrhea is most commonly caused by E. coli, Campylobacter jejuni, Shigella, and Salmonella.

[a] O157, O145, and other Shiga toxin–producing strains.

today most such outbreaks arise from other strains of Shiga toxin–producing *E. coli* (STEC).‡ Outbreaks of severe or fatal STEC illnesses often focus national attention on two important food-safety issues: raw foods routinely contain live, disease-causing organisms, and strict industry controls are essential to make foods safe.[6]

In most cases, STEC disease involves bloody diarrhea, severe intestinal cramps, and dehydration starting a few days after eating tainted meat, raw milk, or contaminated fresh raw produce. In the worst cases, **hemolytic-uremic syndrome** causes a dangerous failure of the kidneys and organ systems that very young, very old, or otherwise vulnerable people may not survive. Antibiotics and self-prescribed antidiarrheal medicines can make the condition worse because they increase absorption and retention of the toxin. Severe cases require hospitalization.

hemolytic-uremic (HEEM-oh-LIT-ic you-REEM-ick) **syndrome** a severe result of infection with Shiga toxin–producing *E. coli*, characterized by abnormal blood clotting with kidney failure, damage to the central nervous system and other organs, and death, especially among children.

Figure 12–1

From Farm to Plate: Make Food Safe

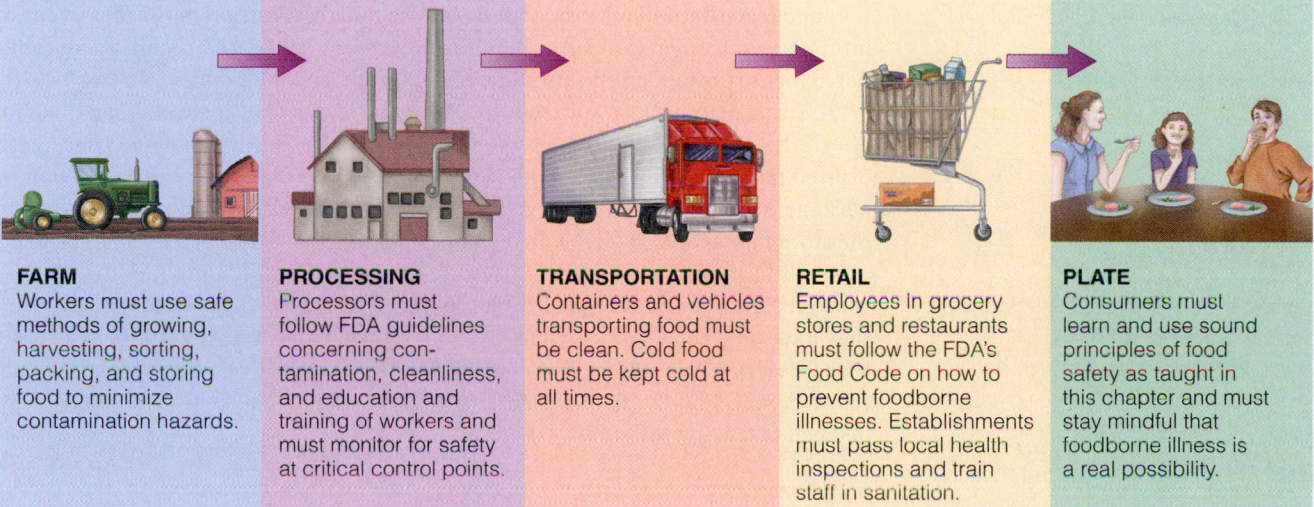

FARM
Workers must use safe methods of growing, harvesting, sorting, packing, and storing food to minimize contamination hazards.

PROCESSING
Processors must follow FDA guidelines concerning contamination, cleanliness, and education and training of workers and must monitor for safety at critical control points.

TRANSPORTATION
Containers and vehicles transporting food must be clean. Cold food must be kept cold at all times.

RETAIL
Employees in grocery stores and restaurants must follow the FDA's Food Code on how to prevent foodborne illnesses. Establishments must pass local health inspections and train staff in sanitation.

PLATE
Consumers must learn and use sound principles of food safety as taught in this chapter and must stay mindful that foodborne illness is a real possibility.

‡ Shiga toxin was named for the Japanese researcher, who discovered the microbial cause of dysentery over 100 years ago.

Table 12–4

Are Your Foods Expiring?

Food manufacturers voluntarily print the following kinds of dates on labels to inform both sellers and consumers of the products' freshness.

- *Sell by:* Specifies the shelf life of the food. After this date, the food may still be safe for consumption if it has been handled and stored properly. Also called *pull date*.
- *Best if used by:* Specifies the last date the food will be of the highest quality. After this date, quality is expected to diminish, although the food may still be safe for consumption if it has been handled and stored properly. Also called *freshness date* or *quality assurance date*.
- *Expiration date:* The last day the food should be consumed. All foods except eggs should be discarded after this date. For eggs, the expiration date refers to the last day the eggs may be sold as "fresh eggs." For safety, purchase eggs before the expiration date, keep them in their original carton in the refrigerator, and use them within 30 days.[a]
- *Open dating:* A general term referring to label dates that are stated in ordinary language that consumers can understand, as opposed to *closed dating*, which refers to dates printed in codes decipherable only by manufacturers. Open dating is used primarily on perishable foods and closed dating on shelf-stable products such as some canned goods.
- *Pack date:* The day the food was packaged or processed. When used on packages of fresh meats, pack dates can provide a general guide to freshness.

[a]*For best quality, use eggs within 3 weeks of purchase.*

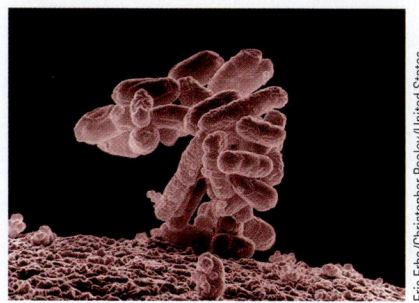

A colony of an *E. coli* bacterium (magnified 7,000 times).

Eric Erbe/Christopher Pooley/United States Department of Agriculture

Food Industry Controls

Inspections of U.S. meat-processing plants, performed every day by USDA inspectors, help to ensure that these facilities meet government standards. Seafood, egg, produce, and processed food facilities are inspected less often, but all food producers must employ a **Hazard Analysis Critical Control Point (HACCP) plan** to help prevent foodborne illnesses at their source. Each slaughterhouse, producer, packer, distributor, and transporter of susceptible foods must identify "critical control points" in its procedures that pose a risk of food contamination and then devise and implement verifiable ways to eliminate or minimize the risk.

The HACCP system has proved a remarkable success. *Salmonella* contamination of U.S. poultry, eggs, ground beef, and pork has been greatly reduced, and *E. coli* infection from meats has dropped dramatically.

Grocery Safety for Consumers

Canned and packaged foods sold in grocery stores are generally safe, but accidents do happen, and foods can become contaminated. FDA scientists track outbreaks of illnesses due to large-scale contamination and trace both likely production sources and distribution paths to prevent or minimize consumer exposure. Batch numbering enables the recall of contaminated foods through public announcements in the media.

You can help protect yourself, too. Shop at stores that look and smell clean. Check the freshness dates printed on many food packages, and avoid those with expired dates (see Table 12–4, above). Inspect all seals and wrappers. If a can or package is bulging, leaking, ragged, soiled, or punctured, don't buy it—turn it in to the store manager. A badly dented can or a mangled package is useless in protecting food from microorganisms, insects, or other spoilage. Many jars have safety "buttons" on the lid, designed to pop up once the jar is opened; make sure that they have not "popped." Frozen foods should be solidly frozen, and those in a chest-type freezer case should be stored below the frost line. Check fresh eggs and reject cracked ones. Finally, shop for frozen and refrigerated foods and fresh meats last, just before leaving the store.

Hazard Analysis Critical Control Point (HACCP) plan a systematic plan to identify and correct potential microbial hazards in the manufacturing, distribution, and commercial use of food products. *HACCP* may be pronounced "HASS-ip."

KEY POINTS

- Farm to plate food safety requires that farmers, processors, transporters, retailers, and consumers use effective food safety methods.
- Consumers should carefully inspect foods before purchasing them.

Safe Food Practices for Individuals

Some people have come to accept a yearly bout or two of intestinal illness as inevitable, but these illnesses can and should be prevented. Take the safety quiz in Table 12–5 (p. 478) to see how well you follow food-safety rules.

Food can provide ideal conditions for bacteria to multiply and to produce toxins. Disease-causing bacteria require these three conditions to thrive:

- Nutrients.
- Moisture.
- Warmth, 40°F to 140°F (4°C to 60°C).§

To defeat bacteria, you must prevent them from contaminating food or deprive them of one of these conditions. Four core practices illustrated in Figure 12–2 can help to achieve these goals.

Any food with an "off" appearance or odor should be thrown away, of course, and not even tasted. However, you cannot rely on your senses of smell, taste, and sight to warn you because most hazards are not detectable by odor, taste, or appearance. As the old saying goes, "When in doubt, throw it out."

Core Practice #1: Clean Keeping your hands and surfaces clean requires using freshly washed utensils and new or disinfected towels and washing your hands properly, not just rinsing them, particularly before and after handling raw food.[7] Normal, healthy skin is covered with bacteria, some of which may cause foodborne illness when deposited on moist, nutrient-rich food and allowed to multiply, as Figure 12–3 illustrates. Remember to use a nailbrush to clean under your fingernails when washing your hands and tend to routine nail care—artificial nails, long nails, chipped polish, and even a hangnail harbor more bacteria than do natural, clean, short, healthy nails. Figure 12–4 (p. 479) delineates steps to thorough hand washing.

For routine cleansing, washing your hands with ordinary soap and warm water is effective; using an alcohol-based hand-sanitizing gel can also provide killing power against many bacteria and most viruses.[8] Following up a good washing with a sanitizer may provide an extra measure of protection that is useful when someone in the house is ill or when preparing food for an infant, an elderly person, or someone with

Figure 12–2

Fight Bac!

Four "core" ways to keep food safe. The Fight Bac! website is at www.fightbac.org.

Clean—keep hands, utensils, and surfaces clean.

Separate—keep raw foods separated from ready-to-eat foods.

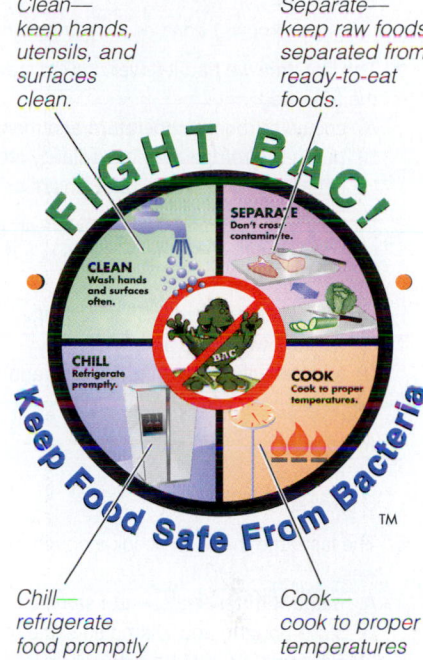

Chill—refrigerate food promptly and keep cold foods cold.

Cook—cook to proper temperatures and keep hot foods hot.

Figure 12–3

Why Wash Your Hands?

The photo on the left shows a person's clean-looking but unwashed hand touching a sterile, moist, nutrient-rich gel in a laboratory dish. After 24 hours in a warm incubator, the large colonies provide visible evidence of the microorganisms that were transferred from the hand to the gel.

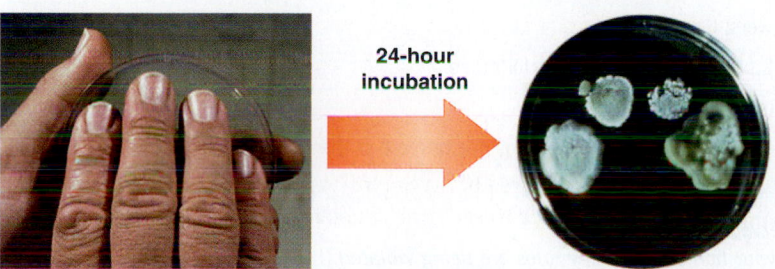

24-hour incubation

Source: Photos courtesy of A. Estes Reynolds, George A. Schuler, James A. Christian, and William C. Hurst.

---

§The FDA suggests these temperatures to consumers at the FDA/CFSAN website; see www.fda.gov. For food industry professionals, the FDA makes other recommendations; see U.S. Public Health Service and Food and Drug Administration, *Food Code* (College Park, Md.: U.S. Department of Health and Human Services, 2013), available at www.fda.gov.

Table 12–5

Can You Pass the Kitchen Food-Safety Quiz?

How food-safety savvy are you? Give yourself 2 points for each correct answer.

1. The temperature of the refrigerator in my home is
   A. 50°F (10°C).
   B. 40°F (4°C).
   C. I don't know; I don't own a refrigerator thermometer.

2. The last time we had leftover cooked stew or other meaty food, the food was
   A. cooled to room temperature and then put in the refrigerator.
   B. put in the refrigerator immediately after the food was served.
   C. left at room temperature overnight or longer.

3. If I use a cutting board to cut raw meat, poultry, or fish and it will be used to chop another food, the board is
   A. reused as is.
   B. wiped with a damp cloth or sponge.
   C. washed with soap and water.
   D. washed with soap and hot water and then sanitized.

4. The last time I had a hamburger, I ate it
   A. rare.
   B. medium.
   C. well-done.

5. The last time there was cookie dough where I live, the dough was
   A. made with raw eggs, and I sampled some of it.
   B. store-bought, and I sampled some of it.
   C. not sampled until baked.

6. I clean my kitchen counters and food preparation areas with
   A. a damp sponge that I rinse and reuse.
   B. a clean sponge or cloth and water.
   C. a clean cloth with hot water and soap.
   D. the same as above and then a bleach solution or other sanitizer.

7. When dishes are washed in my home, they are
   A. cleaned by an automatic dishwasher and then air-dried.
   B. left to soak in the sink for several hours and then washed with soap in the same water.
   C. washed right away with hot water and soap in the sink and then air-dried.
   D. washed right away with hot water and soap in the sink and immediately towel-dried.

8. The last time I handled raw meat, poultry, or fish, I cleaned my hands afterward by
   A. wiping them on a towel.
   B. rinsing them under warm tap water.
   C. washing with soap and water.

9. Meat, poultry, and fish products are defrosted in my home by
   A. setting them on the counter.
   B. placing them in the refrigerator.
   C. microwaving and cooking promptly when thawed.
   D. soaking them in warm water.

10. I realize that eating raw seafood poses special problems for people with
    A. diabetes.
    B. HIV infection.
    C. cancer.
    D. liver disease.

ANSWERS

1. Refrigerators should stay at 40°F or less, so if you chose answer B, give yourself 2 points; 0 for other answers.

2. Answer B is the best practice. Give yourself 2 points if you picked it; 0 for other answers.

3. If answer D best describes your household's practice, give yourself 2 points; if C, 1 point.

4. Give yourself 2 points if you picked answer C; 0 for other answers.

5. If you answered A, you may be putting yourself at risk for infection from bacteria in raw shell eggs. Answer C—eating the baked product—will earn you 2 points; answer B, 1 point. Commercial dough is made with pasteurized eggs, but some bacteria may remain.

6. Answer C or D will earn you 2 points each; answer B, 1 point; answer A, 0.

7. Answers A and C are worth 2 points each; other answers, 0.

8. The only correct practice is answer C. Give yourself 2 points if you picked it; 0 for others.

9. Give yourself 2 points if you picked B or C; 0 for others.

10. This is a trick question: all of the answers apply. Give yourself 2 points for knowing one or more of the risky conditions.

RATING YOUR HOME'S FOOD-SAFETY PRACTICES
20 points: Feel confident about the safety of foods served in your home.
12 to 19 points: Reexamine food-safety practices in your home. Some key rules are being violated.
11 points or below: Take steps immediately to correct food-handling, storage, and cooking techniques used in your home. Current practices are putting you and other members of your household in danger of foodborne illness.

Figure 12–4

Proper Hand Washing Prevents Illness

You can avoid many illnesses by following these hand washing procedures before, during, and after food preparation; before eating; after using the bathroom, changing a diaper, blowing your nose, or touching your hair; after handling animals or their food or waste; or after handling garbage. Wash hands more frequently when someone in the house is sick.

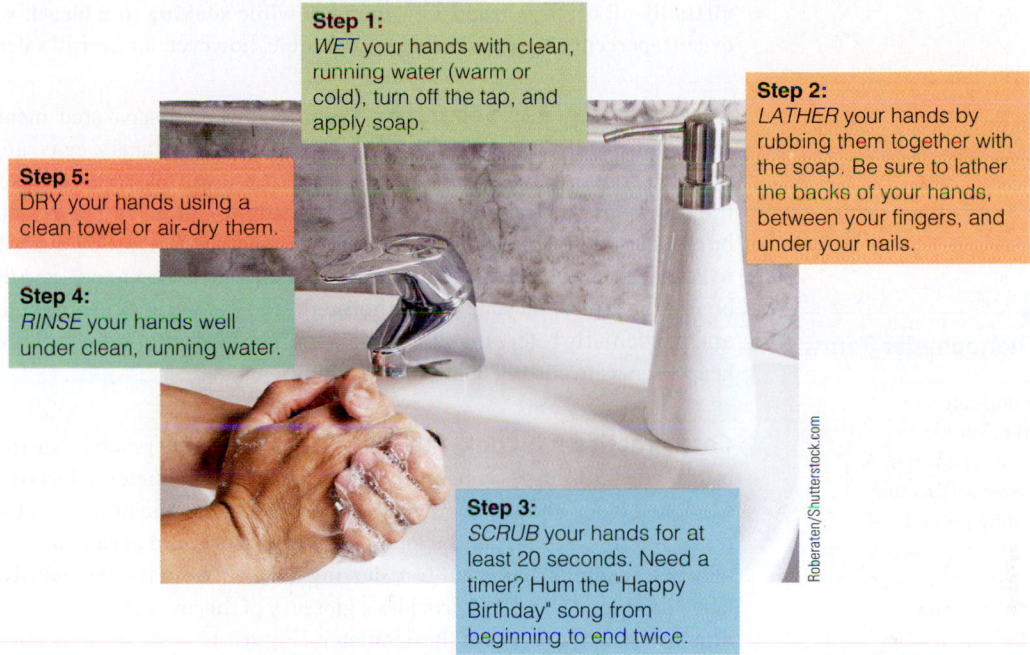

Step 1:
WET your hands with clean, running water (warm or cold), turn off the tap, and apply soap.

Step 2:
LATHER your hands by rubbing them together with the soap. Be sure to lather the backs of your hands, between your fingers, and under your nails.

Step 5:
DRY your hands using a clean towel or air-dry them.

Step 4:
RINSE your hands well under clean, running water.

Step 3:
SCRUB your hands for at least 20 seconds. Need a timer? Hum the "Happy Birthday" song from beginning to end twice.

Roberaten/Shutterstock.com

Source: Centers for Disease Control and Prevention, Handwashing: Clean Hands Save Lives (2014), available at http://www.cdc.gov/handwashing/.

a compromised immune system.** If you are ill or have open cuts or sores, stay away from food preparation.

Antibacterial hand soaps and cleansers possess a chemical additive intended to deter bacterial growth, but regular products work almost as well. The additive is absorbed through human skin and accumulates in the body with unknown consequences; when it drains into wastewater and then into the environment, it can disrupt helpful microbial communities.[9]

Microbes love to nestle down in small, damp spaces, such as the inner cells of sponges or the pores between the fibers of wooden cutting boards. To eliminate them on sponges, surfaces, and utensils, you have four choices, each with benefits and drawbacks:

1. Poison the microbes with highly toxic chemicals such as bleach (one teaspoon per quart of water). Chlorine kills most organisms. However, chlorine is toxic to handle, it can ruin clothing, and when washed down household drains into the water supply, it forms chemicals harmful to people and wildlife.

2. Kill the microbes with heat. Soapy water heated to 140°F kills most harmful organisms and washes most others away. This method takes effort, though, since the water must be truly scalding hot, well beyond the temperature of the tap.

3. Use an automatic dishwasher to combine both methods: it washes in water hotter than hands can tolerate, and most dishwasher detergents contain chlorine.

**Effective hand sanitizers contain between 60 and 70 percent isopropyl alcohol.

4. Use a microwave to kill microbes on sponges. Place the *soaking wet* sponge in a microwave oven, and heat it a minute or two until steaming hot (times vary). Caution: heat only wet sponges in the microwave oven, and watch them carefully; dry sponges or those that contain metal can catch on fire. Also, to prevent scalding your hands, use tongs to remove the steaming-hot sponge.

The third and fourth options—washing in a dishwasher and microwaving —kill virtually all bacteria trapped in sponges, while soaking in a bleach solution misses over 10 percent. The dishwasher is preferable, however, for overall safety.

Core Practice #2: Separate

Keeping raw food separated means preventing **cross-contamination** of foods. Raw foods, especially meats, eggs, and seafood, are likely to contain illness-causing bacteria. To prevent bacteria from spreading, keep the raw foods and their juices away from ready-to-eat foods. For example, if you take burgers out to the grill on a plate, wash that plate in hot, soapy water before using it to retrieve the cooked burgers. If you use a cutting board to cut raw meat, wash the board, the knife, and your hands thoroughly with soap before handling other foods— and particularly before making a salad or other foods that are eaten raw. Many cooks keep a separate cutting board just for raw meats.

Core Practice #3: Cook

Cook foods long enough to reach a safe internal temperature. The USDA urges consumers to use a food thermometer to test the temperatures of cooked foods and not to rely on appearance. Place the probe of a food thermometer in the thickest part of the food, away from bone and gristle, and wash the probe between readings to prevent transferring bacteria from the uncooked food to the finished product. Table 12–6 provides a glossary of thermometer terms, and Figure 12–5 illustrates various types of thermometers. Figure 12–6 (p. 483) specifies safe internal temperatures for cooked foods.

After cooking, hot foods must be held at 140°F or higher until served. A temperature of 140°F on a thermometer feels hot, not just warm. Even well-cooked foods, if handled improperly prior to serving, can cause illness. Delicious-looking meatballs on a buffet may harbor bacteria unless they have been kept steaming hot. After the meal, cooked foods should be refrigerated immediately or within two hours at the maximum (one hour if room temperature approaches 90°F, or 32°C). If food has been left out longer than this, toss it out.

Core Practice #4: Chill

Chilling and keeping cold food cold starts when you leave the grocery store. If you are running errands, shop last so that the groceries do not stay in the car too long. (If ice cream begins to melt, it has been too long.) An ice chest or insulated bag can help to keep foods cold during transit. Upon arrival home, load foods into the refrigerator or freezer immediately. Table 12–7 (p. 482) lists some safe keeping times for foods stored in the refrigerator at or below 40°F. Foods older than this should be discarded, not ingested.

To ensure safety, thaw frozen meats or poultry in the refrigerator, not at room temperature, and marinate meats in the refrigerator, too. To thaw a food more quickly, submerge it in cold (not hot or warm) water in waterproof packaging or use a microwave to thaw food just before cooking it. Most foods can simply be cooked from the frozen state—just increase the cooking time and use a thermometer to ensure that the food reaches a safe internal temperature.

Chill prepared or cooked foods in shallow containers, not in deep ones. A shallow container allows quick chilling throughout; deeper containers take too many hours to chill through to the center, allowing bacteria time to grow.

Cold meats and mixed salads make a convenient buffet, but keep perishable items safe by placing their containers on ice during serving. This applies to all perishable foods, including custards, cream pies, and whipped-cream or cream-cheese treats. Even pumpkin pie, because it contains milk and eggs, should be kept cold.

Table 12–6

Glossary of Thermometer Terms

- **appliance thermometer** a thermometer that verifies the temperature of an appliance. An *oven thermometer* verifies that the oven is heating properly; a *refrigerator/freezer thermometer* tests for proper refrigerator temperature (<40°F, or <4°C) or freezer temperature (0°F, or –17°C).
- **fork thermometer** a utensil combining a meat fork and an instant-read food thermometer.
- **instant-read thermometer** a thermometer that, when inserted into food, measures its temperature within seconds; designed to test temperature of food at intervals.
- **oven-safe thermometer** a thermometer designed to remain in the food to give constant readings during cooking.
- **pop-up thermometer** a disposable timing device commonly used in turkeys. The center of the device contains a spring that "pops up" when food reaches the right temperature.
- **single-use temperature indicator** a disposable instant-read thermometer that changes color to indicate temperature. This type is often used in commercial food establishments to eliminate cross-contamination.

cross-contamination the contamination of a food through exposure to utensils, hands, or other surfaces that were previously in contact with a contaminated food.

Different thermometers do different jobs. To choose the right one, pay attention to its temperature range: Some have high temperature ranges intended to test the doneness of meats and other hot foods (see Figure 12–6). Others have lower ranges for testing temperatures of refrigerators and freezers.

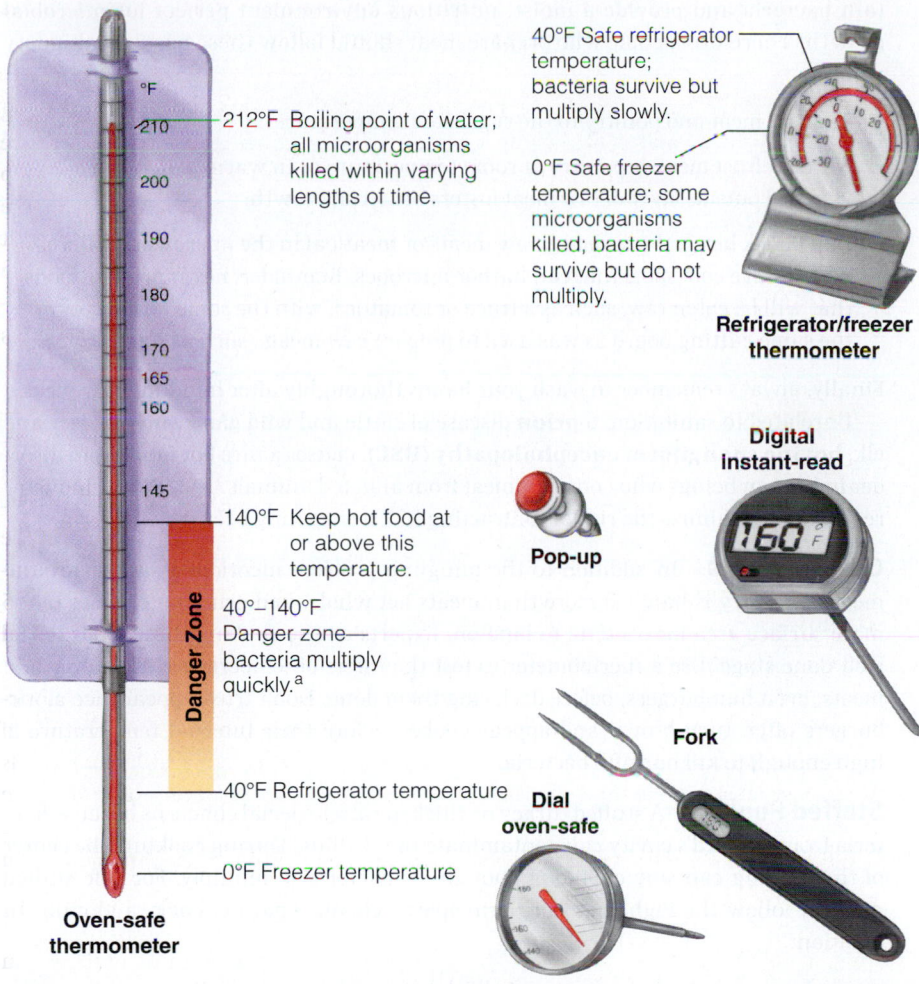

°F

212°F Boiling point of water; all microorganisms killed within varying lengths of time.

40°F Safe refrigerator temperature; bacteria survive but multiply slowly.

0°F Safe freezer temperature; some microorganisms killed; bacteria may survive but do not multiply.

Refrigerator/freezer thermometer

Digital instant-read

Pop-up

Danger Zone

140°F Keep hot food at or above this temperature.

40°–140°F Danger zone— bacteria multiply quickly.[a]

Fork

40°F Refrigerator temperature

Dial oven-safe

0°F Freezer temperature

Oven-safe thermometer

[a]The FDA's food storage danger zone for use by consumers. Food professionals adhere to more specific guidelines as put forth in the FDA's Food Code (College Park, Md.: U.S. Department of Health and Human Services, 2013), available at http://www.fda.gov/Food/GuidanceRegulation/RetailFoodProtection/FoodCode/ucm374275.htm.

Which Foods Are Most Likely to Cause Illness?

LO 12.2 Identify the categories of foods that most often cause foodborne illnesses.

Some foods are more hospitable to microbial growth than others. Foods that are high in moisture and nutrients and those that are chopped or ground are especially favorable hosts. Bacteria in these foods are likely to grow quickly without proper refrigeration.

Table 12–7

Safe Food Storage Times: Refrigerator (≤40°F)

For products with longer shelf lives, rotate them like restaurants do. "First-In-First-Out" means to check dates and use up older products first.

1 to 2 Days

Raw ground meats, breakfast or other raw sausages; raw fish or poultry; gravies

3 to 5 Days

Raw steaks, roasts, or chops; cooked meats, poultry, vegetables, and mixed dishes; lunchmeats (packages opened); mayonnaise salads (chicken, egg, pasta, tuna); fresh vegetables (spinach, green beans, tomatoes)

1 Week

Hard-cooked eggs, bacon, or hot dogs (opened packages); smoked sausages or seafood; milk, cottage cheese

1 to 2 Weeks

Yogurt; carrots, celery, lettuce

2 to 4 Weeks

Fresh eggs (in shells); lunchmeats, bacon, or hot dogs (packages unopened); dry sausages (pepperoni, hard salami); most aged and processed cheeses (Swiss, brick)

2 Months

Mayonnaise (opened jar); most dry cheeses (Parmesan, Romano)

prion a disease agent consisting of an unusually folded protein that disrupts normal cell functioning. Prions cannot be controlled or killed by cooking or disinfecting, and the disease they cause cannot be treated; prevention is the only form of control.

bovine spongiform encephalopathy (BOH-vine SPUNJ-ih-form en-SEH-fal-AH-path-ee) **(BSE)** an often fatal illness of the nerves and brain observed in cattle and wild game and in people who consume affected meats. Also called *mad cow disease.*

Protein Foods

Protein-rich foods require special handling. When produced on an industrial scale, protein foods are often mingled together, such as in tanks of raw milk, vats of raw eggs, or masses of ground meats or poultry.[10] Mingling causes problems when a pathogen from a single source contaminates the whole batch.

Packages of raw meats, for example, bear labels to instruct consumers on meat safety (see Figure 12–6, page 483).[††] Meats in the grocery cooler very often contain bacteria and provide a moist, nutritious environment perfect for microbial growth. Therefore, people who prepare meat should follow these basic meat-safety rules:

- Cook all meat and poultry to the suggested temperatures.

- Never defrost meat or poultry at room temperature or in warm water. The warmed outside layer of raw meat fosters bacterial growth.

- Don't cook large, thick, dense, raw meats or meatloaf in the microwave. Microwaves leave cool spots that can harbor microbes. Reminder: never prepare foods that will be eaten raw, such as lettuce or tomatoes, with the same utensils or on the same cutting board as was used to prepare raw meats, such as hamburgers.

Finally, always remember to wash your hands thoroughly after handling raw meat.

Unrelated to sanitation, a **prion** disease of cattle and wild game such as deer and elk, **bovine spongiform encephalopathy (BSE)**, causes a rare but fatal brain disorder in human beings who consume meat from afflicted animals.[11][‡‡] U.S. beef industry regulations minimize the risk of contracting BSE from eating beef.

Ground Meats   In addition to the mingling problem mentioned earlier, ground meat or poultry is handled more than meats left whole, and grinding exposes much more surface area for bacteria to land on. Experts advise cooking these foods to the well-done stage. Use a thermometer to test the internal temperature of poultry and meats, even hamburgers, before declaring them done. Don't trust appearance alone: burgers often turn brown and appear cooked before their internal temperature is high enough to kill harmful bacteria.

Stuffed Poultry   A stuffed turkey or chicken raises special concerns because bacteria from the bird's cavity can contaminate the stuffing. During cooking, the center of the stuffing can stay cool long enough for bacteria to multiply. For safe stuffed poultry, follow the Fight Bac core principles—clean, separate, cook, and chill. In addition:

- Cook any raw meat, poultry, or shellfish before adding it to stuffing.

- Mix wet and dry ingredients right before stuffing into the cavity and stuff loosely; cook immediately afterward in a preheated oven set no lower than 325°F (use an oven thermometer to make sure).

- Use a meat thermometer to test the center of the stuffing. It should reach 165°F.

To repeat: test the stuffing. Even if the poultry meat itself has reached the safe temperature of 165°F, the center of the stuffing may be cool enough to harbor live bacteria. Better yet, bake the stuffing separately.

Eggs   Eating undercooked eggs at home accounts for about 30 percent of U.S. *Salmonella* infections.[12] Bacteria from the intestinal tract of hens often contaminate eggs as they are laid, and some bacteria may enter the egg itself. All commercially available eggs are washed and sanitized before packing, and some are pasteurized in the shell to make them safer. The FDA requires measures to control *Salmonella* and other bacteria on major egg-producing poultry farms.

[††] The USDA's Food Information Hotline answers questions about meat, poultry, and seafood safety: 1–888-MPHOTLINE.

[‡‡] The human disease is variant Creutzfeldt-Jakob disease (vCJD).

Figure 12-6

Safe Handling Instructions and Cooking Temperatures

Following safe handling instructions for meat and poultry minimizes bacterial growth and cross-contamination. Cooking and cooling foods to proper temperatures also reduces microbial threats.

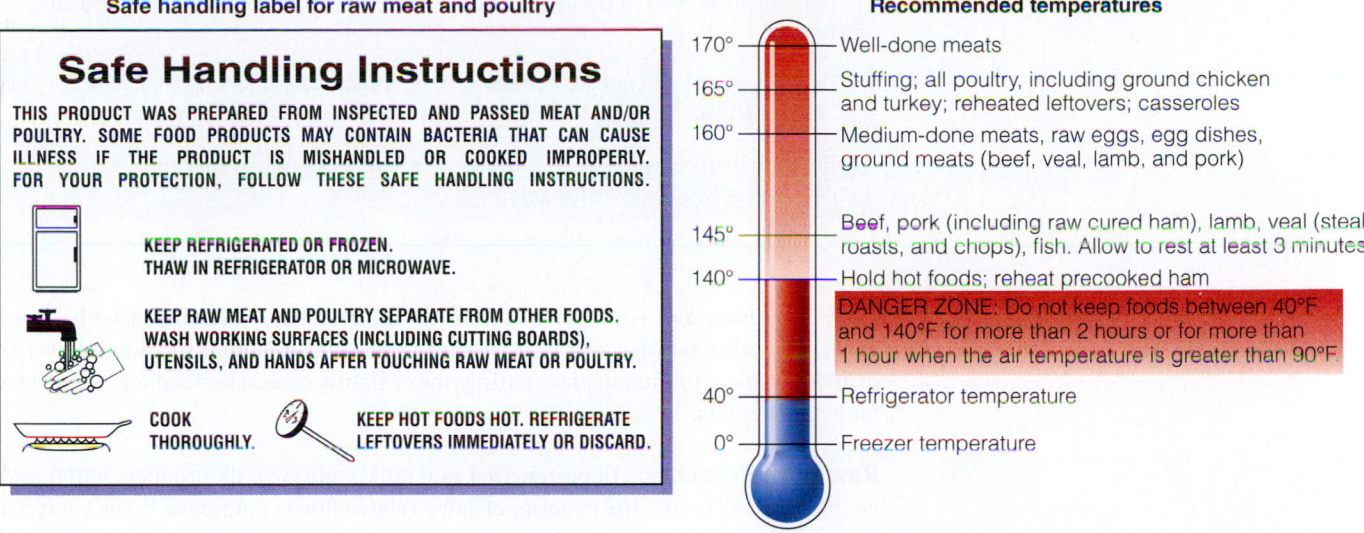

Safe handling label for raw meat and poultry

Safe Handling Instructions

THIS PRODUCT WAS PREPARED FROM INSPECTED AND PASSED MEAT AND/OR POULTRY. SOME FOOD PRODUCTS MAY CONTAIN BACTERIA THAT CAN CAUSE ILLNESS IF THE PRODUCT IS MISHANDLED OR COOKED IMPROPERLY. FOR YOUR PROTECTION, FOLLOW THESE SAFE HANDLING INSTRUCTIONS.

KEEP REFRIGERATED OR FROZEN. THAW IN REFRIGERATOR OR MICROWAVE.

KEEP RAW MEAT AND POULTRY SEPARATE FROM OTHER FOODS. WASH WORKING SURFACES (INCLUDING CUTTING BOARDS), UTENSILS, AND HANDS AFTER TOUCHING RAW MEAT OR POULTRY.

COOK THOROUGHLY.

KEEP HOT FOODS HOT. REFRIGERATE LEFTOVERS IMMEDIATELY OR DISCARD.

Recommended temperatures

- 170° — Well-done meats
- 165° — Stuffing; all poultry, including ground chicken and turkey; reheated leftovers; casseroles
- 160° — Medium-done meats, raw eggs, egg dishes, ground meats (beef, veal, lamb, and pork)
- 145° — Beef, pork (including raw cured ham), lamb, veal (steaks, roasts, and chops), fish. Allow to rest at least 3 minutes.[a]
- 140° — Hold hot foods; reheat precooked ham
- DANGER ZONE: Do not keep foods between 40°F and 140°F for more than 2 hours or for more than 1 hour when the air temperature is greater than 90°F.
- 40° — Refrigerator temperature
- 0° — Freezer temperature

[a]During the 3 minutes after meat is removed from the heat source, its temperature remains constant or continues to rise, which destroys pathogens.

Source: Data from U.S. Department of Agriculture and U.S. Department of Health and Human Services, Scientific report of the 2015 Dietary Guidelines Advisory Committee, 2015, D-5:46–47, available at www.health.gov.

For consumers, egg cartons bear reminders to keep eggs refrigerated, cook eggs until their yolks are firm, and cook egg-containing foods thoroughly before eating them.

What about tempting foods like homemade ice cream, hollandaise sauce, unbaked cake batter, or raw cookie dough that contain raw or undercooked eggs? Healthy adults can enjoy them if they are made safer by replacing regular shell eggs with pasteurized eggs or liquid egg products. Even these products, because they are made from raw eggs, may contain a few live bacteria that survived pasteurization, making them unsafe for pregnant women, the elderly, young children, or people with weakened immunity.

Seafood Properly cooked fish and other seafood sold in the United States are safe from microbial threats. However, even the freshest, most appealing, raw or partly cooked seafood can harbor disease-causing viruses; parasites, such as worms and flukes; and bacteria that cause illnesses ranging from stomach cramps to severe, life-threatening conditions.[13] Table 12–8 (p. 484) lists beliefs about raw seafood that can make people sick.

The dangers posed by seafood are increasing. As burgeoning human populations along the world's shorelines release more contaminants into lakes, rivers, and oceans, the seafood living there becomes less safe to consume. Viruses that cause human diseases have been detected in some 90 percent of the waters off the U.S. coast and easily contaminate filter feeders such as clams and oysters. Government agencies monitor commercial fishing areas and close unsafe waters to harvesters, but illegal harvesting is common.

As for **sushi** or "seared" partially raw fish, even a master chef cannot detect microbial dangers that may lurk within. The marketing term "sushi grade," often applied to seafood to imply wholesomeness, is not legally defined and does not indicate quality, purity, or freshness. Also, freezing does not make raw fish entirely safe to eat. Freezing kills adult parasitic worms, but only cooking can kill all worm eggs and other

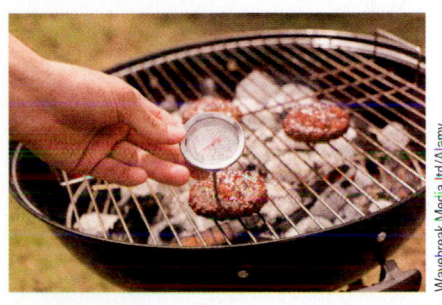

A safe hamburger is cooked well done (internal temperature of 160°F) and has juices that run clear. Place it on a clean plate when it's done.

sushi a Japanese dish that consists of vinegar-flavored rice, seafood, and colorful vegetables, typically wrapped in seaweed. Some sushi contains raw fish; other sushi contains only cooked ingredients.

Table 12–8

Raw Seafood Myths and Truths

Myth	Truth
▪ If a raw seafood was consumed in the past with no ill effect, it is safe to do so today.	▪ Each harvest bears separate risks, and seafood is increasingly contaminated.
▪ Drinking alcohol with raw seafood will "kill the germs."	▪ Alcoholic beverages cannot make contaminated raw seafood safe.
▪ Putting hot sauce on raw oysters and other raw seafood will "kill the germs."	▪ Hot sauce has no effect on microbes in seafood.

microorganisms. Safe sushi is made from cooked seafood, seaweed, vegetables, avocados, and other safe delicacies. Experts unanimously agree that today's high levels of microbial contamination make eating raw or lightly cooked seafood too risky, even for healthy adults.

Raw Milk Products   Unpasteurized raw milk and raw milk products (often sold as "health food") cause the majority of dairy-related illness outbreaks.[14] The bacterial counts of raw milk are unpredictable and even raw milk from a trusted dairy can cause severe illness. Drinking raw milk presents a real risk with no advantages—the nutrients in pasteurized milk and raw milk are identical.

Even in pasteurized milk, a few bacteria may survive, so milk must be refrigerated to hold bacterial growth to a minimum. Shelf-stable milk, often sold in boxes, is sterilized by an **ultra-high temperature** treatment and so needs no refrigeration until it is opened.

KEY POINTS

- Raw meats and poultry pose special microbial threats and so require special handling.
- Consuming raw eggs, milk, or seafood is risky.

Raw Produce

The Dietary Guidelines urge greater intakes of fruits and vegetables, but consumers should also be aware of a risk of illness from contamination.[15] Foods such as lettuce, salad spinach, tomatoes, melons, berries, herbs, and scallions grow close to the ground, making bacterial contamination from the soil, animal waste runoff, and manure fertilizers likely. For example, one farm recalled 300,000 cases of cantaloupe when illness from *Listeria* caused 33 deaths and sickened many more people across 28 states.[16] Other kinds of produce, and even peanut butter, have been responsible for transmitting dangerous foodborne illnesses to consumers. Such problems often spring from sanitation mistakes made by growers and producers.[17]

Washing produce at home to remove dirt and debris is important, and Table 12–9 provides some guidance. However, washing may not entirely remove certain bacterial strains. These strains—*E. coli*, among others—exude a sticky, protective coating that glues microbes to each other and to food surfaces, forming a **biofilm** that can survive home rinsing or even industrial washing.[18] Somewhat more effective is vigorous scrubbing with a vegetable brush to dislodge bacteria; rinsing with vinegar, which may help cut through biofilm; and removing and discarding the outer leaves from heads of leafy vegetables, such as cabbage and lettuce, before washing. Vinegar doesn't sterilize foods, but it can reduce bacterial populations, and it's safe to consume.

ultra-high temperature a process of sterilizing food by exposing it for a short time to temperatures above those normally used in processing.

biofilm a layer of microbes mixed with a sticky, protective coating of proteins and carbohydrates exuded by certain bacteria.

Table 12–9

How to Wash Produce

Follow these steps:

- Wash your hands (see Figure 12–4, p. 479).
- Wash fruits and vegetables (organic, conventional, or homegrown) thoroughly under running water before cutting or peeling.
- Wash produce that will be peeled to remove dirt and bacteria that could be transferred from the peel to the edible parts by the peeler or knife.
- Scrub firm produce, such as melons and cucumbers, with a clean produce brush to dislodge dirt and bacteria.
- Cut away any damaged or bruised parts.
- Dry with a clean cloth.
- Prewashed, ready-to-eat produce needs no further washing; if you choose to rewash it, avoid contamination by following the basic rules of food safety.

Source: U.S. Department of Agriculture and U.S. Department of Health and Human Services, Scientific report of the 2015 Dietary Guidelines Advisory Committee, 2015, D-5:44, available at www.health.gov.

Unpasteurized Juices Unpasteurized or raw juices and ciders pose a special problem. Juice producers mingle fruit from many different trees and orchards, and any bacteria introduced into a batch of juice can multiply rapidly in the sugary fluid. Labels of unpasteurized juices must carry the warning shown in Figure 12–7. Especially infants, children, the elderly, and people with weakened immune systems should never be given raw or unpasteurized juice products. Refrigerated pasteurized juices, reconstituted frozen juices, and shelf-stable juices in boxes, cans, or pouches are generally safe.

Sprouts Sprouts (alfalfa, clover, radish, and others) grow in the warm, moist, nutrient-rich conditions that microbes need to thrive.[19] A few bacteria or spores on sprout seeds can quickly bloom into widespread contamination of the sprouts; both commercial and homegrown raw sprouts pose this risk.[20] Sprouts are often eaten raw, but the only sure way to make sprouts safe is to cook them. The elderly, young children, and those with weakened immunity are particularly vulnerable.

KEY POINTS

- Produce causes many foodborne illnesses each year.
- Proper washing and refrigeration can reduce risks.
- Cooking ensures that sprouts are safe to eat.

Other Foods

Careful handling can reduce microbial threats from other foods, too. Foods in this section are common in the food supply, and their safety is worth considering.

Imported Foods Today, nearly two-thirds of the fruits and vegetables and 80 percent of the seafood consumed in the United States are imported into the United States, as illustrated in Figure 12–8 (p. 486). This poses an enormous food-safety challenge—the methods and standards of many thousands of food producers in far-away countries vary substantially. Cooked, frozen, irradiated, or canned imported foods and foods from developed areas with effective food-safety policies are generally safe. Concerns arise, however, about fresh produce, fish, shrimp, and other susceptible foods that originate in areas where food-safety practices are lax, food handling is unregulated, and contagious diseases are likely. Fields may be irrigated with contaminated water, crops may be fertilized with untreated manure, and produce may be picked by infected farm workers.

To prevent contamination of imported foods at its source, the FDA recently stepped up its routine inspections of the riskiest farms and facilities around the world.[21] Also, to help U.S. consumers distinguish between imported and domestic

Figure 12–7

Warning Label for Unpasteurized Juice

Unpasteurized or untreated juice must bear the following warning on its label:

> **WARNING:** This product has not been pasteurized and therefore may contain harmful bacteria that can cause serious illness in children, the elderly, and persons with weakened immune systems.

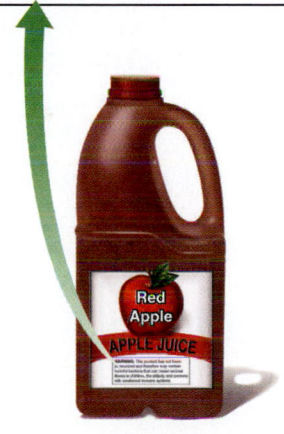

Figure 12–8
How Far Did Your Salad Travel?

A simple salad on a U.S. dinner plate may result from world-wide efforts to provide it.

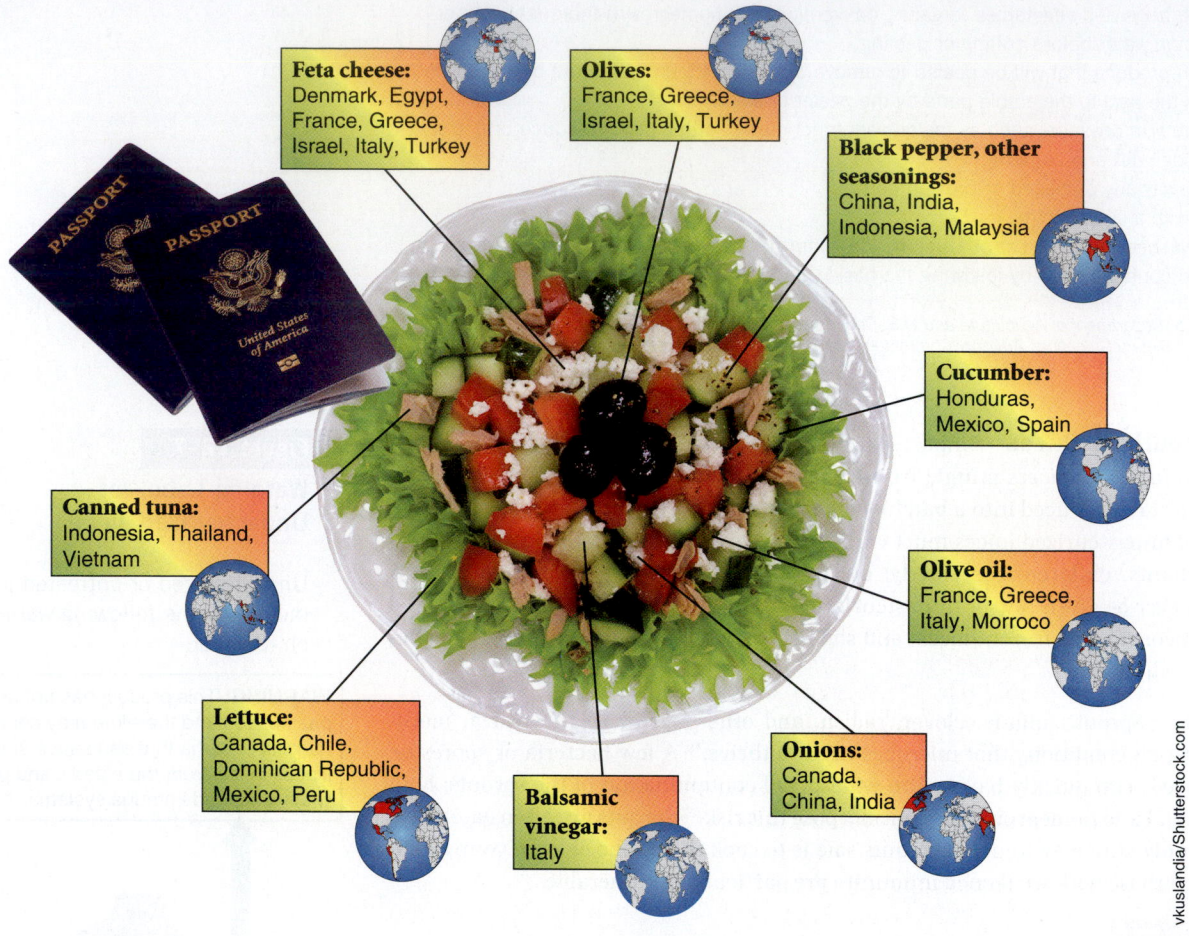

Feta cheese:
Denmark, Egypt, France, Greece, Israel, Italy, Turkey

Olives:
France, Greece, Israel, Italy, Turkey

Black pepper, other seasonings:
China, India, Indonesia, Malaysia

Cucumber:
Honduras, Mexico, Spain

Canned tuna:
Indonesia, Thailand, Vietnam

Olive oil:
France, Greece, Italy, Morroco

Lettuce:
Canada, Chile, Dominican Republic, Mexico, Peru

Onions:
Canada, China, India

Balsamic vinegar:
Italy

vkuslandia/Shutterstock.com

foods, regulators require certain foods, including fish and shellfish, perishable items other than meats or poultry, and some nuts to bear a **country of origin label** specifying where they were produced.[22]

Honey   Honey can contain dormant spores of *Clostridium botulinum* that, when eaten, can germinate and begin to grow and produce their deadly botulinum toxin within the human body. Mature, healthy adults are usually protected against this threat, but infants under one year of age should never be fed honey.

Picnics and Lunch Bags   Picnics can be fun, and packed lunches are a convenience, but to keep them safe, do the following:

- Choose foods that are safe without refrigeration, such as whole fruits and vegetables, breads and crackers, shelf-stable foods, and canned spreads, fish and seafood, and cheeses to open and use on the spot.

- Chill lunch bag foods and pack them in a thermal lunch bag with several reusable ice packs. Food at room temperature in a paper bag may be unsafe to eat by lunchtime.[23]

country of origin label (COOL) the required label stating the country of origination of certain imported fish and shellfish, certain other perishable foods, certain nuts, peanuts, and ginseng. Meats and poultry are no longer subject to COOL labeling.

- Choose well-aged cheeses, such as cheddar and Swiss; skip fresh cheeses, such as cottage cheese and Mexican queso fresco. Aged cheese does well without chilling for an hour or two; for longer times, carry it on ice in a cooler or thermal lunch bag.

A handy tip: freeze beverages, such as juice boxes or pouches, to replace ice packs in a thermal bag. As the beverages thaw in the hours before lunch, they keep the foods cold.

Note that individual servings of cheese or cold cuts prepackaged with crackers and promoted as lunch foods keep well, but they are high in saturated fat and sodium, they cost triple the price of the foods purchased separately. Additionally, their excessive packaging adds to the nation's waste disposal burden.

Mayonnaise, despite its reputation for easy spoilage, is itself somewhat spoilage-resistant because of its acid content. Mayonnaise mixed with chopped ingredients in pasta, meat, or vegetable salads, however, spoils readily. The chopped ingredients have extensive surface areas for bacteria to invade, and cutting boards, hands, and kitchen utensils used in preparation often harbor bacteria. For safe chopped raw foods, start with clean chilled ingredients, and then chill the finished product in shallow containers; keep it chilled before and during serving; and promptly refrigerate any remainder.

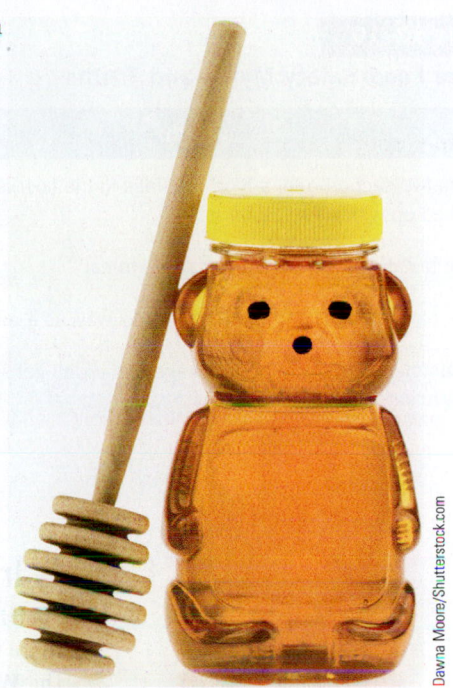

Dawna Moore/Shutterstock.com

Take-Out Foods and Leftovers   Many people rely on take-out foods—rotisserie chicken, pizza, Chinese dishes, and the like—for parties, picnics, or weeknight suppers. When buying these foods, food-safety rules apply: hot foods should be steaming hot, and cold foods should be thoroughly chilled.

Leftovers of all kinds make a convenient later lunch or dinner. However, microbes on serving utensils and in the air can quickly contaminate freshly cooked foods; for safety, refrigerate them promptly and reheat them to steaming hot (165°F) before eating. Discard any portion held at room temperature for longer than 2 hours from the time it was served at the table until you place it in your refrigerator. Follow the 2, 2, and 4 rules of leftover safety: within 2 hours of cooking, refrigerate the food in clean, shallow containers about 2 inches deep, and use it up within 4 days or toss it out. Exceptions: stuffing and gravy must be used within 2 days, and if room temperature reaches 90°F, all cooked foods must be chilled after 1 hour of exposure. Remember to use shallow containers, not deep ones, for quick chilling.

Consumers bear a responsibility for food safety, and an essential step is to cultivate awareness that foodborne illness is likely. They must discard old notions that put them at risk (see Table 12–10, page 488) and adopt an attitude of self-defense to prevent illness.

KEY POINTS

- Many foods are imported, and the FDA is working to improve their safety.
- Honey should never be fed to infants.
- Lunch bags, picnics, and leftovers require safe handling.

Advances in Microbial Food Safety

LO 12.3 Outline technological advances aimed at reducing microbial food contamination.

Advances in technology, such as pasteurization, have dramatically improved the quality and safety of foods over the past century. Today, other technologies promise similar benefits, but some raise concerns among consumers.

Table 12-10

More Food-Safety Myths and Truths

Myth	Truth
■ "The five-second rule: a food that falls to the floor is safe if it is picked up within five seconds."	■ Food dropped on a microbe-laden hard surface, such as a floor, becomes contaminated in far less than five seconds.
■ "If it tastes and smells okay, it's safe to eat."	■ Most microbial contamination is undetectable by human senses.
■ "We have always handled our food this way, so it must be safe."	■ Past generations did not recognize the causes of illness.
■ "I sampled it a couple of hours ago and didn't get sick, so it is safe to eat."	■ Illnesses often take half a day or longer to develop.

Is Irradiation Safe?

Food **irradiation** has been extensively evaluated over the past 50 years. Approved in more than 40 countries, its use is endorsed by numerous health agencies, including the **World Health Organization (WHO)** and the American Medical Association. Food irradiation protects consumers and offers other benefits:

- *Foodborne illnesses.* Irradiation effectively eliminates many organisms that cause foodborne illnesses, such as *Salmonella, E. coli*, and parasites.

- *Preservation.* Irradiation can decrease spoilage and extend the shelf life of foods by destroying or inactivating organisms such as the mold that produces the carcinogenic toxin **aflatoxin**.

- *Control of insects.* Irradiation penetrates tough exoskeletons to destroy insects on imported fruits. Irradiation also decreases the need for other pest-control practices that may harm the fruit.

- *Delay of sprouting and ripening.* Irradiation inhibits the sprouting of onions and potatoes and delays the ripening of many kinds of fruit to increase shelf life.

- *Sterilization.* Irradiation can be used to sterilize some products, such as dried herbs, spices, and teas. In hospitals, other kinds of sterilized foods are useful for patients with severely impaired immunity.[24]

Supporters of irradiation say that if more everyday foods were irradiated, the nation's rates of foodborne illnesses would drop dramatically. All irradiated foods except spices must be identified as such on their labels.

How Irradiation Works
Irradiation exposes foods to controlled doses of gamma rays from the radioactive compound cobalt 60. As the rays pass through living cells, they disrupt internal DNA, protein, and other structures, killing or deactivating the cells. For example, low radiation doses can kill the growing cells in the "eyes" of potatoes, preventing them from sprouting. Low doses also delay the ripening of bananas, avocados, and other fruits. Higher doses easily penetrate tough insect exoskeletons and mold or bacterial cell walls to destroy them. Irradiation works even while food is frozen, making it uniquely useful in protecting foods such as whole frozen turkeys.

Irradiation Effects on Foods
Irradiation does not sterilize most foods because doses high enough to kill all microorganisms also substantially alter the food. In approved doses, irradiation does not noticeably change the taste, texture, or appearance of citrus fruits, eggs, many meats, onions, potatoes, spices, strawberries, and other FDA-approved foods, and it does not make foods radioactive. Some vitamins are destroyed by irradiation, but the losses are comparable to those from other food-processing methods such as canning.

irradiation the application of ionizing radiation to foods to reduce insect infestation or microbial contamination or to slow the ripening or sprouting process. Also called *cold pasteurization*.

World Health Organization (WHO) an agency of the United Nations charged with improving human health and preventing or controlling diseases in the world's people.

aflatoxin (af-lah-TOX-in) a toxin from a mold that grows on corn, grains, peanuts, and tree nuts stored in warm, humid conditions; a cause of liver cancer prevalent in tropical developing nations. (To prevent it, discard shriveled, discolored, or moldy foods.)

Chapter 12 Food Safety and Food Technology

Consumer Concerns about Irradiation Many consumers associate radiation with cancer, birth defects, and mutations, so they respond negatively to the idea of irradiating foods. Some erroneously fear that food will become contaminated with radioactive particles. More realistic fears concern transporting radioactive materials, training workers to handle them safely, and safely disposing of spent wastes, which remain radioactive for many years. The food industry echoes these concerns and strives to safeguard both workers and consumers through compliance with strict operating standards and regulations.

Finally, some worry that unscrupulous manufacturers might irradiate old or bacterially tainted foods, thereby escaping detection by USDA testers. Instead of being seized or destroyed, the food could be passed off as wholesome to unsuspecting consumers. This objection raises an important point: irradiation is intended to complement, not replace, other traditional food-safety methods. Irradiation cannot entirely protect people from poor sanitation on the farm, in industry, or at home.

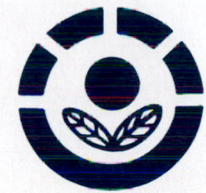

This "radura" logo is the international symbol for foods treated with irradiation.

KEY POINTS

- Food irradiation kills bacteria, insects, molds, and parasites on foods.
- Consumers have concerns about the effects of irradiation on foods, workers, and the environment.

Other Technologies

The FDA and USDA are improving their monitoring techniques for microbial contamination at all levels of food production. In addition, some food-processing and packaging technologies are currently helping to reduce microbial threats to consumers, and others show potential for future use.

Improved Testing and Surveillance Microbial testing of foods before they reach consumers is a critical step toward preventing foodborne illnesses. Automated systems have improved testing accuracy from farms to markets. For example, using a mobile laboratory, FDA scientists can test fresh produce at the growing field and analyze it for many kinds of bacterial contamination. In addition, better detection methods for *E. coli* in water, sediment, and other environmental harbors allow intervention before microbes can contaminate food crops.

Modified Atmosphere Packaging Common packaging methods improve the safety and shelf life of many fresh and prepared foods. Vacuum packaging or **modified atmosphere packaging (MAP)** reduces the oxygen inside a package. This makes it possible for unopened packages of soft pasta noodles, baked goods, prepared foods, fresh and cured meats, seafood, dry beans and other dry products, and ground and whole-bean coffee to stay fresh and safe much longer than they would in conventional packaging. Reducing oxygen:

- Reduces growth of oxygen-dependent microbes.
- Prevents discoloration of cut vegetables and fruits.
- Prevents spoilage of fats by rancidity and development of "off" flavors.
- Slows ripening of fruits and vegetables and enzyme-induced breakdown of vitamins.

Perishable foods packaged with MAP must still be chilled properly, however, to keep them safe from microbes that flourish in anaerobic environments, such as the *Clostridium botulinum* bacterium. Chilling precut salad greens is also a must: temperatures above 50°F cause a dangerous change in *E. coli* bacteria strains present in MAP-bagged lettuces that helps them to survive the eater's stomach acid, increasing their ability to cause infection.

modified atmosphere packaging (MAP) a technique used to extend the shelf life of perishable foods; the food is packaged in a gas-impermeable container from which air is removed or to which an oxygen-free gas mixture, such as carbon dioxide and nitrogen, is added to deprive microbes of oxygen.

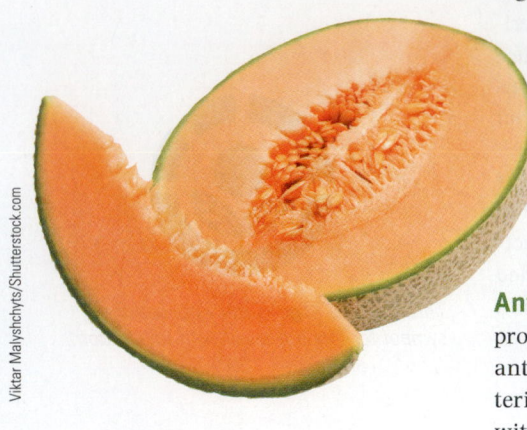

High Pressure and Ultrasound   High-pressure processing (HPP) technology compresses water to create intense pressure that can kill many kinds of disease-causing microbes, including certain viruses. HPP "cold-pasteurizes" applesauce, avocado products, deli meats, orange juice, shellfish, meats, and many prepared foods, making them both safer and longer lasting.[25] However, the equipment is expensive, and not all microbes are destroyed in processing, so continuous refrigeration of most treated foods is a must.

High-powered ultrasound also holds promise as a sanitizer for organic salad greens. It works by sending high-energy shockwaves through water to dislodge pathogens from the small crevices of leafy greens. It may one day replace chlorine rinses but does not sterilize the food.

Antimicrobial Wraps and Films   Bacteria-killing food wraps and films hold promise. One biodegradable wrap made from milk whey protein with a dose of herbal antimicrobial oil may protect perishable foods from both oxidation spoilage and bacterial growth. Other films are made from fungal extract or fruit or vegetable purees with a dose of rosemary or oregano oil or other edible antibacterial agent.[26] In addition to protecting the food, the edible wraps may lend a pleasing flavor.

Microbial foodborne illnesses undoubtedly pose the most immediate threat to consumers, but other factors also affect food safety. The next sections address some of these concerns.

KEY POINTS

- Irradiation controls mold, sterilizes spices and teas, controls insects, extends shelf life, and destroys disease-causing bacteria.
- Scientific advances, such as research on high-pressure processing, continuously improve food safety.

Toxins, Residues, and Contaminants in Foods

LO 12.4 Discuss natural toxins, residues, and contaminants in food.

Nutrition-conscious consumers often wonder if our nation's foods are made unsafe by chemical contamination. The FDA, along with the Environmental Protection Agency (EPA), regulates many chemicals in foods that occur as a result of human activities. A later section describes these substances. First, some toxins produced naturally by the foods themselves are worthy of attention.

Natural Toxins in Foods

Some people think they can eliminate all poisons from their diets by eating only "natural" foods. On the contrary, nature has provided many plants with natural poisons to fend off diseases, insects, and other predators. Humans rarely suffer harm from such poisons, but the *potential* for harm does exist.

Potatoes provide a common example. They contain many natural poisons, including solanine, a powerful, bitter, narcotic-like substance. The small amounts of solanine normally found in potatoes are harmless, but solanine can build up to toxic levels when potatoes are exposed to light during storage. Cooking does not destroy solanine, but most of a potato's solanine develops in a thin green layer just beneath the skin, so it can often be peeled off, making the potato safe to eat. If a potato tastes bitter, however, throw it out.

Solanine, along with other naturally occurring toxins (Table 12–11), serve as a reminder of three principles. First, poisons are poisons, whether made by people or by nature. It's not the source of a compound that makes it hazardous but its chemical structure. Second, any substance—even pure water—can be toxic

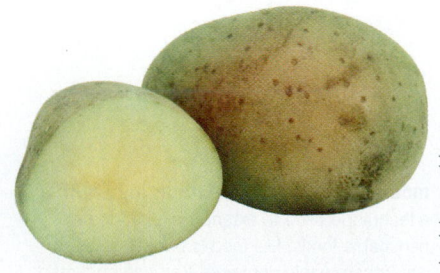

Exposure to light causes the bitter green toxin solanine to form under the skin of potatoes.

Table 12–11

A Sampling of Natural Toxins

Herbs	Belladonna and hemlock are infamous poisonous herbs, but sassafras contains the carcinogen and liver toxin safrole, which is so potent that it is banned from use in foods and beverages.
Cabbages	Cabbage, turnips, mustard greens, and radishes all contain small quantities of harmful goitrogens, compounds that can enlarge the thyroid gland and aggravate thyroid problems. When people have little to eat but cabbages, goitrogens can become a problem, but cooking deactivates the goitrogens.
Foods with Cyanogens	Cyanogens, precursors to the deadly poison cyanide, are found in bitter varieties of cassava, a root vegetable staple for many people. Most cassava contains just traces of cyanogens. An infamous cyanogen from apricot pits is laetrile, a fake cancer cure often passed off as a vitamin.[a] True, the poison laetrile kills cancer cells but only at doses that can kill the person, too. Other fruit pits also contain cyanogens, but an occasional swallowed seed or two presents no danger.
Seafood Red Tide Toxin	At certain times of the year, seafood may become contaminated with the so-called *red tide* toxin that occurs during algae blooms. Eating seafood contaminated with red tide can cause paralysis, so the FDA closes fishing waters when red tide algae appear.

[a]*Also called amygdalin and, erroneously, vitamin B_{17}.*

when consumed in excess. Third, by choosing a variety of foods, toxins present in one food are diluted by the volume of the other foods in the diet.

KEY POINTS

- Natural foods contain natural toxins that can be hazardous under some conditions.
- To avoid harm from toxins, eat all foods in moderation, treat toxins from all sources with respect, and choose a variety of foods.

Pesticides

The use of **pesticides** helps to ensure the survival of food crops, but the damage pesticides do to the environment is considerable and increasing. Moreover, there is some question about whether the widespread use of pesticides has truly increased overall yields of food. Even with extensive pesticide use, the world's farmers lose large quantities of their crops to pests every year.

The use of pesticides on food crops demonstrates a principle inherent to nutrition decision-making: the expected benefits of an action or inaction must be weighed against its risks.[27] In general, agricultural pesticides:

- Protect crops from insect damage.
- Increase potential yield per acre.

But they also:

- Accumulate in the food chain.
- Kill valuable pollinators, such as bees.
- Kill pests' natural predators, including birds and insects.
- Pollute the water, soil, and air.

pesticides chemicals used to control insects, diseases, weeds, fungi, and other pests on crops and around animals. Used broadly, the term includes *herbicides* (to kill weeds), *insecticides* (to kill insects), and *fungicides* (to kill fungi).

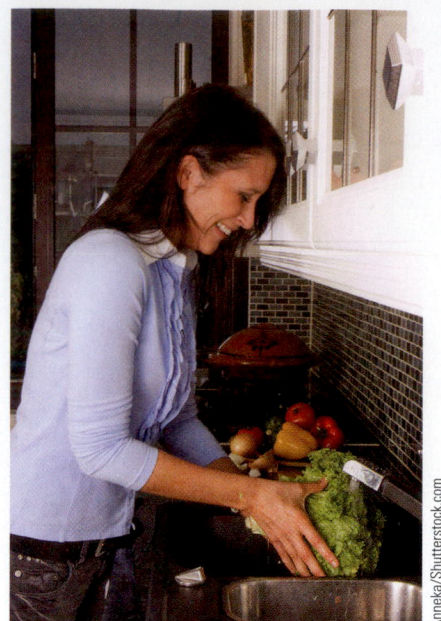
Wash fresh fruits and vegetables to remove pesticide residues.

Scientists, farmers, and consumers must all weigh the risks and benefits to determine their best course of action.

Do Pesticides on Foods Pose a Hazard to Consumers?
Many pesticides are broad-spectrum poisons that damage all living cells, not just those of pests. Their use can harm the plants and animals in natural systems, and they also present risks to people who produce, transport, and apply them. High doses of pesticides in laboratory animals cause birth defects, sterility, tumors, organ damage, and central nervous system impairment. Equivalent doses are extremely unlikely to occur in human beings, however, except through accidental spills. Minute quantities of pesticide **residues** on agricultural products can survive processing, and traces are often present in foods served to people, but these amounts pose negligible risks to most people (see the Consumer's Guide section).

Especially Vulnerable: Infants and Children
Infants and children are more susceptible than adults to the ill effects of pesticides for four reasons. First, the immature human detoxifying system cannot effectively cope with poisons, so they tend to stay longer in the body. Second, the developing brain cannot yet fully exclude pesticides, many of which kill insects by interfering with normal nerve and brain chemistry.

Third, children's bodies are small in size, yet their pesticide exposure is often greater than that of adults. Children pick up pesticides through normal child behaviors, such as playing outdoors on treated soil or lawns; handling sticks, rocks, and other contaminated objects; crawling on treated carpets, furniture, and floors; placing fingers and toys in their mouths; seldom washing their hands; and using fingers instead of utensils to grasp foods.

Fourth, children eat proportionally more food per pound of body weight than do adults, and even the trace amounts of pesticides on foods can contribute to total exposure. Fortunately, these traces rarely exceed allowable limits, and most can be further reduced by washing produce thoroughly and following the other guidelines in Table 12–12.[§§] Another possibility for reducing pesticide exposure is to choose **organic foods**—read the Consumer's Guide for perspective.

Regulation of Pesticides
The EPA sets a **reference dose** for the maximum residue of an approved pesticide allowable in foods. Over 10,000 regulations set reference doses for hundreds of pesticide chemicals approved for use on U.S. crops. These limits generally represent between 1/100th to 1/1,000th of the highest dose

---

[§§] For answers to questions about pesticides, call the 24-hour National Pesticide Information Center: 1–800–858-PEST.

---

residues whatever remains; in the case of pesticides, those amounts that remain on or in foods when people buy and use them.

organic foods foods meeting strict USDA production regulations for *organic*—that is, produced without synthetic pesticides, herbicides, fertilizers, drugs, and preservatives and without genetic engineering or irradiation.

reference dose an estimate of the intake of a substance over a lifetime that is considered to be without appreciable health risk; for pesticides, the maximum amount of a residue permitted in a food. Formerly called *tolerance limit*.

Table 12–12
Ways to Reduce Pesticide Residue Intakes

In addition to these steps, remember to eat a variety of foods to minimize exposure to any one pesticide.

- Trim the fat from meat, and remove the skin from poultry and fish; discard fats and oils in broths and pan drippings. (Pesticide residues concentrate in the animal's fat.)
- Select fruits and vegetables with intact skins.
- Wash fresh produce in warm running water. Use a scrub brush, and rinse thoroughly.
- Use a knife to peel an orange or grapefruit; do not bite into the peel.
- Discard the outer leaves of leafy vegetables such as cabbage and lettuce.
- Peel waxed fruits and vegetables; waxes don't wash off and can seal in pesticide residues.
- Peel vegetables such as carrots and fruits such as apples when appropriate. (Peeling removes not only pesticides that remain in or on the peel but also fibers, vitamins, and minerals.)
- Choose organically grown foods, which generally contain fewer pesticides.

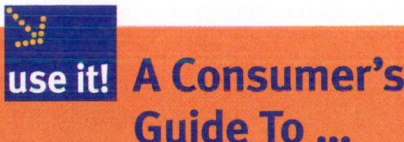

use it! A Consumer's Guide To ...

Understanding Organic Foods

LO 12.5 Compare potential advantages and drawbacks of organic and conventional foods.

Sales of certified organic foods have skyrocketed from under $4 billion in 1997 to $32.3 billion in 2013.[1]* Even at a 10 to 40 percent higher price, organic foods appeal to consumers who believe that they are buying the freshest, best-tasting, most nutrient-packed, chemical-free, non-genetically engineered foods available. Just the word *organic* conjures up positive feelings in some consumers, an effect aptly named "the halo effect."[2] When people were asked to judge two *identical* yogurts, they rated the yogurt bearing an "organic" label as more nutritious, lower in fat, more flavorful, and worth more money than a yogurt labeled "regular"—but in fact only the labels differed. The halo effect held true for identical cookies and potato chips, too—people thought those labeled "organic" were better.

Many people are also willing to pay extra for foods produced with little impact on the earth and with respect for

*Reference notes are in Appendix F.

animals. Are they getting what they are paying for?

Organic Rules

A U.S. farmer or manufacturer selling *certified organic* food must pass USDA inspections at every step of production, from the seed sown in the ground, through the making of compost for fertilizer, to the manufacturing and labeling of the final product. Figure 12–9 describes the meanings of organic food labels. In contrast, foods labeled with "natural," "free-range," "locally grown," or other wholesome-*sounding* words are not held to any standards to bear out such claims.

The National Organic Program develops, implements, and administers production, handling, and labeling standards for organic agricultural products. Enforcement has proved difficult, however, and compliance problems are common. Program officials are working to solve these problems and close open loopholes.

Pesticide Residues— They're Everywhere

When tested, organic foods generally contain no pesticides or lower levels than similar, conventionally grown products.[3] Also, eating a diet of organic foods measurably reduces pesticide exposure.[4] When scientists measured a marker for pesticide exposure in the urine of thousands of people across the United States, they found that people who reported eating organic foods had the lowest levels of the marker—they had been exposed to less pesticide.

Does this mean that an organic diet is better for health than a conventional diet? No strong scientific evidence suggests that conventional foods pose excess health risks or that using organic products reduces risks.[5] The typical pesticide exposure in the United States represents an amount 10,000 times below the level at which risks begin to rise. Children are more sensitive than adults to pesticides, and their risks are

Figure 12–9

Labels on Organic Food Products

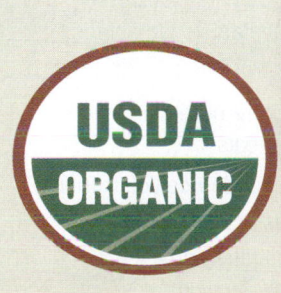
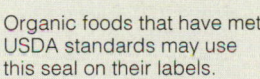
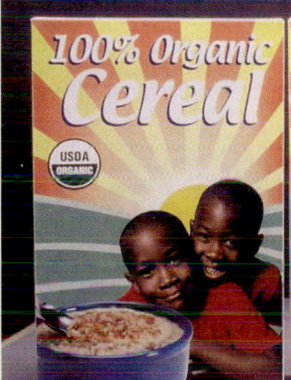
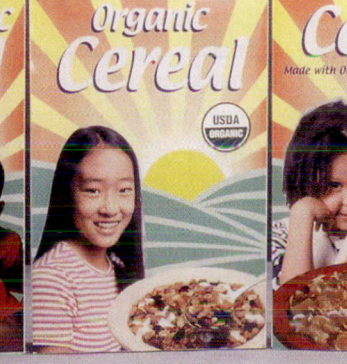

Organic foods that have met USDA standards may use this seal on their labels.

Foods made with 100 percent organic ingredients may claim "100% organic" and use the seal.

Foods made with at least 95 percent organic ingredients may claim "organic" and use the seal.

Foods made with at least 70 percent organic ingredients may list up to three of those ingredients on the front panel.

Foods made with less than 70 percent organic ingredients may list them on the side panel, but cannot make any claims on the front.

less well-defined, so parents may wish to reduce their children's exposure from all sources, including foods.[6]

To Bean or Not To Bean

A popular consumer group advocates choosing organically grown varieties of certain fruits and vegetables. Their list correctly reflects the results of federal tests for pesticide residues on produce—the foods they name test highest for one or more pesticide residues.[7] So far, so good. However, the group then goes on to urge consumers to choose organic varieties of these foods, implying that they can reduce their health risks by doing so. But this doesn't tell the whole story—the health risks from eating conventional varieties of those foods are infinitesimally small.[8]

Still, the risk from pesticide residues is not zero, and many people fear harm from unfamiliar chemicals applied to food in any amount.[9] Such worries are emotional, however, and not scientific, and they can needlessly put consumers in a bind. If people cannot afford organic foods but fear that conventional foods may harm them, they may limit the amount or variety of fruits and vegetables they take in. This choice greatly increases health risks.[10]

Nutrient Composition

Few nutrient differences exist between conventional and organic foods, and these generally fall within expected variations among food crops. Small nutrient differences occur with varying soil types, soil nutrients, seasonal rainfall, or other factors. In contrast to nutrients, organic foods may be higher in certain phytochemicals.[11] This makes sense because plants, unassisted by pesticides, muster their own phytochemical defenses to ward off insects and other dangers. Even so, organic foods appear to offer no apparent nutrition-related benefits.

The most meaningful nutrient comparisons are not between organic and conventional foods but between whole foods and heavily processed ones, a comparison made clear in the Food Feature of this chapter. Organic candy bars, soy desserts, and fried vegetable snack chips

are no more nutritious (or less fattening) than ordinary treats. Likewise, organic main dishes laden with saturated fats and sodium can throw the health-seeking consumer off course.

Environmental Benefits

Growers of organic foods use *sustainable* agricultural techniques (see Chapter 15 and Controversy 15) that minimize harm to the environment. They add composted animal manure or vegetable matter instead of the synthetic, petroleum-based fertilizers that run off into waterways and pollute them. They battle pests and diseases by using a pesticide derived from a bacterial toxin, by rotating crops each season, by introducing predatory insects to kill off pests, or by picking off large insects or diseased plant parts by hand.

Farmers and ranchers who sell organic eggs, dairy products, and meats must keep their animals in surroundings natural to their species with at least some access to the outdoors. Animals raised this way can grow large and stay healthy without growth hormones, daily antibiotics, and the other drugs that become necessary when animals are stressed in overcrowded pens. Without overcrowding, animal waste runoff, a threat to the nation's waterways, is greatly reduced, too.

Organics' Potential Pitfalls

Foods contaminated with untreated manure or feces from fertilizer, runoff, or wild animals can harbor dangerous bacteria, but such contamination is equally likely to occur in organic foods and conventional foods.[12] Proper composting of manure-based fertilizers eliminates disease-causing microbes.

Organic ingredients imported from other countries often cost less than domestic ingredients and so make attractive alternatives to dollar-conscious organic food manufacturers. However, overseas farms and producers are difficult to regulate, and although some adhere to strict standards, others are lax. Also, shipping organic ingredients over long distances violates principles of sustainability.

Moving Ahead

The practical marketplace advice, based on science, is this: buy safe, affordable conventionally grown fruits and vegetables, wash them well, and consume them with confidence. If you prefer the taste of organic fruits and vegetables, if you appreciate extra care of animals and the environment, and if you can afford them, you can choose organics with equal confidence.

If you want organic foods at bargain prices, you might ask for imperfect produce at farmer's markets. Alternatively, try growing some leafy greens, herbs, and tomatoes in pots on a sunny deck—a surprisingly simple and rewarding endeavor. Whatever your choice, choose nutritious fruits and vegetables in abundance.

Review Questions*

1. To be labeled *100% organic*, a food must _____.
   a. be inspected before it is sold
   b. contain at least 95% organic ingredients
   c. be labeled "natural" or "free range"
   d. contain only 100% organic ingredients

2. The risk to health from pesticides in foods is exceedingly small.   T   F

3. Organic candy bars, soy desserts, and fried vegetable snack chips _____.
   a. are not more nutritious than ordinary treats
   b. are superior sources of nutrients for children
   c. are a less-fattening alternative to nonorganic snack foods
   d. can provide an adequate daily intake of important organic minerals

*Answers to Consumer's Guide review questions are found in Appendix G.

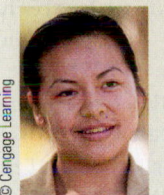
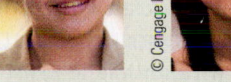
that still causes *no adverse health effects* in laboratory animals.[28] If a pesticide is misused, growers risk fines, lawsuits, and destruction of their crops.

While the EPA sets limits, both the USDA and the FDA occasionally test crop and food product samples for compliance. Over decades of testing, seldom have these agencies found residues above approved limits. This makes sense because growers are not anxious to squander capital on unneeded chemicals.

Pesticide-Resistant Insects   Ironically, some pesticides also promote the survival of the very pests they are intended to wipe out. A pesticide aimed at certain insects may kill almost 100 percent of them, but because of the genetic variability of large populations, a few hardy individuals survive exposure. These resistant insects then multiply free of competition and soon produce offspring with inherited pesticide resistance that attack the crop with enhanced vigor. Controlling resistant insects requires application of different pesticides, which leads to the emergence of a population of insects that survive multiple pesticides. The same biological sequences occur when herbicides and fungicides are repeatedly applied to weeds and fungal pests. One alternative to this destructive series of events is to manage pests using a combination of improved farming techniques and biological controls, as discussed in Controversy 15.

Natural Pesticides   Pesticides are not produced only in laboratories; they also occur in nature. The nicotine in tobacco and phytochemicals of celery are examples.*** Another is known as Bt pesticide, an insecticidal peptide made by a common soil bacterium. (*Peptide* refers to bonds that join amino acids—see Chapter 6.) This pesticide is extracted and sprayed on organic farm crops and **organic gardens**; it is also produced in the tissues of genetically engineered crops (see the Controversy section). Peptide pesticides leave less **persistent** residues in the environment than most others. An ideal pesticide would destroy pests in the field but vanish before consumers ate the food.

KEY POINTS

- Pesticides can be part of a safe food production process but can also be hazardous if mishandled.
- Consumers can take steps to minimize their ingestion of pesticide residues in foods.

Animal Drugs—What Are the Risks?

Consumers often worry about consuming meats that may contain hormones, antibiotics, and drugs that contain **arsenic** compounds. However, the most pressing concern to the world's scientists is the emergence and rapid spread of bacterial strains that no longer respond to antibiotic drugs.[29]

***The celery plant produces psoralens that repel insects.

organic gardens gardens grown with techniques of *sustainable agriculture*, such as using fertilizers made from composts and introducing predatory insects to control pests, in ways that have minimal impact on soil, water, and air quality.

persistent of a stubborn or enduring nature; with respect to food contaminants, the quality of remaining unaltered and unexcreted in plant foods or in the bodies of animals and human beings.

arsenic a poisonous metallic element. In trace amounts, arsenic is believed to be an essential nutrient in some animal species. Arsenic is often added to insecticides and weed killers and, in tiny amounts, to certain animal drugs.

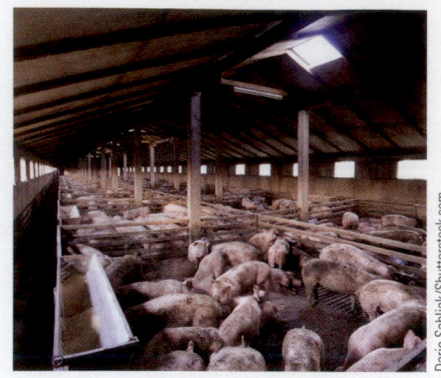
Overcrowding of farm animals makes infection likely.

Dario Sabljak/Shutterstock.com

Livestock and Antibiotic-Resistant Microbes

For a half-century, ranchers and farmers have dosed livestock with antibiotic drugs as part of a daily feeding regimen to ward off infections common in animals living in crowded conditions. These drugs also speed up animal growth and increase feed efficiency. When bacteria too frequently encounter antibiotics, they adapt, losing their sensitivity to the drugs over time.[30] The resulting **antibiotic-resistant bacteria** cause severe infections that do not yield to standard antibiotic therapy, often ending in fatality.

A substantial threat to human health and life arises from antibiotic-resistant bacteria. A limited number of antibiotic drugs exist—the same or related drugs used daily in livestock are also of critical importance for treating illnesses in people. Few treatment options remain for people who become infected with antibiotic-resistant bacteria. So long as antibiotics are overused in animals and people, new resistant strains can be expected to emerge, and once here, they tend to stay.

Federal voluntary guidelines urge farmers to use antibiotics only under veterinary care and only to prevent, control, or treat diseases, but these protections are not mandatory, so no one can predict their effectiveness. One day, new drugs and vaccines now under development may reduce the need for antibiotics in food animals, but progress is slow.[31] Meanwhile, unrestrained global use of antibiotics in livestock threatens to undo a true medical miracle.[32]

Growth Hormone in Meat and Milk

> Genetic engineering of bacteria and food products is discussed in **Controversy 12**.

Cattle producers in the United States commonly inject their herds with a form of **growth hormone—recombinant bovine somatotropin (rbST)**—to increase lean tissue growth, increase milk production, and reduce feed requirements. The hormone, produced by genetically altered bacteria, is identical to growth hormone made in the pituitary gland of the animal's brain. The FDA and WHO deem the use of the drug to be safe, and the FDA does not require testing of food products for traces of it.

Ranchers advocate the use of rbST because more meat and milk on less feed means higher profits. The environment may profit as well. Smaller herds that eat sparingly require less cleared land and fewer resources to produce and transport their feed. Tests of conventional milk, hormone-free milk, and organic milk reveal no differences in terms of antibiotic, bacteria, hormone, or nutrient contents.

Arsenic in Food

Arsenic, a naturally occurring element from the earth's crust and an infamous poison, is administered in tiny amounts to poultry flocks to kill parasites that would otherwise stall their growth. Arsenic thus builds up in poultry meat, wastes, and feathers.[33] This and other human activity add to the natural arsenic content of water and soil, and ultimately increase the arsenic in the food supply.

Foods such as rice and apple juice—even organic apple juice—contain small amounts of arsenic. For apple juice, the FDA is confident in its safety for people who consume normal amounts and vary their choices.[34] No immediate threat exists, but the FDA is investigating the potential for long-term consequences of current levels of consumption.[35] People with gluten sensitivities, especially children, often have unusually high intakes of rice, one of the few gluten-free grains. Some groups are calling for arsenic values to be revealed on labels of rice-based staple foods, such as gluten-free breads and baked goods, cereals, pastas, and rice "milk."[36] Other sources of arsenic include fish and shellfish, eggs, milk products, and drinking water.

antibiotic-resistant bacteria bacterial strains that cause increasingly common and potentially fatal infectious diseases that do not respond to standard antibiotic therapy. An example is MRSA (pronounced MER-suh), a multidrug-resistant *Staphyloccocus aureus* bacterium.

growth hormone a hormone (somatotropin) that promotes growth and that is produced naturally in the pituitary gland of the brain.

recombinant bovine somatotropin (so-mat-oh-TROPE-in) **(rbST)** growth hormone of cattle, which can be produced for agricultural use by way of genetic engineering. A *recombinant* protein arises from genetically engineered DNA (see Controversy 12). Also called *bovine growth hormone (bGH)*.

KEY POINTS

- FDA-approved hormones, antibiotics, and other drugs are used to promote growth or increase milk production in conventionally grown animals.
- Antibiotic-resistant bacteria pose a serious and growing threat.

Figure 12–10

Bioaccumulation of Toxins in the Food Chain

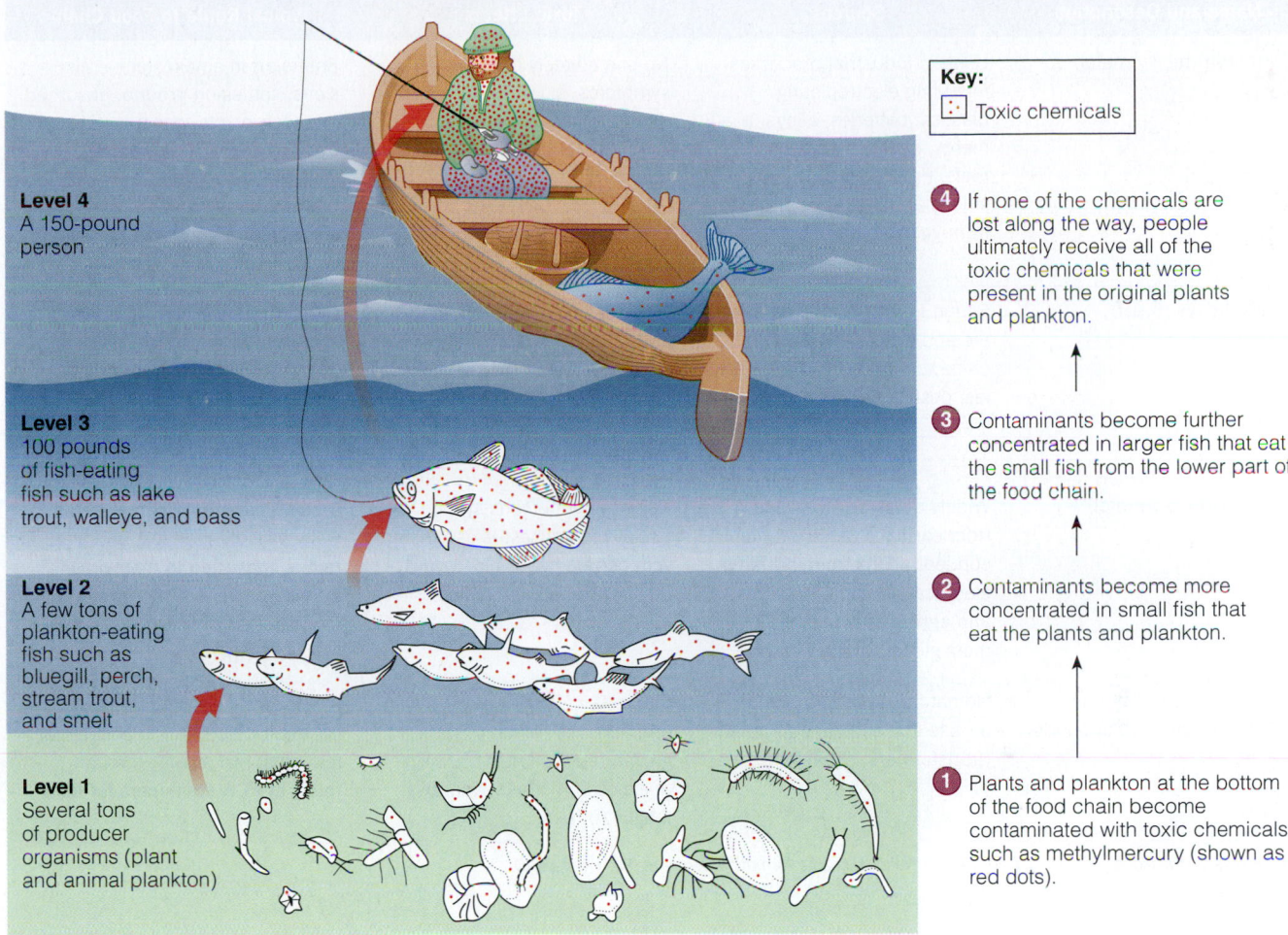

Key:
⬚ Toxic chemicals

Level 4
A 150-pound person

Level 3
100 pounds of fish-eating fish such as lake trout, walleye, and bass

Level 2
A few tons of plankton-eating fish such as bluegill, perch, stream trout, and smelt

Level 1
Several tons of producer organisms (plant and animal plankton)

④ If none of the chemicals are lost along the way, people ultimately receive all of the toxic chemicals that were present in the original plants and plankton.

③ Contaminants become further concentrated in larger fish that eat the small fish from the lower part of the food chain.

② Contaminants become more concentrated in small fish that eat the plants and plankton.

① Plants and plankton at the bottom of the food chain become contaminated with toxic chemicals, such as methylmercury (shown as red dots).

Environmental Contaminants

As world populations increase and become more industrialized, concerns grow about contamination of foods. A **food contaminant** is anything in food that does not belong there.

Harmfulness of Contaminants The potential for harm from a contaminant depends partly on how long it lingers in the environment or in the human body—that is, on how *persistent* it is. Some contaminants are short-lived because microorganisms, sunlight, or oxygen breaks them down. Some contaminants stay in the body for only a short time because the body rapidly excretes or destroys them. Such contaminants present little cause for concern.

Other contaminants linger and resist environmental breakdown, and they interact with the body's systems without being metabolized or excreted. These contaminants can pass from one species to the next and accumulate at higher concentrations in each level of the food chain, a process called **bioaccumulation**—see Figure 12–10.

The toxic effect of a chemical depends largely on two factors: the degree of the chemical's **toxicity** and the degree of human exposure. In small enough amounts, even poisonous substances may be tolerable and of no consequence to health; in larger amounts, even innocuous substances may be dangerous. An old saying, "The dose makes the poison," means that with a large enough dose, normally benign substances, even sand, can kill a person. The reverse is also true: even poisons can be benign in miniscule doses.

food contaminant any substance occurring in food by accident; any food constituent that is not normally present.

bioaccumulation the accumulation of a contaminant in the tissues of living things at higher and higher concentrations along the food chain.

toxicity the ability of a substance to harm living organisms. All substances, even pure water or oxygen, can be toxic in high enough doses.

Table 12–13

Examples of Contaminants in Foods

Name and Description	Sources	Toxic Effects	Typical Route to Food Chain
Cadmium (heavy metal)	Used in industrial processes including electroplating, plastics, batteries, alloys, pigments, smelters, and burning fuels. Present in cigarette smoke and in smoke and ash from volcanic eruptions.	No immediately detectable symptoms; slowly and irreversibly damages kidneys and liver.	Enters air in smokestack emissions, settles on ground, absorbed into food plants, consumed by farm animals, and eaten in vegetables and meat by people. Sewage sludge and fertilizers leave large amounts in soil; runoff contaminates shellfish.
Lead^a (heavy metal)	Found in lead crystal decanters and glassware, painted china, old house paint, batteries, pesticides, old plumbing.	Displaces calcium, iron, zinc, and other minerals from their sites of action in the nervous system, bone marrow, kidneys, and liver, causing failure of function.	Originates from industrial plants and pollutes air, water, and soil. Still present in soil from many years of leaded gasoline use.
Mercury (heavy metal)	Widely dispersed in gases from earth's crust; local high concentrations from industry, electrical equipment, paints, and agriculture; present in most global fishing waters.	Poisons the nervous system, especially in fetuses. Is associated with certain heart, blood, and other tissue abnormalities.	Inorganic mercury is released into waterways by industry, and acid rain is converted to methylmercury by bacteria and ingested by food species of fish (tuna, swordfish, and others).
Polychlorinated biphenyls (PCBs) (organic compounds)	No natural source; produced for use in electrical equipment (transformers, capacitors).	Causes long-lasting skin eruptions, eye irritations, growth retardation in children of exposed mothers, anorexia, fatigue, others.	Is released from discarded electrical equipment, during accidental industrial leakage, or through reuse of PCB containers for food.

^aFor answers to questions concerning lead, call the National Lead Information Center at (800) 424-LEAD.

How much of a threat do environmental contaminants pose to the food supply? It depends on the contaminant. In general, the threat remains small because the FDA monitors contaminants in foods and issues warnings when food contamination is evident. Table 12–13 describes a few contaminants of greatest concern in foods.

Mercury in Seafood   Mercury, **PCBs**, and other hazardous substances are often detected in food fish species worldwide, but the **heavy metal** mercury is of special concern. Scientists learned of mercury's potential for harm through tragedy. In the mid-20th century, more than 120 people, including 23 infants, in Minamata, Japan, became ill with a strange disease. Mortality was high, and the survivors suffered progressive, irreversible blindness, deafness, loss of coordination, and severe mental and physical retardation.[†††]

Finally, the cause of this misery was discovered: manufacturing plants in the region were discharging mercury into the waters of the bay, where aquatic bacteria metabolized it into the nerve poison methylmercury.[37] The fish in the bay were accumulating the poison in their bodies, and townspeople who regularly ate fish from the bay fell ill. The infants had not eaten any fish, but their mothers had during their pregnancies; the mothers were spared because the poison concentrates in the tissues of the fetus.

Today, in the United States, scientists warn that methylmercury concentrations in our nation's ocean and freshwater fisheries, and also in some popular food fish

PCBs (polychlorinated biphenyls) stable oily synthetic chemicals, once used in hundreds of U.S. industrial operations, that persist today in underwater sediments and contaminate fish and shellfish. Now banned from use in the United States, PCBs circulate globally from areas where they are still in use. PCBs cause cancer, nervous system damage, immune dysfunction, and a number of other serious health effects.

heavy metal any of a number of mineral ions such as mercury and lead, so called because they are of relatively high atomic weight; many heavy metals are poisonous.

[†††] Minamata disease was named for the location of the disaster.

species, are unacceptably high and growing higher by the year.[38] The FDA advises all pregnant women, women who may become pregnant, nursing mothers, and young children to avoid certain marine fish species known to be high in methylmercury (Chapter 5 weighs the benefits of eating seafood against the risks).

No one expects the tragic results of the 1950s to occur again, but efforts to lower methylmercury in global fisheries are needed to help protect these valuable and imperiled resources. Methylmercury is persistent in the environment, so today's efforts to reduce pollution of ocean, lake, and river waters will take years to be effective.

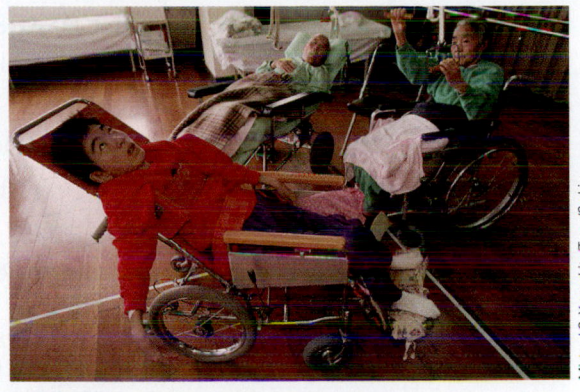

Minimata disease. The effects of mercury contamination can be severe.

KEY POINTS

- Persistent environmental contaminants present in food pose a small but significant risk to U.S. consumers.
- Mercury and other contaminants pose the greatest threat during pregnancy, lactation, and childhood.

Are Food Additives Safe?

LO 12.6 Discuss the uses and safety of food additives.

Many foods contain **additives**, and consumers rightly want to know why they are there and if they are safe to consume. On the FDA's list of food worries, food additives rank low. Thousands of food additives are approved for use in the United States, and most are strictly controlled and well studied for safety. Some common classes of additives and their functions in foods are listed in Table 12–14.

additives substances that are added to foods but are not normally consumed by themselves as foods.

Table 12–14

Selected Food Additives and Their Functions

Agent Type	Function in Foods	Examples
Antimicrobial agents (preservatives)	Prevent food spoilage by mold or bacterial growth.	Acetic acid (vinegar), benzoic acid, nitrates and nitrites, propionic acid, salt, sugar, sorbic acid.
Antioxidants (preservatives)	Prevent oxidative changes and delay rancidity of fats; prevent browning of fruit and vegetable products.	BHA, BHT, propyl gallate, sulfites, vitamin C, vitamin E.
Artificial colors	Add color to foods.	Certified food colors such as dyes from vegetables (beet juice or beta-carotene) or synthetic dyes (tartrazine and others).
Artificial flavors, flavor enhancers	Add flavors; boost natural flavors of foods.	Amyl acetate (artificial banana flavor), artificial sweeteners, MSG (monosodium glutamate), salt, spices, sugars.
Bleaching agents	Whiten foods such as flour or cheese.	Peroxides.
Chelating (KEE-late-ing) agents (preservatives)	Prevent discoloration, off flavors, and rancidity.	Citric acid, malic acid, tartaric acid (cream of tartar).
Nutrient additives	Improve nutritional value.	Vitamins and minerals.
Stabilizing and thickening agents	Maintain emulsion, foams, or suspensions or lend a desirable thick consistency to foods.	Dextrins (short glucose chains), pectin, starch, or gums such as agar, carrageenan, guar, and locust bean.

Regulations Governing Additives

Before using a new additive in food products, a manufacturer must test the additive and satisfy the FDA that:

- It is effective (it does what it is supposed to do).

- It can be detected and measured in the final food product.

Then the manufacturer must provide proof that it is safe (causes no birth defects or other injuries) when fed in large doses to experimental animals.[39] This formal process may take several years. Then manufacturers must comply with a host of other regulations that ensure the proper use and application of the additive as well. For example, additives may *not* be used in any application where they disguise faulty or inferior products, or deceive consumers, or significantly destroy nutrients in foods.

The GRAS List

Many additives are exempted from complying with the procedures just described because they have been used for a long time and their use entails no known hazards. More and more additives are being submitted to the FDA for inclusion on the **generally recognized as safe (GRAS) list**.[40] No additives are permanently approved, however; all are periodically reviewed as new facts emerge.

The Margin of Safety

An important distinction between toxicity and hazard arises during evaluation of an additive's safety. Toxicity is a general property of all substances; hazard is the capacity of a substance to produce injury *under conditions of its use*.[‡‡‡] As mentioned, all substances can be toxic at some level of consumption, but they are called hazardous only if they are toxic in the amounts ordinarily consumed. To determine risk, experimenters feed test animals the substance at different concentrations throughout their lifetimes.

An approved food additive has a wide **margin of safety**. Most additives that involve risk are allowed in foods only at concentrations at least 100 times lower than the highest concentration at which the risk is still zero (1/100). Some *natural* toxins produced in food by plants occur at levels that bring their margins of safety close to 1/10. For some trace elements, it is about 1/5. People commonly consume table salt in daily amounts only three to five times less than those that cause serious toxicity.

Risks and Benefits of Food Additives

Most additives used in foods offer benefits that may outweigh their risks or that may make the risks worth taking. In the case of color additives that only enhance the appearance of foods without improving their health value or safety, no amount of risk may be deemed worth taking. In contrast, the FDA finds it worth taking a small, uncertain risk associated with nitrites on processed meats because nitrites are proven to inhibit harmful bacterial growth in these foods.

KEY POINTS

- Food additives must be safe, effective, and measurable in the final product for FDA approval.
- Approved additives have wide margins of safety.

Additives to Improve Safety and Quality

Some additives improve food safety. They restrict bacterial growth or otherwise enhance food quality in ways many people take for granted.

Salt and Sugar

Since before the dawn of history, salt has been used to preserve meat and fish; sugar, a relative newcomer to the food supply, serves the same purpose in jams, jellies, and canned and frozen fruits. Both salt and sugar work by withdrawing water from the food; microbes cannot grow without sufficient moisture. Safety questions surrounding these two preservatives center on their overuse as flavoring agents—salt and sugar make foods taste delicious and are often added with a liberal hand. Chapters 4 and 8 provided detailed discussions of these issues.

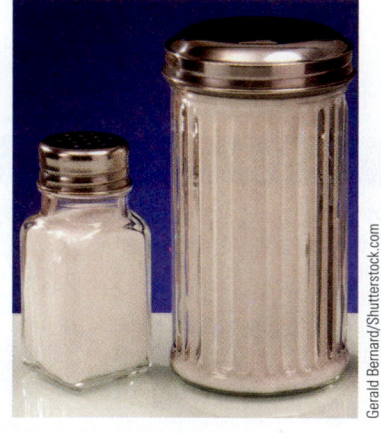

Salt and sugar: two long-used preservatives.

Gerald Bernard/Shutterstock.com

generally recognized as safe (GRAS) list a list, established by the FDA, of food additives long in use and believed to be safe.

margin of safety in reference to food additives, a zone between the concentration normally used and that at which a hazard exists. For common table salt, for example, the margin of safety is 1/5 (five times the amount normally used would be hazardous).

---

‡‡‡ The Delaney Clause, a legal requirement of zero cancer risk for additives, is no longer universally applied.

Nitrites The *nitrites* added to meats and meat products help to preserve their color (especially the pink color of hot dogs and other cured meats) and to inhibit rancidity and thwart bacterial growth. In particular, nitrites prevent the growth of the deadly *Clostridium botulinum* bacterium. Even though nitrites are useful, they raise safety issues. Once in the stomach, nitrites can be converted to nitrosamines, chemicals linked with colon cancer in animals. Other nitrite sources, such as tobacco and beer, may be more significant sources of nitrosamine-related compounds than foods. Still, processed meats are associated with an elevated risk of colon cancer, so the cautious consumer limits intakes of these foods.[41]

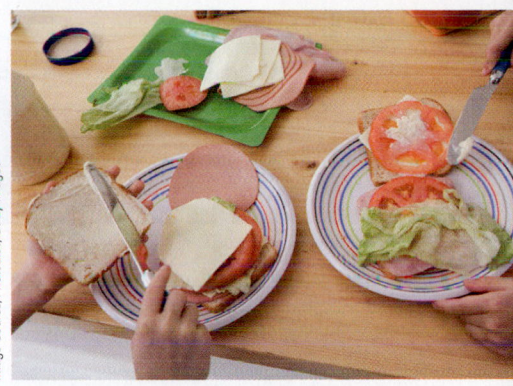

Without additives, bread would quickly mold and salad dressing would go rancid.

Sulfites Sulfites prevent oxidation in many processed foods, in alcoholic beverages (especially wine), and in drugs. Some people experience dangerous allergic reactions to the sulfites, so their use is strictly controlled. The FDA prohibits sulfite use on food meant to be eaten raw (fresh grapes are an exception), and it requires foods and drugs to list on their labels any sulfites that are present. For most people, sulfites do not pose a hazard in the amounts used in products, but they have one other drawback. Because sulfites can destroy a lot of thiamin in foods, you can't count on a food that contains sulfites to contribute to your daily thiamin intake.

> Use of nonnutritive sweeteners in weight control is a topic of **Chapter 9.**

Use of nonnutritive sweeteners in weight control is a topic of **Chapter 9.**

KEY POINTS

- Sugar and salt have the longest history of use as additives to prevent food spoilage.
- Nitrites and sulfites have advantages and drawbacks.

Flavoring Agents

Many additives add desirable flavors to foods. One group, the **nonnutritive sweeteners**, may be added by manufacturers or by consumers at home.

Nonnutritive Sweeteners Nonnutritive sweeteners make foods taste sweet without promoting dental decay or providing the empty calories of sugar. The human taste buds perceive many of them as supersweet, so just tiny amounts are added to foods and beverages to achieve the desired sweet taste.[42] The FDA endorses the use of nonnutritive sweeteners as safe over a lifetime when used within **acceptable daily intake (ADI)** levels. Table 12–15 (p. 502), provides some details about the nonnutritive sweeteners, including ADI levels.

Through the years, questions have emerged about the safety of nonnutritive sweeteners, particularly saccharin and aspartame. For example, early research indicated that large quantities of saccharin caused bladder tumors in laboratory animals, but these issues have since been resolved.

Currently, researchers are investigating links among saccharin intakes, microbial communities in the intestine, and type 2 diabetes.[43] When researchers fed saccharin or glucose to mice, they noted that the saccharin group had developed glucose intolerance—impaired glucose regulation in the body. To test whether the microbiota might be involved, they dosed some of the glucose-intolerant mice with antibiotics, wiping out their intestinal bacteria; these mice regained their glucose tolerance in just a few days. For further evidence, the researchers inoculated a new group of mice with the gut bacteria harvested from the glucose-intolerant saccharin mice. As predicted, the new group also became glucose-intolerant. More research is needed to confirm or refute these findings.

Aspartame, a sweetener made from two amino acids (phenylalanine and aspartic acid) is one of the most thoroughly studied food additives ever approved by FDA. Evidence linking aspartame with chronic diseases is weak or nonexistent, and a recent up-to-date evaluation of the body's biochemical milieu, along with other physical and psychological testing, yielded no evidence of acute adverse physical or psychological effects.[44] However, aspartame's phenylalanine base poses a threat to those with the inherited disease phenylketonuria (PKU), a disease that, without

nonnutritive sweeteners sweet-tasting synthetic or natural food additives that offer sweet flavor but with negligible or no calories per serving; also called *artificial sweeteners, intense sweeteners, noncaloric sweeteners,* and *very low-calorie sweeteners.* Also defined in Chapter 4.

acceptable daily intake (ADI) the estimated amount of a sweetener that can be consumed daily over a person's lifetime without any adverse effects.

Table 12-15

U.S.-Approved Nonnutritive Sweeteners

Sweetener	Chemical Composition	Digestion/ Absorption	Sweetness Relative to Sucrose[a]	Energy (cal/g)	Acceptable Daily Intake (ADI) and Estimated Equivalent[b]	Approved Uses
Acesulfame potassium or acesulfame-K (Sunette, Sweet One)	Potassium salt	Not digested or absorbed	200	0	15 mg/kg body weight[c] (30 cans diet soda)	General use, except in meat and poultry; tabletop sweeteners; heat stable
Advantame	Aspartame derivative, similar to neotame	Rapidly digested; poorly absorbed	20,000	0	32.8 mg/kg body weight (4,000 packets of sweetener)	General use, except in meat and poultry; heat stable at baking temperatures
Aspartame (NutraSweet, Equal, others)	Amino acids (phenylalanine and aspartic acid) and a methyl group	Digested and absorbed	180	4[d]	50 mg/kg body weight[e] (18 cans diet soda)	General use in all foods and beverages; warning to population with PKU; degrades when heated
Luo han guo	Glycosides extracts from monk fruit	Digested and absorbed	150–300	1	No ADI determined	GRAS[f]; general use as a food ingredient and tabletop sweetener
Neotame	Aspartame with an additional side group attached	Not digested or absorbed	7,000	0	18 mg/day	General use, except in meat and poultry
Saccharin (SugarTwin, Sweet'N Low, others)	Benzoic sulfimide	Rapidly absorbed and excreted	300	0	5 mg/kg body weight (10 packets of sweetener)	Tabletop sweeteners, wide range of foods, beverages, cosmetics, and pharmaceutical products
Stevia (Sweetleaf, Truvia, PurVia)	Glycosides extracted from the leaves of the stevia herb	Digested and absorbed	200–300	0	4 mg/kg body weight	GRAS[f]; tabletop sweeteners, a variety of foods and beverages
Sucralose (Splenda)	Sucrose with Cl atoms instead of OH groups	Not digested or absorbed	600	0	5 mg/kg body weight (6 cans diet soda)	Baked goods, carbonated beverages, chewing gum, coffee and tea, dairy products, frozen desserts, fruit spreads, salad dressing, syrups, tabletop sweeteners
Tagatose[g] (Nutralose, Nutrilatose, Tagatesse)	Monosaccharide similar in structure to fructose; naturally occurring or derived from lactose	Not well absorbed	0.9	1.5	7.5 g/day	GRAS[f]; bakery products, beverages, cereals, chewing gum, confections, dairy products, dietary supplements, energy bars, tabletop sweeteners

[a]Relative sweetness is determined by comparing the approximate sweetness of a sugar substitute with the sweetness of pure sucrose, which has been defined as 1.0. Chemical structure, temperature, acidity, and other flavors of the foods in which the substance occurs all influence relative sweetness.

[b]Based on a person weighing 70 kg (154 lb).

[c]Recommendations from the World Health Organization limit acesulfame-K intake to 9 mg/kg of body weight per day.

[d]Aspartame provides 4 cal/g, as does protein, but because so little is used, its energy contribution is negligible. In powdered form, it is sometimes mixed with lactose, however, so a 1-g packet may provide 4 cal.

[e]Recommendations from the World Health Organization and in Europe and Canada limit aspartame intake to 40 mg/kg of body weight per day.

[f]Generally recognized as safe. For stevia, one of its extracts (but not other forms) has GRAS status.

[g]Tagatose is a poorly digested sugar and technically not a nonnutritive sweetener.

Figure 12–11

Nonnutritive Sweeteners on Food Labels

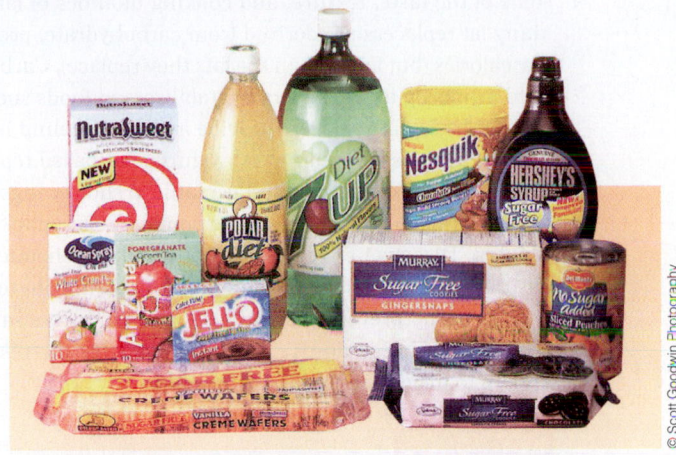

This partial ingredient list is for a sugar-free food.

Products containing aspartame must carry a warning for people with phenylketonuria.

INGREDIENTS: ARTIFICIAL AND NATURAL FLAVORING, TITANIUM DIOXIDE (COLOR), ASPARTAME, ACESULFAME POTASSIUM, STEVIA. **PHENYLKETONURICS: CONTAINS PHENYLALANINE.**

Nutrition Facts	Amount per serving	% DV*
	Total Fat 0g	0%
	Sodium 0mg	0%
Serving Size 8 oz	**Total Carb.** 0g	0%
Servings 6	Sugars 0g	
Calories 0	**Protein** 0g	
*Percent Daily Values (DV) are based on a 2,000 calorie diet.	Not a significant source of other nutrients.	

Products containing less than 0.5 g of sugar per serving can claim to be "sugarless" or "sugar-free."

a low phenylalanine diet, can damage the developing brain in children. Food labels warn people with PKU of the extra phenylalanine in aspartame-sweetened foods (see Figure 12–11). In any case, artificially sweetened foods and drinks have no place in the diets of infants or toddlers. People who believe a sweetener causes symptoms should use a different sweetener.

Monosodium Glutamate (MSG)   MSG, the sodium salt of the amino acid glutamic acid, is used widely in restaurants, especially Asian restaurants.[§§§] In addition to enhancing other flavors, MSG itself presents a basic taste (termed *umami*) independent of the well-known sweet, salty, bitter, and sour tastes.

In a few sensitive individuals, MSG produces adverse reactions known as the **MSG symptom complex**. Plain broth with MSG seems most likely to bring on symptoms in sensitive people, whereas carbohydrate-rich foods, such as rice or noodles, seem to protect against them. Deemed safe for adults, MSG is prohibited in baby foods because huge doses destroy brain cells in developing mice and monkeys.[45] Human brains are thought to be resistant to such effects, however. MSG may even help to protect the brain from the effects of a toxic drug used to treat cancers, and may also increase satiety during a meal.[46] The FDA requires that food labels disclose each additive, including MSG, by its full name.

§§§The MSG trade name is Accent.

MSG symptom complex the acute, temporary, and self-limiting reactions, including burning sensations or flushing of the skin with pain and headache, experienced by sensitive people upon ingesting a large dose of MSG. Formerly called *Chinese restaurant syndrome*.

Fat Replacers and Artificial Fats

Fat replacers and artificial fats, introduced in Chapter 5, are ingredients that provide some of the taste, texture, and cooking qualities of fats but with fewer or no calories. Many fat replacers are derived from carbohydrate, protein, or fat, and these provide a few calories (but fewer than the fats they replace). Carbohydrate-based fat replacers are used primarily as thickeners or stabilizers in foods such as soups and salad dressings. Protein-based fat replacers provide a creamy feeling in the mouth and are often used in foods such as ice creams and yogurts. Fat-based replacers act as emulsifiers and are heat stable, making them most versatile in shortenings used in cake mixes and cookies.

An artificial fat used to make some low-fat snack foods, such as potato chips, is **olestra**. Digestive enzymes cannot break its chemical bonds, so olestra cannot be absorbed. Olestra binds fat-soluble vitamins and phytochemicals, causing their excretion; to partly prevent these losses, manufacturers saturate olestra with vitamins A, D, E, and K. Large doses can cause digestive distress, but no serious problems are known to have occurred with normal use.

> **KEY POINTS**
> - Fat replacers and artificial fats reduce the fat calories in processed foods.
> - Olestra in large amounts can cause digestive distress.

Incidental Food Additives

Consumers are often unaware that many substances can migrate into food during production, processing, storage, packaging, or consumer preparation. These substances, although called indirect or **incidental additives**, are really contaminants because no one intentionally adds them to foods. Examples of incidental additives include compounds released from plastics; tiny bits of glass, paper, metal, and the like from packages; or unavoidable filth, such as tiny amounts of rodent hairs or insect fragments. Incidental additives are well regulated, and once discovered in food, their safety must be confirmed by strict procedures like those governing intentional additives.

BPA   The incidental additive BPA migrate into many foods and beverages from plastic-lined food cans, soft-drink cans, baby formula containers, and certain clear, hard plastic water bottles.**** Manufacturers have replaced BPA in baby bottles, toddler "sippy" cups, and infant formula packaging because some studies raised questions about potential risks. However, BPA replacements have produced similar health problems in laboratory animals.[47]

BPA is rapidly broken down by the human body, and exposures are far lower than once feared, so the FDA generally supports its safety but is continuing to investigate its effects.[48] If you should wish to limit exposure to BPA, avoid hard, clear plastic reusable water bottles stamped with recycle code 3 or 7. In addition:

- Do not use hard, clear plastic containers for very hot foods or beverages, do not wash them in the dishwasher, and do not heat them in the microwave because heat releases BPA from plastics.

- Discard scratched hard plastic bottles, which can harbor bacteria and also release BPA.

Microwave Packages   Some microwave products are sold in "active packaging" that participates in cooking the food. Pizza, for example, may rest on a cardboard pan coated with a thin film of metal that absorbs microwave energy and may heat up to 500°F (260°C). During the intense heat, some particles of the packaging components migrate into the food. This is expected; the particles have been tested for safety.

In contrast, incidental additives from plastic packages may not be entirely safe for consumption. To avoid them, do not reuse disposable plastic margarine tubs or

---

olestra a nonnutritive artificial fat made from sucrose and fatty acids; also called *sucrose polyester*; trade name, *Olean*.

incidental additives substances that can get into food not through intentional introduction but as a result of contact with the food during growing, processing, packaging, storing, or some other stage before the food is consumed. Also called *accidental* or *indirect additives*.

****BPA is an abbreviation of bisphenol A, a plastic hardener and component of epoxy resin.

single-use trays from microwavable meals for microwaving other foods. Use glass or ceramic containers or plastic ones labeled as safe for the microwave. In addition, wrap foods in microwave-safe plastic wraps, waxed paper, cooking bags, parchment paper, or white microwave-safe paper towels instead of ordinary plastic wraps before microwave cooking.

KEY POINTS

- Incidental additives enter food during processing and are regulated; most do not constitute a hazard.
- Consumers should use only microwave-safe containers and wraps for microwaving food.

Conclusion

To sum up the messages of this chapter, the ample U.S. food supply is largely safe, and hazards are rare. Foodborne microbial illnesses pose the greatest threat by far, and an urgent need exists for new preventive technologies and procedures, along with greater consumer awareness. The Food Feature that follows explores the effects of certain food-processing techniques on nutrients in foods.

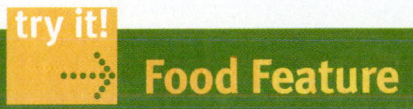

try it!

Food Feature

Processing and the Nutrients in Foods

LO 12.7 Explain how food-processing techniques affect the nutrients in foods.

Nutritionists know that the terms *processed foods* and *junk foods* are not synonymous.[49] Enriched processed foods provide important nutrients that may otherwise be lacking from the U.S. diet, such as calcium, iron, folate, and vitamin D. Processing also makes the food supply safer and more convenient. Thanks to commercial processing, few people in this country must spend their days grinding grains for bread, separating curds from whey to make cheese, or curing ham before making a sandwich.

It is also true, however, that in general terms, the more heavily processed a food, the less nutritious it may be. Heavily processed foods contribute much of the sodium, sugar, saturated fats, and calories found in the U.S. diet. In short, the nutrient value of a processed food depends on the food and the process (Table 12–16 (p. 506) provides examples). Consider the case of orange juice choices and vitamin C.

Choosing Your Juice

Orange juice is available in several forms, each processed in a different way.

- *Fresh squeezed, not from concentrate.* Juice extracted from the fibrous structures of whole oranges is quickly packaged, pasteurized, and refrigerated. These processes make it easy to consume the nutrients and calories of several oranges in a cupful of juice. (8 ounces provides 120 milligrams of vitamin C and 110 calories.)
- *Made from concentrate.* Fluid juice is condensed by heat and pressure, and frozen to be reconstituted later by adding water. Once reconstituted, it can be packaged in cartons and refrigerated. Alternatively, the concentrate may be purchased frozen for reconstituting at home. (8 ounces of reconstituted juice provides 97 milligrams of vitamin C and 110 calories; some vitamin C is destroyed during condensing.)

- *Canned 100% orange juice (not refrigerated).* Fluid juice, most often reconstituted, is treated with sterilizing heat during canning. (8 ounces provides 75 milligrams of vitamin C and 110 calories.)

The numbers in these comparisons seem to indicate that fresh juice is the superior food, but consider this: any of these choices meets or comes close to meeting most people's entire daily need for vitamin C (75 milligrams for women or 90 milligrams for men). Thus, for vitamin C, processing causes negligible nutrient loss, but confers enormous convenience, distribution, and consumer price advantages.

Fresh oranges and fresh-squeezed juice, and in fact all fresh fruits and vegetables, contain active enzymes that continue to break down nutrients and cause significant vitamin losses over time. Canning and concentrating juice require heat that destroys enzymes,

Table 12–16

Effects of Food Processing on Nutrients

Processes affect nutrients by milling or separating food parts; by exposing food to air, light, or heat; or by changing food pH.

Process	Method and Purpose	Typical Foods	Effects on Nutrients
Canning	Boil food to sterilize it and seal it in an impervious can or jar to preserve it.	Fruit, fruit preserves, prepared foods such as soups or pasta dishes, vegetables, and meats.	Prolonged high-temperature heating causes substantial losses of water-soluble vitamins, particularly thiamin and riboflavin; other water-soluble vitamins are dissolved in canning liquid.
Drying	Dehydrate food to eliminate the water that microbes require for growth.	Fruit, vegetables, meats.	Commercial drying (especially freeze-drying) leaves most nutrients intact; home drying may destroy substantial vitamin content due to heat and air exposure; thiamin may be lost in foods treated with sulfur dioxide.
Extruding	Grind, heat, and blend foods with color and flavor additives and push the resulting paste through screens to form various shapes.	Grains or soybeans, particularly as cereals, bacon-like salad toppings, or snack foods in the form of puffs, crisps, or bits.	Loss of food parts and exposure to heat, light, and air cause considerable nutrient losses, notably all vitamins, fiber, and magnesium.
Freezing	Cool food to its frozen state to stop bacterial reproduction and slow enzymatic reactions.	Fruit, vegetables, ready-to-bake doughs, prepared grain products, meats, soy meat replacers, and mixed dishes.	Freezing has negligible effects on nutrients; blanching (momentary boiling) of fresh vegetables before freezing denatures enzymes that break down vitamins.
Modified atmospheric packaging	Package food in a gas-impermeable container from which air is removed or replaced with other gases to preserve food freshness.	Ready-to-eat salads, cut fruits, soft fresh pasta noodles, baked goods, prepared foods, fresh and preserved meats.	Such packaging preserves vitamins by slowing enzymatic breakdown.
Pasteurizing	Expose food to elevated temperature for long enough to reduce bacterial contamination.	Refrigerated foods such as milk, fruit juice, and eggs.	Flash heating causes trivial losses of some vitamins.
Ultra-high-temperature processing	Expose food to high temperatures for a short time to eliminate microbial contamination.	Shelf-stable foods such as boxed milk, boxed fruit juice, shelf-stable entrée dishes for microwaving.	Short-time, high-temperature heating causes trivial losses of some vitamins.

so canned or frozen concentrated juices retain their vitamins and provide convenient, storable options for many people to keep on hand. Oxygen in air also readily destroys vitamin C, however, so whatever the processing method, all vitamin C–rich foods should be stored properly and consumed within a week after opening.

Processing Mischief

Some processing stories are not so rosy. Chapter 8, for instance, explained how processed foods often gain sodium, which people must limit, while needed potassium is leached away. Another misdeed of processors is the addition of sugar and fat—palatable, high-calorie additives that reduce nutrient density. For example, nuts and raisins covered with "natural yogurt" may sound like one healthy food being added to another, but about 75 percent of the weight of the "yogurt" topping is sugar and fat; only 8 percent is yogurt. These sugar- and fat-coated foods taste so good that wishful thinking can take hold, but they are, in reality, candy.

A particularly severe food process involves **extrusion**, used to make many ultra-processed foods (defined in Chapter 1). Extruded foods generally start out as refined corn, rice, potatoes, or starches that have been ground, separated, and cooked (often with high heat and pressure). The food may then be mixed with salt, sugar, flavors, colors, conditioners, and other additives; shaped by being pushed through a die; expanded by puffing with air or frying; and coated with more fat, sugar, salt, colors, and flavors. Typical products are chips and crisps, cereal bits, snacks that resemble sliced vegetables, and puffy tidbits sold for toddlers. Such ultra-processed food may be attractive with bright colors, tasty flavors, and pretty shapes, but it has sustained oxidation and heat losses of about 30 percent of its vitamin A, 50 percent of its vitamin K, and 90 percent of its vitamin C, with similar losses for almost every other vitamin. The manufacturer may spray a few vitamins or minerals on the food during processing, but not all of the nutrients and phytochemicals lost from the original whole foods can be replaced.

extrusion processing techniques that transform grains, legumes, and other foods into fine particles that are cooked, shaped, colored, flavored, and often puffed, producing snacks, breakfast cereals, and other products.

Best Nutrient Buys

The closer the foods you eat are to the farm, the better nourished you are likely to be, but this doesn't mean that you have to live in the fields. You can also opt for nutritious foods that processing has improved by increasing accessibility or convenience, increasing food safety, improving or leaving intact the nutrient profile, or reducing the cost or the potential for waste. Following are a few examples:

- Skimming removes saturated fat from fat-free milk and improves the food's nutrient profile.
- Irradiation destroys disease-causing organisms, making nutritious foods like berries and melons safer to eat.
- Commercial prewashing and cutting of fresh vegetables and salads makes them more accessible and convenient, with less potential for food waste (see Chapter 15).
- Commercial canning of fish and shellfish creates convenient, storable portions, and destroys disease-causing organisms.

Many other examples exist: commercially prepared whole-grain breads, frozen cuts of meats, bags of frozen vegetables, and canned legumes do little disservice to nutrition and provide convenience to consumers. The nutrient density of processed foods exists on a continuum:

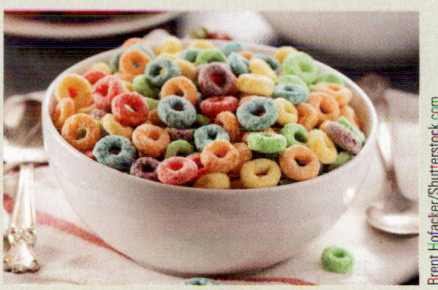
Brent Hofacker/Shutterstock.com

Extrusion is hard on nutrients.

- Whole-grain bread > refined white bread > sugared doughnuts.
- Milk > fruit-flavored yogurt > canned chocolate pudding.
- Corn on the cob > canned creamed corn > caramel popcorn.
- Oranges > canned orange juice > orange-flavored drink.
- Baked pork loin > ham lunch meat> fried bacon.

Making wise food choices is half the story of smart nutrition; skillful food preparation is the other half. In general, short cooking times with little water, such as in microwaving, steaming, or stir frying, best preserve the nutrients of vegetables, whereas long boiling in copious water that is discarded increases nutrient losses. With reasonable care, if you start with foods containing ample amounts of vitamins, you will receive a bounty of the nutrients that they contain.

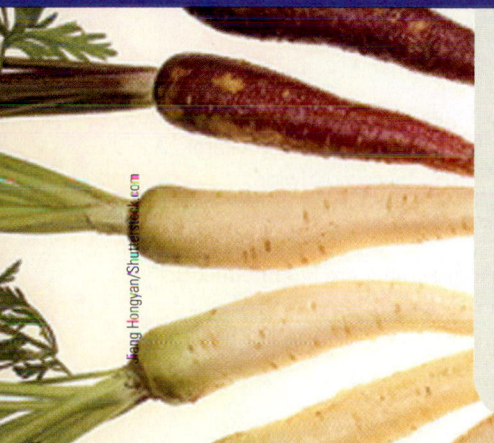
Fang Hongyan/Shutterstock.com

what did you decide?

Are most digestive tract symptoms from "stomach flu"?

Are most foods from grocery stores germ-free?

Should you refrigerate leftover party foods after the guests have gone home?

Which poses the greater risk: raw sushi from a sushi master or food additives?

Self Check

1. (LO 12.1) Microorganisms can cause foodborne illness either by infection or by intoxication.
   T F

2. (LO 12.1) Some microorganisms produce illness-causing _____.
   a. neurotoxins and enterotoxins
   b. neurotransmitters and aflatoxins
   c. enzymes and hormones
   d. none of the above

3. (LO 12.2) To prevent foodborne illnesses, the refrigerator's temperature should be less than _____.
   a. 70°F   **c.** 40°F
   b. 65°F   **d.** 30°F

4. (LO 12.2) Which of the following may be contracted from fresh raw or undercooked seafood?
   a. hepatitis
   b. worms and flukes
   c. viral intestinal disorders
   d. all of the above

5. (LO 12.2) Which of the following organisms can cause hemolytic-uremic syndrome?
   a. *Listeria monocytogenes*
   b. *Campylobacter jejuni*
   c. *Escherichia coli*
   d. *Salmonella*

6. (LO 12.2) The threat of foodborne illness from meats or seafood is serious, but produce causes illness only rarely.
   T F

7. (LO 12.2) Infants under one year of age should never be fed honey because it can contain spores of *Clostridium botulinum*.
   T F

8. (LO 12.3) Which of the following is correct concerning fruits that have been irradiated?
   a. They decay and ripen more slowly.
   b. They lose substantial nutrients.
   c. They lose their sweetness.
   d. They emit gamma radiation.

9. (LO 12.3) Irradiation can
   a. destroy vitamins.
   b. sterilize spices.
   c. make food radioactive.
   d. promote sprouting.

10. (LO 12.3) Food packaging can contribute to food safety.
    T F

11. (LO 12.4) It is possible to eliminate all toxins from your diet by eating only "natural" foods.
    T F

12. (LO 12.4) Pregnant women are advised not to eat certain species of fish because the FDA and the EPA have detected unacceptably high lead levels in them.
    T F

13. (LO 12.5) Evidence does not suggest that conventional foods pose health risks or that using organic products reduces risks.
    T F

14. (LO 12.5) Compared with conventionally grown produce, organic produce is often
    a. lower in pesticides.
    b. higher in phytochemicals.
    c. both a and b.
    d. none of the above

15. (LO 12.6) Incidental food additives
    a. help to preserve foods.
    b. consist mostly of added sugars and salt.
    c. are really contaminants.
    d. none of the above

16. (LO 12.6) Nitrites added to foods
    a. prevent the growth of the deadly *Clostridium botulinum* bacterium.
    b. preserve the pink color of hot dogs.
    c. are linked with colon cancer in animals.
    d. all of the above

17. (LO 12.7) The term *processed foods* is not synonymous with *junk foods*.
    T F

18. (LO 12.7) Food processing can confer a nutritional advantage by
    a. adding yogurt to the candy coating of raisins.
    b. reducing the costs of nutritious foods.
    c. reducing a food's potassium content.
    d. all of the above.

19. (LO 12.8) Selective breeding
    a. involves manipulating an organism's genes in a laboratory.
    b. has been used for thousands of years.
    c. allows scientists to cross species boundaries.
    d. all of the above

20. (LO 12.8) A genetically engineered rice variety in existence today supplies sufficient beta-carotene to fight vitamin A deficiency and childhood blindness worldwide.
    T F

Answers to these Self Check questions are in Appendix G.

Genetically Engineered Foods: What Are the Pros and Cons?

LO 12.8 Summarize the advantages and disadvantages of producing food through genetic engineering.

With or without their awareness, most people in this country consume foods that contain products of **genetic engineering**. As Figure C12–1 illustrates, 90 percent of U.S. soybeans and 88 percent of animal feed corn (*not* sweet corn consumed by people) are **genetically modified organisms (GMOs).** Ubiquitous food additives, such as soy lecithin and high-fructose corn syrup, arise from these genetically engineered plant materials and enter the human food supply in processed foods. Other GMOs, such as papayas, are consumed directly. Some consumers recoil from the idea of eating products from GMOs, and whole countries have banned such foods

outright. Some objections are based on credible ideas; however, many others arise from emotional fears, distrust of technology, and misinformation.[1]* This Controversy sorts the scientific fact from fiction, starting with some definitions of **biotechnology** terms (see Table C12–1 (p. 510).[2]

Advances in biotechnology have raised hopes of solving some of today's most pressing food and energy problems while boosting profits for farmers and other producers. Although **recombinant DNA (rDNA) technology** may seem futuristic, its roots lie in genetic events that have been occurring unaided for

*Reference notes are found in Appendix F.

untold millions of years. Human beings have exploited these processes from the advent of agriculture.

Selective Breeding

Season after season, farmers influence the genetic makeup of food plants and animals by selecting only the best farm animals and plants for breeding. Today's lush, hefty, healthy agricultural crops and animals, from cabbage and squash to pigs and cattle, are the result of thousands of years of **selective breeding**. A consumer of today's large cobs of sweet corn, for example, may not recognize the original wild native corn with its sparse four or five kernels to a stalk (shown in the photo).

Today, accelerated selective breeding techniques involve hundreds of thousands of cross-bred seeds planted on vast acreage. To develop crops with desired traits, DNA data from successful seedlings are analyzed by computer. Seedlings with the right genes are grown to maturity and reproduced to yield new breeds in a relatively short time. Some unusually colorful carrots, including the purple, light yellow, or deep red varieties now seen in some specialty grocery stores, are products of this kind of selective breeding. Selective breeding must stay within the boundaries of a species—a carrot, for example, cannot be crossed with a mosquito. Recombinant DNA technology, however, knows no such limits.

Recombinant DNA Technology

With economy, speed, and precision, rDNA technology can change one or

Figure C12–1

Growth of Selected Genetically Engineered Crops, United States 1996–2014

The economic benefits of growing genetically engineered soybeans, cotton, and corn have led to widespread replacement of conventional crops on U.S. farms.

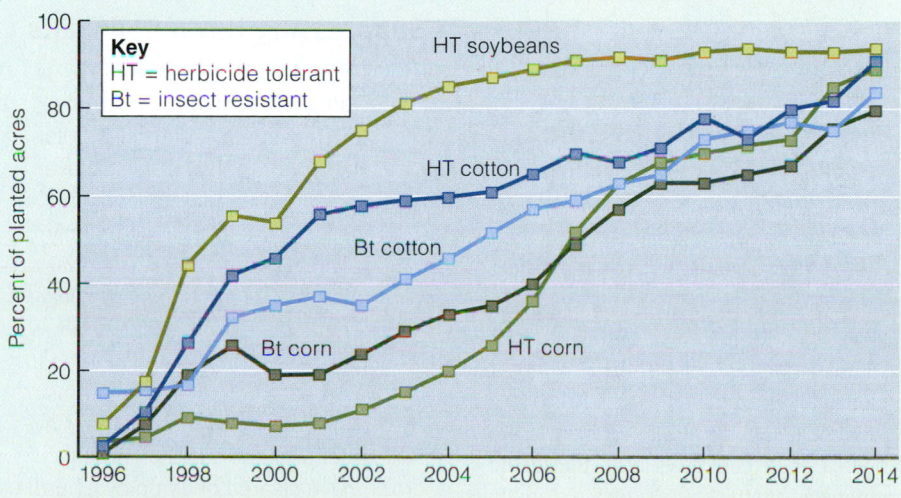

Key
HT = herbicide tolerant
Bt = insect resistant

HT soybeans
HT cotton
Bt cotton
Bt corn
HT corn

Percent of planted acres

Source: U.S. Department of Agriculture, Adoption of genetically engineered crops in the U.S., July 2014, available at www.ers.usda.gov/data-products/adoption-of-genetically-engineered-crops-in-the-us /recenttrends-in-ge-adoption.aspx.

- **biotechnology** the science of manipulating biological systems or organisms to modify their products or components or create new products; biotechnology includes recombinant DNA technology and traditional and accelerated selective breeding techniques.
- **clone** an individual created asexually from a single ancestor, such as a plant grown from a single stem cell; a group of genetically identical individuals descended from a single common ancestor, such as a colony of bacteria arising from a single bacterial cell; in genetics, a replica of a segment of DNA, such as a gene, produced by genetic engineering.
- **genetic engineering** the direct, intentional manipulation of the genetic material of living things in order to obtain some desirable inheritable trait not present in the original organism. Also called *biotechnology*.
- **genetically modified organism (GMO)** popular term referring to an organism produced by genetic engineering; the term *genetically engineered organism (GEO)* is more scientifically accurate.

- **outcrossing** the unintended breeding of a domestic crop with a related wild species.
- **plant pesticides** substances produced within plant tissues that kill or repel attacking organisms.
- **recombinant DNA (rDNA) technology** a technique of genetic modification whereby scientists directly manipulate the genes of living things; includes methods of removing genes, doubling genes, introducing foreign genes, and changing gene positions to influence the growth and development of organisms.
- **selective breeding** a technique of genetic modification whereby organisms are chosen for reproduction based on their desirability for human purposes, such as high growth rate, high food yield, or disease resistance, with the intention of retaining or enhancing these characteristics in their offspring.
- **stem cell** an undifferentiated cell that can mature into any of a number of specialized cell types. A stem cell of bone marrow may mature into one of many kinds of blood cells, for example.
- **transgenic organism** an organism resulting from the growth of an embryonic, stem, or germ cell into which a new gene has been inserted.

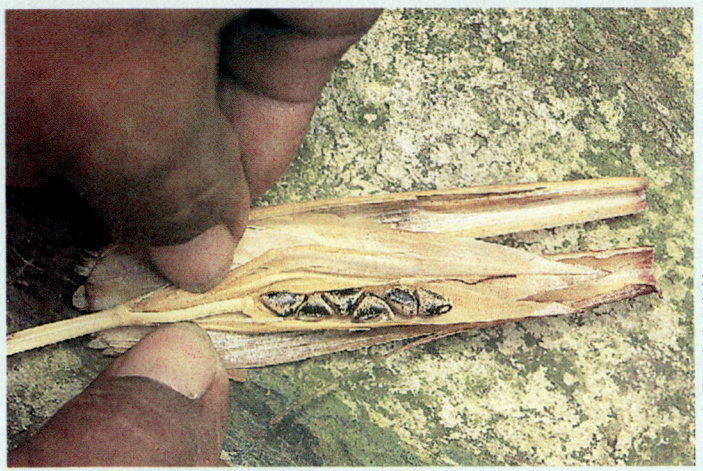

Smithsonian Photo by Antonio Mortaner

This wild corn, with its sparse kernels, bears little resemblance to today's large, full, sweet ears.

more characteristics of a living thing. The genes for a desirable trait in one organism are transferred directly into another organism's DNA. Figure C12–2 (p. 511) compares the genetic results of selective breeding and rDNA technology. Table C12–2 (p. 511) presents examples of biotechnology research directions.

Obtaining Desired Traits

Using rDNA technology, scientists can confer useful traits, such as disease resistance, on food crops. To make a disease-resistant potato plant, for example, the process begins with the DNA of an immature cell, known as a **stem cell**, from the "eye" of a potato. Into that stem cell scientists insert a gene snipped from the DNA of a virus that attacks potato plants (enzymes do the snipping). This gene codes for a harmless viral protein, not the infective part.

The newly created stem cell is then stimulated to replicate itself, creating **clone** cells—exact genetic replicas of the modified cell. With time, what was once a single cell grows into a **transgenic organism**—in this case, a potato plant that makes a piece of viral protein in each of its cells. The presence of the viral protein

stimulates the potato plant to develop resistance against an attack from the real wild virus in the potato field.

Plants make likely candidates for genetic engineering because a single plant cell can often be coaxed into producing an entire new plant. Animals can also be modified by rDNA technology, however. Under development is a line of goats that, thanks to a spider's gene, express spider silk protein in their milk (see the photo). Once processed, the stronger-than-steel silk fiber can be used to make artificial ligaments and bulletproof vests.[3]

Suppressing Unwanted Traits

rDNA technology can also remove an unwanted protein from a plant by silencing the genes responsible for its creation. For example, scientists have created a safer peanut by silencing the genes for proteins that commonly cause allergic reactions.[4] Likewise, a newly approved GE potato may soon be made into safer potato chips and French fries because it is engineered to have less of an amino acid that forms a toxin during frying.[5†] Apples that stay white after slicing instead of turning brown have cleared one approval hurdle

† *The Innate Potato makes less acrylamide when fried.*

Figure C12–2

Comparing Selective Breeding and rDNA Technology

Selective Breeding—DNA is a strand of genes, depicted as a strand of pearls. Traditional selective breeding combines many genes from two individuals of the same species.

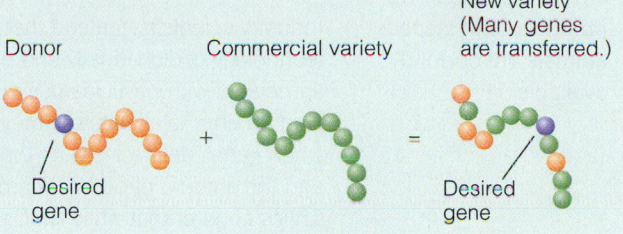

Donor

Desired gene

+

Commercial variety

=

New variety
(Many genes are transferred.)

Desired gene

rDNA Technology—Through rDNA technology, a single gene or several may be transferred to the receiving DNA from the same species or others.

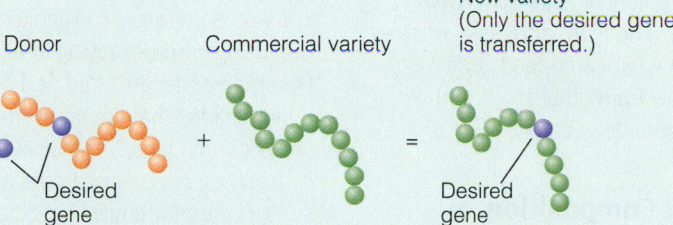

Donor

Desired gene

+

Commercial variety

=

New variety
(Only the desired gene is transferred.)

Desired gene

Table C12–2

Some Examples of Biotechnology Research Directions

Research in genetic engineering is currently directed at creating:

- Crops and animals with added desired traits, such as altered nutrient composition, extended shelf life, freedom from allergy-causing constituents, or resistance to diseases or insect pests.
- Crops that survive harsh conditions, such as applications of herbicides, heavily polluted or salty soils, or drought conditions.
- Microorganisms that produce needed substances, such as pharmaceuticals, hydrocarbon fuels, or other products that do not occur in nature or occur only in limited amounts.

and may soon be available in markets; gluten-free wheat may be next. These "next generation" or "genetically edited" foods contain no foreign genes, so their developers hope that consumers will react positively to them.

The Promises and Problems of rDNA Technology

Supporters hail genetic engineering as nothing short of a revolutionary

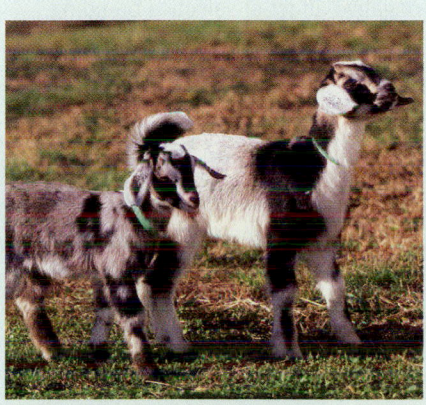

Sean O'Neill/Alamy

Females of this line of GE goats produce spider silk protein in their milk.

means of overcoming many of the planet's pressing problems, such as food shortages, nutrient deficiencies, medicine shortages, dwindling farmland, lack of renewable energy sources, and environmental degradation. A few examples follow.

Human Nutrition

Rice leads the way in a genomic revolution of the world's food supply. A rice (called *Golden Rice*) provides up to 35 micrograms of absorbable beta-carotene per gram of rice (for comparison, carrots have about 80 micrograms), sufficient to fight vitamin A deficiency diseases and childhood blindness worldwide.[6] Other rice varieties, some offering 80 percent more iron and zinc than ordinary rice, could relieve much iron-deficiency anemia and zinc deficiency around the world. Still others may resist drought, floods, or insects and thus provide more food for hungry populations. Not just rice but worldwide staples like cassava roots or potatoes can be "biofortified" with minerals, vitamins, fatty acids, or promising phytochemicals.[7] In the case

of cassava, it can also be made safer by reducing its concentration of naturally occurring toxins.

Molecules from Microbes

The genes of microorganisms have been altered to make pharmaceutical and industrial products. For example, a transgenic bacterial factory now mass-produces the hormone insulin used by people with diabetes. Another bacterium received a bovine gene to make the enzyme rennin, necessary in cheese production. Historically, rennin was harvested from the stomachs of calves, an expensive process. Today, intensive efforts are under way to develop biofuel-producing microbes to supply a more sustainable and price-stable alternative to fossil fuels.[8]

Plants and animals may also play similar roles. Researchers have induced bananas and potatoes to produce a hepatitis vaccine. Animals can be engineered to secrete vaccines in their milk, and herds could provide both nourishment and immunization to villages now lacking both food and medicine.

Controversy 12 Genetically Engineered Foods: What Are the Pros and Cons?

511

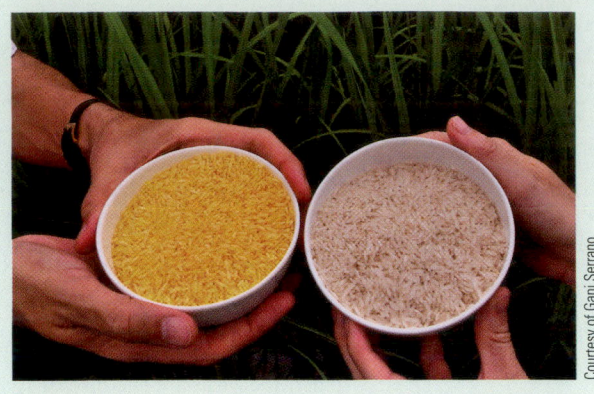

Courtesy of Gani Serrano

Beta-carotene, the vitamin A precursor, gives Golden Rice its yellow hue.

Greater Crop Yields

Most of today's genetically engineered crops are of two types: herbicide-resistant and insect-resistant, both used to improve yields and protect farmed land. Herbicide-resistant crops, for example, offer weed control with less soil tillage by allowing farmers to spray whole fields, not just weeds, with potent herbicides. The weeds die, their roots hold soil in place between the rows, and crops grow normally. After years of such spraying, however, some weeds, such as pigweed, have developed vigorous resistance to today's herbicide. Pigweed grows large and spreads fast despite repeated sprayings, forcing many farmers to return to old tillage methods to control it, thus exposing vast quantities of farm topsoil to wind and water erosion.[‡9]

As for insect-resistant crops, these GMOs make what the EPA calls **plant pesticides**—pesticides made by the plant tissues themselves. For example, a type of feed corn produces a pesticide that kills a common corn-destroying worm, thereby greatly increasing yields per acre of farmland.

In areas where people cannot afford to lose a single morsel of food and where plant diseases and insects can claim up to 80 percent of a season's yield, genetically engineered plants can save the crop. Such innovations promise relief for the world's chronically hungry people.

Food from Cloned Animals

According to the FDA, milk and meat from cloned cattle, pigs, and goats

‡*Pigweed is officially known as Palmer amaranth.*

are as safe as similar conventional foods, but many people have reservations about consuming them, and they are costly to produce. No products from cloned animals are currently available.

Issues Surrounding GMOs

Consumers rightly want to know about any potential risks from rDNA technology. The FDA, also, asks whether genetically engineered foods differ substantially from other foods in their nutrient contents or safety.

Nutrient Composition

In most cases, except for intentional variation created through rDNA technology, the nutrient composition of genetically engineered foods is identical to that of traditional foods. From the body's point of view, therefore, eating Golden Rice, mentioned earlier, would be the same as eating plain rice and taking a beta-carotene supplement—and beta-carotene supplements carry risks (see Controversy 7). Thus, while GMOs may contribute to *overdoses* of nutrients or phytochemicals, they pose no unusual threat of deficiencies.

Accidental Ingestion of Drugs from Foods

Genetically modified corn, soybeans, rice, and other food crops that make human and animal drugs and industrial proteins must be grown indoors in selected locations. Their containment areas, however, often abut farms where conventional food crops are grown. Critics fear that DNA from drug-producing GMOs might contaminate the food supply, despite USDA oversight.[10] Disasters such as tornadoes, floods, or other events could liberate the sequestered plants, and high winds or

water could transport their pollen long distances to mingle undetected with food crops.

Pesticide Residues and Resistance

Industry scientists contend that rDNA technology could virtually end problems associated with pesticide use on foods. Human error is eliminated, they say, when genes determine both the nature and the amount of pesticide produced. Critics counter that while GMOs may be protected from one or two common pests that may or may not be present on a particular field, farmers must still spray for other pests devouring their crops. Also, in a worrisome sign, constant exposure is causing crop-destroying insects to become resistant to plant pesticides.

Pesticides that are sprayed onto crops can be largely removed from food by washing or peeling produce, but consumers cannot remove pesticides that form within the tissues of a GMO. Still, plant pesticides are highly unlikely to cause health problems because they are made of peptide chains (small protein strands) that human digestive enzymes readily denature. Plant pesticides, like other pesticide residues, are approved and regulated by the FDA (see the preceding chapter).

Unintended Health Effects

The possibility exists that GMOs may have unintended and therefore unpredictable effects on human health. A lesson comes from an unexpected negative effect of selective breeding. Over many years, celery growers had crossed their most attractive celery plants because consumers paid a premium for good-looking celery. Unbeknownst to the growers, however, the most beautiful celery was especially high in a natural plant pesticide, and its concentration increased with each breeding cycle. Soon farm and grocery workers who handled the celery began suffering from serious skin rashes until the problem was finally traced to high levels of the natural pesticide in the beautiful plants. Advanced tests to identify such products of metabolism may soon reveal molecules in GMO foods that previously escaped detection.[11]

Another example, this time an unintended *benefit* of genetic engineering, involves a carcinogenic fungus that sometimes grows on corn.§ After several growing seasons, scientists confirmed that corn with plant pesticide suffered much less worm damage than ordinary corn. Surprisingly, the crops also had far less than the expected growth of the dangerous fungus. It turns out that the worms spread the fungus as they burrow into cobs of ordinary corn, but the plant pesticide in the genetically engineered corn killed the worms and stopped the fungus.[12]

Environmental Effects

Between 1996 and 2006, the planting of genetically engineered crops reduced insecticide use by almost 500 million pounds of active ingredients worldwide. At the same time, the use of herbicides to which GMOs are resistant, such as glyphosate (pronounced gly-FOSS-ate), has greatly increased, replacing more highly toxic and persistent herbicides in the fields.[13]** Also, herbicide-resistant crops require far less plowing to kill weeds and so minimize soil erosion (more about soil conservation in Controversy 15).

However, the possibility of **outcrossing**, the accidental cross-pollination of plant pesticide crops with related wild weeds remains a concern. If a weed inherits a pest-resistant trait from a neighboring field of genetically engineered crops, it could gain an enormous survival advantage over other important wild species and crowd them out.

Loss of species is another serious threat. By propagating only a few crop varieties worldwide, humankind

§ *The fungus (Aspergillus flavus) produces the carcinogenic toxin aflatoxin.*

** *Glyphosate is the chemical in a popular herbicide, trade name Roundup.*

becomes vulnerable in a changing environment. Species that teeter on the brink of extinction today may hold critical genetic traits that could help food crops to survive in harsher future conditions.

Concerns for wildlife also exist. In the laboratory, monarch butterfly larvae die when fed pollen from pesticide-producing corn. In real life, wild butterflies do not seem to consume enough toxic corn pollen for populations to be harmed. The new technology may even protect some percentage of the dwindling monarchs and other harmless or beneficial insects that now die when they feed on conventionally sprayed fields.

Ethical Arguments about rDNA Technology

In the end, consumer acceptance determines the applications of genetic engineering. Some people fear that by tampering with the basic blueprint of life, rDNA technology will sooner or later unleash mayhem on an unsuspecting world. Any degree of risk is unjustified, they say, because while it raises profits for biotechnology companies and farmers, its products provide little direct benefit to consumers. Others object to rDNA technology on religious grounds, holding that genetic decisions are best left to nature or a higher power. At the very least, these people want food labels to clearly identify foods that contain GMO ingredients.[14] Table C12–3 (p. 514) summarizes some of these issues.

Proponents of genetic engineering respond that most of the world's people cannot afford the luxury of rejecting the potential benefits of rDNA technology—they lack the abundant foods and fertile lands that protesters take for granted. Delays hurt the poorest of the poor, they say. GMO opponents counter that the scope of world hunger far exceeds simple solutions such as increasing food supplies—it involves war, politics, and education. (Chapter 15 explores the tragedy of world hunger.)

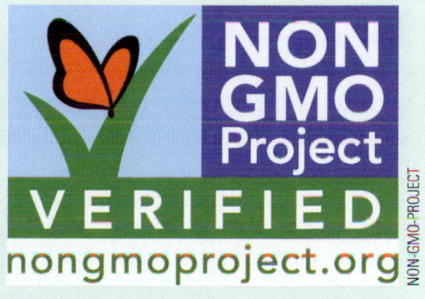

Foods bearing voluntary "non-GMO" labels are gaining popularity among U.S. consumers.

Regulation of GMOs

The FDA evaluates the safety of today's genetically modified fruits, vegetables, and grains for human consumption and takes the position that they are safe unless they differ substantially from similar foods already in use. To help consumers who wish to avoid GMOs, USDA has developed a voluntary certification and labeling system for foods. In application, the system resembles organic food certification (described earlier in this chapter's Consumer's Guide). Food producers pay a fee to certify that their product contains no GMO ingredients; after certification, the product may bear a USDA-approved symbol on its label.

The Final Word

For those who would worry themselves into a diet of crackers and water, abundant evidence supports eating sufficient fruits and vegetables regardless of their source. Stay alert for new information about rDNA technology, food technology, and their effects on our rapidly changing food supply.[15] Armed with scientific knowledge, you can make informed choices about your diet.

Critical Thinking

1. Discuss options and roadblocks to obtaining only non-GMO foods.
2. Outline possible motivations of industry, growers, and consumers for supporting/opposing GMOs.

Table C12–3

Genetic Engineering of Foods: Point, Counterpoint

Arguments in Opposition to Genetic Engineering	Arguments in Support of Genetic Engineering
1. *Ethical and moral issues.* It's immoral to "play God" by mixing genes from organisms unable to do so naturally. Religious and vegetarian groups object to genes from prohibited species occurring in their allowable foods.	1. *Ethical and moral issues.* Scientists throughout history have been persecuted and even put to death by fearful people who accuse them of playing God. Yet today, many of the world's citizens enjoy a long and healthy life of comfort and convenience due to once-feared scientific advances put to practical use.
2. *Imperfect technology.* The technology is young and imperfect; genes rarely function in just one way, their placement is often imprecise, and potential effects are impossible to predict. Toxins are as likely to be produced as the desired trait.	2. *Advanced technology.* Recombinant DNA technology is precise and reliable. Many of the most exciting recent advances in medicine, agriculture, and technology were made possible by the application of this technology.
3. *Environmental concerns.* Environmental side effects are unknown. The power of a genetically modified organism to change the world's environments is unknown until such changes actually occur—then the "genie is out of the bottle." Once out, the genie cannot be put back in the bottle because insects, birds, and the wind distribute genetically altered seed and pollen to points unknown.	3. *Environmental protection.* Genetic engineering may be the only hope of saving rain forest and other habitats from destruction by impoverished people desperate for arable land. Through genetic engineering, farmers can make use of previously unproductive lands such as salt-rich soils and arid areas.
4. *"Genetic pollution."* Other kinds of pollution can often be cleaned up with money, time, and effort. Once genes are spliced into living things, those genes forever bear the imprint of human tampering.	4. *Genetic improvements.* Genetic side effects are more likely to benefit the environment than to harm it.
5. *Crop vulnerability.* Pests and disease can quickly adapt to overtake genetically identical plants or animals around the world. Diversity is key to defense.	5. *Improved crop resistance.* Pests and diseases can be specifically fought on a case-by-case basis. Biotechnology is the key to defense.
6. *Loss of gene pool.* Loss of genetic diversity threatens to deplete valuable gene banks from which scientists can develop new agricultural crops.	6. *Gene pool preserved.* Thanks to advances in genetics, laboratories around the world are able to stockpile the genetic material of millions of species that, without such advances, would have been lost forever.
7. *Profit motive.* Genetic engineering will profit industry more than the world's poor and hungry.	7. *Everyone profits.* Industries benefit from genetic engineering, and a thriving food industry benefits the nation and its people, as witnessed by countries lacking such industries. Genetic engineering promises to provide adequate nutritious food for millions who lack such food today. Developed nations gain cheaper, more attractive, more delicious foods with greater variety and availability year-round.
8. *Unproven safety for people.* Testing of genetically altered products for human safety is generally lacking. The population is an unwitting experimental group in a nationwide laboratory study for the benefit of industry.	8. *Safe for people.* Testing of genetically altered products for human safety is unnecessary because the products are essentially the same as the original foodstuffs.
9. *Increased allergens.* Allergens can unwittingly be transferred into foods.	9. *Control of allergens.* Allergens can be transferred into foods, but these are known and thus can be avoided. Allergen-free peanuts and other foods are under development.
10. *Decreased nutrients.* A fresh-looking tomato or other produce held for several weeks may have lost substantial nutrients.	10. *Increased nutrients.* Genetic modifications can easily enhance the nutrients in foods.

Genetic Engineering of Foods: Point, Counterpoint (*continued*)

Arguments in Opposition to Genetic Engineering	Arguments in Support of Genetic Engineering
11. *No product tracking.* Without labeling, the food industry cannot track problems to the source.	11. *Excellent product tracking.* The identity and location of genetically altered foodstuffs are known, and they can be tracked should problems arise.
12. *Overuse of herbicides.* Farmers, knowing that their crops resist herbicide effects, will use them liberally.	12. *Conservative use of herbicides.* Farmers will not waste expensive herbicides in second or third applications when the prescribed amount gets the job done the first time.
13. *Increased consumption of pesticides.* When a pesticide is produced by the flesh of produce, consumers cannot wash it off the skin of the produce with running water as they can with most ordinary sprays.	13. *Reduced pesticides on foods.* Pesticides produced by plants in tiny amounts known to be safe for consumption are more predictable than applications by agricultural workers who make mistakes. Because other genetic manipulations will eliminate the need for postharvest spraying, fewer pesticides will reach the dinner table.
14. *Lack of oversight.* Government oversight is run by industry people for the benefit of industry—no one is watching out for the consumer.	14. *Sufficient regulation, oversight, and rapid response.* The National Academy of Sciences has established a protocol for the safety testing of GE foods. Government agencies are efficient in identifying and correcting problems as they occur in the industry.

13 Life Cycle Nutrition: Mother and Infant

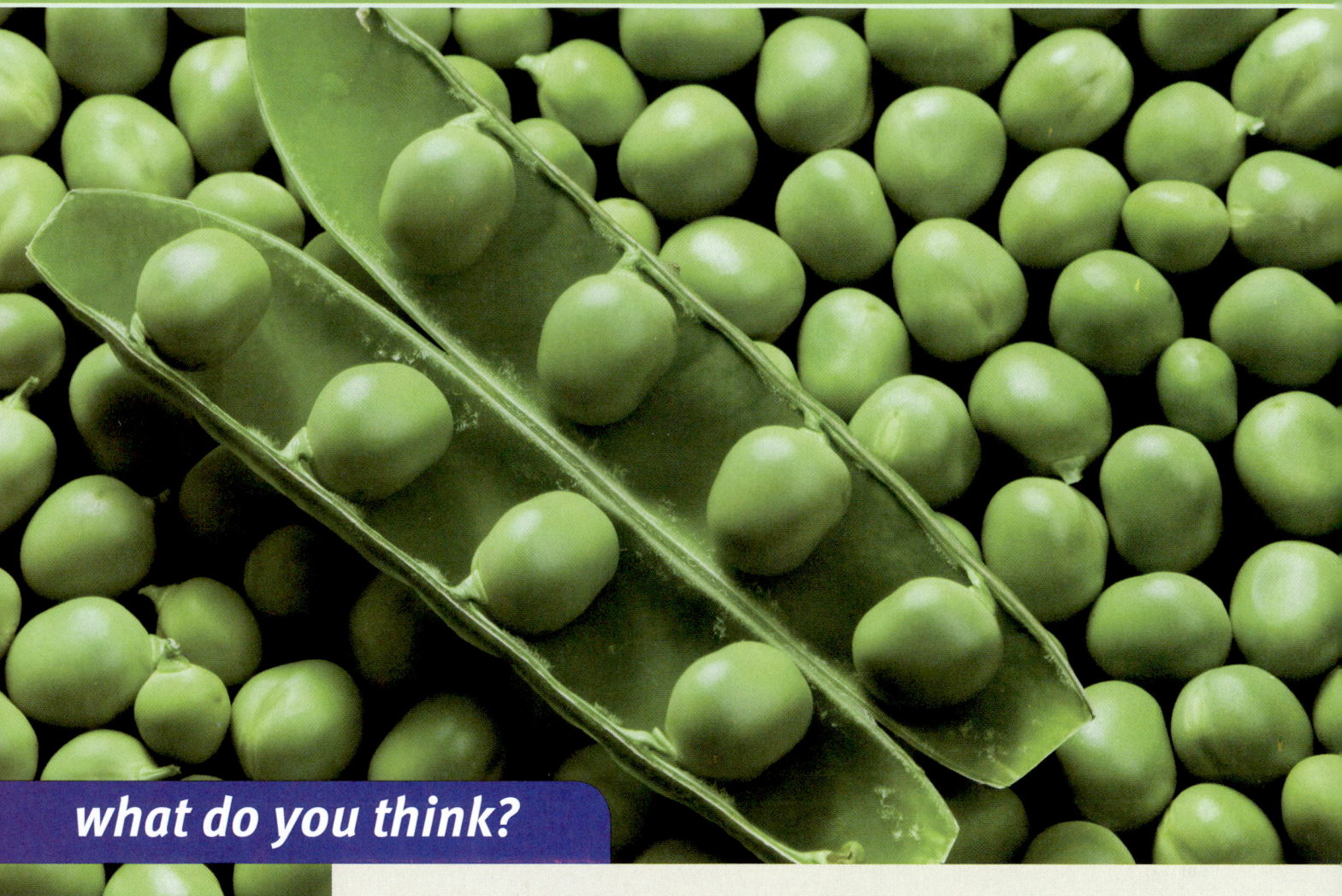

PHB.cz/Richard Semik/Shutterstock.com

what do you think?

what do you think?

Can a man's lifestyle habits affect a future pregnancy?

How much alcohol does it take to harm a developing fetus?

Are breast milk and formula about the same for an infant?

Can infants grow and thrive on only breast milk or formula?

Learning Objectives

After completing this chapter, you should be able to accomplish the following:

LO 13.1 Explain the roles of nutrition before and during pregnancy.

LO 13.2 Summarize the evidence against alcohol intake during pregnancy.

LO 13.3 List the effects of diabetes, hypertension, and preeclampsia on pregnancy.

LO 13.4 Underline the role of nutrition during lactation.

LO 13.5 Identify nutrition practices that promote the infant's well-being.

LO 13.6 List five feeding guidelines that encourage normal eating behaviors and autonomy in the child.

LO 13.7 Recognize the challenges associated with childhood obesity.

All people need the same nutrients but in differing amounts throughout life. This chapter is the first of two on life's changing nutrient needs. It focuses on the two life stages that might be the most important to an individual's life-long health—pregnancy and infancy.

Pregnancy: The Impact of Nutrition on the Future

LO 13.1 Explain the roles of nutrition before and during pregnancy.

People normally think of nutrition as personal, affecting them alone. For the woman who is pregnant, or who soon will be, however, nutrition choices today profoundly affect the health of her future child and the adult that the child will one day become. The nutrient demands of pregnancy are extraordinary.

iStockphoto.com/Squaredpixels

Both parents can prepare in advance for a healthy pregnancy.

Preparing for Pregnancy

Before she becomes pregnant, a woman must establish eating habits that will optimally nourish both the growing **fetus** and herself. She must be well nourished at the outset because early in pregnancy the **embryo** undergoes rapid and significant developmental changes that depend on good nutrition.

Fathers-to-be are also wise to examine their eating and drinking habits. For example, leading a sedentary lifestyle and consuming too few fruits and vegetables may affect men's **fertility** (and the fertility of their children), and men who drink too much alcohol or encounter other toxins in the weeks before conception can sustain damage to their sperm's genetic material.[1]* When both partners adopt healthy habits, they will be better prepared to meet the demands of parenting that lie ahead.

> Some heritable traits do not result from DNA variations but arise from epigenetic influences before or during pregnancy—see **Controversy 11.**

Prepregnancy Weight Before pregnancy, all women, but underweight women in particular, should strive for an appropriate body weight. A woman who begins her pregnancy underweight and who fails to gain sufficiently during pregnancy is very likely to bear a baby with a dangerously **low birthweight**.[2] Infant birthweight is the most potent single indicator of an infant's future health. A low-birthweight baby, defined as one who weighs less than 5½ pounds (2,500 grams), is nearly 40 times more likely to die in the first year of life than a normal-weight baby. To prevent low

fetus (FEET-us) the stage of human gestation from eight weeks after conception until the birth of an infant.

embryo (EM-bree-oh) the stage of human gestation from the third to the eighth week after conception.

fertility the capacity of a woman to produce a normal ovum periodically and of a man to produce normal sperm; the ability to reproduce.

low birthweight a birthweight of less than 5½ pounds (2,500 grams); used as a predictor of probable health problems in the newborn and as a probable indicator of poor nutrition status of the mother before and/or during pregnancy. Low-birthweight infants may be premature (born early) or small for gestational age (suffered growth failure in the uterus).

---

*Reference notes are found in Appendix F.

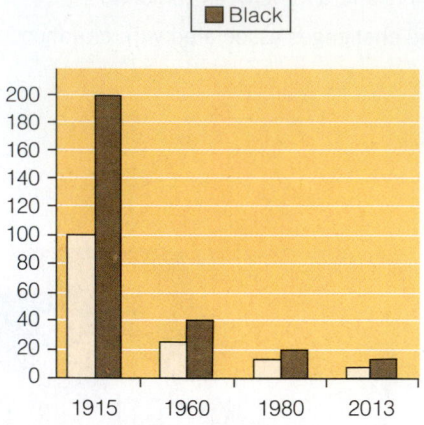

Figure 13–1
Infant Mortality Decline over Time

The graph shows infant deaths per 1,000 live births.

Source: Data from M. J. K. Osterman and coauthors, Annual Summary of vital statistics: 2012–2013, Pediatrics 135 (2015): 1115–1125.

birthweight, underweight women are advised to gain weight before becoming pregnant and to strive to gain adequately thereafter.

When nutrient supplies during pregnancy fail to meet demands, the developing fetus may adapt to the sparse conditions in ways that may make obesity or chronic diseases more likely in later life.[3] Low birthweight is also associated with lower adult IQ and other brain impairments, short stature, and educational disadvantages.[4] Nutrient deficiency coupled with low birthweight is the underlying cause of more than half of all the deaths worldwide of children under 5 years of age. In the United States, the infant mortality rate in 2013 was just under 6.0 deaths per 1,000 live births.[5] This rate, though higher than that of some other developed countries, represents a significant decline over the last two decades and is a tribute to public health efforts aimed at reducing infant deaths (see Figure 13–1).

Low birthweight may also reflect heredity, disease conditions, smoking, and drug (including alcohol) use during pregnancy. Even with optimal nutrition and health during pregnancy, some women give birth to small infants for unknown reasons. Nevertheless, poor nutrition is the major factor in low birthweight—and an avoidable one, as later sections make clear.[6]

Obese women are also urged to strive for healthy weights before pregnancy. Infants born to obese women are more likely to be large for their gestational age, weighing more than 9 pounds.[7] Problems associated with a high birthweight include a difficult labor and delivery, birth trauma, and **cesarean section**.[8] Consequently, these babies have a greater risk of poor health and death than infants of normal weight. Infants of obese mothers may be twice as likely to be born with a neural tube defect, too. The vitamin folate may play a role, but a more likely explanation seems to be poor blood glucose control.[9] Obese women themselves are likely to suffer gestational diabetes, hypertension, and complications during and infections after the birth.[10] In addition, both overweight and obese women have a greater risk of giving birth to infants with heart defects and other abnormalities.[11] The obese woman who strives for a healthier prepregnancy body weight helps protect both herself and her future child.

A Healthy Placenta and Other Organs A woman's nutrition before pregnancy is crucial because it determines whether her **uterus** will be able to support the growth of a healthy **placenta** during the first month of **gestation**. The placenta is both a supply depot and a waste-removal system for the fetus. If the placenta works perfectly, the fetus wants for nothing; if it doesn't, no alternative source of sustenance is available, and the fetus will fail to thrive. Figure 13–2 shows the placenta, a mass of tissue in which maternal and fetal blood vessels intertwine and exchange materials. The two bloods never mix, but the barrier between them is notably thin. Nutrients and oxygen move across this thin barrier from the mother's blood into the fetus's blood, and wastes move out of the fetal blood to be excreted by the mother. Thus, by way of the placenta, the mother's digestive tract, respiratory system, and kidneys serve the needs of the fetus, whose organs are not yet functional, as well as her own. The **umbilical cord** acts like a pipeline, conducting fetal blood to and from the placenta. The **amniotic sac** surrounds and cradles the fetus, which floats inside its cushioning fluids.

The placenta is a highly metabolic organ that actively gathers up hormones, nutrients, and protein molecules such as antibodies and transfers them into the fetal bloodstream.[12] The placenta also produces a broad range of hormones that act in many ways to maintain pregnancy and prepare the mother's breasts for **lactation**. Is it any wonder that a healthy placenta is essential for the developing fetus?

If the mother's nutrient stores are inadequate during placental development, no amount of nutrients later on in pregnancy can make up for the lack. If the placenta fails to form or function properly, the fetus will not receive optimal nourishment. After getting such a poor start on life, the child may be ill equipped, even as an adult, to store sufficient nutrients, and a girl may later be unable to grow an adequate placenta or bear healthy full-term infants. For this and other reasons, a woman's

cesarean (see-ZAIR-ee-un) **section** surgical childbirth, in which the infant is taken through an incision in the woman's abdomen.

uterus (YOO-ter-us) the womb, the muscular organ within which the infant develops before birth.

placenta (pla-SEN-tuh) the organ of pregnancy in which maternal blood and fetal blood circulate in close proximity and exchange nutrients and oxygen (flowing into the fetus) and wastes (picked up by the mother's blood).

gestation the period of about 40 weeks (three trimesters) from conception to birth; the term of a pregnancy.

umbilical (um-BIL-ih-cul) **cord** the rope-like structure through which the fetus's veins and arteries reach the placenta; the route of nourishment and oxygen into the fetus and the route of waste disposal from the fetus.

amniotic (AM-nee-OTT-ic) **sac** the "bag of waters" in the uterus in which the fetus floats.

lactation production and secretion of breast milk for the purpose of nourishing an infant.

Figure 13–2

The Placenta

The placenta is composed of spongy tissue in which fetal blood and maternal blood flow side by side, each in its own vessels. The maternal blood transfers oxygen and nutrients to the fetus's blood and picks up fetal wastes to be excreted by the mother. The placenta performs the nutritive, respiratory, and excretory functions that the fetus's digestive system, lungs, and kidneys will provide after birth.

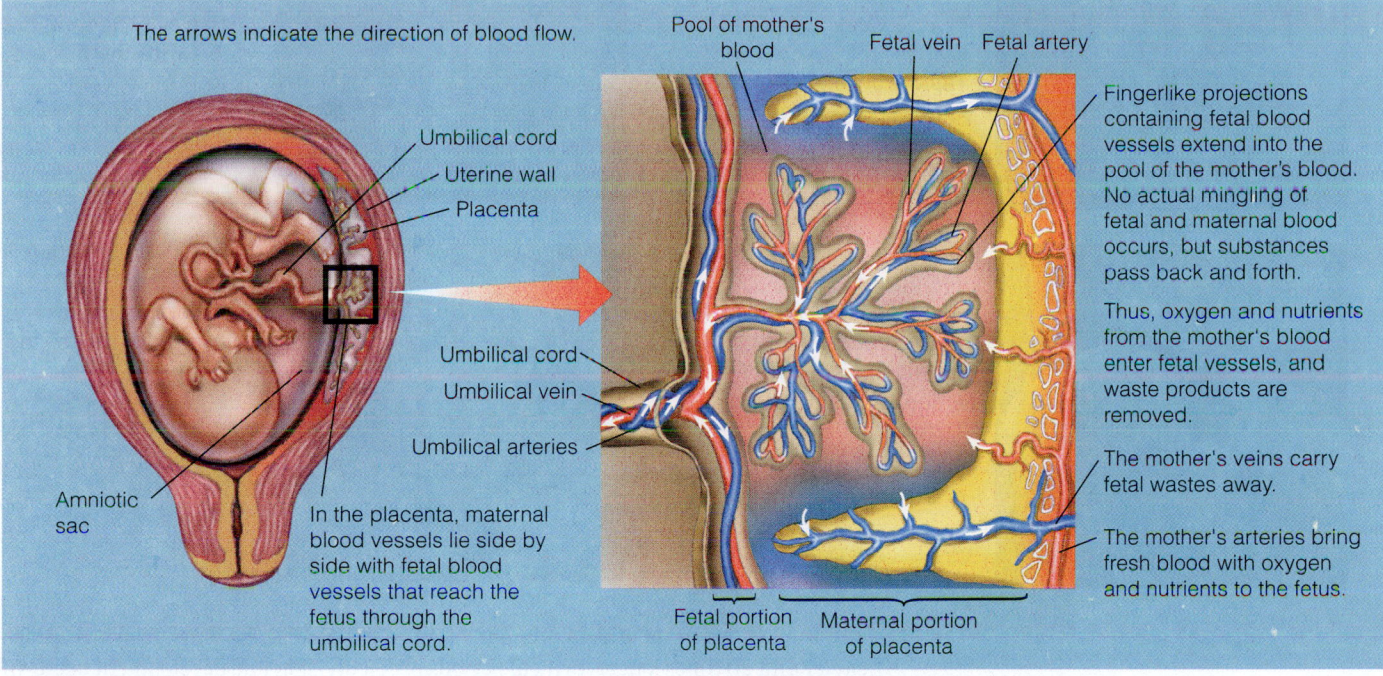

The arrows indicate the direction of blood flow.

Umbilical cord
Uterine wall
Placenta

Amniotic sac

In the placenta, maternal blood vessels lie side by side with fetal blood vessels that reach the fetus through the umbilical cord.

Umbilical cord
Umbilical vein
Umbilical arteries

Pool of mother's blood
Fetal vein   Fetal artery

Fingerlike projections containing fetal blood vessels extend into the pool of the mother's blood. No actual mingling of fetal and maternal blood occurs, but substances pass back and forth.

Thus, oxygen and nutrients from the mother's blood enter fetal vessels, and waste products are removed.

The mother's veins carry fetal wastes away.

The mother's arteries bring fresh blood with oxygen and nutrients to the fetus.

Fetal portion of placenta   Maternal portion of placenta

poor nutrition during her early pregnancy could affect her grandchild as well as her child.

- Adequate nutrition before pregnancy establishes physical readiness and nutrient stores to support placental and fetal growth.
- Both underweight and overweight women should strive for appropriate body weights before pregnancy.
- Newborns who weigh less than 5½ pounds face greater health risks than normal-weight babies.

The Events of Pregnancy

The newly fertilized **ovum** is called a **zygote**. It begins as a single cell and rapidly divides into many cells during the days after fertilization. Within two weeks, if the cluster of cells embeds itself in the uterine wall in a process known as **implantation**, the placenta begins to grow inside the uterus. Minimal growth in size takes place at this time, but it is a crucial period in development. Adverse influences such as smoking, drug abuse, and malnutrition at this time lead to failure to implant or to abnormalities such as neural tube defects that can cause loss of the developing embryo, often before the woman knows she is pregnant.

The Embryo and Fetus   During the next six weeks, the embryo registers astonishing physical changes (see Figure 13–3, p. 520). At eight weeks, the fetus has a complete central nervous system, a beating heart, a fully formed digestive system, well-defined fingers and toes, and the beginnings of facial features.

ovum   the egg, produced by the mother, that unites with a sperm from the father to produce a new individual.

zygote   (ZYE-goat)   the product of the union of ovum and sperm; a fertilized ovum.

implantation   the stage of development, during the first two weeks after conception, in which the fertilized egg (fertilized ovum or zygote) embeds itself in the wall of the uterus and begins to develop.

Figure 13–3

Stages of Embryonic and Fetal Development

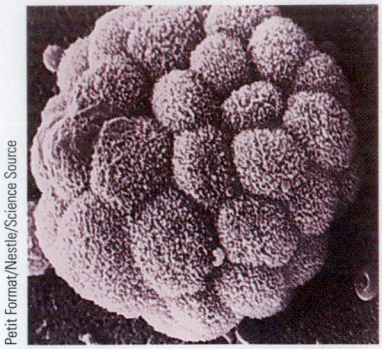

(1) A newly fertilized ovum, called a zygote, is about the size of the period at the end of this sentence. Less than 1 week after fertilization, the zygote has rapidly divided many times and becomes ready for implantation.

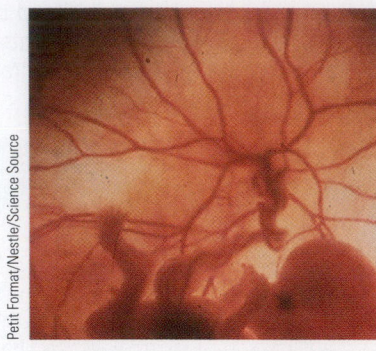

(3) A fetus after 11 weeks of development is just over an inch long. Notice the umbilical cord and blood vessels connecting the fetus with the placenta.

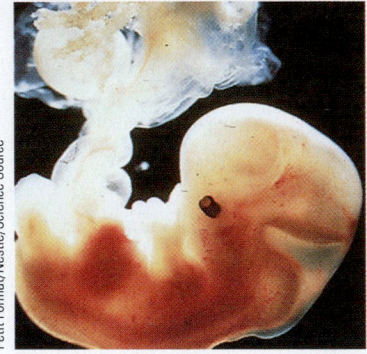

(2) After implantation, the placenta develops and begins to provide nourishment to the developing embryo. An embryo 5 weeks after fertilization is about ½ inch long.

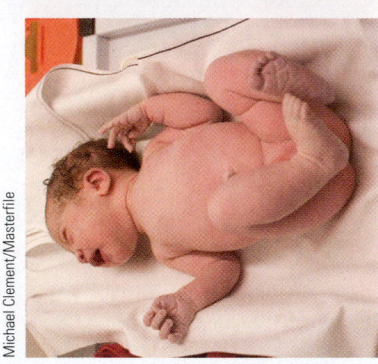

(4) A newborn infant after 9 months of development measures close to 20 inches in length. The average birthweight is about 7½ pounds. From 8 weeks to term, this infant grew 20 times longer and 50 times heavier.

In the last seven months of pregnancy, the fetal period, the fetus grows 50 times heavier and 20 times longer. Critical periods of cell division and development occur in organ after organ. The amniotic sac fills with fluid, and the mother's body changes. The uterus and its supporting muscles increase in size, the breasts may become tender and full, the nipples may darken in preparation for lactation, and the mother's blood volume increases by half to accommodate the added load of materials it must carry. Gestation lasts approximately 40 weeks and ends with the birth of the infant. The 40 or so weeks of pregnancy are divided into thirds, each of which is called a **trimester**.

A Note about Critical Periods   Each organ and tissue type grows with its own characteristic pattern and timing. The development of each takes place only at a certain time—the **critical period**. Whatever nutrients and other environmental conditions are necessary during this period must be supplied on time if the organ is to reach its full potential. If the development of an organ is limited during a critical period, recovery is impossible. For example, the fetus's heart and brain are well developed at 14 weeks; the lungs, 10 weeks later. Therefore, early malnutrition impairs the heart and brain; later malnutrition impairs the lungs.

The effects of malnutrition during critical periods of pregnancy are seen in defects of the nervous system of the embryo (explained later), in the child's poor dental health, and in the adolescent's and adult's vulnerability to infections and possibly higher risks of diabetes, hypertension, stroke, or heart disease.[13] The effects of malnutrition during critical periods are irreversible: abundant and nourishing food, fed after the critical time, cannot remedy harm already done.

Table 13–1 identifies characteristics of a **high-risk pregnancy**. The more factors that apply, the higher the risk. All pregnant women, especially those in high-risk categories, need **prenatal** medical care, including dietary advice.

KEY POINTS

- Implantation, fetal development, and critical period development depend on maternal nutrition status.
- The effects of malnutrition during critical periods are irreversible.

trimester a period representing gestation. A trimester is about 13 to 14 weeks.

critical period a finite period during development in which certain events may occur that will have irreversible effects on later developmental stages. A critical period is usually a period of cell division in a body organ.

high-risk pregnancy a pregnancy characterized by risk factors that make it likely the birth will be complicated by premature delivery, difficult birth, retarded growth, birth defects, and early infant death. A *low-risk pregnancy* has none of these factors.

prenatal (pree-NAY-tal) before birth.

Increased Need for Nutrients

During pregnancy, a woman's nutrient needs increase more for certain nutrients than for others. Figure 13–4 shows the percentage increase in nutrient intakes recommended for pregnant women compared to nonpregnant women. The nutrient demands of pregnancy are high so a woman must make careful food choices, but her body will also do its part by maximizing nutrient absorption and minimizing nutrient losses.

Energy, Carbohydrate, Protein, and Fat Energy needs vary with the progression of pregnancy. In the first trimester, the pregnant woman needs no additional energy, but her energy needs rise as pregnancy progresses. She requires an additional 340 daily calories during the second trimester and an extra 450 calories each day during the third trimester.[14] Well-nourished pregnant women meet these demands for more energy in several ways: some eat more food, some reduce their activity, and some store less of their food energy as fat.[15] A woman can easily meet the need for extra calories by selecting more nutrient-dense foods from the five food groups. Table 13–2 (p. 522) offers a sample menu for pregnant and lactating women.

Ample carbohydrate (ideally, 175 grams or more per day and certainly no less than 135 grams) is necessary to fuel the fetal brain and spare the protein needed for fetal growth. Whole-grain breads and cereals, dark green and other vegetables, legumes, and citrus and other fruit provide carbohydrates, nutrients, and phytochemicals, along with fiber to help alleviate the constipation that many pregnant women experience.

Table 13–1

High-Risk Pregnancy Factors

- Prepregnancy BMI either <18.5 or ≥25
- Insufficient or excessive pregnancy weight gain
- Nutrient deficiencies or toxicities; eating disorders
- Poverty, lack of family support, low level of education, limited food availability
- Smoking, alcohol, or other drug use
- Age, especially 15 years or younger or 35 years or older
- Many previous pregnancies (3 or more to mothers younger than age 20; 4 or more to mothers age 20 or older)
- Short or long intervals between pregnancies (<18 months or >59 months)
- Previous history of problems such as low- or high-birthweight infants
- Twins or triplets
- Pregnancy-related hypertension or gestational diabetes
- Diabetes; heart, respiratory, and kidney disease; certain genetic disorders; special diets and medications

Figure 13–4

Comparison of Selected Nutrient Recommendations for Nonpregnant, Pregnant, and Lactating Women[a]

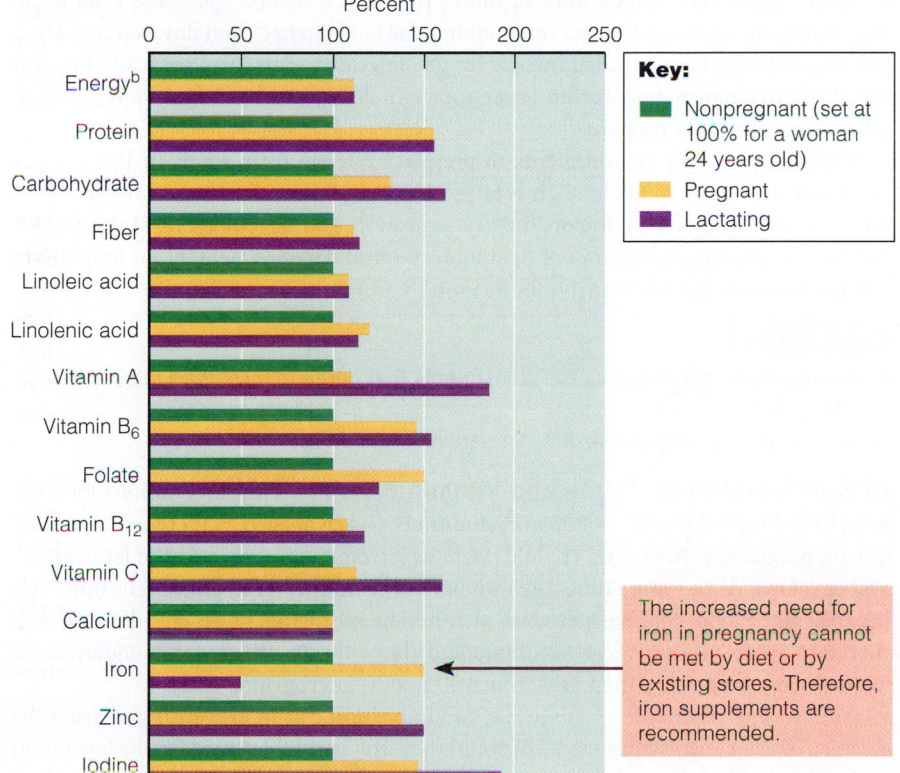

The increased need for iron in pregnancy cannot be met by diet or by existing stores. Therefore, iron supplements are recommended.

[a]Values for other nutrients are listed on the inside front cover, pages A and B.

[b]Energy allowance during pregnancy is for the 2nd trimester; energy allowance during the 3rd trimester is slightly higher; no additional allowance is provided during the 1st trimester. Energy allowance during lactation is for the first 6 months; energy allowance during the second 6 months is slightly higher.

Food Group	Amount	SAMPLE MENU	
Fruits	2 c	**Breakfast** 1 whole-wheat English muffin	**Dinner** Chicken cacciatore
Vegetables	3 c	2 tbs peanut butter 1 c low-fat vanilla yogurt ½ c fresh strawberries 1 c orange juice	3 oz chicken ½ c stewed tomatoes 1 c rice ½ c summer squash
Grains	8 oz	**Midmorning snack** ½ c cranberry juice 1 oz pretzels	1½ c salad (spinach, mushrooms, carrots) 1 tbs salad dressing 1 slice Italian bread
Protein Foods	6½ oz	**Lunch** Sandwich (tuna salad on whole-wheat bread)	2 tsp soft margarine 1 c low-fat milk
Milk	3 c	½ carrot (sticks) 1 c low-fat milk	

Note: This sample meal plan provides about 2,500 calories (55% from carbohydrate, 20% from protein, and 25% from fat) and meets most of the vitamin and mineral needs of pregnant and lactating women.

The protein DRI recommendation for pregnancy is an additional 25 grams per day higher than for nonpregnant women. Most women in the United States, however, need not add protein-rich foods to their diets because they already consume plenty of meats, seafood, poultry and eggs. Low-fat milk and milk products provide protein, calcium, vitamin D, and other nutrients.

Some vegetarian women limit or omit protein-rich meats, eggs, and milk products. For them, meeting the recommendation for food energy each day and including plant-protein foods such as legumes, tofu, whole grains, nuts, and seeds are imperative. Protein supplements during pregnancy can be harmful to infant development, and their use is discouraged.

The high nutrient requirements of pregnancy leave little room in the diet for excess fat, especially solid fats such as fatty meats and butter. The essential fatty acids, however, are particularly important to the growth and development of the fetus.[16] The brain is composed mainly of lipid material and depends heavily on long-chain omega-3 and omega-6 fatty acids for its growth, function, and structure.

KEY POINTS

- Pregnancy brings physiological adjustments that demand increased intakes of energy and nutrients.
- A balanced nutrient-dense diet is essential for meeting nutrient needs.

Of Special Interest: Folate and Vitamin B$_{12}$

Two vitamins famous for their roles in cell reproduction—folate and vitamin B$_{12}$—are needed in increased amounts during pregnancy. New cells are laid down at a tremendous pace as the fetus grows and develops. At the same time, the number of the mother's red blood cells must rise because her blood volume increases, a function requiring more cell division and therefore more vitamins. To accommodate these needs, the recommendation for folate during pregnancy increases from 400 to 600 micrograms a day.

As described in Chapter 7, folate plays an important role in preventing neural tube defects. To review, the early weeks of pregnancy are a critical period for the formation and closure of the **neural tube** that will later develop to form the brain and spinal cord. By the time a woman suspects she is pregnant, usually around the sixth week of pregnancy, the embryo's neural tube normally has closed. A **neural tube defect (NTD)** occurs when the tube fails to close properly. Each year in the United States, an

neural tube the embryonic tissue that later forms the brain and spinal cord.

neural tube defect (NTD) a group of abnormalities of the brain and spinal cord apparent at birth and caused by interruption of the normal early development of the neural tube.

Figure 13–5

Spina Bifida

Spina bifida, a common neural tube defect, occurs when the vertebrae of the spine fail to close around the spinal cord, leaving it unprotected. The B vitamin folate helps prevent spina bifida and other neural tube defects.

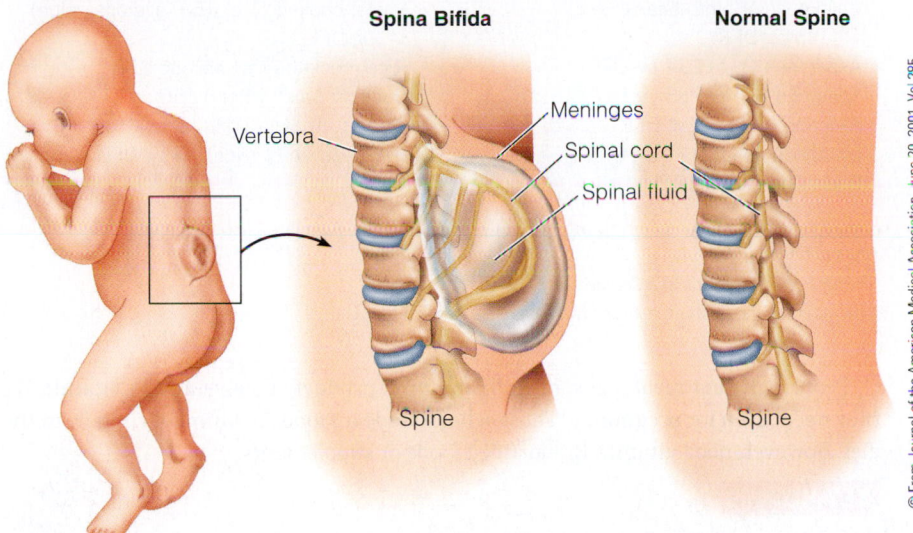

© From Journal of the American Medical Association, June 20, 2001, Vol 285.

estimated 3,000 pregnancies are affected by a NTD.[17] The two most common types of NTDs are anencephaly (no brain) and spina bifida (split spine).

In **anencephaly**, the upper end of the neural tube fails to close. Consequently, the brain is either missing or fails to develop. Pregnancies affected by anencephaly often end in miscarriage; infants born with anencephaly die shortly after birth.

Spina bifida is characterized by incomplete closure of the spinal cord and its bony encasement (see Figure 13–5). The membranes covering the spinal cord and sometimes the cord itself may protrude from the spine as a sac. Spina bifida often produces paralysis in varying degrees, depending on the extent of spinal cord damage. Mild cases may not be noticed. Moderate cases may involve curvature of the spine, muscle weakness, mental handicaps, and other ills; severe cases can result in death. Table 13–3 lists risk factors for neural tube defects.

To reduce the risk of neural tube defects, women who are capable of becoming pregnant are advised to obtain 400 micrograms of folic acid daily from supplements, fortified foods, or both, *in addition* to eating folate-rich foods (see Table 13–4, p. 524). The DRI committee recommends intake of synthetic folate—folic acid—in supplements and fortified foods because it is better absorbed than the folate naturally present in foods. Foods that naturally contain folate are still important, however, because they contribute to folate intakes while providing other needed vitamins, minerals, fiber, and phytochemicals.

The folic acid enrichment of grain products (cereal, grits, pasta, rice, bread, and the like) sold commercially in the United States has improved the folate status of women of childbearing age and lowered the number of neural tube defects that occur each year.[18] Researchers expect to see declines in some other birth defects (cleft lip and cleft palate) and miscarriages as well.[19] A safety concern arises, however. The pregnant woman also needs a greater amount of vitamin B_{12} to assist folate in the manufacture of new cells. Because high intakes of folate complicate the diagnosis of a vitamin B_{12} deficiency, quantities of 1 milligram of folic acid or more require a prescription. Most over-the-counter multivitamin supplements contain 400 micrograms of folic acid; supplements for pregnant women usually contain at least 800 micrograms.

Table 13–3

Risk Factors for Neural Tube Defects

A pregnancy affected by a neural tube defect can occur in any woman, but these factors make it more likely:

- A personal or family history of a pregnancy affected by a neural tube defect.
- Maternal diabetes.
- Maternal use of certain antiseizure medications.
- Mutations in folate-related enzymes.
- Maternal obesity.

anencephaly (an-en-SEFF-ah-lee) an uncommon and always fatal neural tube defect in which the brain fails to form.

spina bifida (SPY-na BIFF-ih-duh) one of the most common types of neural tube defects, in which gaps occur in the bones of the spine. Often the spinal cord bulges and protrudes through the gaps, resulting in a number of motor and other impairments.

Table 13–4

Rich Folate Sources[a]

Natural Folate Sources	Fortified Folic Acid Sources
Liver (3 oz) 221 μg DFE[b]	Highly enriched ready-to-eat cereals
Lentils (½ c) 179 μg DFE	(¾ c) 680 μg DFE[c]
Chickpeas or pinto beans (½ c) 145 μg DFE	Pasta, cooked (1 c) 154 (average value) μg DFE
Asparagus (½ c) 134 μg DFE	Rice, cooked (1 c) 153 μg DFE
Spinach (1 c raw) 58 μg DFE	Bagel (1 small whole) 156 μg DFE
Avocado (½ c) 61 μg DFE	Waffles, frozen (2) 78 μg DFE
Orange juice (1 c) 74 μg DFE	Bread, white (1 slice) 48 μg DFE
Beets (½ c) 68 μg DFE	

[a]Folate amounts for these and thousands of other foods are listed in the Table of Food Composition in Appendix A.

[b]Dietary folate equivalent (see Chapter 7).

[c]Folic acid in cereals varies; read the Nutrition Facts panel of the label.

People who eat meat, eggs, or milk and milk products receive all the vitamin B_{12} they need, even for pregnancy. Those who exclude all foods of animal origin from the diet, however, need vitamin B_{12}–fortified foods or supplements.

KEY POINTS

- Folate and vitamin B_{12} play key roles in cell replication and are needed in large amounts during pregnancy.
- Folate plays an important role in preventing neural tube defects.

Choline   Although not defined as a vitamin, choline is commonly grouped with the B vitamins. Choline is a dietary component that is vital for the structural integrity of cell membranes, the synthesis of an important neurotransmitter, and the metabolism of lipids. During fetal development, choline, like folate, is needed for the closure of the neural tube and for the normal development of the brain and spinal cord.[20] During pregnancy, large amounts of choline are delivered to the fetus via the placenta.[21] This transfer of choline from mother to fetus depletes maternal stores.

The DRI recommendation for choline in pregnancy is set at 450 milligrams per day, which is slightly higher than for nonpregnant women. Because prenatal supplements do not typically contain choline, pregnant women are advised to include choline-rich foods such as eggs, milk and milk products, legumes, and meats and seafood in their eating patterns.

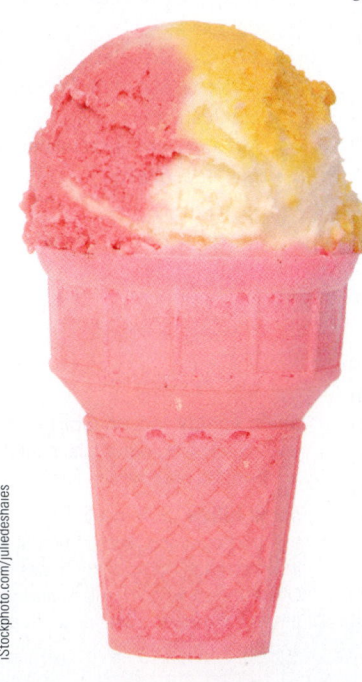

iStockphoto.com/juliedeshaies

Vitamin D and Calcium   Vitamin D and the minerals involved in building the skeleton—calcium, phosphorus, and magnesium—are in great demand during pregnancy. Insufficient intakes may have adverse effects on fetal bone growth and tooth development.[22]

Vitamin D plays a vital role in calcium absorption and use. Severe maternal vitamin D deficiency interferes with normal calcium metabolism and, in rare cases, may cause the vitamin D–deficiency disease rickets in a newborn.[23] Regular exposure to sunlight and consumption of vitamin D–fortified milk are usually sufficient to provide the recommended amount of vitamin D during pregnancy (15 μg), which is the same as for nonpregnant women.[24] The vitamin D in prenatal supplements helps to protect many, but not all, pregnant women from inadequate intakes.[25]

A woman's intestinal absorption of calcium doubles early in pregnancy, and the extra mineral is stored in her bones. Later, as the fetal bones begin to calcify, a dramatic shift of calcium across the placenta occurs. Still unknown is whether the extra calcium added to the mother's bones early in pregnancy is withdrawn later to help meet the fetus's needs.[26] In the final weeks of pregnancy, more than 300 milligrams of calcium a day are transferred to the fetus.[27]

Typically, young women in this country take in too little calcium. Of particular importance, pregnant women younger than age 25, whose own bones are still actively depositing minerals, should strive to meet the DRI recommendation by increasing their intakes of calcium-rich foods. The DRI recommendation for calcium intake is the same for nonpregnant and pregnant women in the same age group. The USDA Eating Patterns suggest consuming 3 cups per day of fat-free or low-fat milk or the equivalent in milk products. Women who exclude milk products need calcium-fortified foods such as soy milk, orange juice, and cereals. Less preferred is a daily supplement of 600 milligrams of calcium.

Iron   A pregnant woman needs iron to help increase her blood volume and to provide for placental and fetal needs. The developing fetus draws heavily on the mother's iron stores to accumulate sufficient stores of its own to last through the first four to six months after birth. The transfer of iron to the fetus is regulated by the placenta, which gives the iron needs of the fetus higher priority. Even a woman with inadequate iron stores transfers a considerable amount of iron to the fetus. In addition, blood losses are inevitable at birth, especially during a delivery by cesarean section, further draining the mother's iron supply. Women who enter pregnancy with iron-deficiency anemia have a greater-than-normal risk of delivering low-birthweight or preterm infants.[28]

During pregnancy, the body makes several adaptations to help meet the exceptionally high need for iron. Menstruation, the major route of iron loss in women, ceases, and absorption of iron increases up to threefold. Even so, to help prevent iron supplies from dwindling during pregnancy, all women capable of becoming pregnant are advised do three things:

1. Choose foods that supply heme iron (meat, fish, and poultry), which is most readily absorbed.

2. Choose additional iron sources, such as iron-rich eggs, vegetables, and legumes.

3. Consume foods that enhance iron absorption, such as vitamin C–rich fruits and vegetables.

Without corrective action, a woman's iron deficit worsens with each subsequent pregnancy. Few women enter pregnancy with adequate iron stores, so a daily 30-milligram iron supplement is recommended early in pregnancy, if not before.[29] A woman with a severe deficiency may need more. To enhance iron absorption, the supplement should be taken between meals and with liquids other than milk, coffee, or tea, which inhibit iron absorption.

Zinc   Zinc is vital for protein synthesis and cell development during pregnancy. Typical zinc intakes of pregnant women are lower than recommendations, but fortunately zinc absorption increases when intakes are low. Large doses of iron can interfere with zinc absorption and metabolism, but most prenatal supplements supply the right balance of these minerals for pregnancy. Zinc is abundant in protein-rich foods such as shellfish, meat, and nuts.

KEY POINTS

- Choline is needed for neural tube closure and for the normal development of the brain and spinal cord.
- Adequate vitamin D and calcium are indispensable for normal bone development of the fetus.
- Iron supplements are recommended for pregnant women.
- Zinc is needed for protein synthesis and cell development during pregnancy.

Prenatal Supplements   A healthy pregnancy and optimal infant development depend heavily on the mother's diet.[30] Pregnant women who make wise food choices can meet most of their nutrient needs, with the possible exception of iron. Even so, physicians routinely recommend daily prenatal multivitamin–mineral supplements for pregnant women. **Prenatal supplements** typically provide more folate, iron, and calcium than regular supplements. Women with poor diets need them urgently, as do women in these high-risk groups: women carrying twins or triplets and women who

prenatal supplements nutrient supplements specifically designed to provide the nutrients needed during pregnancy—particularly folate, iron, and calcium—without excesses or unneeded constituents.

smoke cigarettes, drink alcohol, or abuse drugs.[31] For these women in particular, prenatal supplements may reduce the risks of preterm delivery, low infant birthweights, and birth defects.

KEY POINTS

- Physicians routinely recommend daily prenatal multivitamin–mineral supplements for pregnant women.
- Prenatal supplements are most likely to benefit women who do not eat adequately, who are carrying twins or triplets, or who smoke cigarettes, drink alcohol, or abuse drugs.

Food Assistance Programs

The nationwide **Special Supplemental Nutrition Program for Women, Infants, and Children (WIC)** provides vouchers redeemable for nutritious foods, along with nutrition education and referrals to health and social services, for low-income pregnant and lactating women and their children.[32] WIC-sponsored foods include baby foods, eggs, dried and canned beans and peas, tuna fish, peanut butter, fruits and vegetables and their juices, iron-fortified cereals, milk and cheese, soy-based beverages and tofu, whole-wheat bread, and other whole-grain products. WIC encourages breastfeeding and offers incentives to mothers who do so. For infants given infant formula, WIC also provides iron-fortified formula.

More than 9 million people—most of them infants and young children—receive WIC benefits each month. Proven benefits from WIC participation include improved nutrient status and growth among infants and children, improved iron status among pregnant women, reduced risk of infant mortality and low birthweight, and reduced maternal and newborn medical costs. In addition to WIC, the Supplemental Nutrition Assistance Program (formerly the Food Stamp Program) can help to stretch the low-income family's grocery dollars.

KEY POINTS

- Food assistance programs such as WIC can provide nutritious food for pregnant women of limited financial means.
- Participation in WIC during pregnancy can reduce iron deficiency, infant mortality, low birthweight, and maternal and newborn medical costs.

How Much Weight Should a Woman Gain during Pregnancy?

Women must gain weight during pregnancy—fetal and maternal well-being depends on it. Ideally, a woman will have begun her pregnancy at a healthy weight, and she will gain appropriately for her prepregnancy body mass index (BMI) and the number of fetuses she carries, as shown in Table 13–5. The benefits of proper weight gain include a lower risk of surgical birth, a greater chance of having a healthy birthweight baby, and other positive outcomes for both mothers and infants. Many women exceed the recommended ranges, however, and a few even fall short.[33]

Weight loss during pregnancy is not recommended.[34] Even obese women are advised to gain between 11 and 20 pounds for the best chance of delivering a healthy baby. Ideally, overweight women will achieve a healthy body weight before becoming pregnant, avoid excessive weight gain during pregnancy, and postpone weight loss until after childbirth.

The ideal weight-gain pattern for a woman who begins pregnancy at a healthy weight is 3½ pounds during the first trimester and 1 pound per week thereafter. If a woman gains more than is recommended early in pregnancy, she should not restrict her energy intake later on in order to lose weight. Any sudden, large weight gain is a danger signal, however, because it may indicate the onset of preeclampsia (see the section entitled "Troubleshooting"). The weight the pregnant woman gains is nearly all lean tissue: the placenta, uterus, blood, and milk-producing glands and the fetus itself (see Figure 13–6). The fat she gains is needed later for lactation.

Special Supplemental Nutrition Program for Women, Infants, and Children (WIC) a USDA program offering low-income pregnant and lactating women and those with infants or preschool children coupons redeemable for specific foods that supply the nutrients deemed most necessary for growth and development. For more information, visit www.usda.gov/FoodandNutrition.

Table 13–5

Recommended Weight Gains Based on Prepregnancy Weight

Prepregnancy Weight	RECOMMENDED WEIGHT GAIN	
	For single birth	*For twin birth*
Underweight (BMI <18.5)	28 to 40 lb (12.5 to 18.0 kg)	Insufficient data to make recommendation
Healthy weight (BMI 18.5 to 24.9)	25 to 35 lb (11.5 to 16.0 kg)	37 to 54 lb (17.0 to 25.0 kg)
Overweight (BMI 25.0 to 29.9)	15 to 25 lb (7.0 to 11.5 kg)	31 to 50 lb (14.0 to 23.0 kg)
Obese (BMI ≥30)	11 to 20 lb (5.0 to 9.0 kg)	25 to 42 lb (11.0 to 19.0 kg)

Source: Institute of Medicine, *Weight Gain during Pregnancy: Reexamining the Guidelines* (Washington, D.C.: National Academies Press, 2009).

Weight Loss after Pregnancy

The pregnant woman loses some weight at delivery. In the following weeks, she loses more as her blood volume returns to normal and she loses accumulated fluids. The typical woman does not immediately return to her prepregnancy weight. In general, the more weight a woman gains beyond the needs of pregnancy, the more she retains—mostly as body fat.[35] Even without excessive gain, most women tend to retain a few pounds with each pregnancy. When those few pounds become 7 or more and BMI increases by a unit or more, risks of diabetes and hypertension in future pregnancies, as well as chronic diseases later in life, can increase. Women who achieve a healthy weight prior to the first pregnancy and maintain it between pregnancies best avoid the cumulative weight gain that threatens health later on.

KEY POINTS

- Appropriate weight gain is essential for a healthy pregnancy.
- Weight gain recommendations are influenced by the prepregnancy BMI and number of fetuses in the pregnancy.

Figure 13–6

Components of Weight Gain during Pregnancy

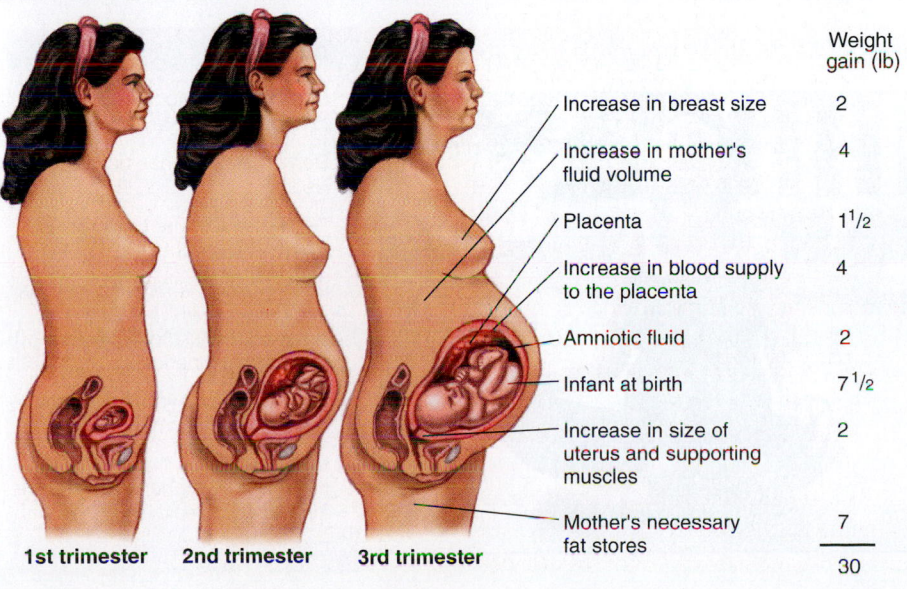

	Weight gain (lb)
Increase in breast size	2
Increase in mother's fluid volume	4
Placenta	1 1/2
Increase in blood supply to the placenta	4
Amniotic fluid	2
Infant at birth	7 1/2
Increase in size of uterus and supporting muscles	2
Mother's necessary fat stores	7
	30

1st trimester   2nd trimester   3rd trimester

Should Pregnant Women Be Physically Active?

An active, physically fit woman experiencing a normal, healthy pregnancy can and should continue to exercise throughout pregnancy, adjusting the intensity and duration as the pregnancy progresses. Staying active improves the fitness of the mother-to-be, facilitates labor, helps to prevent or manage gestational diabetes, and reduces psychological stress.[36] Active women report fewer discomforts throughout their pregnancies and are more likely to meet weight gain recommendations and retain habits that help to lose excess weight and regain fitness later.[37]

Pregnant women should choose "low-impact" activities and avoid sports in which they might fall or be hit by other people or objects (for some safe activity suggestions, see the Think Fitness box). Pregnant women with medical conditions or pregnancy complications should seek medical advice before engaging in physical activity. A few more guidelines are offered in Figure 13–7. Several of the guidelines are aimed at preventing excessively high internal body temperature and dehydration, both of which can harm fetal development. To this end, the pregnant woman should also stay out of saunas, steam rooms, and hot whirlpools.

KEY POINTS

- Physically fit women can continue physical activity throughout pregnancy but should choose activities wisely.
- Pregnant women should avoid sports in which they might fall or be hit and should not become overheated or dehydrated.

Teen Pregnancy

The number of infants born to teenaged mothers has steadily declined during the last 50 years. Despite the long-term decline, however, the U.S. teen birthrate is still one of highest among industrialized nations.[38] In 2013, more than 273,000 infants were born to teenaged mothers.

A pregnant adolescent presents a special case of intense nutrient needs. Young teenage girls have a hard enough time meeting nutrient needs for their own rapid growth and development, let alone those of pregnancy. Many teens enter pregnancy with deficiencies of vitamins B_{12} and D, folate, iron, and calcium that can impair fetal growth.[39] Pregnant adolescents are less likely to receive early prenatal care and are more likely to smoke during pregnancy—two factors that predict low birthweight and

Figure 13–7

Guidelines for Physical Activity during Pregnancy

Pregnant women can enjoy the benefits of physical activity.

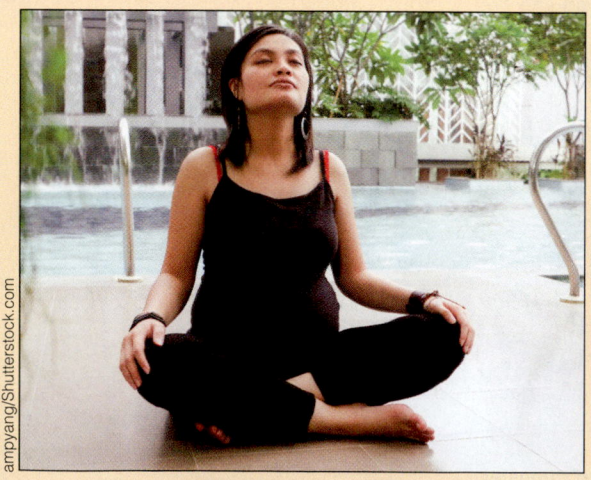

DO	DON'T
Do exercise regularly (most, if not all, days of the week).	Don't exercise vigorously after long periods of inactivity.
Do warm up with 5 to 10 minutes of light activity.	Don't exercise in hot, humid weather.
Do 30 minutes or more of moderate physical activity.	Don't exercise when sick with fever.
Do cool down with 5 to 10 minutes of slow activity and gentle stretching.	Don't exercise while lying on your back after the first trimester of pregnancy or stand motionless for prolonged periods.
Do drink water before, during, and after exercise.	Don't exercise if you experience any pain or discomfort.
Do eat enough to support the additional needs of pregnancy plus exercise.	Don't participate in activities that may harm the abdomen or involve jerky, bouncy movements.
Do rest adequately.	Don't scuba dive.

ampyang/Shutterstock.com

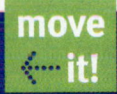
Is there an ideal physical activity for the pregnant woman? There might be. Swimming and water aerobics offer advantages over other activities during pregnancy. Water cools and supports the body, provides a natural resistance, and lessens the impact of the body's movement, especially in the later months. Water aerobics can help to reduce the intensity of back pain during pregnancy. Other activities considered safe and comfortable for pregnant women include walking, light strength training, rowing, yoga, and climbing stairs.

start now! ⋯⟩ Ready to make a change? If you weren't exercising regularly before you became pregnant, talk to your doctor before undertaking an activity. Track your activity daily using the Diet and Wellness Plus Activity Tracker.

---

infant death.[40] The rates of stillbirths, preterm births, and low-birthweight infants are high when either parent is a teen. Adequate nutrition and appropriate weight gain during pregnancy are indispensable components of prenatal care for teenagers and can substantially improve the outlook for both mother and infant.

A pregnant teenager with a healthy body weight is encouraged to gain about 35 pounds. Pregnant and lactating teenagers can follow the eating pattern presented earlier in Table 2–2 (p. 38), choosing a calorie level high enough to support adequate, but not excessive, weight gain.

KEY POINTS

- Pregnant teenage girls have extraordinarily high nutrient needs and an increased likelihood of problem pregnancies.
- Adequate nutrition and appropriate weight gain for pregnant teenagers can substantially improve outcomes for mothers and infants.

Why Do Some Women Crave Pickles and Ice Cream While Others Can't Keep Anything Down?

Does pregnancy give a woman the right to demand pickles and ice cream at 2 a.m.? Perhaps so, but not for nutrition's sake. Food cravings and aversions during pregnancy are common but do not seem to reflect real physiological needs. In other words, a woman who craves pickles is probably not in need of salt. Food cravings and aversions that arise during pregnancy may be due to hormone-induced changes in taste and sensitivities to smells, and they quickly disappear after the birth.

Some pregnant women respond to cravings by eating nonfood items such as laundry starch, clay, soil, or ice—a practice known as pica.[41] Pica may be practiced for cultural reasons that reflect a society's folklore. Chapter 8 provides more details.

The nausea of "morning" (actually, anytime) sickness seems unavoidable and may even be a welcome sign of a healthy pregnancy because it arises from the hormonal changes of early pregnancy. The problem typically peaks at 9 weeks of gestation and resolves within a month or two. Many women complain that odors, especially cooking smells, make them feel nauseated, so minimizing odors may provide some relief. Traditional strategies for quelling nausea are listed in Table 13–6, but little evidence exists to support such advice.[42] Some women do best by simply eating what they desire whenever they feel hungry. Morning sickness can be persistent, however, and if it interferes with normal eating for more than a week or two, the woman should seek medical help to prevent nutrient deficiencies.

As the hormones of pregnancy alter her muscle tone and the thriving fetus crowds her intestinal organs, an expectant mother may complain of heartburn or constipation. Raising the head of the bed with two or three pillows can help to relieve nighttime heartburn. A high-fiber diet, physical activity, and a plentiful fluid intake will

Table 13–6
Tips for Relieving Common Discomforts of Pregnancy

To alleviate the nausea of pregnancy:

- On waking, get up slowly.
- Eat dry toast or crackers.
- Chew gum or suck hard candies.
- Eat small, frequent meals whenever hunger strikes.
- Avoid foods with offensive odors.

To prevent or alleviate constipation:

- Eat foods high in fiber.
- Exercise daily.
- Drink at least 8 cups of liquids a day.
- Respond promptly to the urge to defecate.
- Use laxatives only as prescribed by a physician.

To prevent or relieve heartburn:

- Relax and eat slowly.
- Chew food thoroughly.
- Eat small, frequent meals.
- Drink liquids between meals.
- Avoid spicy or greasy foods.
- Sit up while eating.
- Wait an hour after eating before lying down.
- Wait 2 hours after eating before exercising.

help relieve constipation. The pregnant woman should use laxatives or heartburn medications only if her physician prescribes them.

- Food cravings usually do not reflect physiological needs, and some may interfere with nutrition.
- Nausea arises from normal hormonal changes of pregnancy.

Some Cautions for the Pregnant Woman

Some choices that pregnant women make or substances they encounter can harm the fetus, sometimes severely. Smoking and other threats all deserve consideration, but alcohol constitutes an even greater threat to fetal health and is given a section of its own.

Cigarette Smoking   A surgeon general's warning states that parental smoking can kill an otherwise healthy fetus or newborn. Unfortunately, an estimated 12 percent of pregnant women in the United States smoke, and rates are even higher for unmarried women and those who have not graduated from high school.[43]

Constituents of cigarette smoke, such as nicotine, carbon monoxide, arsenic, and cyanide, are toxic to a fetus.[44] Smoking during pregnancy can damage fetal DNA, which could lead to developmental defects or diseases such as cancer.[45] Smoking restricts the blood supply to the growing fetus and so limits the delivery of oxygen and nutrients and the removal of wastes. It slows fetal growth, can reduce brain size, and may impair the intellectual and behavioral development of the child later in life. Smoking during pregnancy damages fetal blood vessels, an effect that is still apparent at the age of 5 years.[46]

A mother who smokes is more likely to have a complicated birth and a low-birthweight infant. The more a mother smokes, the smaller her baby will be. Of all preventable causes of low birthweight in the United States, smoking has the greatest impact. Table 13–7 lists complications of smoking during pregnancy.

Smoking during pregnancy interferes with fetal lung development and increases the risks of respiratory infections and childhood asthma.[47] Sudden infant death syndrome (SIDS), the unexplained deaths that sometimes occur in otherwise healthy infants, has been linked to the mother's cigarette smoking during pregnancy.[48] Even in nonsmokers, regular exposure to **environmental tobacco smoke** (or secondhand smoke) during pregnancy increases the risk of low birthweight and the likelihood of SIDS.

Alternatives to smoking—such as using snuff, chewing tobacco, or using nicotine-replacement therapy—are not safe during pregnancy. A woman who uses nicotine in any form and who is considering pregnancy or is already pregnant should make every effort to quit.

Medicinal Drugs and Herbal Supplements   Medicinal drugs taken during pregnancy can cause serious birth defects. A pregnant woman should not take over-the-counter drugs or any medications not prescribed by a physician; even then, she should read the labels and take warnings seriously.

Some pregnant women mistakenly consider herbal supplements to be safe alternatives to medicinal drugs and take them to relieve nausea, promote water loss, alleviate depression, or aid sleep or for other reasons. Some herbal products may be safe, but almost none have been tested for safety or effectiveness during pregnancy. Pregnant women should stay away from herbal supplements, teas, or other products unless their safety during pregnancy has been ascertained.[49]

Drugs of Abuse   Drugs of abuse such as methamphetamine and cocaine easily cross the placenta and impair fetal growth and development. Furthermore, such drugs are responsible for preterm births, low-birthweight infants, and sudden infant deaths. If these newborns survive, central nervous system damage is evident: their cries, sleep, and behaviors early in life are abnormal, and their cognitive development

---

Table 13–7

Complications Associated with Smoking during Pregnancy

- Fetal growth restriction
- Preterm birth
- Low birthweight
- Premature separation of the placenta
- Miscarriage
- Stillbirth
- Sudden infant death syndrome
- Congenital malformations

environmental tobacco smoke the combination of exhaled smoke (mainstream smoke) and smoke from lighted cigarettes, pipes, or cigars (sidestream smoke) that enters the air and may be inhaled by other people.

later in life is impaired.[50] They may be hypersensitive or underaroused; many suffer the symptoms of withdrawal. Delays in their growth and development persist throughout childhood and adolescence.[51]

Environmental Contaminants   Pregnant women who are exposed to contaminants such as lead may bear low-birthweight infants with delayed mental and psychomotor development who struggle to survive. During pregnancy, the heavy metal lead readily moves across the placenta, inflicting severe damage on the developing fetal nervous system. For pregnant women, choosing a diet free of contamination takes on extra urgency. Adequate dietary calcium can help to defend against lead toxicity by reducing its absorption.

Fatty fish is a good source of omega-3 fatty acids, but some species contain large amounts of the pollutant mercury that can harm the developing fetal brain and nervous system (described in Chapter 12). The benefits of eating fish and shellfish greatly outweigh the dangers, however, so pregnant and lactating women are urged to consume 8 to 12 ounces of lower-mercury cooked or canned fish and seafood (Table 5-7, p. 180), and to avoid these high-mercury species: shark, swordfish, king mackerel, and tilefish (also called golden snapper or golden bass).[52] White albacore tuna (cooked or canned) contains more mercury than other types, so the U. S. Food and Drug Administration (FDA) also recommends that pregnant or lactating women limit their intake to no more than 6 ounces weekly.[53]

Foodborne Illness   The vomiting and diarrhea caused by many foodborne illnesses can leave a pregnant woman exhausted and dangerously dehydrated. Particularly threatening, however, is **listeriosis**, which can cause miscarriage, stillbirth, or severe brain or other infections in fetuses and newborns. Pregnant women are more likely than other healthy adults to contract listeriosis. A woman with listeriosis may develop symptoms such as fever, vomiting, and diarrhea in about 12 hours after eating a contaminated food; serious symptoms may develop a week to six weeks later. A blood test can reliably detect listeriosis, and antibiotics given promptly to the pregnant sufferer can often prevent infection of the fetus or newborn. To protect herself and her fetus from listeriosis, a pregnant woman should follow all of the food safety advice of Chapter 12, and she should observe the following recommendations:

- Use only pasteurized juices and dairy products; do not eat soft cheeses such as feta, brie, Camembert, panela, "queso blanco," "queso fresco," and blue-veined cheeses such as Roquefort; do not drink raw (unpasteurized) milk or eat foods that contain it.

- Do not eat hot dogs or luncheon or deli meats unless heated until steaming hot.

- Thoroughly cook meat, poultry, eggs, and seafood.

- Wash all fruits and vegetables.

- Avoid refrigerated patés or smoked seafood or fish labeled "nova-style," "lox," or "kippered." Canned varieties are generally safe.

Vitamin–Mineral Overdoses   Many vitamins and minerals are toxic when taken in excess. Excessive vitamin A is widely known for its role in fetal malformations of the cranial nervous system. Intakes before the seventh week of pregnancy appear to be the most damaging. For this reason, vitamin A supplements are not given during pregnancy unless there is specific evidence of deficiency, which is rare.

Restrictive Dieting   Restrictive dieting, even for short periods, can be hazardous during pregnancy. In particular, low-carbohydrate diets or fasts that cause ketosis deprive the growing fetal brain of needed glucose and may impair cognitive development. Such diets are also likely to lack other nutrients vital to fetal growth. Regardless of prepregnancy weight, pregnant women need an adequate diet to support healthy fetal development.

listeriosis a serious foodborne infection that can cause severe brain infection or death in a fetus or a newborn; caused by the bacterium *Listeria monocytogenes*, which is found in soil and water.

Sugar Substitutes　Artificial sweeteners have been studied extensively and found to be acceptable during pregnancy if used within the FDA's guidelines.[54] Women with the inborn error of metabolism known as phenylketonuria should not use the artificial sweetener aspartame.

Caffeine　Caffeine crosses the placenta, and the fetus has only a limited ability to metabolize it. Even so, women can safely consume less than 200 milligrams a day without apparent ill effects on their pregnancy duration or outcome.[55] Limited evidence suggests that heavy use—intake equaling more than three cups of coffee a day—may increase the risk of hypertension and miscarriage.[56] Depending on the quantities consumed and the mother's metabolism, caffeine may also interfere with fetal growth.[57] The most sensible course therefore is to limit caffeine consumption to the equivalent of about two cups of coffee or three 12-ounce cola beverages a day. Caffeine amounts in food and beverages are listed in Controversy 14.

KEY POINTS

- Smoking during pregnancy delivers toxins to the fetus, damages DNA, restricts fetal growth, and limits the delivery of oxygen and nutrients and the removal of wastes.
- Smoking and other drugs, contaminants such as mercury, foodborne illnesses, large supplemental doses of nutrients, weight-loss diets, and excessive use of artificial sweeteners and caffeine should be avoided during pregnancy.

Drinking during Pregnancy

LO 13.2 Summarize the evidence against alcohol intake during pregnancy.

Alcohol is arguably the most hazardous drug to future generations because it is legally available, heavily promoted, and widely abused. Society sends mixed messages concerning alcohol. Beverage companies promote an image of drinkers as healthy and active. Opposing this image, health authorities warn that alcohol can injure health, especially during pregnancy (see Figure 13–8). Every container of beer, wine, liquor, or mixed drinks for sale in the United States is required to warn pregnant women of the dangers of drinking during pregnancy.

Alcohol's Effects

Women of childbearing age need to know about alcohol's harmful effects on a fetus. Alcohol crosses the placenta freely and is directly toxic:

- A sudden dose of alcohol can halt the delivery of oxygen through the umbilical cord. The fetal brain and nervous system are extremely vulnerable to a deficit of oxygen or glucose, and alcohol causes both by disrupting placental functioning. Alcohol slows cell division, reducing the number of cells produced and inflicting abnormalities on those that are produced and all of their progeny.

- During the first month of pregnancy, the fetal brain is growing at the rate of 100,000 new brain cells a minute. Even a few minutes of alcohol exposure during this critical period can exert a major detrimental effect.

- Alcohol interferes with placental transport of nutrients to the fetus and can cause malnutrition in the mother; then all of malnutrition's harmful effects compound the effects of the alcohol.

- Before fertilization, alcohol can damage the ovum or sperm in the mother- or father-to-be, leading to abnormalities in the child.

KEY POINTS

- Alcohol crosses the placenta and is directly toxic to the fetus.
- Alcohol limits oxygen delivery to the fetus, slows cell division, and reduces the number of cells organs produce.

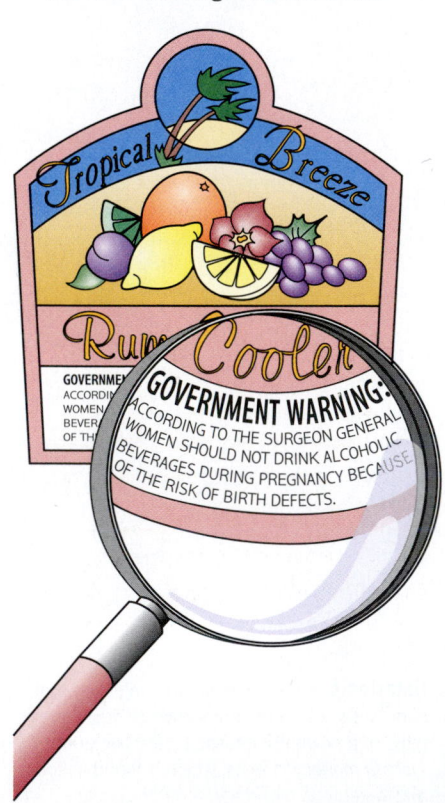

Figure 13–8

Mixed Messages in Alcohol Advertisements

Labels on alcoholic beverages often display "healthy" images, but their warnings tell the truth.

Fetal Alcohol Syndrome

Drinking alcohol during pregnancy threatens the fetus with irreversible brain damage, growth restriction, mental retardation, facial abnormalities, vision abnormalities, and many more health problems—a spectrum of symptoms known as **fetal alcohol spectrum disorders**, or **FASD**. Children at the most severe end of the spectrum (those with all of the symptoms) are defined as having **fetal alcohol syndrome**, or **FAS**. The lifelong mental retardation and other tragedies of FAS can be prevented by abstaining from drinking alcohol during pregnancy. Once the damage is done, however, the child remains impaired. Figure 13–9 shows the facial abnormalities of FAS, which are easy to depict. A visual picture of the internal harm is impossible, but that damage seals the fate of the child. An estimated 5 to 20 of every 10,000 children are victims of FAS, making it one of the leading known preventable causes of mental retardation in the world.[58]

Even when a child does not develop full FAS, prenatal exposure to alcohol can lead to less severe, but nonetheless serious, mental and physical problems. The cluster of mental problems is known as **alcohol-related neurodevelopmental disorder (ARND)**, and the physical malformations are referred to as **alcohol-related birth defects (ARBD)**.[†] Some of these children show no outward sign of impairment, but others are short in stature or display subtle facial abnormalities. Many perform poorly in school and in social interactions and suffer a subtle form of brain damage. Mood disorders and problem behaviors, such as aggression, are common.

A child with FAS.

[†] Formerly, ARND and ARBD were grouped together and called fetal alcohol effects (FAE).

Figure 13–9
Typical Facial Characteristics of FAS

The severe facial abnormalities shown here are just outward signs of severe mental impairments and internal organ damage. These defects, though hidden, may create major health problems later.

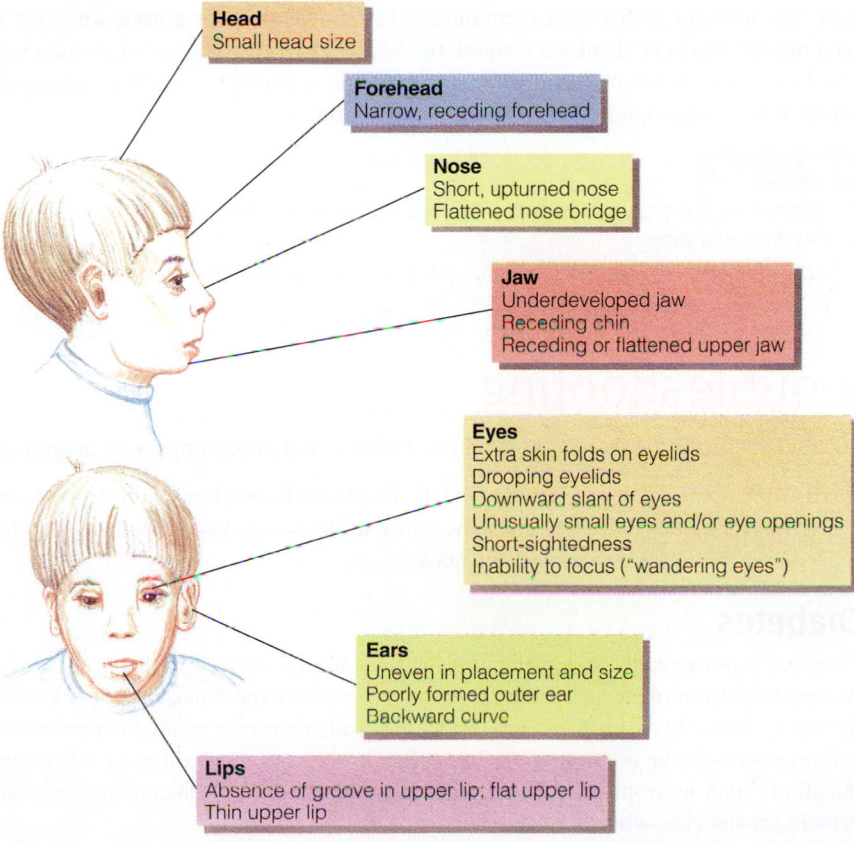

Head
Small head size

Forehead
Narrow, receding forehead

Nose
Short, upturned nose
Flattened nose bridge

Jaw
Underdeveloped jaw
Receding chin
Receding or flattened upper jaw

Eyes
Extra skin folds on eyelids
Drooping eyelids
Downward slant of eyes
Unusually small eyes and/or eye openings
Short-sightedness
Inability to focus ("wandering eyes")

Ears
Uneven in placement and size
Poorly formed outer ear
Backward curve

Lips
Absence of groove in upper lip; flat upper lip
Thin upper lip

fetal alcohol spectrum disorders (FASD) a spectrum of physical, behavioral, and cognitive disabilities caused by prenatal alcohol exposure.

fetal alcohol syndrome (FAS) the cluster of symptoms including brain damage, growth restriction, mental retardation, and facial abnormalities seen in an infant or child whose mother consumed alcohol during her pregnancy.

alcohol-related neurodevelopmental disorder (ARND) behavioral, cognitive, or central nervous system abnormalities associated with prenatal alcohol exposure.

alcohol-related birth defects (ARBD) malformations in the skeletal and organ systems (heart, kidneys, eyes, ears) associated with prenatal alcohol exposure.

© James W. Hanson, M.D./NICHD

Many children with ARND or ARBD go undiagnosed until problems develop in the preschool years. Upon reaching adulthood, such children are ill equipped for employment, relationships, and the other facets of life most adults take for granted. Alcohol exposure before birth may alter the person's later response to alcohol and other mind-altering drugs, making addictions likely.

- The severe birth defects of fetal alcohol syndrome arise from damage to the fetus by alcohol.
- Lesser conditions, ARND and ARBD, also arise from alcohol use in pregnancy.

Experts' Advice

Despite alcohol's potential for harm, 1 out of 13 pregnant women drinks alcohol at some time during pregnancy; 1 out of 71 reports "binge" drinking (four or more drinks on one occasion).[59] Controversy 3 defines binge drinking and other alcohol-related terms.

Women who know they are pregnant and choose to drink alcohol often ask, "How much alcohol is too much?" The damaging effects are dose dependent, becoming greater as the dose increases.[60] Even one drink a day threatens neurological development and behavior. Low birthweight is reported among infants born to women who drink 1 ounce (two drinks) per day during pregnancy, and FAS is also known to occur with as few as two drinks a day. Birth defects have been reliably observed among the children of women who drink 2 ounces (four drinks) of alcohol daily during pregnancy. Compared to women who do not drink, a sizable and significant increase in stillbirths occurs in women who drink five or more drinks per week. The most severe impact is likely to occur in the first two months, when the woman may not even be aware that she is pregnant.

Researchers have looked for a "safe" alcohol intake limit during pregnancy and have found none.[61] Their conclusion: abstinence from alcohol is the best policy for pregnant women. Given such evidence, the Dietary Guidelines for Americans 2015 and the American Academy of Pediatrics (AAP) state that women should stop drinking as soon as they *plan* to become pregnant, an important step for fathers-to-be as well. The authors of this book recommend this choice, too. For a pregnant woman who has already been drinking alcohol, the best advice is "Stop now." A woman who has drunk heavily during the first two-thirds of her pregnancy can still prevent some organ damage by stopping during the third trimester.

- Alcohol's damaging effects on the fetus are dose dependent, becoming greater as the dose increases.
- Abstinence from alcohol in pregnancy is critical to preventing irreversible damage to the fetus.

Troubleshooting

LO 13.3 List the effects of diabetes, hypertension, and preeclampsia on pregnancy.

Disease during pregnancy can endanger the health of the mother and the health and growth of the fetus. If discovered early, many diseases can be controlled—another reason early prenatal care is recommended.

Diabetes

Pregnancy presents special challenges for the management of diabetes. Pregnant women with unmanaged type 1 or type 2 diabetes may experience episodes of severe hypoglycemia or hyperglycemia, preterm labor, and pregnancy-related hypertension. Infants may be large or may suffer physical and mental abnormalities or other complications such as respiratory distress. Signs of fetal health problems are apparent even in prediabetes, when maternal glucose is just above normal.

Excellent glycemic control in the first trimester and throughout the pregnancy is associated with the lowest frequency of maternal, fetal, and newborn complications. Ideally, a woman will receive the prenatal care needed to achieve glucose control before conception and continued glucose control throughout pregnancy. Then continued diabetes management after pregnancy will guard the woman's long-term health.

Some women are prone to develop a pregnancy-related form of diabetes, **gestational diabetes**. Gestational diabetes usually resolves after the birth, but some women develop diabetes (usually type 2) later in life, especially if they are overweight.[62] When gestational diabetes is identified early and managed properly, the most serious risks, fetal and infant illness and mortality, fall dramatically. Gestational diabetes often leads to surgical birth and high infant birthweight. To ensure prompt diagnosis and treatment, at the first prenatal visit physicians screen all women who are overweight (BMI ≥25) and have one or more additional risk factors for type 2 diabetes. Risk factors include high blood pressure, family history of diabetes or heart disease, previous gestational diabetes, and family background that is Hispanic/Latino American, African American, Native American, Asian American, or Pacific Islander. In addition, all pregnant women not previously diagnosed with diabetes are tested for glucose tolerance at 24 to 28 weeks of gestation.[63]

Hypertension

Hypertension during pregnancy may be **chronic hypertension** or **gestational hypertension**.[64] In chronic hypertension, the condition is generally present before and remains after pregnancy. In women with gestational hypertension, blood pressure usually returns to normal during the first few weeks after childbirth.

Both types of hypertension pose risks to the mother and fetus; the higher the blood pressure, the worse the risk. In addition to heart attack and stroke, high blood pressure may increase the likelihood of growth restriction, preterm birth, and separation of the placenta from the wall of the uterus before the birth.[65]

Preeclampsia

Preeclampsia involves not only high blood pressure but also protein in the urine.[66] Preeclampsia usually occurs in first pregnancies (see Table 13–8 for its warning signs), almost always appears after 20 weeks of gestation, and starts to disappear within a few days after delivery.[67] Because delivery is the only known cure, preeclampsia is a leading cause of indicated preterm delivery and accounts for about 15 percent of infants who are growth restricted.[68]

Preeclampsia affects almost all of the mother's organs—the circulatory system, liver, kidneys, and brain. If the condition progresses, she may experience seizures; when this occurs, the condition is called **eclampsia**. Maternal mortality during pregnancy is rare in developed countries, but eclampsia is one of the most common causes.[69] Preeclampsia and eclampsia demand prompt medical attention.

KEY POINTS

- If discovered early, many diseases of pregnancy can be controlled—an important reason early prenatal care is recommended.
- Gestational diabetes, hypertension, and preeclampsia are problems of some pregnancies that must be managed to minimize associated risks.

Lactation

LO 13.4 Underline the role of nutrition during lactation.

As the time of childbirth nears, a woman must decide whether she will feed her baby breast milk, infant formula, or both. These options are the only foods recommended for an infant during the first four to six months of life. A woman who plans to breast-feed her baby should begin to prepare toward the end of her pregnancy. No elaborate or expensive preparations are needed, but the expectant mother can read one of

Table 13–8

Warning Signs of Preeclampsia

- Hypertension.
- Protein in the urine.
- Upper abdominal pain.
- Severe and constant headaches.
- Swelling, especially of the face.
- Dizziness.
- Blurred vision.
- Sudden weight gain (1 lb/day).

gestational diabetes abnormal glucose tolerance appearing during pregnancy.

chronic hypertension in pregnant women, hypertension that is present and documented before pregnancy; in women whose prepregnancy blood pressure is unknown, the presence of sustained hypertension before 20 weeks of gestation.

gestational hypertension high blood pressure that develops in the second half of pregnancy and usually resolves after childbirth.

preeclampsia (PRE-ee-CLAMP-seeah) a potentially dangerous condition during pregnancy characterized by hypertension and protein in the urine.

eclampsia (eh-CLAMP-see-ah) a severe complication during pregnancy in which seizures occur.

the many handbooks available on breastfeeding or consult a **certified lactation consultant**, employed at many hospitals.[‡] Health-care professionals play an important role in providing encouragement and accurate information on breastfeeding. Part of the preparation involves learning what dietary changes are needed because adequate nutrition is essential to successful lactation.

In rare cases, women produce too little milk to nourish their infants adequately. Severe consequences, including infant dehydration, malnutrition, and brain damage, can occur if the condition goes undetected for long. Early warning signs of insufficient milk are dry diapers (a well-fed infant wets about six to eight diapers a day) and infrequent bowel movements.

Nutrition during Lactation

A nursing mother produces about 25 ounces of milk a day, with considerable variation from woman to woman and in the same woman from time to time. The volume produced depends primarily on the infant's demand for milk. The more milk the infant needs, the more the well-nourished mother's body will produce, enough to feed the infant—or even twins—amply.

Energy Cost of Lactation Producing milk costs a woman almost 500 calories per day above her regular need during the first six months of lactation. To meet this energy need, the woman is advised to eat an extra 330 calories of food each day. The other 170 calories can be drawn from the fat stores she accumulated during pregnancy. The food energy consumed by the nursing mother should carry with it abundant nutrients. A lactating woman's nutrient recommendations are listed on the inside front cover; look again at Table 13–2 on page 522 for a sample menu to meet them.

Fluid Need Breast milk contains a lot of water, so the nursing mother is advised to drink plenty of fluid each day (about 13 cups) to protect herself from dehydration.[§] To help themselves remember, many women make a habit of drinking a glass of milk, juice, or water each time the baby nurses, as well as at mealtimes.

Variations in Breast Milk A common question is whether a mother's milk may lack a nutrient if she fails to get enough in her diet. The answer differs from one nutrient to the next, but in general the effect of nutritional deprivation of the mother is to reduce the *quantity* more than the *quality* of her milk.

Women can produce milk with adequate protein, carbohydrate, fat, folate, and most minerals, even when their own supplies are limited, at the expense of maternal stores. This is most evident in the case of calcium: dietary calcium has no effect on the calcium concentration of breast milk, but maternal bones lose some of their density during lactation if calcium intakes are inadequate.[70] Such losses are generally made

certified lactation consultant a health-care provider, often a registered nurse or a registered dietitian nutritionist, with specialized training and certification in breast and infant anatomy and physiology who teaches the mechanics of breastfeeding to new mothers.

[‡]La Leche League is an international organization that helps women with breastfeeding concerns: www.lalecheleague.org.
[§]The DRI recommendation for *total* water intake during lactation is 3.8 L/day. This includes 3.1 L, or about 13 cups, as total beverages, including water.

up quickly when lactation ends, and breastfeeding has no long-term harmful effects on women's bones.

Foods with strong or spicy flavors (such as onions or garlic) may alter the flavor of breast milk. A sudden change in the taste of the milk may annoy some infants. Familiar flavors may enhance enjoyment. Flavors in breast milk from the mother's diet can influence the infant's later food preferences.[71] A mother who is breastfeeding her infant is advised to eat whatever nutritious foods she chooses. If a particular food seems to cause an infant discomfort, the mother can eliminate that food from her diet for a few days to see if the problem goes away.

Generally, infants with a strong family history of food allergies benefit from breastfeeding. Current evidence, however, does not support a major role for maternal dietary restrictions during lactation to prevent or delay the onset of food allergy in infants.[72]

Lactation and Weight Loss

Another common question is whether breastfeeding promotes a more rapid loss of the extra body fat accumulated during pregnancy. Studies on this question have not provided a definitive answer. How much weight a woman retains after pregnancy depends on her gestational weight gain and the duration and intensity of breastfeeding.[73] Many women who follow recommendations for gestational weight gain and breastfeeding can readily return to prepregnancy weight by six months after giving birth. Neither the quality nor the quantity of breast milk is adversely affected by moderate weight loss, and infants grow normally. Physical activity is also compatible with breastfeeding and infant growth.[74] A gradual weight loss (1 pound per week) is safe and does not reduce milk output. Too large an energy deficit, especially soon after birth, will inhibit lactation.

KEY POINTS

- The lactating woman needs extra fluid and adequate energy and nutrients for milk production.
- Malnutrition diminishes the quantity of the milk without altering quality.
- Moderate weight loss during lactation does not adversely affect the quality or quantity of breast milk.

When Should a Woman Not Breastfeed?

Some substances impair maternal milk production or enter breast milk and interfere with infant development, making breastfeeding an unwise choice. Some medical conditions also prohibit breastfeeding.

Alcohol and Illicit Drugs

Alcohol enters breast milk and can adversely affect production, volume, composition, and ejection of breast milk, as well as overwhelming an infant's immature alcohol-degrading system.[75] Alcohol concentration peaks within one hour after ingestion of even moderate amounts (equivalent to a can of beer). This amount may alter the taste of the milk to the disapproval of the nursing infant, who may, in protest, drink less milk than normal. Mothers who use illicit drugs should not breastfeed. Breast milk can deliver such high doses of drugs as to cause irritability, tremors, hallucinations, and even death in infants.

Tobacco and Caffeine

About 40 percent of women who quit smoking during pregnancy relapse after delivery.[76] Lactating women who smoke tobacco produce less milk, and milk of lower fat content, than do nonsmokers.[77] Consequently, infants of smokers gain less weight. A lactating woman who smokes not only transfers nicotine and other chemicals to her infant via her breast milk but also exposes the infant to hazardous sidestream smoke.** Babies who are "smoked over" experience a wide array of health problems—poor growth, hearing impairment, vomiting, breathing difficulties, and even unexplained death.[78]

Excess caffeine can make a breastfed infant jittery and wakeful. As during pregnancy, caffeine consumption should be moderate when breastfeeding.

** Also called *environmental tobacco smoke* or *secondhand smoking.*

Medications Many medications pose no danger during breastfeeding, but others may suppress lactation or may be secreted into breast milk and harm the infant.[79] If a nursing mother must take such a medicine, then breastfeeding must be put on hold for the duration of treatment. Meanwhile, the flow of milk can be sustained by pumping the breasts and discarding the milk. A nursing mother should consult with her physician before taking medicines or even herbal supplements—herbs may have unpredictable effects on breastfeeding infants.

Many women wonder about using oral contraceptives during lactation. One type that combines the hormones estrogen and progestin may suppress milk output and shorten the duration of breastfeeding. In contrast, progestin-only pills have no effect on breast milk or breastfeeding and are considered appropriate for lactating women.

Environmental Contaminants A woman sometimes hesitates to breastfeed because she has heard warnings that contaminants in fish, water, and other foods may enter breast milk and harm her infant. Although some contaminants do enter breast milk, others may be filtered out. Because formula is made with water, formula-fed infants consume any contaminants that may be in the water supply. With the exception of rare massive exposure to a contaminant, the many benefits of breastfeeding far outweigh any small risk from environmental hazards in the United States.

Maternal Illness If a woman has an ordinary cold, she can continue nursing without worry. The infant will probably catch it from her anyway, and thanks to immunological protection, a breastfed baby may be less susceptible than a formula-fed baby. A woman who has active, infectious tuberculosis can breastfeed once she has been treated and it is documented that she is no longer infectious.[80] If a woman has not received treatment, breastfeeding is contraindicated.

The human immunodeficiency virus (HIV), responsible for causing HIV/AIDS, can be passed from an infected mother to her infant during pregnancy, at birth, or through breast milk, especially during the early months of breastfeeding. In developed countries such as the United States, where safe alternatives are available, HIV-positive women should not breastfeed their infants.[81] In developing countries, where feeding inappropriate or contaminated formulas causes more than 1 million infant deaths each year, breastfeeding can be critical to infant survival. For these women, the most appropriate infant-feeding option depends on individual circumstances, including the health status of the mother and the local situation, as well as the health services available. The World Health Organization (WHO) recommends exclusive breastfeeding for infants of HIV-infected women for the first six months of life unless replacement feeding is acceptable, feasible, affordable, sustainable, and safe for mothers and their infants. Alternatively, HIV-exposed infants may be protected by receiving drugs known as antiretrovirals while being breastfed.

> **KEY POINTS**
> - Breastfeeding is not advised if the mother's milk is contaminated with alcohol, drugs, or environmental pollutants.
> - Most ordinary infections such as colds have no effect on breastfeeding infants, but HIV/AIDS may be transmitted through milk.

Feeding the Infant

LO 13.5 Identify nutrition practices that promote the infant's well-being.

Early nutrition affects later development, and early feedings establish eating habits that influence nutrition throughout life. Trends change, and experts may argue the fine points, but nourishing a baby is relatively simple. Common sense and a nurturing, relaxed environment go far to promote the infant's well-being.

Nutrient Needs

A baby grows faster during the first year of life than ever again, as Figure 13–10 shows. Pediatricians carefully monitor the growth of infants and children because growth

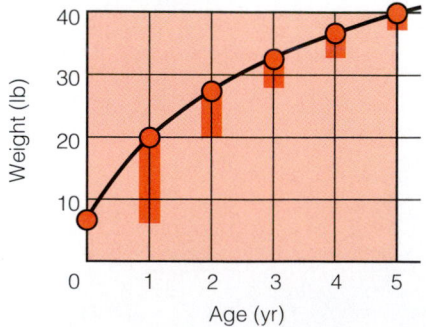

Figure 13–10

Weight Gain of Human Infants and Children in the First Five Years of Life

The colored vertical bars show how the yearly increase in weight gain slows its pace over the years.

Chapter 13 Life Cycle Nutrition: Mother and Infant

directly reflects their nutrition status. An infant's birthweight doubles by about 5 months of age and triples by the age of 1 year. (If a 150-pound adult were to grow like this, the person would weigh 450 pounds after a single year.) The infant's length changes more slowly than weight, increasing about 10 inches from birth to 1 year. By the end of the first year, the growth rate slows considerably; an infant typically gains less than 10 pounds during the second year and grows about 5 inches in height.

Not only do infants grow rapidly, but also their basal metabolic rate is remarkably high—about twice that of an adult's, based on body weight. The rapid growth and metabolism of the infant demand an ample supply of all the nutrients. Of special importance during infancy are the energy nutrients and the vitamins and minerals critical to the growth process, such as vitamin A, vitamin D, and calcium.

Because they are small, babies need smaller *total* amounts of these nutrients than adults do, but as a percentage of body weight, babies need more than twice as much of most nutrients. Infants require about 100 calories per kilogram of body weight per day; most adults require fewer than 40. Figure 13–11 compares a 5-month-old baby's needs (per unit of body weight) with those of an adult man. You can see that differences in vitamin D and iodine, for instance, are extraordinary.

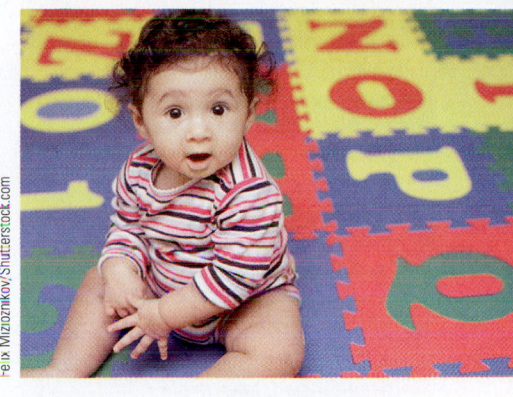

Growth slows in later infancy, but babies become more active.

Figure 13–11

Nutrient Recommendations for a 5-Month-Old Infant and an Adult Male Compared on the Basis of Body Weight

Infants may be relatively small and inactive, but they use large amounts of energy and nutrients in proportion to their body size to keep all their metabolic processes going.

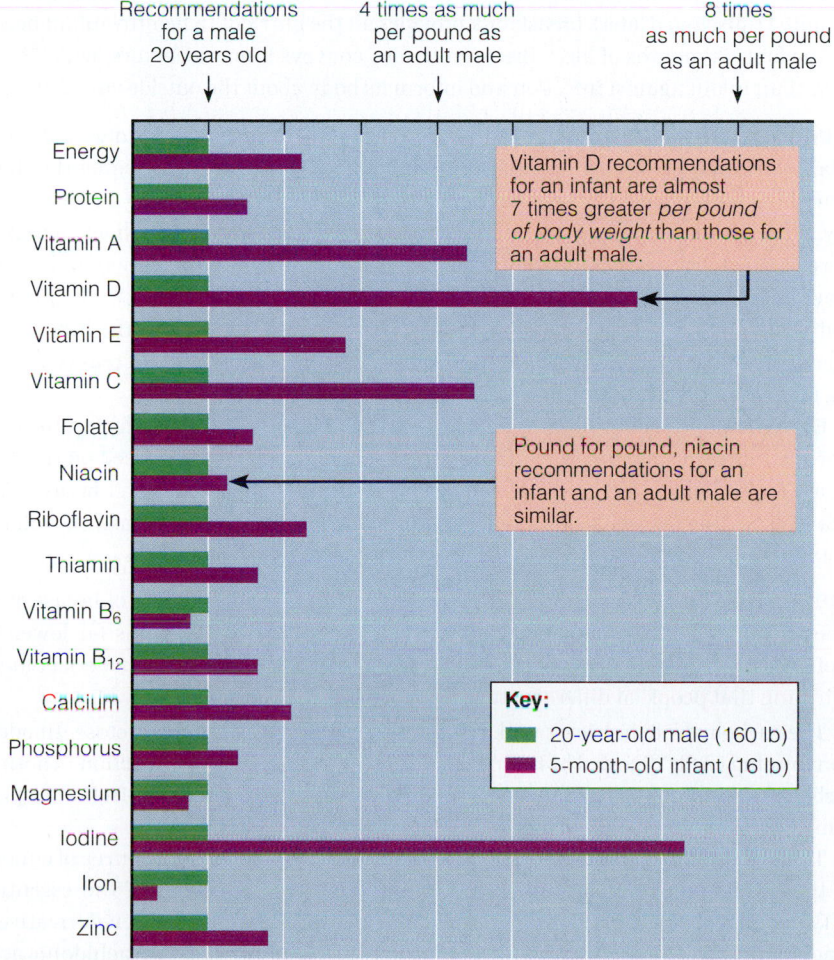

Recommendations for a male 20 years old

4 times as much per pound as an adult male

8 times as much per pound as an adult male

Energy
Protein
Vitamin A
Vitamin D
Vitamin E
Vitamin C
Folate
Niacin
Riboflavin
Thiamin
Vitamin B$_6$
Vitamin B$_{12}$
Calcium
Phosphorus
Magnesium
Iodine
Iron
Zinc

Vitamin D recommendations for an infant are almost 7 times greater *per pound of body weight* than those for an adult male.

Pound for pound, niacin recommendations for an infant and an adult male are similar.

Key:
■ 20-year-old male (160 lb)
■ 5-month-old infant (16 lb)

Table 13–9
Benefits of Breastfeeding
For Infants:
• Provides the appropriate composition and balance of nutrients.
• Provides hormones that promote physiological development.
• Improves cognitive development.
• Protects against a variety of infections.
• May protect against some chronic diseases, such as diabetes and hypertension, later in life.
• Protects against food allergies.
• Reduces the risk of SIDS.
For Mothers:
• Contracts the uterus.
• Delays the return of regular ovulation, thus lengthening birth intervals. (It is not, however, a dependable method of contraception.)
• Conserves iron stores (by prolonging amenorrhea).
• May protect against breast and ovarian cancer.
Other:
• Saves on doctor visits for infant illness.
• Saves costs of formulas, bottles, brushes, etc.
• Is more environmentally sustainable.

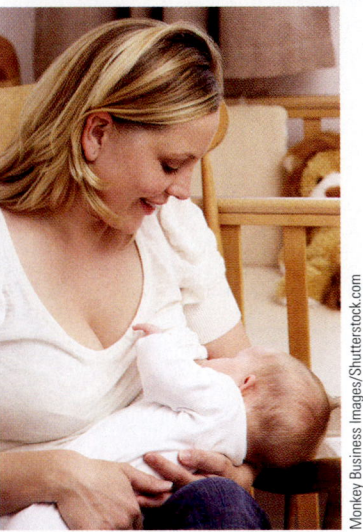

Breastfeeding is a natural extension of pregnancy—the mother's body continues to nourish the infant.

exclusive breastfeeding an infant's consumption of human milk with no supplementation of any type (no water, no juice, no nonhuman milk, and no foods) except for vitamins, minerals, and medications.

Around 6 months of age, energy needs begin to increase less rapidly as the growth rate begins to slow down, but some of the energy saved by slower growth is spent in increased activity. When their growth slows, infants spontaneously reduce their energy intakes. Parents should expect their babies to adjust their food intakes downward when appropriate and should not force or coax them to eat more.

One of the most important nutrients for infants, as for everyone, is water. The younger a child is, the more of its body weight is water. Breast milk or infant formula normally provides enough water to replace fluid losses in a healthy infant. If the environmental temperature is extremely high, however, infants need supplemental water.[82] Much more of an infant's body water is between the cells and in the vascular space, and this water is easy to lose. Conditions that cause rapid fluid loss, such as vomiting or diarrhea, require an electrolyte solution designed for infants.

KEY POINTS

• An infant's birthweight doubles by about 5 months of age and triples by 1 year.
• Infants' rapid growth and development depend on adequate nutrient supplies, including water from breast milk or formula.

Why Is Breast Milk So Good for Babies?

Many medical and professional organizations advocate breastfeeding for the best infant nutrition, as well as for the many other benefits it provides both infant and mother (see Table 13–9).[83] The AAP and the Academy of Nutrition and Dietetics recommend **exclusive breastfeeding** for 6 months and breastfeeding with complementary foods for at least 12 months as an optimal feeding pattern for infants.[84] All legitimate nutrition authorities share this view, but some makers of baby formula try to convince women otherwise—see the Consumer's Guide on page 543.

Breast milk excels as a source of nutrients for the young infant. With the exception of vitamin D (discussed later), breast milk provides all the nutrients a healthy infant needs for the first six months of life.[85] Breast milk also conveys immune factors, which both protect an infant against infection and inform its body about the outside environment.

Breastfeeding Tips Breast milk is more easily and completely digested than infant formula, so breastfed infants usually need to eat more frequently than formula-fed infants do. During the first few weeks, approximately 8 to 12 feedings a day, on demand, as soon as the infant shows early signs of hunger such as increased alertness, activity, or suckling motions, promote optimal milk production and infant growth. Crying is a late indicator of hunger. An infant who nurses every 2 to 3 hours and sleeps contentedly between feedings is adequately nourished. As the infant gets older, stomach capacity enlarges and the mother's milk production increases, allowing for longer intervals between feedings.

Even though the baby obtains about half the milk from the breast during the first 2 or 3 minutes of suckling, the infant should be encouraged to breastfeed on the first breast for as long as he or she wishes, before being offered the second breast. The infant's suckling, as well as the complete removal of milk from the breast, stimulates lactation. Begin each feeding on the breast offered last.

Energy Nutrients in Breast Milk The energy-nutrient balance of breast milk differs dramatically from that recommended for adults; breast milk is far lower in protein but higher in fat. Yet for infants, breast milk is the most nearly perfect food, affirming that people at different stages of life have different nutrient needs.

The carbohydrate in breast milk (and standard infant formula) is lactose. In addition to being easily digested by infants, lactose enhances calcium absorption. Another carbohydrate component of breast milk helps protect the infant from infection by preventing the binding of pathogens to the infant's intestinal cells.[86]

The lipids in breast milk—and infant formula—provide the main source of energy in the infant's diet. Breast milk contains a generous proportion of the essential fatty acids linoleic acid and linolenic acid, as well as their longer-chain derivatives, arachidonic acid and DHA. Most formulas today also contain added arachidonic acid and DHA (read the label). Infants can produce some arachidonic acid and DHA from linoleic and linolenic acid, but some infants may need more than they can make.

DHA is the most abundant fatty acid in the brain and is also present in the retina of the eye. DHA accumulation in the brain is greatest during fetal development and early infancy.[87] Research has focused on the visual and mental development of breast-fed infants and infants fed standard formula with and without DHA added.[88] Results of studies for visual acuity development in term infants have been inconsistent. Factors such as the amount of DHA provided, the sources of the DHA, and the sensitivity of different measures for visual acuity may have contributed to the inconsistent outcomes. As for mental development, a number of studies suggest that DHA supplementation during development can influence certain measures of cognitive function.[89] Still needed are longer-term studies that follow child development beyond infancy.

The protein in breast milk is largely **alpha-lactalbumin**, a protein the human infant can easily digest. Another breast milk protein, **lactoferrin**, is an iron-gathering compound that helps absorb iron into the infant's bloodstream, keeps intestinal bacteria from getting enough iron to grow out of control, and kills certain bacteria.

Vitamins and Minerals in Breast Milk

With one exception—vitamin D—the vitamin content of the breast milk of a well-nourished mother is ample. Even vitamin C, for which cow's milk is a poor source, is supplied generously. The concentration of vitamin D in breast milk is low, however, and vitamin D deficiency impairs bone mineralization.[90] Vitamin D deficiency is most likely in infants who are not exposed to sunlight daily, have darkly pigmented skin, and receive breast milk without vitamin D supplementation.[91] Vitamin D intake recommendations for infants have been increased for two reasons. First, rickets, the vitamin D–deficiency disease, has been diagnosed among U.S. infants. Second, the AAP recommends that infants younger than six months be protected from direct sunlight, eliminating this source of vitamin D.

As for minerals, the calcium content of breast milk is ideal for infant bone growth, and the calcium is well absorbed. Breast milk is also low in sodium. The limited amount of iron in breast milk is highly absorbable, and its zinc, too, is absorbed better than from cow's milk, thanks to the presence of a zinc-binding protein.

Supplements for Infants

Pediatricians may prescribe supplements containing vitamin D, iron, and fluoride (after 6 months of age) as outlined in Table 13–10. Vitamin K nutrition for newborns presents a unique case. A newborn's digestive tract is sterile, and vitamin K–producing bacteria take weeks to establish themselves in the baby's intestines. To prevent bleeding in the newborn, the AAP recommends that a single dose of vitamin K be given at birth.

The AAP currently recommends a vitamin D supplement for all infants who are breast-fed exclusively and for any infants who do not receive at least 1 liter (1,000 milliliters) or 1 quart (32 ounces) of vitamin D–fortified formula daily.[92] Despite such recommendations, most infants in the United States are consuming inadequate amounts of vitamin D.

Immune Factors in Breast Milk

Breast milk offers the infant unsurpassed protection against infection.[93] Its protective factors include antiviral agents, anti-inflammatory agents, antibacterial agents, and infection inhibitors.

During the first two or three days of lactation, the breasts produce **colostrum**, a premilk substance containing antibodies and white cells from the mother's blood. Colostrum (like breast milk) helps protect the newborn infant from infections against which the mother has developed immunity—precisely those in the environment likely to infect the infant. For example, maternal antibodies in colostrum and breast milk inactivate harmful bacteria within the infant's digestive tract before they can start infections.[94] This explains, in part, why breastfed infants have fewer intestinal infections than formula-fed infants.

Breastfeeding also protects against other common illnesses of infancy, such as middle ear infections and respiratory illnesses. In addition, breastfed infants have fewer allergic reactions such as asthma, wheezing, and skin rash.[95] This protection is especially noticeable among infants with a family history of allergies. Even the risk of SIDS

Table 13–10		
Supplements for Full-Term Breastfed Infants		
Birth	4 Months of Age	6 Months of Age
Vitamin D[a]	Iron[b]	Fluoride[c]

[a]Vitamin D supplements are recommended for all infants who are exclusively breastfed and for any infants who do not receive at least 1 L (1,000 ml) or 1 qt (32 oz) of vitamin D–fortified formula per day.

[b]At 4 months of age, 1 mg per kg of body weight per day of supplemental iron is recommended for all infants who are exclusively breastfed and for all infants who are receiving more than one-half of their daily feedings as breast milk and no iron-containing complementary foods. Once iron-containing foods are introduced, iron supplements may not be needed.

[c]At 6 months of age, breastfed infants and formula-fed infants who receive ready-to-use formulas (these are made with water low in fluoride) or formula mixed with water that contains little or no fluoride (less than 0.3 ppm) may need supplements, but this depends on the health-care provider's assessment of the infant's fluoride exposure.

Source: Adapted from American Academy of Pediatrics, Pediatric Nutrition, 7th ed., ed. R. E. Kleinman (Elk Grove Village, Ill.: American Academy of Pediatrics, 2014).

alpha-lactalbumin (lact-AL-byoo-min) the chief protein in human breast milk. The chief protein in cow's milk is *casein* (CAY-seen).

lactoferrin (lack-toe-FERR-in) a factor in breast milk that binds iron and keeps it from supporting the growth of the infant's intestinal bacteria.

colostrum (co-LAHS-trum) a milklike secretion from the breasts during the first day or so after delivery before milk appears; rich in protective factors.

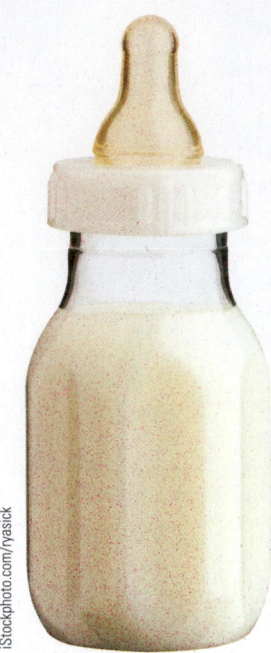

is lower among breastfed infants.[96] This protective effect is stronger when breast-feeding is exclusive, but any amount of breast milk for any duration is protective against SIDS.

In addition to their protective features, colostrum and breast milk contain hormones and other factors that stimulate the development and maintenance of the infant's digestive tract. Clearly, breast milk is a very special substance.

Other Potential Benefits Breastfeeding may offer some protection against excessive weight gain later, although findings are inconsistent.[97] Many other factors—socioeconomic status, other infant- and child-feeding practices, and especially the mother's weight—strongly predict a child's body weight.[98]

The possibility that breastfeeding may positively affect later intelligence is intriguing. Many studies have suggested such benefits, but when subjected to strict standards of methodology (for example, large sample size and appropriate intelligence testing), the evidence is less convincing.[99] Most likely, a combination of factors, such as the DHA in breast milk and the feeding process itself, benefits the infant's development. More large, well-controlled studies are needed to confirm the effects, if any, of breastfeeding on later intelligence.

KEY POINTS

- With the exception of vitamin D, breast milk provides all the nutrients a healthy infant needs for the first 4 months of life.
- Breast milk offers the infant unsurpassed protection against infection—including antiviral agents, anti-inflammatory agents, antibacterial agents, and infection inhibitors.

Formula Feeding

Formula feeding offers an acceptable alternative to breastfeeding. Nourishment for an infant from formula is adequate, and parents can choose this course with confidence. All currently available infant formulas meet all of the energy and nutrient requirements for healthy, full-term infants during the first 6 months of life. After the infant is 6 months of age, formulas, along with a variety of solid foods in the diet, continue to supply a significant part of the infant's nutrient needs. One advantage of formula feeding is that parents can see how much milk the infant drinks during feedings. Another is that other family members can participate in feeding the infant, giving them a chance to develop the special closeness that feeding fosters.

Mothers who return to work soon after giving birth may choose formula for their infants, but they have another option. Breast milk can be pumped into bottles and given to the baby in day care. At home, mothers may breastfeed as usual. Many mothers use both methods—they breastfeed at first but **wean** their children within 1 to 12 months. If infants are less than a year of age, mothers must wean them onto *infant formula*, not onto plain cow's milk of any kind—whole, reduced-fat, low-fat, or fat-free. Infant formula is available as a powdered (least expensive option) or liquid concentrate that must be mixed with water according to label directions and as a ready-to-feed liquid (most expensive option).

Infant Formula Composition The substitution of formula feeding for breast-feeding involves striving to copy nature as closely as possible. Human milk and cow's milk differ; cow's milk is significantly higher in protein, calcium, and phosphorus, for example, to support the calf's faster growth rate. Thus, to prepare a formula from cow's milk, the formula makers must first dilute the milk and then add carbohydrate and nutrients to make the proportions comparable to those of human milk. Figure 13–12 compares the energy–nutrient balances of breast milk, standard infant formula, and

Figure 13–12

Percentages of Energy-Yielding Nutrients in Breast Milk, Infant Formula, and Cow's Milk

The average proportions of energy-yielding nutrients in human breast milk and formula differ slightly. In contrast, cow's milk provides too much protein and too little carbohydrate.

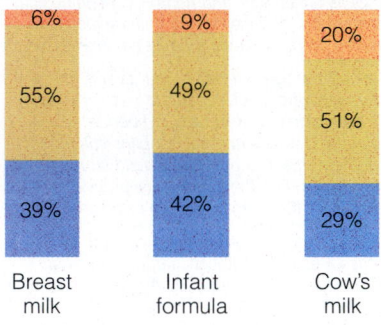

Breast milk	Infant formula	Cow's milk
6%	9%	20%
55%	49%	51%
39%	42%	29%

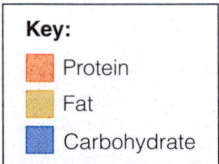

Key:
- Protein
- Fat
- Carbohydrate

wean to gradually replace breast milk with infant formula or other foods appropriate to an infant's diet.

Formula Advertising versus Breastfeeding Advocacy

Formula feed or breastfeed? New mothers must answer this question amidst the whirlwind of physical and emotional changes associated with pregnancy and delivery. For a few women, breastfeeding may be proscribed by illness or physical condition; in a few more cases, special needs of the infant may make breastfeeding impossible. The strong scientific consensus holds, however, that breastfeeding is preferable for all other infants, so why do so many women continue to choose formula? For some, the time and logistics required for breastfeeding compete with work or school schedules; for many others, the decision to forgo breastfeeding is influenced by the aggressive advertising of formulas.

Formula Advertising Claims and Tactics

Advertisements of infant formulas often create the illusion that formula is identical to human milk. No formula can match the nutrients, agents of immunity, and environmental information conveyed to infants through human milk, but the ads are convincing: "Like mother's milk, our formula provides complete nutrition" or "Our brand is scientifically formulated to meet your baby's needs." The ads seem to work: according to one survey, one out of four people of various ages, races, and socioeconomic backgrounds agrees with the statement "Infant formula is as good as breast milk."

Formula manufacturers give coupons and samples of free formula to pregnant women. After childbirth, women in the hospital may receive "goody bags" with more coupons to tempt them to go retrieve their "gifts." More coupons arrive by mail a couple of months later, at a time when many women give up breastfeeding, even though nutrition authorities urge continued breastfeeding for several more months. Aggressive marketing tactics like these can undermine a woman's confidence concerning her choice to breastfeed, and lack of confidence causes many women to quit early.[1]*

*References are found in Appendix F.

- Learn about the benefits of breastfeeding.
- Initiate breastfeeding within 1 hour of birth.
- Ask a health-care professional to explain how to breastfeed and how to maintain lactation.
- Give newborn infants no food or drink other than breast milk unless medically indicated.
- Breastfeed on demand.
- Give no artificial nipples or pacifiers to breastfeeding infants.[a]
- Find breastfeeding support groups, books, or websites to help troubleshoot breastfeeding problems.

[a] *Compared with nonusers, infants who use pacifiers breastfeed less frequently and stop breastfeeding at a younger age.*

Breastfeeding Advocacy

National efforts to promote breastfeeding seem to be working, at least to some extent: the percentage of infants who were ever breastfed rose from 60 percent among those born in 1994 to 79 percent among those born in 2011.[2] This still falls short of national goals, however.[3] Only about 49 percent of infants are still breastfeeding at 6 months of age, and about 27 percent are still doing so at 1 year of age.

Many hospitals employ certified lactation consultants who specialize in helping new mothers establish a healthy breastfeeding relationship with their newborns. Table 13–11 lists tips for successful long-term breastfeeding.

Where Breastfeeding Is Critical

Infant formula is an appropriate substitute when breastfeeding is impossible, but for most infants, the benefits of breast milk outweigh those of formula. Formula-fed infants in developed nations are healthy and grow normally, but they miss out on the breastfeeding advantages described in the text.

In developing nations, however, the consequence of choosing not to breastfeed can be tragic. Feeding formula is often fatal to the infant when poverty limits access to formula mixes, clean water for safe formula preparation, and medical help when needed. Even in developed nations, a woman may easily lose track of a bottle that spoils in a crib within easy reach of an infant. The World Health Organization (WHO) strongly supports breastfeeding for the world's infants in its "babyfriendly" initiative and opposes the marketing of infant formulas to new mothers.

Moving Ahead

Women are free to choose between breast milk and formula. Breast milk is recommended and is a thrifty choice; infant formula, bottles, and paraphernalia are expensive for anyone's wallet, particularly after the initial coupons run out. During pregnancy, parents-to-be should seek out the facts about each feeding method and be aware that sophisticated formula advertisements are designed to make sales and not primarily to help potential customers make the best choice.

Review Questions*

1. Commercial infant formula is more reliable than breast milk because it has been scientifically engineered for complete nutrition. T F

2. About 60 percent of U.S. infants are still breastfeeding at one year of age. T F

3. Lactation consultants are employed by hospitals to help new mothers understand the advantages of feeding their babies with infant formula. T F

*Answers to Consumer's Guide review questions are found in Appendix G.

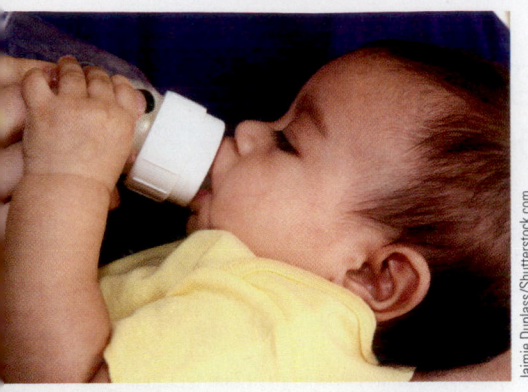

The infant thrives on formula offered with affection.

cow's milk. Notice the higher protein concentration of cow's milk, which can stress the infant's kidneys. The AAP recommends that all formula-fed infants receive iron-fortified infant formulas.[100] Use of iron-fortified formulas has increased in recent decades and is credited with the decline of iron-deficiency anemia in U.S. infants.

Special Formulas Standard cow's milk–based formulas are inappropriate for some infants. Special formulas have been designed to meet the dietary needs of infants with specific conditions such as prematurity or inherited diseases. Most infants allergic to milk protein can drink formulas based on soy protein.[101] Soy formulas also use cornstarch and sucrose instead of lactose and so are recommended for infants with lactose intolerance as well. They are also useful as an alternative to milk-based formulas for vegan families. Some infants who are allergic to cow's milk protein may also be allergic to soy protein.[102] For these infants, special formulas based on hydrolyzed protein are available.

The Transition to Cow's Milk For good reasons, the AAP advises that cow's milk is not appropriate for infants younger than one year old.[103] In some infants, particularly those younger than 6 months of age, cow's milk causes intestinal bleeding, which can lead to iron deficiency. Cow's milk is also a poor source of iron, and its higher calcium and lower vitamin C contents inhibit iron absorption. Consequently, plain cow's milk threatens the infant's iron status in three ways: it causes iron loss, it fails to replace iron, and it reduces the bioavailability of iron from infant cereal and other foods. In short, cow's milk is a poor choice during the first year of life; infants need breast milk or iron-fortified formula.

Once the baby is obtaining at least two-thirds of total daily food energy from a balanced mixture of cereals, vegetables, fruits, and other foods (after 12 months of age), reduced-fat or low-fat cow's milk (in the context of an overall diet that supplies 30 percent of calories from fat) is an acceptable and recommended beverage.[104] After the age of 2, a transition to fat-free milk can take place, but care should be taken to avoid excessive restriction of dietary fat.

> **KEY POINTS**
> - Infant formulas are designed to resemble breast milk in nutrient composition.
> - After the baby's first birthday, reduced-fat or low-fat cow's milk can replace formula.

An Infant's First Solid Foods

Complementary foods can be introduced into the diet as the infant becomes physically ready to handle them. This readiness develops in stages. A newborn can swallow only liquids that are well back in the throat. Later (at 4 months or so), the tongue can move against the palate to swallow semisolid food such as cooked cereal. The stomach and intestines are immature at first; they can digest milk sugar (lactose) but not starch. At about 4 months, most infants can begin to digest starchy foods. Still later, the first teeth erupt, but not until sometime during the second year can a baby begin to handle chewy food.

When to Introduce Solid Food The AAP supports exclusive breastfeeding for 6 months but recognizes that infants are often developmentally ready to accept some solid foods between 4 and 6 months of age.[105] Complementary foods can provide needed nutrients that are no longer supplied adequately by breast milk or formula alone.[106] The foods chosen must be those that the infant is developmentally capable of handling both physically and metabolically. The exact timing depends on the individual infant's needs, developmental readiness (see Table 13–12), and tolerance of the food.

In short, the addition of foods to an infant's diet should be governed by three considerations: the infant's nutrient needs, the infant's physical readiness to handle different forms of foods, and the need to detect and control allergic reactions, as described next. With respect to increased nutrient needs, the nutrients needed first are iron and zinc and then vitamin C.

complementary foods nutrient- and energy-containing solid or semisolid foods (or liquids) fed to infants in addition to breast milk or infant formula.

Table 13–12

Infant Development and Recommended Foods

Note: Because each stage of development builds on the previous stage, the foods from an earlier stage continue to be included in all later stages.

Age (mo)	Feeding Skill	Foods Introduced into the Diet
0–4	Turns head toward any object that brushes cheek. Initially swallows using back of tongue; gradually begins to swallow using front of tongue as well. Strong reflex (extrusion) to push food out during first 2 to 3 months.	Feed breast milk or infant formula.
4–6	Extrusion reflex diminishes, and the ability to swallow nonliquid foods develops. Indicates desire for food by opening mouth and leaning forward. Indicates satiety or disinterest by turning away and leaning back. Sits erect with support at 6 months. Begins chewing action. Brings hand to mouth. Grasps objects with palm of hand.	Begin iron-fortified cereal mixed with breast milk, formula, or water. Begin pureed meats, legumes, vegetables, and fruits.
6–8	Able to feed self with fingers. Develops pincher (finger to thumb) grasp. Begins to drink from cup.	Begin textured vegetables and fruits. Begin plain, unsweetened fruit juices from cup.
8–10	Begins to hold own bottle. Reaches for and grabs food and spoon. Sits unsupported.	Begin breads and cereals from table. Begin yogurt. Begin pieces of soft, cooked vegetables and fruit from table. Gradually begin finely cut meats, fish, casseroles, cheese, eggs, and legumes.
10–12	Begins to master spoon, but still spills some.	Add variety. Gradually increase portion sizes.[a]

[a]Portions of foods for infants and young children are smaller than those for an adult. For example, a grain serving might be ½ slice of bread instead of 1 slice or ¼ cup of rice instead of ½ cup.

Source: Adapted in part from American Academy of Pediatrics, Pediatric Nutrition, 7th ed., ed. R. E. Kleinman (Elk Grove Village, Ill.: American Academy of Pediatrics, 2014), pp. 123–139.

Foods to Provide Iron, Zinc, and Vitamin C Rapid growth demands iron. At about 4 to 6 months, the infant begins to need more iron than body stores plus breast milk or iron-fortified formula can provide. In addition to breast milk or iron-fortified formula, infants can receive iron from iron-fortified cereals and, once they readily accept solid foods, from protein foods such as meat, poultry, seafood, eggs, and legumes (see Figure 13–13). Iron-fortified cereals contribute a significant amount of iron to an infant's diet, but the iron's bioavailability is poor.[107] Caregivers can enhance iron absorption from iron-fortified cereals by serving vitamin C–rich foods with meals.

The concentration of zinc in breast milk is initially high but decreases sharply over the first few months of lactation. Although the infant's ability to absorb the zinc in breast milk is highly efficient, this does not compensate for the low concentration over time. Infant formulas are fortified with zinc at higher levels than breast milk. Thus, breastfed infants depend more on complementary foods to provide adequate zinc intakes than formula-fed infants do.[108] Infant cereals are not routinely fortified with zinc, so the best sources are protein foods such as meats, poultry, seafood, eggs, and legumes. Zinc is not as well absorbed from legumes as it is from other protein foods, however.

The best sources of vitamin C are fruits and vegetables (see Snapshot 7–5 on p. 264). Fruit juice is a source of vitamin C, but excessive juice intake can lead to diarrhea in infants and young children.[109] Furthermore, too much fruit juice contributes excessive calories and displaces other nutrient-rich foods. The AAP recommends limiting juice consumption for infants and young children (1 to 6 years of age) to between 4 and 6 ounces per day.[110] Fruit juices should be diluted and served in a cup, not a bottle, once the infant is 6 months of age or older.

Figure 13–13

Iron Sources for Infants

Foods such as iron-fortified cereals and formulas, mashed legumes, and strained meats provide iron.

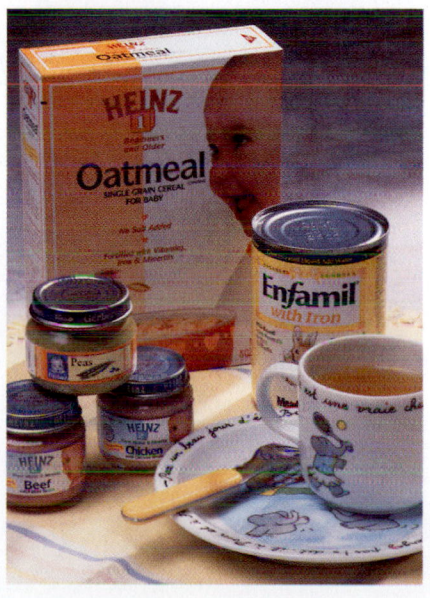

Physical Readiness for Solid Foods Foods introduced at the right times contribute to an infant's physical development. The ability to swallow food develops at around 4 to 6 months, and food offered by spoon helps to develop swallowing ability. At 8 months to a year, a baby can sit up, can handle finger foods, and begins to teethe. At that time, hard crackers and other finger foods may be introduced to promote the development of manual dexterity and control of the jaw muscles. These feedings must occur under the watchful eye of an adult because the baby can also choke on such foods. Babies and young children cannot safely chew and swallow any of the foods listed in Table 13–13; they can easily choke on these foods, a risk not worth taking. Nonfood items of small size should always be kept out of the infant's reach to prevent choking.

Some parents want to feed solids as early as possible on the theory that "stuffing the baby" at bedtime will promote sleeping through the night. There is no proof for this theory. Babies start to sleep through the night when they are ready, no matter when solid foods are introduced.

Preventing Food Allergies To prevent allergy or identify one promptly, experts recommend introducing single-ingredient foods, one at a time, in small portions and waiting three to five days before introducing the next new food.[111] For example, when introducing cereals, try fortified rice cereal first for several days; it causes allergy least often. Try wheat-containing cereal last; it is a common offender. If a food causes an allergic reaction (irritability due to skin rash, digestive upset, or respiratory discomfort), discontinue its use before going on to the next food. If allergies run in your family, use extra caution in introducing new foods. Parents or caregivers who detect allergies early in an infant's life can spare the whole family much grief.

Choice of Infant Foods Infant foods should be selected to provide variety, balance, and moderation. Commercial baby foods in the United States offer a wide variety of palatable, nutritious foods in a safe and convenient form. Brands vary in their use of starch fillers and sugar—check the ingredients lists (Appendix A lists nutrients in many baby foods). Parents or caregivers should not feed directly from the jar—spoon the needed portion into a dish to prevent contamination of the leftovers that will be stored in the jar.

An alternative to commercial baby food is to process a small portion of the family's table food in a blender, food processor, or baby food grinder. This necessitates cooking without salt or sugar, though, as the best baby food manufacturers do. Adults can season their own food after taking out the baby's portion. Pureed food can be frozen in an ice cube tray to yield a dozen or so servings that can be quickly thawed, heated, and served on a busy day.

Foods to Omit Sweets of any kind (including baby food "desserts") have no place in a baby's diet. The added food energy can promote obesity, and such treats convey few or no nutrients to support growth. Products containing sugar alcohols such as sorbitol should also be limited, as these may cause diarrhea. Salty canned vegetables are inappropriate for babies, but unsalted varieties provide a convenient source of well-cooked vegetables. Maintaining an awareness of foodborne illnesses and taking precautions against them are imperative—even a normally mild foodborne illness can cause serious harm to an infant or young child. Infants should not be given unpasteurized milk, milk products, or juices; raw or undercooked eggs, meat, poultry, fish, or shellfish; or raw sprouts. Honey and corn syrup should never be fed to infants because of the risk of botulism. Infants and young children are vulnerable to foodborne illnesses.

Foodborne illnesses and their prevention are topics of **Chapter 12.**

Table 13-14

Sample Meal Plan for a 1-Year-Old

SAMPLE MENU	
BREAKFAST	1 scrambled egg 1 slice whole-wheat toast ½ c whole milk
MORNING SNACK	½ c yogurt ¼ c fruit[a]
LUNCH	½ grilled cheese sandwich: 1 slice whole-wheat bread with 1 slice cheese ½ c vegetables[b] (steamed carrots) ¼ c 100% fruit juice
AFTERNOON SNACK	½ c fruit[a] ½ c toasted oat cereal
DINNER	1 oz chopped meat or ¼ c well-cooked mashed legumes ½ c rice or pasta ½ c vegetables[b] (chopped broccoli) ½ c whole milk

Note: This sample menu provides about 1,000 calories.

[a]Include citrus fruits, melons, and berries.

[b]Include dark green, leafy vegetables and red and orange vegetables.

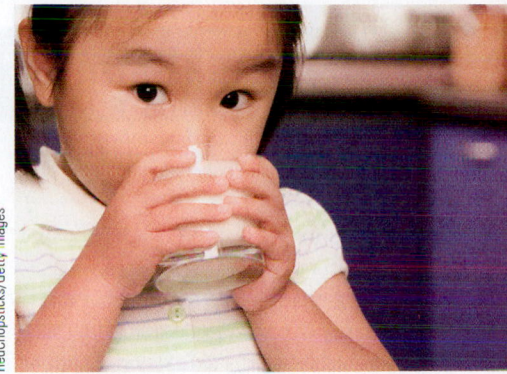

With the first birthday comes the possibility of tasting cow's milk for the first time.

Beverages and Foods at 1 Year At 1 year of age, reduced-fat or low-fat cow's milk can become a primary source of most of the nutrients an infant needs; 2 to 3 cups a day meet those needs. More milk than this displaces iron-rich foods and can lead to the iron-deficiency anemia known as **milk anemia**. A variety of other foods—protein foods such as meat, poultry, seafood, eggs, and legumes; iron-fortified cereal; enriched or whole-grain bread; fruits; and vegetables—should be supplied in amounts sufficient to round out total energy needs. Ideally, the 1-year-old sits at the table, eats many of the same foods everyone else eats, and drinks liquids from a cup, not a bottle. Table 13–14 shows a sample menu that meets the requirements for a 1-year-old.

KEY POINTS

- At 6 months, an infant may be ready to try some solid foods.
- By 1 year, the child should be eating foods from all food groups.

Looking Ahead

The first year of life is the time to lay the foundation for future health. From the nutrition standpoint, the problems most common in later years are obesity and dental disease. Prevention of obesity may also help to prevent the obesity-related diseases: atherosclerosis, diabetes, and cancer.

The most important single measure to undertake during the first year is to encourage eating habits that will support continued normal weight as the child grows. This means introducing a variety of nutritious foods in an inviting way (not forcing the baby to finish the bottle or baby food jar) and avoiding concentrated sweets and empty-calorie foods while encouraging physical activity. Parents should not teach babies to seek food as a reward, to expect food as comfort for unhappiness, or to associate food deprivation with punishment. If they cry for companionship, pick them up—don't feed them. If they are hungry, by all means, feed them appropriately. More pointers are offered in this chapter's Food Feature.

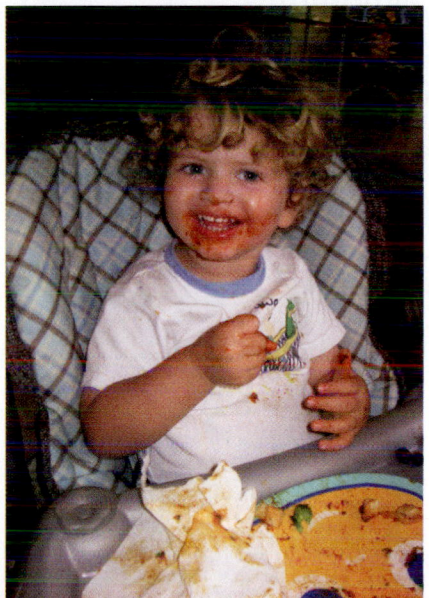

Older babies love to eat what their families eat. Let them enjoy their food.

milk anemia iron-deficiency anemia caused by drinking so much milk that iron-rich foods are displaced from the diet.

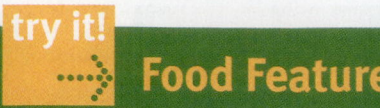
Mealtimes with Infants

LO 13.6 List five feeding guidelines that encourage normal eating behaviors and autonomy in the child.

The nurturing of a young child involves more than nutrition. Those who care for young children are responsible for providing not only nutritious foods, milk, and water but also a safe, loving, secure environment in which the children may grow and develop.

Foster a Sense of Autonomy

The person feeding a 1-year-old has to be aware that the child's exploring and experimenting are normal and desirable behaviors. The child is developing a sense of autonomy that, if allowed to develop, will provide the foundation for later assertiveness in choosing when and how much to eat and when to stop eating.

Some Feeding Guidelines

In light of the developmental and nutrient needs of 1-year-olds and in the face of their often contrary and willful behavior, a few feeding guidelines may be helpful:

- *Discourage unacceptable behavior (such as standing at the table or throwing food) by removing the child from the table to wait until later to eat.* Be consistent and firm, not punitive. For example, instead of saying "You make me mad when you don't sit down," say, "The fruit salad tastes good—please sit down and eat some with me." The child will soon learn to sit and eat.

- *Let young children explore and enjoy food.* This may mean eating with fingers for a while. Learning to use a spoon will come in time. Children who are allowed to touch, mash, and smell their food while exploring it are more likely to accept it.

- *Don't force food on children.* Rejecting new foods is normal, and acceptance is more likely as children become familiar with new foods through repeated opportunities to taste them. Instead of saying "You cannot go outside to play until you taste your carrots," say, "You can try the carrots again another time."

- *Provide nutritious foods, and let children choose which ones, and how much, they will eat.* Gradually, they will acquire a taste for different foods.

- *Limit sweets.* Infants and young children have little room for empty-calorie foods in their daily energy allowance. Do not use sweets as a reward for eating meals.

- *Don't turn the dining table into a battleground.* Make mealtimes enjoyable. Teach healthy food choices and eating habits in a pleasant environment. Mealtimes are not the time to fight, argue, or scold.

These recommendations reflect a spirit of tolerance that best serves the emotional and physical interests of the infant. This attitude, carried throughout childhood, helps the child to develop a healthy relationship with food. The next chapter finishes the story of growth and nutrition.

Figure 13–14

Nursing Bottle Tooth Decay— An Extreme Example

The upper teeth have decayed all the way to the gum line.

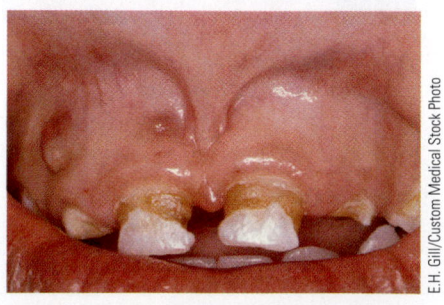

Dentists strongly discourage the practice of giving a baby a bottle as a pacifier and recommend limiting treats. Sucking for long periods of time pushes the normal jaw line out of shape and causes a bucktoothed profile: protruding upper and receding lower teeth. Prolonged sucking on a bottle of milk or juice also bathes the upper teeth in a carbohydrate-rich fluid that favors the growth of acid-producing bacteria, which dissolves tooth material. Babies regularly put to bed with a bottle sometimes have teeth decayed all the way to the gum line, a condition known as nursing bottle tooth decay, shown in Figure 13–14.

KEY POINTS

- The early feeding of the infant lays the foundation for lifelong eating habits.
- The most important single measure to undertake during the first year is to encourage eating habits that will support continued normal weight as the child grows.

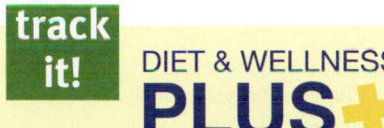
Concepts in Action

Analyze the Adequacy of a Diet for Pregnancy

The purpose of this exercise is to reinforce the importance of good food choices that provide nutrients necessary to support health during the mother's pregnancy and lactation and the infant's growth.

1. To reduce the risk for neural tube defects in infants, women of childbearing age are urged to obtain 400 micrograms (μg DFE) of folic acid daily in addition to a varied diet. Find folic acid among enriched grains and other fortified foods. Select the Track Diet tab from the navigation bar. Select a new date, and enter the foods to create a meal that provides folic acid from enriched sources (see Table 13–4, p. 524). (*Hint:* A good meal to choose is breakfast.) Select the Reports tab; then select Intake vs. Goals. How close did your meal come to providing one-third of the needed 400 μg DFE folic acid? What food might you add to increase your intake?

2. A pregnant teenager's need for calcium is 1,300 mg a day. Many teenagers fail to meet their calcium needs, even before pregnancy. Select the Track Diet tab, and select a new day. Add foods to create a high-calcium meal for a pregnant teen. (For tips, see Snapshot 8–1, p. 311.) Select the Reports tab: then select Source Analysis. Select Calcium from the drop-down box. Which food provided the most calcium in this meal? Select the Reports tab and choose Intake vs. Goals. Did the meal supply at least one-third of the day's calcium need? If not, make substitutions to reach the goal.

3. During lactation, a woman needs an additional 330 calories per day more than her regular need. Create a new profile from the Profile drop-down box on the navigation bar. Make the new profile similar to your own but select "female" and "pregnant, 28+ weeks." To meet this woman's need, choose among nutrient-dense foods (refer to Table 13–2, p. 522), and create a one-day diet to meet her increased energy need. Select the Reports tab and then Energy Balance, and generate a report for the entire day's meals. Did your food choices help this woman to meet her increased energy need?

4. Zinc is required for protein synthesis and cell development. Obtaining zinc poses a challenge to vegetarians. Create a vegetarian meal that includes zinc-rich foods. Select the Track Diet tab, and select the profile for the pregnant woman. Select a new date. Choose some zinc-rich foods to create a meal. Select Reports and then Source Analysis. Select Zinc from the drop-down box, and generate a report. What zinc-rich foods would you advise for a pregnant vegetarian?

5. An infant just beginning to eat solid foods needs iron and vitamin C in particular. From the Profile drop-down box, create a profile for a 30-inch, 24-pound 1-year-old child. Select the Track Diet tab, and create a breakfast and snack that include food sources of iron and vitamin C. Select the Reports tab, then Source Analysis, and finally Iron from the drop-down box, and generate a report. What were the top sources of iron? Do the same for vitamin C, and name the top sources. From the Reports tab, select Intake vs. Goals. Did your food choices supply more than a third of the child's iron and vitamin C requirements? If not, what other foods might you select?

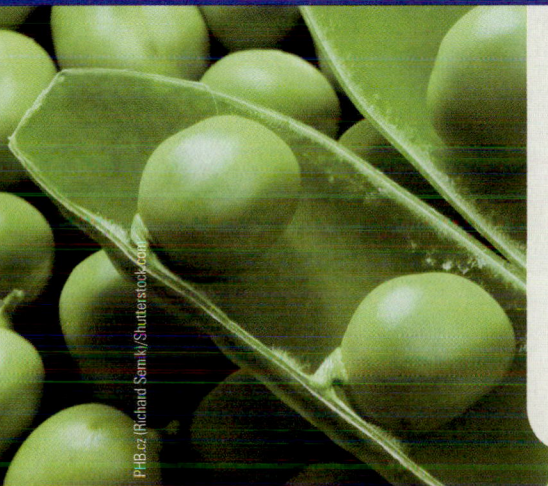

what did you decide?

Can a man's lifestyle habits affect a future pregnancy?

How much alcohol does it take to harm a developing fetus?

Are breast milk and formula about the same for an infant?

Can infants grow and thrive on only breast milk or formula?

Self Check

1. (LO 13.1) A pregnant woman needs an extra 450 calories above the allowance for nonpregnant women during which trimester(s)?

   a. first
   b. second
   c. third
   d. first, second, and third

2. (LO 13.1) A major reason why a woman's nutrition before pregnancy is crucial is that it determines whether her uterus will support the growth of a normal placenta.
   T F

3. (LO 13.1) A deficiency of which nutrient during pregnancy appears to be related to an increased risk of neural tube defects in newborns?

   a. vitamin B_6
   b. folate
   c. calcium
   d. niacin

4. (LO 13.1) The pregnant woman's body helps to conserve iron by

   a. triggering food cravings.
   b. reducing physical activity.
   c. increasing iron excretion.
   d. increasing iron absorption.

5. (LO 13.1) Which of the following preventative measures should a pregnant woman take to avoid contracting listeriosis?

   a. avoid feta cheese
   b. avoid pasteurized milk
   c. thoroughly heat hot dogs
   d. a and c

6. (LO 13.2) Fetal alcohol syndrome (FAS) is one of the leading known preventable causes of mental retardation in the world.
   T F

7. (LO 13.2) Which of the following does not characterize the damage done by alcohol during pregnancy?

   a. halts delivery of oxygen through the umbilical cord
   b. stimulates maternal appetite and therefore increases fetal nutrition
   c. slows cell division
   d. interferes with placental transport of nutrients to the fetus

8. (LO 13.2) The American Academy of Pediatrics urges all women to drink only moderately during pregnancy.
   T F

9. (LO 13.3) Without proper management, type 1 or type 2 diabetes during pregnancy can cause all except

   a. severe nausea.
   b. severe hypoglycemia or hyperglycemia.
   c. preterm labor.
   d. pregnancy-related hypertension.

10. (LO 13.3) When women in developed countries die of pregnancy complications, the cause is often eclampsia.
    T F

11. (LO 13.4) To support lactation, a breastfeeding woman needs more of the following:

    a. fluid
    b. fluoride
    c. energy
    d. a and c

12. (LO 13.4) Maternal dietary calcium intake has no effect on the calcium content of breast milk.
    T F

13. (LO 13.4) Lactating women who smoke tobacco

    a. transfer nicotine and other chemicals to their infants through their breast milk.
    b. produce more milk than nonsmokers.
    c. produce milk with a higher fat content, damaging the infant's arteries.
    d. b and c

14. (LO 13.5) Breastfed infants may need supplements of _____.

    a. fluoride, iron, and vitamin D
    b. zinc, iron, and vitamin C
    c. vitamin E, calcium, and fluoride
    d. vitamin K, magnesium, and potassium

15. (LO 13.5) Protective factors in breast milk include

    a. antiviral agents.
    b. anti-inflammatory agents.
    c. antibacterial agents.
    d. all of the above.

16. (LO 13.5) Which of the following foods poses a choking hazard to infants and small children?

    a. pudding
    b. marshmallows
    c. hot dog slices
    d. b and c

17. (LO 13.5) A sure way to get a baby to sleep through the night is to feed solid foods as soon as the baby can swallow them.
    T F

18. (LO 13.6) Fostering a sense of autonomy in a one-year-old includes allowing the child to explore and experiment with her food.
    T F

19. (LO 13.6) In light of the developmental needs of one-year-olds, parents should allow such behaviors as standing at the table and throwing food.
    T F

20. (LO 13.7) To treat obesity in children, a first goal is to

    a. reduce their weight by 10 percent while they grow taller.
    b. quickly achieve their ideal weight.
    c. slow their rate of gain while they grow taller.
    d. a and b

Answers to these Self Check questions are in Appendix G.

Childhood Obesity and Early Chronic Diseases

LO 13.7 Recognize the challenges associated with childhood obesity.

When most people think of health problems in children and adolescents, they often think of dental caries and acne, not type 2 diabetes and hypertension. Today, however, about a third of U.S. children and adolescents 2 to 19 years of age are overweight or obese.[1]* Serious risk factors and "adult diseases," such as type 2 diabetes, often accompany obesity, even in a child.[2]

Trends in Childhood Obesity

Children in the United States are not alone in these problems—childhood obesity rates are soaring around the globe.[3]

Although no group has fully escaped the national gain in body weight, obese children tend to have these characteristics:

- Are male.[4]
- Are older.
- Are of African American or Hispanic descent.[5]
- Are sedentary.[6]
- Have parents who are obese.[7]

Additionally, low family income predicts obesity among Caucasian, Hispanic, and Asian children.[8]

By some measures, childhood obesity rates appear to have steadied or even fallen slightly in a few areas of the country, leading scientists to hope that a turning point may have been reached. However, childhood obesity remains a national challenge.[9]

*Reference notes are found in Appendix F.

Table C13–1

Physical Complications of Obesity during Childhood

These conditions increase a child's risks for chronic diseases now and into adulthood.

- Abnormal blood lipid profile
  - High total cholesterol
  - High triglycerides
  - High LDL cholesterol
- High blood pressure
- High fasting insulin
- Structural changes to the heart
- Asthma
- Breathing difficulties (sleep apnea)
- Nonalcoholic liver disease

Sources: L. Hurt and coauthors, Diagnosis and screening for obesity-related conditions among children and teens receiving Medicaid—Maryland, 2005–2010, Morbidity and Mortality Weekly Report 63 (2014): 305–308; C. A. Evans and coauthors, Effects of OSA and obesity on exercise function in children, Sleep 37 (2014): 1103–1110; C. Koebnick and coauthors, High blood pressure in overweight and obese youth: Implications for screening, Journal of Clinical Hypertension 15 (2013), epub, doi:10.1111/jch.12199.

The Challenge of Childhood Obesity

Obesity takes a heavy toll on the well-being of a child. Education is urgently needed—most parents do not recognize the development of obesity in their own children, let alone the associated health risks it may pose.[10]

Physical and Emotional Perils

Excessive body weight in the young is more than just a cosmetic problem. Table C13–1 summarizes the physical complications that can accompany obesity in children. The consequences of

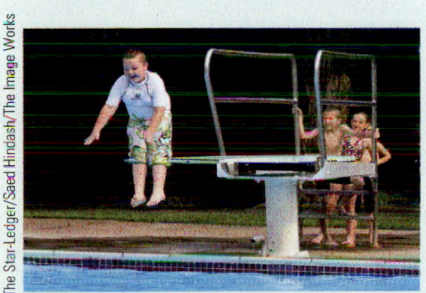

Children with obesity may develop type 2 diabetes, among other illnesses.

childhood obesity can be serious, and they set the stage for future health problems.

Obese children may also suffer psychologically.[11] Adults may discriminate against them, and peers may make thoughtless comments or reject them based on their physical appearance. An obese child may develop a poor self-image, a sense of failure, and a passive approach to life. The emotional perils of childhood obesity are often amplified by the media. More than 75 percent of popular children's movies denigrate or stigmatize the fat person as a social misfit.[12] Social media also abound with negative judgments of overweight people, particularly females. Unfortunately, children have few defenses against these unfair portrayals and quickly internalize negative attitudes toward bulky body sizes.

Overweight or Chubby and Healthy: How Can You Tell?

An accurate assessment of a child's body mass index (BMI) for age is essential and requires a trained individual—guesswork can lead to unneeded lifestyle changes for a healthy-weight child or to a missed opportunity to help a truly overweight child. Physicians, registered dietitian nutritionists, and other health-care providers can accurately assess a child's BMI and interpret it using a growth chart, as Figure C13–1 demonstrates. Because body fat differs between boys and girls and changes with age, BMI-for-age percentiles are calculated for children and teens using gender-specific growth charts.[13] Although cutoffs for children generate controversy, children and adolescents are generally considered *overweight* from the 85th to the 94th percentile on growth charts and *obese* at the 95th percentile and above. Pediatric obesity is underreported—U.S.

physicians report an obesity diagnosis in only 18 percent of obese youth.[14]

Darla and Gabby

Eight-year-old Gabriella and her worried mother Darla tell a typical story of childhood obesity, and they model some appropriate responses. Recently, a note from the school nurse explained that during a routine screening, Gabby's BMI-for-age percentile was found to be too high. The nurse has suggested further testing for risk factors of chronic diseases because Gabby's BMI of 23 places her in the obese weight category (the red dot in Figure C13–1).[15] With Gabby's health in danger, Darla's

concern grows: "I didn't know that a little baby fat at Gabby's age could be a threat. Both my father and his father died of diabetes-related conditions, and I'm worried."

Development of Type 2 Diabetes

An estimated 85 percent of the children with type 2 diabetes are obese. Diabetes is most often diagnosed around the age of puberty, but type 2 diabetes is quickly encroaching on younger age groups as children grow fatter. Ethnicity (being Native American or of African, Asian, or Hispanic descent) increases the risk, as does having a family history of type 2

Figure C13–1

Assessing Body Fatness in Children: An Example

Growth charts reflect population-wide data for children's BMI values as they age. Gabby is female, so this chart is for girls; a chart for boys is offered on the inside back cover.

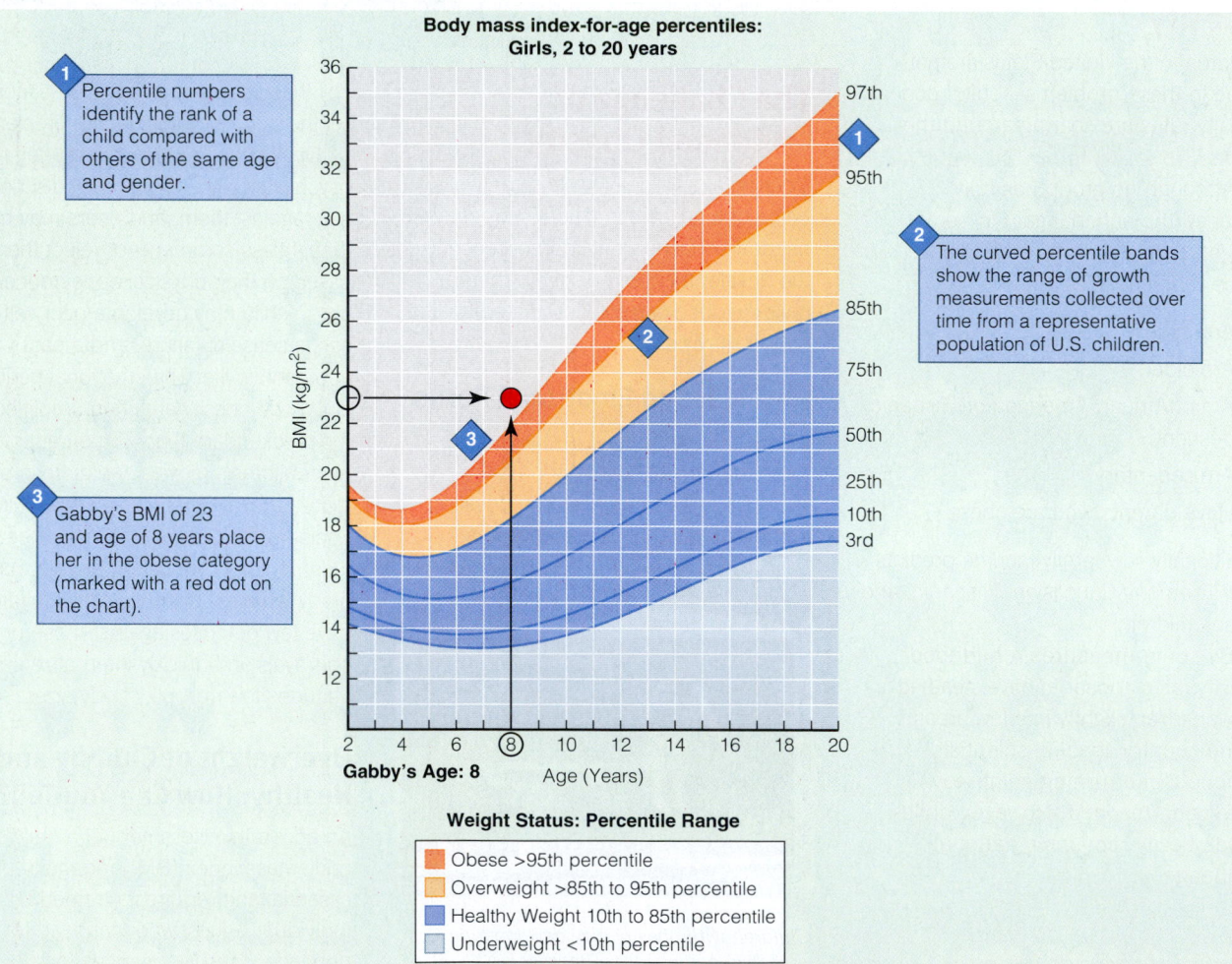

Body mass index-for-age percentiles: Girls, 2 to 20 years

1 Percentile numbers identify the rank of a child compared with others of the same age and gender.

2 The curved percentile bands show the range of growth measurements collected over time from a representative population of U.S. children.

3 Gabby's BMI of 23 and age of 8 years place her in the obese category (marked with a red dot on the chart).

BMI (kg/m²) — Age (Years) — Gabby's Age: 8

Weight Status: Percentile Range

Obese >95th percentile
Overweight >85th to 95th percentile
Healthy Weight 10th to 85th percentile
Underweight <10th percentile

diabetes. Chapter 4 described the risks associated with type 2 diabetes, and Chapter 11 revealed its connection with cardiovascular disease (CVD).

Determining exactly how many children suffer from type 2 diabetes is tricky. The child with type 2 diabetes may lack telltale symptoms, such as glucose in the urine, ketones in the blood, weight loss, or excessive thirst and urination, so diabetes often advances undetected. Without treatment, children with diabetes are left undefended against its ravages.[16]

Development of Heart Disease

Atherosclerosis, first apparent as heart disease in adulthood, begins in youth. By adolescence, most children have formed fatty streaks in their coronary arteries. By early adulthood, the arterial lesions that make heart attacks and strokes likely have formed.

Children with the highest risks of developing heart disease in adulthood are sedentary and obese, and they consume suboptimal diets. They may also have diabetes, high blood pressure, and an abnormal lipid profile.[17] Adolescents who take up smoking greatly compound their risk.

High childhood BMI alone may not always predict increased adulthood heart disease risk, however. Overweight and obese youth who grow into normal-weight adults may reduce their health risks substantially.[18] Still, authorities recommend that all children aged 6 years and older be screened for obesity and that obese children be treated with intensive counseling that includes diet, physical activity, and behavior changes.[19]

The note from Gabby's school nurse prompted medical testing, including a family history, a fasting blood glucose test, a blood lipid profile, and a blood pressure test. Luckily, the results for both glucose and blood pressure were normal.

High Blood Cholesterol

Gabby's blood lipid results, however, confirmed her mother's fears: her LDL cholesterol is 135—too high for optimal health. Cholesterol standards for children

Table C13–2

Cholesterol Values for Children and Adolescents

Disease Risk	Total Cholesterol (mg/dL)	LDL Cholesterol (mg/dL)
Acceptable	<170	<110
Borderline	170–199	110–129
High	≥200	≥130

Note: Adult values appeared in Chapter 11.

and adolescents (ages 2 to 18 years) are in Table C13–2.

Obesity, especially central obesity, and high blood cholesterol often occur together. As children mature into adolescents, they often choose more foods rich in saturated and *trans* fats, and their blood cholesterol levels tend to rise. Further, sedentary children and adolescents have lower HDL, higher LDL, and higher blood pressure than those who are physically active.

Family history sometimes predicts high blood cholesterol. If the parents or grandparents suffered from early heart disease, chances are that a child's blood cholesterol will be higher than average and will remain so through life. Diabetes, smoking, being overweight, and eating diets high in saturated and *trans* fats also raise the risk.[20]

High Blood Pressure

High blood pressure in a child or adolescent is a concern—it can signal the early onset of hypertension. Childhood hypertension, left untreated, tends to worsen with time and can accelerate atherosclerosis.[21] Diagnosing hypertension in children must account for age, gender, and height; simple tables like the ones for adults are useless for children.

Dramatic improvements often occur when children with hypertension take up regular aerobic activity and hold their weight down as they grow taller ("grow into their weight"). Restricting sodium intake also causes an immediate drop in most children's and adolescents' blood pressures.[22]

Early Childhood Influences on Obesity

Children begin to learn behaviors that affect their health from a young age. Parents and other caregivers have a unique opportunity to help children form healthy habits related to the foods they eat, the physical and leisure activities they participate in, and their emotional well-being—all of which will pave the way to becoming healthy adults.

Calories—and Cautions

Gabby, who loves sweets, budgets her pocket money (she's saving for an MP3 player) to join her friends for a chocolate almond bar (250 calories) every day after school.[23] In addition, she knows how to bake peanut butter cookies from a roll of refrigerated dough and enjoys eating two cookies each night at bedtime (another 240 calories). Gabby knows that nuts and peanut butter are better than candy for health, but she doesn't understand that the calories from fat and sugar greatly outweigh the healthy ingredients in her chocolate almond bar and cookies.

Intuitively, Darla would like to eliminate these treats. However, excessive restriction of sweets or calories can intensify cravings, contribute to eating in the absence of hunger, and spark unnecessary battles about food.[24] Worse, children who feel deprived or hungry may begin to sneak banned foods or hide them and binge on them in secret—behaviors that often predict eating disorders.

Figure C13–2 lists frequent high-calorie snacking as a contributing factor in a child's weight gain, but good-tasting snacks and meals are important to all children. A balanced approach may be to include favorite high-calorie treats occasionally in the context of structured, nutritious, and appealing meals and snacks.

Sedentary Behavior

Children who are more sedentary and less physically active are more often overweight.[25] The AAP recommends no TV time before two years of age and a limit of two hours of quality

Factors Affecting Childhood Weight Gain

The more of these factors in a child's life, the greater the likelihood of unhealthy weight gain.

Food Factors
- Frequent snacks consisting of high-energy foods, such as candies, cookies, crackers, fried foods, and ice cream.
- Irregular or sporadic mealtimes; missed meals.
- Eating when not hungry; eating while watching TV or doing homework.
- Fast-food meals more than once per week.
- Frequent meals of fried or sugary foods and beverages.
- Exposure to advertising that promotes high-calorie foods.

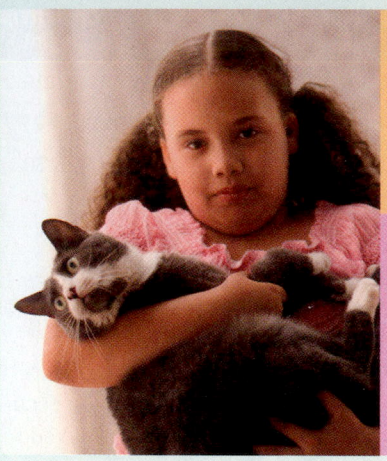

Jose Luis Pelaez Inc./Blend Images/Getty Images

Activity Factors
- More than an hour of sedentary activity, such as television, each day.
- Less than 20 minutes of physical activity, such as outdoor play, each day.
- No access to recreational facilities.

Family and Other Factors
- Overweight family members, particularly parents.
- Low-income family.
- Tall for age.

media entertainment, including TV and computers, for older children to help prevent obesity.[26] However, U.S. children far exceed these recommendations (Figure C13–3).[27] Adolescents in the United States spend more than five hours, on average, each day engaged in screen time, such as TV viewing, video game playing, and computer use.[28]

Currently, most research on the relationship between sedentary behaviors and obesity has focused on TV viewing. A systematic review of studies in young children identified a relation-ship between longer TV viewing times and increased levels of body fatness.[29] However, the child's level of attention during TV watching may influence BMI more than viewing time. A child paying attention to television is exposed to multiple food advertisements that may increase his or her preference for, and ultimately intake of, unhealthy food. The distraction of TV while eating may also cause a child to ignore satiety cues and overeat.[30] Although the exact mechanism linking TV viewing and obesity has not been identified, children are less likely to be active and more likely to snack while watching TV.[31]

Darla recalls, "My sisters and I hit the door on Saturday mornings with sandwiches in a bag. We explored, climbed trees, played softball with our friends, jumped in puddles, and played 'tag.' But Gabby and her friends have 252 television channels to choose from, not to mention video games and the Internet—no wonder they never play outside!"

Food Advertising to Children

Children and youth influence a huge portion of the nation's food spending—up to $200 billion of their own pocket money each year and hundreds of billions more in annual family purchases of foods, beverages, and restaurant meals.[32] To capture these dollars, the food industry loads children's TV programs and games with advertisements for highly processed foods and beverages.[33] Sugar-coated breakfast cereals, salty chips, sugar-sweetened beverages, and fat-laden fast foods dominate these ads. Children and teens view an average of three to five advertisements for fast food *each day*.[34] The food companies target children and youth with sophisticated messages that connect the featured foods with a child's needs for fun, love, and social acceptance.[35]

On the Internet, food marketing agencies develop free, child-attracting "advergames,"—that is, games built around a manufacturer's foods and beverages that spark brand loyalty in young children. Appealing animated "spokescharacters" speak directly to children to increase their desire for the featured low-nutrient-density products.[36] This approach succeeds, partly because young children cannot yet grasp the intent of advertising.[37]

Some food companies have pledged to encourage a healthier lifestyle for children by devoting all advertising to healthier foods, limiting the use of beloved children's characters, and halting the advertisement of foods in elementary schools.[38] However, progress is slow and today's advertisements do not meet the proposed guidelines.[39] Advertising

Prevalence of Obesity by Hours of TV per Day, Children Ages 10–15 Years

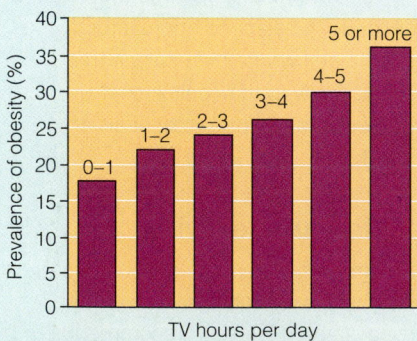

Prevalence of obesity (%)

TV hours per day

Source: Centers for Disease Control and Prevention, Youth Risk Behavior Survey, available at www.cdc.gov.

is protected to some extent by the First Amendment to the U.S. Constitution, protection that is opposed by children's health advocates.[40] In recent years, the American Heart Association has taken a position in support of increased regulation, and the World Health Organization has released guidelines for responsible food marketing to children.[41]

Preventing and Reversing Overweight in Children: A Family Affair

Prevention and treatment of childhood obesity are national priorities.[42] Parents play a critical role in the development of child weight status, from the selection of early feeding practices to the shaping of eating behaviors and attitudes later on.[13]

For a child who is overweight or obese, an initial goal might be to slow the child's rate of gain while the child grows taller. Weight loss ordinarily is not recommended because diet restriction can easily interfere with normal growth, but this may depend on the severity of the obesity or the presence of medical conditions.[44] Family-based efforts that focus on healthy food choices and physical activity can help children grow into their weight, without making them feel singled out.[45]

Gabby's pediatrician has recommended lifestyle changes to improve both her BMI and her blood lipids. Darla is motivated: "I need to take some action!" A warning to Darla: the lifestyle changes may sound easy, but implementing them may prove more difficult than she expects—people's behaviors are notoriously resistant to change. Further, Gabby must be involved at the planning stage for the changes to be successful.

Parents Set an Example

Parents are among the most influential forces shaping the self-concept, weight concerns, and eating habits of children, and young children learn food behaviors largely from their families.[46] Whole families may be eating too much, dieting inappropriately, and exercising too little.[47] Therefore, successful plans for stabilizing a child's weight center on whole-family lifestyle changes (see Table C13–3)

Table C13–3

Family Lifestyle Changes to Help the Overweight Child

The whole family can benefit from health-promoting habits such as these:

- Learn and use appropriate food portions.
- Involve children in shopping for and preparing family meals.
- Set regular mealtimes and dine together frequently.
- For other days, plan and provide a wide variety of nutritious snacks that are low in fat and sugar.
- Provide an appropriate nutritious breakfast every day.
- Provide recommended amounts of fruit juices but no more than this amount.
- Limit high-sugar, high-fat foods, including sugar-sweetened soft drinks and fruit-flavored punches.
- Set a good example and demonstrate positive behaviors for children to imitate.
- Slow down eating and pause to enjoy table companions; stop eating when full.
- Do not use foods to reward or punish behaviors.
- Involve children in daily active outdoor play or structured physical activities, as a family or with friends.
- Limit television time; set a rule to eliminate television-watching during meals.
- Celebrate family special events and holidays with outdoor activities, such as a softball game, a hike, or a summer swim.
- Keep a calendar of scheduled family meals and activity events where everyone can read it.
- Obtain parent and child nutrition and physical activity education and training or family counseling to guide family-based behavioral and other interventions as needed.
- Work with schools to institute school-wide food and activity policies to support a healthy body weight and prevent obesity.

Sources: Centers for Disease Control and Prevention, Healthy weight—It's not a diet, it's a lifestyle!: Tips for parents—Ideas to help children maintain a healthy body weight, 2014, available at www.cdc.gov; WebMD, Healthy eating habits for your child, 2014, available at www.webmd.com/children/guide/kids-healthy-eating-habits.

---

because when parents set patterns for family behaviors, the children will most often follow their lead.[48]

Lifestyle Changes First, Medications Later

A general rule for treating overweight children is "Lifestyle changes first; medications later, if at all." Children with elevated disease risk factors, such as high blood cholesterol or a family history of early heart disease, should still first be treated with diet and physical activity, but if blood cholesterol remains high after 6 to 12 months, then certain drugs may safely be used to lower blood cholesterol without interfering with normal growth or development. Only one obesity drug, orlistat, is approved for limited use in adolescents aged 12 years and older.[49]

Obesity Surgery

Limited research shows that, after weight loss surgery, extremely obese adolescents lose significant weight and reduce their risk factors for type 2 diabetes and CVD.[50] Surgery may be an option for physically mature adolescents with a BMI of 50 or above or a BMI of 40 or above with significant weight-related health problems who have failed at previous lifestyle modifications and who can adhere to the long-term lifestyle changes required after surgery. Physicians disagree about whether surgery is a reasonable option for obese teens, however.[51]

Achievable Goals, Loving Support

To preserve the child's healthy sense of self, setting realistic, specific, and achievable goals is a first priority. Keeping a positive, upbeat attitude is another. The reverse—impossible goals and a critical, blaming adult—may damage the child's developing self-image and may set the stage for eating disorders later on.

Most of all, Darla must let Gabby know that she is loved, regardless of weight. Blame is a useless concept and can trigger emotional withdrawal of the child just when the opposite—active engagement—is needed most. By being supportive, Darla can help Gabby grow into a healthy young woman with positive attitudes about food and herself. Meanwhile, she must make some changes to diet and physical activity—but exactly which ones? And how?

Luckily, some government agencies offer help to anyone with Internet access. Several reliable websites that teach parents and children practical ways to attain a healthy body weight and encourage healthy daily choices include:

- MyPlate (www.choosemyplate.gov)
- Team Nutrition (http://teamnutrition.usda.gov)
- Let's Move: America's Move to Raise a Healthier Generation of Kids (www.letsmove.gov)

Diet Moderation, Not Deprivation

All children should eat an appropriate amount and variety of foods, regardless of body weight (Chapter 14 provides many details). For the health of the heart, children older than 2 years of age benefit from the same diet recommended for older individuals—that is, a diet limited in saturated fat and *trans* fat while rich in nutrients and age-appropriate in calories. Such a diet benefits blood lipids without compromising nutrient adequacy, physical growth, or neurological development.

Darla decides to set some goals for providing nutritious, good-tasting lower-calorie foods at regular mealtimes. She also recognizes that pleasure is important, too. She knows that Gabby loves her daily chocolate treat and the social opportunity it creates with her peers. To give Gabby more healthy alternatives to chocolate, Darla introduces Gabby to some new lower-calorie treats. Gabby now enjoys 100-calorie cereal bars—almost as much as chocolate—and agrees to purchase them when she meets with her friends after school. This simple change saves 150 calories a day. They also decide to replace the evening cookies with apple slices spread with a little peanut butter, which cuts the evening snack calories in half without leaving Gabby feeling hungry or deprived. Table C13–4 outlines diet and physical activity recommendations for preventing obesity in children.

Restaurant Food and Added Sugars

A steady diet of the offerings on most "children's menus" in restaurants, such as fried chicken nuggets, hot dogs, and French fries, invites both nutrient shortages and gains of body fat. Often, better choices can be found among appetizers, soups, salads, and side selections, and the best establishments offer steamed vegetables, fresh fruit, and broiled or grilled poultry on menus for both children and adults.[52]

The 2015–2020 Dietary Guidelines for Americans recommend limiting intake of added sugars to a maximum of 10 percent of daily calories; however, U.S. children and adolescents consume approximately 16 percent of total caloric intake from added sugars.[53] Sugar-sweetened beverages (SSB), including soft drinks, fruit drinks, and energy or water drinks with added sugars, are a main source of added sugar in the American diet.[54] Research has linked SSB consumption with excess body fatness in children and increased risk of chronic diseases in children and adults.[55] Foods and beverages high in added sugar are best enjoyed in moderation.

Physical Activity and Sleep

Physical activity assists with controlling body weight, decreasing blood pressure, increasing HDL cholesterol levels, and improving self-esteem and confidence. Yet children are spending only an average of 30 minutes each day engaged in moderate physical activity, far short of the current recommendations of 60 minutes

---

Table C13–4

Recommended Diet and Physical Activity to Prevent Childhood Obesity

American Heart Association Dietary Recommendations—For Children 2 to 18 Years of Age

- Provide plenty of vegetables, fruits and whole-grain products.
- Include low-fat or non-fat milk or dairy products.
- Choose lean meats, poultry, fish, lentils and beans for protein.
- Serve reasonably sized portions.
- Encourage your family to drink lots of water.
- Limit sugar-sweetened beverages, sugar, sodium and saturated fat.
- Alter recipes to make favorite dishes healthier.
- Remove calorie-rich temptations. Offer fruit and vegetables instead.
- Limit television and other screen time to no more than 2 hours a day.

Physical Activity Guidelines for Americans—For Children 6 to 17 Years of Age

- Children and adolescents should participate in 60 minutes (1 hour) or more of physical activity daily.
- Aerobic: Most of the 60 or more minutes a day should be either moderate- or vigorous-intensity aerobic physical activity and should include vigorous-intensity physical activity at least 3 days a week. Walking, bike riding, practicing martial arts, and dancing are examples.[a]
- Muscle-strengthening: As part of their 60 minutes of daily physical activity, children and adolescents should include muscle-strengthening physical activity on at least 3 days of the week. Resistance can be provided by free weights, weight machines, other objects, or the person's own body weight.
- Bone-strengthening: As part of their 60 or more minutes of daily physical activity, children and adolescents should include bone-strengthening physical activity on at least 3 days of the week. Hopping, skipping, jumping, and running sports including basketball and tennis are examples.

[a]Chapter 10 specified activities that characterize various intensity levels.
Sources: www.heart.org/HEARTORG/GettingHealthy/HealthierKids/ChildhoodObesity/Preventing-Childhood-Obesity-Tips-for-Parents-and-Caretakers_UCM_456118_Article.jsp;www.health.gov/paguidelines/guidelines/chapter3.aspx.

---

a day. Not surprisingly, children reporting longer physical activity times have better cardiovascular profiles than their less active counterparts.[56] Active video games offer some amount of physical activity, but controversy exists over the value of active gaming as an intervention against childhood obesity.[57] The best way for parents to promote physical activity in youth is to set limits on screen time, provide appealing opportunities for active play, and join in the fun.

Parents who establish healthful daily routines often set in place lifelong habits that ultimately influence a child's future health.[58] For example, young children who receive adequate sleep, view minimal TV, and have no TV in the bedroom have lower levels of obesity than others (Figure C13–4).[59] If those children then grow into active adults, their healthy habits may help to ward off obesity and chronic diseases in mid-life and beyond. Therefore, intervention strategies for stabilizing a child's weight should begin with the parents and include the development of healthy patterns for parents and children alike.[60]

Darla's Efforts and Gabby's Future

"Currently, I'm achieving four of our goals," says Darla, "but with Gabby's input, I've planned additional goals. First, Gabby and I are getting up a little earlier in the mornings to eat a nutritious breakfast. Gabby's doctor explained that breakfast is important because it can help Gabby focus at school and reach a healthier weight.[61] Second, I'm packing Gabby a healthy, tasty, lower-calorie lunch for school. It's easy to make ahead whole-grain sandwiches or wraps for the week and freeze them and then toss one into a lunch bag with a low-fat yogurt, or low-fat cheese sticks, and water (not soda!). I'm also including some nutritious snacks that she loves, like baby carrots and raisins, to sustain her energy and tempt her away from higher-calorie snacks on some days.

"Third, because we both have a sweet tooth, I keep ready-to-eat snacks of fresh fruit, like grapes and strawberries, in clear plastic containers on a refrigerator shelf at eye level. Fourth, although I work days and go to school four nights a week, we have started a new tradition: family meal night each Friday at 6:00 sharp. Gabby and I choose the menu during the week and look forward to making dinner together. We also switched from full-sized dinnerware to pretty new luncheon-sized plates and small dessert-sized bowls. Gabby was charmed with the bright colors, and we both find the smaller portions just as satisfying.

"Although my daughter's idea of a good vegetable has always been a fried potato, she's gradually opening up to trying new foods, which is goal number four. During Friday meal preparation, she's tried bites of broccoli, green beans—even squash! French fries are now just an occasional treat when we eat out. Gabby is doing great, and I'm going to keep offering her healthy new foods to try because it takes a while for a child to acquire a taste for a new food.[62]

"Goal number five has proved harder: we must start walking together, but when? I need to let her see that I am serious about my personal fitness, but I'm tired after work, and my studies gobble my time. To get Gabby moving after school, I've offered her credits toward her MP3 player in exchange for physical chores, such as raking, planting flowers, vacuuming, and washing the car—and when she gets her MP3 player, we've agreed to have nightly dance-offs to her favorite songs. Today though, rain or shine, tired or not, I'm going to pull on my running shoes and walk around our neighborhood with Gabby.

"I love my smart, stubborn, sturdy girl—no matter her shape or size! But I know her future will be shaped by what we are doing right now. She will grow into her weight if we can hold the line with our new healthy habits. I see her potential to do great things, and what she is learning today about taking care of herself she can pass on to others—to her own children maybe." Darla smiles, "I am so happy we are in this together, and taking charge of our health."

Critical Thinking

1. Who do you believe is responsible for childhood obesity? Organize a chart listing the changes a family and child can make to combat obesity. Include changes in food intake and activity patterns.

2. Draw a picture that represents the concept of energy balance that you could use as a visual aid in explaining this concept to a 10- to 12-year-old.

Figure C13–4

Sleep and Screen Time Routines Associated with Obesity in Preschoolers

Researchers asked parents whether their children's daily routines included adequate sleep (10 hours), limited screen time (<2 hours), and no television in the bedroom. The results are shown below: the taller bars represent the rates of obesity in children whose parents answered "no" to all of the questions—their children were more often obese. The children whose parents answered "yes" to all the questions were substantially less likely to be obese.

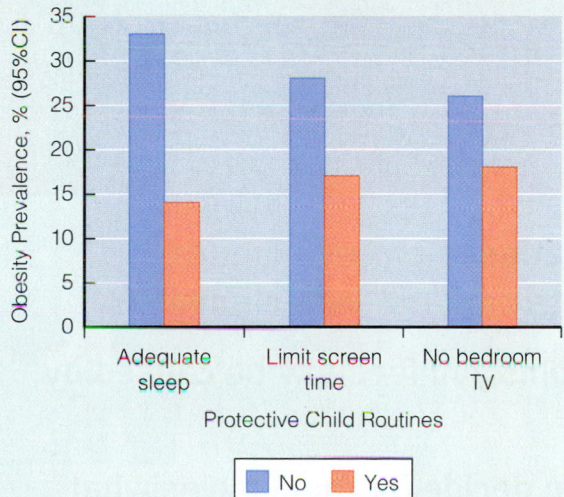

Source: B. L. Jones, B. H. Fiese, and The STRONG Kids Team, Parent routines, child routines, and family demographics associated with obesity in parents and preschool-aged children, Frontiers in Psychology (2014), epub, doi:10.3389/fpsyg.2014.00374.

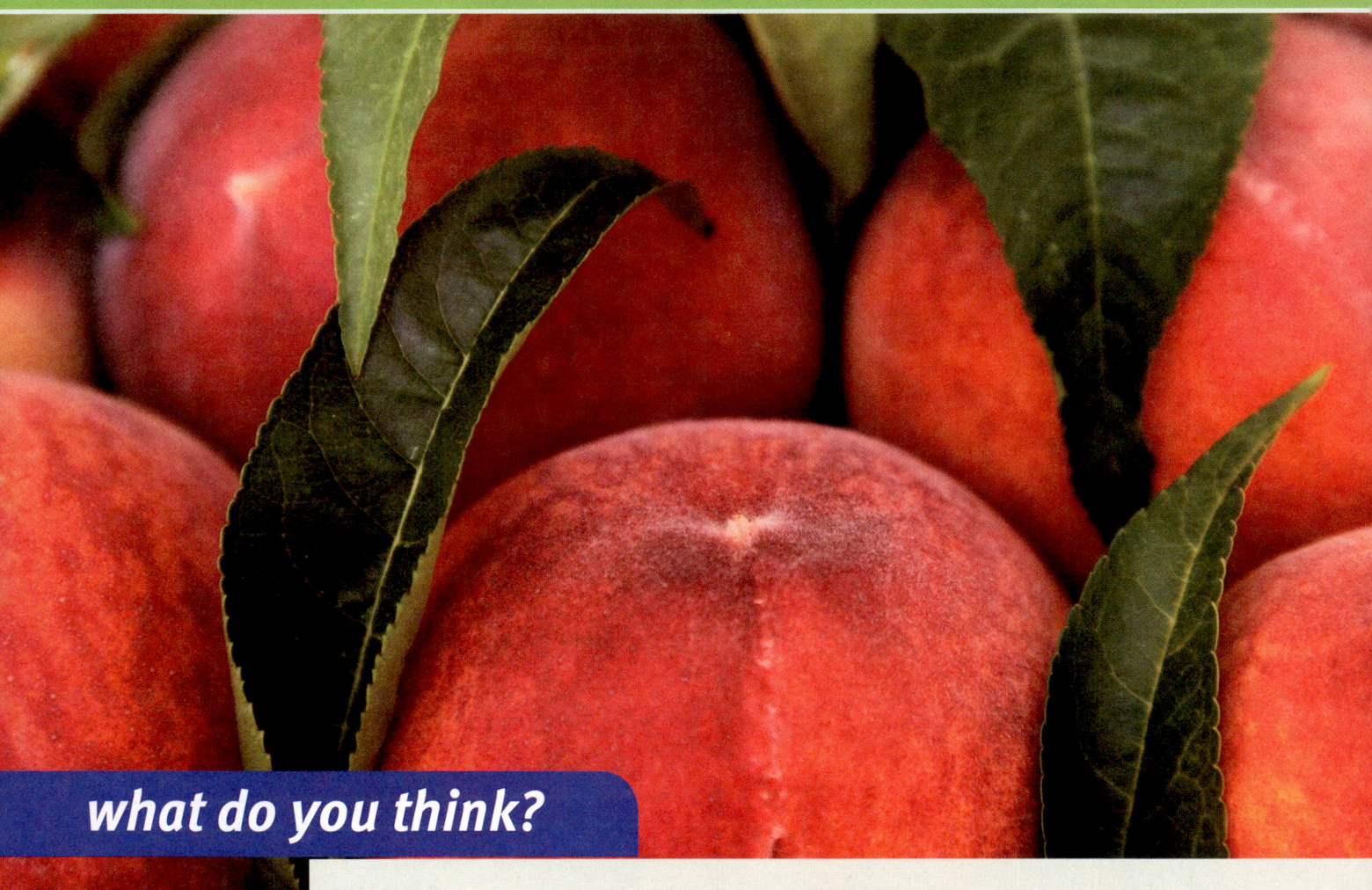

14 Child, Teen, and Older Adult

what do you think?

Do you need **special information** to properly nourish children, or are they like "little adults" in their needs?

Do you suspect that symptoms you feel may be caused by a **food allergy**?

Are **teenagers** old enough to decide for themselves what to eat?

Can good nutrition help you live **better and longer**?

LO 14.1 Discuss nutrient needs, eating habits, and dietary cautions for early and middle childhood.

LO 14.2 Summarize the nutrient needs of adolescents.

LO 14.3 Identify the factors associated with successful and healthy aging.

LO 14.4 Discuss the nutrient needs of older adults.

LO 14.5 Assess the challenges associated with regularly eating alone.

LO 14.6 Summarize the concerns surrounding nutrient–drug interactions.

To grow and to function well in the adult world, children need a firm background of sound eating habits, which begin during the second half of infancy with the introduction of solid foods. At that point, the person's nutrition story has just begun; the plot thickens. Nutrient needs change in childhood and throughout life, depending on the rate of growth, gender, activities, and many other factors. Nutrient needs also vary from individual to individual, but universal recommendations are available and useful.

Most children's diets in the United States fail to meet the recommendations of the Dietary Guidelines for Americans.[*][1] The consequences of such diets may not be evident to the casual observer, but nutritionists know that nutrient deficiencies during growth often have far-reaching effects on physical and mental development. Likewise, dietary excesses during childhood often set up a lifelong struggle against obesity and chronic diseases.

> Childhood obesity and related chronic diseases are so complex and pervasive that **Controversy 13** was devoted to them.

Early and Middle Childhood

LO 14.1 Discuss nutrient needs, eating habits, and dietary cautions for early and middle childhood.

Imagine growing 10 inches taller in just one year, as the average healthy infant does during the first dramatic year of life. At age 1, infants have just learned to stand and toddle, and growth has slowed by half; by 2 years, they can take long strides with solid confidence and are learning to run, jump, and climb. These accomplishments reflect the accumulation of a larger mass, greater density of bone and muscle tissue, and refinement of nervous system coordination. These same growth trends, a lengthening of the long bones and an increase in musculature, continue until adolescence but more slowly.

Mentally, too, the child is making rapid advances, and proper nutrition is critical to normal brain development. The child malnourished at age 3 often demonstrates diminished mental capacities compared with peers at age 11.

Feeding a Healthy Young Child

At no time in life does the human diet change faster than during the second year. From 12 to 24 months, a child's diet changes from infant foods consisting of mostly formula or breast milk to mostly modified adult foods. This doesn't mean, of course, that milk loses its importance in the toddler's diet—it remains a central source of calcium, protein, and other nutrients. Nevertheless, the rapid growth and changing body shape

---

[*]Reference notes are found in Appendix F.

Figure 14–1

Body Shape of 1-Year-Old and 2-Year-Old Compared

The body shape of a 1-year-old (left) changes dramatically by age 2 (right). The 2-year-old has lost much of the baby fat; the muscles (especially in the back, buttocks, and legs) have firmed and strengthened; and the leg bones have lengthened.

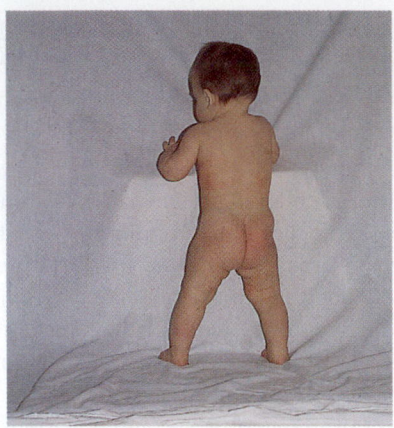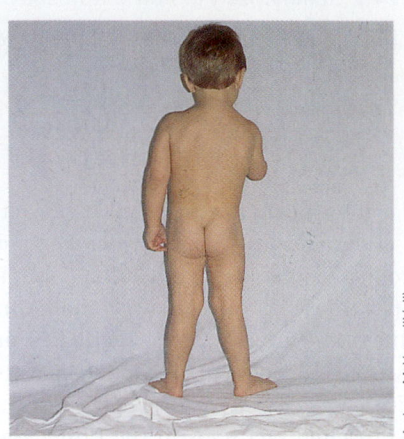

Anthony M. Vannelli (all)

Table 14–1

Estimated Daily Calorie Needs for Children

Age (y)	Sedentary[a]	Active[b]
2 (male/female)	1,000	1,000
3 (male/female)	1,000	1,400
Females		
4	1,200	1,400
5 to 6	1,200	1,600
7	1,200	1,800
8 to 9	1,400	1,800
10	1,400	2,000
11	1,600	2,000
12 to 13	1,600	2,200
Males		
4 to 5	1,200	1,600
6 to 7	1,400	1,800
8	1,400	2,000
9	1,600	2,000
10	1,600	2,200
11	1,800	2,200
12	1,800	2,400
13	2,000	2,600

[a]Sedentary describes a lifestyle that includes only the activities typical of day-to-day life.

[b]Active describes a lifestyle that includes at least 60 minutes per day of moderate physical activity (equivalent to walking more than 3 miles per day at 3 to 4 miles per hour) in addition to the activities of day-to-day life.

Source: U.S. Department of Agriculture and U.S. Department of Health and Human Services, Scientific report of the 2015 Dietary Guidelines Advisory Committee, 2015, D-1:102, available at www.health.gov.

(see Figure 14–1) during this remarkable period demand more nutrients than can be provided by milk alone. Further, the toddler years are marked by bustling activity made possible by new muscle tissue and refined neuromuscular coordination. To support both their activity and their growth, toddlers need nutrients and plenty of them.

Appetite Regulation   An infant's appetite decreases markedly near the first birthday and fluctuates thereafter. At times, children seem insatiable; at other times, they seem to live on air and water. Parents and other caregivers need not worry: given an ample selection of nutritious foods at regular intervals, internal appetite regulation in healthy, normal-weight children guarantees that their overall energy intakes will remain remarkably constant and will be right for each stage of growth.[2]

This ideal situation depends on restriction of low-nutrient, high-calorie foods, however. Today's children too often consume a constant stream of tempting foods high in added sugars, saturated fat, refined grains, and calories throughout the day, short-circuiting normal hunger and satiety cues. Children who receive regularly timed snacks and meals of a variety of nutritious foods, with only occasional special treats, often are those who gain weight appropriately and grow normally.[3] The Dietary Guidelines for Americans are safe and appropriate goals for the diets of children 2 years of age and older to provide nutrients and energy needed for growth without excesses.

Energy   Individual children's energy needs vary widely, depending on their growth and physical activity. On average, though, a 1-year-old child needs about 800 calories a day; at age 6, the child's needs double to about 1,600 daily calories. By age 10, about 1,800 calories a day support normal growth and activity without causing excess storage of body fat. As children age, the total number of calories needed increases, but per pound of body weight, the need declines from the extraordinarily high demand of infancy. Table 14–1 shows that both age and activity level help to determine calorie needs in children.[†]

Some children, notably those fed a vegan diet, may have difficulty meeting their energy needs. Whole grains, many kinds of vegetables, and fruits provide plenty of fiber and nutrients, but their low energy content may make them inadequate to support growth. Soy products, other legumes, and nut or seed butters offer more

[†]DRI estimated energy requirements for infants and children derive from values for weight, age, physical activity, and other parameters.

concentrated sources of energy and nutrients to support optimal growth and development in these children.[4]

Protein   The total amount of protein needed increases somewhat as a child grows larger. On a pound-for-pound basis, however, the older child's need for protein decreases slightly relative to the younger child's need (see the DRI values, inside front cover). Protein needs of children are well covered by typical U.S. diets and well-planned vegetarian diets.

Carbohydrate and Fiber   Glucose use by the brain sets the carbohydrate intake recommendations. A 1-year-old's brain is large relative to the size of the body, so the glucose demanded by the 1-year-old falls in the adult range (see inside front cover).[5] Fiber recommendations derive from adult intakes and should be adjusted downward for children who are picky eaters and take in little energy (see Table 14–2).

Fat and Fatty Acids   Keeping fat intake within bounds helps to control saturated and *trans* fats and so may help protect children from developing early signs of adult diseases. Taken to extremes, however, a low-fat diet can lack the energy and essential nutrients required for growth. The essential fatty acids are critical to proper development of nerve, eye, and other tissues.

Children's small stomachs can hold only so much food, and fat provides a concentrated source of food energy needed for growth. For children, aged 1 to 3 years, dietary fat recommendations are 30–40 percent of energy; older children, aged 4 to 18 years, require 25–35 percent of energy from fat.[6]

The Need for Vitamins and Minerals   As a child grows larger, so does the demand for vitamins and minerals. On a pound-for-pound basis, a 5-year-old's need for, say, vitamin A is about double the need of an adult man. A balanced diet of nutritious foods can meet children's needs for most nutrients, with the exceptions of specific recommendations for fluoride, vitamin D, and iron. Well-nourished children do not need other supplements, and those who receive them typically end up with extra amounts of nutrients already amply provided by their diets.[7] For fluoride, pediatricians may prescribe it for children in areas with fluoride-poor water; vitamin D and iron are discussed next.

Vitamin D   According to the DRI committee, children's intakes of vitamin D–fortified foods—including milk, ready-to-eat cereals, and juices—should provide 15 micrograms of vitamin D each day to maximize their absorption of calcium and ensure normal, healthy bone growth.[8] In the United States, vitamin D intake among children is inadequate, and as a result, vitamin D deficiency is prevalent.[9] Children who do not consume enough vitamin D from fortified foods should receive a vitamin D supplement to make up the shortfall.

Iron   As for iron, iron deficiency is a major problem worldwide and is prevalent in U.S. children aged 1 year and older.[10] Following infancy, children progress from a diet of iron-rich infant foods such as breast milk, iron-fortified formula, and iron-fortified infant cereal to a diet of adult foods and iron-poor cow's milk. Their stores of iron from birth are exhausted, but their rapid growth demands new red blood cells to fill a larger volume of blood. Compounding the problem is the variability in toddlers' appetites: sometimes 2-year-olds are finicky, sometimes they eat voraciously, and sometimes they may enter phases where they opt for milk and juice in place of solid foods. All of these factors—switching to whole milk and unfortified foods, diminished iron stores, and unreliable food consumption—make iron deficiency likely at a time when iron is critically needed for normal brain growth and development. A later section revisits iron deficiency and its consequences for the brain.

To prevent iron deficiency, children's foods must deliver 7 to 10 milligrams of iron per day. To achieve this goal, snacks and meals should include iron-rich foods. Although milk is an important source of dietary calcium, needed for the growth of dense, healthy bones, excessive intake should be avoided, as it can displace iron-rich

Table 14–2	
DRI Recommended Fiber Intakes for Children	
Age (yr)	**Fiber (g)**
1–3	19
4–8	25
9–13	
Boys	31
Girls	26
14–18	
Boys	38
Girls	26

Table 14–3

USDA Eating Patterns for Children (1,000 to 1,800 Calories)

For an estimate of a child's average energy need based on age, gender, and physical activity, access SuperTracker on the MyPlate website (www .choose-myplate.gov/); click on Daily Food Plans and follow the prompts. Height, weight, rate of growth, and other factors also alter energy needs.

Food Group	1,000 cal	1,200 cal	1,400 cal	1,600 cal	1,800 cal
Fruits	1 c	1 c	1½ c	1½ c	1½ c
Vegetables	1 c	1½ c	1½ c	2 c	2½ c
Grains (half whole grains)	3 oz	4 oz	5 oz	5 oz	6 oz
Protein foods	2 oz	3 oz	4 oz	5 oz	5 oz
Milk	2 c	2½ c	2½ c	3 c	3 c

Source: U.S. Department of Health and Human Services and U.S. Department of Agriculture, 2015–2020 Dietary Guidelines for Americans, 8th edition (2015), available at http://health.gov/dietaryguidelines/2015/guidelines/.

foods, including lean meats, fish, poultry, eggs, legumes, and whole-grain or enriched grain products, from the diet.

Planning Children's Meals   To provide all the needed nutrients, children's meals should include a variety of foods from each food group in amounts suited to their appetites and needs. Table 14–3 provides USDA eating patterns for children who need 1,000 to 1,800 calories per day. MyPlate online resources for children, parents, and educators translate eating patterns into messages that can help to promote better nutrition for the nation's children (Figure 14–2).

KEY POINTS

- Other than specific recommendations for fluoride, vitamin D, and iron, well-fed children do not need supplements.
- USDA Eating Patterns provide adequate nourishment for growth without obesity.

Figure 14–2

MyPlate Kids' Place

MyPlate Kids' Place offers nutrition education resources for adults, along with activities, games, songs, and videos for children (www.choosemyplate.gov/kids/).

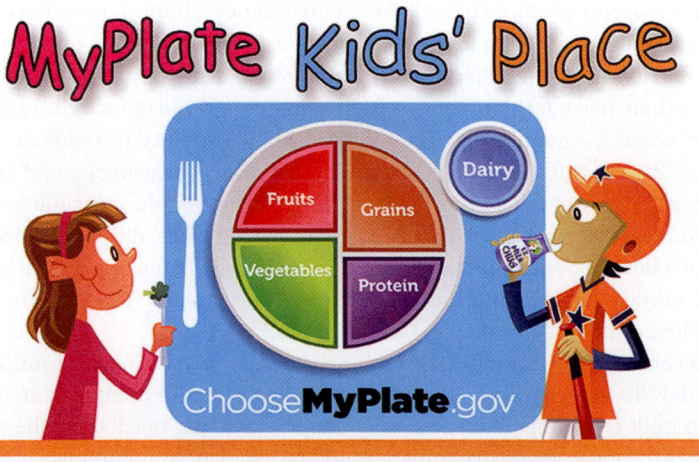

Mealtimes and Snacking

The early childhood years are the parents' greatest chance to influence lifelong food choices that promote the child's health today and reduce chronic disease risks later on.[11] The challenge is to deliver nutrients in the form of meals and snacks that are both nutritious and appealing so that children will learn to enjoy a variety of health-promoting, nutritious foods.

Current U.S. Children's Food Intakes   According to a recent survey, most infants are fed too few fruits and vegetables and on a typical day 16–27 percent of those older than 9 months eat none at all.[12] By age 15 months, one vegetable and one fruit stand out as predominant: French fries and bananas, neither a rich source of many needed nutrients. Sugar-sweetened beverages and desserts are commonly added to the diet during infancy and their intake increases with age.[13] Most children take in too little vitamin E, vitamin D, calcium, magnesium, potassium, and fiber and too much dietary fat and added sugar for health.[14] When children develop preferences for nutrient-poor selections, providing the nutritious foods they need can prove challenging.

Dealing with Children's Preferences   Many children prefer sweet fruits and mild-flavored vegetables served raw or undercooked because they are crunchy and easy to eat. Cooked foods should be served warm, not hot, because a child's mouth is much more sensitive than an adult's. The flavors should be mild because a child has more taste buds.

Little children prefer small portions of food served at little tables. If offered large portions, children may fill up on favorite foods, ignoring others. Toddlers often go on food jags—consecutive days of eating only one or two favored foods. For food jags lasting a week or so, make no response because 2-year-olds regard any form of attention as a reward. After two weeks of serving the favored foods, try serving small portions of many foods, including the favored items. Invite the child's friends to occasional meals, and make other foods as attractive as possible.

Bribing a child to eat certain foods by, for example, allowing extra television time as a reward for eating vegetables often fails to produce the desired effect: the child will likely *not* develop a preference for those foods. Likewise, when children are forbidden to eat favorite foods, they yearn for them more—the reverse of the well-meaning caregiver's goal. Include favorites as occasional treats.

Most children can safely enjoy occasional treats of high-calorie foods, but such treats should also be nutritious. From the milk group, ice cream or pudding is good now and then; from the grains group, whole-grain or enriched cakes, oatmeal cookies, snack crackers, or even small doughnuts are an acceptable occasional addition to a nutritious diet. These foods encourage a child to learn that pleasure in eating is important. A steady diet of these treats, however, leads to nutrient deficiencies, obesity, or both.

Fear of New Foods   A fear of new foods, **food neophobia**, is almost universal among toddlers and preschoolers.[15] Without so much as a taste, the child rejects the new food on sight, but the reason why this occurs is not fully known. The child may remember disliking foods with a similar appearance or aroma. Or it may have evolved as a protective mechanism that prevented curious ancestral toddlers from tasting toxic plants in their environment. In any case, severe food neophobia can harm a child's health, growth, or social interactions and should be evaluated by a pediatrician.[16]

In the meantime, some practical tips can help. First, keep an upbeat but persistent attitude: a child may ignore or reject a food the first 14 times it is offered but on the 15th may suddenly recognize it as a familiar, accepted food in the diet. Parents' negative attention or attempts to force "just a taste" before the child is ready interrupt this learning process. Offering new foods at the beginning of a meal when the child is hungry often works best, as does serving the child samples of the same foods

food neophobia (NEE-oh-FOE-beeah) the fear of trying new foods, common among toddlers.

Table 14–4

Tips for Feeding Picky Eaters

If a child fails to eat enough to support healthy growth and development, consult a registered dietitian nutritionist or physician right away. Otherwise, try these tips.

Get Them Involved

Children are more likely to try foods when they feel a sense of ownership. Include them in

- Meal planning.
- Grocery shopping.
- Food preparation.
- Gardening and harvesting the foods they eat.

Be Creative

- Serve vegetables as finger foods with dips or spreads.
- Use cookie cutters to cut fruits and vegetables into fun shapes.
- Serve traditional meals out of order (for example, breakfast for dinner).
- Encourage (don't force) children's interest and enthusiasm for nutritious foods, such as legumes or whole grains, by using them in craft projects.

Enhance Favorite Recipes

- Blend, slice, or shred vegetables into sauces, casseroles, pancakes, or muffins.
- Serve fruit over cereal, yogurt, or ice cream.
- Bake brownies with black beans or cookies with lentils as an ingredient (find recipes on the Internet).

Model and Share

- Be a role model to children by eating healthy foods yourself. Offer to share your healthy snack with them.
- Children may need multiple exposures to a new food before they accept it, so do continue offering foods that a child initially rejects.
- Encourage children to taste at least one bite of each food served at a meal.

Respect and Relax

- Children tend to eat sporadically. They have small stomachs and so tend to fill up fast and become hungry again soon after eating.
- Focus on the child's overall weekly intake of food and nutrients rather than on daily consumption.

Source: Adapted from Mayo Clinic Staff, Children's nutrition: 10 tips for picky eaters, 2014, available at www.mayoclinic.com/health/childrens-health/HQ01107.

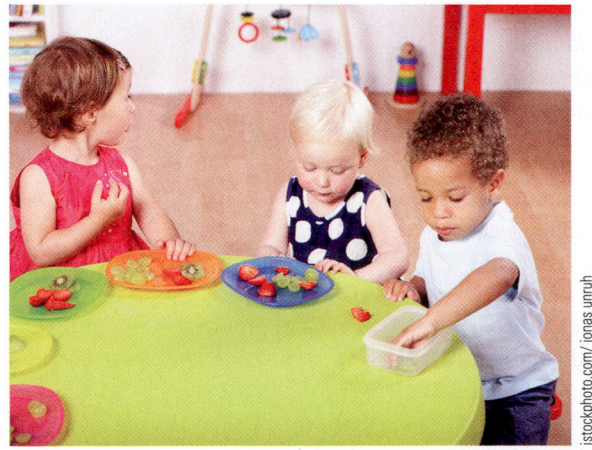

Little children like to eat small portions of food at little tables.

that adults are enjoying; children follow the examples of adults. The tips offered in Table 14–4 can often make mealtimes go more smoothly.

Child Preferences versus Parental Authority   Just as parents are entitled to their likes and dislikes, a child who genuinely and consistently rejects a food should be allowed the same privilege. Also, children should be believed when they say they are full: the "clean-your-plate" dictum should be stamped out for all time.[17] Children who are forced to override their own satiety signals are in training for obesity.

A bright, unhurried atmosphere free of conflict is conducive to good appetite and provides a climate in which a child can learn to enjoy eating. Parents who beg, cajole, and demand that their children eat make power struggles inevitable. A child may find mealtimes unbearable if she is accompanied by a barrage of accusations—"Susie, your hands are filthy . . . your report card . . . and clean your plate!" The child's stomach recoils as both body and mind react to stress of this kind.

Honoring children's preferences does not mean allowing them to dictate the diet, however, because children naturally prefer fatty, sugary, and salty foods, such

Table 14–5

Healthy Snack Ideas from Each Food Group

Well-planned snacks that include two or more food groups, such as yogurt with fruit, a mini bagel with hummus, or whole-grain cereal with milk, provide a wide variety of needed nutrients.

■ **Grains**	Ready-to-eat cereal, whole-grain crackers, mini rice or wheat cakes, sliced bread, mini bagel, graham crackers, whole-wheat tortilla
■ **Vegetables**	Veggie "matchsticks" (thin sticks) made from fresh carrots[a] or zucchini,[a] bell pepper rings, cut cherry tomatoes,[a] green beans, sugar peas, avocados, steamed broccoli
■ **Fruits**	Thin apple slices,[a] tangerine sections, strawberry halves, banana, pineapple, kiwi, peach, mango, nectarine, melon, cut grapes,[a] berries, diced dried apricots[a]
■ **Milk and Milk Products**	Low-fat cheese slices or string cheese, mini yogurt cup, fat-free or low-fat milk or soy milk, low-fat cottage cheese
■ **Protein Foods**	Egg slices or wedges, peanut butter,[a] bean dip, hummus, black beans, thin strips of lean turkey[a] or chicken,[a] shelled pumpkin seeds, soy "burger" or "sausage" slices

[a] These foods can pose a choking hazard unless cut into small pieces. Plain peanut butter by the spoonful can also cause choking; small amounts spread on bread, fruit, or other foods that help to disperse it in the mouth are safer.

Source: Adapted from U.S. Department of Agriculture, Develop healthy eating habits, available at www.choosemyplate.gov/preschoolers/healthy-habits/snack-ideas.html.

as heavily advertised snack chips, cookies, crackers, fast foods, and sugary cereals and drinks. When children's tastes are allowed to rule the family's pantry, everyone's nutrition suffers because busy parents often eat the foods they prepare for children.[18] The responsibility for *what* the child is offered to eat lies squarely with the adult caregiver, but the child should be allowed to decide *how much* and even *whether* to eat.

Many parents overlook perhaps the single most important influence on their children's food habits—their own habits.[19] Parents who don't prepare, serve, and eat carrots shouldn't be surprised when their children refuse to eat carrots. Conversely, parents who share food shopping and cooking tasks with children, and who enjoy nutritious foods at family meals, set healthy patterns for children to follow.

Snacking   Parents often find that their children snack so much that they are not hungry at mealtimes. This is not a problem if children are taught how to snack—nutritious snacks are just as health promoting as small meals. Table 14–5 provides healthy snack ideas from each food group that many children like to eat.

Restaurant Choices   It takes some artful maneuvering to choose nutritious restaurant meals that children can enjoy. Children's menus reliably offer fatty, salty sandwiches, "nuggets," and French fries. For better choices:

- Ask to split a regular meal among several children.

- Choose from appetizers, soups, salads, and side dishes.

- Order vegetable toppings and lean meats on pizza (skip the sausages and hamburger); reduce the saturated fat by requesting half the cheese.

- Request water, fat-free milk, or fruit juice (not punch or soft drinks) for beverages.

Parents who make nutritious restaurant choices for themselves also set good examples for children.

Choking   A child who is choking may make no sound, so an adult should keep an eye on children when they are eating. A child who is coughing most often dislodges the food and recovers without help. To prevent choking, encourage the child to sit when eating—choking is more likely when children are running or reclining. Round foods such as grapes, nuts, hard candies, and pieces of hot dog can become lodged in a child's small windpipe. Other potentially dangerous foods include tough meat

Table 14–6

Food Skills and Developmental Milestones of Preschool Children[a]

Food Skills	Developmental Milestones
Age 1 to 2 years	
<ul><li>Uses a spoon</li><li>Lifts and drinks from a cup</li><li>Helps scrub fruits and vegetables, tear lettuce or greens, snap green beans, or dip foods</li><li>Can be messy; can be easily distracted</li></ul>	<ul><li>Large muscles develop</li><li>Experiences slowed growth and decreased appetite</li><li>Develops likes and dislikes</li><li>May suddenly refuse certain foods</li></ul>
Age 3 years	
<ul><li>Spears food with a fork</li><li>Feeds self independently</li><li>Helps wrap, pour, mix, shake, stir, or spread foods</li><li>Follows simple instructions</li></ul>	<ul><li>Medium hand muscles develop</li><li>May suddenly refuse certain foods</li><li>Begins to request favorite foods</li><li>Makes simple either/or food choices</li></ul>
Age 4 years	
<ul><li>Uses all utensils and napkin</li><li>Helps measure dry ingredients</li><li>Learns table manners</li></ul>	<ul><li>Small finger muscles develop</li><li>Influenced by TV, media, and peers</li><li>May dislike many mixed dishes</li></ul>
Age 5 years	
<ul><li>Measures liquids</li><li>Helps grind, grate, and cut (soft foods with dull knife)</li><li>Uses hand mixer with supervision</li></ul>	<ul><li>Fine coordination of fingers and hands develops</li><li>Usually accepts food that is available</li><li>Eats with minor supervision</li></ul>

[a]These ages are approximate. Healthy, normal children develop at their own pace.

Source: Adapted from MyPlate for Preschoolers, Behavioral milestones, available at www.choosemyplate.gov/preschoolers/healthy-habits/Milestones.pdf.

chunks, popcorn, chips, and peanut butter eaten by the spoonful (more foods and nonfood items that pose a choking hazard were listed in Table 13–14, p. 547).

Food Skills   Children love to be included in meal preparation, and they like to eat foods they helped to prepare (see Table 14–6). A positive experience is most likely when tasks match developmental abilities and are undertaken in a spirit of enthusiasm and enjoyment, not criticism or drudgery. Praise for a job well done (or at least well attempted) expands a child's sense of pride and helps to develop skills and positive feelings toward healthy foods.

KEY POINTS

- Healthy eating habits are learned in childhood, and parents teach best by example.
- Choking can often be avoided by supervising children during meals and avoiding hazardous foods.

How Do Nutrient Deficiencies Affect a Child's Brain?

A child who suffers from nutrient deficiencies exhibits physical and behavioral symptoms: the child feels sick and out of sorts. Such children may be irritable, aggressive, and disagreeable or sad and withdrawn. They may be labeled "hyperactive," "depressed," or "unlikable." Diet–behavior connections are of keen interest to caregivers who both feed children and live with them.

Iron plays key roles in many molecules of the brain and nervous system. An iron deficit in the brain, even before anemia shows up in the blood, has well-known and widespread effects on children's behavior and intellectual performance.[20] The motivation to persist at intellectually challenging tasks is dampened, the attention span is shortened, and the overall intellectual performance is reduced. Administering iron resolves some of the problems, but others may persist for years after treatment.[21] Both iron deficit and the poverty and poor health often associated with it may contribute to these effects.[22] Despite public health efforts to prevent iron deficiency, such as food fortification, iron deficiency remains a key problem among U.S. children and adolescents.

Only a health-care provider, such as a registered dietitian nutritionist, should make the decision to give a child a single-nutrient iron supplement. Iron is toxic, and overdoses can easily injure or even kill a toddler or child who accidentally ingests iron pills. All supplements should be kept out of children's reach.

KEY POINT

- Iron deficiency and toxicity pose a threat to children.

The Problem of Lead

Lead poisoning is a common childhood affliction, caused by environmental lead. Nearly 500,000 children in the United States, most younger than age 6, have blood lead concentrations high enough to cause mental, behavioral, and other health problems.[23] Lead is an indestructible metal element with no fundamental role in the human body; however, once inside, the body cannot alter it or easily excrete it.

Sources of Lead   Babies love to explore and put everything into their mouths, including chips of old lead paint, pieces of metal that contain lead, and other unlikely substances. Lead may also leach into a home's drinking water supply from old lead pipes and end up in a baby's formula and the family's beverages. In older children, lead dust mixed into outdoor soil can stick to clothing and hands and eventually be consumed. Appreciable lead has also been found in chewable vitamins, medications, makeup, and skin creams.[24] Once exposed to lead, infants and young children absorb 5 to 10 times as much of the toxin as adults do.

Harm from Lead   There is virtually no safe level of lead for the developing body. Figure 14–3 identifies several organs affected by elevated blood lead levels. Tragically,

Figure 14–3

Harm from Lead

Lead can build up so silently in a child's body that caregivers may not notice its symptoms until it's too late. Lead toxicity affects every organ in the body. In 2012, the Centers for Disease Control and Prevention reduced the threshold for unacceptably high levels of lead exposure in a child from 10 micrograms per deciliter (µg/dL) to 5 µg/dL.

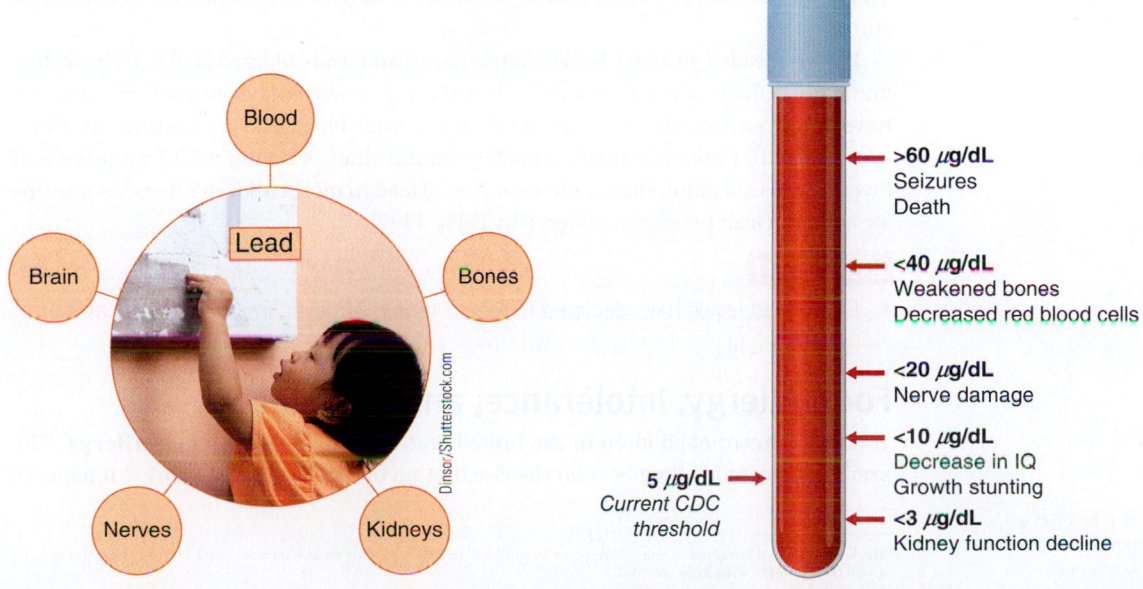

Blood

Brain

Lead

Bones

Nerves

Kidneys

Dinso/Shutterstock.com

>60 µg/dL
Seizures
Death

<40 µg/dL
Weakened bones
Decreased red blood cells

<20 µg/dL
Nerve damage

<10 µg/dL
Decrease in IQ
Growth stunting

<3 µg/dL
Kidney function decline

5 µg/dL →
Current CDC threshold

Table 14–7

Steps to Prevent Lead Poisoning

To protect children:

- If your home was built before 1978, wash floors, windowsills, and other surfaces weekly with warm water and detergent to remove dust released by old lead paint; clean up flaking paint chips immediately.
- Feed children balanced, timely meals with ample iron and calcium.
- Prevent children from chewing on old painted surfaces.
- Wash children's hands, bottles, and toys often.
- Wipe soil off shoes before entering the home.
- Ask a pediatrician whether your child should be tested for lead.

To safeguard yourself:

- Avoid daily use of handmade, imported, or old ceramic mugs or pitchers for hot or acidic beverages, such as juices, coffee, or tea. Commercially made U.S. ceramic, porcelain, and glass dishes or cups are safe. If ceramic dishes or cups become chalky, use them for decorative purposes only.
- Do not use lead crystal decanters for storing alcoholic or other beverages.
- If your home is old and may have lead pipes, run the water for a minute before using, especially before the first use in the morning.

once symptoms set in, medical treatments may not reverse all of the functional damage, some of which may linger long beyond childhood.[25]

The physiological effects of long-term elevated blood lead levels include decreased bone and muscle growth, neurological damage, kidney malfunction, hearing impairment, speech and language difficulty, and developmental delay.[26] Among school-age children, early lead exposure is linked with lower scores on IQ tests and poorer academic performance.[27]

As lead toxicity slowly injures the kidneys, nerves, brain, bone marrow, and other organs, the child may slip into a coma, may have convulsions, and may even die if an accurate diagnosis is not made in time. Older children with high blood lead may be mislabeled as delinquent, aggressive, or learning disabled.

Lead and Nutrient Interactions Poor nutritional status influences the likelihood of a child developing lead poisoning. Children absorb more lead if they lack the minerals iron, calcium, and zinc, which share similar chemical properties with lead. In addition, lead displaces these minerals from their sites of action in the body, limiting their biological functions. Even slight iron, calcium, or zinc deficiencies may open the door to lead toxicity, and a child with iron-deficiency anemia is three times as likely to have elevated blood lead as a child with normal iron status.[28]

Bans on leaded gasoline, leaded house paint, and lead-soldered food cans have dramatically reduced the amount of lead in the U.S. environment in past decades and have produced a steady decline in children's average blood lead concentrations. However, lead still remains a threat in older communities of homes with lead pipes and layers of old lead paint, the primary sources of lead in most children's lives [‡]. Some tips for avoiding lead toxicity are offered in Table 14–7.

KEY POINT

- Blood lead levels have declined in recent times, but even low lead levels can harm children.

Food Allergy, Intolerance, and Aversion

Today, 8 percent of children in the United States are living with a food **allergy**. The prevalence of food allergies is on the rise, but no one knows exactly why.[29] It appears

allergy an immune reaction to a foreign substance, such as a component of food. Also called *hypersensitivity* by researchers.

‡The Environmental Protection Agency (EPA) provides a toll-free telephone hotline for lead information: 1 (800) 424-LEAD [5323], or visit their website: www2.epa.gov/lead.

that many people "grow out" of food allergies, so rates in adults are much lower, at about 1 percent of the population.[30]

Food Allergy   A true food allergy occurs when a food protein or other large molecule enters body tissues and triggers an immune response. Most food proteins are dismantled to smaller fragments in the digestive tract before absorption, but some larger fragments enter the bloodstream. The immune system of an allergic person reacts to the foreign molecules as it does to any other **antigen**: it releases **antibodies**, **histamine**, or other defensive agents to attack the invaders. For some, a food allergy can illicit a life-threatening reaction of **anaphylactic shock**, which can involve symptoms such as tingling of the tongue, throat, or skin or difficulty breathing. Eight foods cause the great majority of food allergy reactions (see Table 14–8).

If a child reacts to allergens with a life-threatening response, two courses of action are required: first, the child's family and school must guard against any ingestion of the allergen. Second, easy-to-administer doses of the life-saving drug **epinephrine** must be kept close at hand.

Allergen Exposure   Avoiding allergens can be tricky because they often sneak into foods in unexpected ways. For example, a pork chop (an innocent food) may be dipped in egg (egg allergy) and breaded (wheat allergy) before being fried in peanut oil (peanut allergy); marshmallow candies may contain egg whites; lunchmeats may contain milk protein binders; and so forth.

Invisible traces of allergen from, say, peanut butter left on tables, chairs, or other surfaces can easily contaminate the hands of a severely allergic child and cause a life-threatening reaction. Scrupulous cleaning of surfaces and regular hand washing by the allergic child can often prevent such an occurrence. Exposure can also occur when the allergen is inhaled. However, the protein allergens of peanuts are not volatile—that is, they do not fly off the food into the air under normal conditions, such as when they are being eaten. The distinctive aroma of peanuts can alert people to their presence, but the aroma itself does not cause allergy—only ingestion of peanut protein can do so.[31]

Caregivers of allergic children must pack safe lunches and snacks at home and ask school officials to strictly enforce a "no-swapping" policy in the lunchroom. To prevent nutrient deficiencies, caregivers must also provide adequate substitutes that supply the essential nutrients in the omitted foods.[32] Nutritional counseling and growth monitoring are recommended for all children with food allergies.[33]

Strictly controlled research studies that feed small amounts of allergen under medical supervision have noted improvements in immune markers of reactivity.[34] However, significant allergic symptoms may also occur, and persons attempting such therapy on their own take a serious risk.

Food Labels   Food labels must announce the presence of common allergens in plain language.[35] For example, a food containing "textured vegetable protein" must say "soy" on its label. Similarly, "casein," a protein in milk, must be identified as "milk." Consumers with food allergies rely heavily on the accuracy of food labels (Figure 14–4 provides an example).[36] Table 14–9 (p. 570) lists symptoms associated with allergic reactions to food.

Detection of Food Allergy   Allergies have one or two components. They always involve antibodies, and they sometimes involve symptoms. Therefore, allergies cannot be diagnosed from symptoms alone. Anyone who has suffered anaphylaxis or other severe symptoms should not reintroduce suspected foods but should undergo medical allergy testing.

An immediate allergic reaction is easy to identify because symptoms correlate with the time of eating the food. A delayed reaction, taking 24 hours or more, is more

---

Table 14–8

Common Food Allergens

Eight foods cause up to 90 percent of all food-allergic reactions.

- Peanuts[a]   - Wheat
- Tree nuts[a]   - Soy
- Milk   - Fish[a]
- Egg   - Shellfish[a]

[a]These foods are most likely to cause anaphylactic shock.

---

antigen   a substance foreign to the body that elicits the formation of antibodies or an inflammation reaction from immune system cells. Food antigens are usually large proteins. Inflammation consists of local swelling and irritation and attracts white blood cells to the site. Also defined in Chapter 3.

antibodies   large protein molecules that are produced in response to the presence of antigens to inactivate them. Also defined in Chapters 3 and 6.

histamine   a substance that participates in causing inflammation; produced by cells of the immune system as part of a local immune reaction to an antigen.

anaphylactic (an-ah-feh-LACK-tick) **shock**   a life-threatening whole-body allergic reaction to an offending substance.

epinephrine (epp-ih-NEFF-rin)   a hormone of the adrenal gland that counteracts anaphylactic shock by opening the airways and maintaining heartbeat and blood pressure.

Figure 14–4

A Food Allergy Warning Label

A food that contains, or could contain, even a trace amount of any of the most common food allergens must clearly say so on its label. For instance, if a product contains the milk protein casein, the label must say "contains milk," or the ingredients list must include "milk." The sunflower seeds below carry a warning about peanut allergy—traces of peanuts may have contaminated the seeds during processing.

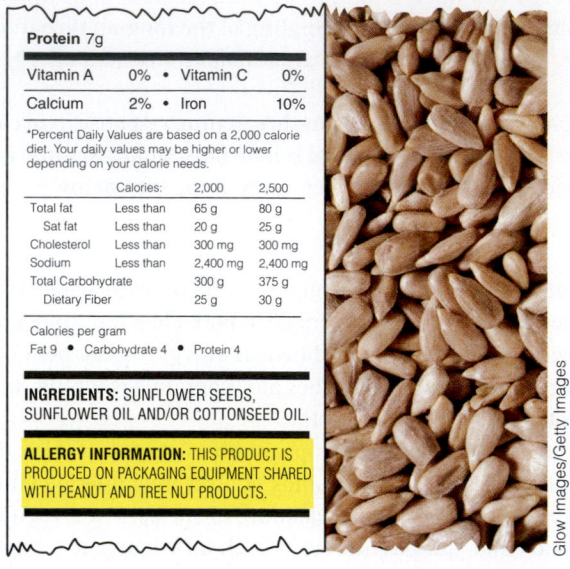

Protein 7g		
Vitamin A	0% • Vitamin C	0%
Calcium	2% • Iron	10%

*Percent Daily Values are based on a 2,000 calorie diet. Your daily values may be higher or lower depending on your calorie needs.

	Calories:	2,000	2,500
Total fat	Less than	65 g	80 g
Sat fat	Less than	20 g	25 g
Cholesterol	Less than	300 mg	300 mg
Sodium	Less than	2,400 mg	2,400 mg
Total Carbohydrate		300 g	375 g
Dietary Fiber		25 g	30 g

Calories per gram
Fat 9 • Carbohydrate 4 • Protein 4

INGREDIENTS: SUNFLOWER SEEDS, SUNFLOWER OIL AND/OR COTTONSEED OIL.

ALLERGY INFORMATION: THIS PRODUCT IS PRODUCED ON PACKAGING EQUIPMENT SHARED WITH PEANUT AND TREE NUT PRODUCTS.

Glow Images/Getty Images

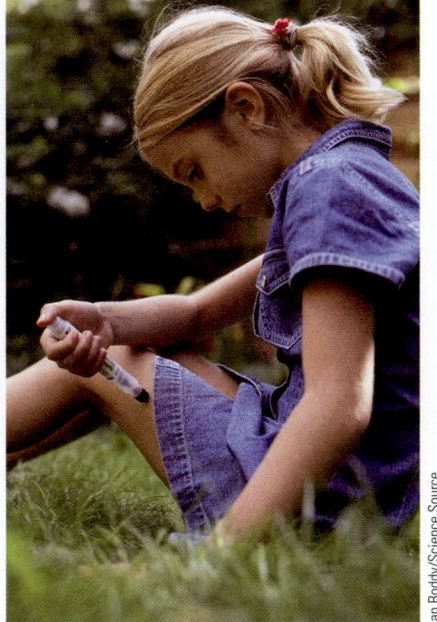

Ian Boddy/Science Source

An epinephrine "pen" can deliver prompt life-saving treatment to a person suffering from anaphylactic shock.

difficult to pinpoint. For mild suspected allergy symptoms, a good starting point is to keep a record of food intakes and symptoms. If the symptoms correlate with a food, then a blood test for elevated levels of food-specific antibodies and a skin prick test, in which a clinician applies droplets of food extracts to the skin and then lightly pricks or scratches the skin, or other tests can confirm the allergy. False positive results can occur, but despite this failing, such tests can support or refute other evidence in making a diagnosis.[37]

Scientific-sounding allergy quackery may deceive people into believing that everything from itchy skin to mental depression is caused by food allergies. Beware of "food sensitivity testing" offered by charlatans on the Internet or elsewhere. It involves fake blood or other tests that supposedly determine for the "patient" which foods to eat and which supplements to buy from the quack to relieve the "allergy."

Technology may soon offer new solutions for those with food allergy. Drugs under development may interfere with the immune response that causes allergic reactions,

Table 14–9

Symptoms of an Allergic Reaction to Food

Any of these symptoms can occur in minutes or hours after ingesting an allergen:

- *Airway.* Difficulty breathing, wheezing, asthma.
- *Digestive tract.* Vomiting, abdominal cramps, diarrhea.
- *Eyes.* Irritated, reddened eyes.
- *Mouth and throat.* Tingling sensation, swelling of the tongue and throat.
- *Skin.* Hives, swelling, rashes.
- *Other.* Drop in blood pressure, loss of consciousness; in extreme reactions, death.

but so far, they remain unavailable.[38] Through genetic engineering, scientists are identifying ways to remove the allergenic proteins from food sources, such as peanuts and soybeans, to make them safer.[39]

Food Intolerance and Aversion   A **food intolerance** is characterized by unpleasant symptoms that reliably occur after consumption of certain foods—lactose intolerance is an example. Unlike allergy, a food intolerance does not involve an immune response. A **food aversion**, an intense dislike of a food, may be a biological response to a food that once caused trouble. Parents are advised to watch for signs of food aversion and to take them seriously. Such a dislike may turn out to be a whim or fancy, but it may turn out to be an allergy or other valid reason to avoid a certain food. Don't prejudge. Test. Then, if an important staple food must be excluded from the diet, find other foods to provide the omitted nutrients.

Foods are often unjustly blamed when behavior problems arise, but children who are sick from any cause are likely to be cranky. The next section singles out one such type of misbehavior.

KEY POINTS

- Food allergy may be diagnosed by the presence of antibodies.
- Food aversions can be related to food allergies or to adverse reactions to food.

Can Diet Make a Child Hyperactive?

Attention-deficit/hyperactivity disorder (ADHD), or **hyperactivity**, is a **learning disability** that occurs in 5 to 10 percent of young, school-aged children—or in 1 to 3 in every classroom of 30 children.[40] ADHD is characterized by the chronic inability to pay attention, along with overly active behavior and poor impulse control. It can delay growth, lead to academic failure, and cause major behavioral problems. Although some children improve with age, many reach the college years or adulthood before they receive a diagnosis and with it the possibility of treatment.

Food Allergies   Food allergies have been blamed for ADHD. Restricting common food allergens and synthetic food additives, or supplementing with omega-3 fatty acids have been reported to reduce symptoms in a few children, but research is insufficient to draw conclusions.[41] Meanwhile, parents who wish to avoid common food allergens or food additives can find them listed with the ingredients on food labels.

Sugar and Behavior   Many teachers, parents, grandparents, and others assert that some children react behaviorally to sugar. Most researchers have dismissed the "sugar-behavior" theory, but in one study of nearly 3,500 European children, those with high intakes of sugary, fatty treats, such as chocolate bars (a source of caffeine) and other candies, were more likely to display emotional symptoms than others.[42] Sugary foods and beverages clearly displace more nutritious choices from the diet, and nutrient deficiencies are known to cause behavioral problems. Sugar itself, however, is unlikely to do so.

Inconsistent Care and Poverty   Common sense says that all children get unruly and "hyper" at times. A child who often fills up on caffeinated colas, "energy" drinks, and chocolate, misses lunch, becomes too cranky to nap, misses out on outdoor play, and spends hours in front of a television or other screen media suffers stresses that can trigger chronic patterns of crankiness.[43] This detrimental cycle resolves itself when the caregivers begin to limit screen time and insist on regular hours of sleep, regular mealtimes, a nutritious diet, and regular outdoor play.

The **Controversy** section of this chapter lists caffeine amounts in common foods and beverages.

---

food intolerance   an adverse reaction to a food or food additive not involving an immune response.

food aversion   an intense dislike of a food, biological or psychological in nature, resulting from an illness or other negative experience associated with that food.

hyperactivity   (in children) a syndrome characterized by inattention, impulsiveness, and excess motor activity; usually diagnosed before age 7, lasts six months or more, and usually does not entail mental illness or mental retardation. Properly called *attention-deficit/ hyperactivity disorder (ADHD)*.

learning disability   a condition resulting in an altered ability to learn basic cognitive skills such as reading, writing, and mathematics.

Figure 14–5
Dental Caries

Caries begin when acid dissolves the enamel that covers the tooth. If not repaired, the decay may penetrate the dentin and spread into the pulp of the tooth, causing inflammation and an abscess.

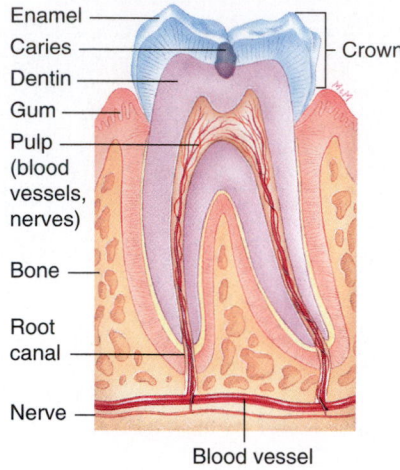

Enamel
Caries
Dentin
Gum
Pulp (blood vessels, nerves)
Bone
Root canal
Nerve
Crown
Blood vessel

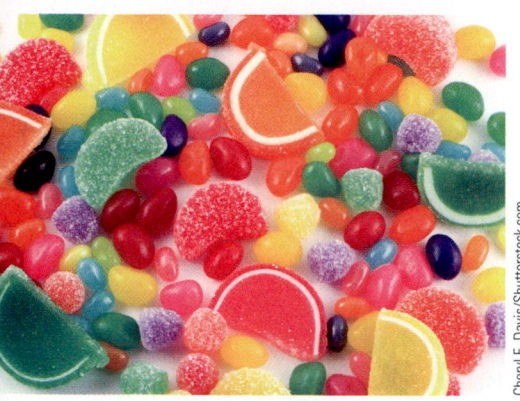

To prevent caries, sticky carbohydrate-rich foods should be removed from the teeth soon after eating.

dental caries decay of the teeth (*caries* means "rottenness"). Also called *cavities*.

plaque (PLACK) a mass of microorganisms and their deposits on the surfaces of the teeth, a forerunner of dental caries and gum disease. The term *plaque* is also used in another connection—arterial plaque in atherosclerosis (see Chapter 11).

Hunger and poverty can influence a child's mental health and subsequent behavior. A long-term study of over 1,500 Canadian youth identified food insecurity as predictive of hyperactive behavior.[44] An estimated 12 million U.S. children are hungry at least some of the time. Such children often lack iron, zinc, or omega-3 polyunsaturated fatty acids, and a link between these nutrient deficiencies and ADHD may be emerging.[45] Once the obvious causes of misbehavior are eliminated, a physician can work with caregivers to provide the best treatment strategies, such as special educational programs or prescription medication.[46]

KEY POINTS

- ADHD is not caused by food allergies or additives.
- Inconsistent care and poverty may cause behavior problems.

Dental Caries

Dental caries are a serious public health problem afflicting many U.S. children, with a prevalence rate of 42 percent among those 2 to 11 years of age.[47] A very lucky few *never* get dental caries because they have an inherited resistance; others have a sealant applied to their teeth during childhood to stop caries before they can begin. Another method used to reduce the incidence of dental decay is fluoridation of community water, considered to be the most effective dental public health measure to date.[48] Perhaps the greatest weapon against caries is simple oral hygiene. But diet has something to do with dental caries, too.

How Caries Develop Caries develop as acids produced by bacterial growth in the mouth eat into tooth enamel (see Figure 14–5). Bacteria form colonies in **plaque**, which sticks more and more firmly to tooth surfaces unless they are brushed, flossed, or scraped away. Eventually, the acid of plaque creates pits that deepen into cavities. The cavities can be treated by a dentist—the decay is removed and replaced with filling material. Scary stories that mercury-containing fillings can harm health are unfounded; the mercury in fillings is present in very small amounts and in a different form from the toxic methylmercury that contaminates many seafoods.[49]

Advanced Dental Disease Left alone, plaque works its way below the gum line until the acid erodes the roots of teeth and the jawbone in which they are embedded, loosening the teeth and leading to infections of the gums. Bacteria from inflamed, infected gums can then migrate by way of the bloodstream to other tissues such as the heart; researchers have identified a link between these bacteria and heart disease.[50] Gum disease severe enough to threaten tooth loss afflicts the majority of our population by their later years.

Food and Caries Bacteria thrive on carbohydrate, producing acid for 20 to 30 minutes after carbohydrate exposure. Of prime importance is the length of time the teeth are exposed to carbohydrate, and this depends to a great extent on whether the teeth are brushed soon afterward as well as on the food's composition, how sticky it is, how long it lasts in the mouth, and the frequency of consumption. Table 14–10 (p. 573) lists foods of both high and low caries potential. Beverages such as soft drinks, orange juice, and sports drinks not only contain sugar but also have a low pH, and their acidic nature can erode the tooth enamel, weakening it. A growing preference for sugary soft drinks or sports drinks instead of water to quench thirst throughout the day may explain why dental erosion is becoming more common.[51] Recent evidence confirms that limiting sugar intake to 10 percent or less of total calories can minimize the development of dental caries throughout life.[52]

KEY POINT

- Carbohydrate-rich foods contribute to dental caries.

Cheryl E. Davis/Shutterstock.com

Table 14–10

The Caries Potential of Foods

Low Caries Potential

These foods are less damaging to teeth:

- Eggs, legumes
- Fresh fruit, fruits packed in water
- Lean meats, fish, poultry
- Milk, cheese, plain yogurt
- Most cooked and raw vegetables

- Pizza
- Popcorn, pretzels
- Sugarless gum and candy,[a] diet soft drinks
- Toast, hard rolls, bagels

High Caries Potential

Brush teeth after eating these foods:

- Cakes, muffins, doughnuts, pies
- Candied sweet potatoes
- Chocolate milk
- Cookies, granola or "energy" bars, crackers
- Dried fruits (raisins, figs, dates)
- Frozen or flavored yogurt
- Fruit juices or drinks
- Fruits in syrup
- Ice cream or ice milk

- Jams, jellies, preserves
- Lunchmeats with added sugar
- Meats or vegetables with sugary glazes
- Oatmeal, oat cereals, oatmeal baked goods[b]
- Peanut butter with added sugar
- Potato and other snack chips
- Ready-to-eat sugared cereals
- Sugared gum, sugar-sweetened soft drinks, candies, honey, sugar, molasses, syrups
- Toaster pastries

[a]Cariogenic bacteria cannot efficiently metabolize the sugar alcohols in these products, so they do not contribute to dental caries.
[b]The soluble fiber in oats makes this grain particularly sticky and therefore cariogenic.

Is Breakfast Really the Most Important Meal of the Day for Children?

A nutritious breakfast is a central feature of a child's diet that supports healthy growth and development.[53] When a child consistently skips breakfast or is allowed to choose sugary foods (candy or marshmallows) in place of nourishing ones (whole-grain cereals), the child will fail to get enough of several nutrients. Nutrients missed from a skipped breakfast are rarely "made up" at lunch and dinner but are most often left out completely that day.

Children who regularly skip breakfast are more likely to be overweight, have difficulty paying attention in the classroom, perform poorly on tasks requiring concentration, and achieve lower test scores.[54] Common sense tells us that it is unreasonable to expect anyone to study and learn when no fuel has been provided, and chronically underfed children suffer most intensely. Table 14–11 (p. 574) offers some ideas for quick breakfasts.

The U.S. government funds nutritious, high-quality meals, including breakfast, for U.S. schoolchildren.[55] For low-income students, such meals are available at no or low cost, ensuring that all schoolchildren have access to the nutrients they need to perform their best. Additionally, when schools participate in federal school meal programs, student attendance improves, and tardiness declines.

KEY POINTS

- Breakfast supports school performance.
- Free or reduced-priced nutritious school meals are available to low-income children.

How Nourishing Are the Meals Served at School?

In the United States today, 50 million children ages 5 to 19 years spend a large portion of each day in school for about nine months of each year. More than 30 million children receive lunches through the National School Lunch Program—more than half of them free or at a reduced price.[56] Ten million children eat breakfast at school

Table 14–11

Breakfast Ideas for Rushed Mornings

With some planning, even a rushed morning can include a nutritious breakfast.

- Make sandwiches or tortilla wraps ahead of time. Freeze, thaw or heat, and serve with juice. Fillings may include peanut butter, low-fat cream cheese or other cheeses, jams, fruit slices, refried beans, or meats.
- Teach school-aged children to help themselves to dry cereals, milk, and juice. Keep unbreakable bowls and cups in low cabinets, and keep milk and juice in small plastic pitchers on a low refrigerator shelf.
- Keep a bowl of fresh fruit and small containers of shelled nuts, trail mix (the kind without candy), or roasted peanuts for grabbing.
- Mix granola or other whole-grain cereal into 8-oz tubs of yogurt.
- Toast whole-grain frozen waffles— no syrup needed—to grab and go.
- *Nontraditional choices:* Carrot sticks served with yogurt or bean dip, or leftover casseroles, stews, or pasta dishes, eaten hot or cold, are nutritious choices.

competitive foods unregulated meals, including fast foods, that compete side by side with USDA-regulated school lunches.

adolescence the period from the beginning of puberty until maturity.

growth spurt the marked rapid gain in physical size usually evident around the onset of adolescence.

---

through the National School Breakfast Program. For many children, particularly those living in poverty, school food programs might constitute their major source of nutrients each day.[57]

The National School Lunch and Breakfast Programs   The USDA-regulated school meals provide age-appropriate servings of needed foods each day (see Table 14–12). The lunches are designed to meet, on average, at least a third of the recommended intake for energy, total and saturated fat, protein, calcium, iron, vitamin A, and vitamin C and are often more nutritious than typical lunches brought from home. Students who regularly eat school lunches have the opportunity to eat more fiber and nutrients than students who do not.[58]

Recent changes to school meal patterns and nutrition standards have resulted in greater availability of fruits, vegetables, whole grains, and fat-free and low-fat milk, and decreased levels of sodium, saturated fat, and *trans* fat in meals served to schoolchildren. Guidelines also specify that nutrient needs must be met within specified calorie ranges based on age/grade groups for children.[59]

Competitive Foods at School   A recent concern focuses on private vendors in school lunchrooms who offer **competitive foods**.[60] Nation-wide, USDA's Smart Snacks in School regulations now require that competitive foods and beverages, including those sold in vending machines, offer students healthier options with more fruit, vegetables, dairy products, and whole grains.[61] They must also meet standards for calories, sodium, fat, saturated fat, trans fat, and added sugars. Each state may also set stricter policies, and in states that do so, children and adolescents stay leaner than in states with weaker polices.[62]

Today's school food environment continues to improve, and the changes promise a generation of healthier children.[63] Realizing this outcome demands the cooperation of everyone—legislators, food vendors, school district officials, administrators, and parents—to ensure full participation for the benefit of children's nutrition.

KEY POINTS

- School meals are designed to provide at least a third of certain nutrients that children need daily. Recent changes to the school breakfast and lunch menus include increased availability of fruits, vegetables, whole grains, and low-fat and fat-free fluid milk; reduced sodium in meals; and reduced levels of saturated and *trans* fats.
- Competitive foods are required to meet specific nutritional standards.

Nutrition in Adolescence

LO 14.2 Summarize the nutrient needs of adolescents.

Teenagers are not fed; they eat. Food choices made during the teen years profoundly affect health, both now and in the future. In the face of new demands on their time, including after-school jobs, social activities, sports, and home responsibilities, older children easily fall into irregular eating habits, relying on quick snacks or fast foods for meals. Within this setting, **adolescence** brings a transforming physical maturation and a psychological search for identity, acquired largely through trial and error.

Parents, peers, and the media are the primary influential forces shaping the adolescent's behaviors and beliefs. Adolescents who frequently eat meals with their families eat more fruits, vegetables, grains, and calcium-rich foods and drink fewer soft drinks than those who seldom eat with their families.[64] They may even be less likely to smoke, drink alcohol, or abuse drugs.[65]

The Adolescent Growth Spurt   The adolescent **growth spurt** brings rapid growth and hormonal changes that affect every organ of the body, including the brain. An average girl's growth spurt begins at 10 or 11 years of age and peaks at about 12 years. Boys' growth spurts begin at 12 or 13 years of age and peak at about 14 years, slowing down at about 19. Two adolescents of the same age may vary in

Table 14–12

School Breakfast and Lunch Patterns for Different Ages

Meal Pattern	Breakfast Meal Pattern			Lunch Meal Pattern		
	Grades K–5[a]	Grades 6–8[a]	Grades 9–12[a]	Grades K–5	Grades 6–8	Grades 9–12
Meal Pattern	Amount of food per week (minimum per day)[b]					
Fruits (c)[c,d]	5 (1)[e]	5 (1)[e]	5 (1)[e]	2½ (½)	2½ (½)	5 (1)
Vegetables (c)[c,d]	0	0	0	3¾ (¾)	3¾ (¾)	5 (1)
Dark green[f]	0	0	0	½	½	½
Red/orange[f]	0	0	0	¾	¾	1¼
Beans/peas (legumes)[f]	0	0	0	½	½	½
Starchy[f]	0	0	0	½	½	½
Other[f,g]	0	0	0	½	½	¾
Additional veg to reach total[h]	0	0	0	1	1	1½
Grains (oz eq)[i]	7–10 (1)[j]	8–10 (1)[j]	9–10 (1)[j]	8–9 (1)	8–10 (1)	10–12 (2)
Meat or meat alternate (oz eq)	0[k]	0[k]	0[k]	8–10 (1)	9–10 (1)	10–12 (2)
Fluid milk (c)[l]	5 (1)	5 (1)	5 (1)	5 (1)	5 (1)	5 (1)
Other Specifications: Daily amount based on the average for a 5-day week						
Calorie range[m,n,o]	350–500	400–500	450–600	550–650	600–700	750–850
Saturated fat (% of total calories)[n,o]	<10	<10	<10	<10	<10	<10
Sodium (mg)[n,p]						
School year 2014–2015	≤540	≤600	≤640	≤1,230	≤1,360	≤1,420
School year 2017–2018	≤485	≤535	≤570	≤935	≤1,035	≤1,080
School year 2022–2023	≤430	≤470	≤500	≤640	≤710	≤740
Trans fat[n,o]	Nutrition label or manufacturer specifications must indicate zero grams of *trans* fat per serving.					

[a] The School Breakfast Program (SBP) adopted these grade groups in 2013.

[b] Minimum creditable serving is ⅛ c.

[c] ¼ c of dried fruit counts as ½ c of fruit; 1 c of leafy greens counts as ½ c of vegetables. No more than half of the fruit or vegetable offerings may be in the form of juice. All juice must be 100% full-strength.

[d] For breakfast, vegetables substitute for fruits, but the first 2 c per week of any such substitution must be from the dark green, red/orange, beans and peas (legumes), or "Other vegetables" subgroups.

[e] The fruit quantity requirement for the SBP (5 c/week and a minimum of 1 c/day) is effective July 1, 2014 (SY 2014–2015).

[f] Larger amounts of these vegetables may be served.

[g] This category consists of "Other vegetables," that is, any additional amounts from the dark green, red/orange, and beans and peas (legumes) vegetable subgroups.

[h] Any vegetable subgroup may be offered to meet the total weekly vegetable requirement.

[i] At least half of the grains offered must be whole grain–rich in the National School Lunch Program (NSLP) beginning July 1, 2012 (SY 2012–2013), and in the SBP beginning July 1, 2013 (SY 2013–2014). All grains must be whole grain–rich in both the NSLP and the SBP beginning July 1, 2014 (SY 2014–2015).

[j] In the SBP, the grain ranges must be offered beginning July 1, 2013 (SY 2013–2014).

[k] There is no separate meat/meat alternate component in the SBP. Beginning July 1, 2013 (SY 2013–2014), schools may substitute 1 oz. eq. of meat/meat alternate for 1 oz. eq. of grains after the minimum daily grains requirement is met.

[l] Fluid milk must be low-fat (1% milk fat or less, unflavored) or fat-free (unflavored or flavored).

[m] The average daily amount of calories for a 5-day school week must be within the range (at least the minimum and no more than the maximum values).

[n] Discretionary sources of calories (solid fats and added sugars) may be added to the meal pattern if within the specifications for calories, saturated fat, trans fat, and sodium. Foods of minimal nutritional value and fluid milk with fat content greater than 1% milk fat are not allowed.

[o] In the SBP, calories and trans fat specifications take effect beginning July 1, 2013 (SY 2013–2014).

[p] Final sodium specifications are to be reached by SY 2022–2023 or July 1, 2022. Intermediate specifications are established for SY 2014–2015 and 2017–2018.

Source: U.S. Department of Agriculture, Food and Nutrition Services, Nutrition standards in the National School Lunch and School Breakfast Programs, Federal Register 77 (2012): 4088–4167.

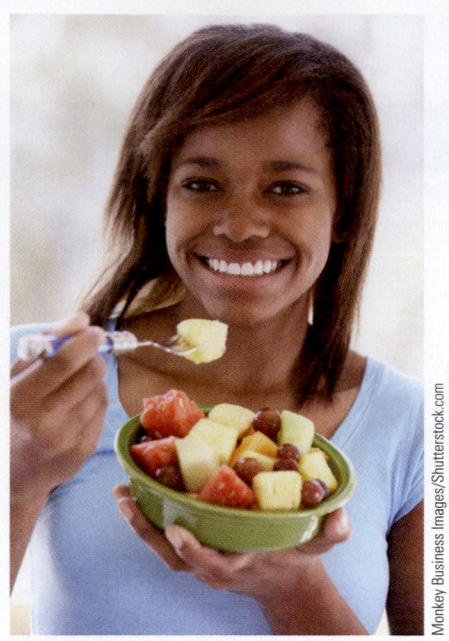

Nutritious snacks play an important role in an active teen's diet.

epiphyseal (eh-PIFF-ih-seal) **plate** a thick, cartilage-like layer that forms new cells that are eventually calcified, lengthening the bone (*epiphysis* means "growing" in Greek).

peak bone mass highest attainable bone density for an individual, developed during the first three decades of life; also defined in Chapter 8.

height by a foot, but if growing steadily, each is fulfilling his or her genetic destiny according to an inborn schedule of events.

Energy Needs and Physical Activity   The energy needs of adolescents vary tremendously depending on growth rate, gender, body composition, and physical activity. An active, growing boy of 15 may need 3,500 calories or more a day just to maintain his weight, but an inactive girl of the same age whose growth has slowed may need fewer than 1,800 calories to avoid unneeded weight gain. Energy balance is often difficult to regulate in this society—an estimated 15 percent of U.S. children and adolescents 6 to 19 years of age are overweight. On the output side, the spontaneous physical activity of childhood diminishes significantly around the age of adolescence, falling well below the recommended levels.[66]

Weight Standards and Body Fatness   Weight standards meant for adults are useless for adolescents. Physicians use growth charts to track height and weight gains in adolescents (as shown in Figure C13–1, p. 552), and parents should monitor progress and guard against comparisons that can diminish the child's self-image.

Girls normally develop a somewhat higher percentage of body fat than boys do, a fact that causes much needless worry about becoming overweight. Teens face tremendous pressures regarding body image, and many readily believe scams that promise slenderness or good-looking muscles through "dietary supplements." Healthy, normal-weight teenagers are often "on diets" and make all sorts of unhealthy weight-loss attempts by fasting or even purging following meals.[67]

Nutrient Needs

Needs for vitamins, minerals, the energy-yielding nutrients, and in fact all nutrients are greater during adolescence than at any other time of life except pregnancy and lactation (see the DRI table on the inside front cover). The need for iron is particularly high, as all teenagers gain body mass and total blood volume and girls begin menstruation.

The Special Case of Iron   The increase in need for iron during adolescence occurs across the genders—but for different reasons. A boy needs more iron at this time to develop extra lean body mass, whereas a girl needs extra iron not only to gain lean body mass but also to support menstruation. In addition, growth spurts increase the need for iron, regardless of the age or gender of the adolescent.[68] This shifting requirement makes pinpointing an adolescent's need tricky, as Table 14–13 demonstrates.

Iron intakes often fail to keep pace with increasing needs, especially for girls, who typically consume fewer iron-rich foods such as meat and fewer total calories than boys. Not surprisingly, iron deficiency is more prevalent among adolescent girls, especially those who are menstruating.[69] Adolescents who live with food insecurity—that is, those who miss meals; eat less nutritious foods; or make other food-related compromises of poverty—have an increased risk for developing iron deficiency compared with food-secure children.[70]

Calcium and the Bones   Adolescence is a crucial time for bone development. The bones are growing longer at a rapid rate (see Figure 14–6) thanks to a special bone structure, the **epiphyseal plate**, which disappears as a teenager reaches adult height. At the same time, the bones are gaining density, laying down the calcium needed later in life. Calcium intakes must be high to support the development of **peak bone mass**.[71]

Among U.S. adolescents, low calcium intakes have reached crisis proportions.[72] Milk is an abundant source of calcium, providing nearly 300 milligrams per cup.

Figure 14–6

Growth of Long Bones

Bones grow longer as new cartilage cells accumulate at the top portion of the epiphyseal plate and older cartilage cells at the bottom of the plate are calcified.

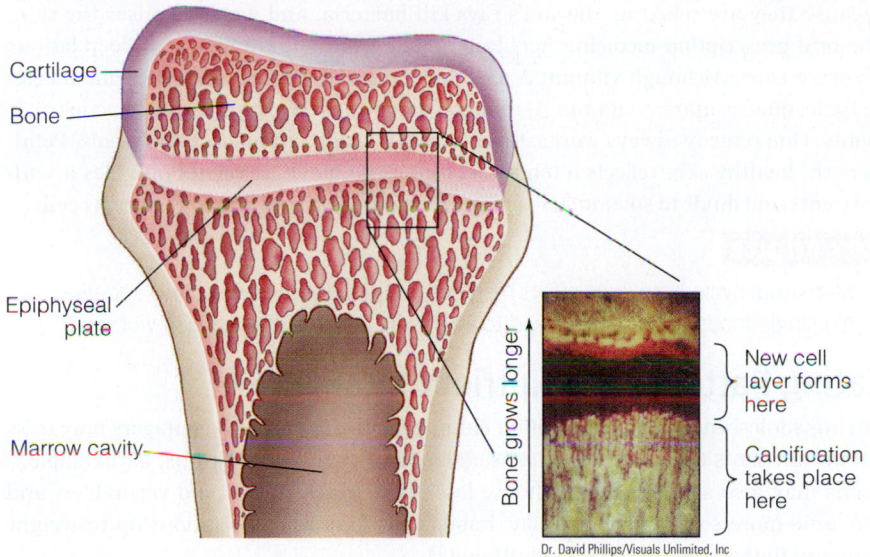

Cartilage

Bone

Epiphyseal plate

Marrow cavity

Bone grows longer

New cell layer forms here

Calcification takes place here

Dr. David Phillips/Visuals Unlimited, Inc

However, U.S. adolescents consume an average of 1 cup of milk each day, far short of the nearly 4.5 cups needed to meet the calcium recommendations.[73] Paired with a lack of physical activity, low calcium intakes can compromise the development of peak bone mass, greatly increasing the risk of osteoporosis later on.

In the United States, 77 percent of adolescents report drinking sugar-sweetened beverages each day (see Figure 14–7). This seemingly harmless choice of a sweetened beverage in place of milk, when repeated time and again, can deprive growing bones of needed nutrients and prevent them from reaching their full attainable density.[74] Conversely, increasing milk consumption can greatly increase bone density.[75]

Vitamin D Vitamin D is also essential for calcium absorption and for proper bone growth and development of bone density. Adolescents who do not receive 15 μg of vitamin D from vitamin D–fortified milk (2.5 μg per cup of fat-free milk) and other vitamin D–fortified foods each day should take vitamin D in a supplement.

KEY POINTS
- The need for iron increases during adolescence in both boys and girls.
- Sufficient calcium and vitamin D intakes are also crucial during adolescence.

Common Concerns

Two other physical changes stand out as important in adolescence. Menstruation and acne pose special concern to many adolescents.

Menstruation Girls face a major change with the onset of menstruation. The hormones that regulate the menstrual cycle affect not just the uterus and the ovaries but the metabolic rate, glucose tolerance, appetite, food intake, and, often, mood and behavior as well. Most women live easily with the cyclic rhythm of the menstrual cycle, but some are afflicted with physical and emotional pain prior to menstruation: **premenstrual syndrome**, or **PMS** (see the Consumer's Guide, p. 579).

Acne Genes clearly play a role in who gets **acne** and who doesn't, but other factors also affect its development.[76] The hormones of adolescence stimulate the oil glands

Figure 14–7

Average Daily Intake of Sugar-Sweetened Beverages

The American Heart Association recommends limiting consumption of sugar-sweetened beverages to 450 calories *per week*, an amount clearly exceeded by many U.S. adolescents.

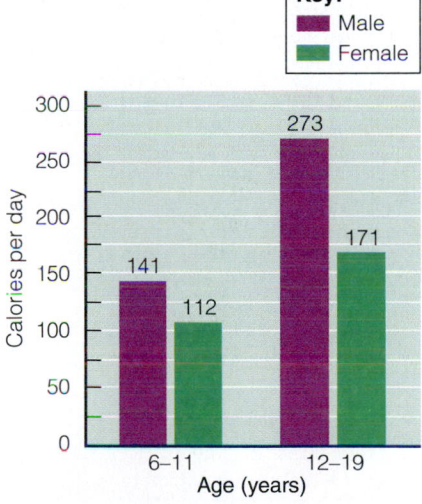

Key:
- Male
- Female

Calories per day

141

112

273

171

6–11   12–19

Age (years)

premenstrual syndrome (PMS) a cluster of symptoms that some women experience prior to and during menstruation. They include, among others, abdominal cramps, back pain, swelling, headache, painful breasts, and mood changes.

acne chronic inflammation of the skin's follicles and oil-producing glands, which leads to an accumulation of oils inside the ducts that surround hairs; usually associated with the maturation of young adults.

deep in the skin. The skin's natural oil is supposed to flow out through tiny ducts at the skin's surface, but in many teens the ducts become clogged, and oily secretions build up in the ducts, causing irritation, inflammation, and breakouts of acne. A "Western" diet high in dairy and refined carbohydrates is associated with acne.[77] Although often accused, chocolate, sugar, French fries, pizza, salt, and iodine do not worsen acne, but psychological stress clearly does.

Vacations from school, sun exposure, and swimming help to relieve acne, perhaps because they are relaxing, the sun's rays kill bacteria, and water cleanses the skin. The oral prescription medicine Accutane, made from vitamin A, cures deep lesions of severe acne. Although vitamin A itself has no effect on acne and supplements can be toxic, quacks market vitamin A–related compounds to young people as acne treatments. One remedy always works: time. While waiting, attend to basic needs. Petal-smooth, healthy skin reflects a tended, cared-for body whose owner provides it with nutrients and fluids to sustain it, exercise to stimulate it, and rest to restore its cells.

KEY POINTS

- Menstrual cycle hormones affect metabolism, glucose tolerance, and appetite.
- No single foods have been proved to aggravate acne, but stress can worsen it.

Eating Patterns and Nutrient Intakes

During adolescence, food habits often change for the worse, and teenagers may miss out on nutrients they need. Few teens choose sufficient whole grains, for example.[78] Teens may also skip breakfast; choose less milk, fruits, juices, and vegetables; and consume more soft drinks each day, habits that may bear a relationship to weight gain and higher disease risks in adulthood.[79]

Roles of Adults   Ideally, the adult becomes a **gatekeeper**, controlling the type and availability of food in the teenager's environment.[80] Teenage sons and daughters and their friends should find plenty of nutritious, easy-to-grab food in the refrigerator (meats for sandwiches, raw vegetables, fruit, milk, and fruit juices) and more in the cabinets (breads, peanut butter, nuts, popcorn, cereals). In reality, in many households today, all the adults work outside the home, and teens perform many of the gatekeeper's roles, such as shopping for groceries or choosing fast foods or prepared foods.

Snacks   On average, about a fourth of a teenager's total daily energy intake comes from snacks, which, if chosen carefully, can contribute needed protein and other nutrients. Nutritious protein-rich snacks may also ward off between-meal hunger, protecting against overeating and obesity.[81]

The gatekeeper can help the teenager choose wisely by delivering nutrition information at "teachable moments." Teens prone to weight gain will often open their ears to news about calories in fast foods. Athletic teens may best attend to information about meal timing and sports performance. Still others are fascinated to learn of the skin's need for vitamins and fluid. The gatekeeper must set a good example, keep lines of communication open, and stand by with plenty of nourishing food and reliable nutrition information, but the rest is up to the teens themselves. Ultimately, they make the choices.

KEY POINT

- The gatekeeper can encourage teens to meet nutrient requirements by providing nutritious snacks.

The Later Years

LO 14.3 Identify the factors associated with successful and healthy aging.

The title of this section may imply it is about older people, but it is relevant even if you are only 20 years old—how you live and think at age 20 affects the quality of your life at 60 or 80. According to an old saying, "As the twig is bent, so grows the tree." Unlike a tree, however, you can bend your own twig.

gatekeeper with respect to nutrition, a key person who controls other people's access to foods and thereby affects their nutrition profoundly. Examples are the spouse who buys and cooks the food, the parent who feeds the children, and the caregiver in a day-care center.

Chapter 14 Child, Teen, and Older Adult

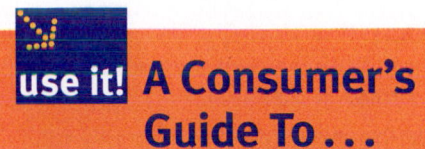
Nutrition for PMS Relief

Jasmine, seeking relief from premenstrual syndrome (PMS) symptoms, found a promise of a cure on an Internet website. All that she needs to do to vanquish her PMS, according to the site, is to triple her vitamin D intake (and buy their "special" variety). Can a vitamin really cure PMS?

Who Has It and What It Is

Internet websites like this are successful because so many women are seeking help for PMS symptoms and so little help is available. Up to 80 percent of menstruating girls and women report uncomfortable menstrual symptoms, and up to 37 percent meet the criteria for PMS.[1]* A great number of possible cyclic symptoms are common, but researchers have isolated six core symptoms useful for diagnosing PMS:

- Anxiety and tension.
- Mood swings.
- Aches and pains.
- Increased appetite and food cravings.
- Abdominal cramps.
- Decreased interest in activities.[2]

Causes

PMS symptoms may arise from an altered response to the two major regulatory hormones of the menstrual cycle: estrogen and progesterone. In particular, the hormone estrogen affects mood by altering the brain's neurotransmitter, serotonin. Taking oral contraceptives, which supply estrogen, often improves mood by eliminating hormonal peaks and valleys. Antidepressant drugs that amplify serotonin's effects also may provide some relief.[3]

Energy Metabolism

Scientists believe that during the two weeks prior to menstruation:

- The basal metabolic rate during sleep speeds up.

*Reference notes are found in Appendix F.

- Appetite, particularly for carbohydrate-rich or fat-rich foods, increases.[4]
- Alcohol consumption may increase, particularly among restrained eaters.[5]
- Cigarette smoking may also increase in women who use tobacco.[6]

For the woman striving to lose weight, then, it may be easier to reduce calorie intakes during the two weeks after menstruation. During the two weeks *before* menstruation, she is fighting a natural, hormone-governed increase in appetite.

Calcium and Vitamin D

Calcium is critical for regulating muscle contraction, and shared symptoms between calcium deficiency and PMS suggest a link, but current research offers little support.[7] Vitamin D shows more promise, although research is mixed and many questions remain unanswered.

Blood levels of vitamin D do not often correlate with overall risk of PMS.[8] Within a group of young women reporting painful menstrual cycles, PMS symptoms were *not* associated with vitamin D status or dairy intake.[9] Countering this, a long-term study revealed a link between higher blood concentrations of vitamin D and a decreased risk of developing some PMS symptoms, including breast tenderness and mental depression.[10] Symptoms of depression commonly correlate with PMS.[11] Vitamin D supplements, however, have no effect on depression in the great majority of studies but may be of some help to a few severely depressed people.[12]

What about the megadoses of vitamin D offered as PMS cures? One small study of Italian women is suggestive.[13] After a single 300,000 IU dose of vitamin D, women with severe PMS reported less pain and less need for painkillers than those given a placebo. The dose used in the study vastly exceeds the DRI Tolerable Upper Intake Level of 4,000 IU. The dose was so high that if it were taken

only once every two months, it would still average about 5,000 IU per day and cannot be recommended.[14]

Many more trials are needed to explore vitamin D's safety and effectiveness. Predictably, however, quacks jump the gun and use preliminary evidence to "prove" that their vitamin D megadoses "cure PMS." Meanwhile, real scientists suggest other possibilities: for example, that the women may have been vitamin D deficient at the start and that the dose of vitamin D may have both reversed the deficiency and reduced their symptoms.[15]

Other Vitamins and Minerals

Years ago, high doses of vitamin B_6 were hawked by vitamin sellers for PMS relief until women who took them developed numb feet and hands, and eventually became unable to walk—symptoms that resolved when the supplements were stopped. Recently, a study suggested that high dietary intakes of non-heme iron (the kind found in plants and supplements), and possibly zinc, may be linked with a decreased risk for PMS.[16] In a surprising twist, the same study linked high intakes of potassium, a mineral generally associated with health, with *increased* risk of PMS.

Ongoing Research

Research has *not* shown these to be useful: taking multivitamins, magnesium, or manganese supplements; cutting down on alcohol or sodium; or taking diuretics to relieve water retention. Sodium and water retention just before menstruation may be normal and desirable; diuretic drugs taken to eliminate excess sodium and water can also cause electrolyte imbalances. Caffeine may worsen PMS symptoms, but how much is too much is not clear. And while adequate sleep, physical activity, and stress reduction strategies may help some women, research in these areas is lacking.

Moving Ahead

The good news for Jasmine and others coping with PMS is that, while a cure may be elusive, PMS symptoms may be lessened with simple daily strategies:

- Eat small, frequent meals.
- Choose a diet pattern that follows the Dietary Guidelines for Americans.

- Meet the need for calcium and vitamin D.
- Minimize caffeine intake.
- Exercise regularly.
- Get enough sleep.
- Reduce stress.

With just these few changes, food cravings, bloating, and stress may improve, and mood often brightens.

Review Questions[†]

1. Taking 300,000 IU per day of vitamin D may alleviate some PMS symptoms, but this amount may not be safe. T F

2. Taking multivitamins, magnesium, manganese, or diuretics can often cure PMS. T F

3. During the two weeks *before* menstruation, women may experience a decreased desire for carbohydrate-rich or fat-rich foods. T F

[†]Answers to Consumer's Guide review questions are found in Appendix G.

As the Twig Is Bent...   Before you will adopt nutrition behaviors to enhance your health in old age, you must accept on a personal level that you, yourself, are aging. Genetics, as well as lifestyle factors, influences aging, but no one escapes the physical, emotional, and social changes that occur. Nutrition has many documented roles that are critical to successful aging, however.[82] In general, people who reach old age in good mental and physical health most often:

- Are nonsmokers.
- Abstain from alcohol or drink only moderately.
- Are physically active (they walk, bike, swim, or otherwise spend more than 150 minutes per week in physical activity).
- Are well nourished and, in particular, consume sufficient fruits and vegetables.[83]
- Maintain a healthy body weight.

They also keep a cheerful attitude and are not often depressed.

Life Expectancy   The "graying" of America is a continuing trend.[84] Since 1950, the population older than age 65 has almost tripled, and numbers of people older than age 85 have increased sevenfold. People reaching and exceeding age 100 have doubled in number in recent decades, a trend evident among many of the world's populations.

How long a person can expect to live depends on several factors. An estimated 70 to 80 percent of the average person's **life expectancy** depends on individual health-related behaviors, with genes determining the remaining 20 to 30 percent. In the United States, an average person can expect to live 78 years. Specifically, life expectancy is 81 years for white women and 78 years for black women; for white men, it is 76 years and for black men, 72 years—all record highs.[85] The racial gap in life expectancy is narrowing, although efforts to reduce cardiovascular diseases, homicide, and infant mortality are needed to reduce it further.[86]

Human Life Span   The biological schedule that we call aging cuts off life at a genetically fixed point in time. The human **life span** is believed to be 125 years. Even this limit may one day be challenged with advances in medical and genetic technologies.[87] One caution: to date, scientists who study the aging process have found no specific diet or nutrient supplement that will increase **longevity**, despite hundreds of dubious claims to the contrary.

KEY POINTS

- Life expectancy for U.S. adults is increasing, but the human life span is set by genetics.
- Life choices can greatly affect how long a person lives and the quality of life in the later years.

life expectancy the average number of years lived by people in a given society.

life span the maximum number of years of life attainable by a member of a species.

longevity long duration of life.

Chapter 14 Child, Teen, and Older Adult

Nutrition in the Later Years

LO 14.4 Discuss the nutrient needs of older adults.

Nutrient needs become more individual with age, depending on genetics and individual medical history. For example, one person's stomach acid secretion, which helps in iron absorption, may decline, so that person may need more iron. Another person may have difficulty storing folate due to past liver damage and therefore have increased folate needs. Table 14–14 lists some changes that can affect nutrition. Because physiological changes advance with age, separate DRI nutrient intake standards are set for people 51 to 70 years old and for those older than age 70 (see inside front cover).

Energy, Activity, and the Muscles

Energy needs often decrease with advancing age. One reason is that the number of active cells in each organ often decreases and the metabolism-controlling hormone thyroxine diminishes, reducing the body's resting metabolic rate.[88] Another reason is that as older people reduce their physical activity, their lean tissue diminishes, resulting in **sarcopenia**, an age-related loss of muscle tissue with serious health implications.[89] Although sarcopenia can be observed in active adults, it is accelerated in the inactive older adult.

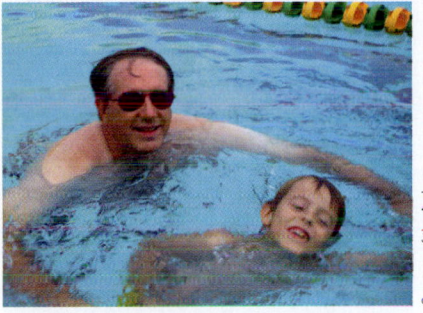

Physical activity yields benefits at all stages of life.

Energy Recommendations   After about the age of 50, the intake recommendation for energy assumes about a 5 percent reduction in energy output per decade. As in other age groups, obesity increasingly poses a problem. For those who must limit energy intake, there is little leeway in the diet for foods of low nutrient density such as added sugars, fats, and alcohol.

Current findings refute the idea that declining energy needs are unavoidable, however. Staying physically active boosts energy needs and contributes to a healthy immune response and sharp mental functioning, too.[90] Physical activity and an adequate diet also oppose a destructive spiral of sedentary behavior and mental and physical losses in the elderly, sometimes called geriatric failure to thrive or "the dwindles."[91] The set of conditions associated with failure to thrive includes:

- Decreased physical ability to function; inability to shop, cook, or prepare meals.

- Depression or anxiety.

Table 14–14

Physical Changes of Aging That Affect Nutrition

DIGESTIVE TRACT	Intestines lose muscle strength, resulting in sluggish motility that leads to constipation. Stomach inflammation, abnormal bacterial growth, and greatly reduced acid output impair digestion and absorption. Pain and fear of choking may cause food avoidance or reduced intake.
HORMONES	Among many hormone changes, the pancreas secretes less insulin and cells become less responsive to it, causing abnormal glucose metabolism.
MOUTH	Tooth loss, gum disease, and reduced salivary output impede chewing and swallowing. Choking may become likely; pain may cause avoidance of hard-to-chew foods.
SENSORY ORGANS	Diminished sight can make food shopping and preparation difficult; diminished senses of smell and taste may reduce appetite, although research is needed to clarify this effect.
BODY COMPOSITION	Weight loss and decline in lean body mass lead to lowered energy requirements. May be preventable or reversible through physical activity.

sarcopenia (SAR-koh-PEE-nee-ah) age-related loss of skeletal muscle mass, muscle strength, and muscle function.

Figure 14–8

Muscle Loss in Aging: Sarcopenia

These photos show cross sections of two women's thighs. They may appear to be about the same size from the outside, but the 20-year-old woman's thigh is dense with muscle tissue (dark areas), while the 64-year-old woman's thigh has lost muscle and gained fat. Such debilitating muscle loss is prevalent in aging but not inevitable. Optimal protein nutrition and strength-building physical activity can oppose its development.

20-year-old woman's thigh

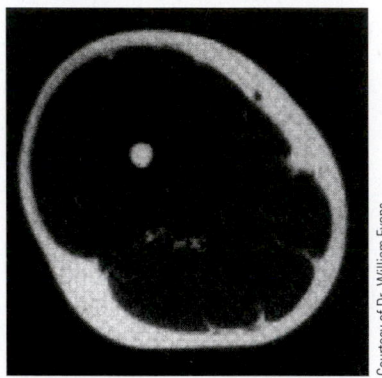

Courtesy of Dr. William Evans

64-year-old woman's thigh

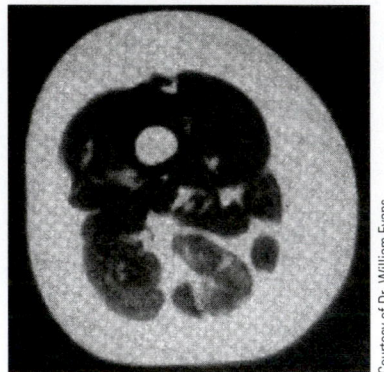

Courtesy of Dr. William Evans

- Malnutrition, with impaired immunity, slow wound healing, slow recovery from surgery, and increased hospitalizations.

- Weight loss and appetite loss with sarcopenia.[92]

Involuntary weight loss deserves immediate attention in the older person. It could be the result of some easily treatable condition, such as ulcers. For people older than 70 years, the best health and lowest risk of death have been observed in those who maintain a body mass index (BMI) between 25 and 32, which is higher than the optimal BMI for younger people. Dealing effectively with weight loss entails finding the causes (physical, psychological, or others) and addressing them. At the same time, offering the person's favorite foods in five or six small, high-calorie meals each day instead of three larger ones often helps stop or reverse weight loss and increases nutrient intakes.[93]

Physical Activity   The Think Fitness feature (p. 583) emphasizes the importance of physical activity to maintaining body tissue integrity throughout life.[94] People spending energy in physical activity can also eat more food, gaining nutrients. Sadly, physical activity declines with aging; approximately 80 percent of older adults fail to meet national exercise objectives, and up to 33 percent are fully inactive, missing the opportunity for more robust health and fitness in their later years.[95] In fact, older adults spend more than 5 hours each day engaged in sedentary behaviors.[96] Any movement seems better than no movement: participating in leisure activities or even performing daily physical chores seems to help the elderly expend energy and improve health outcomes.[97] Some people in their 90s have improved their balance, added pep to their walking steps, and regained some precious independence after just eight weeks of resistance training.

Figure 14–8 emphasizes this point: the photos compare cross sections of the thighs of a young woman and of an older woman to demonstrate the sarcopenia typical of sedentary aging, which brings with it destructive weakness, poor balance, and deterioration of health and vigor. Resistance training through life helps to prevent at least some of this muscle loss, and consuming sufficient protein may help, too.[98]

KEY POINTS

- Energy needs decrease with age.
- Physical activity helps maintain lean tissue during aging.

Protein Needs

Protein DRI recommended intakes remain about the same for older people as for young adults (see inside front cover). However, older adults may not consume enough protein—they often experience a decrease in energy need, a change in food preferences, or barriers to obtaining the protein they need.

Researchers are investigating whether by increasing dietary protein, older people may maintain muscle mass and function.[99] Some findings suggest that a little extra dietary protein, above the DRI recommended level, may stimulate muscle protein synthesis in older adults and shift nitrogen balance toward the positive. However, increased dietary protein does not seem to stave off the muscle loss experienced by older people who become inactive due to injury or illness.[100]

For older people who have lost their teeth, chewing tough, protein-rich meats sufficiently to allow their proper use by the body becomes next to impossible. They need soft-cooked protein sources, such as well-cooked, stewed or chopped meats, milk-based soups, soft cheeses, eggs, or fish. Those with chronic constipation, heart disease, or diabetes may benefit most from fiber-rich, low-fat protein sources, such as legume–whole grain combinations.

As energy needs decrease, lower-calorie protein sources, such as lean tender meats, poultry, fish, boiled eggs, fat-free milk products, and legumes can help hold weight to a healthy level. Underweight or malnourished older adults need the opposite—energy-dense protein sources such as eggs scrambled with margarine, tuna salad with mayonnaise, peanut butter, and milkshakes. Should a flagging appetite reduce food

Benefits of Physical Activity for the Older Adult

The Physical Activity Guidelines for Americans and the American College of Sports Medicine recommend that older adults strive to obtain 150 minutes of physical activity, or whatever amount they can safely and comfortably perform, each week.[101] Older adults who do so have more lean body mass, a better sense of balance, a stronger immune system, and improved sleep quality; they suffer fewer injuries from falls, experience fewer symptoms of arthritis, enjoy better overall health, and even live longer than their less-fit peers.[102] Those at risk of falling can benefit from exercises that improve balance.

At some point, perhaps around 80 years of age, the body struggles to add new muscle tissue in response to resistance training.[103] Some extra protein at each meal may help in this regard by stimulating protein synthesis, even at advanced age.[104] Middle-aged and older people who wish to retain vitality should start now and continue to build and defend their muscle mass through life.

Each elderly person faces different degrees and types of physical limitations. Therefore, each should exercise in his or her own way and pace. Even modest exercise, such as a 10-minute walk a day, a workout of upper body flexibility, or resistance training (even while seated) provides progressive benefits.[105] Great achievements are possible and improvements are inevitable.

start now! ⋯⟩ Ready to make a change? If you are an older person, or if you care for an older person, devise a sensible exercise plan and track your activity in Diet & Wellness Plus for one week. At the end of that week, look at your total physical activity, and decide if you can increase your level of activity in the following week.

---

intake, supplemental nutrient-fortified formulas in liquid, pudding, cookie, or other forms between meals can supply needed energy, protein, and other nutrients.

KEY POINT

- Protein recommendations remain about the same through adult life, but physical conditions change and may affect both protein needs and appropriate sources.

Carbohydrates and Fiber

Ample whole-grain breads, cereals, rice, and pasta provide the steady supply of carbohydrate that the brain demands for optimal functioning. The fiber in these foods takes on extra importance in aging to prevent constipation, a common complaint among older adults and nursing home residents in particular.

Fruits and vegetables supply soluble fibers and other food components to help ward off chronic diseases. With aging, however, come problems of transportation, limited cooking facilities, and chewing disabilities that limit some elderly people's intakes of fresh fruits and vegetables. Even without such problems, most older adults fail to obtain the recommended 25 or so grams of fiber each day (14 grams per 1,000 calories).[106] When low fiber intakes are combined with low fluid intakes, inadequate exercise, and constipating medications, constipation becomes inevitable.

KEY POINT

- Adequate fiber can help older adults to avoid constipation.

Fats and Arthritis

Older adults must attend to fat intakes for several reasons. Consuming enough of the essential fatty acids supports continued good health, and limiting intakes of saturated and *trans* fats is a priority to minimize the risk of heart disease and other conditions of aging.

Osteoarthritis   The common type of **arthritis**, osteoarthritis, often results from being overweight or from unknown causes as people age.[107] During movement, the ends of healthy bones are protected by small sacs of fluid that act as lubricants. With arthritis, the sacs erode, cartilage and bone ends disintegrate, and joints become malformed and painful to move. Loss of body weight often brings relief, particularly in the

arthritis a usually painful inflammation of joints caused by many conditions, including infections, metabolic disturbances, or injury; usually results in altered joint structure and loss of function.

knees; physical activities such as walking, bicycling, and swimming can reduce pain and improve physical function, mental health, and quality of life.[108]

Rheumatoid Arthritis   Rheumatoid arthritis arises from an immune system malfunction—the immune system mistakenly attacks the bone coverings as if they were foreign tissue. The lining around the joints becomes swollen and inflamed, and as a result, joints become painful to move. Drug therapy, including anti-inflammatory or steroidal drugs, and surgery are available; however, some individuals report some relief from consuming plant oils, antioxidants, and the omega-3 fatty acid EPA, found in fish oil.[109] Many ineffective or unproven "cures" are sold for arthritis relief. Research is mixed on whether the popular dietary supplements chondroitin sulfate and glucosamine, both components of cartilage, provide relief, but at least one large, randomized, controlled human study supports the idea.[110] Researchers observed improvements in joint pain, swelling, and function after six months of combined treatment.

Gout   A form of inflammatory arthritis known as gout affects millions of U.S. adults, and its prevalence increases with age. An increased incidence of gout has been observed with "triggers" such as insulin resistance, overweight, elevated blood pressure, heart disease, low-level lead exposure, and higher intakes of meat and seafood, beer and spirits, soft drinks, and fructose.[111] Incidences appear to decline with increased consumption of coffee, milk, and vitamin C.

KEY POINT

- Arthritis causes pain and immobility, and older people with arthritis often fall for quack cures.

Vitamin Needs

Vitamin needs change as people age. Changes in absorption, metabolism, and excretion affect the body's needs.

Vitamin A   Vitamin A stands alone among the vitamins in that its absorption appears to increase with aging. For this reason, some researchers have proposed lowering the vitamin A requirement for aged populations. Others resist this proposal because foods containing vitamin A and its precursor beta-carotene confer health benefits and many, such as green leafy vegetables, are frequently lacking in the diet.

Vitamin D   For people in their 50s and 60s, minimizing bone loss becomes a critical concern, and the DRI vitamin D recommendation of 15 micrograms a day covers their needs.[112] Because individual medical concerns and physiological changes with aging can interfere with vitamin D metabolism, a slightly higher intake of 20 micrograms a day is recommended for people in their 70s and older.[113]

As people age, vitamin D synthesis in the skin declines fourfold, and the kidneys' ability to activate it diminishes, setting the stage for deficiency. Also, many older adults drink little or no vitamin D–fortified milk and get little or no exposure to sunlight. Supplements of vitamin D and calcium are not recommended for preventing bone fractures in healthy postmenopausal women and their use entails some risk.[114] Vitamin D may help prevent falls in elderly people, however, and anyone with osteoporosis should follow the advice of a physician.[115]

Vitamin B$_{12}$ By age 60, reduced stomach acid production in about 6 percent of people reduces their ability to absorb vitamin B$_{12}$ from food, making deficiency likely. Up to 20 percent of elderly people may suffer marginal deficiencies, but most of these cases go unrecognized and untreated.[116] No one yet knows whether dietary insufficiency, malabsorption, or another factor is the primary cause of these deficiencies.[117] Synthetic vitamin B$_{12}$ is reliably absorbed and injections are available, however, and much misery can be averted by preventing deficiencies of vitamin B$_{12}$ in elderly people.

Diet and Vision   A key aspect of healthy aging is maintaining good vision.[118] Loss of vision in the elderly correlates with loss of life that cannot be explained by other risk factors.[119] Dark green, leafy vegetables, which are rich in certain carotenoid phytochemicals, may protect the eyes from one cause of blindness: macular degeneration.[120]§ Carotenoid and other nutrient supplements are unproven for eye protection, although some physicians may prescribe them in cases of advanced macular degeneration.[121]

Another vision problem facing older people is **cataracts**. A cataract is a clouding of the lens that impairs vision and leads to blindness. Only 5 percent of people younger than 50 years have cataracts; afterward, the percentage jumps to between 20 and 30 percent. The lens of the eye is easily oxidized. Some studies suggest that a diet high in *foods* that provide ample antioxidants—carotenoids, vitamin C, and vitamin E— may reduce the risk of early onset and progression of cataracts.[122] High doses of vitamin C or E supplements, conversely, may increase some people's cataract risk.[123]

KEY POINTS
- Vitamin A absorption increases with aging.
- Elderly people are vulnerable to deficiencies of vitamin D and vitamin B$_{12}$.

Water and the Minerals

Dehydration is a major risk for older adults. Total body water decreases with age, so even mild stresses, such as a hot day or a fever, can quickly dehydrate the tissues. The thirst mechanism may diminish, and even healthy older people may go for long periods without drinking. The kidneys also become less efficient in recapturing water before it is lost as urine. Dehydration then leads to problems such as constipation, bladder problems, and mental confusion that is easily mistaken for **senile dementia**, an effect that may occur with a water loss of as little as 2 percent of body weight.[124] In a person with asthma, dehydration thickens mucus in the lungs, blocking airways and leading to pneumonia. In a bedridden person, dehydration can lead to **pressure ulcers**. To prevent dehydration, older adults should consume sufficient fluid each day. The beverage recommendations for adults 51 years and older suggest that women consume 9 cups of fluid each day; for men, recommendations increase to 13 cups.

Fluid choices, strategically made, can improve the nutrition status of an elderly person. For example, a person with diminished appetite and weight loss may be tempted by a smoothie of bananas, frozen strawberries or other frozen fruit, milk or soy milk, and a touch of chocolate syrup or powdered sugar. Hearty, soft-cooked meat and vegetable soups, milk-based seafood or vegetable bisque, puddings, and commercial liquid meal replacers all provide fluid along with calories, protein, and other nutrients essential for health. Conversely, an overweight elderly person needs tempting low- or no-calorie beverages: plain or sparkling water with lemon or lime, broth-based soups, artificially sweetened tea or coffee, and low-sodium vegetable juices.

Iron   Iron status generally improves in later life, especially in women after menstruation ceases and in those who take iron supplements, eat red meat regularly, and include vitamin C–rich fruits in their daily diet. When iron-deficiency anemia does occur, diminished appetite with low food intake is often the cause. Aside from diet, other factors make iron deficiency likely in older people:

- Chronic blood loss from ulcers or hemorrhoids.
- Poor iron absorption due to reduced stomach acid secretion.
- Antacid use, which interferes with iron absorption.
- Use of medicines that cause blood loss, including anticoagulants, aspirin, and arthritis medicines.

§The carotenoids are lutein and zeaxanthin, which help to form pigments of the macula of the eye.

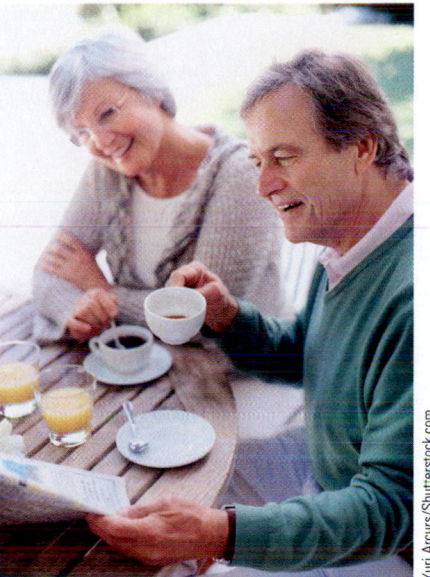

Yuri Arcurs/Shutterstock.com

Adults of all ages need to attend to daily fluid intakes.

cataract (CAT-uh-ract) clouding of the lens of the eye that can lead to blindness. Cataracts can be caused by injury, viral infection, toxic substances, genetic disorders, and possibly some nutrient deficiencies or imbalances.

senile dementia the loss of brain function beyond the normal loss of physical adeptness and memory that occurs with aging.

pressure ulcers damage to the skin and underlying tissues as a result of unrelieved compression and poor circulation to the area; also called *bed sores*.

Table 14–15

Summary of Nutrient Concerns in Aging

Nutrient	Effects of Aging	Comment
Energy	Need decreases.	Physical activity moderates the decline.
Fiber	Low intakes make constipation likely; beneficial for controlling weight and reducing the risk of heart disease and type 2 diabetes.	Inadequate water intakes and physical activity, along with some medications, compound risks of constipation.
Protein	Needs may stay the same or slightly increase; intake often decreases.	Low-fat milk and other high-quality protein foods are appropriate; high-fiber legumes provide protein and other nutrients.
Vitamin A	Absorption increases.	Supplements normally not needed.
Vitamin D	Increased likelihood of inadequate intake; synthesis in skin tissue declines.	Daily moderate exposure to sunlight may be of benefit.
Vitamin B_{12}	Malabsorption of some forms.	Foods fortified with synthetic vitamin B_{12} or a supplement may be of benefit in addition to a balanced diet.
Water	Lack of thirst and increased urine output make dehydration likely.	Mild dehydration is a common cause of confusion.
Iron	In women, status improves after menopause; deficiencies linked to chronic blood losses and low stomach acid output.	Stomach acid is required for absorption; antacid or other medicine use may aggravate iron deficiency; vitamin C and meat enhance absorption.
Zinc	Intakes are often inadequate and absorption may be poor, but needs may also increase.	Medications interfere with absorption; deficiency may depress appetite and sense of taste.
Calcium	Intakes may be low; osteoporosis becomes common.	Lactose intolerance commonly limits milk intake; calcium-rich substitutes or supplements are needed (consider supplements that include vitamin D).
Potassium	Increased intake might decrease the risk of high blood pressure.	Include fruits, vegetables, and low-fat or fat-free milk and yogurt in the diet.
Sodium	Decreasing intake might lower the risk of high blood pressure.	Choose and prepare foods with little to no added salt; consider herbs or salt substitutes to add flavor to foods.
Fat	Increased risk of cardiovascular disease.	Look for foods low in saturated fats, *trans* fats, and cholesterol, and make most fats polyunsaturated or monounsaturated.

Older people take more medicines than others, and drug and nutrient interactions are common.

Zinc Zinc deficiencies, common in older people, are known to impair immune function and may increase the likelihood of infectious diseases, such as pneumonia.[125] Zinc deficiency can also depress the appetite and blunt the sense of taste, thereby reducing food intakes and worsening zinc status. Many medications interfere with the body's absorption or use of zinc, and an older adult's medicine load can worsen zinc deficiency.

Multinutrient Supplements Overall, elderly people often benefit from a single balanced low-dose vitamin and mineral supplement. Older people taking such supplements suffer fewer sicknesses caused by infection. A summary of the effects of aging on nutrient needs appears in Table 14–15.

KEY POINT
- Aging alters vitamin and mineral needs; some rise, while others decline.

Can Nutrition Help People to Live Longer?

Although people cannot alter the year of their birth, they can probably alter the length and quality of their lives. Lifestyle choices make a difference.

Lifestyle Factors   Have you ever noticed that some older adults seem younger than their chronological ages? Research on this observation has focused on health habits of older people and has identified three major factors related to nutrition:

- Abstinence from, or moderation in, alcohol use.
- Regular nutritious meals.
- Weight control.

Three additional factors are regular adequate sleep, abstinence from smoking, and regular physical activity. The physical health of those who engage in all six positive health practices may be comparable to that of people 30 years younger who engage in few or none. Some changes of aging, such as graying hair and reduced senses of smell, taste, and eyesight are inescapable, whereas others may yield to individual life choices (Table 14–16).

Energy Restriction   Evidence that diet might influence the life span emerged decades ago when researchers fed young rats a diet extremely low in energy. The starved rats stopped growing, while a group of control rats ate and grew normally; when the researchers increased food energy in the starved group, growth resumed. Many of the starved rats died young from malnutrition. The few survivors, although permanently deformed from their ordeal, remained alive far beyond the normal life span for such animals and developed diseases of aging much later than normal. Since then, this result has been repeated in many species (see Table 14–17).

With moderate energy restriction, animals also retain youthfulness longer and develop fewer disease risk factors such as high blood pressure, glucose intolerance, and immune system impairments.[126] In monkeys, moderate calorie restriction prolongs life and reduces the incidence of diabetes, cancer, and cardiovascular disease.[127] In contrast, one ongoing study reports no improvement in survival of monkeys.[128] No one can say conclusively whether any of these findings might also apply to human beings.[129]

On the negative side, severely energy-restricted mice are more susceptible to acute infections.[130] And although energy restriction may improve chronic disease risks, it stunts growth and may damage some systems to benefit others. Also, without supplements, calorie-restricted diets lack needed nutrients.[131] Scientists are hoping to discover drugs that mimic the benefits of calorie restriction while minimizing risks.[132] For now, however, any supplement or treatment claiming to prolong human life is a hoax.

KEY POINT

- In rats and other species, food energy deprivation lengthens the lives of individuals.

Table 14–16

What to Expect in Aging

Changes with Age You Probably Can Slow or Prevent

By exercising, eating an adequate diet, reducing stress, and planning ahead, you may be able to slow or prevent:

✓ Wrinkling of skin due to sun damage
✓ Some forms of mental confusion
✓ Elevated blood pressure
✓ Accelerated resting heart rate
✓ Reduced lung capacity and oxygen uptake
✓ Increased body fatness
✓ Elevated blood cholesterol
✓ Slowed energy metabolism
✓ Decreased maximum work rate
✓ Loss of sexual functioning
✓ Loss of joint flexibility
✓ Diminished oral health: loss of teeth, gum disease
✓ Bone loss
✓ Digestive problems, constipation

Changes with Age You Probably Must Accept

These changes are probably beyond your control:

✓ Graying hair
✓ Balding
✓ Some drying and wrinkling of skin
✓ Impairment of near vision
✓ Some loss of hearing
✓ Reduced taste and smell sensitivity
✓ Reduced touch sensitivity
✓ Slowed reactions (reflexes)
✓ Slowed mental function
✓ Diminished visual memory
✓ Menopause (women)
✓ Loss of fertility (men)
✓ Loss of joint elasticity

Table 14–17

Effects of Energy Restriction on Life Span

Differences in maximum life span are observed between animals eating normally and those that are energy-restricted.

	Normal Diet	Energy Restricted
Rats	33 months	47 months
Spiders	100 days	139 days
Single-celled animals (protozoa)	13 days	25 days

Programs That Help Nutrition professionals are calling for improved nutrition-related services for all Americans aged 60 years and older.[146] Currently, several federal programs can provide help for older people. Social Security provides income to retired people older than age 62 who paid into the system during their working years. The Supplemental Nutrition Assistance Program (SNAP), formerly called the Food Stamp Program, assists the very poor by supplementing their monthly food budgets. The Administration on Aging coordinates services governed by the Older Americans Act, including the provision of nutritious meals in a social congregate setting, education and shopping assistance, counseling and referral to other needed services, and transportation to necessary appointments. An estimated 33 percent of the nation's elderly poor benefit from meals provided by the program. For the homebound, Meals on Wheels volunteers deliver meals to the door. Nutritionists are wise not to focus solely on nutrient and food intakes of the elderly because enjoyment and social interactions may be as important as food itself.

Many older people, even able-bodied ones with financial resources, find themselves unable to perform cooking, cleaning, and shopping tasks. For anyone living alone, and particularly for those of advanced age, it is important to work through the problems that food preparation presents. This chapter's Food Feature presents some ideas.

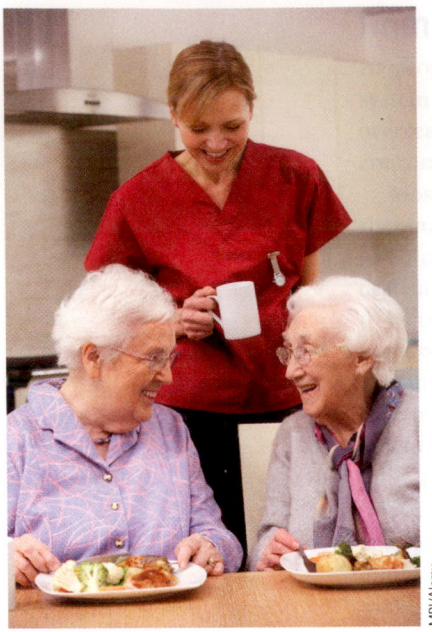

Shared meals can be the high point of the day.

MBI/Alamy

KEY POINTS

- Food choices of the elderly are affected by aging, altered health status, and changed life circumstances.
- Federal programs can help to provide nourishment, transportation, and social interactions.

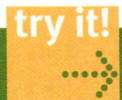

Food Feature

Single Survival and Nutrition on the Run

LO 14.5 Assess the challenges associated with regularly eating alone.

A single person of any age, whether a busy student in a college dormitory, an elderly person in a retirement apartment, or a professional in an efficiency suite, faces challenges in obtaining nourishing meals. People without access to kitchens and freezers find storing foods problematic, so they often eat out. Following is a collection of ideas gathered from single people who have devised ways to nourish themselves despite obstacles.

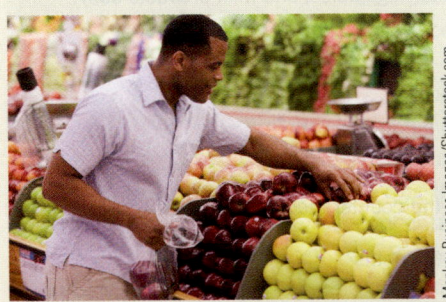

Shopping for and preparing nutritious foods for one person takes some special know-how.

Monkey Business Images/Shutterstock.com

Is Eating in Restaurants the Answer?

Restaurant foods are convenient, but can such foods meet nutrient needs or support health as well as homemade foods? The answer is "perhaps," but making it so takes some effort. A few chefs and restaurant owners are concerned with the nutritional health of their patrons, but more often chefs strive to please the palate. Restaurant foods are often overly endowed with calories, fat, saturated fat, sugar, and salt but often lack fiber, folate, or calcium. Vegetables and fruits may be in short supply, but a single meat or pasta portion may exceed a whole day's recommended intake. To improve restaurant meals, follow these suggestions:

- Restrict your portions to sizes that do not exceed your energy needs.
- Ask that excess portions be placed in take-out containers right away.

- Ask for extra vegetables, fruit, or salad.
- Request whole-grain breads and pasta (more restaurants now supply these, and others may do so with repeated requests).
- Make judicious choices of foods that stay within intake guidelines for solid fats, added sugars, and salt.

The Food Feature of Chapter 5 offered specific suggestions for ordering fast food and other foods with an eye to keeping fat intakes within bounds, and Chapter 8 listed foods high in sodium. Table 14–19 provides tips for single survival in the grocery store and at home.

Managing Loneliness

Loneliness affects many people, young and old alike, and can negatively influence overall health. For nutrition's sake, among many reasons, it is important to attend to loneliness, and mealtimes provide an opportunity to do so.[147] The person who is living alone must learn to connect food with socializing. Invite guests and make enough food so that you can enjoy the leftovers later on. If you know of a friend or acquaintance who frequently eats alone, you can bet that person would love to join you for a meal now and then.

Table 14–19

Smart Shopping and Creative Cooking

Smart Shopper Tips

- Make a list to reduce impulse buying; buy on sale, and use coupons for needed items.
- Watch sizes: gallons of milk may be cheaper than pints per ounce, but the savings are lost if the milk sours. Dry milk and small shelf-stable milk boxes often make sense.
- Bulk staple foods, such as dry milk, oatmeal, ready-to-eat cereals, or rice are cheapest, but they must be stored properly (see Chapter 15 for hints to avoid food waste).
- If freezer space allows, buy whole chickens or "family pack" meats at bargain prices. Divide into single servings, wrap well, mark the date, freeze, and use as needed.
- Ask grocers to break open large packages of fresh foods; buy only the amount you can use up. More expensive but convenient small bags of cut and washed fresh vegetables may be an option.
- Frozen vegetables in large resealable bags are more economical than small boxes.

- Freeze a loaf of whole-grain bread; defrost or toast as needed.
- Eggs keep for weeks in the refrigerator; after their sell-by date, hard-boil and refrigerate them for handy protein servings that last one week longer.
- Buy three pieces of tomatoes, pears, and other fresh fruit in various stages of ripeness: a ripe one to eat right away, a less ripe one to eat soon after, and a green one to ripen in a few days.
- Buy ready-to-heat and eat foods from the grocery store delicatessen section—these cost less than similar foods from restaurants. Choose nutrient-dense items; skip stuffing, macaroni and cheese, meat loaf and gravy, vegetables in sauce, mayonnaise-dressed mixed salads, and fried foods.
- Buy a ready-roasted chicken; use the main pieces for several dinners; simmer the remainder with herbs and vegetables in a broth for soup.

Creative Kitchen Tricks

- Divide a head of cauliflower or broccoli into thirds. Cook one-third right away; marinate one-third in Italian salad dressing to use later in a salad; toss the remainder into a casserole, soup, or stew, or eat it raw with dip for a crunchy snack.
- Stir-fry ready-to-use blends of cabbage, snow peas, and onions; bags of slaw-cut vegetables; or raw vegetables for a delicious dinner. Add Asian seasonings and leftover chicken or seafood. Bonus: one pan to wash.
- Microwavable bags of brown rice cost more but provide a whole-grain food for those less able to cook.

- Treat leftovers with respect: nothing beats a plate of delicious leftovers for speed and convenience—plate, reheat in the microwave, and eat.
- Use nutritious frozen dinners judiciously (caution: these can be very high in solid fats, added sugars, and salt—read Nutrition Facts panels). Round out the meal with a salad, a whole-grain roll, and a glass of fat-free milk.

My Turn watch it! Eating Solo

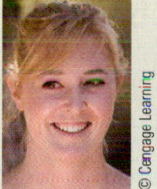
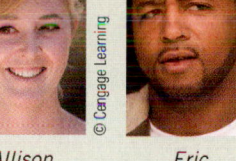

Allison *Eric*

© Cengage Learning

Have you ever felt uninspired by the thought of eating alone? Two students talk about dealing with loneliness, making easy but nutritious meals, and choosing wisely among takeout foods.

Visit www.cengagebrain.com to access MindTap, a complete digital course that includes these videos and other resources.

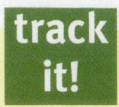 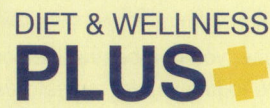

DIET & WELLNESS PLUS+ Concepts in Action

Analyze Three Diets

The purpose of this exercise is to explore food choices and the potential for nutrient deficiencies among young children, teens, and older adults, using three new profiles: a 2-year-old, a 14-year-old, and a 70-year-old.

1. Iron nutrition is required for normal development. Create a new profile for a 2-year-old toddler (32 lbs; 35" tall). Select the Track Diet tab, choose a new day, and then, using Snapshot 8–5 (p. 322), choose foods to create a balanced iron-rich meal to satisfy the needs and tastes of a young child. Once you've entered the foods, select the Reports tab, and select Intake Spreadsheet for that meal. Did the meal supply a third of the iron this toddler needs (consult the DRI table, inside front cover p. B)? Which foods contributed most of the iron?

2. For nutrient adequacy, a child's diet should include a variety of foods from each food group (see Table 14–3, p. 562 and Table 14–5, p. 565). Modify your 2-year-old's meal to provide servings of foods from each group, keeping in mind that children eat small portions and often like colorful, crunchy vegetables and smooth,

bland foods. Enter the foods from the Track Diet tab. Select MyPlate Analysis for this meal. Did your meal provide about a third of the needed foods for the day from all the food groups? If not, what choices can you make in later meals to compensate?

3. Nutrients missed at breakfast often cannot be made up at lunch or dinner. Create a nutritious breakfast for your 2-year-old, using ideas for a rushed morning (Table 14–11, p. 574). Enter the data from the Track Diet tab. Select Intake vs. Goals for that date and meal. Did the breakfast meet a significant portion of the child's nutrient needs? If not, what foods or beverages might improve it?

4. Teens' diets often lack calcium, iron, and vitamin A. From the Profile drop-down box, create a new profile for a 14-year-old girl. Select the Track Diet tab, and choose foods that are excellent sources of calcium, iron, and vitamin A for a lunch meal. Recall that vitamin C helps maximize iron absorption from non-heme (non-meat) sources of iron. Select the Reports tab and then Source Analysis. From the drop-down box, generate reports for Calcium, Iron, Vitamin A, and Vitamin C. Did the meal meet the teen's

needs for calcium and iron? Did meat or non-heme sources of iron predominate? Which foods also supplied vitamin A and vitamin C?

5. Teens often make snack choices with convenience and taste in mind, but nutritious snacks better suit their nutrient needs. Select the teen's profile (already created), and select the Track Diet tab. Plan nutritious snacks for the morning and afternoon. Make each snack supply about 150 calories of nutritious foods. Select the Intake vs. Goals, and evaluate the report for the snacks. Did the snacks provide about 20 percent of nutrients significant for teens? Which? How much saturated fat did the snacks provide?

6. For older people, nutritious meals help to retain good health. From the Profile drop-down box, create a new profile for a 70-year-old single adult. Select the Track Diet tab, and choose foods to create a nutritious, convenient, easy-to-eat dinner for this person. Select the Reports tab and then the Intake vs. Goals for that meal. Did the meal supply enough zinc, protein, vitamin B_{12}, and calcium to meet one-third of the person's need without excessive calories? Did it supply omega-3 fatty acids? If not, suggest ways of improving it.

what did you decide?

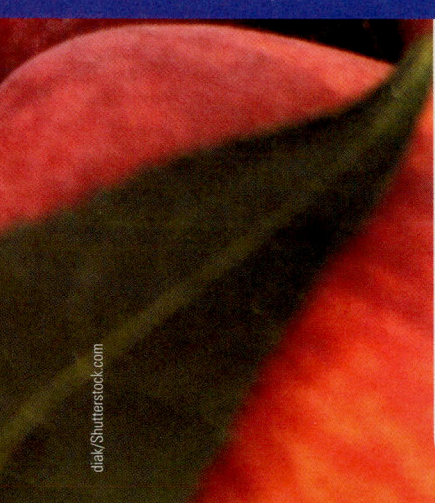

Do you need special information to properly nourish children, or are they like "little adults" in their needs?

Do you suspect that symptoms you feel may be caused by a food allergy?

Are teenagers old enough to decide for themselves what to eat?

Can good nutrition help you live better and longer?

Self Check

1. (LO 14.1) Children often fail to consume adequate amounts of _____.
   a. dairy
   b. meats
   c. vegetables
   d. sugar-sweetened beverages

2. (LO 14.1) A healthy child's normal appetite control system
   a. cannot be trusted to provide the right level of calories for growth.
   b. can be short-circuited by a constant stream of foods high in added sugars, saturated fat, and refined grains.
   c. holds the child's appetite constant, without much fluctuation from day to day.
   d. none of the above

3. (LO 14.1) On a pound-for-pound basis, a 5-year-old's need for vitamin A is about double the need of an adult man.
   T F

4. (LO 14.1) Which of the following can contribute to choking in children?
   a. peanut butter eaten by the spoonful
   b. hot dogs and tough meat
   c. grapes and hard candy
   d. all of the above

5. (LO 14.1) Lead poisoning in young children
   a. is no longer a problem in the United States.
   b. is likely because they absorb 5 to 10 times more lead than do adults.
   c. arises primarily from ingesting of foods packed in metal cans.
   d. all of the above

6. (LO 14.1) Research to date supports the idea that food allergies or intolerances are common causes of hyperactivity in children.
   T F

7. (LO 14.1) A child who ate cream of broccoli soup and became ill now feels ill whenever it is served. The child most likely has a
   a. food allergy.   c. food aversion.
   b. food intolerance.   d. food antibody.

8. (LO 14.2) Which of the following is most commonly deficient in adolescents?
   a. folate   c. iron
   b. zinc   d. vitamin D

9. (LO 14.2) Which of the following may lessen symptoms of depression associated with PMS?
   a. alcohol
   b. caffeine
   c. vitamin D
   d. all of the above

10. (LO 14.2) Which of the following is *not* associated with peak bone mass?
    a. physical activity
    b. scholastic achievement
    c. vitamin D status
    d. calcium intake

11. (LO 14.3) Physical changes of aging that can affect nutrition include _____.
    a. reduced stomach acid
    b. increased saliva output
    c. tooth loss and gum disease
    d. a and c

12. (LO 14.3) In research, which of the following is associated with a longer life span in many species?
    a. energy restriction
    b. superoxide dismutase
    c. omega-3 fatty acids
    d. none of the above

13. (LO 14.4) Nutrition does not seem to play a role in the causation of osteoarthritis.
    T F

14. (LO 14.4) Vitamin A absorption decreases with age.
    T F

15. (LO 14.4) Antioxidant supplements have been shown to slow down the progression of Alzheimer's disease.
    T F

16. (LO 14.4) A person planning a nutritious diet for an elderly person should pay particular attention to providing enough _____.
    a. vitamin A   c. iron
    b. vitamin B$_{12}$ d. b and c

17. (LO 14.4) The word DETERMINE is an acronym used in assessing an elderly person's _____.
    a. risk of malnutrition
    b. bone integrity
    c. degree of independence
    d. all of the above

18. (LO 14.5) Single elderly people who routinely eat alone most often prefer isolation and should be left to themselves.
    T F

19. (LO 14.6) Nutrients and drugs can interact
    a. before ingestion or absorption.
    b. within the body tissues.
    c. at the level of gene expression.
    d. all of the above

Answers to these Self Check questions are in Appendix G.

Nutrient–Drug Interactions: Who Should Be Concerned?

LO 14.6 Summarize the concerns surrounding nutrient–drug interactions.

A 45-year-old Chicago business executive attempts to give up smoking with the help of nicotine gum. She replaces smoking breaks with beverage breaks, drinking frequent servings of tomato juice, coffee, and colas. She is discouraged when her stomach becomes upset and her craving for tobacco continues unabated, despite the nicotine gum. Problem: nutrient–drug interaction.

A 14-year-old girl develops frequent and prolonged respiratory infections. Over the past six months, she has suffered constant fatigue despite adequate sleep, has had trouble completing school assignments, and has given up playing volleyball because she runs out of energy on the court. During the same six months, she has been taking antacid pills several times a day because she heard this was a sure way to lose weight. Her pediatrician has diagnosed iron–deficiency anemia. Problem: nutrient–drug interaction.

A 30-year-old schoolteacher who benefits from antidepressant medication attends a faculty wine and cheese party. After sampling the cheese with a glass or two of red wine, his face becomes flushed. His behavior prompts others to drive him home. In the early morning hours, he awakens with severe dizziness, a migraine headache, vomiting, and trembling. An ambulance delivers him to an emergency room where a physician takes swift action to save his life. Problem: nutrient–drug interaction.

The Potential for Harm

People sometimes think that medical drugs do only good, not harm. As the opening stories illustrate, however, both prescription and over-the-counter (OTC) medicines can have unintended consequences, among which are significant interactions with nutrition.[1]*

As Figure C14–1 shows, drugs can interact with foods, nutrients, and herbs in a number of ways.[2] Each may affect the absorption, action, metabolism, or excretion of the others.

Some drugs are known to interact with specific nutrients (see Table C14–1). In addition, alcohol is infamous for its interactions with nutrients, and the more alcohol ingested, the more likely that a significant nutrient interaction will occur (see Controversy 3).

Reference notes are found in Appendix F.

Figure C14–1

How Foods, Drugs, and Herbs Can Interact

The arrows show that foods, drugs, and herbs can interfere with each other's absorption, actions, metabolism, or excretion. Drugs also often change the appetite, affecting food intake.

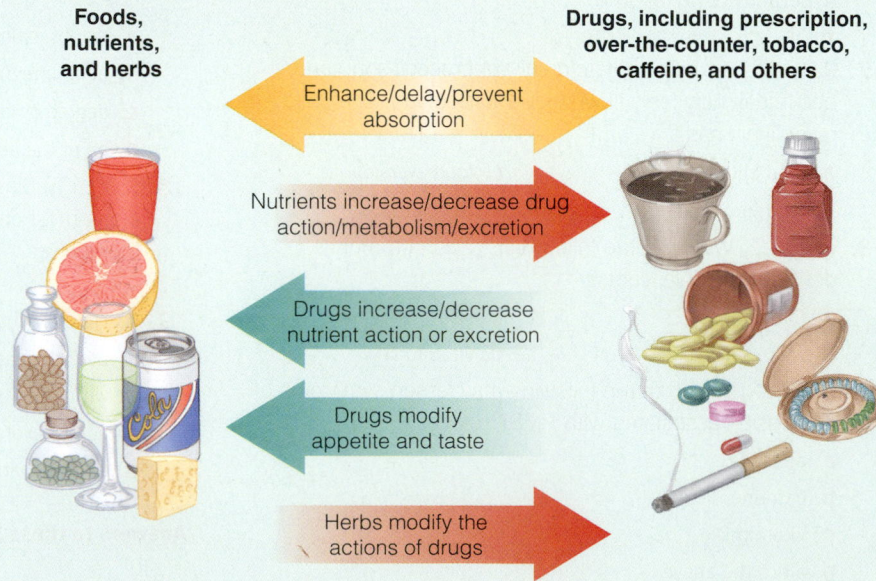

Foods, nutrients, and herbs

Drugs, including prescription, over-the-counter, tobacco, caffeine, and others

Enhance/delay/prevent absorption

Nutrients increase/decrease drug action/metabolism/excretion

Drugs increase/decrease nutrient action or excretion

Drugs modify appetite and taste

Herbs modify the actions of drugs

iStockphoto.com/AvailableLight

Table C14-1

Selected Nutrient-Drug Interactions

Drug	Effects on Nutrient Absorption	Effects on Nutrient Excretion	Effects on Nutrient Metabolism
Antacids (aluminum containing)	Reduce iron absorption	Increase calcium and phosphorus excretion	May accelerate destruction of thiamin
Antibiotics (long-term usage)	Reduce absorption of fats, amino acids, folate, fat-soluble vitamins, vitamin B_{12}, calcium, copper, iron, other minerals	Increase excretion of folate, niacin, potassium, riboflavin, and vitamin C	Destroy vitamin K–producing bacteria and reduce vitamin K production
Antidepressants (monoamine oxidase inhibitors, MAOI)			Slow breakdown of tyramine, with dangerous blood pressure spike and other symptoms on consuming tyramine-rich foods (Table C14-2, p. 596) or alcoholic beverages (sherry, vermouth, red wines, some beers)
Aspirin (large doses, long-term usage)	Lowers blood concentration of folate	Increases excretion of thiamin, vitamin C, and vitamin K; causes iron and potassium losses through gastric blood loss	
Caffeine		Increases excretion of small amounts of calcium and magnesium	Stimulates release of fatty acids into the blood
Cholesterol-lowering "statin" drugs (Zocor, Lipitor)			Grapefruit juice slows drug metabolism, causing buildup of high drug levels; potentially life-threatening muscle toxicity can result.
Diuretics		Raise blood calcium and zinc; lower blood folate, phosphorus, electrolytes, vitamin B_{12}; increase excretion of calcium, water-soluble nutrients	Interfere with storage of zinc
Estrogen replacement therapy	May reduce absorption of folate	Causes sodium retention	May raise blood glucose, triglycerides, vitamin A, vitamin E, copper, and iron; may lower blood vitamin C, folate, vitamin B_6, riboflavin, calcium, magnesium, and zinc
Laxatives (effects vary with type)	Reduce absorption of many nutrients	Increase excretion of all unabsorbed nutrients	
Oral contraceptives	Reduce absorption of folate, may improve absorption of calcium	Cause sodium retention	Raise blood vitamin A, vitamin D, copper, and iron; may lower blood beta-carotene, riboflavin, vitamin B_{12}, and vitamin C; may elevate requirements for riboflavin and vitamin B_6; alter blood lipids

Factors That Make Interactions Likely

Significant nutrient–drug interactions do not occur every time a person takes a drug. The potential for interactions is greatest in those who take a medicine for a long time, who take multiple drugs, who drink alcohol daily, or who are poorly nourished to begin with. Ninety percent of people over the age of 70 receive at least one prescription medication, and some may take as many as 10 drugs at a time.[3] The risk of an adverse effect rises substantially among older people taking five or more daily medications and compounds further when herbs and other supplements are added to the mix.

The details of nutrient–drug interactions are many and far more extensive than can be presented in this section. The following discussions are intended to raise awareness of the most common ones.

Absorption of Drugs and Nutrients

The business executive described earlier felt the effects of chemical incompatibility. Acids from the tomato juice, coffee, and colas she drank before chewing the nicotine gum kept the nicotine from being absorbed into the bloodstream through the lining of her mouth as intended, and so did not quell her craving. Instead, it traveled to her stomach and caused nausea.[‡]

Similarly, dairy products or calcium-fortified juices interfere with the absorption of certain antibiotics. Drug label instructions, such as "Take on an empty stomach" or "Do not combine with dairy products," help to avert most such interactions.

Certain drugs can also interfere with the small intestine's absorption of minerals. This interaction explains the experience of the tired 14-year-old. Her overuse of antacids eliminated the stomach's normal acidity, on which iron absorption depends. The medicine bound tightly to the iron molecules, forming an insoluble, unabsorbable complex. Her iron stores already bordered on deficiency, as iron stores for young girls typically do, so her misuse of antacids pushed her over the edge into iron-deficiency anemia.

Chronic laxative use can also lead to malnutrition. Laxatives can carry nutrients through the intestines so rapidly that many vitamins have no time to be absorbed. Mineral oil, a laxative the body cannot absorb, can rob a person of important fat-soluble vitamins and potentially beneficial phytochemicals by dissolving them and carrying them out in the feces.

Metabolic Interactions

The teacher who landed in the emergency room was taking an antidepressant medicine, one of the monoamine oxidase inhibitors (MAOI). At the party, he suffered a dangerous chemical interaction between the medicine and the compound tyramine in his cheese and wine. Tyramine is produced during the fermenting process in cheese and wine manufacturing. Table C14–2 lists some foods high in tyramine.

The MAOI medication works by depressing the activity of enzymes that destroy the brain neurotransmitter dopamine. With less enzyme activity, more dopamine is left, and depression lifts.

[‡]These items also interfere with the action of nicotine gum: beer; coffee; condiments (ketchup, mustard, and soy sauce); juices (apple, grape, orange, and pineapple); and lemon-lime soda.

Table C14–2

Some Foods High in Tyramine

- Aged cheeses
- Aged meats
- Alcoholic beverages (beer, wine)
- Anchovies
- Caviar
- Fava beans
- Fermented foods (sauerkraut, sausages)
- Feta cheese
- Lima beans
- Mushrooms
- Pickled fish or meat
- Prepared soy foods (miso, tempeh, tofu)
- Smoked fish or meat
- Soy sauce
- Yeast extract (Marmite); yeast supplements

Note: The tyramine content of foods depends on storage conditions and processing; thus, the amounts in similar products can vary substantially.

As a side effect, the drug also depresses enzymes in the liver that destroy tyramine. Ordinarily, the man's liver would have quickly destroyed the tyramine from the cheese and wine, but due to the MAOI medication, tyramine built up and caused the potentially fatal reaction.

Other culprits affecting drug metabolism include food and spice phytochemicals and popular herbal supplements.[4] A chemical constituent of grapefruit juice suppresses an enzyme responsible for breaking down many kinds of medical drugs. With less drug breakdown, doses build up to toxic levels in the body. A person who drinks either grapefruit or cranberry juice and also takes the blood-thinning drug warfarin may exhibit delayed blood clotting with dangerously prolonged bleeding times.[5]

Caffeine and Tobacco

People in every society use caffeine in some form for its well-known "wake-up" effect. Caffeine is a true stimulant drug. Like all stimulants, it increases the respiratory rate, heart rate, and secretion of stress and other hormones. Caffeine also raises the blood pressure, an effect that lasts for hours after consumption.

Caffeine's interactions with foods and nutrients are subtle but may be significant because caffeine is ubiquitous in foods and beverages—see Table C14–3. Chocolate bars, colas, and other foods favored by children contain caffeine, and children are more sensitive to its effects. Many popular cold and headache remedies also offer about a cup of coffee's worth of caffeine per dose because, in addition to being a mild pain reliever in its own right, this amount of caffeine remedies the caffeine-withdrawal headache that no other pain reliever can touch.[6] The 2015 Dietary Guidelines for Americans committee has concluded that excessive intakes of caffeine (>400 milligrams per day for adults) can lead to caffeine toxicity and fatal cardiovascular events.[7] Deaths from pure powered caffeine, sold as a "dietary supplement" but actually a powerful stimulant drug, have triggered FDA warnings to manufacturers and other actions. The powder delivers the caffeine of more than 30 cups of coffee in a single teaspoon.

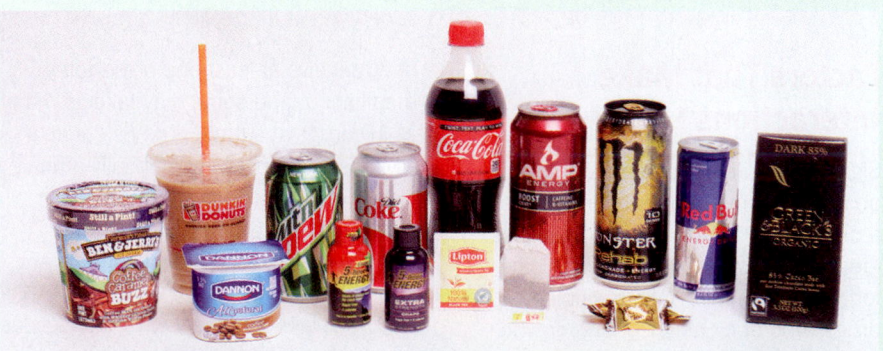

These foods and beverages all contain caffeine, but few, if any, of their labels state how much.

© Sam Kolich/Bill Smith Group/Cengage Learning

Table C14–3

Caffeine Content of Selected Beverages and Foods

Beverages and Foods	Average (mg)
Coffee, Tea, Soft Drinks, Other Beverages[a]	
Brewed coffee, 8 oz	95
Instant coffee, 8 oz	64
Starbucks Frappuccino, 9.5 oz	72
Brewed tea, green, 8 oz	30
Brewed tea, black, 8 oz	47
Instant tea, 8 oz	26
Snapple iced tea (all flavors), 16 oz	42
Colas, Creme Soda, Dr Pepper, Mr. Pibb, Sunkist Orange	30–35
Mello Yello, Mountain Dew, 12 oz	45–50
Chocolate milk or hot cocoa, 8 oz	5
Energy drinks	
5-Hour Energy, 2 oz	138
AMP, Red Bull, 8–8.3 oz	80
Monster, 16 oz	160
No Fear, Rock Star, 16 oz	174
Wired X344, 16 oz	344
Candies, Gum, Other	
Gum, caffeinated, 1 piece	95
Dark chocolate–covered coffee beans, 1 oz	235
Dark chocolate, semisweet, 1 oz	18
Milk chocolate, 1 oz	6
Frozen yogurt, Ben & Jerry's coffee fudge, 1 c	85
Ice cream, Starbucks coffee flavored, 1 c	50
Yogurt, Dannon coffee flavored, 1 c	45
Powdered caffeine, 1 tsp	3,200

[a]Product formulations change often; contact the manufacturer about products you use regularly.

Caffeine is also a diuretic (which causes water loss from the body). However, when taken in moderation, caffeinated beverages can contribute to daily fluid intakes without impairing the body's water balance (see Chapter 8 for details).

As for moderate intakes, research is limited, but it mostly refutes any causative links between daily caffeine and cancer, cardiovascular disease, or birth defects. In fact, observational research suggests that consuming caffeine or coffee, including decaffeinated coffee, may lower the risk of type 2 diabetes.[8] Such correlations cannot establish cause, however. It may be that people who choose coffee over sugar-sweetened soft drinks take in fewer calories and weigh less, factors that reduce diabetes risk. Much more research is needed to clarify these associations.

As for cigarette and other tobacco use, it is a delivery system for the drug nicotine. Tobacco's dangers are well known, and most are beyond the scope of nutrition. Smoking does depress hunger and, in turn, sometimes reduces body fatness; it also accelerates the breakdown of vitamin C, increasing requirements.

Herbal Remedies, Alcohol, Other Drugs

Herbs can also interact with drugs, sometimes dangerously (see Table C14-4, p. 598). For example, people may take ginkgo biloba hoping to improve memory (evidence disproves this effect), but instead experience increased bleeding (ginkgo opposes blood clotting). When combined with other blood-thinning medications, such as aspirin or vitamin E, ginkgo biloba is associated with dangerous hemorrhaging.[9]

People who drink alcohol take note: alcohol interacts with a wide range of medications, including cardiovascular agents, central nervous system agents, and metabolic agents, causing symptoms ranging from nausea and headaches to loss of coordination, internal bleeding, heart problems, and breathing difficulties.[10] When taken with diuretics, alcohol can cause dehydration; when taken with sedatives such as sleeping pills or pain relievers, alcohol can suppress brain areas that maintain breathing, heart rate, and other life-sustaining functions. Always check with the prescribing physician about whether a medication may interact with alcohol.

Compounds in marijuana produce an enhanced enjoyment of eating, especially of sweets. Proposed medical uses of marijuana include increasing food intake among patients with failing appetites with weight loss (in HIV/AIDS and other wasting diseases) and quelling nausea and vomiting caused by diseases or treatments.[11]

In contrast, many drugs of abuse cause loss of appetite, weight loss, and malnutrition among people who abuse them heavily. The stronger the craving for the drug, the less a drug abuser wants nutritious food. Rats given unlimited access to cocaine will choose the drug over food until they die of starvation. Drug abusers face multiple nutrition problems, and an important aspect of

Herb	Drug	Interaction
Bilberry, dong quai, feverfew, garlic, ginger, ginkgo biloba, ginseng, meadowsweet, St. John's wort, turmeric, willow	Warfarin, coumadin (anticlotting drugs, "blood thinners"); aspirin, ibuprofen, and other nonsteroidal anti-inflammatory drugs	Prolonged bleeding time; danger of hemorrhage
Black tea, St. John's wort, saw palmetto	Iron supplement; antianxiety drug	Tannins in herbs inhibit iron absorption; St. John's wort speeds clearance of many drugs.
Borage, evening primrose oil	Anticonvulsants	Seizures
Echinacea (possible immunostimulant)	Cyclosporine and corticosteroids (immunosuppressants)	May reduce drug effectiveness
Feverfew	Aspirin, ibuprofen, and other nonsteroidal anti-inflammatory drugs	Drugs negate the effect of the herb for headaches
Garlic supplements	Protease inhibitors (HIV-AIDS[a]) drug	Decreased blood concentrations of the drug
Ginseng	Estrogens, corticosteroids	Enhanced hormonal response
Ginseng, hawthorn, kyushin, licorice, plantain, St. John's wort, uzara root	Digoxin (cardiac antiarrhythmic drug derived from the herb foxglove)	Interference with drug action and monitoring
Ginseng, karela	Blood glucose regulators	Altered blood glucose level
Kelp (iodine source)	Synthroid or other thyroid hormone replacers	Interference with drug action
Licorice	Corticosteroids (oral and topical)	Overreaction to drug (potentiation)
Panax ginseng	Antidepressants	Overexcitability, mania
St. John's wort	Cyclosporine (immunosuppressant); antiretroviral drugs (HIV/AIDS[a] drugs); warfarin (reduces blood clotting); MAOIs (used to treat depression)[a]	Increased enzymatic destruction of many drugs; decreased drug effectiveness; increased organ transplant rejection; reduced anticoagulant effect. Potentiation, with serotonin syndrome (mild): sweating, chills, blood pressure spike, abnormal heartbeat, seizures
Valerian	Barbiturates (sedatives)	Enhanced sedation

Note: A valuable free resource for reliable online information about herbs is offered by the Memorial Sloan-Kettering Cancer Center at www.mskcc.org/aboutherbs.

[a]MAOI stands for monoamine oxidase inhibitors.

Sources: M. Z. Liu and coauthors, Pharmacogenomics and herb-drug interactions: Merge of future and tradition, Evidence-Based Complementary and Alternative Medicine (2015), epub, doi:10.1155/2015/321091; B. Ge, Z. Zhang, and Z. Zuo, Updates on the clinical evidenced herb–warfarin interactions, Evidence-Based Complementary and Alternative Medicine (2014), epub, doi:10.1155/2014/9573.

addiction recovery is their identification and correction.

Personal Strategy

In conclusion, when you need to take a medicine, do so wisely. Ask your physician, pharmacist, or other health-care provider for specific instructions about the doses, times, and how to take the medication—for example, with meals or on an empty stomach. If you notice new symptoms or if a drug seems not to be working well, consult your physician.

In general, strive to live life with less chemical assistance. If you are sleepy, try a 15-minute nap or 15 minutes of stretching exercises instead of a 15-minute coffee break. The coffee will stimulate your nerves for an hour, but the alternatives will refresh your attitude for the rest of the day. If you suffer constipation, try getting enough exercise, fiber, and water for a few days. Chances are that a laxative will be unnecessary. Given adequate nutrition, rest, exercise, and hygiene, your body's ability to fine-tune itself may surprise you.

Critical Thinking

1. List all of the foods and drinks that you consume in one day that contain caffeine. Calculate your total caffeine intake. Do you think this is an appropriate caffeine intake for you? Why or why not?

2. Choose three nutrient–drug interactions that are a concern to you. Create a chart that lists the interaction and paraphrases how the interaction affects absorption, excretion and metabolism.

15 Hunger and the Future of Food

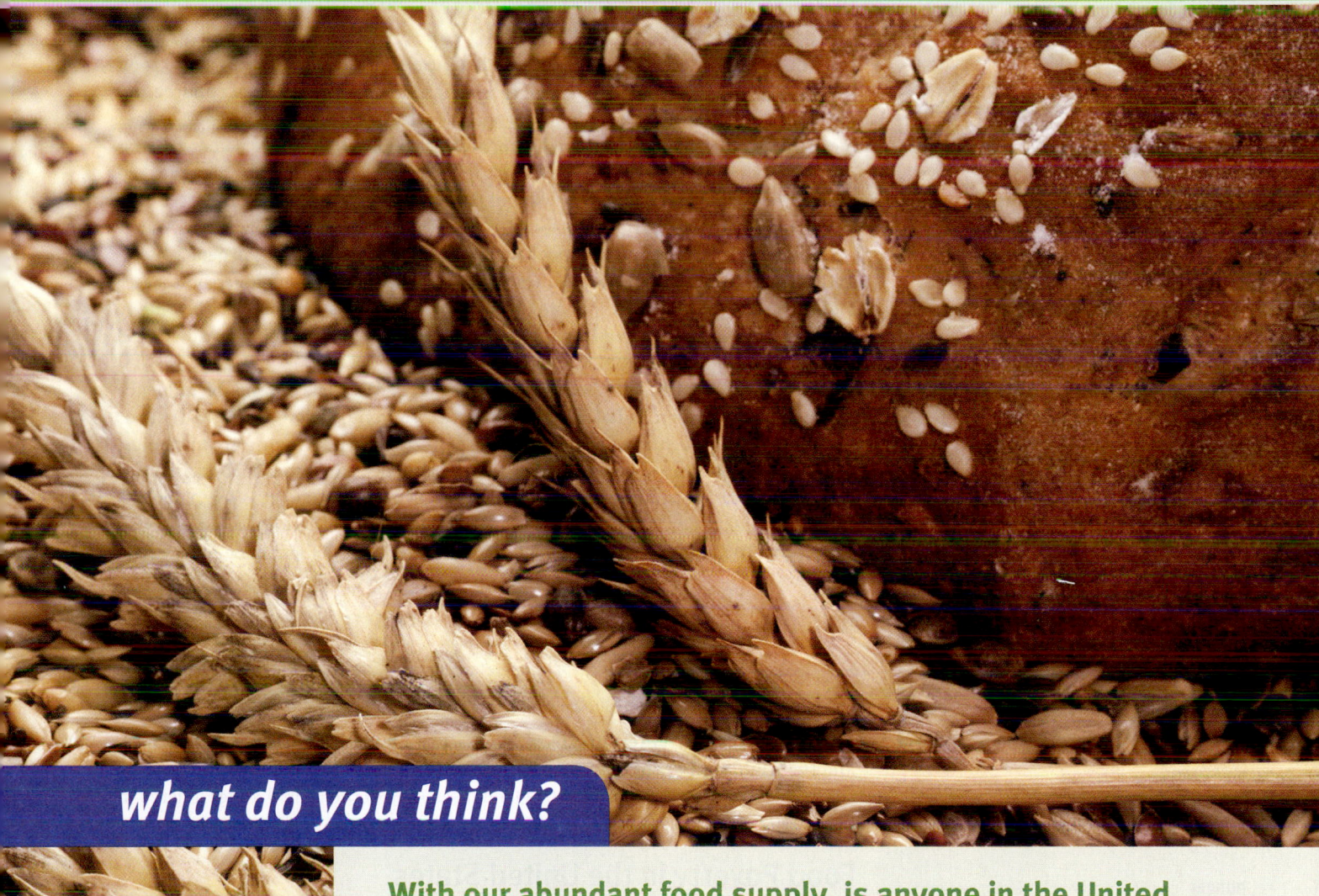

what do you think?

With our abundant food supply, is anyone in the United States **hungry**?

Can **one person** make a difference to the world's problems?

Will the earth yield **enough food** to feed human populations in the future?

Is a meal's **monetary price** its only cost?

Learning Objectives

After completing this chapter, you should be able to accomplish the following:

LO 15.1 Discuss food insecurity in the United States.

LO 15.2 Recognize the severity and extent of poverty and starvation in the developing world.

LO 15.3 Discuss how extreme poverty affects nutrition status in adults and children.

LO 15.4 Discuss the world food supply and the factors that affect it.

LO 15.5 Outline the steps that governments, private enterprises, and individuals can take to ensure a sustainable food supply.

LO 15.6 Describe low-input agriculture and its importance to future food production.

"Never doubt that a small group of thoughtful, committed people can change the world. Indeed, it is the only thing that ever has."

—Margaret Mead

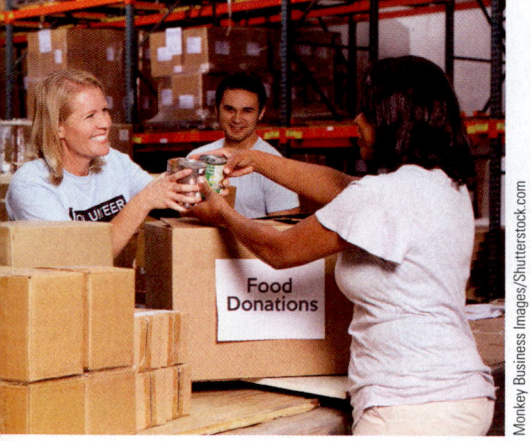

Each person's efforts can help to bring about needed change.

hunger physical discomfort, illness, weakness, or pain beyond a mild uneasy sensation arising from a prolonged involuntary lack of food; a consequence of food insecurity.

food crisis a steep decline in food availability with a proportional rise in hunger and malnutrition at the local, national, or global level.

food poverty hunger occurring when enough food exists in an area but some of the people cannot obtain it because they lack money, are being deprived for political reasons, live in a country at war, or suffer from other problems such as lack of transportation.

In the United States today, 6.8 million households live with **very low food security**—one or more members of these households, many of them children, repeatedly have little or nothing to eat because of a lack of money (Table 15–1 defines terms).[1]* Another 10.7 million food-insecure households experience somewhat less dire conditions. Food insecurity often leads to **hunger**—not the healthy appetite triggered by anticipation of a hearty meal but the pain, illness, or weakness caused by a prolonged and involuntary lack of food.

Worldwide, the problems are much more severe. At least 805 million people living in the poorest developing nations suffer chronic food insufficiency, hunger, and severe malnutrition, while their neighbors are food secure or even overfed.[2] Today, many nations are facing a **food crisis** in which already meager food supplies have dwindled further, and rates of malnutrition have risen sharply.

The tragedy described on these pages may seem at first to be beyond the influence of the ordinary person. What possible difference can one person make? As it turns out, quite a bit. Students in particular play a powerful role in bringing about change. Students everywhere are helping to change governments, support education, improve human predicaments, and solve environmental problems. Students offer major services to communities through soup kitchens, home repair programs, and childhood education. The young people of today are the world's single best hope for a better tomorrow.

U.S. Food Insecurity

LO 15.1 Discuss food insecurity in the United States.

In the United States, poverty and low food security exist side by side with affluence and the **high food security** enjoyed by most U.S. citizens. Survey questions help to determine the existence and degree of food insecurity in the United States (offered in Table 15–2). Figure 15–1 (p. 602) depicts the latest survey results.

Food Poverty in the United States

In the United States and other developed countries, hunger results primarily from **food poverty**. People go without nourishing meals not because there is no food nearby to purchase but because they lack sufficient money to pay both for the food they need and for other necessities, such as clothing, housing, medicines, and utilities. More than 14 percent of the population of the United States, including 20 percent of U.S. children, lives in a general state of poverty.[3] The likelihood of food poverty increases with problems such as abuse of alcohol and other drugs, mental or physical illness, lack of awareness of or access to available food programs, and reluctance to accept what some perceive as "government handouts" or charity.

---

*Reference notes are found in Appendix F.

Table 15–1

U.S. Food Security Terms

Food security exists on a continuum.

Term	Definition	Example
Food Security		
▪ **High food security**	No reported indications of food access problems or limitations.	A family who has a full refrigerator and pantry, without shortages.
▪ **Marginal food security**	One or two reported indications of problems—typically of anxiety over food sufficiency or shortage of food in the house. Little or no indication of changes in diets or food intake.	A parent who worries that the food purchased will not last until the next paycheck.
Food Insecurity		
▪ **Low food security**	Reports of reduced quality, variety, or desirability of diet. Little or no indication of reduced food intake.	A family whose diet centers on inexpensive, low-nutrient foods such as refined grains, processed meats, sweets, and fats.
▪ **Very low food security**	Reports of multiple indications of disrupted eating patterns and reduced food intake.	A family in which one or more members have gone to bed hungry, have lost weight, or have not eaten for a whole day because they did not have enough food.

Source: United States Department of Agriculture, *Economic Research Service, Definitions of food security,* available at http://www.ers.usda.gov/topics/food-nutrition-assistance/food-security-in-the-us/definitions-of-food-security.aspx.

Table 15–2

Food Security Questions for U.S. Households

Questions such as these help to identify households that have trouble meeting their basic food needs. Households reporting two or fewer of these conditions are classified as *food secure*; those with more than two are *food insecure* (for scoring details, visit the website below). For a household with children, additional questions determine their degree of food insecurity as well.

1. "We worried whether our food would run out before we got money to buy more." Was that often, sometimes, or never true for you in the last 12 months?

2. "The food that we bought just didn't last and we didn't have money to get more." Was that often, sometimes, or never true for you in the last 12 months?

3. "We couldn't afford to eat balanced meals." Was that often, sometimes, or never true for you in the last 12 months?

4. In the last 12 months, did you or other adults in the household ever cut the size of your meals or skip meals because there wasn't enough money for food? (Yes/No)

5. (If yes to question 4) How often did this happen—almost every month, some months but not every month, or in only 1 or 2 months?

6. In the last 12 months, did you ever eat less than you felt you should because there wasn't enough money for food? (Yes/No)

7. In the last 12 months, were you ever hungry, but didn't eat, because there wasn't enough money for food? (Yes/No)

8. In the last 12 months, did you lose weight because there wasn't enough money for food? (Yes/No)

9. In the last 12 months, did you or other adults in your household ever not eat for a whole day because there wasn't enough money for food? (Yes/No)

10. (If yes to question 9) How often did this happen—almost every month, some months but not every month, or in only 1 or 2 months?

Source: A. Coleman-Jensen, C. Gregory, and A. Singh, *Household food security in the United States in 2013,* Economic Research Report *173*, September 2014, available at www.ers.usda.gov/publications/err-economic-research-report/err173.aspx.

Figure 15–1

Food Security of U.S.
Households

Most U.S. households are food
secure.

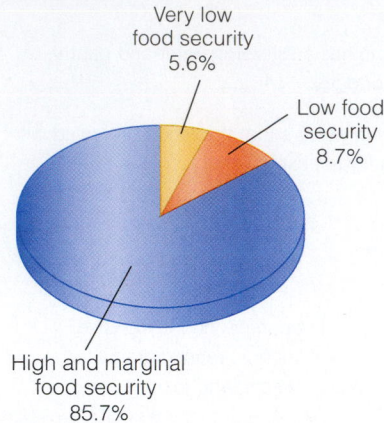

Very low
food security
5.6%

Low food
security
8.7%

High and marginal
food security
85.7%

Source: A. Coleman-Jensen, C. Gregory, and A. Singh,
Economic Research Service report summary:
Household food security in the United States in
2013, September 2014, available at www.ers.usda
.gov/publications/err-economic-research-report
/err173.aspx.

food deserts a term used to describe urban
and rural low-income neighborhoods and communities that have limited access to affordable
and nutritious foods.

Limited Nutritious Food Intakes To stretch meager food supplies, adults may
skip meals or cut their portions. When desperate, they may be forced to break social
rules—begging from strangers, stealing from markets, consuming pet foods, or even
scavenging through garbage cans. In the latter case, such foods may be spoiled or
contaminated and inflict dangerous foodborne illnesses that compound the harm to
health from borderline malnutrition. Children in such families sometimes go hungry
for an entire day until the adults can obtain food.

Significant numbers of U.S. children in families with low food security consume
enough calories each day but from a steady diet of inexpensive, low-nutrient foods,
such as white bread, fats, sugary punches, chips, and snack cakes, with few of the
fruits, vegetables, milk products, and other nutritious foods children need to be
healthy. The more severe their circumstances, the more likely children are to be in
poor or fair health, and the greater their likelihood of hospitalization.

Poverty and Obesity Food insecurity and obesity often exist side by side—
sometimes within the same household or even in the same person.[4] With obesity
comes an increased risk of developing chronic diseases, such as diabetes and hypertension, while poverty worsens the outlook for controlling those diseases.[5]

Some suggest that **food deserts** (first mentioned in Chapter 9) may help to
explain why obesity rates rise as incomes fall. Low-income urban and rural residents often lack access to markets that sell fresh produce, dairy products, lean
meats, and other nutrient-dense foods. Instead, such communities, especially in
urban areas, abound with stores selling doughnuts, packaged sweet cakes, sugary punches, hamburgers, and French fries—high-calorie foods that provide a full
stomach, are affordable, are constantly available, are easily carried, require no
preparation, and taste good.

In response, some communities are building supermarkets, funding fresh produce
trucks, and launching farmers' markets within food deserts, hoping to increase the
fruit and vegetable intakes of residents.[6] These efforts may improve people's diets to
a degree but are unlikely to reverse obesity, a notoriously intractable condition that
pervades well-supplied higher-income neighborhoods, too.[7]

Costs may be a factor for some people—research confirms that certain nutritious
foods cost more than less nutritious choices, particularly among the grains, meats,
oils, and snacks.[8] However, most people choose foods primarily on taste and preference; cost concerns are often secondary.[9]

KEY POINTS

- As poverty in the United States increases, food insecurity does, too.
- Children living in food-insecure households often lack the food they need.
- People with low food security may suffer obesity alongside hunger in the same
  community or family.

What U.S. Food Programs Address Low Food Security?

An extensive network of food assistance programs delivers life-giving food daily to
tens of millions of U.S. citizens living in poverty (see Table 15–3). One of every four
Americans receives food assistance of some kind, at a total cost of over $109 billion
per year.[10] Figure 15–2 shows the distribution of this cost across the programs.

Nationwide Efforts The centerpiece U.S. food program for low-income people is the Supplemental Nutrition Assistance Program (SNAP), administered by the
U.S. Food and Drug Administration (USDA).[†] It provided assistance to more than
46 million people in 2014; about half of the recipients are children. Eligible households receive electronic debit transfer cards through state social services or welfare
agencies. Recipients can use the cards like cash to purchase food and food-bearing
plants and seeds but not tobacco, cleaning items, alcohol, or other nonfood items.

[†] SNAP was formerly known as the Food Stamp Program.

Table 15–3

U.S. Federal and State Food Assistance Programs

This is a sampling of national and state programs aimed at reducing hunger in the United States.

- Commodity Supplemental Food Program
- Child and Adult Care Food Program
- Emergency Food Assistance Program
- Food Distribution Program on Indian Reservations
- National School Lunch and Breakfast Programs (see Chapter 14)
- Special Supplemental Feeding Program for Women, Infants, and Children (WIC; see Chapter 13)
- Supplemental Nutrition Assistance Program (SNAP), formerly called the Food Stamp Program

To help stretch consumer food dollars and SNAP credits, the USDA provides guidance on planning thrifty meals, complete with daily menus and recipes.

Community Efforts To assist where government programs fall short, concerned citizens in many communities work through local agencies and religious organizations to help deliver food to hungry people. National **food recovery** programs, such as Feeding America, coordinate the efforts of **food banks**, **food pantries**, **emergency kitchens**, and homeless shelters that provide food to tens of millions of people a year.[‡]

Many communities are working to promote food security. Table 15–4 (p. 604) presents actions in three stages for developing a hunger-free community. The table also points out that, while food relief for the hungry is critical, developing **sustainable** long-term solutions that attack the underlying problems of limited food access, low wages, and poverty are equally important. To rephrase a well-known adage: If you give a man a fish, he will eat for a day. If you teach him to fish so that he can buy his own gear and bait, he will eat for a lifetime and help to feed you, too.

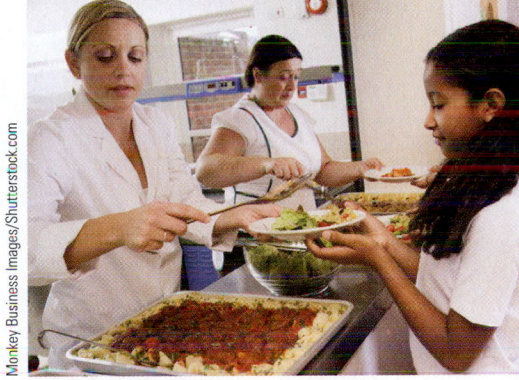

Monkey Business Images/Shutterstock.com

School breakfasts and lunches provide low-income children with nourishment at little or no cost.

Figure 15–2

Percentages of Expenditures for U.S. Food Programs

In 2014, the Supplemental Nutrition Assistance Program (SNAP) accounted for over two-thirds of U.S. food assistance expenditures.

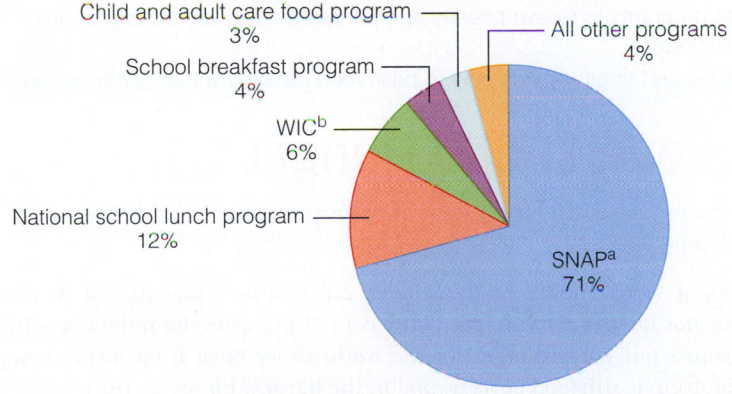

Child and adult care food program 3%
School breakfast program 4%
WIC[b] 6%
National school lunch program 12%
All other programs 4%
SNAP[a] 71%

[a]SNAP = Supplemental Nutrition Assistance Program.
[b]WIC = Special Supplemental Nutrition Program for Women, Infants, and Children.

Source: V. Olivera, U.S. Department of Agriculture, Economic Research Service, The food assistance landscape: FY 2014 annual report (EIB-137), March 2015, available at www.ers.usda.gov/publications /eib-economic-information-bulletin/eib137.aspx.

[‡]For information about food pantries, food banks, and other agencies in your community, call the National Hunger Hotline: (800) GLEAN-IT.

food recovery collecting wholesome surplus food for distribution to low-income people who are hungry.

food banks facilities that collect and distribute food donations to authorized organizations feeding the hungry.

food pantries community food collection programs that provide groceries to be prepared and eaten at home.

emergency kitchens programs that provide prepared meals to be eaten on-site; often called *soup kitchens*.

sustainable able to continue indefinitely; the use of resources in ways that maintain both natural resources and human life into the future; the use of natural resources at a pace that allows the earth to replace them and does not cause pollution to accumulate.

Table 15–4

Addressing Community Hunger

Consistently applied, these goals and actions can help to curtail food insecurity within a community.

Stage 1 Short–Term Goals—Fully Use Resources Currently Available

- Make full use of assistance that is available now. Assess available federal, state, local, and private food organizations and make them known to nutrition and other professionals in the community.
- Find out why people in need are not using the services. In particular, assess accessibility of food organizations to people who need them and assess transportation systems.
- Identify food quality and price inequities in low-income neighborhoods.
- Educate consumers and institutions about using local, organic, and seasonal foods.

Stage 2 Medium–Range Goals—Network and Connect Food Relief Agencies and Others to Identify and Address Problems

- Connect emergency food programs with local urban agriculture projects to encourage collection and distribution of available nutritious foods.
- Coordinate food services with parks and recreation programs and other community outlets, such as churches, to which area residents have easy access.
- Integrate public and private hunger-relief agencies, local businesses, and others to create an emergency food delivery network; include low-income participants for input.
- Take a leadership role by serving on community food councils or homeless-relief organizations; organize workshops to educate others.

Stage 3 Long–Range Goals—Redesign Food and Other Systems for Effectiveness and Longevity

- Mobilize government and community leaders to encourage urban agriculture to foster food self-reliance and improve nutrient intakes.
- Advocate for land-use policies and land grants that allow and encourage urban agriculture, such as community gardens and school gardens.
- Suggest improvements to public transportation to human services agencies and food resources.
- Encourage tax and other financial incentives to attract appropriate food businesses, such as farmer's markets and supermarkets, to low-income neighborhoods.
- Advocate increased minimum wage and more affordable housing.

KEY POINTS

- Government programs to relieve poverty and hunger are crucial to many people, if not fully successful.
- Local agencies and organizations help to build food security within communities.

World Poverty and Hunger

LO 15.2 Recognize the severity and extent of poverty and starvation in the developing world.

In the developing world, poverty and hunger are intense—one person in nine worldwide does not have enough to eat.[11] Table 15–5 presents the numbers, while Figure 15–3 points out which nations of the world suffer most from insufficiency. The primary problem is still food poverty, and in the hardest hit areas, the poverty is extreme.

The Staggering Statistics   Grasping the severity of poverty in the developing world can be difficult, but some statistics may help. One-fifth of the world's people have no land and no possessions *at all*. They survive on less than one U.S. dollar a day, they lack water that is safe to drink, and they cannot read or write.[12] Many spend about 80 percent of all they earn on food, but still they are hungry and malnourished.

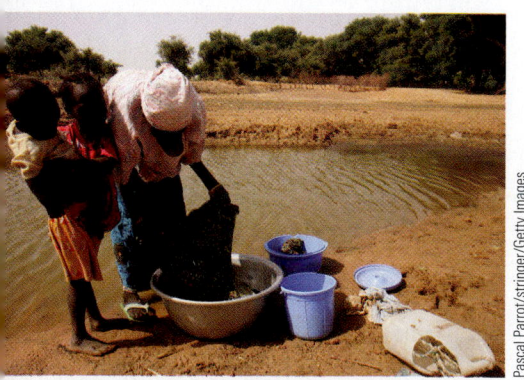

Unclean water and poor sanitation spread parasites and infectious diseases that claim many lives, particularly among the young.

Pascal Parrot/stringer/Getty Images

Figure 15–3

World Hunger Hot Spots

Hunger is most prevalent in the developing world.

Key:

<5% Very low malnutrition	25% – >34.9% - High
5% – >14.9% - Moderately low	35% and over - Very high
15% – >24.9% - Moderately high	Missing or insufficient data

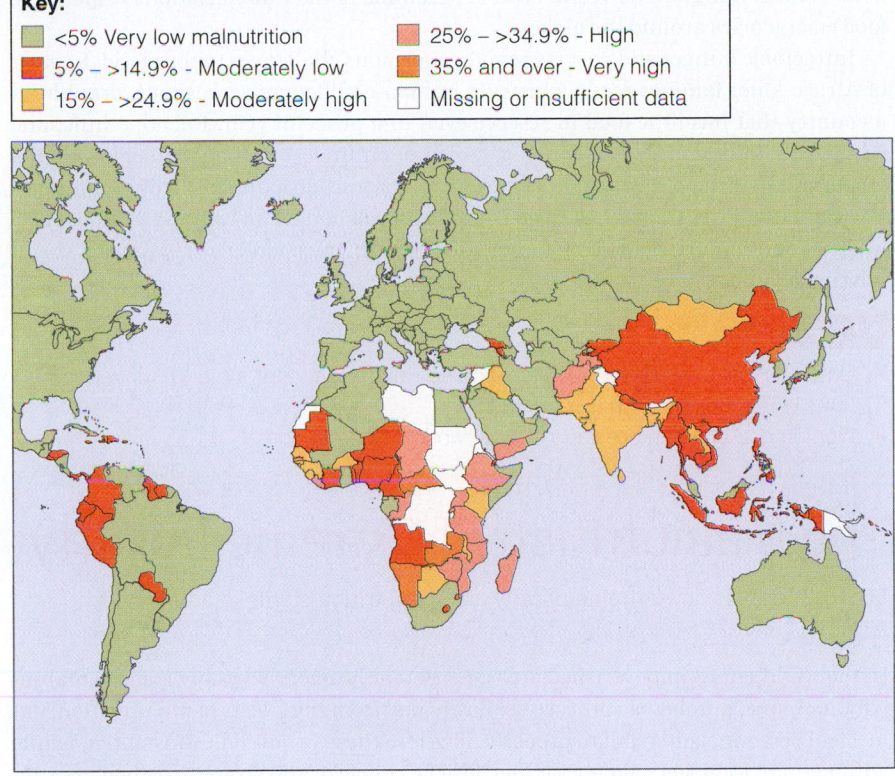

Source: Food and Agriculture Organization of the United Nations, The State of Food Insecurity in the World 2015, available at http://www.fao.org/hunger/en/.

Table 15–5

Global Undernutrition and Overnutrition

Condition	Global Incidence
Hunger, chronic or acute malnutrition	>805 million people
Vitamin and mineral deficiencies[a]	2.0 billion people
Overnutrition, obesity	≥2.1 billion people

[a]Vitamin and mineral deficiencies occur in both underfed and overfed populations.

Sources: Food and Agriculture Organization of the United Nations 2014; World Health Organization 2013.

The average U.S. house cat eats twice as much protein every day as one of these people, and the yearly cost of keeping that cat is greater than that person's annual income.

Some hopeful news also exists within these bleak statistics. Substantial worldwide efforts have reduced today's number of hungry people by some 160 million over the past decade.[13] The improvement is not evenly distributed, however—many Southeast Asian, Latin American, and Caribbean nations have successfully fought hunger within their borders, but Sub-Saharan Africa experienced an increase of 38 million since the early 1990s and is now home to more than a quarter of the world's undernourished people. Progress in this area will require even greater cooperation and resources.

Women and Children The world's "poorest poor" are usually women and children. Many societies around the world undervalue females, providing girls with poorer diets, less or no education, and fewer opportunities than boys. Malnourished girls become malnourished mothers who give birth to low-birthweight infants—so the cycle of hunger, malnutrition, and poverty continues. Worldwide, three-fourths of those who die each year from starvation and related illnesses are children.[14] Those who survive simply cannot work hard enough to get themselves out of poverty. Most have no borrowing power, even if credit were available, and lack the money needed to build even small businesses and incomes.

An irony of poverty is that it drives people, even those without sufficient food, to bear more children. An impoverished family depends on its children to farm the land, haul water, and care for the adults in their old age. However, malnutrition and disease cause many young children to die.[15] Therefore, parents will have many children to ensure that some will survive to adulthood.[16]

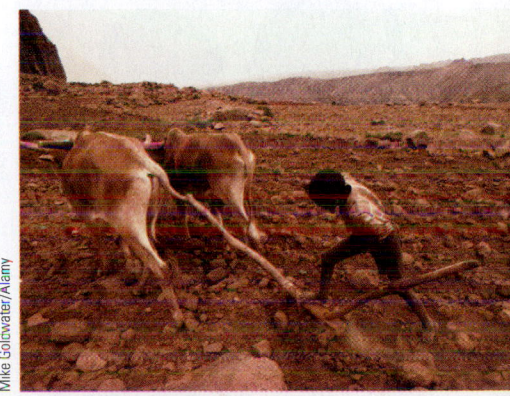

In some countries, every small pair of hands is needed to help feed the family.

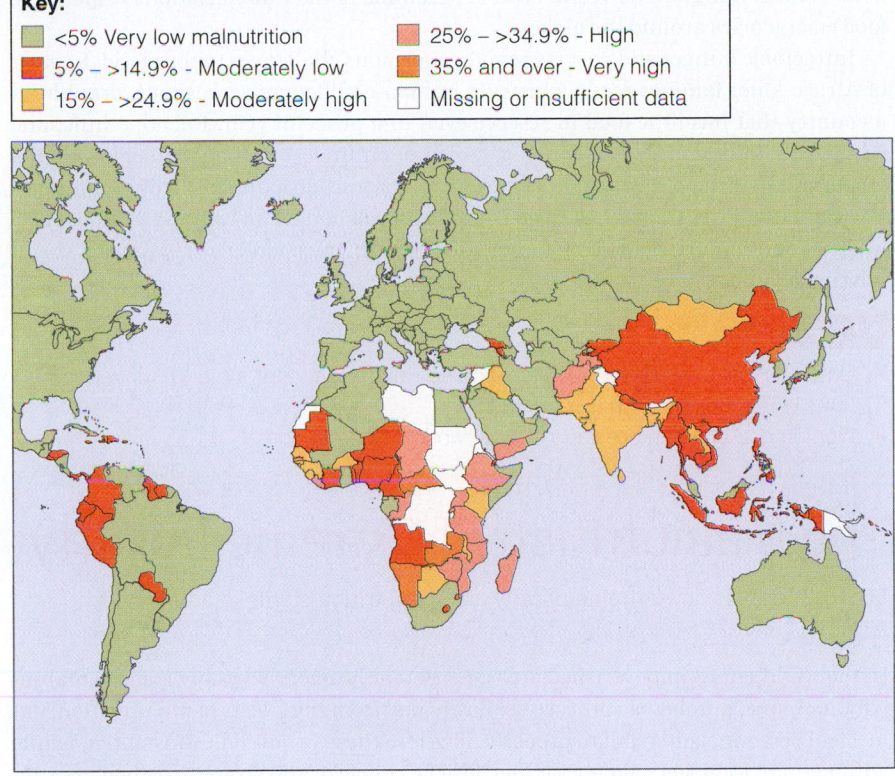 Mike Goldwater/Alamy

Famine The most visible form of hunger is **famine**, a true food crisis in which multitudes of people in an area starve and die. The natural causes of famine—drought, flood, and pests—occur, of course, but they take second place behind the political and social causes.[17] For people of marginal existence, a sudden increase in food prices, a drop in workers' incomes, or a change in government policy can quickly leave millions of them hungry. The World Food Programme of the United Nations responds to food emergencies around the globe.

Intractable hunger and poverty remain enormous challenges to the world. In parts of Africa, killer famines recur whenever human conflict converges with drought in a country that has little food in reserve even in a peaceful year. Racial, ethnic, and religious hatred along with monetary greed often underlies the food deprivation of whole groups of people. Farmers become warriors, and agricultural fields become battlegrounds while citizens starve. Food becomes a weapon when warring factions repel international famine relief in hopes of starving their opponents before they themselves succumb.

KEY POINTS

- Natural causes, along with political and social causes, contribute to hunger and poverty in many developing countries.
- Women and children are generally the world's poorest poor.

The Malnutrition of Extreme Poverty

LO 15.3 Discuss how extreme poverty affects nutrition status in adults and children.

In the world's most impoverished areas, persistent hunger inevitably leads to malnutrition. A huge number of adults suffer day to day from the effects of malnutrition, but medical personnel often fail to properly diagnose these conditions. Most often, adults with malnutrition feel vaguely ill; they lose fat, muscle, and strength—they are thin and getting thinner.[18] Their energy and enthusiasm are sapped away. With unrelenting food shortages, observable nutrient deficiency diseases develop.

Hidden Hunger—Vitamin and Mineral Deficiencies

Almost 2 billion people worldwide who consume sufficient calories still lack the variety and quality of foods needed to provide sufficient vitamins and minerals—they suffer the hidden hunger of deficiencies.[19] Nutrient deficiency diseases emerge as body systems begin to fail. Iron, iodine, vitamin A, and zinc are most commonly lacking, and the results can be severe—learning disabilities, mental retardation, impaired immunity, blindness, incapacity to work, and premature death.

The scope of nutrient deficiencies among adults and children is almost impossible to imagine:

- 40 percent of women in the developing world suffer poor health and debilitating fatigue from iron deficiency. More than 50,000 women a year die during childbirth due to severe anemia.[20]

- 18 million newborns every year have irreversible mental retardation (cretinism) from iodine deficiency.

- Half a million or more children (younger than age 5) become permanently blind from severe vitamin A deficiency.[21] Over 100 million more have marginally poor status that reduces their resistance to infections, such as measles.

- 25 percent of the world's population suffers from zinc deficiency that contributes to growth failure, diarrhea, and pneumonia.

These conditions are devastating not only to individuals but also to entire nations. When people suffer from mental retardation, blindness, infections, and early death

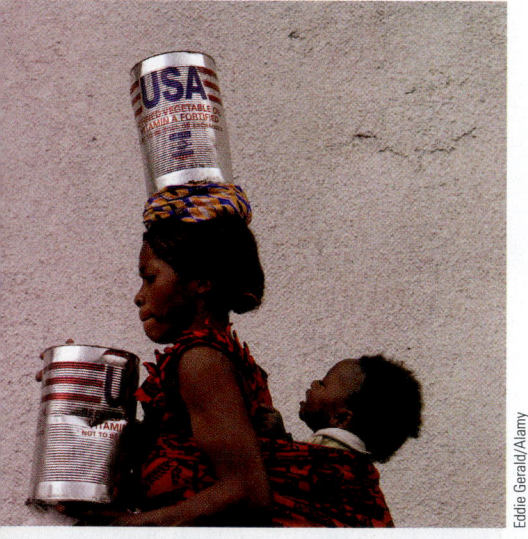

Donated food may temporarily ease hunger for some, but it is usually sporadic and insufficient to prevent nutrient deficiencies or support growth.

Eddie Gerald/Alamy

famine widespread and extreme scarcity of food that causes starvation and death in a large portion of the population in an area.

Table 15-6
Characteristics of Severe Acute Malnutrition and Chronic Malnutrition

	Severe Acute Malnutrition	Chronic Malnutrition
FOOD DEPRIVATION	Current or recent	Long term
PHYSICAL FEATURES	Rapid weight loss Wasting (marasmus: underweight for height; small upper-arm circumference) Edema (kwashiorkor)	Stunting (short for age)

Note: Vitamin and mineral deficiencies are common in both types of malnutrition.

due to malnutrition, national economies decline as productivity ceases and health-care costs soar.

KEY POINTS
- Malnutrition in adults most often appears as general thinness and loss of muscle.
- Vitamin and mineral deficiencies cause much misery worldwide.

Two Faces of Childhood Malnutrition

In contrast to malnourished adults, young impoverished and malnourished children often exhibit specific, more readily identifiable conditions. The form malnutrition takes in a hungry child depends partly on the nature of the food shortage that caused it. The most perilous condition, **severe acute malnutrition (SAM)**, occurs when food suddenly becomes unavailable, such as in drought or war. Less immediately deadly but still damaging to health is **chronic malnutrition**, the unrelenting chronic food deprivation that occurs in areas where food supplies are usually scanty and food quality is low. Table 15–6 compares key features of SAM with those of chronic malnutrition.

SAM   About 10 percent of the world's children suffer from SAM, often diagnosed by their degree of **wasting**. In the form of SAM called **marasmus**, lean and fat tissues have wasted away, burned off to provide energy to stay alive. Children with marasmus weigh too little for their height, and their upper arm circumference measures smaller than normal (see Figure 15–4).[22] Loose skin on the buttocks and thighs often sags down, so these children look as if they are wearing baggy pants. They often feel cold and are obviously ill. Sadly, such children are described as just "skin and bones."

Some starving children face this threat to life by engaging in as little activity as possible—not even crying for food. Others cry inconsolably. All of the muscles, including the heart muscle, are weak and deteriorating. Enzymes are in short supply, and the GI tract lining deteriorates. Consequently, what little food is eaten often cannot be absorbed.

A less common form of SAM is **kwashiorkor**. Its distinguishing feature is edema, a fluid shift out of the blood and into the tissues that causes swelling.[23] Loss of hair color is also common, and telltale patchy and scaly skin develops, often with sores that fail to heal. In a dangerous combination condition—**marasmic kwashiorkor**—muscles waste, but the wasting may not be apparent because the child's face, limbs, and abdomen are swollen with edema. Historically, kwashiorkor was attributed to too little protein in the diet, but today researchers recognize that the meager diets of starving children do not differ much—they all lack protein and many other nutrients.[24]

Each year, 3.1 million children, as many as 6 children *every minute*, die as a result of poor nutrition. Most of them do not starve to death—they die from the diarrhea and dehydration that accompany infections.

Chronic Malnutrition   A much greater number of children worldwide live with chronic malnutrition. They subsist on diluted cereal drinks that supply scant energy

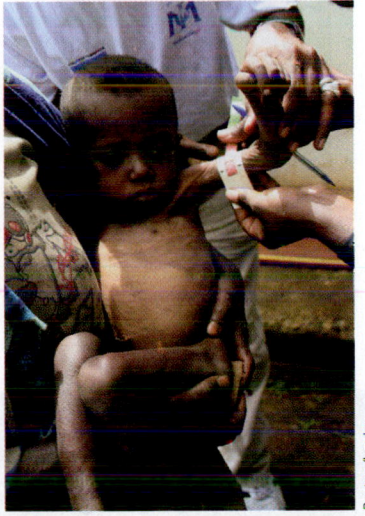

Figure 15–4
Arm Circumference

Measuring a child's mid-upper-arm circumference helps to assess the severity of SAM.

Reuters/Landov

severe acute malnutrition (SAM) malnutrition caused by recent severe food restriction; characterized in children by underweight for height (wasting).

chronic malnutrition malnutrition caused by long-term food deprivation; characterized in children by short height for age (stunting).

wasting in malnutrition, thin for height, indicating recent rapid weight loss or failure to gain, often from severe acute malnutrition.

marasmus (ma-RAZ-mus) severe malnutrition characterized by poor growth, dramatic weight loss, loss of body fat and muscle, and apathy. From the Greek word meaning "dying away."

kwashiorkor (kwash-ee-OR-core, kwash-ee-or-CORE) severe malnutrition characterized by failure to grow and develop, edema, changes in the pigmentation of hair and skin, fatty liver, anemia, and apathy.

marasmic kwashiorkor a particularly lethal form of severe acute malnutrition, in which a child's dangerously reduced lean body tissue is masked by edema, making the condition harder to detect.

and even less protein; such food allows them to survive but not to thrive. Intestinal parasites sap nourishment away, too.[25] Growth ceases because they chronically lack the nutrients required to grow normally—they develop **stunting**, and it is often irreversible.[26] They may appear normal because their bodies are proportionate, but these stunted children may be no larger at age 4 than at age 2, and they often suffer the miseries of malnutrition: increased risks of infection and diarrhea, and vitamin and mineral deficiencies.

A fully nourished developing brain normally grows to almost its full adult size within the first two years of life. When malnutrition occurs during these years, it can impair brain development and learning ability, effects that may become irreversible.

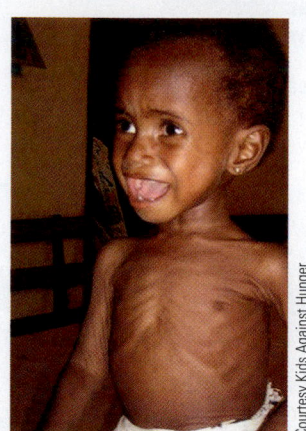

This 2-year-old girl was suffering from severe acute malnutrition.

Courtesy Kids Against Hunger

KEY POINTS

- Malnutrition in adults is widespread but is often overlooked; severe observable deficiency diseases develop as body systems fail.
- Many of the world's children suffer from wasting due to severe acute malnutrition, the deadliest form of malnutrition.
- In many more children, growth is stunted because they chronically lack the nutrients children need to grow normally.

Rehabilitation

Loss of appetite and impaired food assimilation interfere with attempts to provide nourishment to a malnourished child. To restore metabolic balance and promote physical growth, mental development, and recovery from illnesses, malnourished children need specially formulated fluids and foods. SAM often demands hospitalization, intensive nursing care, medical nutrition therapy, and medication.

Children dehydrated from diarrhea need immediate rehydration. With severe fluid and mineral losses, blood pressure drops and the heartbeat weakens. The right fluid, given quickly by knowledgeable providers, can help raise the blood pressure and strengthen the heartbeat, thereby averting disaster. Health-care workers save millions of lives each year by reversing dehydration with **oral rehydration therapy (ORT)**. In addition, such children need adequate sanitation and a safe water supply to prevent infectious diseases.

Once medically stable, malnourished children benefit from **ready-to-use therapeutic food (RUTF)**, commercial products intended to promote rapid reversal of weight loss and nutrient deficiencies.[27] Manufacturers blend smooth pastes of oil and sugars with ground peanuts, powdered milk, or other protein sources and seal premeasured single doses in sterilized pouches. RUTF need not be mixed with water (a plus in areas with unclean water sources) or prepared in any way, and the pouches resist bacterial contamination. Importantly, RUTF can be safely stored for 3 to 4 months without refrigeration, a rare luxury in many impoverished areas.

RUTF's downside is cost: commercial products are expensive to buy and ship to impoverished areas. A child may need to receive daily RUTF for up to 3 months for a full recovery with a low risk of relapse.[28] To lower the cost, RUTF pastes can often be made on site from more affordable local ingredients.[29]

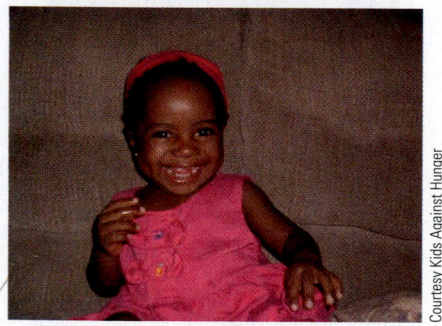

After a few weeks of medical nutrition therapy, she gained substantial weight and health along with a new appetite for living.

Courtesy Kids Against Hunger

KEY POINTS

- Oral rehydration therapy and ready-to-use therapeutic foods, properly applied, can save the life of a starving person.
- Many health and nutrition professionals work to eradicate childhood malnutrition.

The Future Food Supply and the Environment

LO 15.4 Discuss the world food supply and the factors that affect it.

Banishing hunger for all of the world's citizens poses two major challenges. The first is to provide enough food to meet the needs of the earth's expanding population

stunting low height for age, indicating restriction of potential growth in children, often from chronic malnutrition.

oral rehydration therapy (ORT) oral fluid replacement for children with severe diarrhea caused by infectious disease. A simple recipe for ORT: ½ L boiled water, 4 tsp sugar, ½ tsp salt.

ready-to-use therapeutic food (RUTF) highly caloric food products offering carbohydrate, lipid, protein, and micronutrients in a soft-textured paste used to promote rapid weight gain in malnourished people, particularly children.

without destroying natural resources needed to continue producing food. The second challenge is to ensure that all people have access to enough nutritious food to live active, healthy lives.

By all accounts, today's total **world food supply** can abundantly feed the entire current population.[30] For future supplies to remain ample, the world must cope with forces that threaten its food production and distribution.

Threats to the Food Supply

Many forces compound to threaten world food production and distribution, both today and in coming decades. The following list names just some of them.

- *Hunger, poverty, and population growth.* Every 60 seconds, 109 people die in the world, but in that same 60 seconds 255 are born to replace them.[31] Every year, the earth gains another 76,854,987 new residents to feed, most of them born in impoverished areas. By 2050, 1 billion additional tons of grains will be needed to feed the world's population; food increase may not be possible beyond the earth's human **carrying capacity**.

- *Loss of food-producing land.* Food-producing land is becoming saltier, eroding, and being paved over. The world's deserts are expanding.

- *Fossil fuel use.* Fossil fuel use underlies much world economic growth, with associated pollution of air, soil, and water.

- *Atmosphere and global climate change.* That climate change is occurring is no longer a serious academic debate.[32] The National Academies of Science conclude that "there is a strong, credible body of evidence, based on multiple lines of research, documenting that Earth is warming. Strong evidence also indicates that recent warming is largely caused by human activities, especially the release of **greenhouse gases** through the burning of fossil fuels." The associated heat waves, droughts, fires, storms, and floods thwart farmers and destroy crops, particularly in the poorest areas of the world. Arid deserts are projected to expand by 200 million acres in coming years in Sub-Saharan Africa alone. As ocean heat builds up, ocean food chains may fail.

- *Ozone loss from the outer atmosphere.* The outer atmosphere's protective ozone layer is thinning, permitting more harmful radiation from the sun to penetrate. As radiation increases the earth's temperature, polar ice caps are melting, threatening the world's coastlines. Radiation may also directly damage important crops.

- *Fresh water shortages.* Growing food requires great quantities of fresh water. The earth's fresh water supply is unevenly distributed, and too much of it is wasted, polluted, and unsustainably managed. Over a billion people lack access to fresh water today. If climate change continues on its current trajectory, almost half the world's population may be living in areas of high **water stress** in just 20 years from now; water scarcity could displace many millions of people from their homelands.[33]

- *Increased flooding.* Crop-damaging localized heavy storms are expected to become more frequent, causing flash floods that erode large swaths of topsoil from parched land.

- *Ocean pollution.* Ocean pollution, particularly agricultural and industrial runoff, is killing fish in large "dead zones" that form when excessive algal growth depletes water oxygen; dead zones are expected to expand as sea temperatures rise.[34]

The global problems just described are all related, and, often, so are their solutions. To think positively, this means that any initiative a person takes to address one problem will help solve many others.

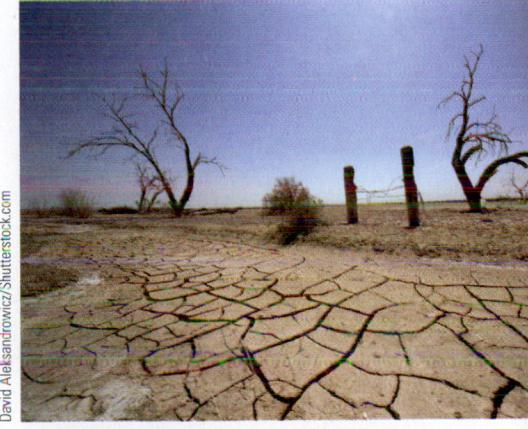

As groundwater is used up, deserts spread.

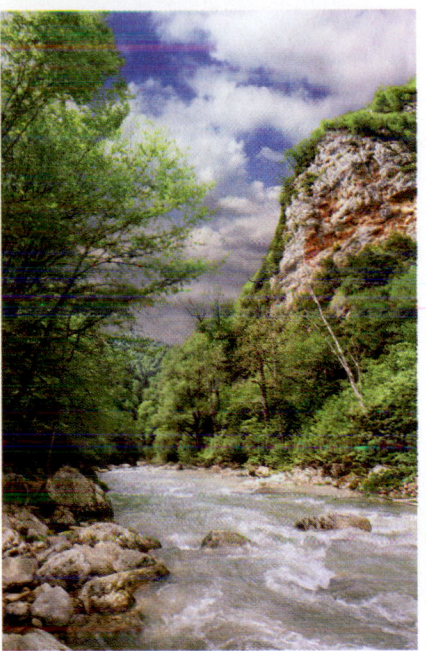

Pure rivers, lakes, and streams represent irreplaceable water resources.

world food supply the quantity of food, including stores from previous harvests, available to the world's people at a given time.

carrying capacity the total number of living organisms that a given environment can support without deteriorating in quality.

greenhouse gases gases that contribute to global climate change by absorbing the sun's infrared radiation and trapping heat; examples of greenhouse gases are carbon dioxide and methane.

water stress a measure of the pressure placed on water resources by human activities such as municipal water supplies, industries, power plants, and agricultural irrigation.

KEY POINTS

- The world's current food supply is sufficient, but distribution remains a problem.
- Future food security is threatened by many forces.

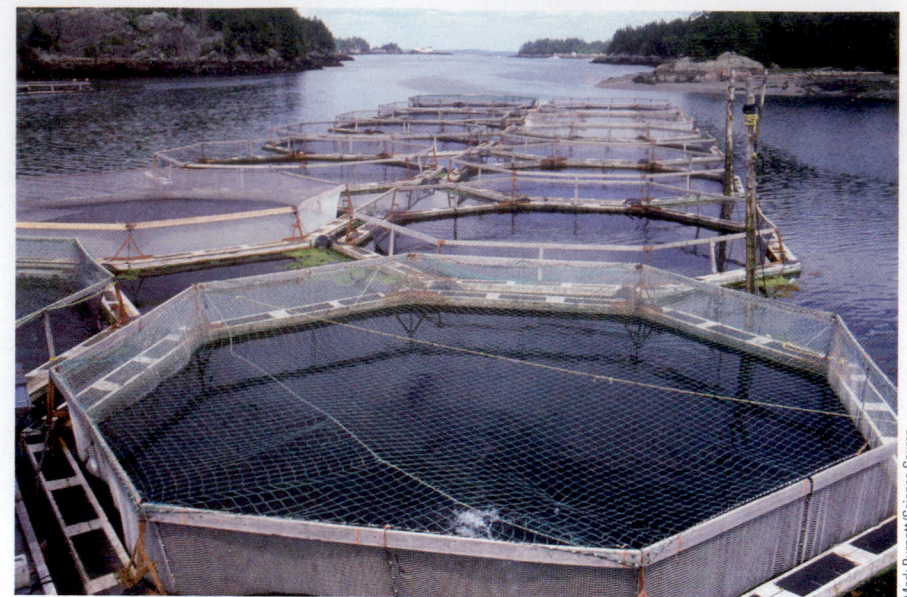

An open net cage houses fish in the ocean or a lake, where natural flow refreshes the cages.

Fisheries and Food Waste

Many other topics of food production and sustainability are worth investigating. This section presents just two more: the changing world supply of fish and seafood and the huge quantities of food, once produced, that are wasted.

Wild Fisheries and Aquaculture People around the world love seafood and demand is rising, but overfishing in past decades caused the near collapse of some species.[35] Today, over 60 percent of the world food fish stocks are fully exploited or overexploited, meaning that harvests cannot expand, despite increasing efforts to catch more—the fish stocks are too small. International efforts to protect important food fish species include seasonal quotas, "no fishing zones" in breeding and recovery areas, and rules against illegal harvesting. Some species have returned from the brink of extinction, but rebuilding wild oceanic fish stocks to a sustainable level will require world-wide cooperation.

Wild fish shortages and large profits have spurred the rapid growth of **aquaculture** businesses, which now provide more than half of the world's food fish and shellfish. Some aquaculture "fish farms" consist of vast net cages that enclose fish in ocean inlets or freshwater lakes, where natural water flow refreshes the cages. Other types house fish in artificial ponds positioned inland close to coast lines. Natural water is diverted through the ponds, bringing in fresh water and washing wastes into streams, lakes, or oceans. Farther inland, pond water is continuously filtered and cleansed. All farmed fish must be fed chow that contains fish, such as sardines, harvested from wild stocks, diverting them from direct human use and from larger wild fish species, such as cod, that depend on them.[36] As for consumer safety and nutrition, the 2015 Dietary Guidelines for Americans committee concluded that consumers can freely choose between wild and farm-raised tuna and salmon because their levels of contamination and nutrients are similar.[37] In general, smaller species are less contaminated and more sustainable.§

Food Loss and Waste In a hungry world, 1.3 billion tons of nourishing food, one-third of total annual production, are lost to spoilage, pests, or waste each year, squandering not just the food but the resources spent to produce, package, and transport it.[38] More than 25 percent of all the fresh water used each year is spent producing food that is ultimately wasted. Similarly, about 300 million barrels of oil are spent to fuel the production of that wasted food.

The scope of U.S. food waste is enormous (see Figure 15–5). Discarded food constitutes the single greatest component of municipal waste—even greater than yard

§For a guide to sustainable species by state, visit www.seafoodwatch.org/seafood-recommendations/consumer-guides.

Figure 15–5

U.S. Food Waste—Calories Per Capita

About 40 percent of the food produced in the United States each year is wasted. For each person, daily food waste amounts to 1,400 calories worth of food, easily enough to cover the energy needs of a hungry child.

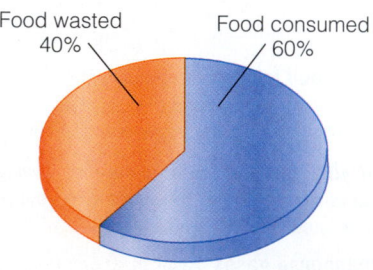

Food wasted 40% Food consumed 60%

aquaculture the farming of aquatic organisms for food, generally fish, mollusks, or crustaceans, that involves such activities as feeding immature organisms, providing habitat, protecting them from predators, harvesting them, and selling or consuming them.

Figure 15–6
Food Recovery Hierarchy

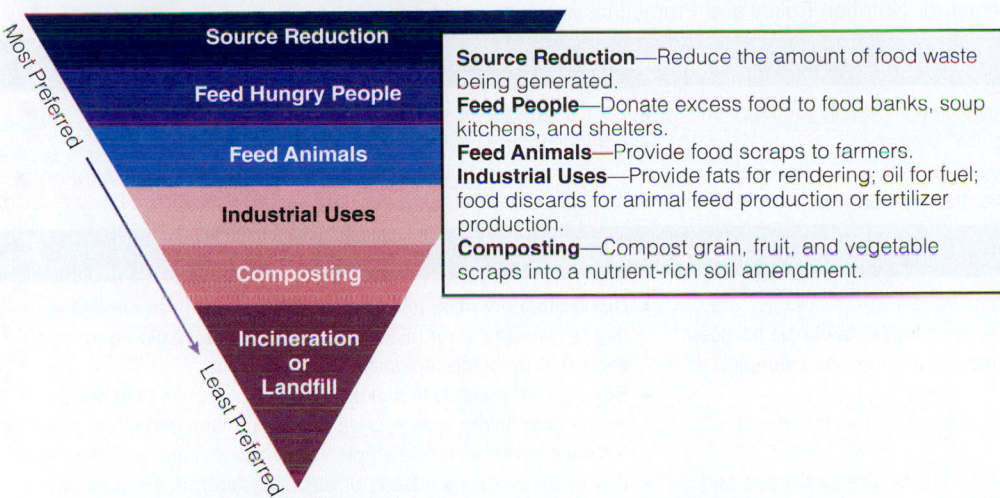

FOOD RECOVERY HIERARCHY

Source Reduction
Feed Hungry People
Feed Animals
Industrial Uses
Composting
Incineration or Landfill

Most Preferred
Least Preferred

Source Reduction—Reduce the amount of food waste being generated.
Feed People—Donate excess food to food banks, soup kitchens, and shelters.
Feed Animals—Provide food scraps to farmers.
Industrial Uses—Provide fats for rendering; oil for fuel; food discards for animal feed production or fertilizer production.
Composting—Compost grain, fruit, and vegetable scraps into a nutrient-rich soil amendment.

Source: Environmental Protection Agency, Generators of food waste, April 26, 2012, available at www.epa.gov.

wastes or plastics.[39] As food waste decomposes, it generates both methane and carbon dioxide, greenhouse gases that contribute to climate change.

The old proverb "Waste not, want not" seems to apply: preventing even half of the current food waste could provide food for huge numbers of people without using a single additional acre of farmland, drop of water, or barrel of oil. In less developed areas of the world, safer storage, better transportation, and more effective packaging are needed to keep food wholesome for human consumption. In this country, better food planning, purchasing, and use by U.S. food service industries and consumers are needed to put food where it belongs: on the plates of hungry people. Figure 15–6 illustrates food recovery methods for food industries, and Table 15–7 (p. 612) provides a guide for individuals in both preventing food waste and saving money.

KEY POINTS

- Unsustainable harvesting threatens the world's wild fish stocks.
- Aquaculture provides a substantial portion of the world's seafood.
- Food loss and waste pose challenges, and reducing them would increase the food supply without additional production inputs.

My Turn watch it!

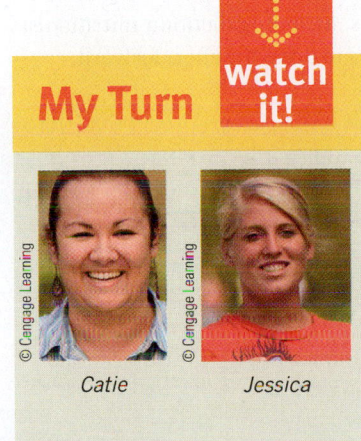

Catie   Jessica

How Responsible Am I?

Listen to two students talk about what they think about individual responsibility with respect to the environment.

Visit www.cengagebrain.com to access MindTap, a complete digital course that includes these videos and other resources.

Table 15–7

How to Reduce Waste and Stretch Food Dollars

Eating well on a budget can pose a challenge, but reducing waste is a good first step. For daily menus and recipes for healthy, thrifty meals, visit the USDA Center for Nutrition Policy and Promotion: www.cnpp.usda.gov.

Plan Ahead

- Plan your menus, write grocery lists, and shop only for foods on your list to avoid expensive "impulse" buying.
- Center meals on whole grains, legumes, and vegetables; use smaller quantities of meat, poultry, fish, or eggs.
- Cook large quantities when time and money allow; freeze portions for convenient later meals.
- Check for sales, and use coupons for products you need; plan meals to take advantage of sale items.

Shop Smart

- Do not shop when hungry.
- Select whole foods instead of convenience foods (raw whole potatoes instead of refrigerated prepared mashed potatoes, for example).
- Try store brands.
- Buy fresh produce in season; buy canned or frozen items at other times.
- Buy large bags of frozen items or dry goods; use as needed and store the remainder.
- Buy cereals to cook, such as oatmeal instead of ready-to-eat breakfast cereals.
- Buy fat-free dry milk; mix and refrigerate quantities needed for a day or two. Buy fresh milk by the gallon or half gallon only if you can use it up before it spoils.
- Buy less red meat. Use inexpensive cuts, such as beef chuck and pork shoulder roasts; cook with liquid long enough to make the meat tender, and add ample vegetables and grains to the meal.
- Buy whole chickens instead of pieces; ask a butcher to show you how to cut them up.
- Frequent discount stores instead of grocery stores for nonfood items such as toilet paper and detergent.

Reduce Waste

- Change your thinking from "what do I want to eat" to "what do I have available to eat." You paid for the food you have on hand, so use it up.
- Buy only the amount of fresh food that you will eat before it spoils. The FDA website offers a refrigerator and freezer storage chart to estimate how long fresh foods will last (see www.fda.gov/Food/FoodborneIllnessContaminants/PeopleAtRisk/ucm182679.htm#storchart).
- Peel away the tough outer layers from stems of asparagus and broccoli; slice and cook the tender stems or add raw to salads.
- Scrub, but don't peel, potatoes before cooking—the skins add color, texture, and nutrients to the dish.
- Before buying food in bulk, plan how to store it properly. If it spoils before use, you'll throw away your savings.
- If your "bargain" bulk food is more than you can use but is still fresh, donate it to your local food bank or homeless shelter. (It won't save you money, but it will provide a wealth of satisfaction.)
- If space permits, compost fruit and vegetable scraps to feed shrubs and other outdoor plants.

How Can People Help?

LO 15.5 Outline the steps that governments, private enterprises, and individuals can take to ensure a sustainable food supply.

Today, the keys to solving the world's poverty, hunger, and environmental problems are within the reach of both poor and rich nations—if they have the will to employ them. In this country, the federal government, the states, local communities, big business and small companies, educators, and all individuals, including dietitian nutritionists and food service managers, have many opportunities to drive the effort forward.

Government Action

Government policies can change to promote sustainability.

- The 2015 Dietary Guidelines for Americans committee focused on sustainability as an essential element of food security for the U.S. population.[40]

- The U.S. government is currently devoting record amounts of tax dollars to subsidizing conservation programs for agricultural lands.

- It also promotes sustainable choices for foods available for purchase at federal facilities, among other initiatives.

However, more can be done.[41]

Private and Community Enterprises

Businesses can take the initiative to help; some already have—AT&T, Prudential, and Kraft General Foods are major supporters of antihunger programs. Restaurants and other food facilities can plan for less food waste and participate in the nation's gleaning effort by giving their fresh leftover foods to community distribution centers and using other food recovery methods. Food producers are more often choosing to produce their goods sustainably to meet a growing demand for products produced with integrity.

Educators and Students

Educators, including nutrition educators, have a crucial role to play. The nation and world look to scientists to solve problems and innovate for the future, so a solid science curriculum is critical for students at every level of education. While still learning, students can share the knowledge they gain with families, friends, and communities and take action in their communities and beyond.

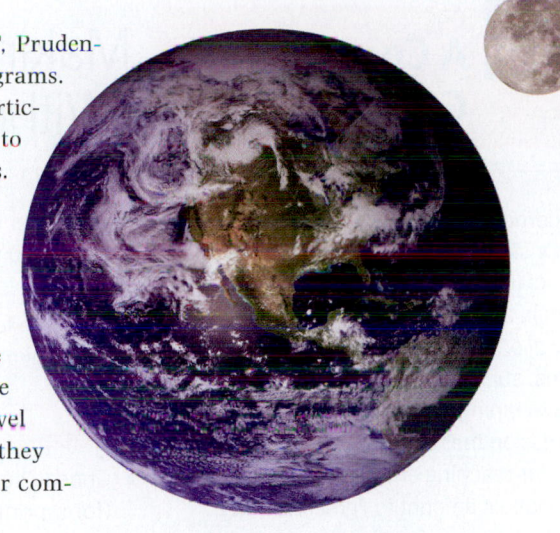

Paul Prescott/Shutterstock.com

Food and Nutrition Professionals

Registered dietitian nutritionists, dietetic technicians, and foodservice managers can make careful, conservative choices in procurement, reuse, recycling, energy use, water use, leadership, and capital improvements both in business and in their personal lives. In addition, the Academy of Nutrition and Dietetics urges its members to work for policy changes in private and government food assistance programs, to intensify education about hunger, and to be advocates on the local, state, and national levels to help end hunger in the United States.[42]

"For every person in the world to reach present U.S. levels of consumption with existing technology would require four more planet Earths."

—E. O. Wilson, 2002

Individuals

All individuals can become involved in these large trends. Many small decisions each day add up to large impacts on the environment. The Consumer's Guide sums up some of these decisions and actions.

Conclusion

No part of the world is safely insulated against future food shortages. Developed countries may be the last to feel the effects, but they will ultimately go as the world goes. To limit the threat will require no less than a major shift in how the world uses its resources. This chapter's Controversy highlights one part of that larger effort: new approaches to continued food abundance through advanced low-input agriculture.

"We do not inherit the earth from our ancestors, we borrow it from our children."

Ascribed to Chief Seattle,
a 19th-century Native American leader

KEY POINT

- Government, business, educators, and individuals have opportunities to promote wise resource use at home and around the world.

Making "Green" Choices (Without Getting "Greenwashed")

Concerned consumers want to shop responsibly. How can they know whether label claims about environmental benefits are truthful? Like the word *natural* on food labels, appealing *green* claims, such as *eco-friendly*, have no legal meaning but may give a false impression that using the product could have far-reaching environmental benefits. Such labels amount to "greenwashing," the shallow use of vague terms or catchy symbols to feign environmental concern and hook unsuspecting consumers.[1]*

Honest manufacturers of "green" products make a sincere effort to mitigate environmental harms from their goods. They make specific, valid claims that are easy to spot: "Made with 60% recycled material," for example. Such labels may also provide a website or phone number for more information. All products have impacts on the environment, however—even the "greenest" ones.

Less Buying, More Doing

As it turns out, the most beneficial choices for the environment often involve less buying and more doing, a trade many consumers are reluctant to make. Viewed from a broader perspective, simple green lifestyle actions such as the following are not purely altruistic—they benefit your health and your budget as well as your planet:

- Ride a bike to work or classes instead of joining a gym to save time and money.
- Shop "carless," to save money on gasoline—use public transportation, bicycle, or walk; carpool when buying bulky items.
- Reduce food waste (review Table 15–7, p. 612).
- Carry clean reusable grocery sacks when biking or driving. Even clean plastic sacks from the store can be reused, and recycled when they wear out.

*Reference notes are found in Appendix F.

- Use fewer electric gadgets. Mix batters, chop vegetables, and open cans by hand.
- Eat more foods from plants, fewer from animals.

Choosing Wisely

- Choose sustainable fish species (for a printable guide, visit www.seafoodwatch.org/seafood-recommendations/consumer-guides).
- Choose minimally packaged items; buy bulk items or those with reusable or recyclable packaging. Packaging uses resources to produce, is bulky to store and handle, and adds substantially to the cost.
- Choose reusable pans, dishes, cups, and utensils, and cloth napkins and kitchen towels rather than disposable ones to save cash and reduce trash.
- Buy reusable plastic food storage containers instead of aluminum foil, plastic wraps, or plastic storage bags. The containers quickly pay for themselves in money *not* spent on disposables.
- Choose coffee and other imported food products labeled "Fair Trade," available at many stores. *Fair Trade* indicates that businesses work toward food security, fair wages for workers, and conservation of natural resources.
- Plant a vegetable or herb garden, or join a community garden. Gardening provides physical activity and food, too. Even a few pots of herbs, lettuces, and radishes in a sunny spot will soon yield a tasty salad.
- Shop at farmers' markets and roadside stands for local foods grown close to home. Locally grown foods require less transportation, packaging, and refrigeration than shipped foods.
- Try picking produce at local farms—it's fun, it's exercise, and it saves money, too.

Bigger Ideas

- Join organizations of like-minded people who work to make things better. You'll enjoy meeting new people and making a difference.
- Buy efficient appliances. ENERGY STAR (see Figure 15–7) appliances rank in the top 25 percent for energy efficiency. These products save money on utility bills year after year.
- Buy from ENERGY STAR–certified manufacturers. They effectively prevent substantial greenhouse gases from entering the air.[2]**
- Insulate the home to save energy and money.

**Find ENERGY STAR–certified partners at www.epa.gov.

Figure 15–7

ENERGY STAR

By choosing ENERGY STAR–certified products, a typical household can save almost $400 per year in energy costs. ENERGY STAR–certified new homes are designed and built to standards that deliver energy savings of up to 30 percent over other new homes. Read more at www.energystar.gov/.

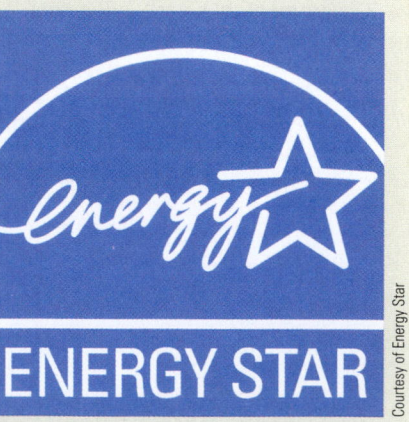

Courtesy of Energy Star

- Consider using solar power, especially to heat water; check with local utilities for reimbursement grants.
- *Reduce.* Save the most money, time, and resources by consuming less. Even recycling has an energy cost.
- *Reuse.* If an item is necessary, go for durable, not disposable.
- *Recycle.* When the last drop of usefulness seems gone, put items into the recycling stream so they can be remade into new useful things.[†]

[†] To help to find out where to recycle common items in your own community, try this website: www.earth911.com.

Moving Ahead

Beyond daily choices, people can make the greatest impact by teaching others and by volunteering with like-minded people in their communities—in local cleanup efforts, in tree-planting projects, and in community gardens. Local food pantries and gleaners also welcome volunteers. If you take action today, you'll soon see the benefits of a "less buying and more doing" lifestyle begin to emerge.

Review Questions[‡]

1. A consumer choosing a product that says "green" on the label can be assured that it is safe for the environment. T F

2. Foods from plants require fewer resources to produce and are generally less expensive to buy than foods from animals. T F

3. Adopting some green lifestyle habits can _____.

   a. save money and benefit personal fitness
   b. reduce household trash
   c. help preserve the environment
   d. all of the above

[‡] Answers to Consumer's Guide review questions are found in Appendix G.

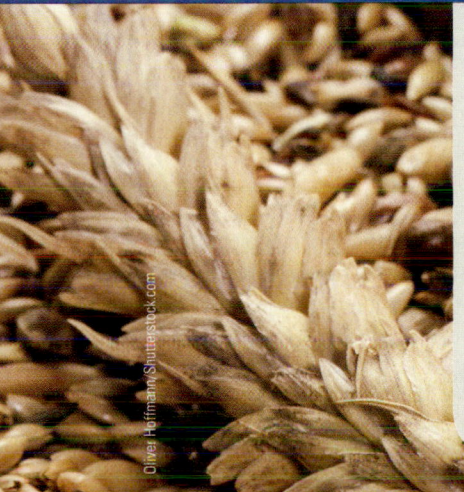

Oliver Hoffmann/Shutterstock.com

what did you decide?

With our abundant food supply, is anyone in the United States hungry?

Can one person make a difference to the world's problems?

Will the earth yield enough food to feed human populations in the future?

Is a meal's monetary price its only cost?

Self Check

1. (LO 15.1) Which of the following is a symptom of food insecurity?
   a. You worry about gaining weight but cannot afford "diet" foods.
   b. You cannot always afford to purchase nutritious foods for balanced meals.
   c. You shop daily to get the best prices and use coupons to stretch your budget.
   d. You buy fresh rather than frozen foods to save money.

2. (LO 15.1) Which of these items can be purchased with electronic debit transfer cards from the Supplemental Nutrition Assistance Program?
   a. hot dogs
   b. cigarettes
   c. dishwashing liquid
   d. red wine

3. (LO 15.1) The primary cause of hunger in the U.S. is
   a. living in food deserts.
   b. a lack of food aid.
   c. a lack of nutrition knowledge.
   d. food poverty.

4. (LO 15.2) Today, famine is most often a result of _____.
   a. global food shortage
   b. drought
   c. social causes such as war
   d. flood

5. (LO 15.2) The world's "poorest poor" spend about 80 percent of their income on food.
   T   F

6. (LO 15.2) Worldwide, _____ of those who die each year from starvation and related illnesses are children.
   a. three-fourths
   b. one-third
   c. one-fourth
   d. none of the above

7. (LO 15.2) Poverty and hunger drive people to bear more children.
   T   F

8. (LO 15.3) The malnutrition of poverty inflicts all of the following except
   a. learning disabilities.
   b. mental retardation.
   c. deafness.
   d. blindness.

9. (LO 15.3) Most children who die of malnutrition starve to death.
   T   F

10. (LO 15.3) The most perilous form of malnutrition, which occurs when food suddenly becomes unavailable, such as in drought or war, is called _____.
    a. severe acute malnutrition (SAM)
    b. chronic malnutrition (CM)
    c. vitamin deficiency malnutrition (VDM)
    d. pericardial abdominal malnutrition (PAM)

11. (LO 15.4) To save a starving child who has a weak heartbeat and low blood pressure, a necessary first step is to quickly administer
    a. protein supplements.
    b. vitamin A supplements.
    c. oral rehydration therapy (ORT).
    d. ready-to-use therapeutic food (RUTF).

12. (LO 15.4) Which of the following is a threat to the future food supply?
    a. fossil fuel use
    b. water shortages
    c. ocean pollution
    d. all of the above

13. (LO 15.4) What percentage of its food supply does the United States waste each year?
    a. 20 percent
    b. 30 percent
    c. 40 percent
    d. 50 percent

14. (LO 15.4) Reducing food waste is a great way to save money.
    T   F

15. (LO 15.5) Today, the keys to solving the world's poverty, hunger, and environmental problems are within the reach of both poor and rich nations.
    T   F

16. (LO 15.5) Only the federal government and large corporations have the resources necessary to make an impact in the fight against poverty, hunger, and environmental degradation.
    T   F

17. (LO 15.6) A vegetarian diet requires just one-third of the energy needed to produce the average meat-containing diet.
    T   F

18. (LO 15.6) The scientific discipline that uses ecological theory to study, design, manage, and evaluate productive agricultural systems to conserve critical resources is known as _____
    a. integrated pest management.
    b. sustainability
    c. agroecology
    d. none of the above

Answers to these Self Check questions are in Appendix G.

How Can We Feed Ourselves Sustainably?

LO 15.6 Describe low-input agriculture and its importance to future food production.

If predictions hold true, the world's farmers will soon face increased pressure to feed a burgeoning world population. To produce this food will require more land, water, and energy, and it must be accomplished while conserving the resources that make growing crops and animals possible into the future. What is needed is nothing short of a second **green revolution**, except that this one must be doubly green: increasing the productivity of available land while protecting or restoring the environment.[1]* In addition, people today are urged to adopt a **sustainable diet**, to ensure that resources are conserved as people are fed.

Costs of Current Food Production Methods

Producing food costs the earth dearly. The environmental impacts of agriculture and the food industry take many forms, such as water use and pollution, greenhouse gas emissions, and resource overuse. Table C15–1 offers definitions of terms relevant to these concepts. Important, but beyond the scope of this discussion, are the costs in terms of human health and other problems associated with farm work, such as overexposure to pesticides.[2]

Reference notes are in Appendix F.

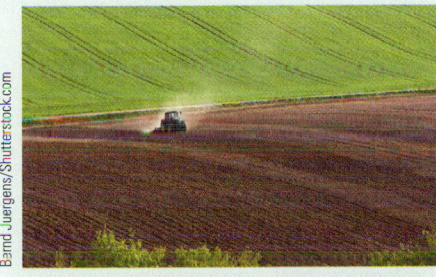

Vast areas under plow are exposed to erosion, and those that must be irrigated can, over time, become salty and unusable.

Impacts on Land and Water

To produce food, first, we clear land—prairie, wetland, or forest—replacing native ecosystems with crops or food animals. Crops pull nutrients from the soil. With each harvest, some of those nutrients are removed, so manufactured fertilizers are applied to replace them. Some of the nitrogen in this fertilizer flies off as gas, contributing to greenhouse gas emissions.

With rain or irrigation, fertilizer from fields and manure from grazing lands and feed lots run off into waterways, causing algae overgrowth. The algae die and decompose, forming ocean **dead zones** as whole areas are depleted of oxygen. Some plowed soil runs off, too, clouding the water and burying aquatic plants and animals. To protect crops, herbicides and pesticides are applied. These poisons also kill native plants, native insects, and animals that eat those plants and insects. Meanwhile, with continued chemical use, weeds and pests grow resistant to their effects.

Finally, we irrigate, a practice that adds salts to the soil—the water evaporates, but the salts do not. As soils become salty, plant growth fails. Irrigation can also deplete the fresh water supply over time because much of the water taken from surface or underground supplies evaporates or runs off. This process, carried to an extreme, can dry up whole rivers and lakes and lower the water table of entire regions.

Soil Depletion

The soil can also be depleted by other agricultural practices, particularly indiscriminate land clearing (deforestation) and overuse by cattle (overgrazing). Traditional farming methods that turn over all topsoil each

Table C15–1
Terms

- **agroecology** a scientific discipline that combines biological, physical, and social sciences with ecological theory to develop methods for producing food sustainably.
- **dead zones** columns of oxygen-depleted ocean water in which marine life cannot survive; often caused by algae blooms that occur when agricultural fertilizers and waste runoff enter natural waterways.
- **farm share** an arrangement in which a farmer offers the public a "subscription" for an allotment of the farm's products throughout the season.
- **green revolution** a series of advances in technology made in the last century that dramatically increased farm yields worldwide. The techniques rely heavily on chemical fertilizers and pesticides, along with large farm machinery.
- **integrated pest management (IPM)** management of pests using a combination of natural and biological controls and minimal or no application of pesticides.
- **low-input agriculture** agriculture practiced on a small scale using individualized approaches that vary with local conditions so as to minimize technological, fuel, and chemical inputs.
- **sustainable diet** a diet with low environmental impact that contributes to food and nutrition security and to healthy life for present and future generations. Sustainable diets are protective and respectful of biodiversity and ecosystems; culturally acceptable; accessible; economically fair and affordable; and nutritionally adequate, safe, and healthy while optimizing natural and human resources.

season expose vast areas to the forces of wind and water. Exposed topsoil blows away on the wind or washes into the sea, leaving an unfertile area behind.

Unsustainable agriculture has already destroyed many once-fertile regions where civilizations formerly flourished. The dry, salty deserts of North Africa were once plowed and irrigated wheat fields, the breadbasket of the Roman Empire. Today's mistreatment of soil and water is causing destruction on an unprecedented scale.

Loss of Species

Agriculture also weakens its own underpinnings when it fails to conserve species diversity. By the year 2050, some 40,000 plant species, existing today, may go extinct. The United Nations Food and Agriculture Organization attributes many of the losses to modern farming practices, as well as to human population growth.

Global eating habits are growing more uniform, a trend that contributes to species loss. As people everywhere eat the same limited array of foods, demand for local, genetically diverse, native plants is insufficient to make them financially worth preserving. Yet, in the future, as the climate warms, those very plants may be needed for food. A wild species of corn that grows in a dry climate, for example, might contain just the genetic information necessary to help make the domestic corn crop resistant to drought. For this and other reasons, protecting biodiversity is a critical human need.

Fuel Use and Energy Sources

Energy and fertilizers from fossil fuels have spurred unprecedented gains in agricultural output, but scientists now recognize that, with limited fossil fuel resources, such gains are not sustainable into the future. Fossil fuel use itself also threatens the future of food production by contributing to pollution and global climate changes.

Biofuels made from renewable corn and soybeans were once hailed as safer alternatives to fossil fuels, but these also carry high environmental costs. Strong world demand for corn or soybean ethanol triggers the conversion of wild native habitats into corn and soybean fields, diverts resources away from growing food crops needed to feed hungry local populations, and increases greenhouse gas emissions.[3] Other materials, such as native grasses and even genetically engineered algae, appear to be more promising materials than food crops for biofuel production.[4] Other potential energy sources, such as wind and solar energy, remain underdeveloped.

Fossil Energy in Food Production

For the roughly 300 calories of food energy available in a can of corn, more than 6,000 calories of fuel (including those needed for the can and transportation) are used to produce it; add 2,000 more calories of fuel to that if the corn comes frozen. Food production represents one-quarter of U.S. fossil energy consumption, mainly for fertilizers, pesticides, and irrigation. Corn and soybeans account for most of the pesticide use.[5] Clearly, food carries an additional cost to the environment—a constellation of inputs not simple to grasp—and not reflected in the price tag. These "hidden" costs must come to account so that our food systems can feed future populations.

The Problems of Livestock

Raising livestock takes an enormous toll on land and energy resources. Like plant crops, herds of livestock occupy land that once maintained itself in a natural state. The land suffers losses of native plants and animals, soil erosion, water depletion, and desert formation.

U.S. Meat Production

If animals are raised in concentrated areas such as cattle feedlots or giant hog "farms," huge masses of manure produced in these overcrowded, factory-style farms leach into local soils and water supplies, polluting them. In an effort to control this source of pollution, the U.S. Environmental Protection Agency (EPA) offers incentives to livestock farmers who agree to clean up

Figure C15–1

Pounds of Grain Needed to Produce One Pound of Bread and One Pound of Animal Weight Gain[a]

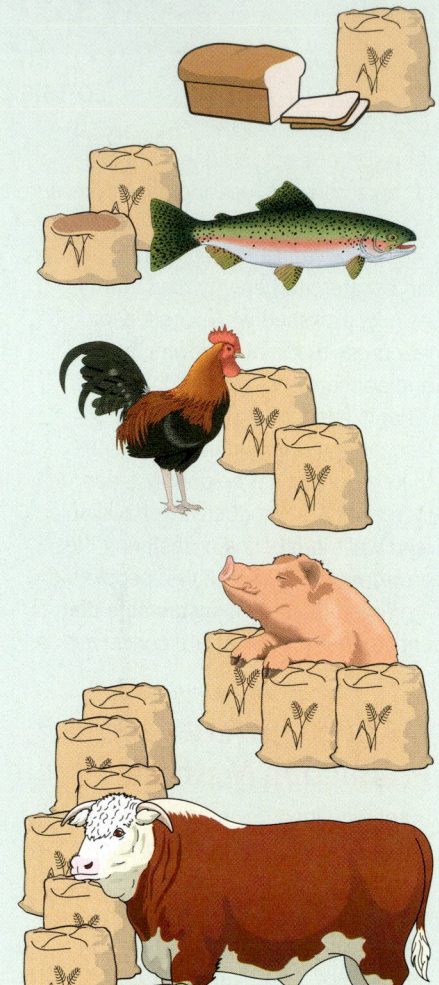

[a]Estimates of grain intakes for beef vary from less than 2.5 to more than 10 pounds of grain depending upon how long the animal is allowed to graze and how long it spends in a feedlot.

their wastes and allow their operations to be monitored for pollution.

In addition, animals in such feedlots must be fed, and grain is grown for them on other land (Figure C15–1, compares the grain required to produce various foods). That grain may require fertilizers, herbicides, pesticides, and irrigation, too. In the United States, one-fifth of all cropland is used to produce feed for livestock—more land than is used to produce grain for people.

World Trends in Meat Consumption

The world is demanding more meat and dairy products, putting pressure on ecological systems.[6] In 1999, for example, meat and milk consumption in East Asia was a little over 100 pounds per person per year; by 2030, yearly consumption will rise to almost 170 pounds per person. This trend has been underestimated in long-term projections of the world's demand for food and energy.

The Future Starts Now

For each of the problems just described, solutions are being devised, and their use is growing worldwide.[7] Across the nation, ideas for sustainable food production are emerging from a new field of study: **agroecology**. This scientific discipline applies ecological theory to develop productive agricultural systems that conserve critical resources.

The crop yields from farms that employ agroecological practices often compare favorably with those from farms using methods of the green revolution. The first of these practices, **low-input agriculture**, emphasizes strategic use of natural processes wherever possible, reducing the need for chemically intensive methods.

Low-Input and Precision Agriculture

Farmers may use low-input agriculture, adopting **integrated pest management (IPM)** strategies, such as rotating crops and introducing natural predators to control pests, rather than depending on pesticides alone. Many low-input techniques are not really new—they would be familiar to our great-grandparents. Many farmers today are rediscovering the benefits of old techniques while also taking advantage of newer technologies, such as precision agriculture, that their predecessors could not have imagined.

The meaning of *precision agriculture* is much the way it sounds: farmers adjust soil and crop management to target the precise needs of various areas

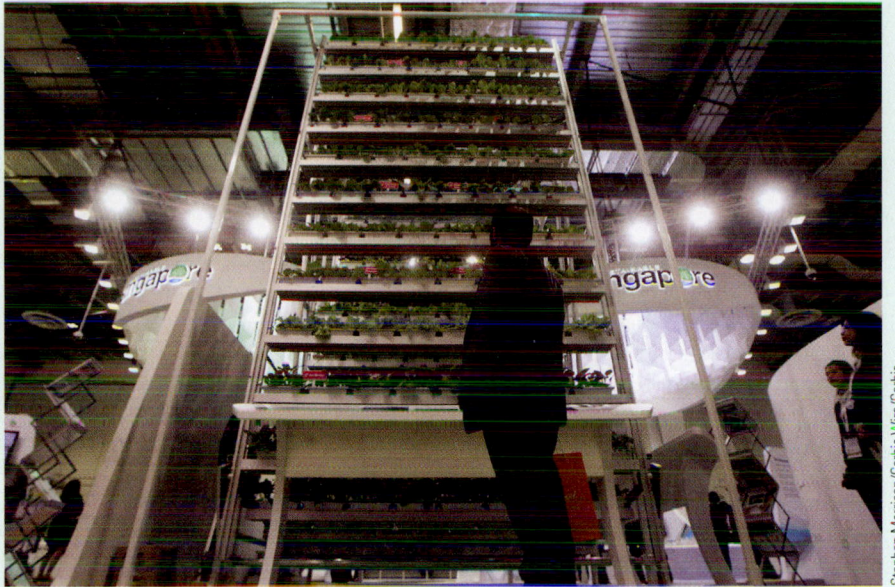

Vertical farms make use of air space instead of acreage. Farming this way requires 95 percent less water than conventional farms, uses no pesticides, and generates no polluting runoff.

of the farm. *Global positioning satellite (GPS)* units in the sky beam data about a field to GPS receiving devices on equipment here on earth. Farmers use the information to target, within a meter's accuracy, land areas that need treatments. The potential dollar and environmental savings in terms of water, fertilizers, and pesticides are enormous. The initial cost of the equipment, however, is high.

Soil Conservation

The U.S. Conservation Reserve Program provides federal assistance to farmers and ranchers who wish to improve their conservation of soil, water, and related natural resources on environmentally sensitive lands.[8] It encourages farmers to plant native grasses, food plants for wildlife, or trees instead of cash crops on highly erodible cropland, wetlands, or other environmentally sensitive acreage. It also encourages conservative techniques such as shallow tilling and the planting of grassy strips to control the flow of water off fields, reducing erosion, and protecting local water quality.

Other programs offer incentives for improving air quality or water quality or for purchasing sensitive lands for conservation. Private foundations or other groups may get help in funding such programs from local, state, or federal agencies.

The Potential of Genetic Engineering

Many farmers worldwide report both financial and conservation benefits from planting genetically engineered crops.[9] Growing herbicide-resistant crops, for example, requires less tilling of the soil to reduce weed growth, decreasing soil loss from wind and water erosion. Pesticide-resistant crops demand less use of both petroleum-based pesticides and the fuel to run the equipment to apply them. Salt-resistant crops can grow in salty areas where conventional crops wither. If approached carefully (see Controversy 12), genetic engineering promises economically feasible, environmentally conservative options for agricultural lands.[10] Table C15–2 (p. 620) provides other approaches to food sustainability. In the struggle to secure global food and energy for the future, no resource can be overlooked and none wasted.

Energy Conservation

Worldwide, the demand for energy increases daily, while fossil fuel supplies dwindle. To conserve energy for the future, our consumption of energy and our means of producing and using it must change. The food industry, for example, is evaluating energy inputs for producing,

Table C15–2

Twelve Steps for the Future of Food

1. **Employ agroforestry.** Planting trees in and around farms reduces soil erosion by providing a natural barrier against strong winds and rainfall, and roots stabilize and nourish soils.

2. **Improve soil management.** Alternating crop species allows soil to rest, restores nutrients, and controls pests. Soil amendments, such as biochar, help soils retain moisture near plant roots.

3. **Increase crop diversity.** Growing many crop varieties reduces pests and diseases and decreases reliance on single varieties, increasing domestic food security.

4. **Increase livestock diversity.** Genetic diversity in food animals strengthens disease resistance. Lesser-known livestock such as North American bison are often hardier and produce richer milk.

5. **Improve food production from existing livestock.** Feeding grass rather than corn or soybeans to animals lowers the demand for feedstuffs and reduces pressure on global human food supplies.

6. **Support "Meatless Mondays."** Forgoing meat on one day a week reduces environmental impacts; the same choice is also widely associated with lower risks of chronic disease in people.

7. **Use smarter irrigation.** Installing water sensors or micro-irrigation technology and planning water-efficient gardens or farms using specific crops and locations can conserve crucial water supplies.

8. **Use integrated farming systems.** Integrated farming systems, such as permaculture, improve soil fertility and agricultural productivity by using natural resources as efficiently as possible. Research on implementation of techniques such as recycling wastewater and planting groups of plants that use the same resources in related ways is expanding rapidly across the United States.

9. **Use organic and agroecological farming.** Organic and agroecological farming methods are designed to build soil quality and promote plant and animal health in harmony with local ecosystems.

10. **Support small-scale farmers.** Small farms often specialize in growing fruits and vegetables for human consumption; large farms often focus on corn and soybeans for industrial uses.

11. **Reevaluate ethanol as fuel.** Encouraging clean energy alternatives to crop-based biofuels will increase the amount of food available for consumption.

12. **Support agricultural research.** Government support for agricultural research and its applications can help address issues such as hunger, malnutrition, and poverty.

Source: Adapted from Worldwatch Institute, 12 innovations to combat drought, improve food security, and stabilize food prices, August 2, 2012, available at www.worldwatch.org/12-innovations-combat -drought-improve-food-security-and-stabilize-food-prices.

processing, packaging, transporting, storing, and preparing foods.

Energy Recycling

A new paradigm for energy calls for converting wastes into energy at many levels of food production. For example:

- Vermont's dairy farmers who join the state-sponsored "Cow Power" program convert methane from cow manure into electricity, which is then sold to utility customers.[11]

- Other farmers turn plant waste into charcoal and bury it, trapping carbon underground and fertilizing the soil, thus avoiding applications of fossil fuel–based fertilizer.[12]

- Some communities capture methane gas, also called "natural gas," produced by decomposing garbage in landfills and use it to fuel vehicles, such as garbage trucks.[13]

Consumer dollars also represent the energy spent to earn them, and they factor into the sustainability equation. Consumers can help by spending their dollars on foods that require low energy inputs from industry, a choice that is described next.

Roles of Consumers

Conscientious consumers can reduce pollution and the use of resources through the choices they make. Some new, fresh ways of thinking about how to obtain foods, and which foods to choose, can enliven the diet and enrich daily life.

Keeping Local Profits Local

Farmers selling their broccoli, carrots, and apples at city farmers' markets and roadside stands often net a higher profit. In addition, families who buy homegrown produce tend to eat a greater quantity and variety of fruits and vegetables, and the health benefits of this outcome are well known. Through a **farm share**, consumers can buy a weekly share of a local farmer's crops, harvested in season and picked up while fresh.

Good for You, Good for the Planet

An often overlooked point: food choices that benefit the environment also benefit human health.[14] A sustainable diet is higher in legumes, whole grains, nuts, seeds, fruit, and vegetables and lower in red meats and highly processed foods. The same kind of diet also reduces risks for chronic diseases.

Overall, a vegetarian diet requires just one-third of the energy needed to produce the average meat-containing diet. As mentioned, meat production entails tremendous amounts of water, grain, and land, thus reducing the resources available to grow staple foods for human beings. An exception is livestock raised on the open range; these animals eat grass and require low energy inputs. So much of our beef is grain-fed, however, that the average energy requirement to produce it is high. Opting for more foods derived from plants and fewer foods derived from animals conserves resources while reducing chronic disease risks.

All in all, our choices as a nation add up to a measurable "ecological footprint"—the productive land and water required to supply all of the resources an individual consumes and to absorb all of the wastes generated using prevailing practices. The footprint of each individual is four times larger in an industrialized country than in a developing one (see Figure C15–2). To help size up your own ecological footprint, take the quiz in Table C15–3 on page 622.

Conclusion

The problems of providing food for future generations are global in scope, yet the actions of individual people lie at the heart of their solutions. Do what you can to tread lightly on the earth. Celebrate changes that are possible today by making them a permanent part of your life, and reap the benefits of increased health and well-being; do the same with changes that become possible tomorrow—and every day thereafter.

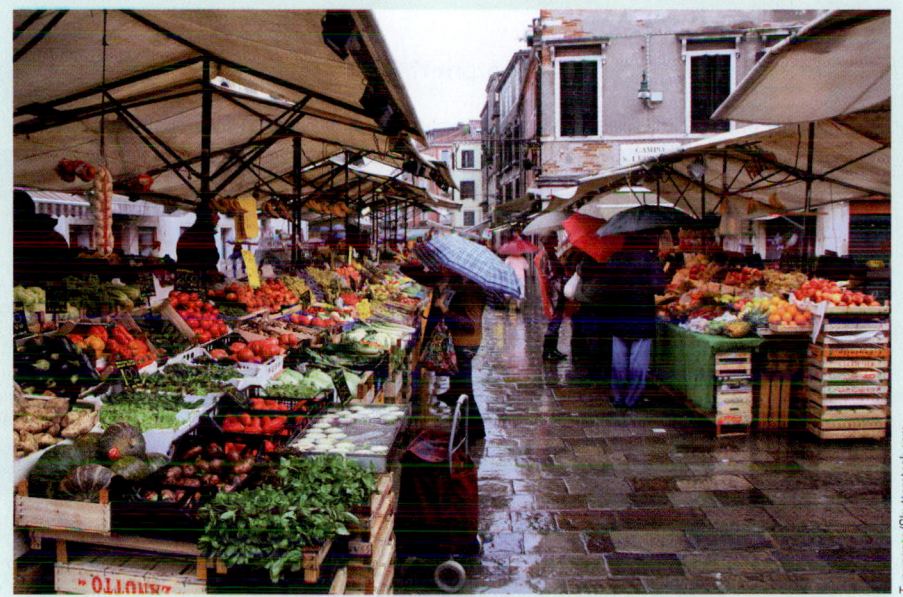

Farmers' markets and farm share arrangements provide fresh foods from local growers.

Figure C15–2

Ecological Footprints

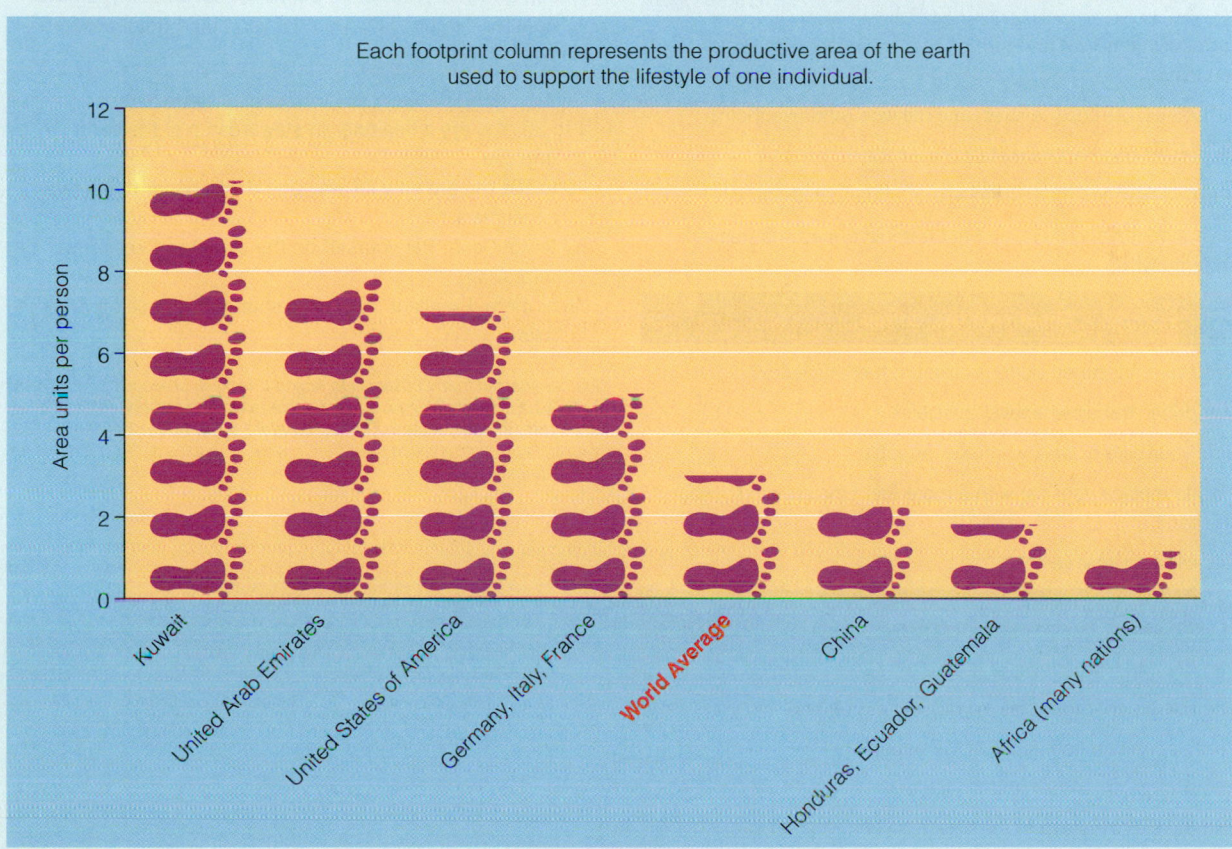

Each footprint column represents the productive area of the earth used to support the lifestyle of one individual.

Source: Data from Global Footprint Network, Footprint by country, 2014, available at www.footprintnetwork.org/index.php.

How Big Is Your Ecological Footprint?

This quiz can help you evaluate your impact on the earth. The higher you score, the smaller your "footprint."

At home, do you

1. Recycle everything you can: newspapers, cans, glass bottles and jars, scrap metal, used oil, etc.?
2. Use cold water in the washer whenever possible?
3. Turn off the tap while you scrub your hands or brush your teeth?
4. Avoid using appliances (such as electric can openers) to do things you can do by hand?
5. Reuse grocery bags to line your wastebasket? Reuse or recycle bread bags, butter tubs, etc.?
6. Store food in reusable containers rather than plastic wrap, disposable bags and containers, or aluminum foil?

In the yard, do you

7. Pull weeds instead of using herbicides?
8. Fertilize with manure and compost, rather than with chemical fertilizers?
9. Compost your leaves and yard debris, rather than burning them?
10. Take extra plastic and rubber pots back to the plant nursery?

On vacation, do you

11. Turn down the heat and turn off the hot water heater before you leave?
12. Carry reusable cups, dishes, and flatware (and use them)?
13. Dispose of trash appropriately (never litter)?
14. Buy no souvenirs made from wild or endangered animals?
15. Stay on roads and trails, and not trample dunes and fragile undergrowth?

About your car, do you

16. Keep your car tuned up for maximum fuel efficiency?
17. Use public transit whenever possible?
18. Ride your bike or walk whenever possible?
19. Plan to replace your car with a more fuel-efficient model when you can?
20. Recycle your engine oil?

At school or work, do you

21. Recycle paper whenever possible?
22. Use scrap paper for notes to yourself and others?
23. Print or copy on both sides of the paper?
24. Reuse large envelopes and file folders?
25. Use the stairs instead of the elevator whenever you can?

When buying, do you

26. Buy as little plastic and foam packaging as possible?
27. Buy permanent, rather than disposable, products?
28. Buy paper rather than plastic, if you must buy disposable products?
29. Buy fresh produce grown locally?
30. Buy in bulk to avoid unnecessary packaging?

In other areas, do you

31. Volunteer your time to conservation projects?
32. Encourage your family, friends, and neighbors to save resources, too?
33. Write letters to support conservation issues?

Scoring

First, give yourself 4 points for answering this quiz: ____
Then, give yourself 1 point each for all the habits you know people should adopt. This is to give you credit for your awareness, even if you haven't acted on it yet (total possible points = 33): ____
Finally, give yourself 2 more points for each habit you have adopted—or honestly would if you could (total possible points = 66): ____

Total score:
1 to 25: You are a beginner in stewardship of the earth. Try to improve.
26 to 50: You are on your way and doing better than many consumers.
51 to 75: Good. Pat yourself on the back, and keep on improving.
76 or more: Excellent. You are a shining example for others to follow.

Source: Adapted from Conservation Action Checklist, produced by the Washington Park Zoo, Portland, Oregon, and available from Conservation International, 1015 18th St. N.W., Suite 1000, Washington, D.C. 20036: 1-800-406-2306 (website: www.conservation.org). Call or write for copies of the original or for more information.

Appendix Table of Contents

Table of Food Composition

This table of food composition is updated periodically to reflect current nutrient data for foods, to remove outdated foods, and to add foods that are new to the marketplace.* The nutrient database for this Appendix is compiled from a variety of sources, including the USDA Nutrient Database and manufacturers' data. The USDA database provides data for a wider variety of foods and nutrients than other sources. Because laboratory analysis for each nutrient can be quite costly, manu-facturers tend to provide data only for those nutrients mandated on food labels. Consequently, data for their foods are often incomplete; any missing information on this table is designated as a dash. Keep in mind that a dash means only that the information is unknown and should not be interpreted as a zero. A zero means that the nutrient is not present in the food.

When using nutrient data, remember that many factors influence the nutri-ent contents of foods. These factors include the mineral content of the soil, the diet fed to the animal or the fertilizer used on the plant, the season of harvest, the method of processing, the length and method of storage, the method of cooking, the method of analysis, and the moisture content of the sample analyzed. With so many influencing factors, users should view nutrient data as a close approximation of the actual amount.

For updates, corrections, and a list of more than 75,000 foods and codes found in the diet analysis software that accompanies this text, visit www.cengagebrain.com and click on Diet & Wellness Plus.

- *Fats* Total fats, as well as the breakdown of total fats to saturated, monounsatu-rated, and polyunsaturated, are listed in the table. The fatty acids seldom add up to the total in part due to rounding but also because values may include some non-fatty acids, such as glycerol, phosphate, or sterols. *Trans*-fatty acids are not listed separately because newer hydrogenated fats generally add less than 0.5 g *trans* fat to a serving of food, an amount often reported as 0.

- *Vitamin A, Vitamin E, and Folate* In keeping with the DRI values for vitamin A, this Appendix presents data for vitamin A in micrograms (μg) RAE. Similarly, because the DRI intake values for vitamin E are based only on the alpha-tocopherol form of vitamin E, this Appendix reports vitamin E data in milligrams (mg) alpha-tocopherol, listed on the table as Vit E (mg α). Folate values are listed in μg DFE, a unit that equalizes the bioavailability of naturally occurring folate and added folic acid in enriched foods.

- *Bioavailability* Keep in mind that the availability of nutrients from foods depends not only on the quantity provided by a food as reflected in this table but also on the amount absorbed and used by the body.

- *Using the Table* The foods and beverages in this table are organized into several categories, which are listed at the head of each right-hand page. Page numbers are provided, and each group is color-coded to make it easier to find individual foods.

---

*This food composition table has been prepared by Cengage Learning. The nutritional data are supplied by Axxya Systems.

Table of Food Composition

(Computer code is for Cengage Diet & Wellness Plus program)

D&W+ Code	Food Description	QTY	Measure	Wt (g)	H₂O (g)	Ener (cal)	Prot (g)	Carb (g)	Fiber (g)	Fat (g)	Fat Breakdown (g)		
											Sat	Mono	Poly
Breads, Baked Goods, Cakes, Cookies, Crackers, Chips, Pies													
	Bagels												
8534	Cinnamon and raisin	1	item(s)	71	22.7	194	7.0	39.2	1.6	1.2	0.2	0.1	0.5
14395	Multi-grain	1	item(s)	61	—	170	6.0	35.0	1.0	1.5	0.5	0.1	0.4
8538	Oat bran	1	item(s)	71	23.4	181	7.6	37.8	2.6	0.9	0.1	0.2	0.3
4910	Plain, enriched	1	item(s)	71	25.8	182	7.1	35.9	1.6	1.2	0.3	0.4	0.5
4911	Plain, enriched, toasted	1	item(s)	66	18.7	190	7.4	37.7	1.7	1.1	0.2	0.3	0.6
	Biscuits												
25008	Biscuits	1	item(s)	41	15.8	121	2.6	16.4	0.5	4.9	1.4	1.4	1.8
16729	Scone	1	item(s)	42	11.5	148	3.8	19.1	0.6	6.2	2.0	2.5	1.3
25166	Wheat biscuits	1	item(s)	55	21.0	162	3.6	21.9	1.4	6.7	1.9	1.9	2.5
	Bread												
325	Boston brown, canned	1	slice(s)	45	21.2	88	2.3	19.5	2.1	0.7	0.1	0.1	0.3
8716	Bread sticks, plain	4	item(s)	24	1.5	99	2.9	16.4	0.7	2.3	0.3	0.9	0.9
25176	Cornbread	1	piece(s)	55	25.9	141	4.7	18.3	0.9	5.4	2.1	1.4	1.5
327	Cracked wheat	1	slice(s)	25	9.0	65	2.2	12.4	1.4	1.0	0.2	0.5	0.2
9079	Croutons, plain	¼	cup(s)	8	0.4	31	0.9	5.5	0.4	0.5	0.1	0.2	0.1
8582	Egg	1	slice(s)	40	13.9	113	3.8	19.1	0.9	2.4	0.6	0.9	0.4
8585	Egg, toasted	1	slice(s)	37	10.5	117	3.9	19.5	0.9	2.4	0.6	1.1	0.4
329	French	1	slice(s)	32	8.9	92	3.8	18.1	0.8	0.6	0.2	0.1	0.3
8591	French, toasted	1	slice(s)	23	4.7	73	3.0	14.2	0.7	0.5	0.1	0.1	0.2
42096	Indian fry, made with lard (Navajo)	3	ounce(s)	85	26.9	281	5.7	41.0	—	10.4	3.9	3.8	0.9
332	Italian	1	slice(s)	30	10.7	81	2.6	15.0	0.8	1.1	0.3	0.2	0.4
1393	Mixed grain	1	slice(s)	26	9.6	69	3.5	11.3	1.9	1.1	0.2	0.2	0.5
8604	Mixed grain, toasted	1	slice(s)	24	7.6	69	3.5	11.3	1.9	1.1	0.2	0.2	0.5
8605	Oat bran	1	slice(s)	30	13.2	71	3.1	11.9	1.4	1.3	0.2	0.5	0.5
8608	Oat bran, toasted	1	slice(s)	27	10.4	70	3.1	11.8	1.3	1.3	0.2	0.5	0.5
8609	Oatmeal	1	slice(s)	27	9.9	73	2.3	13.1	1.1	1.2	0.2	0.4	0.5
8613	Oatmeal, toasted	1	slice(s)	25	7.8	73	2.3	13.2	1.1	1.2	0.2	0.4	0.5
1409	Pita	1	item(s)	60	19.3	165	5.5	33.4	1.3	0.7	0.1	0.1	0.3
7905	Pita, whole wheat	1	item(s)	64	19.6	170	6.3	35.2	4.7	1.7	0.3	0.2	0.7
338	Pumpernickel	1	slice(s)	32	12.1	80	2.8	15.2	2.1	1.0	0.1	0.3	0.4
334	Raisin, enriched	1	slice(s)	26	8.7	71	2.1	13.6	1.1	1.1	0.3	0.6	0.2
8625	Raisin, toasted	1	slice(s)	24	6.7	71	2.1	13.7	1.1	1.2	0.3	0.6	0.2
10168	Rice, white, gluten free, wheat free	1	slice(s)	38	—	130	1.0	18.0	0.5	6.0	0	—	—
8653	Rye	1	slice(s)	32	11.9	83	2.7	15.5	1.9	1.1	0.2	0.4	0.3
8654	Rye, toasted	1	slice(s)	29	9.0	82	2.7	15.4	1.9	1.0	0.2	0.4	0.3
336	Rye, light	1	slice(s)	25	9.3	65	2.0	12.0	1.6	1.0	0.2	0.3	0.3
8588	Sourdough	1	slice(s)	25	7.0	72	2.9	14.1	0.6	0.5	0.1	0.1	0.2
8592	Sourdough, toasted	1	slice(s)	23	4.7	73	3.0	14.2	0.7	0.5	0.1	0.1	0.2
491	Submarine or hoagie roll	1	item(s)	135	40.6	400	11.0	72.0	3.8	8.0	1.8	3.0	2.2
8596	Vienna, toasted	1	slice(s)	23	4.7	73	3.0	14.2	0.7	0.5	0.1	0.1	0.2
8670	Wheat	1	slice(s)	25	8.9	67	2.7	11.9	0.9	0.9	0.2	0.2	0.4
8671	Wheat, toasted	1	slice(s)	23	5.6	72	3.0	12.8	1.1	1.0	0.2	0.2	0.4
340	White	1	slice(s)	25	9.1	67	1.9	12.7	0.6	0.8	0.2	0.2	0.3
1395	Whole wheat	1	slice(s)	46	15.0	128	3.9	23.6	2.8	2.5	0.4	0.5	1.4
	Cakes												
386	Angel food, prepared from mix	1	piece(s)	50	16.5	129	3.1	29.4	0.1	0.2	0	0	0.1
8772	Butter pound, ready to eat, commercially prepared	1	slice(s)	75	18.5	291	4.1	36.6	0.4	14.9	8.7	4.4	0.8
28517	Carrot	1	slice(s)	131	56.6	339	4.8	56.5	1.9	11.1	1.0	5.7	3.8
4931	Chocolate with chocolate icing, commercially prepared	1	slice(s)	64	14.7	235	2.6	34.9	1.8	10.5	3.1	5.6	1.2
8756	Chocolate, prepared from mix	1	slice(s)	95	23.2	352	5.0	50.7	1.5	14.3	5.2	5.7	2.6
393	Devil's food cupcake with chocolate frosting	1	item(s)	35	8.4	120	2.0	20.0	0.7	4.0	1.8	1.6	0.6
8757	Fruitcake, ready to eat, commercially prepared	1	piece(s)	43	10.9	139	1.2	26.5	1.6	3.9	0.5	1.8	1.4
1397	Pineapple upside down, prepared from mix	1	slice(s)	115	37.1	367	4.0	58.1	0.9	13.9	3.4	6.0	3.8
411	Sponge, prepared from mix	1	slice(s)	63	18.5	187	4.6	36.4	0.3	2.7	0.8	1.0	0.4

PAGE KEY: A-4 = Breads/Baked Goods A-10 = Cereal/Rice/Pasta A-14 = Fruit A-20 = Vegetables/Legumes A-30 = Nuts/Seeds A-32 = Vegetarian A-34 = Dairy A-42 = Eggs A-42 = Seafood A-46 = Meats A-50 = Poultry A-50 = Processed Meats A-52 = Beverages A-56 = Fats/Oils A-58 = Sweets A-60 = Spices/Condiments/Sauces A-64 = Mixed Foods/Soups/Sandwiches A-70 = Fast Food A-90 = Convenience A-92 = Baby Foods

CHOL (mg)	CALC (mg)	IRON (mg)	MAGN (mg)	POTA (mg)	SODI (mg)	ZINC (mg)	VIT A (µg)	THIA (mg)	VIT E (mg α)	RIBO (mg)	NIAC (mg)	VIT B6 (mg)	FOLA (µg DFE)	VIT C (mg)	VIT B12 (µg)	SELE (µg)
0	13	2.69	19.9	105.1	228.6	0.80	14.9	0.27	0.22	0.19	2.18	0.04	123.5	0.5	0	22.0
0	60	1.08	—	—	310.0	—	0	—	—	—	2.10	—	—	0	—	—
0	9	2.18	22.0	81.7	360.0	0.63	0.7	0.23	0.23	0.24	2.10	0.03	95.1	0.1	0	24.3
0	63	4.29	15.6	53.3	318.1	1.34	0	0.42	0.07	0.18	2.82	0.04	160.5	0.7	0	16.2
0	65	2.97	15.8	56.1	316.8	0.85	0	0.39	0.07	0.17	2.88	0.04	134.0	0	0	16.6
0	38	0.94	6.0	47.4	206.0	0.20	—	0.16	0.01	0.12	1.20	0.01	46.8	0.1	0.1	7.1
49	79	1.35	7.1	48.7	277.2	0.29	64.7	0.14	0.42	0.15	1.19	0.02	49.1	0	0.1	10.9
0	57	1.21	16.1	81.0	321.1	0.42	—	0.19	0.01	0.14	1.65	0.03	63.2	0.1	0.1	0
0	32	0.94	28.4	143.1	284.0	0.22	11.3	0.01	0.14	0.05	0.50	0.03	6.3	0	0	9.9
0	5	1.02	7.7	29.8	157.7	0.21	0	0.14	0.24	0.13	1.26	0.01	61.0	0	0	9.0
21	94	0.91	10.5	71.5	209.8	0.48	—	0.14	0.32	0.15	1.03	0.04	78.7	1.7	0.2	6.2
0	11	0.70	13.0	44.3	134.5	0.31	0	0.09	—	0.06	0.92	0.08	19.0	0	0	6.3
0	6	0.30	2.3	9.3	52.4	0.06	0	0.04	—	0.02	0.40	0.00	15.7	0	0	2.8
20	37	1.21	7.6	46.0	196.8	0.31	25.2	0.17	0.10	0.17	1.93	0.02	52.0	0	0	12.0
21	38	1.23	7.8	46.6	199.8	0.31	25.5	0.14	0.10	0.16	1.77	0.02	47.7	0	0	12.2
0	14	1.16	9.0	41.0	208.0	0.29	0	0.13	0.05	0.09	1.52	0.03	73.6	0.1	0	8.7
0	11	0.89	7.1	32.2	165.6	0.24	0	0.10	0.04	0.09	1.24	0.02	49.9	0	0	6.8
6	48	3.43	15.3	65.5	279.8	0.29	0	0.36	0.00	0.18	3.91	0.03	166.7	—	0	15.8
0	23	0.88	8.1	33.0	175.2	0.25	0	0.14	0.08	0.08	1.31	0.01	91.2	0	0	8.2
0	27	0.65	20.3	59.8	109.2	0.44	0	0.07	0.09	0.03	1.05	0.06	19.5	0	0	8.6
0	27	0.65	20.4	60.0	109.7	0.44	0	0.06	0.10	0.03	1.05	0.07	16.8	0	0	8.6
0	20	0.93	10.5	44.1	122.1	0.26	0.6	0.15	0.13	0.10	1.44	0.02	36.0	0	0	9.0
0	19	0.92	9.2	33.2	121.0	0.28	0.5	0.12	0.13	0.09	1.29	0.01	28.1	0	0	8.9
0	18	0.72	10.0	38.3	161.7	0.27	1.4	0.10	0.13	0.06	0.84	0.01	23.5	0	0	6.6
0	18	0.74	10.3	38.5	162.8	0.28	1.3	0.09	0.13	0.06	0.77	0.02	18.7	0.1	0	6.7
0	52	1.57	15.6	72.0	321.6	0.50	0	0.35	0.18	0.19	2.77	0.02	99.0	0	0	16.3
0	10	1.95	44.2	108.8	340.5	0.97	0	0.21	0.39	0.05	1.81	0.17	22.4	0	0	28.2
0	22	0.91	17.3	66.6	214.7	0.47	0	0.10	0.13	0.09	0.98	0.04	40.0	0	0	7.8
0	17	0.75	6.8	59.0	101.4	0.18	0	0.08	0.07	0.10	0.90	0.01	40.6	0	0	5.2
0	17	0.76	6.7	59.0	101.8	0.19	0	0.07	0.07	0.09	0.81	0.02	35.5	0.1	0	5.2
0	100	1.08	—	—	140	—	—	0.15	—	0.10	1.20	—	47.5	0	—	—
0	23	0.90	12.8	53.1	211.2	0.36	0	0.13	0.10	0.10	1.21	0.02	48.3	0.1	0	9.9
0	23	0.89	12.5	53.1	210.3	0.36	0	0.11	0.10	0.09	1.09	0.02	42.9	0.1	0	9.9
0	20	0.70	3.9	51.0	175.0	0.18	0	0.10	—	0.08	0.80	0.01	5.3	0	0	8.0
0	11	0.91	7.0	32.0	162.5	0.23	0	0.11	0.05	0.07	1.19	0.03	57.5	0.1	0	6.8
0	11	0.89	7.1	32.2	165.6	0.24	0	0.10	0.04	0.09	1.24	0.02	49.9	0	0	6.8
0	100	3.80	—	128.0	683.0	—	0	0.54	—	0.33	4.50	0.04	—	0	—	42.0
0	11	0.89	7.1	32.2	165.6	0.24	0	0.10	0.04	0.09	1.24	0.02	49.9	0	0	6.8
0	36	0.87	12.0	46.0	130.3	0.30	0	0.09	0.05	0.08	1.30	0.03	24.8	0.1	0	7.2
0	38	0.94	13.6	51.3	140.5	0.34	0	0.10	0.06	0.09	1.44	0.04	23.0	0	0	7.7
0	38	0.94	5.8	25.0	170.3	0.19	0	0.11	0.06	0.08	1.10	0.02	42.8	0	0	4.3
0	15	1.42	37.3	144.4	159.2	0.69	0	0.13	0.35	0.10	1.83	0.09	35.9	0	0	17.8
0	42	0.11	4.0	67.5	254.5	0.06	0	0.04	0.01	0.10	0.08	0.00	14.5	0	0	7.7
166	26	1.03	8.3	89.3	298.5	0.34	111.8	0.10	—	0.17	0.98	0.03	46.5	0	0.2	6.6
0	65	2.18	23.0	279.6	367.7	0.44	—	0.25	0.01	0.19	1.73	0.10	98.2	4.6	0	14.7
27	28	1.40	21.8	128.0	213.8	0.44	16.6	0.01	0.62	0.08	0.36	0.02	14.7	0.1	0.1	2.1
55	57	1.53	30.4	133.0	299.3	0.65	38.0	0.13	—	0.20	1.08	0.03	37.1	0.2	0.2	11.3
19	21	0.70	—	46.0	92.0	—	—	0.04	—	0.05	0.30	—	8.1	0	—	2.0
2	14	0.89	6.9	65.8	116.1	0.11	3.0	0.02	0.38	0.04	0.34	0.02	13.8	0.2	0	0.9
25	138	1.70	15.0	128.8	366.9	0.35	71.3	0.17	—	0.17	1.36	0.03	44.9	1.4	0.1	10.8
107	26	0.99	5.7	88.8	143.6	0.37	48.5	0.10	—	0.19	0.75	0.03	33.4	0	0.2	11.7

TABLE A–1 Table of Food Composition (continued)

(Computer code is for Cengage Diet & Wellness Plus program)

D&W+ Code	Food Description	QTY	Measure	Wt (g)	H₂0 (g)	Ener (cal)	Prot (g)	Carb (g)	Fiber (g)	Fat (g)	Fat Breakdown (g) Sat	Mono	Poly
	BREADS, BAKED GOODS, CAKES, COOKIES, CRACKERS, CHIPS, PIES—CONTINUED												
8817	White with coconut frosting, prepared from mix	1	slice(s)	112	23.2	399	4.9	70.8	1.1	11.5	4.4	4.1	2.4
8819	Yellow with chocolate frosting, ready to eat, commercially prepared	1	slice(s)	64	14.0	243	2.4	35.5	1.2	11.1	3.0	6.1	1.4
8822	Yellow with vanilla frosting, ready to eat, commercially prepared	1	slice(s)	64	14.1	239	2.2	37.6	0.2	9.3	1.5	3.9	3.3
	SNACK CAKES												
8791	Chocolate snack cake, creme filled, with frosting	1	item(s)	50	9.3	200	1.8	30.2	1.6	8.0	2.4	4.3	0.9
25010	Cinnamon coffee cake	1	piece(s)	72	22.6	231	3.6	35.8	0.7	8.3	2.2	2.6	3.0
16777	Funnel cake	1	item(s)	90	37.6	276	7.3	29.1	0.9	14.4	2.7	4.7	6.1
8794	Sponge snack cake, creme filled	1	item(s)	43	8.6	155	1.3	27.2	0.2	4.8	1.1	1.7	1.4
	SNACKS, CHIPS, PRETZELS												
29428	Bagel chips, plain	3	item(s)	29	—	130	3.0	19.0	1.0	4.5	0.5	—	—
29429	Bagel chips, toasted onion	3	item(s)	29	—	130	4.0	20.0	1.0	4.5	0.5	—	—
38192	Chex traditional snack mix	1	cup(s)	45	—	197	3.0	33.3	1.5	6.1	0.8	—	—
654	Potato chips, salted	1	ounce(s)	28	0.6	155	1.9	14.1	1.2	10.6	3.1	2.8	3.5
8816	Potato chips, unsalted	1	ounce(s)	28	0.5	152	2.0	15.0	1.4	9.8	3.1	2.8	3.5
5096	Pretzels, plain, hard, twists	5	item(s)	30	1.0	114	2.7	23.8	1.0	1.1	0.2	0.4	0.4
4632	Pretzels, whole wheat	1	ounce(s)	28	1.1	103	3.1	23.0	2.2	0.7	0.2	0.3	0.2
4641	Tortilla chips, plain	6	item(s)	11	0.2	53	0.8	7.1	0.6	2.5	0.4	0.8	0.5
	COOKIES												
8859	Animal crackers	12	item(s)	30	1.2	134	2.1	22.2	0.3	4.1	1.0	2.3	0.6
8876	Brownie, prepared from mix	1	item(s)	24	3.0	112	1.5	12.0	0.5	7.0	1.8	2.6	2.3
25207	Chocolate chip cookies	1	item(s)	30	3.7	140	2.0	16.2	0.6	7.9	2.1	3.3	2.1
8915	Chocolate sandwich cookie with extra creme filling	1	item(s)	13	0.2	65	0.6	8.9	0.4	3.2	0.7	2.1	0.3
14145	Fig Newtons cookies	1	item(s)	16	—	55	0.5	11.0	0.5	1.3	0	—	—
8920	Fortune cookie	1	item(s)	8	0.6	30	0.3	6.7	0.1	0.2	0.1	0.1	0
25208	Oatmeal cookies	1	item(s)	69	12.3	234	5.7	45.1	3.1	4.2	0.7	1.3	1.8
25213	Peanut butter cookies	1	item(s)	35	4.1	163	4.2	16.9	0.9	9.2	1.7	4.7	2.3
33095	Sugar cookies	1	item(s)	16	4.1	61	1.1	7.4	0.1	3.0	0.6	1.3	0.9
9002	Vanilla sandwich cookie with creme filling	1	item(s)	10	0.2	48	0.5	7.2	0.2	2.0	0.3	0.8	0.8
	CRACKERS												
9012	Cheese cracker sandwich with peanut butter	4	item(s)	28	0.9	139	3.5	15.9	1.0	7.0	1.2	3.6	1.4
9008	Cheese crackers (mini)	30	item(s)	30	0.9	151	3.0	17.5	0.7	7.6	2.8	3.6	0.7
33362	Cheese crackers, low sodium	1	serving(s)	30	0.9	151	3.0	17.5	0.7	7.6	2.9	3.6	0.7
8928	Honey graham crackers	4	item(s)	28	1.2	118	1.9	21.5	0.8	2.8	0.4	1.1	1.1
9016	Matzo crackers, plain	1	item(s)	28	1.2	112	2.8	23.8	0.9	0.4	0.1	0	0.2
9024	Melba toast	3	item(s)	15	0.8	59	1.8	11.5	0.9	0.5	0.1	0.1	0.2
9028	Melba toast, rye	3	item(s)	15	0.7	58	1.7	11.6	1.2	0.5	0.1	0.1	0.2
14189	Ritz crackers	5	item(s)	16	0.5	80	1.0	10.0	0	4.0	1.0	—	—
9014	Rye crispbread crackers	1	item(s)	10	0.6	37	0.8	8.2	1.7	0.1	0	0	0.1
9040	Rye wafer	1	item(s)	11	0.6	37	1.1	8.8	2.5	0.1	0	0	0
432	Saltine crackers	5	item(s)	15	0.8	64	1.4	10.6	0.5	1.7	0.2	1.1	0.2
9046	Saltine crackers, low salt	5	item(s)	15	0.6	65	1.4	10.7	0.5	1.8	0.4	1.0	0.3
9052	Snack cracker sandwich with cheese filling	4	item(s)	28	1.1	134	2.6	17.3	0.5	5.9	1.7	3.2	0.7
9054	Snack cracker sandwich with peanut butter filling	4	item(s)	28	0.8	138	3.2	16.3	0.6	6.9	1.4	3.9	1.3
9048	Snack crackers, round	10	item(s)	30	1.1	151	2.2	18.3	0.5	7.6	1.1	3.2	2.9
9050	Snack crackers, round, low salt	10	item(s)	30	1.1	151	2.2	18.3	0.5	7.6	1.1	3.2	2.9
9044	Soda crackers	5	item(s)	15	0.8	64	1.4	10.6	0.5	1.7	0.2	1.1	0.2
9059	Wheat cracker sandwich with cheese filling	4	item(s)	28	0.9	139	2.7	16.3	0.9	7.0	1.2	2.9	2.6
9061	Wheat cracker sandwich with peanut butter filling	4	item(s)	28	1.0	139	3.8	15.1	1.2	7.5	1.3	3.3	2.5
9055	Wheat crackers	10	item(s)	30	0.9	142	2.6	19.5	1.4	6.2	1.6	3.4	0.8

PAGE KEY: A-4 = Breads/Baked Goods A-10 = Cereal/Rice/Pasta A-14 = Fruit A-20 = Vegetables/Legumes A-30 = Nuts/Seeds A-32 = Vegetarian A-34 = Dairy A-42 = Eggs A-42 = Seafood A-46 = Meats A-50 = Poultry A-50 = Processed Meats A-52 = Beverages A-56 = Fats/Oils A-58 = Sweets A-60 = Spices/Condiments/Sauces A-64 = Mixed Foods/Soups/Sandwiches A-70 = Fast Food A-90 = Convenience A-92 = Baby Foods

A

CHOL (mg)	CALC (mg)	IRON (mg)	MAGN (mg)	POTA (mg)	SODI (mg)	ZINC (mg)	VIT A (µg)	THIA (mg)	VIT E (mg α)	RIBO (mg)	NIAC (mg)	VIT B$_6$ (mg)	FOLA (µg DFE)	VIT C (mg)	VIT B$_{12}$ (µg)	SELE (µg)
1	101	1.29	13.4	110.9	318.1	0.37	13.4	0.14	0.13	0.21	1.19	0.03	57.12	0.1	0.1	12.0
35	24	1.33	19.2	113.9	215.7	0.39	21.1	0.07	—	0.10	0.79	0.02	20.5	0	0.1	2.2
35	40	0.68	3.8	33.9	220.2	0.16	12.2	0.06	—	0.04	0.32	0.01	25.6	0	0.1	3.5
0	58	1.80	18.0	88.0	194.5	0.52	0.5	0.01	0.54	0.03	0.46	0.07	17.5	1.0	0	1.7
26	55	1.36	9.9	91.9	277.6	0.30	—	0.17	0.23	0.16	1.29	0.02	66.1	0.3	0.1	9.6
62	126	1.90	16.2	152.1	269.1	0.65	49.5	0.23	1.54	0.32	1.86	0.04	75.6	0	0.3	17.7
7	19	0.54	3.4	37.0	155.1	0.12	2.1	0.06	0.50	0.05	0.52	0.01	23.0	0	0	1.3
0	0	0.72	—	45.0	70.0	—	0	—	—	—	—	—	—	0	0	—
0	0	0.72	—	50.0	300.0	—	0	—	—	—	—	—	—	0	0	—
0	0	0.55	—	75.8	621.2	—	0	0.09	—	0.05	1.21	—	38.5	0	—	—
0	7	0.45	19.8	465.5	148.8	0.67	0	0.01	1.91	0.06	1.18	0.20	21.3	5.3	0	2.3
0	7	0.46	19.0	361.5	2.3	0.30	0	0.04	2.58	0.05	1.08	0.18	12.8	8.8	0	2.3
0	11	1.29	10.5	43.8	514.5	0.25	0	0.13	0.10	0.18	1.57	0.03	86.0	0	0	1.7
0	8	0.76	8.5	121.9	57.6	0.17	0	0.12	—	0.08	1.85	0.07	15.3	0.3	0	—
0	19	0.25	15.8	23.2	45.5	0.26	0	0.00	0.46	0.01	0.13	0.02	2.2	0	0	0.7
0	13	0.82	5.4	30.0	117.9	0.19	0	0.10	0.03	0.09	1.04	0.01	49.5	0	0	2.1
18	14	0.44	12.7	42.2	82.3	0.23	42.2	0.03	—	0.05	0.24	0.02	9.4	0.1	0	2.8
13	11	0.69	12.4	62.1	108.8	0.24	—	0.08	0.54	0.06	0.87	0.01	14.1	0	0	4.1
0	2	1.01	4.7	17.8	45.6	0.10	0	0.02	0.25	0.02	0.25	0.00	9.0	0	0	1.1
0	10	0.36	—	—	57.5	—	0	—	—	—	—	—	—	0	0	—
0	1	0.12	0.6	3.3	21.9	0.01	0.1	0.01	0.00	0.01	0.15	0.00	8.4	0	0	0.2
0	26	1.93	48.8	176.7	311.1	1.42	—	0.26	0.23	0.13	1.35	0.09	65.6	0.3	0	17.4
13	27	0.65	21.1	112.8	154.1	0.46	—	0.08	0.73	0.09	1.85	0.05	35.0	0	0.1	4.8
18	5	0.30	1.7	12.2	49.4	0.08	—	0.04	0.28	0.05	0.31	0.01	13.1	0	0	3.1
0	3	0.22	1.4	9.1	34.9	0.04	0	0.02	0.16	0.02	0.27	0.00	8.2	0	0	0.3
0	14	0.76	15.7	61.0	198.8	0.29	0.3	0.15	0.66	0.08	1.63	0.04	39.8	0	0.1	2.3
4	45	1.43	10.8	43.5	298.5	0.33	8.7	0.17	0.01	0.12	1.40	0.16	72.3	0	0.1	2.6
4	45	1.43	10.8	31.8	137.4	0.33	5.1	0.17	0.09	0.12	1.40	0.16	40.2	0	0.1	2.6
0	7	1.04	8.4	37.8	169.4	0.22	0	0.06	0.09	0.08	1.15	0.01	18.5	0	0	2.9
0	4	0.89	7.1	31.8	0.6	0.19	0	0.11	0.01	0.08	1.10	0.03	4.8	0	0	10.5
0	14	0.55	8.9	30.3	124.4	0.30	0	0.06	0.06	0.04	0.61	0.01	29.0	0	0	5.2
0	12	0.55	5.9	29.0	134.9	0.20	0	0.07	—	0.04	0.70	0.01	19.4	0	0	5.8
0	20	0.72	—	10.0	135.0	—	0	—	—	—	—	—	—	0	0	—
0	3	0.24	7.8	31.9	26.4	0.23	0	0.02	0.08	0.01	0.10	0.02	6.5	0	0	3.7
0	4	0.65	13.3	54.5	87.3	0.30	0	0.04	0.08	0.03	0.17	0.03	5.0	0	0	2.6
0	10	0.84	3.3	23.1	160.8	0.12	0	0.01	0.14	0.06	0.78	0.01	33.2	0	0	1.5
0	18	0.81	4.1	108.6	95.4	0.11	0	0.08	0.01	0.06	0.78	0.01	33.2	0	0	2.9
1	72	0.66	10.1	120.1	392.3	0.17	4.8	0.12	0.06	0.19	1.05	0.01	44.8	0	0	6.0
0	23	0.77	15.4	60.2	201.0	0.31	0.3	0.13	0.57	0.07	1.71	0.04	34.2	0	0	3.0
0	36	1.08	8.1	39.9	254.1	0.20	0	0.12	0.60	0.10	1.21	0.01	55.8	0	0	2.0
0	36	1.08	8.1	106.5	111.9	0.20	0	0.12	0.60	0.10	1.21	0.01	55.8	0	0	2.0
0	10	0.84	3.3	23.1	160.8	0.12	0	0.01	0.14	0.06	0.78	0.01	33.2	0	0	1.5
2	57	0.73	15.1	85.7	255.6	0.24	4.8	0.10	—	0.12	0.89	0.07	26.0	0.4	0	6.8
0	48	0.74	10.6	83.2	226.0	0.23	0	0.10	—	0.08	1.64	0.03	26.0	0	0	6.1
0	15	1.32	18.6	54.9	238.5	0.48	0	0.15	0.15	0.09	1.48	0.04	56.1	0	0	1.9

A

D&W+ Code	Food Description	QTY	Measure	Wt (g)	H₂O (g)	Ener (cal)	Prot (g)	Carb (g)	Fiber (g)	Fat (g)	Fat Breakdown (g)		
											Sat	Mono	Poly
BREADS, BAKED GOODS, CAKES, COOKIES, CRACKERS, CHIPS, PIES—CONTINUED													
9057	Wheat crackers, low salt	10	item(s)	30	0.9	142	2.6	19.5	1.4	6.2	1.6	3.4	0.8
9022	Whole wheat crackers	7	item(s)	28	0.8	124	2.5	19.2	2.9	4.8	1.0	1.6	1.8
PASTRY													
16754	Apple fritter	1	item(s)	17	6.4	61	1.0	5.5	0.2	3.9	0.9	1.7	1.1
41565	Cinnamon rolls with icing, refrigerated dough	1	serving(s)	44	12.3	145	2.0	23.0	0.5	5.0	1.5	—	—
4945	Croissant, butter	1	item(s)	57	13.2	231	4.7	26.1	1.5	12.0	6.6	3.1	0.6
9096	Danish, nut	1	item(s)	65	13.3	280	4.6	29.7	1.3	16.4	3.8	8.9	2.8
9115	Doughnut with creme filling	1	item(s)	85	32.5	307	5.4	25.5	0.7	20.8	4.6	10.3	2.6
9117	Doughnut with jelly filling	1	item(s)	85	30.3	289	5.0	33.2	0.8	15.9	4.1	8.7	2.0
4947	Doughnut, cake	1	item(s)	47	9.8	198	2.4	23.4	0.7	10.8	1.7	4.4	3.7
9105	Doughnut, cake, chocolate glazed	1	item(s)	42	6.8	175	1.9	24.1	0.9	8.4	2.2	4.7	1.0
437	Doughnut, glazed	1	item(s)	60	15.2	242	3.8	26.6	0.7	13.7	3.5	7.7	1.7
10617	Toaster pastry, brown sugar cinnamon	1	item(s)	50	5.3	210	3.0	35.0	1.0	6.0	1.0	4.0	1.0
30928	Toaster pastry, cream cheese	1	item(s)	54	—	200	3.0	23.0	0	11.0	4.5	—	—
MUFFINS													
25015	Blueberry	1	item(s)	63	29.7	160	3.4	23.0	0.8	6.0	0.9	1.5	3.3
9189	Corn, ready to eat	1	item(s)	57	18.6	174	3.4	29.0	1.9	4.8	0.8	1.2	1.8
9121	English muffin, plain, enriched	1	item(s)	57	24.0	134	4.4	26.2	1.5	1.0	0.1	0.2	0.5
29582	English muffin, toasted	1	item(s)	50	18.6	128	4.2	25.0	1.5	1.0	0.1	0.2	0.5
9145	English muffin, wheat	1	item(s)	57	24.1	127	5.0	25.5	2.6	1.1	0.2	0.2	0.5
8894	Oat bran	1	item(s)	57	20.0	154	4.0	27.5	2.6	4.2	0.6	1.0	2.4
GRANOLA BARS													
38161	Kudos milk chocolate granola bars w/fruit and nuts	1	item(s)	28	—	90	2.0	15.0	1.0	3.0	1.0	—	—
38196	Nature Valley banana nut crunchy granola bars	2	item(s)	42	—	190	4.0	28.0	2.0	7.0	1.0	—	—
38187	Nature Valley fruit 'n' nut trail mix bar	1	item(s)	35	—	140	3.0	25.0	2.0	4.0	0.5	—	—
1383	Plain, hard	1	item(s)	25	1.0	115	2.5	15.8	1.3	4.9	0.6	1.1	3.0
4606	Plain, soft	1	item(s)	28	1.8	126	2.1	19.1	1.3	4.9	2.1	1.1	1.5
PIES													
454	Apple pie, prepared from home recipe	1	slice(s)	155	73.3	411	3.7	57.5	2.3	19.4	4.7	8.4	5.2
470	Pecan pie, prepared from home recipe	1	slice(s)	122	23.8	503	6.0	63.7	—	27.1	4.9	13.6	7.0
33356	Pie crust mix, prepared, baked	1	slice(s)	20	2.1	100	1.3	10.1	0.4	6.1	1.5	3.5	0.8
9007	Pie crust, ready to bake, frozen, enriched, baked	1	slice(s)	16	1.8	82	0.7	7.9	0.2	5.2	1.7	2.5	0.6
472	Pumpkin pie, prepared from home recipe	1	slice(s)	155	90.7	316	7.0	40.9	—	14.4	4.9	5.7	2.8
ROLLS													
8555	Crescent dinner roll	1	item(s)	28	9.7	78	2.7	13.8	0.6	1.2	0.3	0.3	0.6
489	Hamburger roll or bun, plain	1	item(s)	43	14.9	120	4.1	21.3	0.9	1.9	0.5	0.5	0.8
490	Hard roll	1	item(s)	57	17.7	167	5.6	30.0	1.3	2.5	0.3	0.6	1.0
5127	Kaiser roll	1	item(s)	57	17.7	167	5.6	30.0	1.3	2.5	0.3	0.6	1.0
5130	Whole wheat roll or bun	1	item(s)	28	9.4	75	2.5	14.5	2.1	1.3	0.2	0.3	0.6
SPORT BARS													
37026	Balance original chocolate bar	1	item(s)	50	—	200	14.0	22.0	0.5	6.0	3.5	—	—
37024	Balance original peanut butter bar	1	item(s)	50	—	200	14.0	22.0	1.0	6.0	2.5	—	—
36580	Clif Bar chocolate brownie energy bar	1	item(s)	68	—	240	10.0	45.0	5.0	4.5	1.5	—	—
36583	Clif Bar crunchy peanut butter energy bar	1	item(s)	68	—	250	12.0	40.0	5.0	6.0	1.5	—	—
36589	Clif Luna Nutz over Chocolate energy bar	1	item(s)	48	—	180	10.0	25.0	3.0	4.5	2.5	—	—
12005	PowerBar apple cinnamon	1	item(s)	65	—	230	9.0	45.0	3.0	2.5	0.5	1.5	0.5
16078	PowerBar banana	1	item(s)	65	—	230	9.0	45.0	3.0	2.5	0.5	1.0	0.5
16080	PowerBar chocolate	1	item(s)	65	6.4	230	10.0	45.0	3.0	2.0	0.5	0.5	1.0
29092	PowerBar peanut butter	1	item(s)	65	—	240	10.0	45.0	3.0	3.5	0.5	—	—
TORTILLAS													
1391	Corn tortillas, soft	1	item(s)	26	11.9	57	1.5	11.6	1.6	0.7	0.1	0.2	0.4
1669	Flour tortilla	1	item(s)	32	9.7	100	2.7	16.4	1.0	2.5	0.6	1.2	0.5
1390	Taco shells, hard	1	item(s)	13	1.0	62	0.9	8.3	0.6	2.8	0.6	1.6	0.5

PAGE KEY: A-4 = Breads/Baked Goods A-10 = Cereal/Rice/Pasta A-14 = Fruit A-20 = Vegetables/Legumes A-30 = Nuts/Seeds A-32 = Vegetarian A-34 = Dairy A-42 = Eggs A-42 = Seafood A-46 = Meats A-50 = Poultry A-50 = Processed Meats A-52 = Beverages A-56 = Fats/Oils A-58 = Sweets A-60 = Spices/Condiments/Sauces A-64 = Mixed Foods/Soups/Sandwiches A-70 = Fast Food A-90 = Convenience A-92 = Baby Foods

CHOL (mg)	CALC (mg)	IRON (mg)	MAGN (mg)	POTA (mg)	SODI (mg)	ZINC (mg)	VIT A (µg)	THIA (mg)	VIT E (mg α)	RIBO (mg)	NIAC (mg)	VIT B6 (mg)	FOLA (µg DFE)	VIT C (mg)	VIT B12 (µg)	SELE (µg)
0	15	1.32	18.6	60.9	84.9	0.48	0	0.15	0.15	0.09	1.48	0.04	21.6	0	0	10.1
0	14	0.86	27.7	83.2	184.5	0.60	0	0.05	0.24	0.02	1.26	0.05	7.8	0	0	4.1
14	9	0.26	2.2	22.4	6.8	0.09	7.1	0.03	0.07	0.04	0.23	0.01	9.2	0.2	0.1	2.6
0	—	0.72	—	—	340.1	—	0	—	—	—	—	—	—	—	—	—
38	21	1.15	9.1	67.3	424.1	0.42	117.4	0.22	0.47	0.13	1.24	0.03	74.1	0.1	0.1	12.9
30	61	1.17	20.8	61.8	236.0	0.56	5.9	0.14	0.53	0.15	1.49	0.06	79.3	1.1	0.1	9.2
20	21	1.55	17.0	68.0	262.7	0.68	9.4	0.28	0.24	0.12	1.90	0.05	92.7	0	0.1	9.2
22	21	1.49	17.0	67.2	249.1	0.63	14.5	0.26	0.36	0.12	1.81	0.08	88.4	0	0.2	10.6
17	21	0.91	9.4	59.7	256.6	0.25	17.9	0.10	0.90	0.11	0.87	0.02	32.9	0.1	0.1	4.4
24	89	0.95	14.3	44.5	142.8	0.23	5.0	0.01	0.08	0.02	0.19	0.01	27.3	0	0	1.7
4	26	0.36	13.2	64.8	205.2	0.46	2.4	0.53	—	0.04	0.39	0.03	13.2	0.1	0.1	5.0
0	0	1.80	—	70.0	190.0	—	0	0.15	—	0.17	2.00	0.20	21.0	0	0	—
10	100	1.80	—	—	220.0	—	0	0.15	—	0.17	2.00	—	21.0	0	0.6	—
20	56	1.02	7.8	70.2	289.4	0.28	—	0.17	0.75	0.15	1.25	0.02	62.5	0.4	0.1	8.8
15	42	1.60	18.2	39.3	297.0	0.30	29.6	0.15	0.45	0.18	1.16	0.04	63.8	0	0.1	8.7
0	30	1.42	12.0	74.7	264.5	0.39	0	0.25	—	0.16	2.21	0.02	57.0	0	0	—
0	95	1.36	11.0	71.5	252.0	0.38	0	0.19	0.16	0.14	1.90	0.02	62.5	0.1	0	13.5
0	101	1.63	21.1	106.0	217.7	0.61	0	0.24	0.25	0.16	1.91	0.05	46.7	0	0	16.6
0	36	2.39	89.5	289.0	224.0	1.04	0	0.14	0.37	0.05	0.23	0.09	79.2	0	0	6.3
0	200	0.36	—	—	60.0	—	0	—	—	—	—	—	—	0	0	—
0	20	1.08	—	120.0	160.0	—	0	—	—	—	—	—	—	0	—	—
0	0	0.00	—	—	95.0	—	0	—	—	—	—	—	—	0	—	—
0	15	0.72	23.8	82.3	72.0	0.50	0	0.06	—	0.03	0.39	0.02	5.8	0.2	0	4.0
0	30	0.72	21.0	92.3	79.0	0.42	0	0.08	—	0.04	0.14	0.02	6.8	0	0.1	4.6
0	11	1.73	10.9	122.5	327.1	0.29	17.1	0.22	—	0.16	1.90	0.05	58.9	2.6	0	12.1
106	39	1.80	31.7	162.3	319.6	1.24	100.0	0.22	—	0.22	1.03	0.07	41.5	0.2	0.2	14.6
0	12	0.43	3.0	12.4	145.8	0.07	0	0.06	—	0.03	0.47	0.01	22.2	0	0	4.4
0	3	0.36	2.9	17.6	103.5	0.05	0	0.04	0.42	0.06	0.39	0.01	16.3	0	0	0.5
65	146	1.96	29.5	288.3	348.8	0.71	660.3	0.14	—	0.31	1.21	0.07	43.4	2.6	0.1	11.0
0	39	0.93	5.9	26.3	134.1	0.18	0	0.11	0.02	0.09	1.16	0.02	47.6	0	0.1	5.5
0	59	1.42	9.0	40.4	206.0	0.28	0	0.17	0.03	0.13	1.78	0.03	73.5	0	0	8.4
0	54	1.87	15.4	61.6	310.1	0.53	0	0.27	0.23	0.19	2.41	0.02	86.1	0	0	22.3
0	54	1.86	15.4	61.6	310.1	0.53	0	0.27	0.23	0.19	2.41	0.01	86.1	0	0	22.3
0	30	0.69	24.1	77.1	135.5	0.57	0	0.07	0.26	0.04	1.04	0.06	8.5	0	0	14.0
3	100	4.50	40.0	160.0	180.0	3.75	—	0.37	—	0.42	5.00	0.50	102.0	60.0	1.5	17.5
3	100	4.50	40.0	130.0	230.0	3.75	—	0.37	—	0.42	5.00	0.50	102.0	60.0	1.5	17.5
0	250	4.50	100.0	370.0	150.0	3.00	—	0.37	—	0.25	3.00	0.40	80.0	60.0	0.9	14.0
0	250	4.50	100.0	230.0	250.0	3.00	—	0.37	—	0.25	3.00	0.40	80.0	60.0	0.9	14.0
0	350	5.40	80.0	190.0	190.0	5.25	—	1.20	—	1.36	16.00	2.00	400.0	60.0	6.0	24.5
0	300	6.30	140.0	125.0	100.0	5.25	—	1.50	—	1.70	20.00	2.00	400.0	60.0	6.0	—
0	300	6.30	140.0	190.0	100.0	5.25	0	1.50	—	1.70	20.00	2.00	400.0	60.0	6.0	—
0	300	6.30	140.0	200.0	95.0	5.25	0	1.50	—	1.70	20.00	2.00	400.0	60.0	6.0	5.1
0	300	6.30	140.0	140.0	120.0	5.25	0	1.50	—	1.70	20.00	2.00	400.0	60.0	6.0	—
0	21	0.32	18.7	48.4	11.7	0.34	0	0.02	0.07	0.02	0.39	0.06	1.3	0	0	1.6
0	41	1.06	7.0	49.6	203.5	0.17	0	0.17	0.06	0.08	1.14	0.01	64.3	0	0	7.1
0	13	0.25	11.3	29.7	51.7	0.21	0.1	0.03	0.09	0.01	0.25	0.03	11.1	0	0	0.6

(Computer code is for Cengage Diet & Wellness Plus program)

D&W+ Code	Food Description	QTY	Measure	Wt (g)	H₂0 (g)	Ener (cal)	Prot (g)	Carb (g)	Fiber (g)	Fat (g)	Sat	Mono	Poly

Fat Breakdown (g): Sat, Mono, Poly

BREADS, BAKED GOODS, CAKES, COOKIES, CRACKERS, CHIPS, PIES—CONTINUED

PANCAKES, WAFFLES

D&W+ Code	Food Description	QTY	Measure	Wt (g)	H₂0 (g)	Ener (cal)	Prot (g)	Carb (g)	Fiber (g)	Fat (g)	Sat	Mono	Poly
8926	Pancakes, blueberry, prepared from recipe	3	item(s)	114	60.6	253	7.0	33.1	0.8	10.5	2.3	2.6	4.7
5037	Pancakes, prepared from mix with egg and milk	3	item(s)	114	60.3	249	8.9	32.9	2.1	8.8	2.3	2.4	3.3
30311	Waffle, 100% whole grain	1	item(s)	75	32.3	200	6.9	25.0	1.9	8.4	2.3	3.3	2.1
9219	Waffle, plain, frozen, toasted	2	item(s)	66	20.2	206	4.7	32.5	1.6	6.3	1.1	3.2	1.5
500	Waffle, plain, prepared from recipe	1	item(s)	75	31.5	218	5.9	24.7	1.7	10.6	2.1	2.6	5.1

CEREAL, FLOUR, GRAIN, PASTA, NOODLES, POPCORN

GRAIN

D&W+ Code	Food Description	QTY	Measure	Wt (g)	H₂0 (g)	Ener (cal)	Prot (g)	Carb (g)	Fiber (g)	Fat (g)	Sat	Mono	Poly
2861	Amaranth, dry	½	cup(s)	98	9.6	365	14.1	64.5	9.1	6.3	1.6	1.4	2.8
1953	Barley, pearled, cooked	½	cup(s)	79	54.0	97	1.8	22.2	3.0	0.3	0.1	0	0.2
1956	Buckwheat groats, cooked, roasted	½	cup(s)	84	63.5	77	2.8	16.8	2.3	0.5	0.1	0.2	0.2
1957	Bulgur, cooked	½	cup(s)	91	70.8	76	2.8	16.9	4.1	0.2	0	0	0.1
1963	Couscous, cooked	½	cup(s)	79	57.0	88	3.0	18.2	1.1	0.1	0	0	0.1
1967	Millet, cooked	½	cup(s)	120	85.7	143	4.2	28.4	1.6	1.2	0.2	0.2	0.6
1969	Oat bran, dry	½	cup(s)	47	3.1	116	8.1	31.1	7.2	3.3	0.6	1.1	1.3
1972	Quinoa, dry	½	cup(s)	85	11.3	313	12.0	54.5	5.9	5.2	0.6	1.4	2.8

RICE

D&W+ Code	Food Description	QTY	Measure	Wt (g)	H₂0 (g)	Ener (cal)	Prot (g)	Carb (g)	Fiber (g)	Fat (g)	Sat	Mono	Poly
129	Brown, long grain, cooked	½	cup(s)	98	71.3	108	2.5	22.4	1.8	0.9	0.2	0.3	0.3
2863	Brown, medium grain, cooked	½	cup(s)	98	71.1	109	2.3	22.9	1.8	0.8	0.2	0.3	0.3
37488	Jasmine, saffroned, cooked	½	cup(s)	280	—	340	8.0	78.0	0	0	0	0	0
30280	Pilaf, cooked	½	cup(s)	103	74.0	129	2.1	22.2	0.6	3.3	0.6	1.5	1.0
28066	Spanish, cooked	½	cup(s)	244	184.2	241	5.7	50.2	3.3	1.9	0.4	0.6	0.7
2867	White glutinous, cooked	½	cup(s)	87	66.7	84	1.8	18.3	0.9	0.2	0	0.1	0.1
484	White, long grain, boiled	½	cup(s)	79	54.1	103	2.1	22.3	0.3	0.2	0.1	0.1	0.1
482	White, long grain, enriched, instant, boiled	½	cup(s)	83	59.4	97	1.8	20.7	0.5	0.4	0	0.1	0
486	White, long grain, enriched, par-boiled, cooked	½	cup(s)	79	55.6	97	2.3	20.6	0.7	0.3	0.1	0.1	0.1
1194	Wild brown, cooked	½	cup(s)	82	60.6	83	3.3	17.5	1.5	0.3	0	0	0.2

FLOUR AND GRAIN FRACTIONS

D&W+ Code	Food Description	QTY	Measure	Wt (g)	H₂0 (g)	Ener (cal)	Prot (g)	Carb (g)	Fiber (g)	Fat (g)	Sat	Mono	Poly
505	All purpose flour, self-rising, enriched	½	cup(s)	63	6.6	221	6.2	46.4	1.7	0.6	0.1	0	0.2
503	All purpose flour, white, bleached, enriched	½	cup(s)	63	7.4	228	6.4	47.7	1.7	0.6	0.1	0	0.2
1643	Barley flour	½	cup(s)	56	5.5	198	4.2	44.7	2.1	0.8	0.2	0.1	0.4
383	Buckwheat flour, whole groat	½	cup(s)	60	6.7	201	7.6	42.3	6.0	1.9	0.4	0.6	0.6
504	Cake wheat flour, enriched	½	cup(s)	69	8.6	248	5.6	53.5	1.2	0.6	0.1	0.1	0.3
426	Cornmeal, degermed, enriched	½	cup(s)	69	7.8	255	5.0	54.6	2.8	1.2	0.1	0.2	0.5
424	Cornmeal, yellow whole grain	½	cup(s)	61	6.2	221	4.9	46.9	4.4	2.2	0.3	0.6	1.0
1978	Dark rye flour	½	cup(s)	64	7.1	207	9.0	44.0	14.5	1.7	0.2	0.2	0.8
1644	Masa corn flour, enriched	½	cup(s)	57	5.1	208	5.3	43.5	5.5	2.1	0.3	0.6	1.0
1976	Rice flour, brown	½	cup(s)	79	9.4	287	5.7	60.4	3.6	2.2	0.4	0.8	0.8
1645	Rice flour, white	½	cup(s)	79	9.4	289	4.7	63.3	1.9	1.1	0.3	0.3	0.3
1980	Semolina, enriched	½	cup(s)	84	10.6	301	10.6	60.8	3.2	0.9	0.1	0.1	0.4
2827	Soy flour, raw	½	cup(s)	42	2.2	185	14.7	14.9	4.1	8.8	1.3	1.9	4.9
1990	Wheat germ, crude	2	tablespoon(s)	14	1.6	52	3.3	7.4	1.9	1.4	0.2	0.2	0.9
506	Whole wheat flour	½	cup(s)	60	6.2	203	8.2	43.5	7.3	1.1	0.2	0.1	0.5

BREAKFAST BARS

D&W+ Code	Food Description	QTY	Measure	Wt (g)	H₂0 (g)	Ener (cal)	Prot (g)	Carb (g)	Fiber (g)	Fat (g)	Sat	Mono	Poly
39230	Atkins Morning Start apple crisp breakfast bar	1	item(s)	37	—	170	11.0	12.0	6.0	9.0	4.0	—	—
10571	Nutri-Grain apple cinnamon cereal bar	1	item(s)	37	—	140	2.0	27.0	1.0	3.0	0.5	2.0	0.5
10647	Nutri-Grain blueberry cereal bar	1	item(s)	37	5.4	140	2.0	27.0	1.0	3.0	0.5	2.0	0.5
10648	Nutri-Grain raspberry cereal bar	1	item(s)	37	5.4	140	2.0	27.0	1.0	3.0	0.5	2.0	0.5
10649	Nutri-Grain strawberry cereal bar	1	item(s)	37	5.4	140	2.0	27.0	1.0	3.0	0.5	2.0	0.5

BREAKFAST CEREALS, HOT

D&W+ Code	Food Description	QTY	Measure	Wt (g)	H₂0 (g)	Ener (cal)	Prot (g)	Carb (g)	Fiber (g)	Fat (g)	Sat	Mono	Poly
1260	Cream of Wheat, instant, prepared	½	cup(s)	121	—	388	12.9	73.3	4.3	0	0	0	0
365	Farina, enriched, cooked w/water and salt	½	cup(s)	117	102.4	56	1.7	12.2	0.3	0.1	0	0	0

PAGE KEY: A-4 = Breads/Baked Goods A-10 = Cereal/Rice/Pasta A-14 = Fruit A-20 = Vegetables/Legumes A-30 = Nuts/Seeds A-32 = Vegetarian A-34 = Dairy A-42 = Eggs A-42 = Seafood A-46 = Meats A-50 = Poultry A-50 = Processed Meats A-52 = Beverages A-56 = Fats/Oils A-58 = Sweets A-60 = Spices/Condiments/Sauces A-64 = Mixed Foods/Soups/Sandwiches A-70 = Fast Food A-90 = Convenience A-92 = Baby Foods

CHOL (mg)	CALC (mg)	IRON (mg)	MAGN (mg)	POTA (mg)	SODI (mg)	ZINC (mg)	VIT A (µg)	THIA (mg)	VIT E (mg α)	RIBO (mg)	NIAC (mg)	VIT B$_6$ (mg)	FOLA (µg DFE)	VIT C (mg)	VIT B$_{12}$ (µg)	SELE (µg)
64	235	1.96	18.2	157.3	469.7	0.61	57.0	0.22	—	0.31	1.73	0.05	60.4	2.5	0.2	16.0
81	245	1.48	25.1	226.9	575.7	0.85	82.1	0.22	—	0.35	1.40	0.12	61.6	0.7	0.4	—
71	194	1.60	28.5	171.0	371.3	0.87	48.8	0.15	0.32	0.25	1.47	0.08	38.3	0	0.4	20.0
10	203	4.56	15.8	95.0	481.8	0.35	262.7	0.34	0.64	0.46	5.86	0.68	78.5	0	1.9	8.3
52	191	1.73	14.3	119.3	383.3	0.51	48.8	0.19	—	0.26	1.55	0.04	51.0	0.3	0.2	34.7
0	149	7.40	259.3	356.8	20.5	3.10	0	0.06	—	0.20	1.24	0.20	47.8	4.1	0	—
0	9	1.04	17.3	73.0	2.4	0.64	0	0.06	0.01	0.04	1.61	0.09	12.6	0	0	6.8
0	6	0.67	42.8	73.9	3.4	0.51	0	0.03	0.07	0.03	0.79	0.06	11.8	0	0	1.8
0	9	0.87	29.1	61.9	4.6	0.51	0	0.05	0.01	0.02	0.91	0.07	16.4	0	0	0.5
0	6	0.30	6.3	45.5	3.9	0.20	0	0.05	0.10	0.02	0.77	0.04	11.8	0	0	21.6
0	4	0.75	52.8	74.4	2.4	1.09	0	0.12	0.02	0.09	1.59	0.13	22.8	0	0	1.1
0	27	2.54	110.5	266.0	1.9	1.46	0	0.55	0.47	0.10	0.43	0.07	24.4	0	0	21.2
0	40	3.88	167.4	478.5	4.2	2.62	0.8	0.30	2.06	0.26	1.28	0.40	156.4	0	0	7.2
0	10	0.41	41.9	41.9	4.9	0.61	0	0.09	0.02	0.02	1.49	0.14	3.9	0	0	9.6
0	10	0.51	42.9	77.0	1.0	0.60	0	0.09	—	0.01	1.29	0.14	3.9	0	0	38.0
0	—	2.16	—	—	780.0	—	—	—	—	—	—	—	—	—	—	—
0	11	1.16	9.3	54.6	390.4	0.37	33.0	0.13	0.28	0.02	1.23	0.06	73.1	0.4	0	4.3
0	37	1.52	95.4	330.5	97.1	1.40	—	0.27	0.12	0.05	3.24	0.38	89.9	22.6	0	14.3
0	2	0.12	4.4	8.7	4.4	0.35	0	0.01	0.03	0.01	0.25	0.02	0.9	0	0	4.9
0	8	0.94	9.5	27.7	0.8	0.38	0	0.12	0.03	0.01	1.16	0.07	76.6	0	0	5.9
0	7	1.46	4.1	7.4	3.3	0.40	0	0.06	0.01	0.01	1.43	0.04	97.4	0	0	4.0
0	15	1.43	7.1	44.2	1.6	0.29	0	0.16	0.01	0.01	1.82	0.12	107.4	0	0	7.3
0	2	0.49	26.2	82.8	2.5	1.09	0	0.04	0.19	0.07	1.05	0.11	21.3	0	0	0.7
0	211	2.90	11.9	77.5	793.7	0.38	0	0.42	0.02	0.24	3.64	0.02	193.4	0	0	21.5
0	9	2.90	13.7	66.9	1.2	0.42	0	0.48	0.02	0.30	3.68	0.02	183.3	0	0	21.2
0	16	0.70	45.4	185.9	4.5	1.04	0	0.06	—	0.02	2.56	0.14	4.5	0	0	2.0
0	25	2.42	150.6	346.2	6.6	1.86	0	0.24	0.18	0.10	3.68	0.34	32.4	0	0	3.4
0	10	5.01	11.0	71.9	1.4	0.42	0	0.61	0.01	0.29	4.65	0.02	194.6	0	0	3.4
0	2	2.98	24.1	104.9	4.8	0.48	7.6	0.42	0.10	0.28	3.66	0.12	231.1	0	0	8.0
0	4	2.10	77.5	175.1	21.3	1.10	6.7	0.22	0.24	0.12	2.20	0.18	15.2	0	0	9.4
0	36	4.12	158.7	467.2	0.6	3.58	0.6	0.20	0.90	0.16	2.72	0.28	21.1	0	0	22.8
0	80	4.10	62.7	169.9	2.8	1.00	0	0.80	0.08	0.42	5.60	0.20	190.9	0	0	8.5
0	9	1.56	88.5	228.3	6.3	1.92	0	0.34	0.94	0.06	5.00	0.58	12.6	0	0	—
0	8	0.26	27.6	60.0	0	0.62	0	0.10	0.08	0.02	2.04	0.34	3.2	0	0	11.9
0	14	3.64	39.2	155.3	0.8	0.86	0	0.66	0.20	0.46	5.00	0.08	219.2	0	0	74.6
0	87	2.70	182.0	1067.0	5.5	1.65	2.5	0.24	0.82	0.48	1.83	0.18	146.4	0	0	3.2
0	6	0.90	34.4	128.2	1.7	1.76	0	0.27	—	0.07	0.97	0.18	40.4	0	0	11.4
0	20	2.32	82.8	243.0	3.0	1.74	0	0.26	0.48	0.12	3.82	0.20	26.4	0	0	42.4
0	200	—	—	90.0	70.0	—	—	0.22	—	0.25	3.00	—	—	9.0	—	—
0	200	1.80	8.0	75.0	110.0	1.50	—	0.37	—	0.42	5.00	0.50	40.0	0	—	—
0	200	1.80	8.0	75.0	110.0	1.50	—	0.37	—	0.42	5.00	0.50	40.0	0	0	—
0	200	1.80	8.0	70.0	110.0	1.50	—	0.37	—	0.42	5.00	0.50	40.0	0	0	—
0	200	1.80	8.0	55.0	110.0	1.50	—	0.37	—	0.42	5.00	0.50	40.0	0	0	—
0	862	34.91	21.4	150.8	732.6	0.86	—	1.59	—	1.47	21.55	2.15	122.2	0	0	—
0	5	0.58	2.3	15.1	383.3	0.09	0	0.07	0.01	0.05	0.57	0.01	139.2	0	0	10.6

(Computer code is for Cengage Diet & Wellness Plus program)

D&W+ Code	Food Description	QTY	Measure	Wt (g)	H₂O (g)	Ener (cal)	Prot (g)	Carb (g)	Fiber (g)	Fat (g)	Sat	Mono	Poly
											\<Fat Breakdown (g)\>		

CEREAL, FLOUR, GRAIN, PASTA, NOODLES, POPCORN—CONTINUED

D&W+ Code	Food Description	QTY	Measure	Wt (g)	H₂O (g)	Ener (cal)	Prot (g)	Carb (g)	Fiber (g)	Fat (g)	Sat	Mono	Poly
363	Grits, white corn, regular and quick, enriched, cooked w/water and salt	½	cup(s)	121	103.3	71	1.7	15.6	0.4	0.2	0	0.1	0.1
8636	Grits, yellow corn, regular and quick, enriched, cooked w/salt	½	cup(s)	121	103.3	71	1.7	15.6	0.4	0.2	0	0.1	0.1
8657	Oatmeal, cooked w/water	½	cup(s)	117	97.8	83	3.0	14.0	2.0	1.8	0.4	0.5	0.7
5500	Oatmeal, maple and brown sugar, instant, prepared	1	item(s)	198	150.2	200	4.8	40.4	2.4	2.2	0.4	0.7	0.8
5510	Oatmeal, ready to serve, packet, prepared	1	item(s)	186	158.7	112	4.1	19.8	2.7	2.0	0.4	0.7	0.8

BREAKFAST CEREALS, READY TO EAT

D&W+ Code	Food Description	QTY	Measure	Wt (g)	H₂O (g)	Ener (cal)	Prot (g)	Carb (g)	Fiber (g)	Fat (g)	Sat	Mono	Poly
1197	All-Bran	1	cup(s)	62	1.3	160	8.1	46.0	18.2	2.0	0.4	0.4	1.3
1200	All-Bran Buds	1	cup(s)	91	2.7	212	6.4	72.7	39.1	1.9	0.4	0.5	1.2
1199	Apple Jacks	1	cup(s)	33	0.9	130	1.0	30.0	0.5	0.5	0	—	—
1204	Cap'n Crunch	1	cup(s)	36	0.9	147	1.3	30.7	1.3	2.0	0.5	0.4	0.3
1205	Cap'n Crunch Crunchberries	1	cup(s)	35	0.9	133	1.3	29.3	1.3	2.0	0.5	0.4	0.3
1206	Cheerios	1	cup(s)	30	1.0	110	3.0	22.0	3.0	2.0	0	0.5	0.5
3415	Cocoa Puffs	1	cup(s)	30	0.6	120	1.0	26.0	0.2	1.0	—	—	—
1207	Cocoa Rice Krispies	1	cup(s)	41	1.0	160	1.3	36.0	1.3	1.3	0.7	0	0
5522	Complete wheat bran flakes	1	cup(s)	39	1.4	120	4.0	30.7	6.7	0.7	—	—	—
1211	Corn Flakes	1	cup(s)	28	0.9	100	2.0	24.0	1.0	0	0	0	0
1247	Corn Pops	1	cup(s)	31	0.9	120	1.0	28.0	0.3	0	0	0	0
1937	Cracklin' Oat Bran	1	cup(s)	65	2.3	267	5.3	46.7	8.0	9.3	4.0	4.7	1.3
1220	Froot Loops	1	cup(s)	32	0.8	120	1.0	28.0	1.0	1.0	0.5	0	0
38214	Frosted Cheerios	1	cup(s)	37	—	149	2.5	31.1	1.2	1.2	—	—	—
372	Frosted Flakes	1	cup(s)	41	1.1	160	1.3	37.3	1.3	0	0	0	0
38215	Frosted Mini Chex	1	cup(s)	40	—	147	1.3	36.0	0	0	0	0	0
10268	Frosted Mini-Wheats	1	cup(s)	59	3.1	208	5.8	47.4	5.8	1.2	0	0	0.6
38216	Frosted Wheaties	1	cup(s)	40	—	147	1.3	36.0	0.3	0	0	0	0
1223	Granola, prepared	½	cup(s)	61	3.3	298	9.1	32.5	5.5	14.7	2.5	5.8	5.6
2415	Honey Bunches of Oats honey roasted	1	cup(s)	40	0.9	160	2.7	33.3	1.3	2.0	0.7	1.2	0.1
1227	Honey Nut Cheerios	1	cup(s)	37	0.9	149	3.7	29.9	2.5	1.9	0	0.6	0.6
2424	Honeycomb	1	cup(s)	22	0.3	83	1.5	19.5	0.8	0.4	0	—	—
10286	Kashi whole grain puffs	1	cup(s)	19	—	70	2.0	15.0	1.0	0.5	0	—	—
41142	Kellogg's Mueslix	1	cup(s)	83	7.2	298	7.6	60.8	6.1	4.6	0.7	2.4	1.5
1231	Kix	1	cup(s)	24	0.5	96	1.6	20.8	0.8	0.4	—	—	—
30569	Life	1	cup(s)	43	1.7	160	4.0	33.3	2.7	2.0	0.3	0.6	0.6
1233	Lucky Charms	1	cup(s)	24	0.6	96	1.6	20.0	0.8	0.8	—	—	—
38220	Multi Grain Cheerios	1	cup(s)	30	—	110	3.0	24.0	3.0	1.0	—	—	—
1201	Multi-Bran Chex	1	cup(s)	63	1.3	216	4.3	52.9	8.6	1.6	0	0	0.5
13633	Post Bran Flakes	1	cup(s)	40	1.5	133	4.0	32.0	6.7	0.7	0	—	—
1241	Product 19	1	cup(s)	30	1.0	100	2.0	25.0	1.0	0	0	0	0
32432	Puffed rice, fortified	1	cup(s)	14	0.4	56	0.9	12.6	0.2	0.1	0	—	—
32433	Puffed wheat, fortified	1	cup(s)	12	0.4	44	1.8	9.6	0.5	0.1	0	—	—
13334	Quaker 100% natural granola oats and honey	½	cup(s)	48	—	220	5.0	31.0	3.0	9.0	3.8	4.1	1.2
13335	Quaker 100% natural granola oats, honey, and raisins	½	cup(s)	51	—	230	5.0	34.0	3.0	9.0	3.6	3.8	1.1
2420	Raisin Bran	1	cup(s)	59	5.0	190	4.0	46.0	8.0	1.0	0	0.1	0.4
1244	Rice Chex	1	cup(s)	31	0.8	120	2.0	27.0	0.3	0	0	0	0
1245	Rice Krispies	1	cup(s)	26	0.8	96	1.6	23.2	0	0	0	0	0
5593	Shredded Wheat	1	cup(s)	49	0.4	177	5.8	40.9	6.9	1.1	0.1	0	0.2
1248	Smacks	1	cup(s)	36	1.1	133	2.7	32.0	1.3	0.7	—	—	—
1246	Special K	1	cup(s)	31	0.9	110	7.0	22.0	0.5	0	0	0	0
3428	Total corn flakes	1	cup(s)	23	0.6	83	1.5	18.0	0.6	0	0	0	0
1253	Total whole grain	1	cup(s)	40	1.1	147	2.7	30.7	4.0	1.3	—	—	—
1254	Trix	1	cup(s)	30	0.6	120	1.0	27.0	1.0	1.0	—	—	—
382	Wheat germ, toasted	2	tablespoon(s)	14	0.8	54	4.1	7.0	2.1	1.5	0.3	0.2	0.9
1257	Wheaties	1	cup(s)	36	1.2	132	3.6	28.8	3.6	1.2	—	—	—

PASTA, NOODLES

D&W+ Code	Food Description	QTY	Measure	Wt (g)	H₂O (g)	Ener (cal)	Prot (g)	Carb (g)	Fiber (g)	Fat (g)	Sat	Mono	Poly
449	Chinese chow mein noodles, cooked	½	cup(s)	23	0.2	119	1.9	12.9	0.9	6.9	1.0	1.7	3.9
1995	Corn pasta, cooked	½	cup(s)	70	47.8	88	1.8	19.5	3.4	0.5	0.1	0.1	0.2

PAGE KEY: A-4 = Breads/Baked Goods A-10 = Cereal/Rice/Pasta A-14 = Fruit A-20 = Vegetables/Legumes A-30 = Nuts/Seeds A-32 = Vegetarian A-34 = Dairy A-42 = Eggs A-42 = Seafood A-46 = Meats A-50 = Poultry A-50 = Processed Meats A-52 = Beverages A-56 = Fats/Oils A-58 = Sweets A-60 = Spices/Condiments/Sauces A-64 = Mixed Foods/Soups/Sandwiches A-70 = Fast Food A-90 = Convenience A-92 = Baby Foods

A

CHOL (mg)	CALC (mg)	IRON (mg)	MAGN (mg)	POTA (mg)	SODI (mg)	ZINC (mg)	VIT A (µg)	THIA (mg)	VIT E (mg α)	RIBO (mg)	NIAC (mg)	VIT B6 (mg)	FOLA (µg DFE)	VIT C (mg)	VIT B12 (µg)	SELE (µg)
0	4	0.73	6.1	25.4	269.8	0.08	0	0.10	0.02	0.07	0.87	0.03	46.0	0	0	3.8
0	4	0.73	6.1	25.4	269.8	0.08	2.4	0.10	0.02	0.07	0.87	0.03	44.8	0	0	3.3
0	11	1.05	31.6	81.9	4.7	1.17	0	0.09	0.09	0.02	0.26	0.01	7.0	0	0	6.3
0	26	6.83	49.9	126.4	403.5	1.03	0	1.02	—	0.05	1.56	0.30	42.2	0	0	11.1
0	21	3.96	44.7	112.4	240.9	0.92	0	0.60	—	0.04	0.77	0.18	18.7	0	0	3.8
0	241	10.90	224.4	632.4	150.0	3.00	300.1	1.40	—	1.68	9.16	7.44	1362.8	12.4	12.0	5.8
0	57	13.64	186.4	909.1	614.5	4.55	464.5	1.09	1.42	1.27	15.45	6.09	2054.8	18.2	18.2	26.3
0	0	4.50	8.0	30.0	130.0	1.50	150.2	0.37	—	0.42	5.00	0.50	196.0	15.0	1.5	2.4
0	5	6.80	20.0	73.3	266.7	5.00	2.5	0.51	—	0.57	6.68	0.67	946.8	0	0	6.7
0	7	6.53	18.7	73.3	240.0	5.13	2.4	0.51	—	0.57	6.68	0.67	910.7	0	0	6.7
0	100	8.10	40.0	95.0	280.0	3.75	150.3	0.37	—	0.42	5.00	0.50	493.2	6.0	1.5	11.3
0	100	4.50	8.0	50.0	170.0	3.75	0	0.37	—	0.42	5.00	0.50	165.9	6.0	1.5	2.0
0	53	6.00	10.7	66.7	253.3	2.00	200.1	0.49	—	0.56	6.67	0.67	442.8	20.0	2.0	5.8
0	0	24.00	53.3	226.7	280.0	20.00	300.1	2.00	—	2.27	26.67	2.67	909.1	80.0	8.0	4.1
0	0	8.10	3.4	25.0	200.0	0.16	149.8	0.37	—	0.42	5.00	0.50	221.8	6.0	1.5	1.4
0	0	1.80	2.5	25.0	120.0	1.50	150.0	0.37	—	0.42	5.00	0.50	174.7	6.0	1.5	2.0
0	27	2.40	80.0	293.3	200.0	2.00	299.9	0.49	—	0.56	6.67	0.67	217.1	20.0	2.0	14.4
0	0	4.50	8.0	35.0	150.0	1.50	150.1	0.37	—	0.42	5.00	0.50	166.1	15.0	1.5	2.3
0	124	5.60	19.9	68.4	261.3	4.67	—	0.46	—	0.52	6.22	0.62	444.4	7.5	1.9	—
0	0	6.00	3.7	26.7	200.0	0.20	200.1	0.49	—	0.56	6.67	0.67	260.4	8.0	2.0	1.8
0	133	12.00	—	33.3	266.7	4.00	—	0.49	—	0.56	6.67	0.67	266.7	8.0	2.0	—
0	0	16.66	69.4	196.7	5.8	1.74	0	0.43	—	0.49	5.78	0.58	193.5	0	1.7	2.4
0	133	10.80	0	46.7	266.7	10.00	—	1.00	—	1.13	13.33	1.33	901.2	8.0	4.0	—
0	48	2.58	106.8	329.4	15.3	2.45	0.6	0.44	6.77	0.17	1.30	0.17	50.0	0.7	0	17.0
0	0	10.80	21.3	0	253.3	0.40	—	0.49	—	0.56	6.67	0.67	549.6	0	2.0	—
0	124	5.60	39.8	112.0	336.0	4.67	—	0.46	—	0.52	6.22	0.62	444.4	7.5	1.9	8.8
0	0	2.03	6.0	26.3	165.4	1.13	—	0.28	—	0.32	3.74	0.37	126.1	0	1.1	—
0	0	0.36	—	60.0	0	—	0	0.03	—	0.03	0.80	0.00	—	0	—	—
0	48	6.83	74.2	363.3	257.5	5.67	136.7	0.67	6.00	0.67	8.33	3.08	1030.0	0.3	9.2	14.4
0	120	6.48	6.4	28.0	216.0	3.00	120.2	0.30	—	0.34	4.00	0.40	317.8	4.8	1.2	4.8
0	149	11.87	41.3	120.0	213.3	5.33	0.9	0.53	—	0.60	7.12	0.71	607.6	0	0	10.7
0	80	3.60	12.8	48.0	168.0	3.00	—	0.30	—	0.34	4.00	0.40	300.7	4.8	1.2	4.8
0	100	18.00	24.0	85.0	200.0	15.00	—	1.50	—	1.70	20.00	2.00	699.3	15.0	6.0	—
0	108	17.50	64.8	237.7	410.6	4.05	171.1	0.40	—	0.45	5.40	0.54	893.3	6.5	1.6	4.9
0	0	10.80	80.0	266.7	280.0	2.00	—	0.49	—	0.56	6.67	0.67	453.3	0	2.0	—
0	0	18.00	16.0	50.0	210.0	15.00	225.3	1.50	—	1.70	20.00	2.00	675.9	60.0	6.0	3.6
0	1	4.43	3.5	15.8	0.4	0.14	0	0.36	—	0.25	4.94	0.01	2.7	0	0	1.5
0	3	3.80	17.4	41.8	0.5	0.28	0	0.31	—	0.21	4.23	0.02	3.8	0	0	14.8
0	61	1.20	51.0	220.0	20.0	1.05	0.5	0.13	—	0.12	0.82	0.07	16.8	0.2	0.1	8.3
0	59	1.20	49.0	250.0	20.0	0.99	0.5	0.13	—	0.12	0.80	0.08	15.8	0.4	0.1	8.8
0	20	10.80	80.0	360.0	360.0	2.25	—	0.37	—	0.42	5.00	0.50	248.4	0	2.1	—
0	100	9.00	9.3	35.0	290.0	3.75	—	0.37	—	0.42	5.00	0.50	389.4	6.0	1.5	1.2
0	0	1.44	12.8	32.0	256.0	0.48	120.1	0.30	—	0.34	4.80	0.40	237.4	4.8	1.2	4.1
0	18	2.90	60.3	179.3	1.1	1.37	0	0.14	—	0.12	3.47	0.18	21.1	0	0	2.0
0	0	0.48	10.7	53.3	66.7	0.40	200.2	0.49	—	0.56	6.67	0.67	224.6	8.0	2.0	17.5
0	0	8.10	16.0	60.0	220.0	0.90	225.1	0.52	—	0.59	7.00	2.00	675.8	21.0	6.0	7.0
0	752	13.53	0	22.6	157.9	11.28	112.8	1.13	22.56	1.28	15.04	1.50	518.2	45.1	4.5	1.2
0	1333	24.00	32.0	120.0	253.3	20.00	200.4	2.00	31.32	2.27	26.67	2.67	901.2	80.0	8.0	1.9
0	100	4.50	0	15.0	190.0	3.75	150.3	0.37	—	0.42	5.00	0.50	155.4	6.0	1.5	6.0
0	6	1.28	45.2	133.8	0.6	2.35	0.7	0.23	2.25	0.11	0.79	0.13	49.7	0.8	0	9.2
0	24	9.72	38.4	126.0	264.0	9.00	180.4	0.90	—	1.02	12.00	1.20	403.6	7.2	3.6	1.7
0	5	1.06	11.7	27.0	98.8	0.31	0	0.13	0.78	0.09	1.33	0.02	31.1	0	0	9.7
0	1	0.18	25.2	21.7	0	0.44	2.1	0.04	—	0.02	0.39	0.04	4.2	0	0	2.0

Table of Food Composition (continued)

(Computer code is for Cengage Diet & Wellness Plus program)

D&W+ Code	Food Description	QTY	Measure	Wt (g)	H₂O (g)	Ener (cal)	Prot (g)	Carb (g)	Fiber (g)	Fat (g)	Fat Breakdown (g) Sat	Mono	Poly
CEREAL, FLOUR, GRAIN, PASTA, NOODLES, POPCORN—CONTINUED
448	Egg noodles, enriched, cooked	½	cup(s)	80	54.2	110	3.6	20.1	1.0	1.7	0.3	0.5	0.4
1563	Egg noodles, spinach, enriched, cooked	½	cup(s)	80	54.8	106	4.0	19.4	1.8	1.3	0.3	0.4	0.3
440	Macaroni, enriched, cooked	½	cup(s)	70	43.5	111	4.1	21.6	1.3	0.7	0.1	0.1	0.2
2000	Macaroni, tricolor vegetable, enriched, cooked	½	cup(s)	67	45.8	86	3.0	17.8	2.9	0.1	0	0	0
1996	Plain pasta, fresh-refrigerated, cooked	½	cup(s)	64	43.9	84	3.3	16.0	—	0.7	0.1	0.1	0.3
1725	Ramen noodles, cooked	½	cup(s)	114	94.5	104	3.0	15.4	1.0	4.3	0.2	0.2	0.2
2878	Soba noodles, cooked	½	cup(s)	95	69.4	94	4.8	20.4	—	0.1	0	0	0
2879	Somen noodles, cooked	½	cup(s)	88	59.8	115	3.5	24.2	—	0.2	0	0	0.1
493	Spaghetti, al dente, cooked	½	cup(s)	65	41.6	95	3.5	19.5	1.0	0.5	0.1	0.1	0.2
2884	Spaghetti, whole wheat, cooked	½	cup(s)	70	47.0	87	3.7	18.6	3.2	0.4	0.1	0.1	0.1
	POPCORN
476	Air popped	1	cup(s)	8	0.3	31	1.0	6.2	1.2	0.4	0	0.1	0.2
4619	Caramel	1	cup(s)	35	1.0	152	1.3	27.8	1.8	4.5	1.3	1.0	1.6
4620	Cheese flavored	1	cup(s)	36	0.9	188	3.3	18.4	3.5	11.8	2.3	3.5	5.5
477	Popped in oil	1	cup(s)	11	0.1	64	0.8	5.0	0.9	4.8	0.8	1.1	2.6
FRUIT AND FRUIT JUICES
	APPLES
952	Juice, prepared from frozen concentrate	½	cup(s)	120	105.0	56	0.2	13.8	0.1	0.1	0	0	0
225	Juice, unsweetened, canned	½	cup(s)	124	109.0	58	0.1	14.5	0.1	0.1	0	0	0
224	Slices	½	cup(s)	55	47.1	29	0.1	7.6	1.3	0.1	0	0	0
946	Slices without skin, boiled	½	cup(s)	86	73.1	45	0.2	11.7	2.1	0.3	0	0	0.1
223	Raw medium, with peel	1	item(s)	138	118.1	72	0.4	19.1	3.3	0.2	0	0	0.1
948	Dried, sulfured	¼	cup(s)	22	6.8	52	0.2	14.2	1.9	0.1	0	0	0
226	Applesauce, sweetened, canned	½	cup(s)	128	101.5	97	0.2	25.4	1.5	0.2	0	0	0.1
227	Applesauce, unsweetened, canned	½	cup(s)	122	107.8	52	0.2	13.8	1.5	0.1	0	0	0
38492	Crabapples	1	item(s)	35	27.6	27	0.1	7.0	0.9	0.1	0	0	0
	APRICOT
228	Fresh without pits	4	item(s)	140	120.9	67	2.0	15.6	2.8	0.5	0	0.2	0.1
229	Halves with skin, canned in heavy syrup	½	cup(s)	129	100.1	107	0.7	27.7	2.1	0.1	0	0	0
230	Halves, dried, sulfured	¼	cup(s)	33	10.1	79	1.1	20.6	2.4	0.2	0	0	0
	AVOCADO
233	California, whole, without skin or pit	½	cup(s)	115	83.2	192	2.2	9.9	7.8	17.7	2.4	11.3	2.1
234	Florida, whole, without skin or pit	½	cup(s)	115	90.6	138	2.5	9.0	6.4	11.5	2.2	6.3	1.9
2998	Pureed	¹⁄₈	cup(s)	28	20.2	44	0.5	2.4	1.8	4.0	0.6	2.7	0.5
	BANANA
4580	Dried chips	¼	cup(s)	55	2.4	285	1.3	32.1	4.2	18.5	15.9	1.1	0.3
235	Fresh whole, without peel	1	item(s)	118	88.4	105	1.3	27.0	3.1	0.4	0.1	0	0.1
	BLACKBERRIES
237	Raw	½	cup(s)	72	63.5	31	1.0	6.9	3.8	0.4	0	0	0.2
958	Unsweetened, frozen	½	cup(s)	76	62.1	48	0.9	11.8	3.8	0.3	0	0	0.2
	BLUEBERRIES
959	Canned in heavy syrup	½	cup(s)	128	98.3	113	0.8	28.2	2.0	0.4	0	0.1	0.2
238	Raw	½	cup(s)	73	61.1	41	0.5	10.5	1.7	0.2	0	0	0.1
960	Unsweetened, frozen	½	cup(s)	78	67.1	40	0.3	9.4	2.1	0.5	0	0.1	0.2
	BOYSENBERRIES
961	Canned in heavy syrup	½	cup(s)	128	97.6	113	1.3	28.6	3.3	0.2	0	0	0.1
962	Unsweetened, frozen	½	cup(s)	66	56.7	33	0.7	8.0	3.5	0.2	0	0	0.1
35576	**BREADFRUIT**	1	item(s)	384	271.3	396	4.1	104.1	18.8	0.9	0.2	0.1	0.3
	CHERRIES
967	Sour red, canned in water	½	cup(s)	122	109.7	44	0.9	10.9	1.3	0.1	0	0	0
3000	Sour red, raw	½	cup(s)	78	66.8	39	0.8	9.4	1.2	0.2	0.1	0.1	0.1
3004	Sweet, canned in heavy syrup	½	cup(s)	127	98.2	105	0.8	26.9	1.9	0.2	0	0.1	0.1
969	Sweet, canned in water	½	cup(s)	124	107.9	57	1.0	14.6	1.9	0.2	0	0	0
240	Sweet, raw	½	cup(s)	73	59.6	46	0.8	11.6	1.5	0.1	0	0	0

PAGE KEY: A-4 = Breads/Baked Goods A-10 = Cereal/Rice/Pasta A-14 = Fruit A-20 = Vegetables/Legumes A-30 = Nuts/Seeds A-32 = Vegetarian A-34 = Dairy A-42 = Eggs A-42 = Seafood A-46 = Meats A-50 = Poultry A-50 = Processed Meats A-52 = Beverages A-56 = Fats/Oils A-58 = Sweets A-60 = Spices/Condiments/Sauces A-64 = Mixed Foods/Soups/Sandwiches A-70 = Fast Food A-90 = Convenience A-92 = Baby Foods

A

CHOL (mg)	CALC (mg)	IRON (mg)	MAGN (mg)	POTA (mg)	SODI (mg)	ZINC (mg)	VIT A (µg)	THIA (mg)	VIT E (mg α)	RIBO (mg)	NIAC (mg)	VIT B6 (mg)	FOLA (µg DFE)	VIT C (mg)	VIT B12 (µg)	SELE (µg)
23	10	1.17	16.8	30.4	4.0	0.52	4.8	0.23	0.13	0.11	1.66	0.03	110.4	0	0.1	19.1
26	15	0.87	19.2	29.6	9.6	0.50	8.0	0.19	0.46	0.09	1.17	0.09	75.2	0	0.1	17.4
0	5	0.90	12.6	30.8	0.7	0.36	0	0.19	0.04	0.10	1.18	0.03	83.3	0	0	18.5
0	7	0.33	12.7	20.8	4.0	0.30	3.4	0.08	0.14	0.04	0.72	0.02	71.0	0	0	13.3
21	4	0.73	11.5	15.4	3.8	0.36	3.8	0.13	—	0.10	0.64	0.02	66.6	0	0.1	—
18	9	0.89	8.5	34.5	414.5	0.30	—	0.08	—	0.04	0.71	0.03	4.0	0.1	0	—
0	4	0.45	8.5	33.2	57.0	0.11	0	0.09	—	0.02	0.48	0.03	6.6	0	0	—
0	7	0.45	1.8	25.5	141.7	0.19	0	0.01	—	0.03	0.08	0.01	1.8	0	0	—
0	7	1.00	12.4	51.5	0.5	0.35	0	0.12	0.04	0.07	0.90	0.04	77.4	0	0	40.0
0	11	0.74	21.0	30.8	2.1	0.57	0	0.08	0.21	0.03	0.50	0.06	3.5	0	0	18.1
0	1	0.25	11.5	26.3	0.6	0.25	0.8	0.01	0.02	0.01	0.18	0.01	2.5	0	0	0
2	15	0.61	12.3	38.4	72.5	0.20	0.7	0.02	0.42	0.02	0.77	0.01	1.8	0	0	1.3
4	40	0.79	32.5	93.2	317.4	0.71	13.6	0.04	—	0.08	0.52	0.08	3.9	0.2	0.2	4.3
0	0	0.22	8.7	20.0	116.4	0.34	0.9	0.01	0.27	0.00	0.13	0.01	2.8	0	0	0.2
0	7	0.31	6.0	150.6	8.4	0.05	0	0.00	0.01	0.02	0.05	0.04	0	0.7	0	0.1
0	9	0.46	3.7	147.6	3.7	0.04	0	0.03	0.01	0.02	0.12	0.04	0	1.1	0	0.1
0	3	0.06	2.7	58.8	0.5	0.02	1.6	0.01	0.10	0.01	0.05	0.02	1.6	2.5	0	0
0	4	0.16	2.6	75.2	0.9	0.03	1.7	0.01	0.04	0.01	0.08	0.04	0.9	0.2	0	0.3
0	8	0.16	6.9	147.7	1.4	0.05	4.1	0.02	0.24	0.03	0.12	0.05	4.1	6.3	0	0
0	3	0.30	3.4	96.8	18.7	0.04	0	0.00	0.11	0.03	0.20	0.03	0	0.8	0	0.3
0	5	0.44	3.8	77.8	3.8	0.05	1.3	0.01	0.26	0.03	0.24	0.03	1.3	2.2	0	0.4
0	4	0.14	3.7	91.5	2.4	0.03	1.2	0.01	0.25	0.03	0.22	0.03	1.2	1.5	0	0.4
0	6	0.12	2.5	67.9	0.4	—	0.7	0.01	0.20	0.01	0.03	—	2.0	2.8	0	—
0	18	0.54	14.0	362.6	1.4	0.28	134.4	0.04	1.24	0.05	0.84	0.07	12.6	14.0	0	0.1
0	12	0.38	9.0	180.6	5.2	0.14	80.0	0.02	0.77	0.02	0.48	0.07	2.6	4.0	0	0.1
0	18	0.87	10.5	381.5	3.3	0.12	59.1	0.00	1.42	0.02	0.85	0.05	3.3	0.3	0	0.7
0	15	0.66	33.3	583.0	9.2	0.78	8.0	0.08	2.23	0.16	2.19	0.31	102.3	10.1	0	0.4
0	12	0.19	27.6	403.6	2.3	0.45	8.0	0.02	3.03	0.04	0.76	0.08	40.3	20.0	0	—
0	3	0.14	8.0	134.1	1.9	0.17	1.9	0.01	0.57	0.03	0.48	0.07	22.4	2.8	0	0.1
0	10	0.69	41.8	294.8	3.3	0.40	2.2	0.04	0.13	0.01	0.39	0.14	7.7	3.5	0	0.8
0	6	0.30	31.9	422.4	1.2	0.17	3.5	0.03	0.11	0.08	0.78	0.43	23.6	10.3	0	1.2
0	21	0.45	14.4	116.6	0.7	0.38	7.9	0.01	0.84	0.02	0.47	0.02	18.0	15.1	0	0.3
0	22	0.60	16.6	105.7	0.8	0.19	4.5	0.02	0.88	0.03	0.91	0.05	25.7	2.3	0	0.3
0	6	0.42	5.1	51.2	3.8	0.09	2.6	0.04	0.49	0.07	0.14	0.05	2.6	1.4	0	0.1
0	4	0.20	4.4	55.8	0.7	0.12	2.2	0.03	0.41	0.03	0.30	0.04	4.4	7.0	0	0.1
0	6	0.14	3.9	41.9	0.8	0.05	1.6	0.03	0.37	0.03	0.40	0.05	5.4	1.9	0	0.1
0	23	0.55	14.1	115.2	3.8	0.24	2.6	0.03	—	0.04	0.29	0.05	43.5	7.9	0	0.5
0	18	0.56	10.6	91.7	0.7	0.15	2.0	0.04	0.57	0.02	0.51	0.04	41.6	2.0	0	0.1
0	65	2.07	96.0	1881.6	7.7	0.46	0	0.42	0.38	0.11	3.45	0.38	53.8	111.4	0	2.3
0	13	1.67	7.3	119.6	8.5	0.09	46.4	0.02	0.28	0.05	0.22	0.05	9.8	2.6	0	0
0	12	0.25	7.0	134.1	2.3	0.08	49.6	0.02	0.05	0.03	0.31	0.03	6.2	7.8	0	0
0	11	0.44	11.4	183.4	3.8	0.12	10.1	0.02	0.29	0.05	0.50	0.03	5.1	4.6	0	0
0	14	0.45	11.2	162.4	1.2	0.10	9.9	0.03	0.29	0.05	0.51	0.04	5.0	2.7	0	0
0	9	0.26	8.0	161.0	0	0.05	2.2	0.02	0.05	0.02	0.11	0.04	2.9	5.1	0	0

A

D&W+ Code	Food Description	QTY	Measure	Wt (g)	H₂0 (g)	Ener (cal)	Prot (g)	Carb (g)	Fiber (g)	Fat (g)	Sat	Mono	Poly
											Fat Breakdown (g)		

Fruit and Fruit Juices—continued

D&W+ Code	Food Description	QTY	Measure	Wt (g)	H₂0 (g)	Ener (cal)	Prot (g)	Carb (g)	Fiber (g)	Fat (g)	Sat	Mono	Poly
	CRANBERRIES												
3007	Chopped, raw	½	cup(s)	55	47.9	25	0.2	6.7	2.5	0.1	0	0	0
1717	Cranberry apple juice drink	½	cup(s)	123	102.6	77	0	19.4	0	0.1	0	0	0.1
1638	Cranberry juice cocktail	½	cup(s)	127	109.0	68	0	17.1	0	0.1	0	0	0.1
241	Cranberry juice cocktail, low calorie, with saccharin	½	cup(s)	119	112.8	23	0	5.5	0	0	0	0	0
242	Cranberry sauce, sweetened, canned	¼	cup(s)	69	42.0	105	0.1	26.9	0.7	0.1	0	0	0
	DATES												
244	Domestic, chopped	¼	cup(s)	45	9.1	125	1.1	33.4	3.6	0.2	0	0	0
243	Domestic, whole	¼	cup(s)	45	9.1	125	1.1	33.4	3.6	0.2	0	0	0
	FIGS												
975	Canned in heavy syrup	½	cup(s)	130	98.8	114	0.5	29.7	2.8	0.1	0	0	0.1
974	Canned in water	½	cup(s)	124	105.7	66	0.5	17.3	2.7	0.1	0	0	0.1
973	Raw, medium	2	item(s)	100	79.1	74	0.7	19.2	2.9	0.3	0.1	0.1	0.1
	FRUIT COCKTAIL AND SALAD												
245	Fruit cocktail, canned in heavy syrup	½	cup(s)	124	99.7	91	0.5	23.4	1.2	0.1	0	0	0
978	Fruit cocktail, canned in juice	½	cup(s)	119	103.6	55	0.5	14.1	1.2	0	0	0	0
977	Fruit cocktail, canned in water	½	cup(s)	119	107.6	38	0.5	10.1	1.2	0.1	0	0	0
979	Fruit salad, canned in water	½	cup(s)	123	112.1	37	0.4	9.6	1.2	0.1	0	0	0
	GOOSEBERRIES												
982	Canned in light syrup	½	cup(s)	126	100.9	92	0.8	23.6	3.0	0.3	0	0	0.1
981	Raw	½	cup(s)	75	65.9	33	0.7	7.6	3.2	0.4	0	0	0.2
	GRAPEFRUIT												
251	Juice, pink, sweetened, canned	½	cup(s)	125	109.1	57	0.7	13.9	0.1	0.1	0	0	0
249	Juice, white	½	cup(s)	124	111.2	48	0.6	11.4	0.1	0.1	0	0	0
3022	Pink or red, raw	½	cup(s)	114	100.8	48	0.9	12.2	1.8	0.2	0	0	0
248	Sections, canned in light syrup	½	cup(s)	127	106.2	76	0.7	19.6	0.5	0.1	0	0	0
983	Sections, canned in water	½	cup(s)	122	109.6	44	0.7	11.2	0.5	0.1	0	0	0
247	White, raw	½	cup(s)	115	104.0	38	0.8	9.7	1.3	0.1	0	0	0
	GRAPES												
255	American, slip skin	½	cup(s)	46	37.4	31	0.3	7.9	0.4	0.2	0.1	0	0
256	European, red or green, adherent skin	½	cup(s)	76	60.8	52	0.5	13.7	0.7	0.1	0	0	0
3159	Grape juice drink, canned	½	cup(s)	125	106.6	71	0	18.2	0.1	0	0	0	0
259	Grape juice, sweetened, with added vitamin C, prepared from frozen concentrate	½	cup(s)	125	108.6	64	0.2	15.9	0.1	0.1	0	0	0
3060	Raisins, seeded, packed	¼	cup(s)	41	6.8	122	1.0	32.4	2.8	0.2	0.1	0	0.1
987	**GUAVA, RAW**	1	item(s)	55	44.4	37	1.4	7.9	3.0	0.5	0.2	0	0.2
35593	**GUAVAS, STRAWBERRY**	1	item(s)	6	4.8	4	0	1.0	0.3	0	0	0	0
3027	**JACKFRUIT**	½	cup(s)	83	60.4	78	1.2	19.8	1.3	0.2	0	0	0.1
990	**KIWI FRUIT OR CHINESE GOOSEBERRIES**	1	item(s)	76	63.1	46	0.9	11.1	2.3	0.4	0	0	0.2
	LEMON												
262	Juice	1	tablespoon(s)	15	13.8	4	0.1	1.3	0.1	0	0	0	0
993	Peel	1	teaspoon(s)	2	1.6	1	0	0.3	0.2	0	0	0	0
992	Raw	1	item(s)	108	94.4	22	1.3	11.6	5.1	0.3	0	0	0.1
	LIME												
269	Juice	1	tablespoon(s)	15	14.0	4	0.1	1.3	0.1	0	0	0	0
994	Raw	1	item(s)	67	59.1	20	0.5	7.1	1.9	0.1	0	0	0
995	**LOGANBERRIES, FROZEN**	½	cup(s)	74	62.2	40	1.1	9.6	3.9	0.2	0	0	0.1
	MANDARIN ORANGE												
1038	Canned in juice	½	cup(s)	125	111.4	46	0.8	11.9	0.9	0	0	0	0
1039	Canned in light syrup	½	cup(s)	126	104.7	77	0.6	20.4	0.9	0.1	0	0	0
999	**MANGO**	½	cup(s)	83	67.4	54	0.4	14.0	1.5	0.2	0.1	0.1	0
	MELONS												
271	Cantaloupe	½	cup(s)	80	72.1	27	0.7	6.5	0.7	0.1	0	0	0.1
1000	Casaba melon	½	cup(s)	85	78.1	24	0.9	5.6	0.8	0.1	0	0	0

PAGE KEY: A-4 = Breads/Baked Goods A-10 = Cereal/Rice/Pasta A-14 = Fruit A-20 = Vegetables/Legumes A-30 = Nuts/Seeds A-32 = Vegetarian A-34 = Dairy A-42 = Eggs A-42 = Seafood A-46 = Meats A-50 = Poultry A-50 = Processed Meats A-52 = Beverages A-56 = Fats/Oils A-58 = Sweets A-60 = Spices/Condiments/Sauces A-64 = Mixed Foods/Soups/Sandwiches A-70 = Fast Food A-90 = Convenience A-92 = Baby Foods

A

CHOL (mg)	CALC (mg)	IRON (mg)	MAGN (mg)	POTA (mg)	SODI (mg)	ZINC (mg)	VIT A (µg)	THIA (mg)	VIT E (mg α)	RIBO (mg)	NIAC (mg)	VIT B6 (mg)	FOLA (µg DFE)	VIT C (mg)	VIT B12 (µg)	SELE (µg)
0	4	0.13	3.3	46.8	1.1	0.05	1.7	0.01	0.66	0.01	0.05	0.03	0.6	7.3	0	0.1
0	4	0.09	1.2	20.8	2.5	0.02	0	0.00	0.15	0.00	0.00	0.00	0	48.4	0	0
0	4	0.13	1.3	17.7	2.5	0.04	0	0.00	0.28	0.00	0.05	0.00	0	53.5	0	0.3
0	11	0.05	2.4	29.6	3.6	0.02	0	0.00	0.06	0.00	0.00	0.00	0	38.2	0	0
0	3	0.15	2.1	18.0	20.1	0.03	1.4	0.01	0.57	0.01	0.06	0.01	0.7	1.4	0	0.2
0	17	0.45	19.1	291.9	0.9	0.12	0	0.02	0.02	0.02	0.56	0.07	8.5	0.2	0	1.3
0	17	0.45	19.1	291.9	0.9	0.12	0	0.02	0.02	0.02	0.56	0.07	8.5	0.2	0	1.3
0	35	0.36	13.0	128.2	1.3	0.14	2.6	0.03	0.16	0.05	0.55	0.09	2.6	1.3	0	0.3
0	35	0.36	12.4	127.7	1.2	0.15	2.5	0.03	0.10	0.05	0.55	0.09	2.5	1.2	0	0.1
0	35	0.36	17.0	232.0	1.0	0.14	7.0	0.06	0.10	0.04	0.40	0.10	6.0	2.0	0	0.2
0	7	0.36	6.2	109.1	7.4	0.09	12.4	0.02	0.49	0.02	0.46	0.06	3.7	2.4	0	0.6
0	9	0.25	8.3	112.6	4.7	0.11	17.8	0.01	0.47	0.02	0.48	0.06	3.6	3.2	0	0.6
0	6	0.30	8.3	111.4	4.7	0.11	15.4	0.02	0.47	0.02	0.43	0.06	3.6	2.5	0	0.6
0	9	0.37	6.1	95.6	3.7	0.10	27.0	0.02	—	0.03	0.46	0.04	3.7	2.3	0	1.0
0	20	0.42	7.6	97.0	2.5	0.14	8.8	0.03	—	0.07	0.19	0.02	3.8	12.6	0	0.5
0	19	0.23	7.5	148.5	0.8	0.09	11.3	0.03	0.28	0.02	0.23	0.06	4.5	20.8	0	0.5
0	10	0.45	12.5	202.2	2.5	0.08	0	0.05	0.05	0.03	0.40	0.03	12.5	33.6	0	0.1
0	11	0.25	14.8	200.1	1.2	0.06	1.2	0.05	0.27	0.02	0.25	0.05	12.4	46.9	0	0.1
0	25	0.09	10.3	154.5	0	0.07	66.4	0.04	0.14	0.03	0.23	0.06	14.9	35.7	0	0.1
0	18	0.50	12.7	163.8	2.5	0.10	0	0.04	0.11	0.02	0.30	0.02	11.4	27.1	0	1.1
0	18	0.50	12.2	161.0	2.4	0.11	0	0.05	0.11	0.03	0.30	0.02	11.0	26.6	0	1.1
0	14	0.07	10.4	170.2	0	0.08	2.3	0.04	0.15	0.02	0.30	0.05	11.5	38.3	0	1.6
0	6	0.13	2.3	87.9	0.9	0.02	2.3	0.04	0.09	0.02	0.14	0.05	1.8	1.8	0	0
0	8	0.27	5.3	144.2	1.5	0.05	2.3	0.05	0.14	0.05	0.14	0.07	1.5	8.2	0	0.1
0	9	0.16	7.5	41.3	11.3	0.04	0	0.28	0.00	0.44	0.18	0.04	1.3	33.1	0	0.1
0	5	0.13	5.0	26.3	2.5	0.05	0	0.02	0.00	0.03	0.16	0.05	1.3	29.9	0	0.1
0	12	1.06	12.4	340.3	11.6	0.07	0	0.04	—	0.07	0.46	0.07	1.2	2.2	0	0.2
0	10	0.14	12.1	229.4	1.1	0.12	17.1	0.03	0.40	0.02	0.59	0.06	27.0	125.6	0	0.3
0	1	0.01	1.0	17.5	2.2	—	0.3	0.00	—	0.00	0.03	0.00	—	2.2	0	0
0	28	0.49	30.5	250.0	2.5	0.35	12.4	0.02	—	0.09	0.33	0.09	11.5	5.5	0	0.5
0	26	0.23	12.9	237.1	2.3	0.10	3.0	0.02	1.11	0.01	0.25	0.04	19.0	70.5	0	0.2
0	1	0.00	0.9	18.9	0.2	0.01	0.2	0.00	0.02	0.00	0.02	0.01	2.0	7.0	0	0
0	3	0.01	0.3	3.2	0.1	0.01	0.1	0.00	0.01	0.00	0.01	0.00	0.3	2.6	0	0
0	66	0.75	13.0	156.6	3.2	0.10	2.2	0.05	—	0.04	0.21	0.11	—	83.2	0	1.0
0	2	0.02	1.2	18.0	0.3	0.01	0.3	0.00	0.03	0.00	0.02	0.01	1.5	4.6	0	0
0	22	0.40	4.0	68.3	1.3	0.07	1.3	0.02	0.14	0.01	0.13	0.02	5.4	19.5	0	0.3
0	19	0.47	15.4	106.6	0.7	0.25	1.5	0.04	0.64	0.03	0.62	0.05	19.1	11.2	0	0.1
0	14	0.34	13.7	165.6	6.2	0.64	53.5	0.10	0.12	0.04	0.55	0.05	6.2	42.6	0	0.5
0	9	0.47	10.1	98.3	7.6	0.30	52.9	0.07	0.13	0.06	0.56	0.05	6.3	24.9	0	0.5
0	8	0.10	7.4	128.7	1.7	0.03	31.4	0.05	0.92	0.04	0.48	0.11	11.6	22.8	0	0.5
0	7	0.17	9.6	213.6	12.8	0.14	135.2	0.03	0.04	0.01	0.59	0.05	16.8	29.4	0	0.3
0	9	0.29	9.4	154.7	7.7	0.06	0	0.01	0.04	0.03	0.20	0.14	6.8	18.5	0	0.3

A

D&W+ Code	Food Description	QTY	Measure	Wt (g)	H₂0 (g)	Ener (cal)	Prot (g)	Carb (g)	Fiber (g)	Fat (g)	Fat Breakdown (g) Sat	Mono	Poly
	FRUIT AND FRUIT JUICES—CONTINUED												
272	Honeydew	½	cup(s)	89	79.5	32	0.5	8.0	0.7	0.1	0	0	0
318	Watermelon	½	cup(s)	76	69.5	23	0.5	5.7	0.3	0.1	0	0	0
1005	**NECTARINE, RAW, SLICED**	½	cup(s)	69	60.4	30	0.7	7.3	1.2	0.2	0	0.1	0.1
	ORANGE												
14412	Juice with calcium and vitamin D	½	cup(s)	120	—	55	1.0	13.0	0	0	0	0	0
29630	Juice, fresh squeezed	½	cup(s)	124	109.5	56	0.9	12.9	0.2	0.2	0	0	0
14411	Juice, not from concentrate	½	cup(s)	120	—	55	1.0	13.0	0	0	0	0	0
278	Juice, unsweetened, prepared from frozen concentrate	½	cup(s)	125	109.7	56	0.8	13.4	0.2	0.1	0	0	0
3040	Peel	1	teaspoon(s)	2	1.5	2	0	0.5	0.2	0	0	0	0
273	Raw	1	item(s)	131	113.6	62	1.2	15.4	3.1	0.2	0	0	0
274	Sections	½	cup(s)	90	78.1	42	0.8	10.6	2.2	0.1	0	0	0
	PAPAYA, RAW												
16830	Dried, strips	2	item(s)	46	12.0	119	1.9	29.9	5.5	0.4	0.1	0.1	0.1
282	Papaya	½	cup(s)	70	62.2	27	0.4	6.9	1.3	0.1	0	0	0
35640	**PASSION FRUIT, PURPLE**	1	item(s)	18	13.1	17	0.4	4.2	1.9	0.1	0	0	0.1
	PEACH												
285	Halves, canned in heavy syrup	½	cup(s)	131	103.9	97	0.6	26.1	1.7	0.1	0	0	0.1
286	Halves, canned in water	½	cup(s)	122	113.6	29	0.5	7.5	1.6	0.1	0	0	0
290	Slices, sweetened, frozen	½	cup(s)	125	93.4	118	0.8	30.0	2.3	0.2	0	0.1	0.1
283	Raw, medium	1	item(s)	150	133.3	59	1.4	14.3	2.3	0.4	0	0.1	0.1
	PEAR												
8672	Asian	1	item(s)	122	107.7	51	0.6	13.0	4.4	0.3	0	0.1	0.1
293	D'Anjou	1	item(s)	200	168.0	120	1.0	30.0	5.2	1.0	0	0.2	0.2
294	Halves, canned in heavy syrup	½	cup(s)	133	106.9	98	0.3	25.5	2.1	0.2	0	0	0
1012	Halves, canned in juice	½	cup(s)	124	107.2	62	0.4	16.0	2.0	0.1	0	0	0
291	Raw	1	item(s)	166	139.0	96	0.6	25.7	5.1	0.2	0	0	0
1017	**PERSIMMON**	1	item(s)	25	16.1	32	0.2	8.4	—	0.1	0	0	0
	PINEAPPLE												
3053	Canned in extra heavy syrup	½	cup(s)	130	101.0	108	0.4	28.0	1.0	0.1	0	0	0
1019	Canned in juice	½	cup(s)	125	104.0	75	0.5	19.5	1.0	0.1	0	0	0
296	Canned in light syrup	½	cup(s)	126	108.0	66	0.5	16.9	1.0	0.2	0	0	0.1
1018	Canned in water	½	cup(s)	123	111.7	39	0.5	10.2	1.0	0.1	0	0	0
299	Juice, unsweetened, canned	½	cup(s)	125	108.0	66	0.5	16.1	0.3	0.2	0	0	0.1
295	Raw, diced	½	cup(s)	78	66.7	39	0.4	10.2	1.1	0.1	0	0	0
1024	**PLANTAIN, COOKED**	½	cup(s)	77	51.8	89	0.6	24.0	1.8	0.1	0.1	0	0
300	**PLUM, RAW, LARGE**	1	item(s)	66	57.6	30	0.5	7.5	0.9	0.2	0	0.1	0
1027	**POMEGRANATE**	1	item(s)	154	124.7	105	1.5	26.4	0.9	0.5	0.1	0.1	0.1
	PRUNES												
5644	Dried	2	item(s)	17	5.2	40	0.4	10.7	1.2	0.1	0	0	0
305	Dried, stewed	½	cup(s)	124	86.5	133	1.2	34.8	3.8	0.2	0	0.1	0
306	Juice, canned	1	cup(s)	256	208.0	182	1.6	44.7	2.6	0.1	0	0.1	0
	RASPBERRIES												
309	Raw	½	cup(s)	62	52.7	32	0.7	7.3	4.0	0.4	0	0	0.2
310	Red, sweetened, frozen	½	cup(s)	125	90.9	129	0.9	32.7	5.5	0.2	0	0	0.1
311	**RHUBARB, COOKED WITH SUGAR**	½	cup(s)	120	81.5	140	0.5	37.5	2.7	0.1	0	0	0.1
	STRAWBERRIES												
313	Raw	½	cup(s)	72	65.5	23	0.5	5.5	1.4	0.2	0	0	0.1
315	Sweetened, frozen, thawed	½	cup(s)	128	99.5	99	0.7	26.8	2.4	0.2	0	0	0.1
16828	**TANGELO**	1	item(s)	95	82.4	45	0.9	11.2	2.3	0.1	0	0	0
	TANGERINE												
1040	Juice	½	cup(s)	124	109.8	53	0.6	12.5	0.2	0.2	0	0	0
316	Raw	1	item(s)	88	74.9	47	0.7	11.7	1.6	0.3	0	0.1	0.1

PAGE KEY: A-4 = Breads/Baked Goods A-10 = Cereal/Rice/Pasta A-14 = Fruit A-20 = Vegetables/Legumes A-30 = Nuts/Seeds A-32 = Vegetarian A-34 = Dairy A-42 = Eggs A-42 = Seafood A-46 = Meats A-50 = Poultry A-50 = Processed Meats A-52 = Beverages A-56 = Fats/Oils A-58 = Sweets A-60 = Spices/Condiments/Sauces A-64 = Mixed Foods/Soups/Sandwiches A-70 = Fast Food A-90 = Convenience A-92 = Baby Foods

A

CHOL (mg)	CALC (mg)	IRON (mg)	MAGN (mg)	POTA (mg)	SODI (mg)	ZINC (mg)	VIT A (µg)	THIA (mg)	VIT E (mg α)	RIBO (mg)	NIAC (mg)	VIT B₆ (mg)	FOLA (µg DFE)	VIT C (mg)	VIT B₁₂ (µg)	SELE (µg)
0	5	0.15	8.8	201.8	15.9	0.07	2.7	0.03	0.01	0.01	0.37	0.07	16.8	15.9	0	0.6
0	5	0.18	7.6	85.1	0.8	0.07	21.3	0.02	0.04	0.01	0.13	0.03	2.3	6.2	0	0.3
0	4	0.19	6.2	138.7	0	0.12	11.7	0.02	0.53	0.02	0.78	0.02	3.5	3.7	0	0
0	175	0.00	12.0	225.0	0	—	0	0.08	—	0.03	0.40	0.06	30.0	36.0	0	—
0	14	0.25	13.6	248.0	1.2	0.06	12.4	0.11	0.05	0.04	0.50	0.05	37.2	62.0	0	0.1
0	10	0.00	12.5	225.0	0	0.06	0	0.08	—	0.03	0.40	0.06	30.0	36.0	0	0.1
0	11	0.12	12.5	236.6	1.2	0.06	6.2	0.10	0.25	0.02	0.25	0.06	54.8	48.4	0	0.1
0	3	0.01	0.4	4.2	0.1	0.01	0.4	0.00	0.01	0.00	0.01	0.00	0.6	2.7	0	0
0	52	0.13	13.1	237.1	0	0.09	14.4	0.11	0.23	0.05	0.36	0.07	39.3	69.7	0	0.7
0	36	0.09	9.0	162.9	0	0.06	9.9	0.07	0.16	0.03	0.25	0.05	27.0	47.9	0	0.4
0	73	0.30	30.4	782.9	9.2	0.21	83.7	0.06	2.22	0.08	0.93	0.05	58.0	37.7	0	1.8
0	17	0.07	7.0	179.9	2.1	0.05	38.5	0.02	0.51	0.02	0.24	0.01	26.6	43.3	0	0.4
0	2	0.28	5.2	62.6	5.0	0.01	11.5	0.00	0.00	0.02	0.27	0.01	2.5	5.4	0	0.1
0	4	0.35	6.6	120.5	7.9	0.11	22.3	0.01	0.64	0.03	0.80	0.02	3.9	3.7	0	0.4
0	2	0.39	6.1	120.8	3.7	0.11	32.9	0.01	0.59	0.02	0.63	0.02	3.7	3.5	0	0.4
0	4	0.46	6.3	162.5	7.5	0.06	17.5	0.01	0.77	0.04	0.81	0.02	3.8	117.8	0	0.5
0	9	0.37	13.5	285.0	0	0.25	24.0	0.03	1.09	0.04	1.20	0.03	6.0	9.9	0	0.2
0	5	0.00	9.8	147.6	0	0.02	0	0.01	0.14	0.01	0.26	0.02	9.8	4.6	0	0.1
0	22	0.50	12.0	250.0	0	0.24	—	0.04	1.00	0.08	0.20	0.03	14.6	8.0	0	1.0
0	7	0.29	5.3	86.5	6.7	0.10	0	0.01	0.10	0.02	0.32	0.01	1.3	1.5	0	0
0	11	0.36	8.7	119.0	5.0	0.11	0	0.01	0.10	0.01	0.25	0.02	1.2	2.0	0	0
0	15	0.28	11.6	197.5	1.7	0.16	1.7	0.02	0.19	0.04	0.26	0.04	11.6	7.0	0	0.2
0	7	0.62	—	77.5	0.3	—	0	—	—	—	—	—	—	16.5	0	—
0	18	0.49	19.5	132.6	1.3	0.14	1.3	0.11	—	0.03	0.36	0.09	6.5	9.5	0	—
0	17	0.35	17.4	151.9	1.2	0.12	2.5	0.12	0.01	0.02	0.35	0.09	6.2	11.8	0	0.5
0	18	0.49	20.2	132.3	1.3	0.15	2.5	0.11	0.01	0.03	0.36	0.09	6.3	9.5	0	0.5
0	18	0.49	22.1	156.2	1.2	0.15	2.5	0.11	0.01	0.03	0.37	0.09	6.2	9.5	0	0.5
0	16	0.39	15.0	162.5	2.5	0.14	0	0.07	0.03	0.03	0.25	0.13	22.5	12.5	0	0.1
0	10	0.22	9.3	84.5	0.8	0.09	2.3	0.06	0.02	0.03	0.39	0.09	14.0	37.0	0	0.1
0	2	0.45	24.6	358.1	3.9	0.10	34.7	0.04	0.10	0.04	0.58	0.19	20.0	8.4	0	1.1
0	4	0.11	4.6	103.6	0	0.06	11.2	0.02	0.17	0.02	0.27	0.02	3.3	6.3	0	0
0	5	0.46	4.6	398.9	4.6	0.18	7.7	0.04	0.92	0.04	0.46	0.16	9.2	9.4	0	0.9
0	7	0.16	6.9	123.0	0.3	0.07	6.6	0.01	0.07	0.03	0.32	0.03	0.7	0.1	0	0
0	24	0.51	22.3	398.0	1.2	0.24	21.1	0.03	0.24	0.12	0.90	0.27	0	3.6	0	0.1
0	31	3.02	35.8	706.6	10.2	0.53	0	0.04	0.30	0.17	2.01	0.55	0	10.5	0	1.5
0	15	0.42	13.5	92.9	0.6	0.26	1.2	0.02	0.54	0.02	0.37	0.03	12.9	16.1	0	0.1
0	19	0.81	16.3	142.5	1.3	0.22	3.8	0.02	0.90	0.05	0.28	0.04	32.5	20.6	0	0.4
0	174	0.25	16.2	115.0	1.0	—	—	0.02	—	0.03	0.25	—	—	4.0	0	—
0	12	0.30	9.4	110.2	0.7	0.10	0.7	0.02	0.21	0.02	0.28	0.03	17.3	42.3	0	0.3
0	14	0.59	7.7	125.0	1.3	0.06	1.3	0.01	0.30	0.09	0.37	0.03	5.1	50.4	0	0.9
0	38	0.09	9.5	172.0	0	0.06	10.5	0.08	0.17	0.03	0.26	0.05	28.5	50.5	0	0.5
0	22	0.25	9.9	219.8	1.2	0.04	16.1	0.07	0.16	0.02	0.12	0.05	6.2	38.3	0	0.1
0	33	0.13	10.6	146.1	1.8	0.06	29.9	0.05	0.18	0.03	0.33	0.07	14.1	23.5	0	0.1

D&W+ Code	Food Description	QTY	Measure	Wt (g)	H₂O (g)	Ener (cal)	Prot (g)	Carb (g)	Fiber (g)	Fat (g)	Sat	Mono	Poly
												Fat Breakdown (g)	
VEGETABLES, LEGUMES													
	AMARANTH												
1043	Leaves, boiled, drained	½	cup(s)	66	60.4	14	1.4	2.7	—	0.1	0	0	0.1
1042	Leaves, raw	1	cup(s)	28	25.7	6	0.7	1.1	—	0.1	0	0	0
	ARTICHOKE												
1044	Boiled, drained	1	item(s)	120	100.9	64	3.5	14.3	10.3	0.4	0.1	0	0.2
2885	Hearts, boiled, drained	½	cup(s)	84	70.6	45	2.4	10.0	7.2	0.3	0.1	0	0.1
8683	**ARUGULA LEAVES, RAW**	1	cup(s)	20	18.3	5	0.5	0.7	0.3	0.1	0	0	0.1
	ASPARAGUS												
566	Boiled, drained	½	cup(s)	90	83.4	20	2.2	3.7	1.8	0.2	0	0	0.1
568	Canned, drained	½	cup(s)	121	113.7	23	2.6	3.0	1.9	0.8	0.2	0	0.3
565	Tips, frozen, boiled, drained	½	cup(s)	90	84.7	16	2.7	1.7	1.4	0.4	0.1	0	0.2
	BAMBOO SHOOTS												
1048	Boiled, drained	½	cup(s)	60	57.6	7	0.9	1.2	0.6	0.1	0	0	0.1
1049	Canned, drained	½	cup(s)	66	61.8	12	1.1	2.1	0.9	0.3	0.1	0	0.1
	BEANS												
1801	Adzuki beans, boiled	½	cup(s)	115	76.2	147	8.6	28.5	8.4	0.1	0	—	—
511	Baked beans with franks, canned	½	cup(s)	130	89.8	184	8.7	19.9	8.9	8.5	3.0	3.7	1.1
513	Baked beans with pork in sweet sauce, canned	½	cup(s)	127	89.3	142	6.7	26.7	5.3	1.8	0.6	0.6	0.5
512	Baked beans with pork in tomato sauce, canned	½	cup(s)	127	93.0	119	6.5	23.6	5.1	1.2	0.5	0.7	0.3
1805	Black beans, boiled	½	cup(s)	86	56.5	114	7.6	20.4	7.5	0.5	0.1	0	0.2
14597	Chickpeas, garbanzo beans or Bengal gram, boiled	½	cup(s)	82	49.4	134	7.3	22.5	6.2	2.1	0.2	0.5	0.9
569	Fordhook lima beans, frozen, boiled, drained	½	cup(s)	85	62.0	88	5.2	16.4	4.9	0.3	0.1	0	0.1
1806	French beans, boiled	½	cup(s)	89	58.9	114	6.2	21.3	8.3	0.7	0.1	0	0.4
2773	Great northern beans, boiled	½	cup(s)	89	61.1	104	7.4	18.7	6.2	0.4	0.1	0	0.2
2736	Hyacinth beans, boiled, drained	½	cup(s)	44	37.8	22	1.3	4.0	—	0.1	0.1	0.1	0
570	Lima beans, baby, frozen, boiled, drained	½	cup(s)	90	65.1	95	6.0	17.5	5.4	0.3	0.1	0	0.1
515	Lima beans, boiled, drained	½	cup(s)	85	57.1	105	5.8	20.1	4.5	0.3	0.1	0	0.1
579	Mung beans, sprouted, boiled, drained	½	cup(s)	62	57.9	13	1.3	2.6	0.5	0.1	0	0	0
510	Navy beans, boiled	½	cup(s)	91	58.1	127	7.5	23.7	9.6	0.6	0.1	0.1	0.4
32816	Pinto beans, boiled, drained, no salt added	½	cup(s)	63	58.8	14	1.2	2.6	—	0.2	0	0	0.1
1052	Pinto beans, frozen, boiled, drained	½	cup(s)	47	27.3	76	4.4	14.5	4.0	0.2	0	0	0.1
514	Red kidney beans, canned	½	cup(s)	128	99.0	108	6.7	19.9	6.9	0.5	0.1	0.2	0.2
1810	Refried beans, canned	½	cup(s)	127	96.1	119	6.9	19.6	6.7	1.6	0.6	0.7	0.2
1053	Shell beans, canned	½	cup(s)	123	111.1	37	2.2	7.6	4.2	0.2	0	0	0.1
1670	Soybeans, boiled	½	cup(s)	86	53.8	149	14.3	8.5	5.2	7.7	1.1	1.7	4.4
1108	Soybeans, green, boiled, drained	½	cup(s)	90	61.7	127	11.1	9.9	3.8	5.8	0.7	1.1	2.7
1807	White beans, small, boiled	½	cup(s)	90	56.6	127	8.0	23.1	9.3	0.6	0.1	0.1	0.2
575	Yellow snap, string or wax beans, boiled, drained	½	cup(s)	63	55.8	22	1.2	4.9	2.1	0.2	0	0	0.1
576	Yellow snap, string or wax beans, frozen, boiled, drained	½	cup(s)	68	61.7	19	1.0	4.4	2.0	0.1	0	0	0.1
	BEETS												
584	Beet greens, boiled, drained	½	cup(s)	72	64.2	19	1.9	3.9	2.1	0.1	0	0	0.1
2730	Pickled, canned with liquid	½	cup(s)	114	92.9	74	0.9	18.5	3.0	0.1	0	0	0
581	Sliced, boiled, drained	½	cup(s)	85	74.0	37	1.4	8.5	1.7	0.2	0	0	0.1
583	Sliced, canned, drained	½	cup(s)	85	77.3	26	0.8	6.1	1.5	0.1	0	0	0
580	Whole, boiled, drained	2	item(s)	100	87.1	44	1.7	10.0	2.0	0.2	0	0	0.1
16848	**BROCCOFLOWER, RAW, CHOPPED**	½	cup(s)	32	28.7	10	0.9	1.9	1.0	0.1	0	0	0
	BROCCOLI												
588	Chopped, boiled, drained	½	cup(s)	78	69.6	27	1.9	5.6	2.6	0.3	0.1	0	0.1
590	Frozen, chopped, boiled, drained	½	cup(s)	92	83.5	26	2.9	4.9	2.8	0.1	0	0	0.1
587	Raw, chopped	½	cup(s)	46	40.6	15	1.3	3.0	1.2	0.2	0	0	0

PAGE KEY: A-4 = Breads/Baked Goods A-10 = Cereal/Rice/Pasta A-14 = Fruit A-20 = Vegetables/Legumes A-30 = Nuts/Seeds A-32 = Vegetarian A-34 = Dairy A-42 = Eggs A-42 = Seafood A-46 = Meats A-50 = Poultry A-50 = Processed Meats A-52 = Beverages A-56 = Fats/Oils A-58 = Sweets A-60 = Spices/Condiments/Sauces A-64 = Mixed Foods/Soups/Sandwiches A-70 = Fast Food A-90 = Convenience A-92 = Baby Foods

A

CHOL (mg)	CALC (mg)	IRON (mg)	MAGN (mg)	POTA (mg)	SODI (mg)	ZINC (mg)	VIT A (µg)	THIA (mg)	VIT E (mg α)	RIBO (mg)	NIAC (mg)	VIT B$_6$ (mg)	FOLA (µg DFE)	VIT C (mg)	VIT B$_{12}$ (µg)	SELE (µg)
0	138	1.49	36.3	423.1	13.9	0.58	91.7	0.01	—	0.09	0.37	0.12	37.6	27.1	0	0.6
0	60	0.65	15.4	171.1	5.6	0.25	40.9	0.01	—	0.04	0.18	0.05	23.8	12.1	0	0.3
0	25	0.73	50.4	343.2	72.0	0.48	1.2	0.06	0.22	0.10	1.33	0.09	106.8	8.9	0	0.2
0	18	0.51	35.3	240.2	50.4	0.33	0.8	0.04	0.16	0.07	0.93	0.06	74.8	6.2	0	0.2
0	32	0.29	9.4	73.8	5.4	0.09	23.8	0.01	0.09	0.02	0.06	0.01	19.4	3.0	0	0.1
0	21	0.81	12.6	201.6	12.6	0.54	45.0	0.14	1.35	0.12	0.97	0.07	134.1	6.9	0	5.5
0	19	2.21	12.1	208.1	347.3	0.48	49.6	0.07	1.47	0.12	1.15	0.13	116.2	22.3	0	2.1
0	16	0.50	9.0	154.8	2.7	0.36	36.0	0.05	1.08	0.09	0.93	0.01	121.5	22.0	0	3.5
0	7	0.14	1.8	319.8	2.4	0.28	0	0.01	—	0.03	0.18	0.06	1.2	0	0	0.2
0	5	0.21	2.6	52.4	4.6	0.43	0.7	0.02	0.41	0.02	0.09	0.09	2.0	0.7	0	0.3
0	32	2.30	59.8	611.8	9.2	2.03	0	0.13	—	0.07	0.82	0.11	139.2	0	0	1.4
8	62	2.24	36.3	304.3	556.9	2.42	5.2	0.08	0.21	0.07	1.17	0.06	38.9	3.0	0.4	8.4
9	75	2.08	41.7	326.4	422.5	1.73	0	0.05	0.03	0.07	0.44	0.07	10.1	3.5	0	6.3
9	71	4.09	43.0	373.2	552.8	6.93	5.1	0.06	0.12	0.05	0.62	0.08	19.0	3.8	0	5.9
0	23	1.80	60.2	305.3	0.9	0.96	0	0.21	—	0.05	0.43	0.05	128.1	0	0	1.0
0	40	2.36	39.4	238.6	5.7	1.25	0.8	0.09	0.28	0.05	0.43	0.11	141.0	1.1	0	3.0
0	26	1.54	35.7	258.4	58.7	0.62	8.5	0.06	0.24	0.05	0.90	0.10	17.9	10.9	0	0.5
0	56	0.95	49.6	327.5	5.3	0.56	0	0.11	—	0.05	0.48	0.09	66.4	1.1	0	1.1
0	60	1.88	44.3	346.0	1.8	0.77	0	0.14	—	0.05	0.60	0.10	90.3	1.2	0	3.6
0	18	0.33	18.3	114.0	0.9	0.16	3.0	0.02	—	0.03	0.20	0.01	20.4	2.2	0	0.7
0	25	1.76	50.4	369.9	26.1	0.49	7.2	0.06	0.57	0.04	0.69	0.10	14.4	5.2	0	1.5
0	27	2.08	62.9	484.5	14.5	0.67	12.8	0.11	0.11	0.08	0.88	0.16	22.1	8.6	0	1.7
0	7	0.40	8.7	62.6	6.2	0.29	0.6	0.03	0.04	0.06	0.51	0.03	18.0	7.1	0	0.4
—	63	2.14	48.2	354.0	0	0.93	0	0.21	0.01	0.06	0.59	0.12	127.4	0.8	0	2.6
0	9	0.41	11.3	61.7	32.1	0.10	0	0.04	—	0.03	0.45	0.03	18.3	3.8	0	0.4
0	24	1.27	25.4	303.6	39.0	0.32	0	0.12	—	0.05	0.29	0.09	16.0	0.3	0	0.7
0	32	1.62	35.8	327.7	330.2	2.09	0	0.13	0.02	0.11	0.57	0.10	25.6	1.4	0	0.6
10	44	2.10	41.7	337.8	378.2	1.48	0	0.03	0.00	0.02	0.39	0.18	13.9	7.6	0	1.6
0	36	1.21	18.4	133.5	409.2	0.33	13.5	0.04	0.04	0.07	0.25	0.06	22.1	3.8	0	2.6
0	88	4.42	74.0	442.9	0.9	0.98	0	0.13	0.30	0.24	0.34	0.20	46.4	1.5	0	6.3
0	131	2.25	54.0	485.1	12.6	0.82	7.2	0.23	—	0.14	1.13	0.05	99.9	15.3	0	1.3
0	65	2.54	60.9	414.4	1.8	0.97	0	0.21	—	0.05	0.24	0.11	122.6	0	0	1.2
0	29	0.80	15.6	186.9	1.9	0.23	2.5	0.05	0.28	0.06	0.38	0.04	20.6	6.1	0	0.3
0	33	0.59	16.2	85.1	6.1	0.32	4.1	0.02	0.03	0.06	0.26	0.04	15.5	2.8	0	0.3
0	82	1.36	49.0	654.5	173.5	0.36	275.8	0.08	1.30	0.20	0.35	0.09	10.1	17.9	0	0.6
0	12	0.46	17.0	168.0	299.6	0.29	1.1	0.01	—	0.05	0.28	0.05	30.6	2.6	0	1.1
0	14	0.67	19.6	259.3	65.5	0.30	1.7	0.02	0.03	0.03	0.28	0.05	68.0	3.1	0	0.6
0	13	1.54	14.5	125.8	164.9	0.17	0.9	0.01	0.02	0.03	0.13	0.04	25.5	3.5	0	0.4
0	16	0.79	23.0	305.0	77.0	0.35	2.0	0.02	0.04	0.04	0.33	0.06	80.0	3.6	0	0.7
0	11	0.23	6.4	96.0	7.4	0.20	2.6	0.02	0.01	0.03	0.23	0.07	18.2	28.2	0	0.2
0	31	0.52	16.4	228.5	32.0	0.35	60.1	0.04	1.13	0.09	0.43	0.15	84.2	50.6	0	1.2
0	30	0.56	12.0	130.6	10.1	0.25	46.9	0.05	1.21	0.07	0.42	0.12	51.5	36.9	0	0.6
0	21	0.33	9.6	143.8	15.0	0.19	14.1	0.03	0.36	0.05	0.29	0.08	28.7	40.6	0	1.1

D&W+ Code	Food Description	QTY	Measure	Wt (g)	H₂O (g)	Ener (cal)	Prot (g)	Carb (g)	Fiber (g)	Fat (g)	Fat Breakdown (g) Sat	Mono	Poly
	Vegetables, Legumes—continued												
585	Black-eyed peas or cowpeas, boiled, drained	½	cup(s)	83	62.3	80	2.6	16.8	4.1	0.3	0.1	0	0.1
	Brussels sprouts												
591	Boiled, drained	½	cup(s)	78	69.3	28	2.0	5.5	2.0	0.4	0.1	0	0.2
592	Frozen, boiled, drained	½	cup(s)	78	67.2	33	2.8	6.4	3.2	0.3	0.1	0	0.2
	Cabbage												
595	Boiled, drained, no salt added	1	cup(s)	150	138.8	35	1.9	8.3	2.8	0.1	0	0	0
35611	Chinese (pak choi or bok choy), boiled with salt, drained	1	cup(s)	170	162.4	20	2.6	3.0	1.7	0.3	0	0	0.1
16869	Kimchi	1	cup(s)	150	137.5	32	2.5	6.1	1.8	0.3	0	0	0.2
594	Raw, shredded	1	cup(s)	70	64.5	17	0.9	4.1	1.7	0.1	0	0	0
596	Red, shredded, raw	1	cup(s)	70	63.3	22	1.0	5.2	1.5	0.1	0	0	0.1
597	Savoy, shredded, raw	1	cup(s)	70	63.7	19	1.4	4.3	2.2	0.1	0	0	0
35417	**Capers**	1	teaspoon(s)	4	—	2	0	0	0	0	0	0	0
	Carrots												
8691	Baby, raw	8	item(s)	80	72.3	28	0.5	6.6	2.3	0.1	0	0	0.1
601	Grated	½	cup(s)	55	48.6	23	0.5	5.3	1.5	0.1	0	0	0.1
1055	Juice, canned	½	cup(s)	118	104.9	47	1.1	11.0	0.9	0.2	0	0	0.1
600	Raw	½	cup(s)	61	53.9	25	0.6	5.8	1.7	0.1	0	0	0.1
602	Sliced, boiled, drained	½	cup(s)	78	70.3	27	0.6	6.4	2.3	0.1	0	0	0.1
32725	**Cassava or Manioc**	½	cup(s)	103	61.5	165	1.4	39.2	1.9	0.3	0.1	0.1	0
	Cauliflower												
606	Boiled, drained	½	cup(s)	62	57.7	14	1.1	2.5	1.4	0.3	0	0	0.1
607	Frozen, boiled, drained	½	cup(s)	90	84.6	17	1.4	3.4	2.4	0.2	0	0	0.1
605	Raw, chopped	½	cup(s)	50	46.0	13	1.0	2.6	1.2	0	0	0	0
	Celery												
609	Diced	½	cup(s)	51	48.2	8	0.3	1.5	0.8	0.1	0	0	0
608	Stalk	2	item(s)	80	76.3	13	0.6	2.4	1.3	0.1	0	0	0.1
	Chard												
1057	Swiss chard, boiled, drained	½	cup(s)	88	81.1	18	1.6	3.6	1.8	0.1	0	0	0
1056	Swiss chard, raw	1	cup(s)	36	33.4	7	0.6	1.3	0.6	0.1	0	0	0
	Collard Greens												
610	Boiled, drained	½	cup(s)	95	87.3	25	2.0	4.7	2.7	0.3	0	0	0.2
611	Frozen, chopped, boiled, drained	½	cup(s)	85	75.2	31	2.5	6.0	2.4	0.3	0.1	0	0.2
	Corn												
29614	Yellow corn, fresh, cooked	1	item(s)	100	69.2	107	3.3	25.0	2.8	1.3	0.2	0.4	0.6
615	Yellow creamed sweet corn, canned	½	cup(s)	128	100.8	92	2.2	23.2	1.5	0.5	0.1	0.2	0.3
612	Yellow sweet corn, boiled, drained	½	cup(s)	82	57.0	89	2.7	20.6	2.3	1.1	0.2	0.3	0.5
614	Yellow sweet corn, frozen, boiled, drained	½	cup(s)	82	63.2	66	2.1	15.8	2.0	0.5	0.1	0.2	0.3
618	**Cucumber**	¼	item(s)	75	71.7	11	0.5	2.7	0.4	0.1	0	0	0
16870	**Cucumber, Kimchi**	½	cup(s)	75	68.1	16	0.8	3.6	1.1	0.1	0	0	0
	Dandelion Greens												
620	Chopped, boiled, drained	½	cup(s)	53	47.1	17	1.1	3.4	1.5	0.3	0.1	0	0.1
2734	Raw	1	cup(s)	55	47.1	25	1.5	5.1	1.9	0.4	0.1	0	0.2
1066	**Eggplant, Boiled, Drained**	½	cup(s)	50	44.4	17	0.4	4.3	1.2	0.1	0	0	0
621	**Endive or Escarole, chopped, raw**	1	cup(s)	50	46.9	8	0.6	1.7	1.5	0.1	0	0	0
8784	**Jicama or Yam Bean**	½	cup(s)	65	116.5	49	0.9	11.4	6.3	0.1	0	0	0.1
	Kale												
623	Frozen, chopped, boiled, drained	½	cup(s)	65	58.8	20	1.8	3.4	1.3	0.3	0	0	0.2
29313	Raw	1	cup(s)	67	56.6	33	2.2	6.7	1.3	0.5	0.1	0	0.2
	Kohlrabi												
1072	Boiled, drained	½	cup(s)	83	74.5	24	1.5	5.5	0.9	0.1	0	0	0
1071	Raw	1	cup(s)	135	122.9	36	2.3	8.4	4.9	0.1	0	0	0.1

PAGE KEY: A-4 = Breads/Baked Goods A-10 = Cereal/Rice/Pasta A-14 = Fruit A-20 = Vegetables/Legumes A-30 = Nuts/Seeds A-32 = Vegetarian A-34 = Dairy A-42 = Eggs A-42 = Seafood A-46 = Meats A-50 = Poultry A-50 = Processed Meats A-52 = Beverages A-56 = Fats/Oils A-58 = Sweets A-60 = Spices/Condiments/Sauces A-64 = Mixed Foods/Soups/Sandwiches A-70 = Fast Food A-90 = Convenience A-92 = Baby Foods

CHOL (mg)	CALC (mg)	IRON (mg)	MAGN (mg)	POTA (mg)	SODI (mg)	ZINC (mg)	VIT A (µg)	THIA (mg)	VIT E (mg α)	RIBO (mg)	NIAC (mg)	VIT B6 (mg)	FOLA (µg DFE)	VIT C (mg)	VIT B12 (µg)	SELE (µg)
0	106	0.92	42.9	344.9	3.3	0.85	33.0	0.08	0.18	0.12	1.15	0.05	104.8	1.8	0	2.1
0	28	0.93	15.6	247.3	16.4	0.25	30.4	0.08	0.33	0.06	0.47	0.13	46.8	48.4	0	1.2
0	20	0.37	14.0	224.8	11.6	0.18	35.7	0.08	0.39	0.08	0.41	0.22	78.3	35.4	0	0.5
0	72	0.24	22.5	294.0	12.0	0.30	6.0	0.08	0.20	0.04	0.36	0.16	45.0	56.2	0	0.9
0	158	1.76	18.7	630.7	459.0	0.28	360.4	0.04	0.14	0.10	0.72	0.28	69.7	44.2	0	0.7
0	144	1.26	27.0	379.5	996.0	0.36	288.0	0.06	0.36	0.10	0.80	0.32	88.5	79.6	0	1.5
0	28	0.33	8.4	119.0	12.6	0.12	3.5	0.04	0.10	0.02	0.16	0.08	30.1	25.6	0	0.2
0	31	0.56	11.2	170.1	18.9	0.15	39.2	0.04	0.07	0.05	0.29	0.14	12.6	39.9	0	0.4
0	24	0.28	19.6	161.0	19.6	0.18	35.0	0.05	0.11	0.02	0.21	0.13	56.0	21.7	0	0.6
0	0	0.00	—	—	140	—	0	—	—	—	—	—	—	0	—	—
0	26	0.71	8.0	189.6	62.4	0.13	552.0	0.02	—	0.02	0.44	0.08	21.6	2.1	0	0.7
0	18	0.16	6.6	176.0	37.9	0.13	459.2	0.03	0.36	0.03	0.54	0.07	10.4	3.2	0	0.1
0	28	0.54	16.5	344.6	34.2	0.21	1128.1	0.11	1.37	0.07	0.46	0.26	4.7	10.0	0	0.7
0	20	0.18	7.3	195.2	42.1	0.15	509.4	0.04	0.40	0.04	0.60	0.08	11.6	3.6	0	0.1
0	23	0.26	7.8	183.3	45.2	0.15	664.6	0.05	0.80	0.03	0.50	0.11	10.9	2.8	0	0.5
0	16	0.27	21.6	279.1	14.4	0.35	1.0	0.08	0.19	0.04	0.87	0.09	27.8	21.2	0	0.7
0	10	0.19	5.6	88.0	9.3	0.10	0.6	0.02	0.04	0.03	0.25	0.10	27.3	27.5	0	0.4
0	15	0.36	8.1	125.1	16.2	0.11	0	0.03	0.05	0.04	0.27	0.07	36.9	28.2	0	0.5
0	11	0.22	7.5	151.5	15.0	0.14	0.5	0.03	0.04	0.03	0.26	0.11	28.5	23.2	0	0.3
0	20	0.10	5.6	131.3	40.4	0.07	11.1	0.01	0.14	0.03	0.16	0.04	18.2	1.6	0	0.2
0	32	0.16	8.8	208.0	64.0	0.10	17.6	0.01	0.21	0.04	0.25	0.05	28.8	2.5	0	0.3
0	51	1.98	75.3	480.4	156.6	0.29	267.8	0.03	1.65	0.08	0.32	0.07	7.9	15.8	0	0.8
0	18	0.64	29.2	136.4	76.7	0.13	110.2	0.01	0.68	0.03	0.14	0.03	5.0	10.8	0	0.3
0	133	1.10	19.0	110.2	15.2	0.21	385.7	0.03	0.83	0.10	0.54	0.12	88.4	17.3	0	0.5
0	179	0.95	25.5	213.4	42.5	0.22	488.8	0.04	1.06	0.09	0.54	0.09	64.6	22.4	0	1.3
0	2	0.61	32.0	248.0	242.0	0.48	13.0	0.20	0.09	0.07	1.60	0.06	46.0	6.2	0	0.2
0	4	0.48	21.8	171.5	364.8	0.67	5.1	0.03	0.09	0.06	1.22	0.08	57.6	5.9	0	0.5
0	2	0.36	21.3	173.8	0	0.50	10.7	0.17	0.07	0.05	1.32	0.04	37.7	5.1	0	0.2
0	2	0.38	23.0	191.1	0.8	0.51	8.2	0.02	0.05	0.05	1.07	0.08	28.7	2.9	0	0.6
0	12	0.20	9.8	110.6	1.5	0.14	3.8	0.01	0.01	0.01	0.07	0.03	5.3	2.1	0	0.2
0	7	3.61	6.0	87.8	765.8	0.38	—	0.02	—	0.02	0.34	0.08	17.3	2.6	0	—
0	74	0.95	12.6	121.8	23.1	0.15	179.6	0.07	1.28	0.09	0.27	0.08	6.8	9.5	0	0.2
0	103	1.70	19.8	218.3	41.8	0.22	279.4	0.10	1.89	0.14	0.44	0.13	14.8	19.2	0	0.3
0	3	0.12	5.4	60.9	0.5	0.06	1.0	0.04	0.20	0.01	0.30	0.04	6.9	0.6	0	0
0	26	0.41	7.5	157.0	11.0	0.39	54.0	0.04	0.22	0.03	0.20	0.01	71.0	3.2	0	0.1
0	16	0.78	15.5	194.0	5.2	0.20	1.3	0.02	0.59	0.04	0.25	0.05	15.5	26.1	0	0.9
0	90	0.61	11.7	208.7	9.8	0.11	477.8	0.02	0.59	0.07	0.43	0.05	9.1	16.4	0	0.6
0	90	1.14	22.8	299.5	28.8	0.29	515.2	0.07	—	0.08	0.66	0.18	19.4	80.4	0	0.6
0	21	0.33	15.7	280.5	17.3	0.26	1.7	0.03	0.43	0.02	0.32	0.13	9.9	44.6	0	0.7
0	32	0.54	25.7	472.5	27.0	0.04	2.7	0.06	0.64	0.02	0.54	0.20	21.6	83.7	0	0.9

TABLE A–1 Table of Food Composition *(continued)*

(Computer code is for Cengage Diet & Wellness Plus program)

D&W+ Code	Food Description	QTY	Measure	Wt (g)	H₂O (g)	Ener (cal)	Prot (g)	Carb (g)	Fiber (g)	Fat (g)	Sat	Mono	Poly
												Fat Breakdown (g)	
VEGETABLES, LEGUMES—CONTINUED													
	LEEKS												
1074	Boiled, drained	½	cup(s)	52	47.2	16	0.4	4.0	0.5	0.1	0	0	0
1073	Raw	1	cup(s)	89	73.9	54	1.3	12.6	1.6	0.3	0	0	0.1
	LENTILS												
522	Boiled	¼	cup(s)	50	34.5	57	4.5	10.0	3.9	0.2	0	0	0.1
1075	Sprouted	1	cup(s)	77	51.9	82	6.9	17.0	—	0.4	0	0.1	0.2
	LETTUCE												
625	Butterhead leaves	11	piece(s)	83	78.9	11	1.1	1.8	0.9	0.2	0	0	0.1
624	Butterhead, Boston or Bibb	1	cup(s)	55	52.6	7	0.7	1.2	0.6	0.1	0	0	0.1
626	Iceberg	1	cup(s)	55	52.6	8	0.5	1.6	0.7	0.1	0	0	0
628	Iceberg, chopped	1	cup(s)	55	52.6	8	0.5	1.6	0.7	0.1	0	0	0
629	Looseleaf	1	cup(s)	36	34.2	5	0.5	1.0	0.5	0.1	0	0	0
1665	Romaine, shredded	1	cup(s)	56	53.0	10	0.7	1.8	1.2	0.2	0	0	0.1
	MUSHROOMS												
15585	Crimini (about 6)	3	ounce(s)	85	—	28	3.7	2.8	1.9	0	0	0	0
8700	Enoki	30	item(s)	90	79.7	40	2.3	6.9	2.4	0.3	0	0	0.1
1079	Mushrooms, boiled, drained	½	cup(s)	78	71.0	22	1.7	4.1	1.7	0.4	0	0	0.1
1080	Mushrooms, canned, drained	½	cup(s)	78	71.0	20	1.5	4.0	1.9	0.2	0	0	0.1
630	Mushrooms, raw	½	cup(s)	48	44.4	11	1.5	1.6	0.5	0.2	0	0	0.1
15587	Portabella, raw	1	item(s)	84	—	30	3.0	3.9	3.0	0	0	0	0
2743	Shiitake, cooked	½	cup(s)	73	60.5	41	1.1	10.4	1.5	0.2	0	0.1	0
	MUSTARD GREENS												
2744	Frozen, boiled, drained	½	cup(s)	75	70.4	14	1.7	2.3	2.1	0.2	0	0.1	0
29319	Raw	1	cup(s)	56	50.8	15	1.5	2.7	1.8	0.1	0	0	0
	OKRA												
16866	Batter coated, fried	11	piece(s)	83	55.6	156	2.1	12.7	2.0	11.2	1.5	3.7	5.5
32742	Frozen, boiled, drained, no salt added	½	cup(s)	92	83.8	26	1.9	5.3	2.6	0.3	0.1	0	0.1
632	Sliced, boiled, drained	½	cup(s)	80	74.1	18	1.5	3.6	2.0	0.2	0	0	0
	ONIONS												
635	Chopped, boiled, drained	½	cup(s)	105	92.2	46	1.4	10.7	1.5	0.2	0	0	0.1
2748	Frozen, boiled, drained	½	cup(s)	106	97.8	30	0.8	7.0	1.9	0.1	0	0	0
1081	Onion rings, breaded and pan fried, frozen, heated	10	piece(s)	71	20.2	289	3.8	27.1	0.9	19.0	6.1	7.7	3.6
633	Raw, chopped	½	cup(s)	80	71.3	32	0.9	7.5	1.4	0.1	0	0	0
16850	Red onions, sliced, raw	½	cup(s)	57	50.7	24	0.5	5.8	0.8	0	0	0	0
636	Scallions, green or spring onions	2	item(s)	30	26.9	10	0.5	2.2	0.8	0.1	0	0	0
16860	**PALM HEARTS, COOKED**	½	cup(s)	73	50.7	84	2.0	18.7	1.1	0.1	0	0	0.1
637	**PARSLEY, CHOPPED**	1	tablespoon(s)	4	3.3	1	0.1	0.2	0.1	0	0	0	0
638	**PARSNIPS, SLICED, BOILED, DRAINED**	½	cup(s)	78	62.6	55	1.0	13.3	2.8	0.2	0	0.1	0
	PEAS												
639	Green peas, canned, drained	½	cup(s)	85	69.4	59	3.8	10.7	3.5	0.3	0.1	0	0.1
641	Green peas, frozen, boiled, drained	½	cup(s)	80	63.6	62	4.1	11.4	4.4	0.2	0	0	0.1
35694	Pea pods, boiled with salt, drained	½	cup(s)	80	71.1	32	2.6	5.2	2.2	0.2	0	0	0.1
1082	Peas and carrots, canned with liquid	½	cup(s)	128	112.4	48	2.8	10.8	2.6	0.3	0.1	0	0.2
1083	Peas and carrots, frozen, boiled, drained	½	cup(s)	80	68.6	38	2.5	8.1	2.5	0.3	0.1	0	0.2
2750	Snow or sugar peas, frozen, boiled, drained	½	cup(s)	80	69.3	42	2.8	7.2	2.5	0.3	0.1	0	0.1
640	Snow or sugar peas, raw	½	cup(s)	32	28.0	13	0.9	2.4	0.8	0.1	0	0	0
29324	Split peas, sprouted	½	cup(s)	60	37.4	77	5.3	16.9	—	0.4	0.1	0	0.2
	PEPPERS												
644	Green bell or sweet, boiled, drained	½	cup(s)	68	62.5	19	0.6	4.6	0.8	0.1	0	0	0.1
643	Green bell or sweet, raw	½	cup(s)	75	69.9	15	0.6	3.5	1.3	0.1	0	0	0
1664	Green hot chili	1	item(s)	45	39.5	18	0.9	4.3	0.7	0.1	0	0	0
1663	Green hot chili, canned with liquid	½	cup(s)	68	62.9	14	0.6	3.5	0.9	0.1	0	0	0
1086	Jalapeño, canned with liquid	½	cup(s)	68	60.4	18	0.6	3.2	1.8	0.6	0.1	0	0.3
8703	Yellow bell or sweet	1	item(s)	186	171.2	50	1.9	11.8	1.7	0.4	0.1	0	0.2

PAGE KEY: A-4 = Breads/Baked Goods   A-10 = Cereal/Rice/Pasta   A-14 = Fruit   A-20 = Vegetables/Legumes   A-30 = Nuts/Seeds   A-32 = Vegetarian
A-34 = Dairy   A-42 = Eggs   A-42 = Seafood   A-46 = Meats   A-50 = Poultry   A-50 = Processed Meats   A-52 = Beverages   A-56 = Fats/Oils   A-58 = Sweets
A-60 = Spices/Condiments/Sauces   A-64 = Mixed Foods/Soups/Sandwiches   A-70 = Fast Food   A-90 = Convenience   A-92 = Baby Foods

A

CHOL (mg)	CALC (mg)	IRON (mg)	MAGN (mg)	POTA (mg)	SODI (mg)	ZINC (mg)	VIT A (µg)	THIA (mg)	VIT E (mg α)	RIBO (mg)	NIAC (mg)	VIT B6 (mg)	FOLA (µg DFE)	VIT C (mg)	VIT B12 (µg)	SELE (µg)
0	16	0.56	7.3	45.2	5.2	0.02	1.0	0.01	—	0.01	0.10	0.04	12.5	2.2	0	0.3
0	53	1.86	24.9	160.2	17.8	0.10	73.9	0.05	0.81	0.02	0.35	0.20	57.0	10.7	0	0.9
0	9	1.65	17.8	182.7	1.0	0.63	0	0.08	0.05	0.04	0.52	0.09	89.6	0.7	0	1.4
0	19	2.47	28.5	247.9	8.5	1.16	1.5	0.17	—	0.09	0.86	0.14	77.0	12.7	0	0.5
0	29	1.02	10.7	196.4	4.1	0.16	137.0	0.04	0.14	0.05	0.29	0.06	60.2	3.1	0	0.5
0	19	0.68	7.1	130.9	2.7	0.11	91.3	0.03	0.09	0.03	0.19	0.04	40.1	2.0	0	0.3
0	10	0.22	3.8	77.5	5.5	0.08	13.7	0.02	0.09	0.01	0.07	0.02	15.9	1.5	0	0.1
0	10	0.22	3.8	77.5	5.5	0.08	13.7	0.02	0.09	0.01	0.07	0.02	15.9	1.5	0	0.1
0	13	0.31	4.7	69.8	10.1	0.06	133.2	0.02	0.10	0.02	0.13	0.03	13.7	6.5	0	0.2
0	18	0.54	7.8	138.3	4.5	0.13	162.4	0.04	0.07	0.03	0.17	0.04	76.2	13.4	0	0.2
0	0	0.67	—	—	32.6	—	0	—	—	—	—	—	—	0	0	—
0	1	0.98	14.4	331.2	2.7	0.54	0	0.16	0.01	0.14	5.31	0.07	46.8	0	0	2.0
0	5	1.35	9.4	277.7	1.6	0.67	0	0.05	0.01	0.23	3.47	0.07	14.0	3.1	0	9.3
0	9	0.61	11.7	100.6	331.5	0.56	0	0.06	0.01	0.01	1.24	0.04	9.4	0	0	3.2
0	1	0.24	4.3	152.6	2.4	0.25	0	0.04	0.01	0.19	1.73	0.05	7.7	1.0	0	4.5
0	39	0.35	—	—	9.9	—	0	—	—	—	—	—	—	0	0	—
0	2	0.31	10.2	84.8	2.9	0.96	0	0.02	0.02	0.12	1.08	0.11	15.2	0.2	0	18.0
0	76	0.84	9.8	104.3	18.8	0.15	265.5	0.03	1.01	0.04	0.19	0.08	52.5	10.4	0	0.5
0	58	0.81	17.9	198.2	14.0	0.11	294.0	0.04	1.12	0.06	0.45	0.10	104.7	39.2	0	0.5
2	54	1.13	32.2	170.8	109.7	0.44	14.0	0.16	1.50	0.12	1.29	0.11	43.7	9.2	0	3.6
0	88	0.61	46.9	215.3	2.8	0.57	15.6	0.09	0.29	0.11	0.72	0.04	134.3	11.2	0	0.6
0	62	0.22	28.8	108.0	4.8	0.34	11.2	0.10	0.21	0.04	0.69	0.15	36.8	13.0	0	0.3
0	23	0.24	11.5	174.3	3.1	0.21	0	0.03	0.02	0.02	0.17	0.12	15.7	5.5	0	0.6
0	17	0.32	6.4	114.5	12.7	0.06	0	0.02	0.01	0.02	0.14	0.06	13.8	2.8	0	0.4
0	22	1.20	13.5	91.6	266.3	0.29	7.8	0.19	—	0.09	2.56	0.05	73.1	1.0	0	2.5
0	18	0.16	8.0	116.8	3.2	0.13	0	0.03	0.01	0.02	0.09	0.09	15.2	5.9	0	0.4
0	13	0.10	5.7	82.4	1.7	0.09	0	0.02	0.01	0.01	0.04	0.08	10.9	3.7	0	0.3
0	22	0.44	6.0	82.8	4.8	0.11	15.0	0.01	0.16	0.02	0.15	0.01	19.2	5.6	0	0.2
0	13	1.23	7.3	1318.4	10.2	2.72	2.2	0.03	0.36	0.12	0.62	0.53	14.6	5.0	0	0.5
0	5	0.23	1.9	21.1	2.1	0.04	16.0	0.00	0.02	0.00	0.05	0.00	5.8	5.1	0	0
0	29	0.45	22.6	286.3	7.8	0.20	0	0.06	0.78	0.04	0.56	0.07	45.2	10.1	0	1.3
0	17	0.80	14.5	147.1	214.2	0.60	23.0	0.10	0.02	0.06	0.62	0.05	37.4	8.2	0	1.4
0	19	1.21	17.6	88.0	57.6	0.53	84.0	0.22	0.02	0.08	1.18	0.09	47.2	7.9	0	0.8
0	34	1.57	20.8	192.0	192.0	0.29	41.6	0.10	0.31	0.06	0.43	0.11	23.2	38.3	0	0.6
0	29	0.96	17.9	127.5	331.5	0.74	368.5	0.09	—	0.07	0.74	0.11	23.0	8.4	0	1.1
0	18	0.75	12.8	126.4	54.4	0.36	380.8	0.18	0.41	0.05	0.92	0.07	20.8	6.5	0	0.9
0	47	1.92	22.4	173.6	4.0	0.39	52.8	0.05	0.37	0.09	0.45	0.13	28.0	17.6	0	0.6
0	14	0.65	7.6	63.0	1.3	0.08	17.0	0.04	0.12	0.02	0.19	0.05	13.2	18.9	0	0.2
0	22	1.34	33.6	228.6	12.0	0.62	4.8	0.12	—	0.08	1.84	0.14	86.4	6.2	0	0.4
0	6	0.31	6.8	112.9	1.4	0.08	15.6	0.04	0.34	0.02	0.32	0.15	10.9	50.6	0	0.2
0	7	0.25	7.5	130.4	2.2	0.09	13.4	0.04	0.27	0.02	0.35	0.16	7.5	59.9	0	0
0	8	0.54	11.3	153.0	3.2	0.13	26.6	0.04	0.31	0.04	0.42	0.12	10.4	109.1	0	0.2
0	5	0.34	9.5	127.2	797.6	0.10	24.5	0.01	0.46	0.02	0.54	0.10	6.8	46.2	0	0.2
0	16	1.28	10.2	131.2	1136.3	0.23	57.8	0.03	0.47	0.03	0.27	0.13	9.5	6.8	0	0.3
0	20	0.85	22.3	394.3	3.7	0.31	18.6	0.05	—	0.04	1.65	0.31	48.4	341.3	0	0.6

(Computer code is for Cengage Diet & Wellness Plus program)

D&W+ Code	Food Description	QTY	Measure	Wt (g)	H₂O (g)	Ener (cal)	Prot (g)	Carb (g)	Fiber (g)	Fat (g)	Sat	Mono	Poly
											Fat Breakdown (g)		

VEGETABLES, LEGUMES—CONTINUED

D&W+ Code	Food Description	QTY	Measure	Wt (g)	H₂O (g)	Ener (cal)	Prot (g)	Carb (g)	Fiber (g)	Fat (g)	Sat	Mono	Poly
1087	Poi	½	cup(s)	120	86.0	134	0.5	32.7	0.5	0.2	0	0	0.1
	Potatoes												
1090	Au gratin mix, prepared with water, whole milk and butter	½	cup(s)	124	97.7	115	2.8	15.9	1.1	5.1	3.2	1.5	0.2
1089	Au gratin, prepared with butter	½	cup(s)	123	90.7	162	6.2	13.8	2.2	9.3	5.8	2.6	0.3
5791	Baked, flesh and skin	1	item(s)	202	151.3	188	5.1	42.7	4.4	0.3	0.1	0	0.1
645	Baked, flesh only	½	cup(s)	61	46.0	57	1.2	13.1	0.9	0.1	0	0	0
1088	Baked, skin only	1	item(s)	58	27.4	115	2.5	26.7	4.6	0.1	0	0	0
5795	Boiled in skin, flesh only, drained	1	item(s)	136	104.7	118	2.5	27.4	2.1	0.1	0	0	0.1
5794	Boiled, drained, skin and flesh	1	item(s)	150	115.9	129	2.9	29.8	2.5	0.2	0	0	0.1
647	Boiled, flesh only	½	cup(s)	78	60.4	67	1.3	15.6	1.4	0.1	0	0	0
648	French fried, deep fried, prepared from raw	14	item(s)	70	32.8	187	2.7	23.5	2.9	9.5	1.9	4.2	3.0
649	French fried, frozen, heated	14	item(s)	70	43.7	94	1.9	19.4	2.0	3.7	0.7	2.3	0.2
1091	Hashed brown	½	cup(s)	78	36.9	207	2.3	27.4	2.5	9.8	1.5	4.1	3.7
652	Mashed with margarine and whole milk	½	cup(s)	105	79.0	119	2.1	17.7	1.6	4.4	1.0	2.0	1.2
653	Mashed, prepared from dehydrated granules with milk, water, and margarine	½	cup(s)	105	79.8	122	2.3	16.9	1.4	5.0	1.3	2.1	1.4
2759	Microwaved	1	item(s)	202	145.5	212	4.9	49.0	4.6	0.2	0.1	0	0.1
2760	Microwaved in skin, flesh only	½	cup(s)	78	57.1	78	1.6	18.1	1.2	0.1	0	0	0
5804	Microwaved, skin only	1	item(s)	58	36.8	77	2.5	17.2	4.2	0.1	0	0	0
1097	Potato puffs, frozen, heated	½	cup(s)	64	38.2	122	1.3	17.8	1.6	5.5	1.2	3.9	0.3
1094	Scalloped mix, prepared with water, whole milk and butter	½	cup(s)	124	98.4	116	2.6	15.9	1.4	5.3	3.3	1.5	0.2
1093	Scalloped, prepared with butter	½	cup(s)	123	99.2	108	3.5	13.2	2.3	4.5	2.8	1.3	0.2
	Pumpkin												
1773	Boiled, drained	½	cup(s)	123	114.8	25	0.9	6.0	1.3	0.1	0	0	0
656	Canned	½	cup(s)	123	110.2	42	1.3	9.9	3.6	0.3	0.2	0	0
	Radicchio												
8731	Leaves, raw	1	cup(s)	40	37.3	9	0.6	1.8	0.4	0.1	0	0	0
2498	Raw	1	cup(s)	40	37.3	9	0.6	1.8	0.4	0.1	0	0	0
657	**Radishes**	6	item(s)	27	25.7	4	0.2	0.9	0.4	0	0	0	0
1099	**Rutabaga, Boiled, Drained**	½	cup(s)	85	75.5	33	1.1	7.4	1.5	0.2	0	0	0.1
658	**Sauerkraut, Canned**	½	cup(s)	118	109.2	22	1.1	5.1	3.4	0.2	0	0	0.1
	Seaweed												
1102	Kelp	½	cup(s)	40	32.6	17	0.6	3.8	0.5	0.2	0.1	0	0
1104	Spirulina, dried	½	cup(s)	8	0.4	22	4.3	1.8	0.3	0.6	0.2	0.1	0.2
1106	**Shallots**	3	tablespoon(s)	30	23.9	22	0.8	5.0	—	0	0	0	0
	Soybeans												
1670	Boiled	½	cup(s)	86	53.8	149	14.3	8.5	5.2	7.7	1.1	1.7	4.4
2825	Dry roasted	½	cup(s)	86	0.7	388	34.0	28.1	7.0	18.6	2.7	4.1	10.5
2824	Roasted, salted	½	cup(s)	86	1.7	405	30.3	28.9	15.2	21.8	3.2	4.8	12.3
8739	Sprouted, stir fried	½	cup(s)	63	42.3	79	8.2	5.9	0.5	4.5	0.6	1.0	2.5
	Soy products												
1813	Soy milk	1	cup(s)	240	211.3	130	7.8	15.1	1.4	4.2	0.5	1.0	2.3
2838	Tofu, dried, frozen (koyadofu)	3	ounce(s)	85	4.9	408	40.8	12.4	6.1	25.8	3.7	5.7	14.6
13844	Tofu, extra firm	3	ounce(s)	85	—	86	8.6	2.2	1.1	4.3	0.5	0.9	2.8
13843	Tofu, firm	3	ounce(s)	85	—	75	7.5	2.2	0.5	3.2	0	0.9	2.3
1816	Tofu, firm, with calcium sulfate and magnesium chloride (nigari)	3	ounce(s)	85	72.2	60	7.0	1.4	0.8	3.5	0.7	1.0	1.5
1817	Tofu, fried	3	ounce(s)	85	43.0	230	14.6	8.9	3.3	17.2	2.5	3.8	9.7
13841	Tofu, silken	3	ounce(s)	85	—	42	3.7	1.9	0	2.3	0.5	—	—
13842	Tofu, soft	3	ounce(s)	85	—	65	6.5	1.1	0.5	3.2	0.5	1.1	2.2
1671	Tofu, soft, with calcium sulfate and magnesium chloride (nigari)	3	ounce(s)	85	74.2	52	5.6	1.5	0.2	3.1	0.5	0.7	1.8

PAGE KEY: A-4 = Breads/Baked Goods A-10 = Cereal/Rice/Pasta A-14 = Fruit A-20 = Vegetables/Legumes A-30 = Nuts/Seeds A-32 = Vegetarian
A-34 = Dairy A-42 = Eggs A-42 = Seafood A-46 = Meats A-50 = Poultry A-50 = Processed Meats A-52 = Beverages A-56 = Fats/Oils A-58 = Sweets
A-60 = Spices/Condiments/Sauces A-64 = Mixed Foods/Soups/Sandwiches A-70 = Fast Food A-90 = Convenience A-92 = Baby Foods

A

CHOL (mg)	CALC (mg)	IRON (mg)	MAGN (mg)	POTA (mg)	SODI (mg)	ZINC (mg)	VIT A (µg)	THIA (mg)	VIT E (mg α)	RIBO (mg)	NIAC (mg)	VIT B6 (mg)	FOLA (µg DFE)	VIT C (mg)	VIT B12 (µg)	SELE (µg)
0	19	1.06	28.8	219.6	14.4	0.26	3.6	0.16	2.76	0.05	1.32	0.33	25.2	4.8	0	0.8
19	103	0.39	18.6	271.0	543.3	0.29	64.4	0.02	—	0.10	1.16	0.05	8.7	3.8	0	3.3
28	146	0.78	24.5	485.1	530.4	0.85	78.4	0.08	—	0.14	1.22	0.21	16.0	12.1	0	3.3
0	30	2.18	56.6	1080.7	20.2	0.72	2.0	0.12	0.08	0.09	2.84	0.62	56.6	19.4	0	0.8
0	3	0.21	15.3	238.5	3.1	0.18	0	0.06	0.02	0.01	0.85	0.18	5.5	7.8	0	0.2
0	20	4.08	24.9	332.3	12.2	0.28	0.6	0.07	0.02	0.06	1.77	0.35	12.8	7.8	0	0.4
0	7	0.42	29.9	515.4	5.4	0.40	0	0.14	0.01	0.02	1.95	0.40	13.6	17.7	0	0.4
0	13	1.27	34.1	572.0	7.4	0.46	0	0.14	0.01	0.03	2.13	0.44	15.0	18.4	0	—
0	6	0.24	15.6	255.8	3.9	0.21	0	0.07	0.01	0.01	1.02	0.21	7.0	5.8	0	0.2
0	16	1.05	30.8	567.0	8.4	0.39	0	0.08	0.09	0.03	1.34	0.37	16.1	21.2	0	0.4
0	8	0.51	18.2	315.7	271.6	0.26	0	0.09	0.07	0.02	1.55	0.12	19.6	9.3	0	0.1
0	11	0.43	27.3	449.3	266.8	0.37	0	0.13	0.01	0.03	1.80	0.37	12.5	10.1	0	0.4
1	23	0.27	19.9	344.4	349.6	0.31	43.0	0.09	0.44	0.04	1.23	0.25	9.4	11.0	0.1	0.8
2	36	0.21	21.0	164.8	179.5	0.26	49.3	0.09	0.53	0.09	0.90	0.16	8.4	6.8	0.1	5.9
0	22	2.50	54.5	902.9	16.2	0.72	0	0.24	—	0.06	3.46	0.69	24.2	30.5	0	0.8
0	4	0.31	19.4	319.0	5.4	0.25	0	0.10	—	0.01	1.26	0.25	9.3	11.7	0	0.3
0	27	3.44	21.5	377.0	9.3	0.29	0	0.04	0.01	0.04	1.28	0.28	9.9	8.9	0	0.3
0	9	0.41	10.9	199.7	307.2	0.21	0	0.08	0.15	0.02	0.97	0.08	9.0	4.0	0	0.4
14	45	0.47	17.4	252.2	423.7	0.31	43.5	0.02	—	0.06	1.28	0.05	12.4	4.1	0	2.0
15	70	0.70	23.3	463.1	410.4	0.49	0	0.08	—	0.11	1.29	0.22	16.0	13.0	0	2.0
0	18	0.69	11.0	281.8	1.2	0.28	306.3	0.03	0.98	0.09	0.50	0.05	11.0	5.8	0	0.2
0	32	1.70	28.2	252.4	6.1	0.20	953.1	0.02	1.29	0.06	0.45	0.06	14.7	5.1	0	0.5
0	8	0.23	5.2	120.8	8.8	0.25	0.4	0.01	0.90	0.01	0.10	0.02	24.0	3.2	0	0.4
0	8	0.23	5.2	120.8	8.8	0.25	0.4	0.01	0.90	0.01	0.10	0.02	24.0	3.2	0	0.4
0	7	0.09	2.7	62.9	10.5	0.07	0	0.00	0.00	0.01	0.06	0.01	6.8	4.0	0	0.2
0	41	0.45	19.6	277.1	17.0	0.30	0	0.07	0.27	0.04	0.61	0.09	12.8	16.0	0	0.6
0	35	1.73	15.3	200.6	780.0	0.22	1.2	0.03	0.17	0.03	0.17	0.15	28.3	17.3	0	0.7
0	67	1.12	48.4	35.6	93.2	0.48	2.4	0.02	0.32	0.04	0.16	0.00	72.0	1.2	0	0.3
0	9	2.14	14.6	102.2	78.6	0.15	2.2	0.18	0.38	0.28	0.96	0.03	7.1	0.8	0	0.5
0	11	0.36	6.3	100.2	3.6	0.12	18.0	0.02	—	0.01	0.06	0.09	10.2	2.4	—	0.4
0	88	4.42	74.0	442.9	0.9	0.98	0	0.13	0.30	0.24	0.34	0.20	46.4	1.5	0	6.3
0	120	3.39	196.1	1173.0	1.7	4.10	0	0.36	—	0.64	0.90	0.19	176.3	4.0	0	16.6
0	119	3.35	124.7	1264.2	140.2	2.70	8.6	0.08	0.78	0.12	1.21	0.17	181.5	1.9	0	16.4
0	52	0.25	60.4	356.6	8.8	1.32	0.6	0.26	—	0.12	0.69	0.10	79.9	7.5	0	0.4
0	60	1.53	60.0	283.2	122.4	0.28	0	0.14	0.26	0.16	1.23	0.18	43.2	0	0	11.5
0	310	8.27	50.2	17.0	5.1	4.16	22.1	0.42	—	0.27	1.01	0.24	78.2	0.6	0	46.2
0	65	1.16	84.1	—	0	—	0	—	—	—	—	—	—	0	0	—
0	108	1.16	56.1	—	0	—	0	—	—	—	—	—	—	0	0	—
0	171	1.36	31.5	125.9	10.2	0.70	0	0.05	0.01	0.05	0.08	0.06	16.2	0.2	0	8.4
0	316	4.14	51.0	124.2	13.6	1.69	0.9	0.14	0.03	0.04	0.08	0.08	23.0	0	0	24.2
0	56	0.34	33.1	—	4.7	—	0	—	—	—	—	—	—	0	1.7	—
0	108	1.16	35.5	—	0	—	0	—	—	—	—	—	—	0	1.9	—
0	94	0.94	23.0	102.1	6.8	0.54	0	0.04	0.01	0.03	0.45	0.04	37.4	0.2	0	7.6

TABLE A–1 Table of Food Composition (continued)

(Computer code is for Cengage Diet & Wellness Plus program)

D&W+ Code	Food Description	QTY	Measure	Wt (g)	H₂O (g)	Ener (cal)	Prot (g)	Carb (g)	Fiber (g)	Fat (g)	Sat	Mono	Poly
											Fat Breakdown (g)		

VEGETABLES, LEGUMES—CONTINUED

SPINACH

663	Canned, drained	½	cup(s)	107	98.2	25	3.0	3.6	2.6	0.5	0.1	0	0.2
660	Chopped, boiled, drained	½	cup(s)	90	82.1	21	2.7	3.4	2.2	0.2	0	0	0.1
661	Chopped, frozen, boiled, drained	½	cup(s)	95	84.5	32	3.8	4.6	3.5	0.8	0.1	0	0.4
662	Leaf, frozen, boiled, drained	½	cup(s)	95	84.5	32	3.8	4.6	3.5	0.8	0.1	0	0.4
659	Raw, chopped	1	cup(s)	30	27.4	7	0.9	1.1	0.7	0.1	0	0	0
8470	Trimmed leaves	1	cup(s)	32	27.5	3	0.9	0	2.8	0.1	—	—	—

SQUASH

1662	Acorn winter, baked	½	cup(s)	103	85.0	57	1.1	14.9	4.5	0.1	0	0	0.1
29702	Acorn winter, boiled, mashed	½	cup(s)	123	109.9	42	0.8	10.8	3.2	0.1	0	0	0
29451	Butternut, frozen, boiled	½	cup(s)	122	106.9	47	1.5	12.2	1.8	0.1	0	0	0
1661	Butternut winter, baked	½	cup(s)	102	89.5	41	0.9	10.7	3.4	0.1	0	0	0
32773	Butternut winter, frozen, boiled, mashed, no salt added	½	cup(s)	121	106.4	47	1.5	12.2	—	0.1	0	0	0
29700	Crookneck and straightneck summer, boiled, drained	½	cup(s)	65	60.9	12	0.6	2.6	1.2	0.1	0	0	0.1
29703	Hubbard winter, baked	½	cup(s)	102	86.8	51	2.5	11.0	—	0.6	0.1	0	0.3
1660	Hubbard winter, boiled, mashed	½	cup(s)	118	107.5	35	1.7	7.6	3.4	0.4	0.1	0	0.2
29704	Spaghetti winter, boiled, drained, or baked	½	cup(s)	78	71.5	21	0.5	5.0	1.1	0.2	0	0	0.1
664	Summer, all varieties, sliced, boiled, drained	½	cup(s)	90	84.3	18	0.8	3.9	1.3	0.3	0.1	0	0.1
665	Winter, all varieties, baked, mashed	½	cup(s)	103	91.4	38	0.9	9.1	2.9	0.4	0.1	0	0.2
1112	Zucchini summer, boiled, drained	½	cup(s)	90	85.3	14	0.6	3.5	1.3	0	0	0	0
1113	Zucchini summer, frozen, boiled, drained	½	cup(s)	112	105.6	19	1.3	4.0	1.4	0.1	0	0	0.1

SWEET POTATOES

666	Baked, peeled	½	cup(s)	100	75.8	90	2.0	20.7	3.3	0.2	0	0	0.1
667	Boiled, mashed	½	cup(s)	164	131.4	125	2.2	29.1	4.1	0.2	0.1	0	0.1
668	Candied, home recipe	½	cup(s)	91	61.1	132	0.8	25.4	2.2	3.0	1.2	0.6	0.1
670	Canned, vacuum pack	½	cup(s)	100	76.0	91	1.7	21.1	1.8	0.2	0	0	0.1
2765	Frozen, baked	½	cup(s)	88	64.5	88	1.5	20.5	1.6	0.1	0	0	0
1136	Yams, baked or boiled, drained	½	cup(s)	68	47.7	79	1.0	18.7	2.7	0.1	0	0	0

TOMATILLO

| 8774 | Raw | 2 | item(s) | 68 | 62.3 | 22 | 0.7 | 4.0 | 1.3 | 0.7 | 0.1 | 0.1 | 0.3 |
| 8777 | Raw, chopped | ½ | cup(s) | 66 | 60.5 | 21 | 0.6 | 3.9 | 1.3 | 0.7 | 0.1 | 0.1 | 0.3 |

TOMATO

16846	Cherry, fresh	5	item(s)	85	80.3	15	0.7	3.3	1.0	0.2	0	0	0.1
671	Fresh, ripe, red	1	item(s)	123	116.2	22	1.1	4.8	1.5	0.2	0	0	0.1
675	Juice, canned	½	cup(s)	122	114.1	21	0.9	5.2	0.5	0.1	0	0	0
75	Juice, no salt added	½	cup(s)	122	114.1	21	0.9	5.2	0.5	0.1	0	0	0
1699	Paste, canned	2	tablespoon(s)	33	24.1	27	1.4	6.2	1.3	0.2	0	0	0.1
1700	Puree, canned	¼	cup(s)	63	54.9	24	1.0	5.6	1.2	0.1	0	0	0.1
1118	Red, boiled	½	cup(s)	120	113.2	22	1.1	4.8	0.8	0.1	0	0	0.1
3952	Red, diced	½	cup(s)	90	85.1	16	0.8	3.5	1.1	0.2	0	0	0.1
1120	Red, stewed, canned	½	cup(s)	128	116.7	33	1.2	7.9	1.3	0.2	0	0	0.1
1125	Sauce, canned	¼	cup(s)	61	55.6	15	0.8	3.3	0.9	0.1	0	0	0
8778	Sun dried	½	cup(s)	27	3.9	70	3.8	15.1	3.3	0.8	0.1	0.1	0.3
8783	Sun dried in oil, drained	¼	cup(s)	28	14.8	59	1.4	6.4	1.6	3.9	0.5	2.4	0.6
32785	**TARO SHOOTS, COOKED, NO SALT ADDED**	½	cup(s)	70	66.7	10	0.5	2.2	—	0.1	0	0	0

TURNIPS

678	Turnip greens, chopped, boiled, drained	½	cup(s)	72	67.1	14	0.8	3.1	2.5	0.2	0	0	0.1
679	Turnip greens, frozen, chopped, boiled, drained	½	cup(s)	82	74.1	24	2.7	4.1	2.8	0.3	0.1	0	0.1
677	Turnips, cubed, boiled, drained	½	cup(s)	78	73.0	17	0.6	3.9	1.6	0.1	0	0	0

VEGETABLES, MIXED

| 1132 | Canned, drained | ½ | cup(s) | 82 | 70.9 | 40 | 2.1 | 7.5 | 2.4 | 0.2 | 0 | 0 | 0.1 |
| 680 | Frozen, boiled, drained | ½ | cup(s) | 91 | 75.7 | 59 | 2.6 | 11.9 | 4.0 | 0.1 | 0 | 0 | 0.1 |

PAGE KEY: A-4 = Breads/Baked Goods A-10 = Cereal/Rice/Pasta A-14 = Fruit A-20 = Vegetables/Legumes A-30 = Nuts/Seeds A-32 = Vegetarian
A-34 = Dairy A-42 = Eggs A-42 = Seafood A-46 = Meats A-50 = Poultry A-50 = Processed Meats A-52 = Beverages A-56 = Fats/Oils A-58 = Sweets
A-60 = Spices/Condiments/Sauces A-64 = Mixed Foods/Soups/Sandwiches A-70 = Fast Food A-90 = Convenience A-92 = Baby Foods

A

CHOL (mg)	CALC (mg)	IRON (mg)	MAGN (mg)	POTA (mg)	SODI (mg)	ZINC (mg)	VIT A (µg)	THIA (mg)	VIT E (mg α)	RIBO (mg)	NIAC (mg)	VIT B$_6$ (mg)	FOLA (µg DFE)	VIT C (mg)	VIT B$_{12}$ (µg)	SELE (µg)
0	136	2.45	81.3	370.2	28.9	0.48	524.3	0.02	2.08	0.14	0.41	0.11	104.8	15.3	0	1.5
0	122	3.21	78.3	419.4	63.0	0.68	471.6	0.08	1.87	0.21	0.44	0.21	131.4	8.8	0	1.4
0	145	1.86	77.9	286.9	92.2	0.46	572.9	0.07	3.36	0.16	0.41	0.12	115.0	2.1	0	5.2
0	145	1.86	77.9	286.9	92.2	0.46	572.9	0.07	3.36	0.16	0.41	0.12	115.0	2.1	0	5.2
0	30	0.81	23.7	167.4	23.7	0.16	140.7	0.02	0.61	0.06	0.22	0.06	58.2	8.4	0	0.3
0	25	2.13	25.5	134.1	38.0	0.18	—	0.03	—	0.05	0.18	0.07	0	7.5	0	—
0	45	0.95	44.1	447.9	4.1	0.17	21.5	0.17	—	0.01	0.90	0.19	19.5	11.1	0	0.7
0	32	0.68	31.9	322.2	3.7	0.13	50.2	0.12	—	0.01	0.65	0.14	13.5	8.0	0	0.5
0	23	0.70	10.9	161.9	2.4	0.14	203.3	0.06	0.14	0.05	0.56	0.08	19.5	4.3	0	0.6
0	42	0.61	29.6	289.6	4.1	0.13	569.1	0.07	1.31	0.01	0.99	0.12	19.4	15.4	0	0.5
0	23	0.70	10.9	161.2	2.4	0.14	202.4	0.06	—	0.05	0.56	0.08	19.4	4.2	0	0.6
0	14	0.31	13.6	137.1	1.3	0.19	5.2	0.03	—	0.02	0.29	0.07	14.9	5.4	0	0.1
0	17	0.48	22.4	365.1	8.2	0.15	308.0	0.07	—	0.04	0.57	0.17	16.3	9.7	0	0.6
0	12	0.33	15.3	252.5	5.9	0.11	236.0	0.05	0.14	0.03	0.39	0.12	11.8	7.7	0	0.4
0	16	0.26	8.5	90.7	14.0	0.15	4.7	0.02	0.09	0.01	0.62	0.07	6.2	2.7	0	0.2
0	24	0.32	21.6	172.8	0.9	0.35	9.9	0.04	0.12	0.03	0.46	0.05	18.0	5.0	0	0.2
0	23	0.45	13.3	247.0	1.0	0.23	267.5	0.02	0.12	0.07	0.51	0.17	20.5	9.8	0	0.4
0	12	0.32	19.8	227.7	2.7	0.16	50.4	0.04	0.11	0.04	0.39	0.07	15.3	4.1	0	0.2
0	19	0.54	14.5	216.3	2.2	0.22	10	0.05	0.13	0.04	0.43	0.05	8.9	4.1	0	0.2
0	38	0.69	27.0	475.0	36.0	0.32	961.0	0.10	0.71	0.10	1.48	0.28	6.0	19.6	0	0.2
0	44	1.18	29.5	377.2	44.3	0.33	1290.7	0.09	1.54	0.08	0.88	0.27	9.8	21.0	0	0.3
7	24	1.03	10.0	172.6	63.9	0.13	0	0.01	—	0.03	0.36	0.03	10.0	6.1	0	0.7
0	22	0.89	22.0	312.0	53.0	0.18	399.0	0.04	1.00	0.06	0.74	0.19	17.0	26.4	0	0.7
0	31	0.47	18.4	330.1	7.0	0.26	913.3	0.05	0.67	0.04	0.49	0.16	19.3	8.0	0	0.5
0	10	0.35	12.2	455.6	5.4	0.13	4.1	0.06	0.23	0.01	0.37	0.15	10.9	8.2	0	0.5
0	5	0.42	13.6	182.2	0.7	0.15	4.1	0.03	0.25	0.02	1.25	0.03	4.8	8.0	0	0.3
0	5	0.41	13.2	176.9	0.7	0.15	4.0	0.03	0.25	0.02	1.22	0.04	4.6	7.7	0	0.3
0	9	0.22	9.4	201.5	4.3	0.14	35.7	0.03	0.45	0.01	0.50	0.06	12.8	10.8	0	0
0	12	0.33	13.5	291.5	6.2	0.20	51.7	0.04	0.66	0.02	0.73	0.09	18.5	15.6	0	0
0	12	0.52	13.4	278.2	326.8	0.18	27.9	0.06	0.39	0.04	0.82	0.14	24.3	22.2	0	0.4
0	12	0.52	13.4	278.2	12.2	0.18	27.9	0.06	0.39	0.04	0.82	0.14	24.3	22.2	0	0.4
0	12	0.97	13.8	332.6	259.1	0.20	24.9	0.02	1.41	0.05	1.00	0.07	3.9	7.2	0	1.7
0	11	1.11	14.4	274.4	249.4	0.22	16.3	0.01	1.23	0.05	0.91	0.07	6.9	6.6	0	0.4
0	13	0.82	10.8	261.6	13.2	0.17	28.8	0.04	0.67	0.03	0.64	0.10	15.6	27.4	0	0.6
0	9	0.24	9.9	213.3	4.5	0.15	37.8	0.03	0.48	0.01	0.53	0.07	13.5	11.4	0	0
0	43	1.70	15.3	263.9	281.8	0.22	11.5	0.06	1.06	0.04	0.91	0.02	6.4	10.1	0	0.8
0	8	0.62	9.8	201.9	319.6	0.12	10.4	0.01	0.87	0.04	0.59	0.06	6.7	4.3	0	0.1
0	30	2.45	52.4	925.3	565.7	0.53	11.9	0.14	0.00	0.13	2.44	0.09	18.4	10.6	0	1.5
0	13	0.73	22.3	430.4	73.2	0.21	17.6	0.05	—	0.10	0.99	0.08	6.3	28.0	0	0.8
0	10	0.28	5.6	240.8	1.4	0.37	2.1	0.02	—	0.03	0.56	0.07	2.1	13.2	0	0.7
0	99	0.58	15.8	146.2	20.9	0.10	274.3	0.03	1.35	0.05	0.30	0.13	85.0	19.7	0	0.6
0	125	1.59	21.3	183.7	12.3	0.34	441.2	0.04	2.18	0.06	0.38	0.06	32.0	17.9	0	1.0
0	26	0.14	7.0	138.1	12.5	0.09	0	0.02	0.02	0.02	0.23	0.05	7.0	9.0	0	0.2
0	22	0.86	13.0	237.2	121.4	0.33	475.1	0.04	0.24	0.04	0.47	0.06	19.6	4.1	0	0.2
0	23	0.74	20.0	153.8	31.9	0.44	194.7	0.06	0.34	0.10	0.77	0.06	17.3	2.9	0	0.3

(Computer code is for Cengage Diet & Wellness Plus program)

D&W+ Code	Food Description	QTY	Measure	Wt (g)	H₂0 (g)	Ener (cal)	Prot (g)	Carb (g)	Fiber (g)	Fat (g)	Fat Breakdown (g)		
											Sat	Mono	Poly
Vegetables, Legumes—continued													
7489	V8 100% vegetable juice	½	cup(s)	120	—	25	1.0	5.0	1.0	0	0	0	0
7490	V8 low sodium vegetable juice	½	cup(s)	120	—	25	0	6.5	1.0	0	0	0	0
7491	V8 spicy hot vegetable juice	½	cup(s)	120	—	25	1.0	5.0	0.5	0	0	0	0
	Water chestnuts												
31073	Sliced, drained	½	cup(s)	75	70.0	20	0	5.0	1.0	0	0	0	0
31087	Whole	½	cup(s)	75	70.0	20	0	5.0	1.0	0	0	0	0
1135	**Watercress**	1	cup(s)	34	32.3	4	0.8	0.4	0.2	0	0	0	0
Nuts, seeds, and Products													
	Almonds												
32940	Almond butter with salt added	1	tablespoon(s)	16	0.2	101	2.4	3.4	0.6	9.5	0.9	6.1	2.0
1137	Almond butter, no salt added	1	tablespoon(s)	16	0.2	101	2.4	3.4	0.6	9.5	0.9	6.1	2.0
32886	Blanched	¼	cup(s)	36	1.6	211	8.0	7.2	3.8	18.3	1.4	11.7	4.4
32887	Dry roasted, no salt added	¼	cup(s)	35	0.9	206	7.6	6.7	4.1	18.2	1.4	11.6	4.4
29724	Dry roasted, salted	¼	cup(s)	35	0.9	206	7.6	6.7	4.1	18.2	1.4	11.6	4.4
29725	Oil roasted, salted	¼	cup(s)	39	1.1	238	8.3	6.9	4.1	21.7	1.7	13.7	5.3
508	Slivered	¼	cup(s)	27	1.3	155	5.7	5.9	3.3	13.3	1.0	8.3	3.3
1138	**Beechnuts, dried**	¼	cup(s)	57	3.8	328	3.5	19.1	5.3	28.5	3.3	12.5	11.4
517	**Brazil nuts, dried, unblanched**	¼	cup(s)	35	1.2	230	5.0	4.3	2.6	23.3	5.3	8.6	7.2
1166	**Breadfruit seeds, roasted**	¼	cup(s)	57	28.3	118	3.5	22.8	3.4	1.5	0.4	0.2	0.8
1139	**Butternuts, dried**	¼	cup(s)	30	1.0	184	7.5	3.6	1.4	17.1	0.4	3.1	12.8
	Cashews												
32931	Cashew butter with salt added	1	tablespoon(s)	16	0.5	94	2.8	4.4	0.3	7.9	1.6	4.7	1.3
32889	Cashew butter, no salt added	1	tablespoon(s)	16	0.5	94	2.8	4.4	0.3	7.9	1.6	4.7	1.3
1140	Dry roasted	¼	cup(s)	34	0.6	197	5.2	11.2	1.0	15.9	3.1	9.4	2.7
518	Oil roasted	¼	cup(s)	32	1.1	187	5.4	9.6	1.1	15.4	2.7	8.4	2.8
	Chestnuts												
1152	Chinese, roasted	¼	cup(s)	36	14.6	87	1.6	19.0	—	0.4	0.1	0.2	0.1
32895	European, boiled and steamed	¼	cup(s)	46	31.3	60	0.9	12.8	—	0.6	0.1	0.2	0.2
32911	European, roasted	¼	cup(s)	36	14.5	88	1.1	18.9	1.8	0.8	0.1	0.3	0.3
32922	Japanese, boiled and steamed	¼	cup(s)	36	31.0	20	0.3	4.5	—	0.1	0	0	0
32923	Japanese, roasted	¼	cup(s)	36	18.1	73	1.1	16.4	—	0.3	0	0.1	0.1
	Coconut, shredded												
32896	Dried, not sweetened	¼	cup(s)	23	0.7	152	1.6	5.4	3.8	14.9	13.2	0.6	0.2
1153	Dried, shredded, sweetened	¼	cup(s)	23	2.9	116	0.7	11.1	1.0	8.3	7.3	0.4	0.1
520	Shredded	¼	cup(s)	20	9.4	71	0.7	3.0	1.8	6.7	5.9	0.3	0.1
4958	**Flax seeds or linseeds**	¼	cup(s)	43	3.3	225	8.4	12.3	11.9	17.7	1.7	3.2	12.6
32904	**Ginkgo nuts, dried**	¼	cup(s)	39	4.8	136	4.0	28.3	—	0.8	0.1	0.3	0.3
	Hazelnuts or filberts												
32901	Blanched	¼	cup(s)	30	1.7	189	4.1	5.1	3.3	18.3	1.4	14.5	1.7
32902	Dry roasted, no salt added	¼	cup(s)	30	0.8	194	4.5	5.3	2.8	18.7	1.3	14.0	2.5
1156	**Hickory nuts, dried**	¼	cup(s)	30	0.8	197	3.8	5.5	1.9	19.3	2.1	9.8	6.6
	Macadamias												
32905	Dry roasted, no salt added	¼	cup(s)	34	0.5	241	2.6	4.5	2.7	25.5	4.0	19.9	0.5
32932	Dry roasted with salt added	¼	cup(s)	34	0.5	240	2.6	4.3	2.7	25.5	4.0	19.9	0.5
1157	Raw	¼	cup(s)	34	0.5	241	2.6	4.6	2.9	25.4	4.0	19.7	0.5
	Mixed nuts												
1159	With peanuts, dry roasted	¼	cup(s)	34	0.6	203	5.9	8.7	3.1	17.6	2.4	10.8	3.7
32933	With peanuts, dry roasted, with salt added	¼	cup(s)	34	0.6	203	5.9	8.7	3.1	17.6	2.4	10.8	3.7
32906	Without peanuts, oil roasted, no salt added	¼	cup(s)	36	1.1	221	5.6	8.0	2.0	20.2	3.3	11.9	4.1
	Peanuts												
2807	Dry roasted	¼	cup(s)	37	0.6	214	8.6	7.9	2.9	18.1	2.5	9.0	5.7
2806	Dry roasted, salted	¼	cup(s)	37	0.6	214	8.6	7.9	2.9	18.1	2.5	9.0	5.7

CHOL (mg)	CALC (mg)	IRON (mg)	MAGN (mg)	POTA (mg)	SODI (mg)	ZINC (mg)	VIT A (µg)	THIA (mg)	VIT E (mg α)	RIBO (mg)	NIAC (mg)	VIT B6 (mg)	FOLA (µg DFE)	VIT C (mg)	VIT B12 (µg)	SELE (µg)
0	20	0.36	12.9	260.0	310.0	0.24	100.0	0.05	—	0.03	0.87	0.17	—	30.0	0	—
0	20	0.36	—	450.0	70.0	—	100.0	0.02	—	0.02	0.75	—	—	30.0	0	—
0	20	0.36	12.9	240.0	360.0	0.24	50.0	0.05	—	0.03	0.88	0.17	—	15.0	0	—
0	7	0.00	—	—	5.0	0	—	—	—	—	—	—	—	2.0	—	—
0	7	0.00	—	—	5.0	0	—	—	—	—	—	—	—	2.0	—	—
0	41	0.06	7.1	112.2	13.9	0.03	54.4	0.03	0.34	0.04	0.06	0.04	3.1	14.6	0	0.3
0	43	0.59	48.5	121.3	72.0	0.49	0	0.02	4.16	0.10	0.46	0.01	10.4	0.1	0	0.8
0	43	0.59	48.5	121.3	1.8	0.48	0	0.02	—	0.09	0.46	0.01	10.4	0.1	0	—
0	78	1.34	99.7	249.0	10.2	1.13	0	0.07	8.95	0.20	1.32	0.04	10.9	0	0	1.0
0	92	1.55	98.7	257.4	0.3	1.22	0	0.02	8.97	0.29	1.32	0.04	11.4	0	0	1.0
0	92	1.55	98.7	257.4	117.0	1.22	0	0.02	8.97	0.29	1.32	0.04	11.4	0	0	1.0
0	114	1.44	107.5	274.4	133.1	1.20	0	0.03	10.19	0.30	1.43	0.04	10.6	0	0	1.1
0	71	1.00	72.4	190.4	0.3	0.83	0	0.05	7.07	0.27	0.91	0.03	13.5	0	0	0.7
0	1	1.39	0	579.7	21.7	0.20	0	0.16	—	0.20	0.48	0.38	64.4	8.8	0	4.0
0	56	0.85	131.6	230.7	1.1	1.42	0	0.21	2.00	0.01	0.10	0.03	7.7	0.2	0	671.0
0	49	0.50	35.3	616.7	15.9	0.58	8.5	0.22	—	0.12	4.20	0.22	33.6	4.3	0	8.0
0	16	1.21	71.1	126.3	0.3	0.94	1.8	0.12	—	0.04	0.31	0.17	19.8	1.0	0	5.2
0	7	0.81	41.3	87.4	98.2	0.83	0	0.05	0.15	0.03	0.26	0.04	10.9	0	0	1.8
0	7	0.81	41.3	87.4	2.4	0.83	0	0.05	—	0.03	0.26	0.04	10.9	0	0	1.8
0	15	2.06	89.1	193.5	5.5	1.92	0	0.07	0.32	0.07	0.48	0.09	23.6	0	0	4.0
0	14	1.95	88.0	203.8	4.2	1.73	0	0.12	0.30	0.07	0.56	0.10	8.1	0.1	0	6.5
0	7	0.54	32.6	173.0	1.4	0.33	0	0.05	—	0.03	0.54	0.15	26.1	13.9	0	2.6
0	21	0.80	24.8	328.9	12.4	0.11	0.5	0.06	—	0.03	0.32	0.10	17.5	12.3	0	—
0	10	0.32	11.8	211.6	0.7	0.20	0.4	0.08	0.18	0.05	0.48	0.18	25.0	9.3	0	0.4
0	4	0.19	6.5	42.8	1.8	0.14	0.4	0.04	—	0.01	0.19	0.03	6.1	3.4	0	—
0	13	0.75	23.2	154.8	6.9	0.51	1.4	0.15	—	—	0.24	0.14	21.4	10.1	0	—
0	6	0.76	20.7	125.2	8.5	0.46	0	0.01	0.10	0.02	0.13	0.07	2.1	0.3	0	4.3
0	3	0.45	11.6	78.4	60.9	0.42	0	0.01	0.09	0.00	0.11	0.06	1.9	0.2	0	3.9
0	3	0.48	6.4	71.2	4.0	0.21	0	0.01	0.04	0.00	0.11	0.01	5.2	0.7	0	2.0
0	142	2.13	156.1	354.0	11.9	1.83	0	0.06	0.14	0.06	0.59	0.39	118.4	0.5	0	2.3
0	8	0.62	20.7	390.2	5.1	0.26	21.5	0.17	—	0.07	4.58	0.25	41.4	11.4	0	—
0	45	0.98	48.0	197.4	0	0.66	0.6	0.14	5.25	0.03	0.46	0.17	23.4	0.6	0	1.2
0	37	1.31	51.9	226.5	0	0.74	0.9	0.10	4.58	0.03	0.61	0.18	26.4	1.1	0	1.2
0	18	0.64	51.9	130.8	0.3	1.29	2.1	0.26	—	0.04	0.27	0.06	12.0	0.6	0	2.4
0	23	0.88	39.5	121.6	1.3	0.43	0	0.23	0.19	0.02	0.76	0.12	3.4	0.2	0	3.9
0	23	0.88	39.5	121.6	88.8	0.43	0	0.23	0.19	0.02	0.76	0.12	3.4	0.2	0	3.9
0	28	1.24	43.6	123.3	1.7	0.44	0	0.40	0.18	0.05	0.83	0.09	3.7	0.4	0	1.2
0	24	1.27	77.1	204.5	4.1	1.30	0.3	0.07	—	0.07	1.61	0.10	17.1	0.1	0	1.0
0	24	1.26	77.1	204.5	229.1	1.30	0	0.06	3.74	0.06	1.61	0.10	17.1	0.1	0	2.6
0	38	0.92	90.4	195.8	4.0	1.67	0.4	0.18	—	0.17	0.70	0.06	20.2	0.2	0	—
0	20	0.82	64.2	240.2	2.2	1.20	0	0.16	2.52	0.03	4.93	0.09	52.9	0	0	2.7
0	20	0.82	64.2	240.2	296.7	1.20	0	0.16	2.84	0.03	4.93	0.09	52.9	0	0	2.7

(Computer code is for Cengage Diet & Wellness Plus program)

D&W+ Code	Food Description	QTY	Measure	Wt (g)	H₂O (g)	Ener (cal)	Prot (g)	Carb (g)	Fiber (g)	Fat (g)	Fat Breakdown (g) Sat	Mono	Poly
NUTS, SEEDS, AND PRODUCTS—CONTINUED														
1763	Oil roasted, salted	¼	cup(s)	36	0.5	216	10.1	5.5	3.4	18.9	3.1	9.4	5.5
1884	Peanut butter, chunky	1	tablespoon(s)	16	0.2	94	3.8	3.5	1.3	8.0	1.3	3.9	2.4
30303	Peanut butter, low sodium	1	tablespoon(s)	16	0.2	95	4.0	3.1	0.9	8.2	1.8	3.9	2.2
30305	Peanut butter, reduced fat	1	tablespoon(s)	18	0.2	94	4.7	6.4	0.9	6.1	1.3	2.9	1.8
524	Peanut butter, smooth	1	tablespoon(s)	16	0.3	94	4.0	3.1	1.0	8.1	1.7	3.9	2.3
2804	Raw	¼	cup(s)	37	2.4	207	9.4	5.9	3.1	18.0	2.5	8.9	5.7
	PECANS												
32907	Dry roasted, no salt added	¼	cup(s)	28	0.3	198	2.6	3.8	2.6	20.7	1.8	12.3	5.7
32936	Dry roasted with salt added	¼	cup(s)	27	0.3	192	2.6	3.7	2.5	20.0	1.7	11.9	5.6
1162	Oil roasted	¼	cup(s)	28	0.3	197	2.5	3.6	2.6	20.7	2.0	11.3	6.5
526	Raw	¼	cup(s)	27	1.0	188	2.5	3.8	2.6	19.6	1.7	11.1	5.9
12973	**PINE NUTS OR PIGNOLIA, DRIED**	1	tablespoon(s)	9	0.2	58	1.2	1.1	0.3	5.9	0.4	1.6	2.9
	PISTACHIOS												
1164	Dry roasted	¼	cup(s)	31	0.6	176	6.6	8.5	3.2	14.1	1.7	7.4	4.3
32938	Dry roasted with salt added	¼	cup(s)	32	0.6	182	6.8	8.6	3.3	14.7	1.8	7.7	4.4
1167	**PUMPKIN OR SQUASH SEEDS, ROASTED**	¼	cup(s)	57	4.0	296	18.7	7.6	2.2	23.9	4.5	7.4	10.9
	SESAME												
32912	Sesame butter paste	1	tablespoon(s)	16	0.3	94	2.9	3.8	0.9	8.1	1.1	3.1	3.6
32941	Tahini or sesame butter	1	tablespoon(s)	15	0.5	89	2.6	3.2	0.7	8.0	1.1	3.0	3.5
1169	Whole, roasted, toasted	3	tablespoon(s)	10	0.3	54	1.6	2.4	1.3	4.6	0.6	1.7	2.0
	SOY NUTS												
34173	Deep sea salted	¼	cup(s)	28	—	119	11.9	8.9	4.9	4.0	1.0	—	—
34174	Unsalted	¼	cup(s)	28	—	119	11.9	8.9	4.9	4.0	0	—	—
	SUNFLOWER SEEDS												
528	Kernels, dried	1	tablespoon(s)	9	0.4	53	1.9	1.8	0.8	4.6	0.4	1.7	2.1
29721	Kernels, dry roasted, salted	1	tablespoon(s)	8	0.1	47	1.5	1.9	0.7	4.0	0.4	0.8	2.6
29723	Kernels, toasted, salted	1	tablespoon(s)	8	0.1	52	1.4	1.7	1.0	4.8	0.5	0.9	3.1
32928	Sunflower seed butter with salt added	1	tablespoon(s)	16	0.2	93	3.1	4.4	—	7.6	0.8	1.5	5.0
	TRAIL MIX												
4646	Trail mix	¼	cup(s)	38	3.5	173	5.2	16.8	2.0	11.0	2.1	4.7	3.6
4647	Trail mix with chocolate chips	¼	cup(s)	38	2.5	182	5.3	16.8	—	12.0	2.3	5.1	4.2
4648	Tropical trail mix	¼	cup(s)	35	3.2	142	2.2	23.0	—	6.0	3.0	0.9	1.8
	WALNUTS												
529	Dried black, chopped	¼	cup(s)	31	1.4	193	7.5	3.1	2.1	18.4	1.1	4.7	11.0
531	English or Persian	¼	cup(s)	29	1.2	191	4.5	4.0	2.0	19.1	1.8	2.6	13.8
VEGETARIAN FOODS														
	PREPARED												
34222	Brown rice and tofu stir-fry (vegan)	8	ounce(s)	227	244.4	302	16.5	18.0	3.2	21.0	1.7	4.7	13.4
34368	Cheese enchilada casserole (lacto)	8	ounce(s)	227	80.3	385	16.6	38.4	4.1	17.8	9.5	6.1	1.1
34247	Five bean casserole (vegan)	8	ounce(s)	227	175.8	178	5.9	26.6	6.0	5.8	1.1	2.5	1.9
34261	Lentil stew (vegan)	8	ounce(s)	227	227.9	188	11.5	35.9	11.0	0.7	0.1	0.1	0.3
34397	Macaroni and cheese (lacto)	8	ounce(s)	227	352.1	391	18.1	37.1	1.0	18.7	9.8	6.0	1.8
34238	Steamed rice and vegetables (vegan)	8	ounce(s)	227	222.9	587	11.2	87.9	5.8	23.1	4.1	8.7	9.1
34308	Tofu rice burgers (ovo-lacto)	1	piece(s)	218	77.6	435	22.4	68.6	5.6	8.4	1.7	2.4	3.5
34276	Vegan spinach enchiladas (vegan)	1	piece(s)	82	59.2	93	4.9	14.5	1.8	2.4	0.3	0.6	1.3
34243	Vegetable chow mein (vegan)	8	ounce(s)	227	163.3	166	6.5	22.1	2.0	6.4	0.7	2.7	2.5
34454	Vegetable lasagna (lacto)	8	ounce(s)	227	178.9	208	13.7	29.9	2.6	4.1	2.3	1.1	0.3
34339	Vegetable marinara (vegan)	8	ounce(s)	252	200.7	104	3.0	16.7	1.4	3.1	0.4	1.4	1.0
34356	Vegetable rice casserole (lacto)	8	ounce(s)	227	178.9	238	9.7	24.4	4.0	12.5	4.9	3.5	3.1
34311	Vegetable strudel (ovo-lacto)	8	ounce(s)	227	63.1	478	12.0	32.4	2.5	33.8	11.5	16.7	3.9
34371	Vegetable taco (lacto)	1	item(s)	85	46.5	117	4.2	13.6	2.9	5.6	2.1	1.9	1.3
34282	Vegetarian chili (vegan)	8	ounce(s)	227	191.4	115	5.6	21.4	7.1	1.5	0.2	0.3	0.7
34367	Vegetarian vegetable soup (vegan)	8	ounce(s)	227	257.9	111	3.2	16.0	3.2	5.0	1.0	2.1	1.6
	BOCA BURGER												
32067	All American flame grilled patty	1	item(s)	71	—	90	14.0	4.0	3.0	3.0	1.0	—	—
32074	Boca chik'n nuggets	4	item(s)	87	—	180	14.0	17.0	3.0	7.0	1.0	—	—

PAGE KEY: A-4 = Breads/Baked Goods A-10 = Cereal/Rice/Pasta A-14 = Fruit A-20 = Vegetables/Legumes A-30 = Nuts/Seeds A-32 = Vegetarian A-34 = Dairy A-42 = Eggs A-42 = Seafood A-46 = Meats A-50 = Poultry A-50 = Processed Meats A-52 = Beverages A-56 = Fats/Oils A-58 = Sweets A-60 = Spices/Condiments/Sauces A-64 = Mixed Foods/Soups/Sandwiches A-70 = Fast Food A-90 = Convenience A-92 = Baby Foods

A

CHOL (mg)	CALC (mg)	IRON (mg)	MAGN (mg)	POTA (mg)	SODI (mg)	ZINC (mg)	VIT A (µg)	THIA (mg)	VIT E (mg α)	RIBO (mg)	NIAC (mg)	VIT B6 (mg)	FOLA (µg DFE)	VIT C (mg)	VIT B12 (µg)	SELE (µg)
0	22	0.54	63.4	261.4	115.2	1.18	0	0.03	2.49	0.03	4.97	0.16	43.2	0.3	0	1.2
0	7	0.30	25.6	119.2	77.8	0.45	0	0.02	1.01	0.02	2.19	0.07	14.7	0	0	1.3
0	6	0.29	25.4	107.0	2.7	0.47	0	0.01	1.23	0.02	2.14	0.07	11.8	0	0	1.2
0	6	0.34	30.6	120.4	97.2	0.50	0	0.05	1.20	0.01	2.63	0.06	10.8	0	0	1.4
0	7	0.30	24.6	103.8	73.4	0.47	0	0.01	1.44	0.02	2.14	0.09	11.8	0	0	0.9
0	34	1.67	61.3	257.3	6.6	1.19	0	0.23	3.04	0.04	4.40	0.12	87.6	0	0	2.6
0	20	0.78	36.8	118.3	0.3	1.41	1.9	0.12	0.35	0.03	0.32	0.05	4.5	0.2	0	1.1
0	19	0.75	35.6	114.5	103.4	1.36	1.9	0.11	0.34	0.03	0.31	0.05	4.3	0.2	0	1.1
0	18	0.68	33.3	107.8	0.3	1.23	1.4	0.13	0.70	0.03	0.33	0.05	4.1	0.2	0	1.7
0	19	0.69	33.0	111.7	0	1.23	0.8	0.18	0.38	0.04	0.32	0.06	6.0	0.3	0	1.0
0	1	0.47	21.6	51.3	0.2	0.55	0.1	0.03	0.80	0.02	0.37	0.01	2.9	0.1	0	0.1
0	34	1.29	36.9	320.4	3.1	0.71	4.0	0.26	0.59	0.05	0.44	0.39	15.4	0.7	0	2.9
0	35	1.34	38.4	333.4	129.6	0.73	4.2	0.26	0.61	0.05	0.45	0.40	16.0	0.7	0	3.0
0	24	8.48	303.0	457.4	10.2	4.22	10.8	0.12	0.00	0.18	0.99	0.05	32.3	1.0	0	3.2
0	154	3.07	57.9	93.1	1.9	1.17	0.5	0.04	—	0.03	1.07	0.13	16.0	0	0	0.9
0	21	0.66	14.3	68.9	5.3	0.69	0.5	0.24	—	0.02	0.85	0.02	14.7	0.6	0	0.3
0	94	1.40	33.8	45.1	1.0	0.68	0	0.07	—	0.02	0.43	0.07	9.3	0	0	0.5
0	59	1.07	—	—	148.1	—	0	—	—	—	—	—	—	0	—	—
0	59	1.07	—	—	9.9	—	0	—	—	—	—	—	—	0	—	—
0	7	0.47	29.3	58.1	0.8	0.45	0.3	0.13	2.99	0.03	0.75	0.12	20.4	0.1	0	4.8
0	6	0.30	10.3	68.0	32.8	0.42	0	0.01	2.09	0.02	0.56	0.06	19.0	0.1	0	6.3
0	5	0.57	10.8	41.1	51.3	0.44	0	0.03	—	0.02	0.35	0.07	19.9	0.1	0	5.2
0	20	0.76	59.0	11.5	83.2	0.85	0.5	0.05	—	0.05	0.85	0.13	37.9	0.4	0	—
0	29	1.14	59.3	256.9	85.9	1.20	0.4	0.17	—	0.07	1.76	0.11	26.6	0.5	0	—
2	41	1.27	60.4	243.0	45.4	1.17	0.8	0.15	—	0.08	1.65	0.09	24.4	0.5	0	—
0	20	0.92	33.6	248.2	3.5	0.41	0.7	0.15	—	0.04	0.51	0.11	14.7	2.7	0	—
0	19	0.97	62.8	163.4	0.6	1.05	0.6	0.01	0.56	0.04	0.14	0.18	9.7	0.5	0	5.3
0	29	0.85	46.2	129.0	0.6	0.90	0.3	0.10	0.20	0.04	0.32	0.15	28.7	0.4	0	1.4
0	353	6.34	118.3	501.4	142.2	2.03	—	0.23	0.07	0.14	1.49	0.36	51.8	24.8	0	14.8
39	441	2.44	34.6	191.2	1139.7	1.84	—	0.31	0.05	0.35	2.23	0.11	118.3	20.4	0.4	20.0
0	48	1.78	40.8	364.1	613.6	0.61	—	0.10	0.52	0.07	0.93	0.11	64.5	8.3	0	3.3
0	34	3.23	50.0	548.8	436.5	1.42	—	0.24	0.14	0.16	2.31	0.29	202.7	26.4	0	12.1
43	415	1.71	45.4	267.8	1641.0	2.32	—	0.32	0.27	0.48	2.18	0.13	162.7	0.9	0.8	33.3
0	91	3.31	153.1	810.1	3117.8	2.04	—	0.37	3.03	0.21	6.16	0.64	70.1	35.2	0	18.8
52	467	9.01	89.7	455.6	2449.5	2.06	—	0.27	0.12	0.26	3.43	0.29	167.7	2.0	0.1	43.0
0	117	1.13	40.4	170.5	134.2	0.68	—	0.07	—	0.07	0.53	0.10	20.3	1.8	0	5.1
0	189	3.70	28.0	310.3	372.7	0.76	—	0.13	0.05	0.11	1.43	0.14	76.8	8.0	0	6.5
10	176	1.86	41.9	470.0	759.4	1.14	—	0.26	0.05	0.25	2.49	0.22	124.5	19.0	0.4	21.8
0	17	0.94	19.1	189.9	439.6	0.42	—	0.15	0.55	0.08	1.36	0.12	88.4	23.5	0	10.8
17	190	1.28	29.3	414.2	626.0	1.24	—	0.16	0.35	0.29	2.00	0.19	154.8	56.0	0.2	5.8
29	200	2.15	24.5	181.0	512.1	1.24	—	0.28	0.20	0.31	2.88	0.11	111.4	17.4	0.2	19.7
7	77	0.88	26.3	174.1	280.7	0.59	—	0.08	0.04	0.06	0.49	0.08	38.7	4.6	0	3.0
0	65	1.98	41.0	543.1	390.7	0.74	—	0.14	0.15	0.10	1.31	0.18	47.7	20.3	0	4.4
0	46	1.87	34.9	550.3	729.5	0.56	—	0.13	0.55	0.09	1.99	0.27	49.9	29.9	0	1.4
5	150	1.80	—	—	280.0	—	0	—	—	—	—	—	—	0	—	—
0	40	1.44	—	—	500.0	—	—	—	—	—	—	—	—	0	—	—

Table of Food Composition *(continued)*

(Computer code is for Cengage Diet & Wellness Plus program)

D&W+ Code	Food Description	QTY	Measure	Wt (g)	H₂0 (g)	Ener (cal)	Prot (g)	Carb (g)	Fiber (g)	Fat (g)	Sat	Mono	Poly

Fat Breakdown (g): Sat, Mono, Poly

VEGETARIAN FOODS—CONTINUED

D&W+ Code	Food Description	QTY	Measure	Wt (g)	H₂0 (g)	Ener (cal)	Prot (g)	Carb (g)	Fiber (g)	Fat (g)	Sat	Mono	Poly
32075	Boca meatless ground burger	½	cup(s)	57	—	60	13.0	6.0	3.0	0.5	0	—	—
32072	Breakfast links	2	item(s)	45	—	70	8.0	5.0	2.0	3.0	0.5	—	—
32071	Breakfast patties	1	item(s)	38	—	60	7.0	5.0	2.0	2.5	0	—	—
35780	Cheeseburger meatless burger patty	1	item(s)	71	—	100	12.0	5.0	3.0	5.0	1.5	—	—
33958	Original meatless chik'n patties	1	item(s)	71	—	160	11.0	15.0	2.0	6.0	1.0	—	—
32066	Original patty	1	item(s)	71	—	70	13.0	6.0	4.0	0.5	0	—	—
32068	Roasted garlic patty	1	item(s)	71	—	70	12.0	6.0	4.0	1.5	0	—	—
37814	Roasted onion meatless burger patty	1	item(s)	71	—	70	11.0	7.0	4.0	1.0	0	—	—
	GARDENBURGER												
37810	BBQ chik'n with sauce	1	item(s)	142	—	250	14.0	30.0	5.0	8.0	1.0	—	—
39661	Black bean burger	1	item(s)	71	—	80	8.0	11.0	4.0	2.0	0	—	—
39666	Buffalo chik'n wing	3	item(s)	95	—	180	9.0	8.0	5.0	12.0	1.5	—	—
39665	Country fried chicken with creamy pepper gravy	1	item(s)	142	—	190	9.0	16.0	2.0	9.0	1.0	—	—
37808	Flamed grilled chik'n	1	item(s)	71	—	100	13.0	5.0	3.0	2.5	0	—	—
37803	Garden vegan	1	item(s)	71	—	100	10.0	12.0	2.0	1.0	—	—	—
39663	Homestyle classic burger	1	item(s)	71	—	110	12.0	6.0	4.0	5.0	0.5	—	—
37807	Meatless breakfast sausage	1	item(s)	43	—	50	5.0	2.0	2.0	3.5	0	—	—
37809	Meatless meatballs	6	item(s)	85	—	110	12.0	8.0	4.0	4.5	1.0	—	—
37806	Meatless riblets with sauce	1	item(s)	142	—	160	17.0	11.0	4.0	5.0	0	—	—
29913	Original	1	item(s)	71	—	90	10.0	8.0	3.0	2.0	0.5	—	—
39662	Sun-dried tomato basil burger	1	item(s)	71	—	80	10.0	11.0	3.0	1.5	0.5	—	—
29915	Veggie medley	1	item(s)	71	—	90	9.0	11.0	4.0	2.0	0	—	—
	LOMA LINDA												
9311	Big franks, canned	1	item(s)	51	—	110	11.0	3.0	2.0	6.0	1.0	1.5	3.5
9323	Fried chik'n with gravy	2	piece(s)	80	45.9	150	12.0	5.0	2.0	10	1.5	2.5	5.0
9326	Linketts, canned	1	item(s)	35	21.0	70	7.0	1.0	1.0	4.0	0.5	1.0	2.5
9336	Redi-Burger patties, canned	1	slice(s)	85	50.5	120	18.0	7.0	4.0	2.5	0.5	0.5	1.5
9350	Swiss Stake pattie with gravy, frozen	1	piece(s)	92	65.7	130	9.0	9.0	3.0	6.0	1.0	1.5	3.5
9354	Tender Rounds meatball substitute, canned in gravy	6	piece(s)	80	53.9	120	13.0	6.0	1.0	4.5	0.5	1.5	2.5
	MORNINGSTAR FARMS												
33707	America's Original Veggie Dog links	1	item(s)	57	—	80	11.0	6.0	1.0	0.5	0	—	—
9362	Better'n Eggs egg substitute	¼	cup(s)	57	50.3	20	5.0	0	0	0	0	0	0
9371	Breakfast bacon strips	2	item(s)	16	6.8	60	2.0	2.0	0.5	4.5	0.5	1.0	3.0
9368	Breakfast sausage links	2	item(s)	45	26.8	80	9.0	3.0	2.0	3.0	0.5	1.5	1.0
33705	Chik'n nuggets	4	piece(s)	86	—	190	12.0	18.0	2.0	7.0	1.0	2.0	4.0
11587	Chik patties	1	item(s)	71	36.3	150	9.0	16.0	2.0	6.0	1.0	1.5	2.5
2531	Garden veggie patties	1	item(s)	67	40.1	100	10.0	9.0	4.0	2.5	0.5	0.5	1.5
33702	Spicy black bean veggie burger	1	item(s)	78	—	140	12.0	15.0	3.0	4.0	0.5	1.0	2.5
9412	Vegetarian chili, canned	1	cup(s)	230	172.6	180	16.0	25.0	10.0	1.5	0.5	0.5	0.5
	WORTHINGTON												
9424	Chili, canned	1	cup(s)	230	167.0	280	24.0	25.0	8.0	10.0	1.5	1.5	7.0
9436	Diced chik, canned	¼	cup(s)	55	42.7	50	9.0	2.0	1.0	0	0	0	0
9440	Dinner roast, frozen	1	slice(s)	85	53.2	180	14.0	6.0	3.0	11.0	1.5	4.5	5.0
9420	Meatless chicken slices, frozen	3	slice(s)	57	38.9	90	9.0	2.0	0.5	4.5	1.0	1.0	2.5
36702	Meatless chicken style roll, frozen	1	slice(s)	55	—	90	9.0	2.0	1.0	4.5	1.0	1.0	2.5
9428	Meatless corned beef, sliced, frozen	3	slice(s)	57	31.2	140	10.0	5.0	0	9.0	1.0	2.0	5.0
9470	Meatless salami, sliced, frozen	3	slice(s)	57	32.4	120	12.0	3.0	2.0	7.0	1.0	1.0	5.0
9480	Meatless smoked turkey, sliced	3	slice(s)	57	—	140	10.0	4.0	0	9.0	1.5	2.0	5.0
9462	Prosage links	2	item(s)	45	26.8	80	9.0	3.0	2.0	3.0	0.5	0.5	2.0
9484	Stakelets patty beef steak substitute, frozen	1	piece(s)	71	41.5	150	14.0	7.0	2.0	7.0	1.0	2.5	3.5
9486	Stripples bacon substitute	2	item(s)	16	6.8	60	2.0	2.0	0.5	4.5	0.5	1.0	3.0
9496	Vegetable Skallops meat substitute, canned	½	cup(s)	85	—	90	17.0	4.0	3.0	1.0	0	0	0.5

DAIRY

D&W+ Code	Food Description	QTY	Measure	Wt (g)	H₂0 (g)	Ener (cal)	Prot (g)	Carb (g)	Fiber (g)	Fat (g)	Sat	Mono	Poly
	CHEESE												
1433	Blue, crumbled	1	ounce(s)	28	12.0	100	6.1	0.7	0	8.1	5.3	2.2	0.2
884	Brick	1	ounce(s)	28	11.7	105	6.6	0.8	0	8.4	5.3	2.4	0.2

PAGE KEY: A-4 = Breads/Baked Goods A-10 = Cereal/Rice/Pasta A-14 = Fruit A-20 = Vegetables/Legumes A-30 = Nuts/Seeds A-32 = Vegetarian
A-34 = Dairy A-42 = Eggs A-42 = Seafood A-46 = Meats A-50 = Poultry A-50 = Processed Meats A-52 = Beverages A-56 = Fats/Oils A-58 = Sweets
A-60 = Spices/Condiments/Sauces A-64 = Mixed Foods/Soups/Sandwiches A-70 = Fast Food A-90 = Convenience A-92 = Baby Foods

CHOL (mg)	CALC (mg)	IRON (mg)	MAGN (mg)	POTA (mg)	SODI (mg)	ZINC (mg)	VIT A (µg)	THIA (mg)	VIT E (mg α)	RIBO (mg)	NIAC (mg)	VIT B6 (mg)	FOLA (µg DFE)	VIT C (mg)	VIT B12 (µg)	SELE (µg)
0	60	1.80	—	—	270.0	—	0	—	—	—	—	—	—	0	—	—
0	20	1.44	—	—	330.0	—	0	—	—	—	—	—	—	0	—	—
0	20	1.08	—	—	280.0	—	0	—	—	—	—	—	—	0	—	—
5	80	1.80	—	—	360.0	—	—	—	—	—	—	—	—	0	—	—
0	40	1.80	—	—	430.0	—	—	—	—	—	—	—	—	0	—	—
0	60	1.80	—	—	280.0	—	0	—	—	—	—	—	—	0	—	—
0	60	1.80	—	—	370.0	—	0	—	—	—	—	—	—	0	—	—
0	100	2.70	—	—	300.0	—	—	—	—	—	—	—	—	0	—	—
0	150	1.08	—	—	890.0	—	—	—	—	—	—	—	—	0	—	—
0	40	1.44	—	—	330.0	—	—	—	—	—	—	—	—	0	—	—
0	40	0.72	—	—	1000.0	—	—	—	—	—	—	—	—	0	—	—
5	40	1.44	—	—	550.0	—	—	—	—	—	—	—	—	0	—	—
0	60	3.60	—	—	360.0	—	—	—	—	—	—	—	—	0	—	—
0	40	4.50	—	—	230.0	—	—	—	—	—	—	—	—	0	—	—
0	80	1.44	—	—	380.0	—	—	—	—	—	—	—	—	0	—	—
0	20	0.72	—	—	120.0	—	—	—	—	—	—	—	—	0	—	—
0	60	1.80	—	—	400.0	—	—	—	—	—	—	—	—	0	—	—
0	60	1.80	—	—	720.0	—	—	—	—	—	—	—	—	3.6	—	—
0	80	1.08	30.4	193.4	490.0	0.89	—	0.10	—	0.15	1.08	0.08	10.1	1.2	0.1	7.0
5	60	1.44	—	—	260.0	—	—	—	—	—	—	—	—	3.6	—	—
0	40	1.44	27.0	182.0	290.0	0.46	—	0.07	—	0.08	0.90	0.09	10.6	9.0	0	4.0
0	0	0.77	—	50.0	220.0	—	0	0.22	—	0.10	2.00	0.70	—	0	2.4	—
0	20	1.80	—	70.0	430.0	0.33	0	1.05	—	0.34	4.00	0.30	—	0	2.4	—
0	0	0.36	—	20.0	160.0	0.46	0	0.12	—	0.20	0.80	0.16	—	0	0.9	—
0	0	1.06	—	140.0	450.0	—	0	0.15	—	0.25	4.00	0.40	—	0	1.2	—
0	0	0.72	—	200.0	430.0	—	0	0.45	—	0.25	10.00	1.00	—	0	5.4	—
0	20	1.08	—	80.0	340.0	0.66	0	0.75	—	0.17	2.00	0.16	—	0	1.2	—
0	0	0.72	—	60.0	580.0	—	0	—	—	—	—	—	—	0	—	—
0	20	0.72	—	75.0	90.0	0.60	37.5	0.03	—	0.34	0.00	0.08	24.0	—	0.6	—
0	0	0.36	—	15.0	220.0	0.05	0	0.75	—	0.04	0.40	0.07	—	0	0.2	—
0	0	1.80	—	50.0	300.0	—	0	0.37	—	0.17	7.00	0.50	—	0	3.0	—
0	20	2.70	—	320.0	490.0	—	0	0.52	—	0.25	5.00	0.30	—	0	1.5	—
0	0	1.80	—	210.0	540.0	—	0	1.80	—	0.17	2.00	0.20	—	0	1.2	—
0	40	0.72	—	180.0	350.0	—	—	—	—	—	—	—	—	0	—	—
0	40	1.80	—	320.0	470.0	—	0	—	—	—	0.00	—	—	0	—	—
0	40	3.60	—	660.0	900.0	—	—	—	—	—	—	—	—	0	—	—
0	40	3.60	—	330.0	1130.0	—	0	0.30	—	0.13	2.00	0.70	—	0	1.5	—
0	0	1.08	—	100.0	220.0	0.24	0	0.06	—	0.10	4.00	0.08	—	0	0.2	—
0	20	1.80	—	120.0	580.0	0.64	0	1.80	—	0.25	6.00	0.60	—	0	1.5	—
0	250	1.80	—	250.0	250.0	0.26	0	0.37	—	0.13	4.00	0.30	—	0	1.8	—
0	100	1.08	—	240.0	240.0	—	0	0.37	—	0.13	4.00	0.30	—	0	1.8	—
0	0	1.80	—	130.0	460.0	0.26	0	0.45	—	0.17	5.00	0.30	—	0	1.8	—
0	0	1.08	—	95.0	800.0	0.30	0	0.75	—	0.17	4.00	0.20	—	0	0.6	—
0	60	2.70	—	60.0	450.0	0.23	0	1.80	—	0.17	6.00	0.40	—	0	3.0	—
0	0	1.44	—	50.0	320.0	0.36	0	1.80	—	0.17	2.00	0.30	—	0	3.0	—
0	40	1.08	—	130.0	480.0	0.50	0	1.20	—	0.13	3.00	0.30	—	0	1.5	—
0	0	0.36	—	15.0	220.0	0.05	0	0.75	—	0.03	0.40	0.08	—	0	0.2	—
0	0	0.36	—	10.0	390.0	0.67	0	0.03	—	0.03	0.00	0.01	—	0	0	—
21	150	0.08	6.5	72.6	395.5	0.75	56.1	0.01	0.07	0.10	0.28	0.04	10.2	0	0.3	4.1
27	191	0.12	6.8	38.6	158.8	0.73	82.8	0.00	0.07	0.10	0.03	0.01	5.7	0	0.4	4.1

D&W+ Code	Food Description	QTY	Measure	Wt (g)	H₂0 (g)	Ener (cal)	Prot (g)	Carb (g)	Fiber (g)	Fat (g)	Sat	Mono	Poly
											\(Fat Breakdown (g)\)		
DAIRY—CONTINUED													
885	Brie	1	ounce(s)	28	13.7	95	5.9	0.1	0	7.8	4.9	2.3	0.2
34821	Camembert	1	ounce(s)	28	14.7	85	5.6	0.1	0	6.9	4.3	2.0	0.2
5	Cheddar, shredded	¼	cup(s)	28	10.4	114	7.0	0.4	0	9.4	6.0	2.7	0.3
888	Cheddar or colby	1	ounce(s)	28	10.8	112	6.7	0.7	0	9.1	5.7	2.6	0.3
32096	Cheddar or colby, low fat	1	ounce(s)	28	17.9	49	6.9	0.5	0	2.0	1.2	0.6	0.1
889	Edam	1	ounce(s)	28	11.8	101	7.1	0.4	0	7.9	5.0	2.3	0.2
890	Feta	1	ounce(s)	28	15.7	75	4.0	1.2	0	6.0	4.2	1.3	0.2
891	Fontina	1	ounce(s)	28	10.8	110	7.3	0.4	0	8.8	5.4	2.5	0.5
8527	Goat cheese, soft	1	ounce(s)	28	17.2	76	5.3	0.3	0	6.0	4.1	1.4	0.1
893	Gouda	1	ounce(s)	28	11.8	101	7.1	0.6	0	7.8	5.0	2.2	0.2
894	Gruyere	1	ounce(s)	28	9.4	117	8.5	0.1	0	9.2	5.4	2.8	0.5
895	Limburger	1	ounce(s)	28	13.7	93	5.7	0.1	0	7.7	4.7	2.4	0.1
896	Monterey jack	1	ounce(s)	28	11.6	106	6.9	0.2	0	8.6	5.4	2.5	0.3
13	Mozzarella, part skim milk	1	ounce(s)	28	15.2	72	6.9	0.8	0	4.5	2.9	1.3	0.1
12	Mozzarella, whole milk	1	ounce(s)	28	14.2	85	6.3	0.6	0	6.3	3.7	1.9	0.2
897	Muenster	1	ounce(s)	28	11.8	104	6.6	0.3	0	8.5	5.4	2.5	0.2
898	Neufchatel	1	ounce(s)	28	17.6	74	2.8	0.8	0	6.6	4.2	1.9	0.2
14	Parmesan, grated	1	tablespoon(s)	5	1.0	22	1.9	0.2	0	1.4	0.9	0.4	0.1
17	Provolone	1	ounce(s)	28	11.6	100	7.3	0.6	0	7.5	4.8	2.1	0.2
19	Ricotta, part skim milk	¼	cup(s)	62	45.8	85	7.0	3.2	0	4.9	3.0	1.4	0.2
18	Ricotta, whole milk	¼	cup(s)	62	44.1	107	6.9	1.9	0	8.0	5.1	2.2	0.2
20	Romano	1	tablespoon(s)	5	1.5	19	1.6	0.2	0	1.3	0.9	0.4	0
900	Roquefort	1	ounce(s)	28	11.2	105	6.1	0.6	0	8.7	5.5	2.4	0.4
21	Swiss	1	ounce(s)	28	10.5	108	7.6	1.5	0	7.9	5.0	2.1	0.3
IMITATION CHEESE													
42245	Imitation American cheddar cheese	1	ounce(s)	28	15.1	68	4.7	3.3	0	4.0	2.5	1.2	0.1
53914	Imitation cheddar	1	ounce(s)	28	15.1	68	4.7	3.3	0	4.0	2.5	1.2	0.1
COTTAGE CHEESE													
9	Low fat, 1% fat	½	cup(s)	113	93.2	81	14.0	3.1	0	1.2	0.7	0.3	0
8	Low fat, 2% fat	½	cup(s)	113	89.6	102	15.5	4.1	0	2.2	1.4	0.6	0.1
CREAM CHEESE													
11	Cream cheese	2	tablespoon(s)	29	15.6	101	2.2	0.8	0	10.1	6.4	2.9	0.4
17366	Fat-free cream cheese	2	tablespoon(s)	30	22.7	29	4.3	1.7	0	0.4	0.3	0.1	0
10438	Tofutti Better than Cream Cheese	2	tablespoon(s)	30	—	80	1.0	1.0	0	8.0	2.0	—	6.0
PROCESSED CHEESE													
24	American cheese food, processed	1	ounce(s)	28	12.3	94	5.2	2.2	0	7.1	4.2	2.0	0.3
25	American cheese spread, processed	1	ounce(s)	28	13.5	82	4.7	2.5	0	6.0	3.8	1.8	0.2
22	American cheese, processed	1	ounce(s)	28	11.1	106	6.3	0.5	0	8.9	5.6	2.5	0.3
9110	Kraft deluxe singles pasteurized process American cheese	1	ounce(s)	28	—	108	5.4	0	0	9.5	5.4	—	—
23	Swiss cheese, processed	1	ounce(s)	28	12.0	95	7.0	0.6	0	7.1	4.5	2.0	0.2
SOY CHEESE													
10437	Galaxy Foods vegan grated parmesan cheese alternative	1	tablespoon(s)	8	—	23	3.0	1.5	0	0	0	0	0
10430	Nu Tofu cheddar flavored cheese alternative	1	ounce(s)	28	—	70	6.0	1.0	0	4.0	0.5	2.5	1.0
CREAM													
26	Half and half cream	1	tablespoon(s)	15	12.1	20	0.4	0.6	0	1.7	1.1	0.5	0.1
32	Heavy whipping cream, liquid	1	tablespoon(s)	15	8.7	52	0.3	0.4	0	5.6	3.5	1.6	0.2
28	Light coffee or table cream, liquid	1	tablespoon(s)	15	11.1	29	0.4	0.5	0	2.9	1.8	0.8	0.1
30	Light whipping cream, liquid	1	tablespoon(s)	15	9.5	44	0.3	0.4	0	4.6	2.9	1.4	0.1
34	Whipped cream topping, pressurized	1	tablespoon(s)	3	1.8	8	0.1	0.4	0	0.7	0.4	0.2	0
SOUR CREAM													
30556	Fat-free sour cream	2	tablespoon(s)	32	25.8	24	1.0	5.0	0	0	0	0	0
36	Sour cream	2	tablespoon(s)	24	17.0	51	0.8	1.0	0	5.0	3.1	1.5	0.2
IMITATION CREAM													
3659	Coffeemate nondairy creamer, liquid	1	tablespoon(s)	15	—	20	0	2.0	0	1.0	0	0.5	0
40	Cream substitute, powder	1	teaspoon(s)	2	0	11	0.1	1.1	0	0.7	0.7	0	0
904	Imitation sour cream	2	tablespoon(s)	29	20.5	60	0.7	1.9	0	5.6	5.1	0.2	0

PAGE KEY: A-4 = Breads/Baked Goods A-10 = Cereal/Rice/Pasta A-14 = Fruit A-20 = Vegetables/Legumes A-30 = Nuts/Seeds A-32 = Vegetarian A-34 = Dairy A-42 = Eggs A-42 = Seafood A-46 = Meats A-50 = Poultry A-50 = Processed Meats A-52 = Beverages A-56 = Fats/Oils A-58 = Sweets A-60 = Spices/Condiments/Sauces A-64 = Mixed Foods/Soups/Sandwiches A-70 = Fast Food A-90 = Convenience A-92 = Baby Foods

A

CHOL (mg)	CALC (mg)	IRON (mg)	MAGN (mg)	POTA (mg)	SODI (mg)	ZINC (mg)	VIT A (µg)	THIA (mg)	VIT E (mg α)	RIBO (mg)	NIAC (mg)	VIT B6 (mg)	FOLA (µg DFE)	VIT C (mg)	VIT B12 (µg)	SELE (µg)
28	52	0.14	5.7	43.1	178.3	0.67	49.3	0.02	0.06	0.14	0.10	0.06	18.4	0	0.5	4.1
20	110	0.09	5.7	53.0	238.7	0.67	68.3	0.01	0.06	0.14	0.18	0.06	17.6	0	0.4	4.1
30	204	0.19	7.9	27.7	175.4	0.87	74.9	0.01	0.08	0.10	0.02	0.02	5.1	0	0.2	3.9
27	194	0.21	7.4	36.0	171.2	0.87	74.8	0.00	0.07	0.10	0.02	0.02	5.1	0	0.2	4.1
6	118	0.11	4.5	18.7	173.5	0.51	17.0	0.00	0.01	0.06	0.01	0.01	3.1	0	0.1	4.1
25	207	0.12	8.5	53.3	273.6	1.06	68.9	0.01	0.06	0.11	0.02	0.02	4.5	0	0.4	4.1
25	140	0.18	5.4	17.6	316.4	0.81	35.4	0.04	0.05	0.23	0.28	0.12	9.1	0	0.5	4.3
33	156	0.06	4.0	18.1	226.8	0.99	74.0	0.01	0.07	0.05	0.04	0.02	1.7	0	0.5	4.1
13	40	0.53	4.5	7.4	104.3	0.26	81.6	0.02	0.05	0.10	0.12	0.07	3.4	0	0.1	0.8
32	198	0.06	8.2	34.3	232.2	1.10	46.8	0.01	0.06	0.09	0.01	0.02	6.0	0	0.4	4.1
31	287	0.04	10.2	23.0	95.3	1.10	76.8	0.01	0.07	0.07	0.03	0.02	2.8	0	0.5	4.1
26	141	0.03	6.0	36.3	226.8	0.59	96.4	0.02	0.06	0.14	0.04	0.02	16.4	0	0.3	4.1
25	211	0.20	7.7	23.0	152.0	0.85	56.1	0.00	0.07	0.11	0.02	0.02	5.1	0	0.2	4.1
18	222	0.06	6.5	23.8	175.5	0.78	36.0	0.01	0.04	0.08	0.03	0.02	2.6	0	0.2	4.1
22	143	0.12	5.7	21.5	177.8	0.82	50.7	0.01	0.05	0.08	0.02	0.01	2.0	0	0.6	4.8
27	203	0.11	7.7	38.0	178.0	0.79	84.5	0.00	0.07	0.09	0.02	0.01	3.4	0	0.4	4.1
22	21	0.07	2.3	32.3	113.1	0.14	84.5	0.00	—	0.05	0.03	0.01	3.1	0	0.1	0.9
4	55	0.04	1.9	6.3	76.5	0.19	6.0	0.00	0.01	0.02	0.01	0.00	0.5	0	0.1	0.9
20	214	0.14	7.9	39.1	248.3	0.91	66.9	0.01	0.06	0.09	0.04	0.02	2.8	0	0.4	4.1
19	167	0.27	9.2	76.9	76.9	0.82	65.8	0.01	0.04	0.11	0.04	0.01	8.0	0	0.2	10.3
31	127	0.23	6.8	64.6	51.7	0.71	73.8	0.01	0.06	0.12	0.06	0.02	7.4	0	0.2	8.9
5	53	0.03	2.1	4.3	60	0.12	4.8	0.00	0.01	0.01	0.00	0.00	0.4	0	0.1	0.7
26	188	0.15	8.5	25.8	512.9	0.59	83.3	0.01	—	0.16	0.20	0.03	13.9	0	0.2	4.1
26	224	0.05	10.8	21.8	54.4	1.23	62.4	0.01	0.10	0.08	0.02	0.02	1.7	0	0.9	5.2
10	159	0.08	8.2	68.6	381.3	0.73	32.3	0.01	0.07	0.12	0.03	0.03	2.0	0	0.1	4.3
10	159	0.09	8.2	68.6	381.3	0.73	32.3	0.01	0.07	0.12	0.04	0.03	2.0	0	0.1	4.3
5	69	0.15	5.7	97.2	458.8	0.42	12.4	0.02	0.01	0.18	0.14	0.07	13.6	0	0.7	10.2
9	78	0.18	6.8	108.5	458.8	0.47	23.7	0.02	0.02	0.20	0.16	0.08	14.7	0	0.8	11.5
32	23	0.34	1.7	34.5	85.8	0.15	106.1	0.01	0.08	0.05	0.02	0.01	3.8	0	0.1	0.7
2	56	0.05	4.2	48.9	163.5	0.26	83.7	0.01	0.00	0.05	0.04	0.01	11.1	0	0.2	1.5
0	0	0.00	—	—	135.0	—	0	—	—	—	—	—	—	0	—	—
23	162	0.16	8.8	82.5	358.6	0.90	57.0	0.01	0.06	0.14	0.04	0.02	2.0	0	0.4	4.6
16	159	0.09	8.2	68.6	381.3	0.73	49.0	0.01	0.05	0.12	0.03	0.03	2.0	0	0.1	3.2
27	156	0.05	7.7	47.9	422.1	0.80	72.0	0.01	0.07	0.10	0.02	0.02	2.3	0	0.2	4.1
27	338	0.00	0	33.8	459.0	1.22	114.0	—	—	0.14	—	—	—	0	0.2	—
24	219	0.17	8.2	61.2	388.4	1.02	56.1	0.00	0.09	0.07	0.01	0.01	1.7	0	0.3	4.5
0	60	0.00	—	75.0	97.5	—	—	—	—	—	—	—	—	—	—	—
0	200	0.36	—	—	190.0	—	—	—	—	—	—	—	—	0	—	—
6	16	0.01	1.5	19.5	6.2	0.08	14.6	0.01	0.05	0.02	0.01	0.01	0.5	0.1	0	0.3
21	10	0.00	1.1	11.3	5.7	0.03	61.7	0.00	0.15	0.01	0.01	0.00	0.6	0.1	0	0.1
10	14	0.01	1.4	18.3	6.0	0.04	27.2	0.01	0.08	0.02	0.01	0.01	0.3	0.1	0	0.1
17	10	0.00	1.1	14.6	5.1	0.03	41.9	0.00	0.13	0.01	0.01	0.00	0.6	0.1	0	0.1
2	3	0.00	0.3	4.4	3.9	0.01	5.6	0.00	0.01	0.00	0.00	0.00	0.1	0	0	0
3	40	0.00	3.2	41.3	45.1	0.16	23.4	0.01	0.00	0.04	0.02	0.01	3.5	0	0.1	1.7
11	28	0.01	2.6	34.6	12.7	0.06	42.5	0.01	0.14	0.03	0.01	0.00	2.6	0.2	0.1	0.5
0	0	0.00	—	30.0	0	—	0	0.01	—	0.01	0.20	—	—	0	—	—
0	0	0.02	0.1	16.2	3.6	0.01	0	0.00	0.01	0.00	0.00	0.00	0	0	0	0
0	1	0.11	1.7	46.3	29.3	0.34	0	0.00	0.21	0.00	0.00	0.00	0	0	0	0.7

TABLE A–1 Table of Food Composition *(continued)*

(Computer code is for Cengage Diet & Wellness Plus program)

D&W+ Code	Food Description	QTY	Measure	WT (g)	H₂O (g)	ENER (cal)	PROT (g)	CARB (g)	FIBER (g)	FAT (g)	Fat Breakdown (g) SAT	MONO	POLY
	DAIRY—CONTINUED												
35972	Nondairy coffee whitener, liquid, frozen	1	tablespoon(s)	15	11.7	21	0.2	1.7	0	1.5	0.3	1.1	0
35976	Nondairy dessert topping, frozen	1	tablespoon(s)	5	2.4	15	0.1	1.1	0	1.2	1.0	0.1	0
35975	Nondairy dessert topping, pressurized	1	tablespoon(s)	4	2.7	12	0	0.7	0	1.0	0.8	0.1	0
	FLUID MILK												
60	Buttermilk, low fat	1	cup(s)	245	220.8	98	8.1	11.7	0	2.2	1.3	0.6	0.1
54	Low fat, 1%	1	cup(s)	244	219.4	102	8.2	12.2	0	2.4	1.5	0.7	0.1
55	Low fat, 1%, with nonfat milk solids	1	cup(s)	245	220.0	105	8.5	12.2	0	2.4	1.5	0.7	0.1
57	Nonfat, skim or fat free	1	cup(s)	245	222.6	83	8.3	12.2	0	0.2	0.1	0.1	0
58	Nonfat, skim or fat free with nonfat milk solids	1	cup(s)	245	221.4	91	8.7	12.3	0	0.6	0.4	0.2	0
51	Reduced fat, 2%	1	cup(s)	244	218.0	122	8.1	11.4	0	4.8	3.1	1.4	0.2
52	Reduced fat, 2%, with nonfat milk solids	1	cup(s)	245	217.7	125	8.5	12.2	0	4.7	2.9	1.4	0.2
50	Whole, 3.3%	1	cup(s)	244	215.5	146	7.9	11.0	0	7.9	4.6	2.0	0.5
	CANNED MILK												
62	Nonfat or skim evaporated	2	tablespoon(s)	32	25.3	25	2.4	3.6	0	0.1	0	0	0
63	Sweetened condensed	2	tablespoon(s)	38	10.4	123	3.0	20.8	0	3.3	2.1	0.9	0.1
61	Whole evaporated	2	tablespoon(s)	32	23.3	42	2.1	3.2	0	2.4	1.4	0.7	0.1
	DRIED MILK												
64	Buttermilk	¼	cup(s)	30	0.9	117	10.4	14.9	0	1.8	1.1	0.5	0.1
65	Instant nonfat with added vitamin A	¼	cup(s)	17	0.7	61	6.0	8.9	0	0.1	0.1	0	0
5234	Skim milk powder	¼	cup(s)	17	0.7	62	6.1	9.1	0	0.1	0.1	0	0
907	Whole dry milk	¼	cup(s)	32	0.8	159	8.4	12.3	0	8.5	5.4	2.5	0.2
909	**GOAT MILK**	1	cup(s)	244	212.4	168	8.7	10.9	0	10.1	6.5	2.7	0.4
	CHOCOLATE MILK												
33155	Chocolate syrup, prepared with milk	1	cup(s)	282	227.0	254	8.7	36.0	0.8	8.3	4.7	2.1	0.5
33184	Cocoa mix with aspartame, added sodium and vitamin A, no added calcium or phosphorus, prepared with water	1	cup(s)	192	177.4	56	2.3	10.8	1.2	0.4	0.3	0.1	0
908	Hot cocoa, prepared with milk	1	cup(s)	250	206.4	193	8.8	26.6	2.5	5.8	3.6	1.7	0.1
69	Low fat	1	cup(s)	250	211.3	158	8.1	26.1	1.3	2.5	1.5	0.8	0.1
68	Reduced fat	1	cup(s)	250	205.4	190	7.5	30.3	1.8	4.8	2.9	1.1	0.2
67	Whole	1	cup(s)	250	205.8	208	7.9	25.9	2.0	8.5	5.3	2.5	0.3
70	**EGGNOG**	1	cup(s)	254	188.9	343	9.7	34.4	0	19.0	11.3	5.7	0.9
	BREAKFAST DRINKS												
10093	Carnation Instant Breakfast classic chocolate malt, prepared with skim milk, no sugar added	1	cup(s)	243	—	142	11.1	21.3	0.7	1.3	0.7	—	—
10092	Carnation Instant Breakfast classic French vanilla, prepared with skim milk, no sugar added	1	cup(s)	273	—	150	12.9	24.0	0	0.4	0.4	—	—
10094	Carnation Instant Breakfast strawberry sensation, prepared with skim milk, no sugar added	1	cup(s)	243	—	142	11.1	21.3	0	0.4	0.4	—	—
10091	Carnation Instant Breakfast strawberry sensation, prepared with skim milk	1	cup(s)	273	—	220	12.5	38.8	0	0.4	0.4	—	—
1417	Ovaltine rich chocolate flavor, prepared with skim milk	1	cup(s)	258	—	170	8.5	31.0	0	0	0	0	0
8539	**MALTED MILK, CHOCOLATE MIX, FORTIFIED, PREPARED WITH MILK**	1	cup(s)	265	215.8	223	8.9	28.9	1.1	8.6	5.0	2.2	0.5
	MILKSHAKES												
73	Chocolate	1	cup(s)	227	164.0	270	6.9	48.1	0.7	6.1	3.8	1.8	0.2
3163	Strawberry	1	cup(s)	226	167.8	256	7.7	42.8	0.9	6.3	3.9	—	—
74	Vanilla	1	cup(s)	227	169.2	254	8.8	40.3	0	6.9	4.3	2.0	0.3

PAGE KEY: A-4 = Breads/Baked Goods A-10 = Cereal/Rice/Pasta A-14 = Fruit A-20 = Vegetables/Legumes A-30 = Nuts/Seeds A-32 = Vegetarian A-34 = Dairy A-42 = Eggs A-42 = Seafood A-46 = Meats A-50 = Poultry A-50 = Processed Meats A-52 = Beverages A-56 = Fats/Oils A-58 = Sweets A-60 = Spices/Condiments/Sauces A-64 = Mixed Foods/Soups/Sandwiches A-70 = Fast Food A-90 = Convenience A-92 = Baby Foods

A

CHOL (mg)	CALC (mg)	IRON (mg)	MAGN (mg)	POTA (mg)	SODI (mg)	ZINC (mg)	VIT A (µg)	THIA (mg)	VIT E (mg α)	RIBO (mg)	NIAC (mg)	VIT B_6 (mg)	FOLA (µg DFE)	VIT C (mg)	VIT B_{12} (µg)	SELE (µg)
0	1	0.00	0	28.9	12.0	0.00	0.2	0.00	0.12	0.00	0.00	0.00	0	0	0	0.2
0	0	0.00	0.1	0.9	1.2	0.00	0.3	0.00	0.05	0.00	0.00	0.00	0	0	0	0.1
0	0	0.00	0	0.8	2.8	0.00	0.2	0.00	0.04	0.00	0.00	0.00	0	0	0	0.1
10	284	0.12	27.0	370.0	257.3	1.02	17.2	0.08	0.12	0.37	0.14	0.08	12.3	2.5	0.5	4.9
12	290	0.07	26.8	366.0	107.4	1.02	141.5	0.04	0.02	0.45	0.22	0.09	12.2	0	1.1	8.1
10	314	0.12	34.3	396.9	127.4	0.98	144.6	0.09	—	0.42	0.22	0.11	12.3	2.5	0.9	5.6
5	306	0.07	27.0	382.2	102.9	1.02	149.5	0.11	0.02	0.44	0.23	0.09	12.3	0	1.3	7.6
5	316	0.12	36.8	419.0	129.9	1.00	149.5	0.10	0.00	0.42	0.22	0.11	12.3	2.5	1.0	5.4
20	285	0.07	26.8	366.0	100.0	1.04	134.2	0.09	0.07	0.45	0.22	0.09	12.2	0.5	1.1	6.1
20	314	0.12	34.3	396.9	127.4	0.98	137.2	0.09	—	0.42	0.22	0.11	12.3	2.5	0.9	5.6
24	276	0.07	24.4	348.9	97.6	0.97	68.3	0.10	0.14	0.44	0.26	0.08	12.2	0	1.1	9.0
1	93	0.09	8.6	105.9	36.7	0.28	37.6	0.01	0.00	0.09	0.05	0.01	2.9	0.4	0.1	0.8
13	109	0.07	9.9	141.9	48.6	0.36	28.3	0.03	0.06	0.16	0.08	0.02	4.2	1.0	0.2	5.7
9	82	0.06	7.6	95.4	33.4	0.24	20.5	0.01	0.04	0.10	0.06	0.01	2.5	0.6	0.1	0.7
21	359	0.09	33.3	482.5	156.7	1.21	14.9	0.11	0.03	0.48	0.27	0.10	14.2	1.7	1.2	6.2
3	209	0.05	19.9	289.9	93.3	0.75	120.5	0.07	0.00	0.30	0.15	0.06	8.5	1.0	0.7	4.6
3	214	0.05	20.3	296.0	95.3	0.76	123.1	0.07	0.00	0.30	0.15	0.06	8.7	1.0	0.7	4.7
31	292	0.15	27.2	425.6	118.7	1.06	82.2	0.09	0.15	0.38	0.20	0.09	11.8	2.8	1.0	5.2
27	327	0.12	34.2	497.8	122.0	0.73	139.1	0.11	0.17	0.33	0.67	0.11	2.4	3.2	0.2	3.4
25	251	0.90	50.8	408.9	132.5	1.21	70.5	0.11	0.14	0.46	0.38	0.09	14.1	0	1.1	9.6
0	92	0.74	32.6	405.1	138.2	0.51	0	0.04	0.00	0.20	0.16	0.04	1.9	0	0.2	2.5
20	263	1.20	57.5	492.5	110.0	1.57	127.5	0.09	0.07	0.45	0.33	0.10	12.5	0.5	1.1	6.8
8	288	0.60	32.5	425.0	152.5	1.02	145.0	0.09	0.05	0.41	0.31	0.10	12.5	2.3	0.9	4.8
20	273	0.60	35.0	422.5	165.0	0.97	160.0	0.11	0.10	0.45	0.41	0.06	5.0	0	0.8	8.5
30	280	0.60	32.5	417.5	150.0	1.02	65.0	0.09	0.15	0.40	0.31	0.10	12.5	2.3	0.8	4.8
150	330	0.50	48.3	419.1	137.2	1.16	116.8	0.08	0.50	0.48	0.26	0.12	2.5	3.8	1.1	10.7
9	444	4.00	88.9	631.1	195.6	3.38	—	0.33	—	0.45	4.44	0.44	4.0	26.7	1.3	8.0
9	500	4.50	100.0	665.0	192.0	3.75	—	0.37	—	0.51	5.00	0.49	100.0	30.0	1.5	9.0
9	444	4.00	88.9	568.9	186.7	3.38	—	0.33	—	0.45	4.44	0.44	88.9	26.7	1.3	8.0
9	500	4.47	100.0	665.0	288.0	3.75	—	0.37	—	0.51	5.07	0.50	100.0	30.0	1.5	8.8
5	350	3.60	100.0	—	270.0	3.75	—	0.37	—	—	4.00	0.40	—	12.0	1.2	—
27	339	3.76	45.1	577.7	230.6	1.16	903.7	0.75	0.15	1.31	11.08	1.01	13.3	31.8	1.1	12.5
25	300	0.70	36.4	508.9	252.2	1.09	40.9	0.10	0.11	0.50	0.28	0.05	11.4	0	0.7	4.3
25	256	0.24	29.4	412.0	187.9	0.81	58.9	0.10	—	0.44	0.39	0.10	6.8	1.8	0.7	4.8
27	332	0.22	27.3	415.8	215.8	0.88	56.8	0.06	0.11	0.44	0.33	0.09	15.9	0	1.2	5.2

Table of Food Composition *(continued)*

(Computer code is for Cengage Diet & Wellness Plus program)

D&W+ Code	Food Description	QTY	Measure	Wt (g)	H₂0 (g)	Ener (cal)	Prot (g)	Carb (g)	Fiber (g)	Fat (g)	Fat Breakdown (g)		
											Sat	Mono	Poly
Dairy—Continued													
	Ice Cream												
4776	Chocolate	½	cup(s)	66	36.8	143	2.5	18.6	0.8	7.3	4.5	2.1	0.3
12137	Chocolate fudge, no sugar added	½	cup(s)	71	—	100	3.0	16.0	2.0	3.0	1.5	—	—
16514	Chocolate, soft serve	½	cup(s)	87	49.9	177	3.2	24.1	0.7	8.4	5.2	2.4	0.3
16523	Sherbet, all flavors	½	cup(s)	97	63.8	139	1.1	29.3	3.2	1.9	1.1	0.5	0.1
4778	Strawberry	½	cup(s)	66	39.6	127	2.1	18.2	0.6	5.5	3.4	—	—
76	Vanilla	½	cup(s)	72	43.9	145	2.5	17.0	0.5	7.9	4.9	2.1	0.3
12146	Vanilla chocolate swirl, fat-free, no sugar added	½	cup(s)	71	—	100	3.0	14.0	2.0	3.0	2.0	—	—
82	Vanilla, light	½	cup(s)	76	48.3	125	3.6	19.6	0.2	3.7	2.2	1.0	0.2
78	Vanilla, light, soft serve	½	cup(s)	88	61.2	111	4.3	19.2	0	2.3	1.4	0.7	0.1
	Soy Desserts												
10694	Tofutti low fat vanilla fudge nondairy frozen dessert	½	cup(s)	70	—	140	2.0	24.0	0	4.0	1.0	—	—
15721	Tofutti premium chocolate supreme nondairy frozen dessert	½	cup(s)	70	—	180	3.0	18.0	0	11.0	2.0	—	—
15720	Tofutti premium vanilla nondairy frozen dessert	½	cup(s)	70	—	190	2.0	20.0	0	11.0	2.0	—	—
	Ice Milk												
16517	Chocolate	½	cup(s)	66	42.9	94	2.8	16.9	0.3	2.1	1.3	0.6	0.1
16516	Flavored, not chocolate	½	cup(s)	66	41.4	108	3.5	17.5	0.2	2.6	1.7	0.6	0.1
	Pudding												
25032	Chocolate	½	cup(s)	144	109.7	155	5.1	22.7	0.7	5.4	3.1	1.7	0.2
1923	Chocolate, sugar free, prepared with 2% milk	½	cup(s)	133	—	100	5.0	14.0	0.3	3.0	1.5	—	—
1722	Rice	½	cup(s)	113	75.6	151	4.1	29.9	0.5	1.9	1.1	0.5	0.1
4747	Tapioca, ready to eat	1	item(s)	142	102.0	185	2.8	30.8	0	5.5	1.4	3.6	0.1
25031	Vanilla	½	cup(s)	136	109.7	116	4.7	17.6	0	2.8	1.6	0.9	0.2
1924	Vanilla, sugar free, prepared with 2% milk	½	cup(s)	133	—	90	4.0	12.0	0.2	2.0	1.5	—	—
	Frozen Yogurt												
4785	Chocolate, soft serve	½	cup(s)	72	45.9	115	2.9	17.9	1.6	4.3	2.6	1.3	0.2
1747	Fruit varieties	½	cup(s)	113	80.5	144	3.4	24.4	0	4.1	2.6	1.1	0.1
4786	Vanilla, soft serve	½	cup(s)	72	47.0	117	2.9	17.4	0	4.0	2.5	1.1	0.2
	Milk Substitutes												
	Lactose Free												
16081	Fat-free, calcium fortified [milk]	1	cup(s)	240	—	80	8.0	13.0	0	0	0	0	0
36486	Low fat milk	1	cup(s)	240	—	110	8.0	13.0	0	2.5	1.5	—	—
36487	Reduced fat milk	1	cup(s)	240	—	130	8.0	12.0	0	5.0	3.0	—	—
36488	Whole milk	1	cup(s)	240	—	150	8.0	12.0	0	8.0	5.0	—	—
	Rice												
10083	Rice Dream carob rice beverage	1	cup(s)	240	—	150	1.0	32.0	0	2.5	0	—	—
17089	Rice Dream original rice beverage, enriched	1	cup(s)	240	—	120	1.0	25.0	0	2.0	0	—	—
10087	Rice Dream vanilla enriched rice beverage	1	cup(s)	240	—	130	1.0	28.0	0	2.0	0	—	—
	Soy												
34750	Soy Dream chocolate enriched soy beverage	1	cup(s)	240	—	210	7.0	37.0	1.0	3.5	0.5	—	—
34749	Soy Dream vanilla enriched soy beverage	1	cup(s)	240	—	150	7.0	22.0	0	4.0	0.5	—	—
13840	Vitasoy light chocolate soymilk	1	cup(s)	240	—	100	4.0	17.0	0	2.0	0.5	0.5	1.0
13839	Vitasoy light vanilla soymilk	1	cup(s)	240	—	70	4.0	10.0	0	2.0	0.5	0.5	1.0
13836	Vitasoy rich chocolate soymilk	1	cup(s)	240	—	160	7.0	24.0	1.0	4.0	0.5	1.0	2.5
13835	Vitasoy vanilla delite soymilk	1	cup(s)	240	—	120	7.0	13.0	1.0	4.0	0.5	1.0	2.5
	Yogurt												
3615	Custard style, fruit flavors	6	ounce(s)	170	127.1	190	7.0	32.0	0	3.5	2.0	—	—
3617	Custard style, vanilla	6	ounce(s)	170	134.1	190	7.0	32.0	0	3.5	2.0	0.9	0.1
32101	Fruit, low fat	1	cup(s)	245	184.5	243	9.8	45.7	0	2.8	1.8	0.8	0.1

PAGE KEY: A-4 = Breads/Baked Goods A-10 = Cereal/Rice/Pasta A-14 = Fruit A-20 = Vegetables/Legumes A-30 = Nuts/Seeds A-32 = Vegetarian A-34 = Dairy A-42 = Eggs A-42 = Seafood A-46 = Meats A-50 = Poultry A-50 = Processed Meats A-52 = Beverages A-56 = Fats/Oils A-58 = Sweets A-60 = Spices/Condiments/Sauces A-64 = Mixed Foods/Soups/Sandwiches A-70 = Fast Food A-90 = Convenience A-92 = Baby Foods

A

CHOL (mg)	CALC (mg)	IRON (mg)	MAGN (mg)	POTA (mg)	SODI (mg)	ZINC (mg)	VIT A (µg)	THIA (mg)	VIT E (mg α)	RIBO (mg)	NIAC (mg)	VIT B6 (mg)	FOLA (µg DFE)	VIT C (mg)	VIT B12 (µg)	SELE (µg)
22	72	0.61	19.1	164.3	50.2	0.38	77.9	0.02	0.19	0.12	0.14	0.03	10.6	0.5	0.2	1.7
10	100	0.36	—	—	65.0	—	—	—	—	—	—	—	—	0	—	—
22	103	0.32	19.0	192.0	43.3	0.45	66.6	0.03	0.22	0.13	0.11	0.03	4.3	0.5	0.3	2.5
0	52	0.13	7.7	92.6	44.4	0.46	9.7	0.02	0.02	0.08	0.07	0.02	6.8	5.6	0.1	1.3
19	79	0.13	9.2	124.1	39.6	0.22	63.4	0.03	—	0.16	0.11	0.03	7.9	5.1	0.2	1.3
32	92	0.06	10.1	143.3	57.6	0.49	85.0	0.03	0.21	0.17	0.08	0.03	3.6	0.4	0.3	1.3
10	100	0.00	—	—	65.0	—	—	—	—	—	—	—	—	0	—	—
21	122	0.14	10.6	158.1	56.2	0.55	97.3	0.04	0.09	0.19	0.10	0.03	4.6	0.9	0.4	1.5
11	138	0.05	12.3	194.5	61.6	0.46	25.5	0.04	0.05	0.17	0.10	0.04	4.4	0.8	0.4	3.2
0	0	0.00	—	8.0	90.0	—	0	—	—	—	—	—	—	0	—	—
0	0	0.00	—	7.0	180.0	—	0	—	—	—	—	—	—	0	—	—
0	0	0.00	—	2.0	210.0	—	0	—	—	—	—	—	—	0	—	—
6	94	0.15	13.1	155.2	40.6	0.36	15.7	0.03	0.05	0.11	0.08	0.02	3.9	0.5	0.3	2.2
16	76	0.05	9.2	136.2	48.5	0.47	90.4	0.02	0.05	0.11	0.06	0.01	3.3	0.1	0.2	1.3
35	149	0.46	31.3	226.7	137.0	0.71	—	0.05	0.00	0.22	0.15	0.06	8.3	1.2	0.5	4.9
10	150	0.72	—	330.0	310.0	—	—	0.06	—	0.26	—	—	—	0	—	—
7	113	0.28	15.8	201.4	66.4	0.52	41.6	0.03	0.05	0.17	0.34	0.06	4.5	0.2	0.2	4.8
1	101	0.15	8.5	130.6	205.9	0.31	0	0.03	0.21	0.13	0.09	0.03	4.3	0.4	0.3	0
35	146	0.17	17.2	188.9	136.4	0.52	—	0.04	0.00	0.22	0.10	0.05	8.0	1.2	0.5	4.6
10	150	0.00	—	190.0	380.0	—	—	0.03	—	0.17	—	—	—	0	—	—
4	106	0.90	19.4	187.9	70.6	0.35	31.7	0.02	—	0.15	0.22	0.05	7.9	0.2	0.2	1.7
15	113	0.52	11.3	176.3	71.2	0.31	55.4	0.04	0.10	0.20	0.07	0.04	4.5	0.8	0.1	2.1
1	103	0.21	10.1	151.9	62.6	0.30	42.5	0.02	0.07	0.16	0.20	0.05	4.3	0.6	0.2	2.4
3	500	0.00	—	—	125.0	—	100.0	—	—	—	—	—	—	0	0	—
10	300	0.00	—	—	125.0	—	100.0	—	—	—	—	—	—	0	—	—
20	300	0.00	—	—	125.0	—	98.2	—	—	—	—	—	—	0	—	—
35	300	0.00	—	—	125.0	—	58.1	—	—	—	—	—	—	0	—	—
0	20	0.72	—	82.5	100.0	—	—	—	—	—	—	—	—	1.2	—	—
0	300	0.00	13.3	60.0	90.0	0.24	—	0.06	—	0.00	0.84	0.07	—	0	1.5	—
0	300	0.00	—	53.0	90.0	—	—	—	—	—	—	—	—	0	1.5	—
0	300	1.80	60.0	350.0	160.0	0.60	33.3	0.15	—	0.06	0.80	0.12	60.0	0	3.0	—
0	300	1.80	40.0	260.0	140.0	0.60	33.3	0.15	—	0.06	0.80	0.12	60.0	0	3.0	—
0	300	0.72	24.0	200.0	140.0	0.90	—	0.09	—	0.34	—	—	24.0	0	0.9	—
0	300	0.72	24.0	200.0	120.0	0.90	—	0.09	—	0.34	—	—	24.0	0	0.9	—
0	300	1.08	40.0	320.0	150.0	0.90	—	0.15	—	0.34	—	—	60.0	0	0.9	—
0	40	0.72	—	320.0	115.0	—	0	—	—	—	—	—	—	0	—	—
15	300	0.00	16.0	310.0	100.0	—	—	—	—	0.25	—	—	—	0	—	—
15	300	0.00	16.0	310.0	100.0	—	—	—	—	0.25	—	—	—	0	—	—
12	338	0.14	31.9	433.7	129.9	1.64	27.0	0.08	0.04	0.39	0.21	0.09	22.1	1.5	1.1	6.9

D&W+ Code	Food Description	QTY	Measure	Wt (g)	H₂0 (g)	Ener (cal)	Prot (g)	Carb (g)	Fiber (g)	Fat (g)	Fat Breakdown (g)		
											Sat	Mono	Poly
Dairy—continued													
29638	Fruit, nonfat, sweetened with low-calorie sweetener	1	cup(s)	241	208.3	123	10.6	19.4	1.2	0.4	0.2	0.1	0
93	Plain, low fat	1	cup(s)	245	208.4	154	12.9	17.2	0	3.8	2.5	1.0	0.1
94	Plain, nonfat	1	cup(s)	245	208.8	137	14.0	18.8	0	0.4	0.3	0.1	0
32100	Vanilla, low fat	1	cup(s)	245	193.6	208	12.1	33.8	0	3.1	2.0	0.8	0.1
5242	Yogurt beverage	1	cup(s)	245	199.8	172	6.2	32.8	0	2.2	1.4	0.6	0.1
38202	Yogurt smoothie, nonfat, all flavors	1	item(s)	325	—	290	10.0	60.0	6.0	0	0	0	0
	Soy yogurt												
34617	Stonyfield Farm O'Soy strawberry-peach pack organic cultured soy yogurt	1	item(s)	113	—	100	5.0	16.0	3.0	2.0	0	—	—
34616	Stonyfield Farm O'Soy vanilla organic cultured soy yogurt	1	item(s)	170	—	150	7.0	26.0	4.0	2.0	0	—	—
10453	White Wave plain silk cultured soy yogurt	8	ounce(s)	227	—	140	5.0	22.0	1.0	3.0	0.5	—	—
Eggs													
	Eggs												
99	Fried	1	item(s)	46	31.8	90	6.3	0.4	0	7.0	2.0	2.9	1.2
100	Hard boiled	1	item(s)	50	37.3	78	6.3	0.6	0	5.3	1.6	2.0	0.7
101	Poached	1	item(s)	50	37.8	71	6.3	0.4	0	5.0	1.5	1.9	0.7
97	Raw, white	1	item(s)	33	28.9	16	3.6	0.2	0	0.1	0	0	0
96	Raw, whole	1	item(s)	50	37.9	72	6.3	0.4	0	5.0	1.5	1.9	0.7
98	Raw, yolk	1	item(s)	17	8.9	54	2.7	0.6	0	4.5	1.6	2.0	0.7
102	Scrambled, prepared with milk and butter	2	item(s)	122	89.2	204	13.5	2.7	0	14.9	4.5	5.8	2.6
	Egg substitute												
4028	Egg Beaters	¼	cup(s)	61	—	30	6.0	1.0	0	0	0	0	0
920	Frozen	¼	cup(s)	60	43.9	96	6.8	1.9	0	6.7	1.2	1.5	3.7
918	Liquid	¼	cup(s)	63	51.9	53	7.5	0.4	0	2.1	0.4	0.6	1.0
Seafood													
	Cod												
6040	Atlantic cod or scrod, baked or broiled	3	ounce(s)	85	64.6	89	19.4	0	0	0.7	0.1	0.1	0.2
1573	Atlantic cod, cooked, dry heat	3	ounce(s)	85	64.6	89	19.4	0	0	0.7	0.1	0.1	0.2
2905	**Eel, raw**	3	ounce(s)	85	58.0	156	15.7	0	0	9.9	2.0	6.1	0.8
	Fish fillets												
25079	Baked	3	ounce(s)	84	79.9	99	21.7	0	0	0.7	0.1	0.1	0.3
8615	Batter coated or breaded, fried	3	ounce(s)	85	45.6	197	12.5	14.4	0.4	10.5	2.4	2.2	5.3
25082	Broiled fish steaks	3	ounce(s)	85	68.1	128	24.2	0	0	2.6	0.4	0.9	0.8
25083	Poached fish steaks	3	ounce(s)	85	67.1	111	21.1	0	0	2.3	0.3	0.8	0.7
25084	Steamed	3	ounce(s)	85	72.2	79	17.2	0	0	0.6	0.1	0.1	0.2
25089	**Flounder, baked**	3	ounce(s)	85	64.4	113	14.8	0.4	0.1	5.5	1.1	2.2	1.4
1825	**Grouper, cooked, dry heat**	3	ounce(s)	85	62.4	100	21.1	0	0	1.1	0.3	0.2	0.3
	Haddock												
6049	Baked or broiled	3	ounce(s)	85	63.2	95	20.6	0	0	0.8	0.1	0.1	0.3
1578	Cooked, dry heat	3	ounce(s)	85	63.1	95	20.6	0	0	0.8	0.1	0.1	0.3
1886	**Halibut, Atlantic and Pacific, cooked, dry heat**	3	ounce(s)	85	61.0	119	22.7	0	0	2.5	0.4	0.8	0.8
1582	**Herring, Atlantic, pickled**	4	piece(s)	60	33.1	157	8.5	5.8	0	10.8	1.4	7.2	1.0
1587	**Jack mackerel, solids, canned, drained**	2	ounce(s)	57	39.2	88	13.1	0	0	3.6	1.1	1.3	0.9

CHOL (mg)	CALC (mg)	IRON (mg)	MAGN (mg)	POTA (mg)	SODI (mg)	ZINC (mg)	VIT A (µg)	THIA (mg)	VIT E (mg α)	RIBO (mg)	NIAC (mg)	VIT B6 (mg)	FOLA (µg DFE)	VIT C (mg)	VIT B12 (µg)	SELE (µg)
5	369	0.62	41.0	549.5	139.8	1.83	4.8	0.10	0.16	0.44	0.49	0.10	31.3	26.5	1.1	7.0
15	448	0.19	41.7	573.3	171.5	2.18	34.3	0.10	0.07	0.52	0.27	0.12	27.0	2.0	1.4	8.1
5	488	0.22	46.6	624.8	188.7	2.37	4.9	0.11	0.00	0.57	0.30	0.13	29.4	2.2	1.5	8.8
12	419	0.17	39.2	536.6	161.7	2.03	29.4	0.10	0.04	0.49	0.26	0.11	27.0	2.0	1.3	12.0
13	260	0.22	39.2	399.4	98.0	1.10	14.7	0.11	0.00	0.51	0.30	0.14	29.4	2.1	1.5	—
5	300	2.70	100.0	580.0	290.0	2.25	—	0.37	—	0.42	5.00	0.50	100.0	15.0	1.5	
0	100	1.08	24.0	5.0	20.0	—	0	0.22	—	0.10	—	0.04	—	0	0	—
0	150	1.44	40.0	15.0	40.0	—	—	0.30	—	0.13	—	0.08	—	0	0	—
0	400	1.44	—	0	30.0	—	0	—	—	—	—	—	—	0		—
210	27	0.91	6.0	67.6	93.8	0.55	91.1	0.03	0.56	0.23	0.03	0.07	23.5	0	0.6	15.7
212	25	0.59	5.0	63.0	62.0	0.52	84.5	0.03	0.51	0.25	0.03	0.06	22.0	0	0.6	15.4
211	27	0.91	6.0	66.5	147.0	0.55	69.5	0.02	0.48	0.20	0.03	0.06	17.5	0	0.6	15.8
0	2	0.02	3.6	53.8	54.8	0.01	0	0.00	0.00	0.14	0.03	0.00	1.3	0	0	6.6
212	27	0.91	6.0	67.0	70.0	0.55	70.0	0.03	0.48	0.23	0.03	0.07	23.5	0	0.6	15.9
210	22	0.46	0.9	18.5	8.2	0.39	64.8	0.03	0.43	0.09	0.00	0.06	24.8	0	0.3	9.5
429	87	1.46	14.6	168.4	341.6	1.22	174.5	0.06	1.33	0.53	0.09	0.14	36.6	0.2	0.9	27.5
0	20	1.08	4.0	85.0	115.0	0.60	112.5	0.15	—	0.85	0.20	0.08	60.0	0	1.2	—
1	44	1.18	9.0	127.8	119.4	0.58	6.6	0.07	0.95	0.23	0.08	0.08	9.6	0.3	0.2	24.8
1	33	1.32	5.6	207.1	111.1	0.82	11.3	0.07	0.17	0.19	0.07	0.00	9.4	0	0.2	15.6
47	12	0.41	35.7	207.5	66.3	0.49	11.9	0.07	0.68	0.06	2.13	0.24	6.8	0.8	0.9	32.0
47	12	0.41	35.7	207.5	66.3	0.49	11.9	0.07	0.68	0.06	2.13	0.24	6.8	0.9	0.9	32.0
107	17	0.42	17.0	231.3	43.4	1.37	887.0	0.13	3.40	0.03	2.97	0.05	12.8	1.5	2.6	5.5
44	8	0.31	29.1	489.0	86.1	0.48	—	0.02	—	0.05	2.47	0.46	8.1	3.0	1.0	44.3
29	15	1.79	20.4	272.2	452.5	0.37	9.4	0.09	—	0.09	1.78	0.08	17.0	0	0.9	7.7
37	55	0.97	96.7	524.3	62.9	0.49	—	0.05	—	0.08	6.47	0.36	12.6	0	1.2	42.5
32	48	0.85	84.0	455.6	54.7	0.42	—	0.05	—	0.07	5.92	0.33	11.5	0	1.1	37.0
41	12	0.29	24.7	319.3	41.7	0.34	—	0.06	—	0.06	1.89	0.21	6.1	0.8	0.8	32.0
44	19	0.34	47.3	224.7	280.2	0.20	—	0.06	0.40	0.07	2.02	0.18	7.4	2.8	1.6	33.5
40	18	0.96	31.5	404.0	45.1	0.43	42.5	0.06	—	0.01	0.32	0.29	8.5	0	0.6	39.8
63	36	1.15	42.5	339.4	74.0	0.40	16.2	0.03	0.42	0.03	3.94	0.29	6.8	0	1.2	34.4
63	36	1.14	42.5	339.3	74.0	0.40	16.2	0.03	—	0.03	3.93	0.29	11.1	0	1.2	34.4
35	51	0.91	91.0	489.9	58.7	0.45	45.9	0.05	—	0.07	6.05	0.33	11.9	0	1.2	39.8
8	46	0.73	4.8	41.4	522.0	0.31	154.8	0.02	1.02	0.08	1.98	0.10	1.2	0	2.6	35.1
45	137	1.15	21.0	110.0	214.9	0.57	73.7	0.02	0.58	0.12	3.50	0.11	2.8	0.5	3.9	21.4

D&W+ Code	Food Description	QTY	Measure	WT (g)	H₂O (g)	Ener (cal)	Prot (g)	Carb (g)	Fiber (g)	Fat (g)	Sat	Mono	Poly
											Fat Breakdown (g)		

SEAFOOD—CONTINUED

D&W+ Code	Food Description	QTY	Measure	WT (g)	H₂O (g)	Ener (cal)	Prot (g)	Carb (g)	Fiber (g)	Fat (g)	Sat	Mono	Poly
8580	Octopus, common, cooked, moist heat	3	ounce(s)	85	51.5	139	25.4	3.7	0	1.8	0.4	0.3	0.4
1592	Rockfish Pacific, cooked, dry heat	3	ounce(s)	85	62.4	103	20.4	0	0	1.7	0.4	0.4	0.5
1831	Perch, mixed species, cooked, dry heat	3	ounce(s)	85	62.3	100	21.1	0	0	1.0	0.2	0.2	0.4
	Salmon												
2938	Coho, farmed, raw	3	ounce(s)	85	59.9	136	18.1	0	0	6.5	1.5	2.8	1.6
1594	Broiled or baked with butter	3	ounce(s)	85	53.9	155	23.0	0	0	6.3	1.2	2.3	2.3
29727	Smoked Chinook (lox)	2	ounce(s)	57	40.8	66	10.4	0	0	2.4	0.5	1.1	0.6
154	Sardine, Atlantic with bones, canned in oil	3	ounce(s)	85	50.7	177	20.9	0	0	9.7	1.3	3.3	4.4
	Scallops												
155	Mixed species, breaded, fried	3	item(s)	47	27.2	100	8.4	4.7	—	5.1	1.2	2.1	1.3
1599	Steamed	3	ounce(s)	85	64.8	90	13.8	2.0	0	2.6	0.4	1.0	0.8
1839	Snapper, mixed species, cooked, dry heat	3	ounce(s)	85	59.8	109	22.4	0	0	1.5	0.3	0.3	0.5
	Squid												
1868	Mixed species, fried	3	ounce(s)	85	54.9	149	15.3	6.6	0	6.4	1.6	2.3	1.8
16617	Steamed or boiled	3	ounce(s)	85	63.3	89	15.2	3.0	0	1.3	0.4	0.1	0.5
1570	Striped bass, cooked, dry heat	3	ounce(s)	85	62.4	105	19.3	0	0	2.5	0.6	0.7	0.9
1601	Sturgeon, steamed	3	ounce(s)	85	59.4	111	17.0	0	0	4.3	1.0	2.0	0.7
1840	Surimi, formed	3	ounce(s)	85	64.9	84	12.9	5.8	0	0.8	0.2	0.1	0.4
1842	Swordfish, cooked, dry heat	3	ounce(s)	85	58.5	132	21.6	0	0	4.4	1.2	1.7	1.0
1846	Tuna, yellowfin or ahi, raw	3	ounce(s)	85	60.4	92	19.9	0	0	0.8	0.2	0.1	0.2
	Tuna, canned												
159	Light, canned in oil, drained	2	ounce(s)	57	33.9	112	16.5	0	0	4.6	0.9	1.7	1.6
355	Light, canned in water, drained	2	ounce(s)	57	42.2	66	14.5	0	0	0.5	0.1	0.1	0.2
33211	Light, no salt, canned in oil, drained	2	ounce(s)	57	33.9	112	16.5	0	0	4.7	0.9	1.7	1.6
33212	Light, no salt, canned in water, drained	2	ounce(s)	57	42.6	66	14.5	0	0	0.5	0.1	0.1	0.2
2961	White, canned in oil, drained	2	ounce(s)	57	36.3	105	15.0	0	0	4.6	0.7	1.8	1.7
351	White, canned in water, drained	2	ounce(s)	57	41.5	73	13.4	0	0	1.7	0.4	0.4	0.6
33213	White, no salt, canned in oil, drained	2	ounce(s)	57	36.3	105	15.0	0	0	4.6	0.9	1.4	1.9
33214	White, no salt, canned in water, drained	2	ounce(s)	57	42.0	73	13.4	0	0	1.7	0.4	0.4	0.6
	Yellowtail												
8548	Mixed species, cooked, dry heat	3	ounce(s)	85	57.3	159	25.2	0	0	5.7	1.4	2.2	1.5
2970	Mixed species, raw	2	ounce(s)	57	42.2	83	13.1	0	0	3.0	0.7	1.1	0.8
	Shellfish, meat only												
1857	Abalone, mixed species, fried	3	ounce(s)	85	51.1	161	16.7	9.4	0	5.8	1.4	2.3	1.4
16618	Abalone, steamed or poached	3	ounce(s)	85	40.7	177	28.8	10.1	0	1.3	0.3	0.2	0.2
1860	Clams, cooked, moist heat	3	ounce(s)	85	54.1	126	21.7	4.4	0	1.7	0.2	0.1	0.5
	Crab												
1851	Blue crab, canned	2	ounce(s)	57	43.2	56	11.6	0	0	0.7	0.1	0.1	0.2
1852	Blue crab, cooked, moist heat	3	ounce(s)	85	65.9	87	17.2	0	0	1.5	0.2	0.2	0.6
8562	Dungeness crab, cooked, moist heat	3	ounce(s)	85	62.3	94	19.0	0.8	0	1.1	0.1	0.2	0.3
1853	Crayfish, farmed, cooked, moist heat	3	ounce(s)	85	68.7	74	14.9	0	0	1.1	0.2	0.2	0.4

PAGE KEY: A-4 = Breads/Baked Goods A-10 = Cereal/Rice/Pasta A-14 = Fruit A-20 = Vegetables/Legumes A-30 = Nuts/Seeds A-32 = Vegetarian A-34 = Dairy A-42 = Eggs A-42 = Seafood A-46 = Meats A-50 = Poultry A-50 = Processed Meats A-52 = Beverages A-56 = Fats/Oils A-58 = Sweets A-60 = Spices/Condiments/Sauces A-64 = Mixed Foods/Soups/Sandwiches A-70 = Fast Food A-90 = Convenience A-92 = Baby Foods

A

CHOL (mg)	CALC (mg)	IRON (mg)	MAGN (mg)	POTA (mg)	SODI (mg)	ZINC (mg)	VIT A (µg)	THIA (mg)	VIT E (mg α)	RIBO (mg)	NIAC (mg)	VIT B$_6$ (mg)	FOLA (µg DFE)	VIT C (mg)	VIT B$_{12}$ (µg)	SELE (µg)
82	90	8.11	51.0	535.8	391.2	2.85	76.5	0.04	1.02	0.06	3.21	0.55	20.4	6.8	30.6	76.2
37	10	0.45	28.9	442.3	65.5	0.45	60.4	0.03	1.32	0.07	3.33	0.22	8.5	0	1.0	39.8
98	87	0.98	32.3	292.6	67.2	1.21	8.5	0.06	—	0.10	1.61	0.11	5.1	1.4	1.9	13.7
43	10	0.29	26.4	382.7	40.0	0.36	47.6	0.08	—	0.09	5.79	0.56	11.1	0.9	2.3	10.7
40	15	1.02	26.9	376.6	98.6	0.56	—	0.13	1.14	0.05	8.33	0.18	4.2	1.8	2.3	41.0
13	6	0.48	10.2	99.2	1134.0	0.17	14.7	0.01	—	0.05	2.67	0.15	1.1	0	1.8	21.6
121	325	2.48	33.2	337.6	429.5	1.10	27.2	0.04	1.70	0.18	4.43	0.14	10.2	0	7.6	44.8
28	20	0.38	27.4	154.8	215.8	0.49	10.7	0.02	—	0.05	0.70	0.06	23.3	1.1	0.6	12.5
27	20	0.22	45.9	238.0	358.7	0.78	32.3	0.01	0.16	0.05	0.84	0.11	10.2	2.0	1.1	18.2
40	34	0.20	31.5	444.0	48.5	0.37	29.8	0.04	—	0.00	0.29	0.39	5.1	1.4	3.0	41.7
221	33	0.85	32.3	237.3	260.3	1.48	9.4	0.04	—	0.39	2.21	0.04	11.9	3.6	1.0	44.1
227	31	0.62	28.9	192.1	356.2	1.49	8.5	0.01	1.17	0.32	1.69	0.04	3.4	3.2	1.0	43.7
88	16	0.91	43.4	279.0	74.8	0.43	26.4	0.09	—	0.03	2.17	0.29	8.5	0	3.8	39.8
63	11	0.59	29.8	239.7	388.5	0.35	198.9	0.06	0.52	0.07	8.30	0.19	14.5	0	2.2	13.3
26	8	0.22	36.6	95.3	121.6	0.28	17.0	0.01	0.53	0.01	0.18	0.02	1.7	0	1.4	23.9
43	5	0.88	28.9	313.8	97.8	1.25	34.9	0.03	—	0.09	10.02	0.32	1.7	0.9	1.7	52.5
38	14	0.62	42.5	377.6	31.5	0.44	15.3	0.37	0.42	0.04	8.33	0.77	1.7	0.8	0.4	31.0
10	7	0.79	17.6	117.3	200.6	0.51	13.0	0.02	0.49	0.07	7.03	0.06	2.8	0	1.2	43.1
17	6	0.87	15.3	134.3	191.5	0.43	9.6	0.01	0.19	0.04	7.52	0.19	2.3	0	1.7	45.6
10	7	0.78	17.6	117.4	28.3	0.51	0	0.02	—	0.06	7.03	0.06	2.8	0	1.2	43.1
17	6	0.86	15.3	134.4	28.3	0.43	0	0.01	—	0.04	7.52	0.19	2.3	0	1.7	45.6
18	2	0.36	19.3	188.8	224.5	0.26	2.8	0.01	1.30	0.04	6.63	0.24	2.8	0	1.2	34.1
24	8	0.55	18.7	134.3	213.6	0.27	3.4	0.00	0.48	0.02	3.28	0.12	1.1	0	0.7	37.2
18	2	0.36	19.3	188.8	28.3	0.26	0	0.01	—	0.04	6.63	0.24	2.8	0	1.2	34.1
24	8	0.54	18.7	134.4	28.3	0.27	3.4	0.00	—	0.02	3.28	0.12	1.1	0	0.7	37.3
60	25	0.53	32.3	457.6	42.5	0.56	26.4	0.14	—	0.04	7.41	0.15	3.4	2.5	1.1	39.8
31	13	0.28	17.0	238.1	22.1	0.29	16.4	0.08	—	0.02	3.86	0.09	2.3	1.6	0.7	20.7
80	31	3.23	47.6	241.5	502.6	0.80	1.7	0.18	—	0.11	1.61	0.12	11.9	1.5	0.6	44.1
144	50	4.84	68.9	295.0	980.1	1.38	3.4	0.28	6.74	0.12	1.89	0.21	6.0	2.6	0.7	75.6
57	78	23.78	15.3	534.1	95.3	2.32	145.4	0.12	—	0.36	2.85	0.09	24.7	18.8	84.1	54.4
50	57	0.47	22.1	212.1	188.8	2.27	1.1	0.04	1.04	0.04	0.77	0.08	24.4	1.5	0.3	18.0
85	88	0.77	28.1	275.6	237.3	3.58	1.7	0.08	1.56	0.04	2.80	0.15	43.4	2.8	6.2	34.2
65	50	0.36	49.3	347.0	321.5	4.65	26.4	0.04	—	0.17	3.08	0.14	35.7	3.1	8.8	40.5
117	43	0.94	28.1	202.4	82.5	1.25	12.8	0.03	—	0.06	1.41	0.11	9.4	0.4	2.6	29.1

(Computer code is for Cengage Diet & Wellness Plus program)

D&W+ Code	Food Description	QTY	Measure	Wt (g)	H₂O (g)	Ener (cal)	Prot (g)	Carb (g)	Fiber (g)	Fat (g)	Fat Breakdown (g)		
											Sat	Mono	Poly
SEAFOOD—CONTINUED													
1854	LOBSTER, NORTHERN, COOKED, MOIST HEAT	3	ounce(s)	85	64.7	83	17.4	1.1	0	0.5	0.1	0.1	0.1
1862	MUSSELS, BLUE, COOKED, MOIST HEAT	3	ounce(s)	85	52.0	146	20.2	6.3	0	3.8	0.7	0.9	1.0
	OYSTERS												
8720	Baked or broiled	3	ounce(s)	85	68.6	89	5.6	3.2	0	5.8	1.3	2.1	1.9
152	Eastern, farmed, raw	3	ounce(s)	85	73.3	50	4.4	4.7	0	1.3	0.4	0.1	0.5
8715	Eastern, wild, cooked, moist heat	3	ounce(s)	85	59.8	117	12.0	6.7	0	4.2	1.3	0.5	1.6
8584	Pacific, cooked, moist heat	3	ounce(s)	85	54.5	139	16.1	8.4	0	3.9	0.9	0.7	1.5
1865	Pacific, raw	3	ounce(s)	85	69.8	69	8.0	4.2	0	2.0	0.4	0.3	0.8
	SHRIMP												
158	Mixed species, breaded, fried	3	ounce(s)	85	44.9	206	18.2	9.8	0.3	10.4	1.8	3.2	4.3
1855	Mixed species, cooked, moist heat	3	ounce(s)	85	65.7	84	17.8	0	0	0.9	0.2	0.2	0.4
BEEF, LAMB, PORK													
	BEEF												
4450	Breakfast strips, cooked	2	slice(s)	23	5.9	101	7.1	0.3	0	7.8	3.2	3.8	0.4
174	Corned beef, canned	3	ounce(s)	85	49.1	213	23.0	0	0	12.7	5.3	5.1	0.5
33147	Cured, thin siced	2	ounce(s)	57	32.9	100	15.9	3.2	0	2.2	0.9	1.0	0.1
4581	Jerky	1	ounce(s)	28	6.6	116	9.4	3.1	0.5	7.3	3.1	3.2	0.3
	GROUND BEEF												
5898	Lean, broiled, medium	3	ounce(s)	85	50.4	202	21.6	0	0	12.2	4.8	5.3	0.4
5899	Lean, broiled, well done	3	ounce(s)	85	48.4	214	23.8	0	0	12.5	5.0	5.7	0.3
5914	Regular, broiled, medium	3	ounce(s)	85	46.1	246	20.5	0	0	17.6	6.9	7.7	0.6
5915	Regular, broiled, well done	3	ounce(s)	85	43.8	259	21.6	0	0	18.4	7.5	8.5	0.5
	BEEF RIB												
4241	Rib, small end, separable lean, 0" fat, broiled	3	ounce(s)	85	53.2	164	25.0	0	0	6.4	2.4	2.6	0.2
4183	Rib, whole, lean and fat, ¼" fat, roasted	3	ounce(s)	85	39.0	320	18.9	0	0	26.6	10.7	11.4	0.9
	BEEF ROAST												
16981	Bottom round, choice, separable lean and fat, ⅛" fat, braised	3	ounce(s)	85	46.2	216	27.9	0	0	10.7	4.1	4.6	0.4
16979	Bottom round, separable lean and fat, ⅛" fat, roasted	3	ounce(s)	85	52.4	185	22.5	0	0	9.9	3.8	4.2	0.4
16924	Chuck, arm pot roast, separable lean and fat, ⅛" fat, braised	3	ounce(s)	85	42.9	257	25.6	0	0	16.3	6.5	7.0	0.6
16930	Chuck, blade roast, separable lean and fat, ⅛" fat, braised	3	ounce(s)	85	40.5	290	22.8	0	0	21.4	8.5	9.2	0.8
5853	Chuck, blade roast, separable lean, 0" trim, pot roasted	3	ounce(s)	85	47.4	202	26.4	0	0	9.9	3.9	4.3	0.3
4296	Eye of round, choice, separable lean, 0" fat, roasted	3	ounce(s)	85	56.5	138	24.4	0	0	3.7	1.3	1.5	0.1
16989	Eye of round, separable lean and fat, ⅛" fat, roasted	3	ounce(s)	85	52.2	180	24.2	0	0	8.5	3.2	3.6	0.3
	BEEF STEAK												
4348	Short loin, t-bone steak, lean and fat, ¼" fat, broiled	3	ounce(s)	85	43.2	274	19.4	0	0	21.2	8.3	9.6	0.8
4349	Short loin, t-bone steak, lean, ¼" fat, broiled	3	ounce(s)	85	52.3	174	22.8	0	0	8.5	3.1	4.2	0.3
4360	Top loin, prime, lean and fat, ¼" fat, broiled	3	ounce(s)	85	42.7	275	21.6	0	0	20.3	8.2	8.6	0.7
	BEEF VARIETY												
188	Liver, pan fried	3	ounce(s)	85	52.7	149	22.6	4.4	0	4.0	1.3	0.5	0.5
4447	Tongue, simmered	3	ounce(s)	85	49.2	242	16.4	0	0	19.0	6.9	8.6	0.6
	LAMB CHOP												
3275	Loin, domestic, lean and fat, ¼" fat, broiled	3	ounce(s)	85	43.9	269	21.4	0	0	19.6	8.4	8.3	1.4

PAGE KEY: A-4 = Breads/Baked Goods A-10 = Cereal/Rice/Pasta A-14 = Fruit A-20 = Vegetables/Legumes A-30 = Nuts/Seeds A-32 = Vegetarian
A-34 = Dairy A-42 = Eggs A-42 = Seafood A-46 = Meats A-50 = Poultry A-50 = Processed Meats A-52 = Beverages A-56 = Fats/Oils A-58 = Sweets
A-60 = Spices/Condiments/Sauces A-64 = Mixed Foods/Soups/Sandwiches A-70 = Fast Food A-90 = Convenience A-92 = Baby Foods

A

CHOL (mg)	CALC (mg)	IRON (mg)	MAGN (mg)	POTA (mg)	SODI (mg)	ZINC (mg)	VIT A (µg)	THIA (mg)	VIT E (mg α)	RIBO (mg)	NIAC (mg)	VIT B6 (mg)	FOLA (µg DFE)	VIT C (mg)	VIT B12 (µg)	SELE (µg)
61	52	0.33	29.8	299.4	323.2	2.48	22.1	0.01	0.85	0.05	0.91	0.06	9.4	0	2.6	36.3
48	28	5.71	31.5	227.9	313.8	2.27	77.4	0.25	—	0.35	2.55	0.08	64.6	11.6	20.4	76.2
43	36	5.30	37.4	125.0	403.8	72.22	60.4	0.07	0.98	0.06	1.04	0.04	7.7	2.8	14.7	50.7
21	37	4.91	28.1	105.4	151.3	32.23	6.8	0.08	—	0.05	1.07	0.05	15.3	4.0	13.8	54.1
89	77	10.19	80.8	239.0	358.9	154.45	45.9	0.16	—	0.15	2.11	0.10	11.9	5.1	29.8	60.9
85	14	7.82	37.4	256.8	180.3	28.27	124.2	0.10	0.72	0.37	3.07	0.07	12.8	10.9	24.5	131.0
43	7	4.34	18.7	142.9	90.1	14.13	68.9	0.05	—	0.20	1.70	0.04	8.5	6.8	13.6	65.5
150	57	1.07	34.0	191.3	292.4	1.17	0	0.11	—	0.11	2.60	0.08	33.2	1.3	1.6	35.4
166	33	2.62	28.9	154.8	190.5	1.32	57.8	0.02	1.17	0.02	2.20	0.10	3.4	1.9	1.3	33.7
27	2	0.71	6.1	93.1	509.2	1.44	0	0.02	0.06	0.05	1.46	0.07	1.8	0	0.8	6.1
73	10	1.76	11.9	115.7	855.6	3.03	0	0.01	0.12	0.12	2.06	0.11	7.7	0	1.4	36.5
23	6	1.53	10.8	243.2	815.9	2.25	0	0.04	0.00	0.10	2.98	0.19	6.2	0	1.5	16.0
14	6	1.53	14.5	169.2	627.4	2.29	0	0.04	0.13	0.04	0.49	0.05	38.0	0	0.3	3.0
58	6	2.00	17.9	266.2	59.5	4.63	0	0.05	—	0.23	4.21	0.23	7.6	0	1.8	16.0
69	12	2.21	18.4	250.0	62.4	5.86	0	0.08	—	0.23	5.10	0.16	9.4	0	1.7	19.0
62	9	2.07	17.0	248.3	70.6	4.40	0	0.02	—	0.16	4.90	0.23	7.6	0	2.5	16.2
71	12	2.30	18.5	242.4	72.4	5.18	0	0.08	—	0.23	4.93	0.17	8.5	0	1.6	18.0
65	16	1.59	21.3	319.8	51.9	4.64	0	0.06	0.34	0.12	7.15	0.53	8.5	0	1.4	29.2
72	9	1.96	16.2	251.7	53.6	4.45	0	0.06	—	0.14	2.85	0.19	6.0	0	2.1	18.7
68	6	2.29	17.9	223.7	35.7	4.59	0	0.05	0.41	0.15	5.05	0.36	8.5	0	1.7	29.3
64	5	1.83	14.5	182.0	29.8	3.76	0	0.05	0.34	0.12	3.92	0.29	6.8	0	1.3	23.0
67	14	2.15	17.0	205.8	42.5	5.93	0	0.05	0.45	0.15	3.63	0.25	7.7	0	1.9	24.1
88	11	2.66	16.2	198.2	55.3	7.15	0	0.06	0.17	0.20	2.06	0.22	4.3	0	1.9	20.9
73	11	3.12	19.6	223.7	60.4	8.73	0	0.06	—	0.23	2.27	0.24	5.1	0	2.1	22.7
49	5	2.16	16.2	200.7	32.3	4.28	0	0.05	0.30	0.15	4.69	0.34	8.5	0	1.4	28.0
54	5	1.98	15.3	193.1	31.5	3.95	0	0.05	0.34	0.13	4.37	0.31	7.7	0	1.5	25.2
58	7	2.56	17.9	233.9	57.8	3.56	0	0.07	0.18	0.17	3.29	0.27	6.0	0	1.8	10.0
50	5	3.11	22.1	278.1	65.5	4.34	0	0.09	0.11	0.21	3.93	0.33	6.8	0	1.9	8.5
67	8	1.88	19.6	294.3	53.6	3.85	0	0.06	—	0.15	3.96	0.31	6.0	0	1.6	19.5
324	5	5.24	18.7	298.5	65.5	4.44	6586.3	0.15	0.39	2.91	14.86	0.87	221.1	0.6	70.7	27.9
112	4	2.22	12.8	156.5	55.3	3.47	0	0.01	0.25	0.25	2.96	0.13	6.0	1.1	2.7	11.2
85	17	1.53	20.4	278.1	65.5	2.96	0	0.08	0.11	0.21	6.03	0.11	15.3	0	2.1	23.3

D&W+ Code	FOOD DESCRIPTION	QTY	MEASURE	W_T (g)	H₂O (g)	ENER (cal)	PROT (g)	CARB (g)	FIBER (g)	FAT (g)	SAT	MONO	POLY
											FAT BREAKDOWN (g)		

BEEF, LAMB, PORK—CONTINUED

D&W+ Code	FOOD DESCRIPTION	QTY	MEASURE	W_T (g)	H₂O (g)	ENER (cal)	PROT (g)	CARB (g)	FIBER (g)	FAT (g)	SAT	MONO	POLY
	LAMB LEG												
3264	Domestic, lean and fat, ¼″ fat, cooked	3	ounce(s)	85	45.7	250	20.9	0	0	17.8	7.5	7.5	1.3
	LAMB RIB												
182	Domestic, lean and fat, ¼″ fat, broiled	3	ounce(s)	85	40.0	307	18.8	0	0	25.2	10.8	10.3	2.0
183	Domestic, lean, ¼″ fat, broiled	3	ounce(s)	85	50.0	200	23.6	0	0	11.0	4.0	4.4	1.0
	LAMB SHOULDER												
186	Shoulder, arm and blade, domestic, choice, lean and fat, ¼″ fat, roasted	3	ounce(s)	85	47.8	235	19.1	0	0	17.0	7.2	6.9	1.4
187	Shoulder, arm and blade, domestic, choice, lean, ¼″ fat, roasted	3	ounce(s)	85	53.8	173	21.2	0	0	9.2	3.5	3.7	0.8
3287	Shoulder, arm, domestic, lean and fat, ¼″ fat, braised	3	ounce(s)	85	37.6	294	25.8	0	0	20.4	8.4	8.7	1.5
3290	Shoulder, arm, domestic, lean, ¼″ fat, braised	3	ounce(s)	85	41.9	237	30.2	0	0	12.0	4.3	5.2	0.8
	LAMB VARIETY												
3375	Brain, pan fried	3	ounce(s)	85	51.6	232	14.4	0	0	18.9	4.8	3.4	1.9
3406	Tongue, braised	3	ounce(s)	85	49.2	234	18.3	0	0	17.2	6.7	8.5	1.1
	PORK, CURED												
29229	Bacon, Canadian style, cured	2	ounce(s)	57	37.9	89	11.7	1.0	0	4.0	1.3	1.8	0.4
161	Bacon, cured, broiled, pan fried or roasted	2	slice(s)	16	2.0	87	5.9	0.2	0	6.7	2.2	3.0	0.7
35422	Breakfast strips, cured, cooked	3	slice(s)	34	9.2	156	9.8	0.4	0	12.5	4.3	5.6	1.9
189	Ham, cured, boneless, 11% fat, roasted	3	ounce(s)	85	54.9	151	19.2	0	0	7.7	2.7	3.8	1.2
29215	Ham, cured, extra lean, 4% fat, canned	2	2 ounce(s)	57	41.7	68	10.5	0	0	2.6	0.9	1.3	0.2
1316	Ham, cured, extra lean, 5% fat, roasted	3	ounce(s)	85	57.6	123	17.8	1.3	0	4.7	1.5	2.2	0.5
16561	Ham, smoked or cured, lean, cooked	1	slice(s)	42	27.6	66	10.5	0	0	2.3	0.8	1.1	0.3
	PORK CHOP												
32671	Loin, blade, chops, lean and fat, pan fried	3	ounce(s)	85	42.5	291	18.3	0	0	23.6	8.6	10	2.6
32672	Loin, center cut, chops, lean and fat, pan fried	3	ounce(s)	85	45.1	236	25.4	0	0	14.1	5.1	6.0	1.6
32682	Loin, center rib, chops, boneless, lean and fat, braised	3	ounce(s)	85	49.5	217	22.4	0	0	13.4	5.2	6.1	1.1
32603	Loin, center rib, chops, lean, broiled	3	ounce(s)	85	55.4	158	21.9	0	0	7.1	2.4	3.0	0.8
32478	Loin, whole, lean and fat, braised	3	ounce(s)	85	49.6	203	23.2	0	0	11.6	4.3	5.2	1.0
32481	Loin, whole, lean, braised	3	ounce(s)	85	52.2	174	24.3	0	0	7.8	2.9	3.5	0.6
	PORK LEG OR HAM												
32471	Pork leg or ham, rump portion, lean and fat, roasted	3	ounce(s)	85	48.3	214	24.6	0	0	12.1	4.5	5.4	1.2
32468	Pork leg or ham, whole, lean and fat, roasted	3	ounce(s)	85	46.8	232	22.8	0	0	15.0	5.5	6.7	1.4
	PORK RIBS												
32693	Loin, country style, lean and fat, roasted	3	ounce(s)	85	43.3	279	19.9	0	0	21.6	7.8	9.4	1.7
32696	Loin, country style, lean, roasted	3	ounce(s)	85	49.5	210	22.6	0	0	12.6	4.5	5.5	0.9
	PORK SHOULDER												
32626	Shoulder, arm picnic, lean and fat, roasted	3	ounce(s)	85	44.3	270	20.0	0	0	20.4	7.5	9.1	2.0
32629	Shoulder, arm picnic, lean, roasted	3	ounce(s)	85	51.3	194	22.7	0	0	10.7	3.7	5.1	1.0
	RABBIT												
3366	Domesticated, roasted	3	ounce(s)	85	51.5	168	24.7	0	0	6.8	2.0	1.8	1.3
3367	Domesticated, stewed	3	ounce(s)	85	50.0	175	25.8	0	0	7.2	2.1	1.9	1.4

PAGE KEY: A-4 = Breads/Baked Goods A-10 = Cereal/Rice/Pasta A-14 = Fruit A-20 = Vegetables/Legumes A-30 = Nuts/Seeds A-32 = Vegetarian A-34 = Dairy A-42 = Eggs A-42 = Seafood A-46 = Meats A-50 = Poultry A-50 = Processed Meats A-52 = Beverages A-56 = Fats/Oils A-58 = Sweets A-60 = Spices/Condiments/Sauces A-64 = Mixed Foods/Soups/Sandwiches A-70 = Fast Food A-90 = Convenience A-92 = Baby Foods

CHOL (mg)	CALC (mg)	IRON (mg)	MAGN (mg)	POTA (mg)	SODI (mg)	ZINC (mg)	VIT A (µg)	THIA (mg)	VIT E (mg α)	RIBO (mg)	NIAC (mg)	VIT B_6 (mg)	FOLA (µg DFE)	VIT C (mg)	VIT B_{12} (µg)	SELE (µg)
82	14	1.59	19.6	263.7	61.2	3.79	0	0.08	0.11	0.21	5.66	0.11	15.3	0	2.2	22.5
84	16	1.59	19.6	229.5	64.6	3.40	0	0.07	0.10	0.18	5.95	0.09	11.9	0	2.2	20.3
77	14	1.87	24.7	266.1	72.3	4.47	0	0.08	0.15	0.21	5.56	0.12	17.9	0	2.2	26.4
78	17	1.67	19.6	213.4	56.1	4.44	0	0.07	0.11	0.20	5.22	0.11	17.9	0	2.2	22.3
74	16	1.81	21.3	225.3	57.8	5.13	0	0.07	0.15	0.22	4.89	0.12	21.3	0	2.3	24.2
102	21	2.03	22.1	260.3	61.2	5.17	0	0.06	0.12	0.21	5.66	0.09	15.3	0	2.2	31.6
103	22	2.29	24.7	287.5	64.6	6.20	0	0.06	0.15	0.23	5.38	0.11	18.7	0	2.3	32.1
2130	18	1.73	18.7	304.5	133.5	1.70	0	0.14	—	0.31	3.87	0.19	6.0	19.6	20.5	10.2
161	9	2.23	13.6	134.4	57.0	2.54	0	0.06	—	0.35	3.13	0.14	2.6	6.0	5.4	23.8
28	5	0.38	9.6	195.0	798.9	0.78	0	0.42	0.11	0.09	3.53	0.22	2.3	0	0.4	14.2
18	2	0.22	5.3	90.4	369.6	0.56	1.8	0.06	0.04	0.04	1.76	0.04	0.3	0	0.2	9.9
36	5	0.67	8.8	158.4	713.7	1.25	0	0.25	0.08	0.12	2.58	0.11	1.4	0	0.6	8.4
50	7	1.13	18.7	347.7	1275.0	2.09	0	0.62	0.26	0.28	5.22	0.26	2.6	0	0.6	16.8
22	3	0.53	9.6	206.4	711.6	1.09	0	0.47	0.09	0.13	3.00	0.25	3.4	0	0.5	8.2
45	7	1.25	11.9	244.1	1023.1	2.44	0	0.64	0.21	0.17	3.42	0.34	2.6	0	0.6	16.6
23	3	0.39	9.2	132.7	557.3	1.07	0	0.28	0.10	0.10	2.10	0.19	1.7	0	0.3	10.7
72	26	0.74	17.9	282.4	57.0	2.71	1.7	0.52	0.17	0.25	3.35	0.28	3.4	0.5	0.7	29.7
78	23	0.77	24.7	361.5	68.0	1.96	1.7	0.96	0.21	0.25	4.76	0.39	5.1	0.9	0.6	33.2
62	4	0.78	14.5	329.1	34.0	1.76	1.7	0.44	—	0.20	3.66	0.26	3.4	0.3	0.4	28.4
56	22	0.57	21.3	291.7	48.5	1.91	0	0.48	0.08	0.18	6.68	0.57	0	0.5	0.4	38.6
68	18	0.91	16.2	318.1	40.8	2.02	1.7	0.53	0.20	0.21	3.75	0.31	2.6	0.5	0.5	38.5
67	15	0.96	17.0	329.1	42.5	2.10	1.7	0.56	0.17	0.22	3.90	0.32	3.4	0.5	0.5	41.0
82	10	0.89	23.0	318.1	52.7	2.39	2.6	0.63	0.18	0.28	3.95	0.26	2.6	0.2	0.6	39.8
80	12	0.85	18.7	299.4	51.0	2.51	2.6	0.54	0.18	0.26	3.89	0.34	8.5	0.3	0.6	38.5
78	21	0.90	19.6	292.6	44.2	2.00	2.6	0.75	—	0.29	3.67	0.37	4.3	0.3	0.7	31.6
79	25	1.09	20.4	296.8	24.7	3.24	1.7	0.48	—	0.29	3.96	0.37	4.3	0.3	0.7	36.0
80	16	1.00	14.5	276.4	59.5	2.93	1.7	0.44	—	0.25	3.33	0.29	3.4	0.2	0.6	28.6
81	8	1.20	17.0	298.5	68.0	3.46	1.7	0.49	—	0.30	3.66	0.34	4.3	0.3	0.7	32.7
70	16	1.93	17.9	325.7	40.0	1.93	0	0.07	—	0.17	7.17	0.40	9.4	0	7.1	32.7
73	17	2.01	17.0	255.1	31.5	2.01	0	0.05	0.37	0.14	6.09	0.28	7.7	0	5.5	32.7

TABLE A–1 Table of Food Composition (continued)

(Computer code is for Cengage Diet & Wellness Plus program)

D&W+ Code	Food Description	QTY	Measure	Wt (g)	H₂0 (g)	Ener (cal)	Prot (g)	Carb (g)	Fiber (g)	Fat (g)	Sat	Mono	Poly
											\<Fat Breakdown (g)\>		

D&W+ Code	Food Description	QTY	Measure	Wt (g)	H₂0 (g)	Ener (cal)	Prot (g)	Carb (g)	Fiber (g)	Fat (g)	Sat	Mono	Poly
BEEF, LAMB, PORK—CONTINUED													
	VEAL												
3391	Liver, braised	3	ounce(s)	85	50.9	163	24.2	3.2	0	5.3	1.7	1.0	0.9
3319	Rib, lean only, roasted	3	ounce(s)	85	55.0	151	21.9	0	0	6.3	1.8	2.3	0.6
	DEER OR VENISON												
1732	Roasted	3	ounce(s)	85	55.5	134	25.7	0	0	2.7	1.1	0.7	0.5
POULTRY													
	CHICKEN												
29562	Flaked, canned	2	ounce(s)	57	39.3	97	10.3	0.1	0	5.8	1.6	2.3	1.3
	CHICKEN, FRIED												
29632	Breast, meat only, breaded, baked or fried	3	ounce(s)	85	44.3	193	25.3	6.9	0.2	6.6	1.6	2.7	1.7
35327	Broiler breast, meat only, fried	3	ounce(s)	85	51.2	159	28.4	0.4	0	4.0	1.1	1.5	0.9
36413	Broiler breast, meat and skin, flour coated, fried	3	ounce(s)	85	48.1	189	27.1	1.4	0.1	7.5	2.1	3.0	1.7
36414	Broiler drumstick, meat and skin, flour coated, fried	3	ounce(s)	85	48.2	208	22.9	1.4	0.1	11.7	3.1	4.6	2.7
35389	Broiler drumstick, meat only, fried	3	ounce(s)	85	52.9	166	24.3	0	0	6.9	1.8	2.5	1.7
35406	Broiler leg, meat only, fried	3	ounce(s)	85	51.5	177	24.1	0.6	0	7.9	2.1	2.9	1.9
35484	Broiler wing, meat only, fried	3	ounce(s)	85	50.9	179	25.6	0	0	7.8	2.1	2.6	1.8
29580	Patty, fillet or tenders, breaded, cooked	3	ounce(s)	85	40.2	256	14.5	12.2	0	16.5	3.7	8.4	3.7
	CHICKEN, ROASTED, MEAT ONLY												
35409	Broiler leg, meat only, roasted	3	ounce(s)	85	55.0	162	23.0	0	0	7.2	1.9	2.6	1.7
35486	Broiler wing, meat only, roasted	3	ounce(s)	85	53.4	173	25.9	0	0	6.9	1.9	2.2	1.5
35138	Roasting chicken, dark meat, meat only, roasted	3	ounce(s)	85	57.0	151	19.8	0	0	7.4	2.1	2.8	1.7
35136	Roasting chicken, light meat, meat only, roasted	3	ounce(s)	85	57.7	130	23.1	0	0	3.5	0.9	1.3	0.8
35132	Roasting chicken, meat only, roasted	3	ounce(s)	85	57.3	142	21.3	0	0	5.6	1.5	2.1	1.3
	CHICKEN, STEWED												
1268	Gizzard, simmered	3	ounce(s)	85	57.8	124	25.8	0	0	2.3	0.6	0.4	0.3
1270	Liver, simmered	3	ounce(s)	85	56.8	142	20.8	0.7	0	5.5	1.8	1.2	1.7
3174	Meat only, stewed	3	ounce(s)	85	56.8	151	23.2	0	0	5.7	1.6	2.0	1.3
	DUCK												
1286	Domesticated, meat and skin, roasted	3	ounce(s)	85	44.1	287	16.2	0	0	24.1	8.2	11.0	3.1
1287	Domesticated, meat only, roasted	3	ounce(s)	85	54.6	171	20.0	0	0	9.5	3.5	3.1	1.2
	GOOSE												
35507	Domesticated, meat and skin, roasted	3	ounce(s)	85	44.2	259	21.4	0	0	18.6	5.8	8.7	2.1
35524	Domesticated, meat only, roasted	3	ounce(s)	85	48.7	202	24.6	0	0	10.8	3.9	3.7	1.3
1297	Liver pate, smoked, canned	4	tablespoon(s)	52	19.3	240	5.9	2.4	0	22.8	7.5	13.3	0.4
	TURKEY												
3256	Ground turkey, cooked	3	ounce(s)	85	50.5	200	23.3	0	0	11.2	2.9	4.2	2.7
3263	Patty, batter coated, breaded, fried	1	item(s)	94	46.7	266	13.2	14.8	0.5	16.9	4.4	7.0	4.4
219	Roasted, dark meat, meat only	3	ounce(s)	85	53.7	159	24.3	0	0	6.1	2.1	1.4	1.8
222	Roasted, fryer roaster breast, meat only	3	ounce(s)	85	58.2	115	25.6	0	0	0.6	0.2	0.1	0.2
220	Roasted, light meat, meat only	3	ounce(s)	85	56.4	134	25.4	0	0	2.7	0.9	0.5	0.7
1303	Turkey roll, light and dark meat	2	slice(s)	57	39.8	84	10.3	1.2	0	4.0	1.2	1.3	1.0
1302	Turkey roll, light meat	2	slice(s)	57	42.5	56	8.4	2.9	0	0.9	0.2	0.2	0.1
PROCESSED MEATS													
	BEEF												
1331	Corned beef loaf, jellied, sliced	2	slice(s)	57	39.2	87	13.0	0	0	3.5	1.5	1.5	0.2
	BOLOGNA												
13459	Beef	1	slice(s)	28	15.1	90	3.0	1.0	0	8.0	3.5	4.3	0.3
13461	Light, made with pork and chicken	1	slice(s)	28	18.2	60	3.0	2.0	0	4.0	1.0	2.0	0.4
13458	Made with chicken and pork	1	slice(s)	28	15.0	90	3.0	1.0	0	8.0	3.0	4.1	1.1
13565	Turkey bologna	1	slice(s)	28	19.0	50	3.0	1.0	0	4.0	1.0	1.1	1.0
	CHICKEN												
7125	Breast, smoked	1	slice(s)	10	—	10	1.8	0.3	0	0.2	0	—	—

PAGE KEY: A-4 = Breads/Baked Goods A-10 = Cereal/Rice/Pasta A-14 = Fruit A-20 = Vegetables/Legumes A-30 = Nuts/Seeds A-32 = Vegetarian A-34 = Dairy A-42 = Eggs A-42 = Seafood A-46 = Meats A-50 = Poultry A-50 = Processed Meats A-52 = Beverages A-56 = Fats/Oils A-58 = Sweets A-60 = Spices/Condiments/Sauces A-64 = Mixed Foods/Soups/Sandwiches A-70 = Fast Food A-90 = Convenience A-92 = Baby Foods

A

CHOL (mg)	CALC (mg)	IRON (mg)	MAGN (mg)	POTA (mg)	SODI (mg)	ZINC (mg)	VIT A (µg)	THIA (mg)	VIT E (mg α)	RIBO (mg)	NIAC (mg)	VIT B6 (mg)	FOLA (µg DFE)	VIT C (mg)	VIT B12 (µg)	SELE (µg)
435	5	4.34	17.0	279.8	66.3	9.55	8026	0.15	0.57	2.43	11.18	0.78	281.5	0.9	72.0	16.4
98	10	0.81	20.4	264.5	82.5	3.81	0	0.05	0.30	0.24	6.37	0.23	11.9	0	1.3	9.4
95	6	3.80	20.4	284.9	45.9	2.33	0	0.15	—	0.51	5.70	—	—	0	—	11.0
35	8	0.89	6.8	147.4	408.2	0.79	19.3	0.01	—	0.07	3.58	0.19	2.3	0	0.2	—
67	19	1.05	24.7	222.6	450.2	0.84	—	0.08	—	0.09	10.97	0.46	4.3	0	0.3	—
77	14	0.96	26.4	234.7	67.2	0.91	6.0	0.06	0.35	0.10	12.57	0.54	3.4	0	0.3	22.3
76	14	1.01	25.5	220.3	64.6	0.93	12.8	0.06	0.39	0.11	11.68	0.49	6.0	0	0.3	20.3
77	10	1.13	19.6	194.8	75.7	2.45	21.3	0.06	0.65	0.19	5.13	0.29	9.4	0	0.3	15.6
80	10	1.12	20.4	211.8	81.6	2.73	15.3	0.06	—	0.20	5.22	0.33	7.7	0	0.3	16.7
84	11	1.19	21.3	216.0	81.6	2.53	17.0	0.07	0.38	0.21	5.68	0.33	7.7	0	0.3	16.0
71	13	0.96	17.9	176.9	77.4	1.80	15.3	0.03	0.40	0.10	6.15	0.50	3.4	0	0.3	21.6
49	11	0.75	19.6	244.8	411.4	0.79	4.3	0.09	1.04	0.12	5.99	0.24	35.7	0	0.2	13.9
80	10	1.11	20.4	205.8	77.4	2.43	16.2	0.06	0.22	0.19	5.37	0.31	6.8	0	0.3	18.8
72	14	0.98	17.9	178.6	78.2	1.82	15.3	0.03	0.22	0.10	6.21	0.50	3.4	0	0.3	21.0
64	9	1.13	17.0	190.5	80.8	1.81	13.6	0.05	—	0.16	4.87	0.26	6.0	0	0.3	16.7
64	11	0.91	19.6	200.7	43.4	0.66	6.8	0.05	0.22	0.07	8.90	0.45	2.6	0	0.3	21.9
64	10	1.02	17.9	194.8	63.8	1.29	10.2	0.05	—	0.12	6.70	0.34	4.3	0	0.2	20.9
315	14	2.71	2.6	152.2	47.6	3.75	0	0.02	0.17	0.17	2.65	0.06	4.3	0	0.9	35.0
479	9	9.89	21.3	223.7	64.6	3.38	3385.8	0.24	0.69	1.69	9.39	0.64	491.6	23.7	14.3	70.1
71	12	0.99	17.9	153.1	59.5	1.69	12.8	0.04	0.22	0.13	5.20	0.22	5.1	0	0.2	17.8
71	9	2.29	13.6	173.5	50.2	1.58	53.6	0.14	0.59	0.22	4.10	0.15	5.1	0	0.3	17.0
76	10	2.29	17.0	214.3	55.3	2.21	19.6	0.22	0.59	0.39	4.33	0.21	8.5	0	0.3	19.1
77	11	2.40	18.7	279.8	59.5	2.22	17.9	0.06	1.47	0.27	3.54	0.31	1.7	0	0.3	18.5
82	12	2.44	21.3	330.0	64.6	2.69	10.2	0.07	—	0.33	3.47	0.39	10.2	0	0.4	21.7
78	36	2.86	6.8	71.8	362.4	0.47	520.5	0.04	—	0.15	1.30	0.03	31.2	0	4.9	22.9
87	21	1.64	20.4	229.6	91.0	2.43	0	0.04	0.28	0.14	4.09	0.33	6.0	0	0.3	31.6
71	13	2.06	14.1	258.5	752.0	1.35	9.4	0.09	0.87	0.17	2.16	0.18	57.3	0	0.2	20.8
72	27	1.98	20.4	246.6	67.2	3.79	0	0.05	0.54	0.21	3.10	0.30	7.7	0	0.3	34.8
71	10	1.30	24.7	248.3	44.2	1.48	0	0.03	0.07	0.11	6.37	0.47	5.1	0	0.3	27.3
59	16	1.14	23.8	259.4	54.4	1.73	0	0.05	0.07	0.11	5.81	0.45	5.1	0	0.3	27.3
31	18	0.76	10.2	153.1	332.3	1.13	0	0.05	0.19	0.16	2.72	0.15	2.8	0	0.1	16.6
19	4	0.21	10.8	242.1	590.8	0.50	0	0.01	0.07	0.08	4.05	0.23	2.3	0	0.2	7.4
27	6	1.15	6.2	57.3	540.4	2.31	0	0.00	—	0.06	0.99	0.06	4.5	0	0.7	9.8
20	0	0.36	3.9	47.0	310.0	0.56	0	0.01	—	0.03	0.67	0.04	3.6	0	0.4	—
20	40	0.36	5.6	45.6	300.0	0.45	0	—	—	—	—	—	—	0	—	—
30	20	0.36	5.9	43.1	300.0	0.39	0	—	—	—	—	—	—	0	—	—
20	40	0.36	6.2	42.6	270.0	0.51	0	—	—	—	—	—	—	0	—	—
4	0	0.00	—	—	100.0	—	0	—	—	—	—	—	—	0	—	—

TABLE A–1 Table of Food Composition (continued)

(Computer code is for Cengage Diet & Wellness Plus program)

D&W+ Code	Food Description	QTY	Measure	Wt (g)	H₂O (g)	Ener (cal)	Prot (g)	Carb (g)	Fiber (g)	Fat (g)	Sat	Mono	Poly
											Fat Breakdown (g)		

PROCESSED MEATS—CONTINUED

HAM

D&W+ Code	Food Description	QTY	Measure	Wt (g)	H₂O (g)	Ener (cal)	Prot (g)	Carb (g)	Fiber (g)	Fat (g)	Sat	Mono	Poly
7127	Deli-sliced, honey	1	slice(s)	10	—	10	1.7	0.3	0	0.3	0.1	—	—
7126	Deli-sliced, smoked	1	slice(s)	10	—	10	1.7	0.2	0	0.3	0.1	—	—
8614	MORTADELLA, BEEF AND PORK, SLICED	2	slice(s)	46	24.1	143	7.5	1.4	0	11.7	4.4	5.2	1.4
1323	PORK OLIVE LOAF	2	slice(s)	57	33.1	133	6.7	5.2	0	9.4	3.3	4.5	1.1
1324	PORK PICKLE AND PIMENTO LOAF	2	slice(s)	57	34.2	128	6.4	4.8	0.9	9.1	3.0	4.0	1.6
	SAUSAGES AND FRANKFURTERS												
37296	Beerwurst beef, beer salami (bierwurst)	1	slice(s)	29	16.6	74	4.1	1.2	0	5.7	2.5	2.7	0.2
37257	Beerwurst pork, beer salami	1	slice(s)	21	12.9	50	3.0	0.4	0	4.0	1.3	1.9	0.5
35338	Berliner, pork and beef	1	ounce(s)	28	17.3	65	4.3	0.7	0	4.9	1.7	2.3	0.4
37298	Bratwurst pork, cooked	1	piece(s)	74	42.3	181	10.4	1.9	0	14.3	5.1	6.7	1.5
37299	Braunschweiger pork liver sausage	1	slice(s)	15	8.2	51	2.0	0.3	0	4.5	1.5	2.1	0.5
1329	Cheesefurter or cheese smokie, beef and pork	1	item(s)	43	22.6	141	6.1	0.6	0	12.5	4.5	5.9	1.3
1330	Chorizo, beef and pork	2	ounce(s)	57	18.1	258	13.7	1.1	0	21.7	8.2	10.4	2.0
8600	Frankfurter, beef	1	item(s)	45	23.4	149	5.1	1.8	0	13.3	5.3	6.4	0.5
202	Frankfurter, beef and pork	1	item(s)	45	25.2	137	5.2	0.8	0	12.4	4.8	6.2	1.2
1293	Frankfurter, chicken	1	item(s)	45	28.1	100	7.0	1.2	0.2	7.3	1.7	2.7	1.7
3261	Frankfurter, turkey	1	item(s)	45	28.3	100	5.5	1.7	0	7.8	1.8	2.6	1.8
37275	Italian sausage, pork, cooked	1	item(s)	68	32.0	234	13.0	2.9	0.1	18.6	6.5	8.1	2.2
37307	Kielbasa or kolbassa, pork and beef	1	slice(s)	30	18.5	67	5.0	1.0	0	4.7	1.7	2.2	0.5
1333	Knockwurst or knackwurst, beef and pork	2	ounce(s)	57	31.4	174	6.3	1.8	0	15.7	5.8	7.3	1.7
37285	Pepperoni, beef and pork	1	slice(s)	11	3.4	51	2.2	0.4	0.2	4.4	1.8	2.1	0.3
37313	Polish sausage, pork	1	slice(s)	21	11.4	60	2.8	0.7	0	5.0	1.8	2.3	0.5
206	Salami, beef, cooked, sliced	2	slice(s)	52	31.2	136	6.5	1.0	0	11.5	5.1	5.5	0.5
37272	Salami, pork, dry or hard	1	slice(s)	13	4.6	52	2.9	0.2	0	4.3	1.5	2.0	0.5
40987	Sausage, turkey, cooked	2	ounce(s)	57	36.9	111	13.5	0	0	5.9	1.3	1.7	1.5
8620	Smoked sausage, beef and pork	2	ounce(s)	57	30.6	181	6.8	1.4	0	16.3	5.5	6.9	2.2
8619	Smoked sausage, pork	2	ounce(s)	57	32.0	178	6.8	1.2	0	16.0	5.3	6.4	2.1
37273	Smoked sausage, pork link	1	piece(s)	76	29.8	295	16.8	1.6	0	24.0	8.6	11.1	2.8
1336	Summer sausage, thuringer, or cervelat, beef and pork	2	ounce(s)	57	25.6	205	9.9	1.9	0	17.3	6.5	7.4	0.7
37294	Vienna sausage, cocktail, beef and pork, canned	1	piece(s)	16	10.4	37	1.7	0.4	0	3.1	1.1	1.5	0.2
	SPREADS												
1318	Ham salad spread	¼	cup(s)	60	37.6	130	5.2	6.4	0	9.3	3.0	4.3	1.6
32419	Pork and beef sandwich spread	4	tablespoon(s)	60	36.2	141	4.6	7.2	0.1	10.4	3.6	4.6	1.5
	TURKEY												
13604	Breast, fat free, oven roasted	1	slice(s)	28	—	25	4.0	1.0	0	0	0	0	0
13606	Breast, hickory smoked fat free	1	slice(s)	28	—	25	4.0	1.0	0	0	0	0	0
16049	Breast, hickory smoked slices	1	slice(s)	56	—	50	11.0	1.0	0	0	0	0	0
16047	Breast, honey roasted slices	1	slice(s)	56	—	60	11.0	3.0	0	0	0	0	0
16048	Breast, oven roasted slices	1	slice(s)	56	—	50	11.0	1.0	0	0	0	0	0
7124	Breast, oven roasted	1	slice(s)	10	—	10	1.8	0.3	0	0.1	0	0	0
13567	Turkey ham, 10% water added	2	slice(s)	56	40.9	70	10.0	2.0	0	3.0	0	0.4	0.6
37270	Turkey pastrami	1	slice(s)	28	20.3	35	4.6	1.0	0	1.2	0.3	0.4	0.3
3262	Turkey salami	2	slice(s)	57	39.1	98	10.9	0.9	0.1	5.2	1.6	1.8	1.4
37318	Turkey salami, cooked	1	slice(s)	28	20.4	43	4.3	0.1	0	2.7	0.8	0.9	0.7

BEVERAGES

BEER

D&W+ Code	Food Description	QTY	Measure	Wt (g)	H₂O (g)	Ener (cal)	Prot (g)	Carb (g)	Fiber (g)	Fat (g)	Sat	Mono	Poly
866	Ale, mild	12	fluid ounce(s)	360	332.3	148	1.1	13.3	0.4	0	0	0	0
686	Beer	12	fluid ounce(s)	356	327.7	153	1.6	12.7	0	0	0	0	0
16886	Beer, nonalcoholic	12	fluid ounce(s)	360	328.1	133	0.8	29.0	0	0.4	0.1	0	0.2
31609	Bud Light beer	12	fluid ounce(s)	355	335.5	110	0.9	6.6	0	0	0	0	0
31608	Budweiser beer	12	fluid ounce(s)	355	327.7	145	1.3	10.6	0	0	0	0	0

A

CHOL (mg)	CALC (mg)	IRON (mg)	MAGN (mg)	POTA (mg)	SODI (mg)	ZINC (mg)	VIT A (µg)	THIA (mg)	VIT E (mg α)	RIBO (mg)	NIAC (mg)	VIT B6 (mg)	FOLA (µg DFE)	VIT C (mg)	VIT B12 (µg)	SELE (µg)
4	0	0.12	—	—	100.0	—	0	—	—	—	—	—	—	0.6	—	—
4	0	0.12	—	—	103.3	—	0	—	—	—	—	—	—	0.6	—	—
26	8	0.64	5.1	75.0	573.2	0.96	0	0.05	0.10	0.07	1.23	0.06	1.4	0	0.7	10.4
22	62	0.30	10.8	168.7	842.9	0.78	34.1	0.16	0.14	0.14	1.04	0.13	1.1	0	0.7	9.3
33	62	0.75	19.3	210.7	740.7	0.95	44.3	0.22	0.22	0.06	1.41	0.23	21.0	4.4	0.3	4.5
18	3	0.44	3.5	66.5	264.9	0.71	0	0.02	0.05	0.03	0.98	0.04	0.9	0	0.6	4.7
12	2	0.15	2.7	53.3	261.0	0.36	0	0.11	0.03	0.04	0.68	0.07	0.6	0	0.2	4.4
13	3	0.32	4.3	80.2	367.7	0.70	0	0.10	—	0.06	0.88	0.05	1.4	0	0.8	4.0
44	33	0.95	11.1	156.9	412.2	1.70	0	0.37	0.01	0.13	2.36	0.15	1.5	0.7	0.7	15.7
24	1	1.42	1.7	27.5	131.5	0.42	641.0	0.03	0.05	0.23	1.27	0.05	6.7	0	3.1	8.8
29	25	0.46	5.6	88.6	465.3	0.96	20.2	0.10	0.10	0.06	1.24	0.05	1.3	0	0.7	6.8
50	5	0.90	10.2	225.7	700.2	1.93	0	0.35	0.12	0.17	2.90	0.30	1.1	0	1.1	12.0
24	6	0.67	6.3	70.2	513.0	1.10	0	0.01	0.09	0.06	1.06	0.04	2.3	0	0.8	3.7
23	5	0.51	4.5	75.2	504.0	0.82	8.1	0.09	0.11	0.05	1.18	0.05	1.8	0	0.6	6.2
43	33	0.52	9.0	90.9	379.8	0.50	0	0.02	0.09	0.11	2.10	0.14	3.2	0	0.2	10.4
35	67	0.66	6.3	176.4	485.1	0.82	0	0.01	0.27	0.08	1.65	0.06	4.1	0	0.4	6.8
39	14	0.97	12.2	206.7	820.8	1.62	6.8	0.42	0.17	0.15	2.83	0.22	3.4	0.1	0.9	15.0
20	13	0.44	4.9	84.4	283.0	0.61	0	0.06	0.06	0.06	0.87	0.05	1.5	0	0.5	5.4
34	6	0.37	6.2	112.8	527.3	0.94	0	0.19	0.32	0.07	1.55	0.09	1.1	0	0.7	7.7
13	2	0.15	2.0	34.7	196.7	0.30	0	0.05	0.00	0.02	0.59	0.04	0.7	0.1	0.2	2.4
15	2	0.29	2.9	37.3	199.3	0.40	0	0.10	0.04	0.03	0.71	0.03	0.4	0.2	0.2	3.7
37	3	1.14	6.8	97.8	592.8	0.92	0	0.04	0.08	0.08	1.68	0.08	1.0	0	1.6	7.6
10	2	0.16	2.8	48.4	289.3	0.53	0	0.11	0.02	0.04	0.71	0.07	0.3	0	0.4	3.3
52	12	0.84	11.9	169.0	377.1	2.19	7.4	0.04	0.10	0.14	3.24	0.18	3.4	0.4	0.7	0
33	7	0.42	7.4	101.5	516.5	0.71	7.4	0.10	0.07	0.06	1.66	0.09	1.1	0	0.3	0
35	6	0.33	6.2	273.9	468.9	0.74	0	0.12	0.14	0.10	1.59	0.10	0.6	0	0.4	10.4
52	23	0.87	14.4	254.6	1136.6	2.13	0	0.53	0.18	0.19	3.43	0.26	3.8	1.5	1.2	16.4
42	5	1.15	7.9	147.4	737.1	1.45	0	0.08	0.12	0.18	2.44	0.14	1.1	9.4	3.1	11.5
14	2	0.14	1.1	16.2	155.0	0.25	0	0.01	0.03	0.01	0.25	0.01	0.6	0	0.2	2.7
22	5	0.35	6.0	90.0	547.2	0.66	0	0.26	1.04	0.07	1.25	0.09	0.6	0	0.5	10.7
23	7	0.47	4.8	66.0	607.8	0.61	15.6	0.10	1.04	0.08	1.03	0.07	1.2	0	0.7	5.8
10	0	0.00	—	—	340.0	—	0	—	—	—	—	—	—	0	—	—
10	0	0.00	—	—	300.0	—	0	—	—	—	—	—	—	0	—	—
25	0	0.72	—	—	720.0	—	0	—	—	—	—	—	—	0	—	—
20	0	0.72	—	—	660.0	—	0	—	—	—	—	—	—	0	—	—
20	0	0.72	—	—	660.0	—	0	—	—	—	—	—	—	0	—	—
4	0	0.06	—	—	103.3	—	0	—	—	—	—	—	—	0	—	—
40	0	0.72	12.3	162.4	700.0	1.44	0	—	—	—	—	—	—	0	—	—
19	3	1.19	4.0	97.8	278.1	0.61	1.1	0.01	0.06	0.07	1.00	0.07	1.4	4.6	0.1	4.6
43	23	0.70	12.5	122.5	569.3	1.31	1.1	0.24	0.13	0.17	2.25	0.24	5.7	0	0.6	15.0
22	11	0.35	6.2	61.2	284.6	0.65	0.6	0.12	0.06	0.08	1.12	0.12	2.8	0	0.3	7.5
0	18	0.07	21.6	90.0	14.4	0.03	0	0.03	0.00	0.10	1.62	0.18	21.6	0	0.1	2.5
0	14	0.07	21.4	96.2	14.3	0.03	0	0.01	0.00	0.08	1.82	0.16	21.4	0	0.1	2.1
0	25	0.21	25.2	28.8	46.8	0.07	—	0.07	0.00	0.18	3.99	0.10	50.4	1.8	0.1	4.3
0	18	0.14	17.8	63.9	9.0	0.10	0	0.03	—	0.10	1.39	0.12	14.6	0	0	4.0
0	18	0.10	21.3	88.8	9.0	0.07	0	0.02	—	0.09	1.60	0.17	21.3	0	0.1	4.0

(Computer code is for Cengage Diet & Wellness Plus program)

D&W+ Code	Food Description	QTY	Measure	Wt (g)	H₂0 (g)	Ener (cal)	Prot (g)	Carb (g)	Fiber (g)	Fat (g)	Sat	Mono	Poly
											Fat Breakdown (g)		
BEVERAGES—CONTINUED													
869	Light beer	12	fluid ounce(s)	354	335.9	103	0.9	5.8	0	0	0	0	0
31613	Michelob beer	12	fluid ounce(s)	355	323.4	155	1.3	13.3	0	0	0	0	0
31614	Michelob Light beer	12	fluid ounce(s)	355	329.8	134	1.1	11.7	0	0	0	0	0
	GIN, RUM, VODKA, WHISKEY												
857	Distilled alcohol, 100 proof	1	fluid ounce(s)	28	16.0	82	0	0	0	0	0	0	0
687	Distilled alcohol, 80 proof	1	fluid ounce(s)	28	18.5	64	0	0	0	0	0	0	0
688	Distilled alcohol, 86 proof	1	fluid ounce(s)	28	17.8	70	0	0	0	0	0	0	0
689	Distilled alcohol, 90 proof	1	fluid ounce(s)	28	17.3	73	0	0	0	0	0	0	0
856	Distilled alcohol, 94 proof	1	fluid ounce(s)	28	16.8	76	0	0	0	0	0	0	0
	LIQUEURS												
33187	Coffee liqueur, 53 proof	1	fluid ounce(s)	35	10.8	113	0	16.3	0	0.1	0	0	0
3142	Coffee liqueur, 63 proof	1	fluid ounce(s)	35	14.4	107	0	11.2	0	0.1	0	0	0
736	Cordials, 54 proof	1	fluid ounce(s)	30	8.9	106	0	13.3	0	0.1	0	0	0
	WINE												
861	California red wine	5	fluid ounce(s)	150	133.4	125	0.3	3.7	0	0	0	0	0
858	Domestic champagne	5	fluid ounce(s)	150	—	105	0.3	3.8	0	0	0	0	0
690	Sweet dessert wine	5	fluid ounce(s)	147	103.7	235	0.3	20.1	0	0	0	0	0
1481	White wine	5	fluid ounce(s)	148	128.1	121	0.1	3.8	0	0	0	0	0
1811	Wine cooler	10	fluid ounce(s)	300	267.4	159	0.3	20.2	0	0.1	0	0	0
	CARBONATED												
31898	7 Up	12	fluid ounce(s)	360	321.0	140	0	39.0	0	0	0	0	0
692	Club soda	12	fluid ounce(s)	355	354.8	0	0	0	0	0	0	0	0
12010	Coca-Cola Classic cola soda	12	fluid ounce(s)	360	319.4	146	0	40.5	0	0	0	0	0
693	Cola	12	fluid ounce(s)	368	332.7	136	0.3	35.2	0	0.1	0	0	0
2391	Cola or pepper-type soda, low calorie with saccharin	12	fluid ounce(s)	355	354.5	0	0	0.3	0	0	0	0	0
9522	Cola soda, decaffeinated	12	fluid ounce(s)	372	333.4	153	0	39.3	0	0	0	0	0
9524	Cola, decaffeinated, low calorie with aspartame	12	fluid ounce(s)	355	354.3	4	0.4	0.5	0	0	0	0	0
1415	Cola, low calorie with aspartame	12	fluid ounce(s)	355	353.6	7	0.4	1.0	0	0.1	0	0	0
1412	Cream soda	12	fluid ounce(s)	371	321.5	189	0	49.3	0	0	0	0	0
31899	Diet 7 Up	12	fluid ounce(s)	360	—	0	0	0	0	0	0	0	0
12031	Diet Coke cola soda	12	fluid ounce(s)	360	—	2	0	0.2	0	0	0	0	0
29392	Diet Mountain Dew soda	12	fluid ounce(s)	360	—	0	0	0	0	0	0	0	0
29389	Diet Pepsi cola soda	12	fluid ounce(s)	360	—	0	0	0	0	0	0	0	0
12034	Diet Sprite soda	12	fluid ounce(s)	360	—	4	0	0	0	0	0	0	0
695	Ginger ale	12	fluid ounce(s)	366	333.9	124	0	32.1	0	0	0	0	0
694	Grape soda	12	fluid ounce(s)	372	330.3	160	0	41.7	0	0	0	0	0
1876	Lemon lime soda	12	fluid ounce(s)	368	330.8	147	0.2	37.4	0	0.1	0	0	0
29391	Mountain Dew soda	12	fluid ounce(s)	360	314.0	170	0	46.0	0	0	0	0	0
3145	Orange soda	12	fluid ounce(s)	372	325.9	179	0	45.8	0	0	0	0	0
1414	Pepper-type soda	12	fluid ounce(s)	368	329.3	151	0	38.3	0	0.4	0.3	0	0
29388	Pepsi regular cola soda	12	fluid ounce(s)	360	318.9	150	0	41.0	0	0	0	0	0
696	Root beer	12	fluid ounce(s)	370	330.0	152	0	39.2	0	0	0	0	0
12044	Sprite soda	12	fluid ounce(s)	360	321.0	144	0	39.0	0	0	0	0	0
	COFFEE												
731	Brewed	8	fluid ounce(s)	237	235.6	2	0.3	0	0	0	0	0	0
9520	Brewed, decaffeinated	8	fluid ounce(s)	237	234.3	5	0.3	1.0	0	0	0	0	0
16882	Cappuccino	8	fluid ounce(s)	240	224.8	79	4.1	5.8	0.2	4.9	2.3	1.0	0.2
16883	Cappuccino, decaffeinated	8	fluid ounce(s)	240	224.8	79	4.1	5.8	0.2	4.9	2.3	1.0	0.2
16880	Espresso	8	fluid ounce(s)	237	231.8	21	0	3.6	0	0.4	0.2	0	0.2
16881	Espresso, decaffeinated	8	fluid ounce(s)	237	231.8	21	0	3.6	0	0.4	0.2	0	0.2
732	Instant, prepared	8	fluid ounce(s)	239	236.5	5	0.2	0.8	0	0	0	0	0
	FRUIT DRINKS												
29357	Crystal Light sugar-free lemonade drink	8	fluid ounce(s)	240	—	5	0	0	0	0	0	0	0
6012	Fruit punch drink with added vitamin C, canned	8	fluid ounce(s)	248	218.2	117	0	29.7	0.5	0	0	0	0
31143	Gatorade Thirst Quencher, all flavors	8	fluid ounce(s)	240	—	50	0	14.0	0	0	0	0	0
260	Grape drink, canned	8	fluid ounce(s)	250	210.5	153	0	39.4	0	0	0	0	0

PAGE KEY: A-4 = Breads/Baked Goods A-10 = Cereal/Rice/Pasta A-14 = Fruit A-20 = Vegetables/Legumes A-30 = Nuts/Seeds A-32 = Vegetarian
A-34 = Dairy A-42 = Eggs A-42 = Seafood A-46 = Meats A-50 = Poultry A-50 = Processed Meats A-52 = Beverages A-56 = Fats/Oils A-58 = Sweets
A-60 = Spices/Condiments/Sauces A-64 = Mixed Foods/Soups/Sandwiches A-70 = Fast Food A-90 = Convenience A-92 = Baby Foods

A

CHOL (mg)	CALC (mg)	IRON (mg)	MAGN (mg)	POTA (mg)	SODI (mg)	ZINC (mg)	VIT A (µg)	THIA (mg)	VIT E (mg α)	RIBO (mg)	NIAC (mg)	VIT B$_6$ (mg)	FOLA (µg DFE)	VIT C (mg)	VIT B$_{12}$ (µg)	SELE (µg)
0	14	0.10	17.7	74.3	14.2	0.03	0	0.01	0.00	0.05	1.38	0.12	21.2	0	0.1	1.4
0	18	0.10	21.3	88.8	9.0	0.07	0	0.02	—	0.09	1.60	0.17	21.3	0	0.1	4.0
0	18	0.14	17.8	63.9	9.0	0.10	0	0.03	—	0.10	1.39	0.12	14.6	0	0	4.0
0	0	0.01	0	0.6	0.3	0.01	0	0.00	—	0.00	0.00	0.00	0	0	0	0
0	0	0.01	0	0.6	0.3	0.01	0	0.00	0.00	0.00	0.00	0.00	0	0	0	0
0	0	0.01	0	0.6	0.3	0.01	0	0.00	0.00	0.00	0.00	0.00	0	0	0	0
0	0	0.01	0	0.6	0.3	0.01	0	0.00	—	0.00	0.00	0.00	0	0	0	0
0	0	0.02	1.0	10.4	2.8	0.01	0	0.00	0.00	0.00	0.05	0.00	0	0	0	0.1
0	0	0.02	1.0	10.4	2.8	0.01	0	0.00		0.00	0.05	0.00	0	0	0	0.1
0	0	0.02	0.6	4.5	2.1	0.01	0	0.00	0.00	0.00	0.02	0.00	0	0	0	0.1
0	12	1.43	16.2	170.6	15.0	0.14	0	0.01	0.00	0.04	0.11	0.05	1.5	0	0	—
0	—	—	—	—	—	—	0	—	—	—	—	—	—	—	0	—
0	12	0.34	13.2	135.4	13.2	0.10	0	0.01	0.00	0.01	0.30	0.00	0	0	0	0.7
0	13	0.39	14.8	104.7	7.4	0.18	0	0.01	0.00	0.01	0.15	0.06	1.5	0	0	0.1
0	18	0.75	15.0	129.0	24.0	0.18	—	0.01	0.03	0.03	0.13	0.03	3.0	5.4	0	0.6
0	—	—	—	0.6	75.0	—	—	—	—	—	—	—	—	—	—	—
0	18	0.03	3.5	7.1	74.6	0.35	0	0.00	0.00	0.00	0.00	0.00	0	0	0	0
0	—	—	—	0	49.5	—	0	—	—	—	—	—	—	0	—	—
0	7	0.41	0	7.4	14.7	0.06	0	0.00	0.00	0.00	0.00	0.00	0	0	0	0.4
0	14	0.06	3.5	14.2	56.8	0.11	0	0.00	0.00	0.00	0.00	0.00	0	0	0	0.3
0	7	0.08	0	11.2	14.9	0.03	0	0.00	0.00	0.00	0.00	0.00	0	0	0	0.4
0	11	0.06	0	24.9	14.2	0.03	0	0.02	0.00	0.08	0.00	0.00	0	0	0	0.3
0	11	0.39	3.5	28.4	28.4	0.03	0	0.02	0.00	0.08	0.00	0.00	0	0	0	0
0	19	0.18	3.7	3.7	44.5	0.26	0	0.00	0.00	0.00	0.00	0.00	0	0	0	0
0	—	—	—	77.0	45.0	—	—	—	—	—	—	—	—	—	—	—
0	—	—	—	18.0	42.0	—	0	—	—	—	—	—	—	0	—	—
0	—	—	—	70.0	35.0	—	—	—	—	—	—	—	—	—	—	—
0	—	—	—	30.0	35.0	—	—	—	—	—	—	—	—	—	—	—
0	—	—	—	109.5	36.0	—	0	—	—	—	—	—	—	0	—	—
0	11	0.65	3.7	3.7	25.6	0.18	0	0.00	0.00	0.00	0.00	0.00	0	0	0	0.4
0	11	0.29	3.7	3.7	55.8	0.26	0	0.00	—	0.00	0.00	0.00	0	0	0	0
0	7	0.41	3.7	3.7	33.2	0.14	0	0.00	0.00	0.00	0.05	0.00	0	0	0	0
0	—	—	—	0	70.0	—	0	—	—	—	—	—	—	0	—	—
0	19	0.21	3.7	7.4	44.6	0.36	0	0.00	—	0.00	0.00	0.00	0	0	0	0
0	11	0.14	0	3.7	36.8	0.14	0	0.00	—	0.00	0.00	0.00	0	0	0	0.4
0	—	—	—	0	35.0	—	—	—	—	—	—	—	—	—	—	—
0	18	0.18	3.7	3.7	48.0	0.26	0	0.00	0.00	0.00	0.00	0.00	0	0	0	0.4
0	—	—	—	0	70.5	—	0	—	—	—	—	—	—	0	—	—
0	5	0.02	7.1	116.1	4.7	0.04	0	0.03	0.02	0.18	0.45	0.00	4.7	0	0	0
0	7	0.14	11.8	108.9	4.7	0.00	0	0.00	0.00	0.03	0.66	0.00	0	0	0	0.5
12	144	0.19	14.4	232.8	50.4	0.50	33.6	0.04	0.09	0.27	0.13	0.04	7.2	0	0.4	4.6
12	144	0.19	14.4	232.8	50.4	0.50	33.6	0.04	0.09	0.27	0.13	0.04	7.2	0	0.4	4.6
0	5	0.30	189.6	272.6	33.2	0.11	0	0.00	0.04	0.42	12.34	0.00	2.4	0.5	0	0
0	5	0.30	189.6	272.6	33.2	0.11	0	0.00	0.04	0.42	12.34	0.00	2.4	0.5	0	0
0	10	0.09	9.5	71.6	9.5	0.01	0	0.00	0.00	0.00	0.56	0.00	0	0	0	0.2
0	0	0.00	—	160.0	40.0	—	0	—	—	—	—	—	—	0	—	—
0	20	0.22	7.4	62.0	94.2	0.02	5.0	0.05	0.04	0.05	0.05	0.02	9.9	89.3	0	0.5
0	0	0.00	—	30.0	110.0	—	0	—	—	—	—	—	—	0	—	—
0	130	0.17	2.5	30.0	40.0	0.30	0	0.00	0.00	0.01	0.02	0.01	0	78.5	0	0.3

(Computer code is for Cengage Diet & Wellness Plus program)

D&W+ Code	Food Description	QTY	Measure	Wt (g)	H₂0 (g)	Ener (cal)	Prot (g)	Carb (g)	Fiber (g)	Fat (g)	Sat	Mono	Poly
											Fat Breakdown (g)		
Beverages—continued													
17372	Kool-Aid (lemonade/punch/fruit drink)	8	fluid ounce(s)	248	220.0	108	0.1	27.8	0.2	0	0	0	0
17225	Kool-Aid sugar free, low calorie tropical punch drink mix, prepared	8	fluid ounce(s)	240	—	5	0	0	0	0	0	0	0
266	Lemonade, prepared from frozen concentrate	8	fluid ounce(s)	248	221.6	99	0.2	25.8	0	0.1	0	0	0
268	Limeade, prepared from frozen concentrate	8	fluid ounce(s)	247	212.6	128	0	34.1	0	0	0	0	0
14266	Odwalla strawberry C monster smoothie blend	8	fluid ounce(s)	240	—	160	2.0	38.0	0	0	0	0	0
10080	Odwalla strawberry lemonade quencher	8	fluid ounce(s)	240	—	110	0	28.0	0	0	0	0	0
10099	Snapple fruit punch fruit drink	8	fluid ounce(s)	240	—	110	0	29.0	0	0	0	0	0
10096	Snapple kiwi strawberry fruit drink	8	fluid ounce(s)	240	211.2	110	0	28.0	0	0	0	0	0
SlimFast ready-to-drink shake													
16054	French vanilla ready to drink shake	11	fluid ounce(s)	325	—	220	10.0	40.0	5.0	2.5	0.5	1.5	0.5
40447	Optima rich chocolate royal ready-to-drink shake	11	fluid ounce(s)	330	—	180	10.0	24.0	5.0	5.0	1.0	3.5	0.5
16055	Strawberries n' cream ready to drink shake	11	fluid ounce(s)	325	—	220	10.0	40.0	5.0	2.5	0.5	1.5	0.5
Tea													
33179	Decaffeinated, prepared	8	fluid ounce(s)	237	236.3	2	0	0.7	0	0	0	0	0
1877	Herbal, prepared	8	fluid ounce(s)	237	236.1	2	0	0.5	0	0	0	0	0
735	Instant tea mix, lemon flavored with sugar, prepared	8	fluid ounce(s)	259	236.2	91	0	22.3	0.3	0.2	0	0	0
734	Instant tea mix, unsweetened, prepared	8	fluid ounce(s)	237	236.1	2	0.1	0.4	0	0	0	0	0
733	Tea, prepared	8	fluid ounce(s)	237	236.3	2	0	0.7	0	0	0	0	0
Water													
1413	Mineral water, carbonated	8	fluid ounce(s)	237	236.8	0	0	0	0	0	0	0	0
33183	Poland spring water, bottled	8	fluid ounce(s)	237	237.0	0	0	0	0	0	0	0	0
1821	Tap water	8	fluid ounce(s)	237	236.8	0	0	0	0	0	0	0	0
1879	Tonic water	8	fluid ounce(s)	244	222.3	83	0	21.5	0	0	0	0	0
Fats and Oils													
Butter													
104	Butter	1	tablespoon(s)	14	2.3	102	0.1	0	0	11.5	7.3	3.0	0.4
2522	Butter Buds, dry butter substitute	1	teaspoon(s)	2	—	5	0	2.0	0	0	0	0	0
921	Unsalted	1	tablespoon(s)	14	2.5	102	0.1	0	0	11.5	7.3	3.0	0.4
107	Whipped	1	tablespoon(s)	9	1.5	67	0.1	0	0	7.6	4.7	2.2	0.3
944	Whipped, unsalted	1	tablespoon(s)	11	2.0	82	0.1	0	0	9.2	5.9	2.4	0.3
Fats, cooking													
2671	Beef tallow, semisolid	1	tablespoon(s)	13	0	115	0	0	0	12.8	6.4	5.4	0.5
922	Chicken fat	1	tablespoon(s)	13	0	115	0	0	0	12.8	3.8	5.7	2.7
5454	Household shortening with vegetable oil	1	tablespoon(s)	13	0	115	0	0	0	13.0	3.4	5.5	2.7
111	Lard	1	tablespoon(s)	13	0	115	0	0	0	12.8	5.0	5.8	1.4
Margarine													
114	Margarine	1	tablespoon(s)	14	2.3	101	0	0.1	0	11.4	2.1	5.5	3.4
5439	Soft	1	tablespoon(s)	14	2.3	103	0.1	0.1	0	11.6	1.7	4.4	2.1
32329	Soft, unsalted, with hydrogenated soybean and cottonseed oils	1	tablespoon(s)	14	2.5	101	0.1	0.1	0	11.3	2.0	5.4	3.5
928	Unsalted	1	tablespoon(s)	14	2.6	101	0.1	0.1	0	11.3	2.1	5.2	3.5
119	Whipped	1	tablespoon(s)	9	1.5	64	0.1	0.1	0	7.2	1.2	3.2	2.5
Spreads													
54657	I Can't Believe It's Not Butter!, tub, soya oil (non-hydrogenated)	1	tablespoon(s)	14	2.3	103	0.1	0.1	0	11.6	2.8	2.0	5.1
2708	Mayonnaise with soybean and safflower oils	1	tablespoon(s)	14	2.1	99	0.2	0.4	0	11.0	1.2	1.8	7.6
16157	Promise vegetable oil spread, stick	1	tablespoon(s)	14	4.2	90	0	0	0	10.0	2.5	2.0	4.0

PAGE KEY: A-4 = Breads/Baked Goods A-10 = Cereal/Rice/Pasta A-14 = Fruit A-20 = Vegetables/Legumes A-30 = Nuts/Seeds A-32 = Vegetarian
A-34 = Dairy A-42 = Eggs A-42 = Seafood A-46 = Meats A-50 = Poultry A-50 = Processed Meats A-52 = Beverages A-56 = Fats/Oils A-58 = Sweets
A-60 = Spices/Condiments/Sauces A-64 = Mixed Foods/Soups/Sandwiches A-70 = Fast Food A-90 = Convenience A-92 = Baby Foods

CHOL (mg)	CALC (mg)	IRON (mg)	MAGN (mg)	POTA (mg)	SODI (mg)	ZINC (mg)	VIT A (µg)	THIA (mg)	VIT E (mg α)	RIBO (mg)	NIAC (mg)	VIT B6 (mg)	FOLA (µg DFE)	VIT C (mg)	VIT B12 (µg)	SELE (µg)
0	14	0.45	5.0	49.6	31.0	0.19	—	0.03	—	0.05	0.04	0.01	4.3	41.6	0	1.0
0	0	0.00	—	10.1	10.1	—	0	—	—	—	—	—	—	6.0	—	—
0	10	0.39	5.0	37.2	9.9	0.05	0	0.01	0.02	0.05	0.04	0.01	2.5	9.7	0	0.2
0	5	0.00	4.9	24.7	7.4	0.02	0	0.01	0.00	0.01	0.02	0.01	2.5	7.7	0	0.2
0	20	0.72	—	0	20.0	—	0	—	—	—	—	—	—	600.0	0	—
0	0	0.00	—	70.0	10.0	—	0	—	—	—	—	—	—	54.0	0	—
0	0	0.00	—	20.0	10.0	—	0	—	—	—	—	—	—	0	0	—
0	0	0.00	—	40.0	10.0	—	0	—	—	—	—	—	—	0	0	—
5	400	2.70	140.0	600.0	220.0	2.25	—	0.52	—	0.59	7.00	0.70	120.0	60.0	2.1	17.5
5	1000	2.70	140.0	600.0	220.0	2.25	—	0.52	—	0.59	7.00	0.70	120.0	30.0	2.1	17.5
5	400	2.70	140.0	600.0	220.0	2.25	—	0.52	—	0.59	7.00	0.70	120.0	60.0	2.1	17.5
0	0	0.04	7.1	87.7	7.1	0.04	0	0.00	0.00	0.03	0.00	0.00	11.9	0	0	0
0	5	0.18	2.4	21.3	2.4	0.09	0	0.02	0.00	0.01	0.00	0.00	2.4	0	0	0
0	5	0.05	2.6	38.9	5.2	0.02	0	0.00	0.00	0.00	0.02	0.00	0	0	0	0.3
0	7	0.02	4.7	42.7	9.5	0.02	0	0.00	0.00	0.01	0.07	0.00	0	0	0	0
0	0	0.04	7.1	87.7	7.1	0.04	0	0.00	0.00	0.03	0.00	0.00	11.9	0	0	0
0	33	0.00	0	0	2.4	0.00	0	0.00	—	0.00	0.00	0.00	0	0	0	0
0	2	0.02	2.4	0	2.4	0.00	0	0.00	—	0.00	0.00	0.00	0	0	0	0
0	7	0.00	2.4	2.4	7.1	0.00	0	0.00	0.00	0.00	0.00	0.00	0	0	0	0
0	2	0.02	0	0	29.3	0.24	0	0.00	0.00	0.00	0.00	0.00	0	0	0	0
31	3	0.00	0.3	3.4	81.8	0.01	97.1	0.00	0.32	0.01	0.01	0.00	0.4	0	0	0.1
0	0	0.00	0	1.6	120.0	0.00	0	0.00	0.00	0.00	0.00	0.00	0	0	0	—
31	3	0.00	0.3	3.4	1.6	0.01	97.1	0.00	0.32	0.01	0.01	0.00	0.4	0	0	0.1
21	2	0.01	0.2	2.4	77.7	0.01	64.3	0.21	0.00	0.00	0.00	0.00	0.3	0	0	0.1
25	3	0.00	0.2	2.7	1.3	0.01	78.0	0.00	0.26	0.00	0.00	0.00	0.3	0	0	0.1
14	0	0.00	0	0	0	0.00	0	0.00	0.34	0.00	0.00	0.00	0	0	0	0
11	0	0.00	0	0	0	0.00	0	0.00	0.34	0.00	0.00	0.00	0	0	0	0
0	0	0.00	0	0	0	0.00	0	0.00	—	0.00	0.00	0.00	0	0	0	—
12	0	0.00	0	0	0	0.01	0	0.00	0.07	0.00	0.00	0.00	0	0	0	0
0	4	0.01	0.4	5.9	133.0	0.00	115.5	0.00	1.26	0.01	0.00	0.00	0.1	0	0	0
0	4	0.00	0.3	5.5	155.4	0.00	142.7	0.00	1.00	0.00	0.00	0.00	0.1	0	0	0
0	4	0.00	0.3	5.4	3.9	0.00	103.1	0.00	0.98	0.00	0.00	0.00	0.1	0	0	0
0	2	0.00	0.3	3.5	0.3	0.00	115.5	0.00	1.80	0.00	0.00	0.00	0.1	0	0	0
0	2	0.00	0.2	3.4	97.1	0.00	73.7	0.00	0.45	0.00	0.00	0.00	0.1	0	0	0
0	4	0.00	0.3	5.5	155.3	0.00	142.6	0.00	0.72	0.00	0.00	0.00	0.1	0	0	0
8	2	0.06	0.1	4.7	78.4	0.01	11.6	0.00	3.03	0.00	0.00	0.08	1.1	0	0	0.2
0	10	0.18	—	8.7	90.0	—	—	0.00	—	0.00	0.00	—	—	0.6	—	—

A

D&W+ Code	Food Description	QTY	Measure	Wt (g)	H₂0 (g)	Ener (cal)	Prot (g)	Carb (g)	Fiber (g)	Fat (g)	Fat Breakdown (g)		
											Sat	Mono	Poly
Fats and Oils—continued													
	Oils												
2681	Canola	1	tablespoon(s)	14	0	120	0	0	0	13.6	1.0	8.6	3.8
120	Corn	1	tablespoon(s)	14	0	120	0	0	0	13.6	1.8	3.8	7.4
122	Olive	1	tablespoon(s)	14	0	119	0	0	0	13.5	1.9	9.9	1.4
124	Peanut	1	tablespoon(s)	14	0	119	0	0	0	13.5	2.3	6.2	4.3
2693	Safflower	1	tablespoon(s)	14	0	120	0	0	0	13.6	0.8	10.2	2.0
923	Sesame	1	tablespoon(s)	14	0	120	0	0	0	13.6	1.9	5.4	5.7
128	Soybean, hydrogenated	1	tablespoon(s)	14	0	120	0	0	0	13.6	2.0	5.8	5.1
130	Soybean, with soybean and cotton-seed oil	1	tablespoon(s)	14	0	120	0	0	0	13.6	2.4	4.0	6.5
2700	Sunflower	1	tablespoon(s)	14	0	120	0	0	0	13.6	1.8	6.3	5.0
357	**Pam original no-stick cooking spray**	1	serving(s)	0	0.2	0	0	0	0	0	0	0	0
	Salad Dressing												
132	Blue cheese	2	tablespoon(s)	30	9.7	151	1.4	2.2	0	15.7	3.0	3.7	8.3
133	Blue cheese, low calorie	2	tablespoon(s)	32	25.4	32	1.6	0.9	0	2.3	0.8	0.6	0.8
1764	Caesar	2	tablespoon(s)	30	10.3	158	0.4	0.9	0	17.3	2.6	4.1	9.9
29654	Creamy, reduced calorie, fat-free, cholesterol-free, sour cream and/or buttermilk and oil	2	tablespoon(s)	32	23.9	34	0.4	6.4	0	0.9	0.2	0.2	0.5
29617	Creamy, reduced calorie, sour cream and/or buttermilk and oil	2	tablespoon(s)	30	22.2	48	0.5	2.1	0	4.2	0.6	1.0	2.4
134	French	2	tablespoon(s)	32	11.7	146	0.2	5.0	0	14.3	1.8	2.7	6.7
135	French, low fat	2	tablespoon(s)	32	17.4	74	0.2	9.4	0.4	4.3	0.4	1.9	1.6
136	Italian	2	tablespoon(s)	29	16.6	86	0.1	3.1	0	8.3	1.3	1.9	3.8
137	Italian, diet	2	tablespoon(s)	30	25.4	23	0.1	1.4	0	1.9	0.1	0.7	0.5
139	Mayonnaise-type	2	tablespoon(s)	29	11.7	115	0.3	7.0	0	9.8	1.4	2.6	5.3
942	Oil and vinegar	2	tablespoon(s)	32	15.2	144	0	0.8	0	16.0	2.9	4.7	7.7
1765	Ranch	2	tablespoon(s)	30	11.6	146	0.1	1.6	0	15.8	2.3	5.2	7.6
3666	Ranch, reduced calorie	2	tablespoon(s)	30	20.5	62	0.1	2.2	0	6.1	1.1	1.8	2.9
940	Russian	2	tablespoon(s)	30	11.6	107	0.5	9.3	0.7	7.8	1.2	1.8	4.4
939	Russian, low calorie	2	tablespoon(s)	32	20.8	45	0.2	8.8	0.1	1.3	0.2	0.3	0.7
941	Sesame seed	2	tablespoon(s)	30	11.8	133	0.9	2.6	0.3	13.6	1.9	3.6	7.5
142	Thousand Island	2	tablespoon(s)	32	14.9	118	0.3	4.7	0.3	11.2	1.6	2.5	5.8
143	Thousand Island, low calorie	2	tablespoon(s)	30	18.2	61	0.3	6.7	0.4	3.9	0.2	1.9	0.8
	Sandwich Spreads												
138	Mayonnaise with soybean oil	1	tablespoon(s)	14	2.1	99	0.1	0.4	0	11.0	1.6	2.7	5.8
140	Mayonnaise, low calorie	1	tablespoon(s)	16	10.0	37	0	2.6	0	3.1	0.5	0.7	1.7
141	Tartar sauce	2	tablespoon(s)	28	8.7	144	0.3	4.1	0.1	14.4	2.2	3.8	7.7
Sweets													
4799	**Butterscotch or caramel topping**	2	tablespoon(s)	41	13.1	103	0.6	27.0	0.4	0	0	0	0
	Candy												
1786	Almond Joy candy bar	1	item(s)	45	4.3	220	2.0	27.0	2.0	12.0	8.0	3.3	0.7
1785	Bit-O-Honey candy	6	item(s)	40	—	190	1.0	39.0	0	3.5	2.5	—	—
33375	Butterscotch candy	2	piece(s)	12	0.6	47	0	10.8	0	0.4	0.2	0.1	0
1701	Chewing gum, stick	1	item(s)	3	0.1	7	0	2.0	0.1	0	0	0	0
33378	Chocolate fudge with nuts, prepared	2	piece(s)	38	2.9	175	1.7	25.8	1.0	7.2	2.5	1.5	2.9
1787	Jelly beans	15	item(s)	43	2.7	159	0	39.8	0	0	0	0	0
1784	Kit Kat wafer bar	1	item(s)	42	0.8	210	3.0	27.0	0.5	11.0	7.0	3.5	0.3
4674	Krackel candy bar	1	item(s)	41	0.6	210	2.0	28.0	0.5	10.0	6.0	3.9	0.4
4934	Licorice	4	piece(s)	44	7.3	154	1.1	35.1	0	1.0	0	0.1	0
1780	Life Savers candy	1	item(s)	2	—	8	0	2.0	0	0	0	0	0
1790	Lollipop	1	item(s)	28	—	108	0	28.0	0	0	0	0	0
4679	M & Ms peanut chocolate candy, small bag	1	item(s)	49	0.9	250	5.0	30.0	2.0	13.0	5.0	5.4	2.1
1781	M&M'S plain chocolate candy, small bag	1	item(s)	48	0.8	240	2.0	34.0	1.0	10.0	6.0	3.3	0.3
4673	Milk chocolate bar, Symphony	1	item(s)	91	0.9	483	7.7	52.8	1.5	27.8	16.7	7.2	0.6

PAGE KEY: A-4 = Breads/Baked Goods A-10 = Cereal/Rice/Pasta A-14 = Fruit A-20 = Vegetables/Legumes A-30 = Nuts/Seeds A-32 = Vegetarian
A-34 = Dairy A-42 = Eggs A-42 = Seafood A-46 = Meats A-50 = Poultry A-50 = Processed Meats A-52 = Beverages A-56 = Fats/Oils A-58 = Sweets
A-60 = Spices/Condiments/Sauces A-64 = Mixed Foods/Soups/Sandwiches A-70 = Fast Food A-90 = Convenience A-92 = Baby Foods

A

Chol (mg)	Calc (mg)	Iron (mg)	Magn (mg)	Pota (mg)	Sodi (mg)	Zinc (mg)	Vit A (µg)	Thia (mg)	Vit E (mg α)	Ribo (mg)	Niac (mg)	Vit B6 (mg)	Fola (µg DFE)	Vit C (mg)	Vit B12 (µg)	Sele (µg)
0	0	0.00	0	0	0	0.00	0	0.00	2.37	0.00	0.00	0.00	0	0	0	0
0	0	0.00	0	0	0	0.00	0	0.00	1.94	0.00	0.00	0.00	0	0	0	0
0	0	0.07	0	0.1	0.3	0.00	0	0.00	1.93	0.00	0.00	0.00	0	0	0	0
0	0	0.00	0	0	0	0.00	0	0.00	2.11	0.00	0.00	0.00	0	0	0	0
0	0	0.00	0	0	0	0.00	0	0.00	4.63	0.00	0.00	0.00	0	0	0	0
0	0	0.00	0	0	0	0.00	0	0.00	0.19	0.00	0.00	0.00	0	0	0	0
0	0	0.00	0	0	0	0.00	0	0.00	1.10	0.00	0.00	0.00	0	0	0	0
0	0	0.00	0	0	0	0.00	0	0.00	1.64	0.00	0.00	0.00	0	0	0	0
0	0	0.00	0	0	0	0.00	0	0.00	5.58	0.00	0.00	0.00	0	0	0	0
0	0	0.00	0	0.3	1.5	0.01	0.1	0.00	0.00	0.00	0.00	0.00	0	0	0	0
5	24	0.06	0	11.1	328.2	0.08	20.1	0.00	1.80	0.03	0.03	0.01	7.8	0.6	0.1	0.3
0	28	0.16	2.2	1.6	384.0	0.08	—	0.01	0.08	0.03	0.01	0.01	1.0	0.1	0.1	0.5
1	7	0.05	0.6	8.7	323.4	0.03	0.6	0.00	1.56	0.00	0.01	0.00	0.9	0	0	0.5
0	12	0.08	1.6	42.6	320.0	0.05	0.3	0.00	0.21	0.01	0.01	0.01	1.9	0	0	0.5
0	2	0.03	0.6	10.8	306.9	0.01	—	0.00	0.71	0.00	0.01	0.01	0	0.1	0	0.5
0	8	0.25	1.6	21.4	267.5	0.09	7.4	0.01	1.60	0.01	0.06	0.00	0	0	0	0
0	4	0.27	2.6	34.2	257.3	0.06	8.6	0.01	0.09	0.01	0.14	0.01	0.6	0	0	0.5
0	2	0.18	0.9	14.1	486.3	0.03	0.6	0.00	1.47	0.01	0.00	0.01	0	0	0	0.6
2	3	0.19	1.2	25.5	409.8	0.05	0.3	0.00	0.06	0.00	0.00	0.02	0	0	0	2.4
8	4	0.05	0.6	2.6	209.0	0.05	6.2	0.00	0.60	0.01	0.00	0.01	1.8	0	0.1	0.5
0	0	0.00	0	2.6	0.3	0.00	0	0.00	1.46	0.00	0.00	0.00	0	0	0	0.5
1	4	0.03	1.2	8.4	354.0	0.01	5.4	0.00	1.84	0.01	0.00	0.00	0.3	0.1	0	0.1
0	5	0.01	1.5	8.4	413.7	0.01	0.9	0.00	0.72	0.01	0.00	0.00	0.3	0.1	0	0.1
0	6	0.20	3.0	51.9	282.3	0.06	13.2	0.01	0.98	0.01	0.16	0.02	1.5	1.4	0	0.5
2	6	0.18	0	50.2	277.8	0.02	0.6	0.00	0.12	0.00	0.00	0.00	1.0	1.9	0	0.5
0	6	0.18	0	47.1	300.0	0.02	0.6	0.00	1.50	0.00	0.00	0.00	0	0	0	0.5
8	5	0.37	2.6	34.2	276.2	0.08	4.5	0.46	1.28	0.01	0.13	0.00	0	0	0	0.5
0	5	0.27	2.1	60.6	249.3	0.05	4.8	0.01	0.30	0.01	0.13	0.00	0	0	0	0
5	1	0.03	0.1	1.7	78.4	0.02	11.2	0.01	0.72	0.01	0.00	0.08	0.7	0	0	0.2
4	0	0.00	0	1.6	79.5	0.01	0	0.00	0.32	0.00	0.00	0.00	0	0	0	0.3
8	6	0.20	0.8	10.1	191.5	0.05	20.2	0.00	0.97	0.00	0.01	0.07	2.0	0.1	0.1	0.5
0	22	0.08	2.9	34.4	143.1	0.07	11.1	0.01	—	0.03	0.01	0.01	0.8	0.1	0	0
0	18	0.33	30.3	126.5	65.0	0.36	0	0.01	—	0.06	0.21	—	0	0	—	—
0	20	0.00	—	—	150.0	—	0	—	—	—	—	—	—	0	—	—
1	0	0.00	0	0.4	46.9	0.01	3.4	0.00	0.01	0.00	0.00	0.00	0	0	0	0.1
0	0	0.00	0	0.1	0	0.00	0	0.00	0.00	0.00	0.00	0.00	0	0	0	0
5	22	0.74	20.9	69.5	14.8	0.54	14.4	0.02	0.09	0.03	0.12	0.03	6.1	0.1	0	1.1
0	1	0.05	0.9	15.7	21.3	0.02	0	0.00	0.00	0.01	0.00	0.00	0	0	0	0.5
3	60	0.36	16.4	126.0	30.0	0.51	0	0.07	—	0.22	1.07	0.05	59.6	0	0.1	2.0
3	40	0.36	—	168.8	50.0	—	0	—	—	—	—	—	—	0	—	—
0	0	0.22	2.6	28.2	126.3	0.07	0	0.01	0.07	0.01	0.04	0.00	0	0	0	—
0	0	0.00	—	0	0	0.00	0	0.00	—	0.00	0.00	—	—	0	—	0
0	0	0.00	—	—	10.8	—	0	0.00	—	0.00	0.00	—	—	0	—	1.0
5	40	0.36	36.5	170.6	25.0	1.13	14.8	0.03	—	0.06	1.60	0.04	17.3	0.6	0.1	1.9
5	40	0.36	19.6	127.4	30.0	0.46	14.8	0.02	—	0.06	0.10	0.01	2.9	0.6	0.1	1.4
22	228	0.82	61.0	398.6	91.9	1.00	0	0.06	—	0.25	0.14	0.10	10.9	2.0	0.4	—

D&W+ Code	Food Description	QTY	Measure	Wt (g)	H₂O (g)	Ener (cal)	Prot (g)	Carb (g)	Fiber (g)	Fat (g)	Fat Breakdown (g)		
											Sat	Mono	Poly
Sweets—continued													
1783	Milky Way bar	1	item(s)	58	3.7	270	2.0	41.0	1.0	10.0	5.0	3.5	0.3
1788	Peanut brittle	1½	ounce(s)	43	0.3	207	3.2	30.3	1.1	8.1	1.8	3.4	1.9
1789	Reese's peanut butter cups	2	piece(s)	51	0.8	280	6.0	19.0	2.0	15.5	6.0	7.2	2.7
4689	Reese's pieces candy, small bag	1	item(s)	43	1.1	220	5.0	26.0	1.0	11.0	7.0	0.9	0.4
33399	Semisweet chocolate candy, made with butter	½	ounce(s)	14	0.1	68	0.6	9.0	0.8	4.2	2.5	1.4	0.1
1782	Snickers bar	1	item(s)	59	3.2	280	4.0	35.0	1.0	14.0	5.0	6.1	2.9
4694	Special Dark chocolate bar	1	item(s)	41	0.4	220	2.0	25.0	3.0	12.0	8.0	4.6	0.4
4695	Starburst fruit chews, original fruits	1	package(s)	59	3.9	240	0	48.0	0	5.0	1.0	2.1	1.8
4698	Taffy	3	piece(s)	45	2.2	179	0	41.2	0	1.5	0.9	0.4	0.1
4699	Three Musketeers bar	1	item(s)	60	3.5	260	2.0	46.0	1.0	8.0	4.5	2.6	0.3
4702	Twix caramel cookie bars	2	item(s)	58	2.4	280	3.0	37.0	1.0	14.0	5.0	7.7	0.5
4705	York peppermint pattie	1	item(s)	39	3.9	160	0.5	32.0	0.5	3.0	1.5	1.2	0.1
	Frosting, icing												
4760	Chocolate frosting, ready to eat	2	tablespoon(s)	31	5.2	122	0.3	19.4	0.3	5.4	1.7	2.8	0.6
4771	Creamy vanilla frosting, ready to eat	2	tablespoon(s)	28	4.2	117	0	19.0	0	4.5	0.8	1.4	2.2
17291	Dec-A-Cake variety pack candy decoration	1	teaspoon(s)	4	—	15	0	3.0	0	0.5	0	—	—
536	White icing	2	tablespoon(s)	40	3.6	162	0.1	31.8	0	4.2	0.8	2.0	1.2
	Gelatin												
13697	Gelatin snack, all flavors	1	item(s)	99	96.8	70	1.0	17.0	0	0	0	0	0
2616	Sugar free, low calorie mixed fruit gelatin mix, prepared	½	cup(s)	121	—	10	1.0	0	0	0	0	0	0
548	**Honey**	1	tablespoon(s)	21	3.6	64	0.1	17.3	0	0	0	0	0
	Jams, jellies												
550	Jam or preserves	1	tablespoon(s)	20	6.1	56	0.1	13.8	0.2	0	0	0	0
42199	Jams, preserves, dietetic, all flavors, w/sodium saccharin	1	tablespoon(s)	14	6.4	18	0	7.5	0.4	0	0	0	0
552	Jelly	1	tablespoon(s)	21	6.3	56	0	14.7	0.2	0	0	0	0
545	**Marshmallows**	4	item(s)	29	4.7	92	0.5	23.4	0	0.1	0	0	0
4800	**Marshmallow cream topping**	2	tablespoon(s)	40	7.9	129	0.3	31.6	0	0.1	0	0	0
555	**Molasses**	1	tablespoon(s)	20	4.4	58	0	14.9	0	0	0	0	0
4780	**Popsicle or ice pop**	1	item(s)	59	47.5	47	0	11.3	0	0.1	0	0	0
	Sugar												
559	Brown sugar, packed	1	teaspoon(s)	5	0.1	17	0	4.5	0	0	0	0	0
563	Powdered sugar, sifted	⅓	cup(s)	33	0.1	130	0	33.2	0	0	0	0	0
561	White granulated sugar	1	teaspoon(s)	4	0	16	0	4.2	0	0	0	0	0
	Sugar substitute												
1760	Equal sweetener, packet size	1	item(s)	1	—	0	0	0.9	0	0	0	0	0
13029	Splenda granular no calorie sweetener	1	teaspoon(s)	1	—	0	0	0.5	0	0	0	0	0
1759	Sweet N Low sugar substitute, packet	1	item(s)	1	0.1	4	0	0.5	0	0	0	0	0
	Syrup												
3148	Chocolate syrup	2	tablespoon(s)	38	11.6	105	0.8	24.4	1.0	0.4	0.2	0.1	0
29676	Maple syrup	¼	cup(s)	80	25.7	209	0	53.7	0	0.2	0	0.1	0.1
4795	Pancake syrup	¼	cup(s)	80	30.4	187	0	49.2	0	0	0	0	0
Spices, Condiments, Sauces													
	Spices												
807	Allspice, ground	1	teaspoon(s)	2	0.2	5	0.1	1.4	0.4	0.2	0	0	0
1171	Anise seeds	1	teaspoon(s)	2	0.2	7	0.4	1.1	0.3	0.3	0	0.2	0.1
729	Bakers' yeast, active	1	teaspoon(s)	4	0.3	12	1.5	1.5	0.8	0.2	0	0.1	0
683	Baking powder, double acting with phosphate	1	teaspoon(s)	5	0.2	2	0	1.1	0	0	0	0	0
1611	Baking soda	1	teaspoon(s)	5	0	0	0	0	0	0	0	0	0
8552	Basil	1	teaspoon(s)	1	0.8	0	0	0	0	0	0	0	0
34959	Basil, fresh	1	piece(s)	1	0.5	0	0	0	0	0	0	0	0

PAGE KEY: A-4 = Breads/Baked Goods A-10 = Cereal/Rice/Pasta A-14 = Fruit A-20 = Vegetables/Legumes A-30 = Nuts/Seeds A-32 = Vegetarian A-34 = Dairy A-42 = Eggs A-42 = Seafood A-46 = Meats A-50 = Poultry A-50 = Processed Meats A-52 = Beverages A-56 = Fats/Oils A-58 = Sweets A-60 = Spices/Condiments/Sauces A-64 = Mixed Foods/Soups/Sandwiches A-70 = Fast Food A-90 = Convenience A-92 = Baby Foods

A

CHOL (mg)	CALC (mg)	IRON (mg)	MAGN (mg)	POTA (mg)	SODI (mg)	ZINC (mg)	VIT A (µg)	THIA (mg)	VIT E (mg α)	RIBO (mg)	NIAC (mg)	VIT B6 (mg)	FOLA (µg DFE)	VIT C (mg)	VIT B12 (µg)	SELE (µg)
5	60	0.18	19.8	140.1	95.0	0.41	15.1	0.02	—	0.06	0.20	0.02	5.8	0.6	0.2	3.3
5	11	0.51	17.9	71.4	189.2	0.37	16.6	0.05	1.08	0.01	1.12	0.03	19.6	0	0	1.1
3	40	0.72	45.4	217.4	180.0	0.93	0	0.12	—	0.08	2.35	0.07	28.1	0	0.1	2.3
0	20	0.00	18.9	169.9	80.0	0.32	0	0.04	—	0.06	1.22	0.03	12.0	0	0.1	0.8
3	5	0.44	16.3	51.7	1.6	0.23	0.4	0.01	—	0.01	0.06	0.01	0.4	0	0	0.5
5	40	0.36	42.3	—	140.0	1.37	15.3	0.03	—	0.06	1.60	0.05	23.5	0.6	0.1	2.7
0	0	1.80	45.5	136.0	50.0	0.59	0	0.01	—	0.02	0.16	0.01	0.8	0	0	1.2
0	10	0.18	0.6	1.2	0	0.00	—	0.00	—	0.00	0.00	0.00	0	30	0	0.5
4	4	0.00	0	1.4	23.4	0.09	12.2	0.01	0.04	0.01	0.00	0.00	0	0	0	0.3
5	20	0.36	17.5	80.3	110.0	0.33	14.5	0.01	—	0.03	0.20	0.01	0	0.6	0.1	1.5
5	40	0.36	18.5	116.8	115.0	0.45	15.0	0.09	—	0.13	0.69	0.01	13.9	0.6	0.1	1.2
0	0	0.33	23.4	66.1	10.0	0.28	0	0.01	—	0.03	0.31	0.01	1.5	0	0	—
0	2	0.44	6.4	60.0	56.1	0.09	0	0.00	0.48	0.00	0.03	0.00	0.3	0	0	0.2
0	1	0.04	0.3	9.5	51.5	0.01	0	0.00	0.43	0.08	0.06	0.00	2.2	0	0	0
0	0	0.00	—	—	15.0	—	0	—	—	—	—	—	—	0	—	—
0	4	0.01	0.4	5.6	76.4	0.01	44.4	0.00	0.32	0.01	0.00	0.00	0	0	0	0.3
0	0	0.00	—	0	40.0	—	0	—	—	—	—	—	—	0	—	—
0	0	0.00	0	0	50.0	0.00	0	0.00	0.00	0.00	0.00	0.00	0	0	0	—
0	1	0.08	0.4	10.9	0.8	0.04	0	0.00	0.00	0.01	0.02	0.01	0.4	0.1	0	0.2
0	4	0.10	0.8	15.4	6.4	0.01	0	0.00	0.02	0.02	0.01	0.00	2.2	1.8	0	0.4
0	1	0.56	0.7	9.7	0	0.01	0	0.00	0.01	0.00	0.00	0.00	1.3	0	0	0.2
0	1	0.04	1.3	11.3	6.3	0.01	0	0.00	0.00	0.00	0.01	0.00	0.4	0.2	0	0.1
0	1	0.06	0.6	1.4	23.0	0.01	0	0.00	0.00	0.00	0.02	0.00	0.3	0	0	0.5
0	1	0.08	0.8	2.0	32.0	0.01	0	0.00	0.00	0.00	0.03	0.00	0.4	0	0	0.7
0	41	0.94	48.4	292.8	7.4	0.05	0	0.01	0.00	0.00	0.18	0.13	0	0	0	3.6
0	0	0.31	0.6	8.9	4.1	0.08	0	0.00	0.00	0.00	0.00	0.00	0	0.4	0	0.1
0	4	0.03	0.4	6.1	1.3	0.00	0	0.00	0.00	0.00	0.01	0.00	0	0	0	0.1
0	0	0.01	0	0.7	0.3	0.00	0	0.00	0.00	0.00	0.00	0.00	0	0	0	0.2
0	0	0.00	0	0.1	0	0.00	0	0.00	0.00	0.00	0.00	0.00	0	0	0	0
0	0	0.00	0	0	0	0.00	0	0.00	0.00	0.00	0.00	0.00	0	0	0	0
0	0	0.00	—	—	0	—	—	0.00	—	0.00	0.00	—	—	0	0	—
0	0	0.00	—	—	0	—	0	—	—	0.00	—	—	—	0	0	—
0	5	0.79	24.4	84.0	27.0	0.27	0	0.00	0.01	0.01	0.12	0.00	0.8	0.1	0	0.5
0	54	0.96	11.2	163.2	7.2	3.32	0	0.01	0.00	0.01	0.02	0.00	0	0	0	0.5
0	2	0.02	1.6	12.0	65.6	0.06	0	0.01	0.00	0.01	0.00	0.00	0	0	0	0
0	13	0.13	2.6	19.8	1.5	0.01	0.5	0.00	—	0.00	0.05	0.00	0.7	0.7	0	0.1
0	14	0.77	3.6	30.3	0.3	0.11	0.3	0.01	—	0.01	0.06	0.01	0.2	0.4	0	0.1
0	3	0.66	3.9	80.0	2.0	0.25	0	0.09	0.00	0.21	1.59	0.06	93.6	0	0	1.0
0	339	0.51	1.8	0.2	363.1	0.00	0	0.00	0.00	0.00	0.00	0.00	0	0	0	0
0	0	0.00	0	0	1258.6	0.00	0	0.00	0.00	0.00	0.00	0.00	0	0	0	0
0	2	0.02	0.6	2.6	0	0.01	2.3	0.00	0.01	0.00	0.01	0.00	0.6	0.2	0	0
0	1	0.01	0.4	2.3	0	0.00	1.3	0.00	—	0.00	0.00	0.00	0.3	0.1	0	0

A

D&W+ Code	Food Description	QTY	Measure	Wt (g)	H₂0 (g)	Ener (cal)	Prot (g)	Carb (g)	Fiber (g)	Fat (g)	Fat Breakdown (g) Sat	Mono	Poly
	SPICES, CONDIMENTS, SAUCES—CONTINUED												
808	Basil, ground	1	teaspoon(s)	1	0.1	4	0.2	0.9	0.6	0.1	0	0	0
809	Bay leaf	1	teaspoon(s)	1	0	2	0	0.5	0.2	0.1	0	0	0
11720	Betel leaves	1	ounce(s)	28	—	17	1.8	2.4	0	0	—	—	—
730	Brewers' yeast	1	teaspoon(s)	3	0.1	8	1.0	1.0	0.8	0	0	0	0
11710	Capers	1	teaspoon(s)	5	—	0	0	0	0	0	0	0	0
1172	Caraway seeds	1	teaspoon(s)	2	0.2	7	0.4	1.0	0.8	0.3	0	0.2	0.1
1173	Celery seeds	1	teaspoon(s)	2	0.1	8	0.4	0.8	0.2	0.5	0	0.3	0.1
1174	Chervil, dried	1	teaspoon(s)	1	0	1	0.1	0.3	0.1	0	0	0	0
810	Chili powder	1	teaspoon(s)	3	0.2	8	0.3	1.4	0.9	0.4	0.1	0.1	0.2
8553	Chives, chopped	1	teaspoon(s)	1	0.9	0	0	0	0	0	0	0	0
51420	Cilantro (coriander)	1	teaspoon(s)	0	0.3	0	0	0	0	0	0	0	0
811	Cinnamon, ground	1	teaspoon(s)	2	0.2	6	0.1	1.9	1.2	0	0	0	0
812	Cloves, ground	1	teaspoon(s)	2	0.1	7	0.1	1.3	0.7	0.4	0.1	0	0.1
1175	Coriander leaf, dried	1	teaspoon(s)	1	0	2	0.1	0.3	0.1	0	0	0	0
1176	Coriander seeds	1	teaspoon(s)	2	0.2	5	0.2	1.0	0.8	0.3	0	0.2	0
1706	Cornstarch	1	tablespoon(s)	8	0.7	30	0	7.3	0.1	0	0	0	0
1177	Cumin seeds	1	teaspoon(s)	2	0.2	8	0.4	0.9	0.2	0.5	0	0.3	0.1
11729	Cumin, ground	1	teaspoon(s)	5	—	11	0.4	0.8	0.8	0.4	—	—	—
1178	Curry powder	1	teaspoon(s)	2	0.2	7	0.3	1.2	0.7	0.3	0	0.1	0.1
1179	Dill seeds	1	teaspoon(s)	2	0.2	6	0.3	1.2	0.4	0.3	0	0.2	0
1180	Dill weed, dried	1	teaspoon(s)	1	0.1	3	0.2	0.6	0.1	0	0	0	0
34949	Dill weed, fresh	5	piece(s)	1	0.9	0	0	0.1	0	0	0	0	0
4949	Fennel leaves, fresh	1	teaspoon(s)	1	0.9	0	0	0.1	0	0	—	—	—
1181	Fennel seeds	1	teaspoon(s)	2	0.2	7	0.3	1.0	0.8	0.3	0	0.2	0
1182	Fenugreek seeds	1	teaspoon(s)	4	0.3	12	0.9	2.2	0.9	0.2	0.1	—	—
11733	Garam masala, powder	1	ounce(s)	28	—	107	4.4	12.8	0	4.3	—	—	—
1067	Garlic clove	1	item(s)	3	1.8	4	0.2	1.0	0.1	0	0	0	0
813	Garlic powder	1	teaspoon(s)	3	0.2	9	0.5	2.0	0.3	0	0	0	0
1068	Ginger root	2	teaspoon(s)	4	3.1	3	0.1	0.7	0.1	0	0	0	0
1183	Ginger, ground	1	teaspoon(s)	2	0.2	6	0.2	1.3	0.2	0.1	0	0	0
35497	Leeks, bulb and lower-leaf, freeze-dried	¼	cup(s)	1	0	3	0.1	0.6	0.1	0	0	0	0
1184	Mace, ground	1	teaspoon(s)	2	0.1	8	0.1	0.9	0.3	0.6	0.2	0.2	0.1
1185	Marjoram, dried	1	teaspoon(s)	1	0	2	0.1	0.4	0.2	0	0	0	0
1186	Mustard seeds, yellow	1	teaspoon(s)	3	0.2	15	0.8	1.2	0.5	0.9	0	0.7	0.2
814	Nutmeg, ground	1	teaspoon(s)	2	0.1	12	0.1	1.1	0.5	0.8	0.6	0.1	0
2747	Onion flakes, dehydrated	1	teaspoon(s)	2	0.1	6	0.1	1.4	0.2	0	0	0	0
1187	Onion powder	1	teaspoon(s)	2	0.1	7	0.2	1.7	0.1	0	0	0	0
815	Oregano, ground	1	teaspoon(s)	2	0.1	5	0.2	1.0	0.6	0.2	0	0	0.1
816	Paprika	1	teaspoon(s)	2	0.2	6	0.3	1.2	0.8	0.3	0	0	0.2
817	Parsley, dried	1	teaspoon(s)	0	0	1	0.1	0.2	0.1	0	0	0	0
818	Pepper, black	1	teaspoon(s)	2	0.2	5	0.2	1.4	0.6	0.1	0	0	0
819	Pepper, cayenne	1	teaspoon(s)	2	0.1	6	0.2	1.0	0.5	0.3	0.1	0	0.2
1188	Pepper, white	1	teaspoon(s)	2	0.3	7	0.3	1.6	0.6	0.1	0	0	0
1189	Poppy seeds	1	teaspoon(s)	3	0.2	15	0.5	0.7	0.3	1.3	0.1	0.2	0.9
1190	Poultry seasoning	1	teaspoon(s)	2	0.1	5	0.1	1.0	0.2	0.1	0	0	0
1191	Pumpkin pie spice, powder	1	teaspoon(s)	2	0.1	6	0.1	1.2	0.3	0.2	0.1	0	0
1192	Rosemary, dried	1	teaspoon(s)	1	0.1	4	0.1	0.8	0.5	0.2	0.1	0	0
11723	Rosemary, fresh	1	teaspoon(s)	1	0.5	1	0	0.1	0.1	0	0	0	0
2722	Saffron powder	1	teaspoon(s)	1	0.1	2	0.1	0.5	0	0	0	0	0
11724	Sage	1	teaspoon(s)	1	—	1	0	0.3	0	0	—	—	—
1193	Sage, ground	1	teaspoon(s)	1	0.1	2	0.1	0.4	0.3	0.1	0	0	0
30189	Salt substitute	¼	teaspoon(s)	1	—	0	0	0	0	0	0	0	0
30190	Salt substitute, seasoned	¼	teaspoon(s)	1	—	1	0	0.1	0	0	0	—	—
822	Salt, table	¼	teaspoon(s)	2	0	0	0	0	0	0	0	0	0
1194	Savory, ground	1	teaspoon(s)	1	0.1	4	0.1	1.0	0.6	0.1	0	—	—
820	Sesame seed kernels, toasted	1	teaspoon(s)	3	0.1	15	0.5	0.7	0.5	1.3	0.2	0.5	0.6
11725	Sorrel	1	teaspoon(s)	3	—	1	0.1	0.1	0	0	—	—	—
11721	Spearmint	1	teaspoon(s)	2	1.6	1	0.1	0.2	0.1	0	0	0	0
35498	Sweet green peppers, freeze-dried	¼	cup(s)	2	0	5	0.3	1.1	0.3	0	0	0	0
11726	Tamarind leaves	1	ounce(s)	28	—	33	1.6	5.2	0	0.6	—	—	—
11727	Tarragon	1	ounce(s)	28	—	14	1.0	1.8	0	0.3	—	—	—

PAGE KEY: A-4 = Breads/Baked Goods A-10 = Cereal/Rice/Pasta A-14 = Fruit A-20 = Vegetables/Legumes A-30 = Nuts/Seeds A-32 = Vegetarian A-34 = Dairy A-42 = Eggs A-42 = Seafood A-46 = Meats A-50 = Poultry A-50 = Processed Meats A-52 = Beverages A-56 = Fats/Oils A-58 = Sweets A-60 = Spices/Condiments/Sauces A-64 = Mixed Foods/Soups/Sandwiches A-70 = Fast Food A-90 = Convenience A-92 = Baby Foods

A

CHOL (mg)	CALC (mg)	IRON (mg)	MAGN (mg)	POTA (mg)	SODI (mg)	ZINC (mg)	VIT A (µg)	THIA (mg)	VIT E (mg α)	RIBO (mg)	NIAC (mg)	VIT B_6 (mg)	FOLA (µg DFE)	VIT C (mg)	VIT B_{12} (µg)	SELE (µg)
0	30	0.58	5.9	48.1	0.5	0.08	6.6	0.00	0.10	0.00	0.09	0.03	3.8	0.9	0	0
0	5	0.25	0.7	3.2	0.1	0.02	1.9	0.00	—	0.00	0.01	0.01	1.1	0.3	0	0
0	110	2.29	—	155.9	2.0	—	—	0.04	—	0.07	0.19	—	—	0.9	0	0
0	6	0.46	6.1	50.7	3.3	0.21	0	0.41	—	0.11	1.00	0.06	104.3	0	0	0
0	—	—	—	—	105.0	—	—	—	—	—	—	—	—	—	0	—
0	14	0.34	5.4	28.4	0.4	0.11	0.4	0.01	0.05	0.01	0.07	0.01	0.2	0.4	0	0.3
0	35	0.89	8.8	28.0	3.2	0.13	0.1	0.01	0.02	0.01	0.06	0.01	0.2	0.3	0	0.2
0	8	0.19	0.8	28.4	0.5	0.05	1.8	0.00	—	0.00	0.03	0.01	1.6	0.3	0	0.2
0	7	0.37	4.4	49.8	26.3	0.07	38.6	0.01	0.75	0.02	0.20	0.09	2.6	1.7	0	0.2
0	1	0.01	0.4	3.0	0	0.01	2.2	0.00	0.01	0.00	0.01	0.00	1.1	0.6	0	0
0	0	0.01	0.1	1.7	0.2	0.00	1.1	0.00	0.01	0.00	0.00	0.00	0.2	0.1	0	0
0	23	0.19	1.4	9.9	0.2	0.04	0.3	0.00	0.05	0.00	0.03	0.00	0.1	0.1	0	0.1
0	14	0.18	5.5	23.1	5.1	0.02	0.6	0.00	0.17	0.01	0.03	0.01	2.0	1.7	0	0.1
0	7	0.25	4.2	26.8	1.3	0.02	1.8	0.01	0.01	0.01	0.01	0.00	1.6	3.4	0	0.2
0	13	0.29	5.9	22.8	0.6	0.08	0	0.00	—	0.01	0.03	—	0	0.4	0	0.5
0	0	0.03	0.2	0.2	0.7	0.01	0	0.00	—	0.00	0.00	0.00	0	0	0	0.2
0	20	1.39	7.7	37.5	3.5	0.10	1.3	0.01	0.07	0.01	0.09	0.01	0.2	0.2	0	0.1
0	20	—	—	43.6	4.8	—	—	—	—	—	—	—	—	—	—	—
0	10	0.59	5.1	30.9	1.0	0.08	1.0	0.01	0.44	0.01	0.06	0.02	3.1	0.2	0	0.3
0	32	0.34	5.4	24.9	0.4	0.10	0.1	0.00	—	0.01	0.05	0.01	0.2	0.4	0	0.3
0	18	0.48	4.5	33.1	2.1	0.03	2.9	0.00	—	0.00	0.02	0.01	1.5	0.5	0	0
0	2	0.06	0.6	7.4	0.6	0.01	3.9	0.00	0.01	0.00	0.01	0.00	1.5	0.9	0	—
0	1	0.02	—	4.0	0.1	—	0	0.00	—	0.00	0.01	0.00	—	0.3	0	—
0	24	0.37	7.7	33.9	1.8	0.07	0.1	0.01	—	0.01	0.12	0.01	—	0.4	0	—
0	7	1.24	7.1	28.5	2.5	0.09	0.1	0.01	—	0.01	0.06	0.02	2.1	0.1	0	0.2
0	215	9.24	93.6	411.1	27.5	1.07	—	0.09	—	0.09	0.70	—	0	0	0	—
0	5	0.05	0.8	12.0	0.5	0.03	0	0.01	0.00	0.00	0.02	0.03	0.1	0.9	0	0.4
0	2	0.07	1.6	30.8	0.7	0.07	0	0.01	0.01	0.01	0.01	0.08	0.1	0.5	0	1.1
0	1	0.02	1.7	16.6	0.5	0.01	0	0.00	0.01	0.00	0.02	0.01	0.4	0.2	0	0
0	2	0.20	3.3	24.2	0.6	0.08	0.1	0.00	0.32	0.00	0.09	0.01	0.7	0.1	0	0.7
0	3	0.06	1.3	19.2	0.3	0.01	0.1	0.01	—	0.00	0.02	0.01	2.9	0.9	0	0
0	4	0.23	2.8	7.9	1.4	0.03	0.7	0.01	—	0.01	0.02	0.00	1.3	0.4	0	0
0	12	0.49	2.1	9.1	0.5	0.02	2.4	0.00	0.01	0.00	0.02	0.01	1.6	0.3	0	0
0	17	0.32	9.8	22.5	0.2	0.18	0.1	0.01	0.09	0.01	0.26	0.01	2.5	0.1	0	4.4
0	4	0.06	4.0	7.7	0.4	0.04	0.1	0.01	0.00	0.00	0.02	0.00	1.7	0.1	0	0.1
0	4	0.02	1.5	27.1	0.4	0.03	0	0.01	0.00	0.00	0.01	0.02	2.8	1.3	0	0.1
0	8	0.05	2.6	19.8	1.1	0.04	0	0.01	0.01	0.00	0.01	0.02	3.5	0.2	0	0
0	24	0.66	4.1	25.0	0.2	0.06	5.2	0.01	0.28	0.01	0.09	0.01	4.1	0.8	0	0.1
0	4	0.49	3.9	49.2	0.7	0.08	55.4	0.01	0.62	0.03	0.32	0.08	2.2	1.5	0	0.1
0	4	0.29	0.7	11.4	1.4	0.01	1.5	0.00	0.02	0.00	0.02	0.00	0.5	0.4	0	0.1
0	9	0.60	4.1	26.4	0.9	0.03	0.3	0.00	—	0.01	0.02	0.01	0.2	0.4	0	0.1
0	3	0.14	2.7	36.3	0.5	0.04	37.5	0.01	0.53	0.01	0.15	0.04	1.9	1.4	0	0.2
0	6	0.34	2.2	1.8	0.1	0.02	0	0.00	—	0.00	0.01	0.00	0.2	0.5	0	0.1
0	41	0.26	9.3	19.6	0.6	0.28	0	0.02	0.03	0.01	0.02	0.01	1.6	0.1	0	0
0	15	0.53	3.4	10.3	0.4	0.04	2.0	0.00	0.02	0.00	0.04	0.02	2.1	0.2	0	0.1
0	12	0.33	2.3	11.3	0.9	0.04	0.2	0.00	—	0.00	0.03	0.00	0.9	0.4	0	0.2
0	15	0.35	2.6	11.5	0.6	0.03	1.9	0.01	—	0.01	0.01	0.02	3.7	0.7	0	0.1
0	2	0.04	0.6	4.7	0.2	0.01	1.0	0.00	—	0.00	0.01	0.00	0.8	0.2	0	—
0	1	0.07	1.8	12.1	1.0	0.01	0.2	0.00	—	0.00	0.01	0.01	0.7	0.6	0	0
0	4	—	1.1	2.7	0	0.01	—	0.00	—	—	—	—	—	—	0	—
0	12	0.19	3.0	7.5	0.1	0.03	2.1	0.01	0.05	0.00	0.04	0.01	1.9	0.2	0	0
0	7	0.00	0	603.6	0.1	—	0	—	—	—	0.05	—	—	0	—	—
0	0	0.00	—	476.3	0.1	—	0	—	—	—	—	—	—	0	—	—
0	0	0.01	0	0.1	581.4	0.00	0	0.00	0.00	0.00	0.00	0.00	0	0	0	0
0	30	0.53	5.3	14.7	0.3	0.06	3.6	0.01	—	0.00	0.05	0.02	—	0.7	0	0.1
0	3	0.21	9.2	10.8	1.0	0.27	0.1	0.03	0.01	0.01	0.15	0.00	2.6	0	0	0
0	—	—	—	—	0.1	—	—	—	—	—	—	—	—	0	—	—
0	4	0.22	1.2	8.7	0.6	0.02	3.9	0.00	—	0.00	0.01	0.00	2.0	0.3	0	—
0	2	0.16	3.0	50.7	3.1	0.03	4.5	0.01	0.06	0.01	0.11	0.03	3.7	30.4	0	0.1
0	85	1.48	20.2	—	—	—	—	0.06	—	0.02	1.16	—	—	0.9	0	—
0	48	—	14.5	128.1	2.6	0.17	—	0.04	—	—	—	—	—	0.6	0	—

Table of Food Composition *(continued)*

(Computer code is for Cengage Diet & Wellness Plus program)

D&W+ Code	Food Description	QTY	Measure	Wt (g)	H₂O (g)	Ener (cal)	Prot (g)	Carb (g)	Fiber (g)	Fat (g)	Sat	Mono	Poly
											Fat Breakdown (g)		

SPICES, CONDIMENTS, SAUCES—CONTINUED

1195	Tarragon, ground	1	teaspoon(s)	2	0.1	5	0.4	0.8	0.1	0.1	0	0	0.1
11728	Thyme, fresh	1	teaspoon(s)	1	0.5	1	0	0.2	0.1	0	0	0	0
821	Thyme, ground	1	teaspoon(s)	1	0.1	4	0.1	0.9	0.5	0.1	0	0	0
1196	Turmeric, ground	1	teaspoon(s)	2	0.3	8	0.2	1.4	0.5	0.2	0.1	0	0
11995	Wasabi	1	tablespoon(s)	14	10.7	10	0.7	2.3	0.2	0	—	—	—

CONDIMENTS

674	Catsup or ketchup	1	tablespoon(s)	15	10.4	15	0.3	3.8	0	0	0	0	0
703	Dill pickle	1	ounce(s)	28	26.7	3	0.2	0.7	0.3	0	0	0	0
138	Mayonnaise with soybean oil	1	tablespoon(s)	14	2.1	99	0.1	0.4	0	11.0	1.6	2.7	5.8
140	Mayonnaise, low calorie	1	tablespoon(s)	16	10.0	37	0	2.6	0	3.1	0.5	0.7	1.7
1682	Mustard, brown	1	teaspoon(s)	5	4.1	5	0.3	0.3	0	0.3	—	—	—
700	Mustard, yellow	1	teaspoon(s)	5	4.1	3	0.2	0.3	0.2	0.2	0	0.1	0
706	Sweet pickle relish	1	tablespoon(s)	15	9.3	20	0.1	5.3	0.2	0.1	0	0	0
141	Tartar sauce	2	tablespoon(s)	28	8.7	144	0.3	4.1	0.1	14.4	2.2	3.8	7.7

SAUCES

685	Barbecue sauce	2	tablespoon(s)	31	18.9	47	0	11.3	0.2	0.1	0	0	0.1
834	Cheese sauce	¼	cup(s)	63	44.4	110	4.2	4.3	0.3	8.4	3.8	2.4	1.6
32123	Chili enchilada sauce, green	2	tablespoon(s)	57	53.0	15	0.6	3.1	0.7	0.3	0	0	0.1
32122	Chili enchilada sauce, red	2	tablespoon(s)	32	24.5	27	1.1	5.0	2.1	0.8	0.1	0	0.4
29688	Hoisin sauce	1	tablespoon(s)	16	7.1	35	0.5	7.1	0.4	0.5	0.1	0.2	0.3
1641	Horseradish sauce, prepared	1	teaspoon(s)	5	3.3	10	0.1	0.2	0	1.0	0.6	0.3	0
16670	Mole poblano sauce	½	cup(s)	133	102.7	156	5.3	11.4	2.7	11.3	2.6	5.1	3.0
29689	Oyster sauce	1	tablespoon(s)	16	12.8	8	0.2	1.7	0	0	0	0	0
1655	Pepper sauce or Tabasco	1	teaspoon(s)	5	4.8	1	0.1	0	0	0	0	0	0
347	Salsa	2	tablespoon(s)	32	28.8	9	0.5	2.0	0.5	0.1	0	0	0
52206	Soy sauce, tamari	1	tablespoon(s)	18	12.0	11	1.9	1.0	0.1	0	0	0	0
839	Sweet and sour sauce	2	tablespoon(s)	39	29.8	37	0.1	9.1	0.1	0	0	0	0
1613	Teriyaki sauce	1	tablespoon(s)	18	12.2	16	1.1	2.8	0	0	0	0	0
25294	Tomato sauce	½	cup(s)	150	132.8	63	2.2	11.9	2.6	1.8	0.2	0.4	0.9
728	White sauce, medium	¼	cup(s)	63	46.8	92	2.4	5.7	0.1	6.7	1.8	2.8	1.8
1654	Worcestershire sauce	1	teaspoon(s)	6	4.5	4	0	1.1	0	0	0	0	0

VINEGAR

30853	Balsamic	1	tablespoon(s)	15	—	10	0	2.0	0	0	0	0	0
727	Cider	1	tablespoon(s)	15	14.0	3	0	0.1	0	0	0	0	0
1673	Distilled	1	tablespoon(s)	15	14.3	2	0	0.8	0	0	0	0	0
12948	Tarragon	1	tablespoon(s)	15	13.8	2	0	0.1	0	0	0	0	0

MIXED FOODS, SOUPS, SANDWICHES

MIXED DISHES

16652	Almond chicken	1	cup(s)	242	186.8	281	21.8	15.8	3.4	14.7	1.8	6.3	5.6
25224	Barbecued chicken	1	serving(s)	177	99.3	327	27.1	15.7	0.5	17.1	4.8	6.8	3.8
25227	Bean burrito	1	item(s)	149	81.8	326	16.1	33.0	5.6	14.8	8.3	4.7	0.9
9516	Beef and vegetable fajita	1	item(s)	223	143.9	397	22.4	35.3	3.1	18.0	5.9	8.0	2.5
16796	Beef or pork egg roll	2	item(s)	128	85.2	225	9.9	18.4	1.4	12.4	2.9	6.0	2.6
177	Beef stew with vegetables, prepared	1	cup(s)	245	201.0	220	16.0	15.0	3.2	11.0	4.4	4.5	0.5
30233	Beef stroganoff with noodles	1	cup(s)	256	190.1	343	19.7	22.8	1.5	19.1	7.4	5.7	4.4
16651	Cashew chicken	1	cup(s)	242	186.8	281	21.8	15.8	3.4	14.7	1.8	6.3	5.6
30274	Cheese pizza with vegetables, thin crust	2	slice(s)	140	76.6	298	12.7	35.4	2.5	12.0	4.9	4.7	1.6
30330	Cheese quesadilla	1	item(s)	54	18.3	190	7.7	15.3	1.0	10.8	5.2	3.6	1.3
215	Chicken and noodles, prepared	1	cup(s)	240	170.0	365	22.0	26.0	1.3	18.0	5.1	7.1	3.9
30239	Chicken and vegetables with broccoli, onion, bamboo shoots in soy-based sauce	1	cup(s)	162	125.5	180	15.8	9.3	1.8	8.6	1.7	3.0	3.1
25093	Chicken cacciatore	1	cup(s)	244	175.7	284	29.9	5.7	1.3	15.3	4.3	6.2	3.3
28020	Chicken fried turkey steak	3	ounce(s)	492	276.2	706	77.1	68.7	3.6	12.0	3.4	2.9	3.9
218	Chicken pot pie	1	cup(s)	252	154.6	542	22.6	41.4	3.5	31.3	9.8	12.5	7.1
30240	Chicken teriyaki	1	cup(s)	244	158.3	364	51.0	15.2	0.7	7.0	1.8	2.0	1.7
25119	Chicken Waldorf salad	½	cup(s)	100	67.2	179	14.0	6.8	1.0	10.8	1.8	3.1	5.2
25099	Chili con carne	¾	cup(s)	215	174.4	198	13.7	21.4	7.5	6.9	2.5	2.8	0.5
1062	Coleslaw	¾	cup(s)	90	73.4	70	1.2	11.2	1.4	2.3	0.3	0.6	1.2

PAGE KEY: A-4 = Breads/Baked Goods A-10 = Cereal/Rice/Pasta A-14 = Fruit A-20 = Vegetables/Legumes A-30 = Nuts/Seeds A-32 = Vegetarian A-34 = Dairy A-42 = Eggs A-42 = Seafood A-46 = Meats A-50 = Poultry A-50 = Processed Meats A-52 = Beverages A-56 = Fats/Oils A-58 = Sweets A-60 = Spices/Condiments/Sauces A-64 = Mixed Foods/Soups/Sandwiches A-70 = Fast Food A-90 = Convenience A-92 = Baby Foods

A

CHOL (mg)	CALC (mg)	IRON (mg)	MAGN (mg)	POTA (mg)	SODI (mg)	ZINC (mg)	VIT A (µg)	THIA (mg)	VIT E (mg α)	RIBO (mg)	NIAC (mg)	VIT B₆ (mg)	FOLA (µg DFE)	VIT C (mg)	VIT B₁₂ (µg)	SELE (µg)
0	18	0.51	5.6	48.3	1.0	0.06	3.4	0.00	—	0.02	0.14	0.03	4.4	0.8	0	0.1
0	3	0.14	1.3	4.9	0.1	0.01	1.9	0.00	—	0.00	0.01	0.00	0.4	1.3	0	—
0	26	1.73	3.1	11.4	0.8	0.08	2.7	0.01	0.10	0.01	0.06	0.01	3.8	0.7	0	0.1
0	4	0.91	4.2	55.6	0.8	0.09	0	0.00	0.06	0.01	0.11	0.04	0.9	0.6	0	0.1
0	13	0.11	—	—	—	—	—	0.02	—	0.01	0.07	—	—	11.2	0	—
0	3	0.07	2.9	57.3	167.1	0.03	7.1	0.00	0.21	0.02	0.21	0.02	1.5	2.3	0	0
0	12	0.10	2.0	26.1	248.1	0.03	2.6	0.01	0.02	0.01	0.03	0.01	0.3	0.2	0	0
5	1	0.03	0.1	1.7	78.4	0.02	11.2	0.01	0.72	0.01	0.00	0.08	0.7	0	0	0.2
4	0	0.00	0	1.6	79.5	0.01	0	0.00	0.32	0.00	0.00	0.00	0	0	0	0.3
0	6	0.09	1.0	6.8	68.1	0.01	0	0.00	0.09	0.00	0.01	0.00	0.2	0.1	0	—
0	3	0.07	2.5	6.9	56.8	0.03	0.2	0.01	0.01	0.00	0.02	0.00	0.4	0.1	0	1.6
0	0	0.13	0.8	3.8	121.7	0.02	9.2	0.00	0.08	0.00	0.03	0.00	0.2	0.2	0	0
8	6	0.20	0.8	10.1	191.5	0.05	20.2	0.00	0.97	0.00	0.01	0.07	2.0	0.1	0.1	0.5
0	4	0.06	3.8	65.0	349.7	0.04	3.8	0.00	0.20	0.01	0.15	0.01	0.6	0.2	0	0.4
18	116	0.13	5.7	18.9	521.6	0.61	50.4	0.00	—	0.07	0.01	0.01	2.5	0.3	0.1	2.0
0	5	0.36	9.5	125.7	61.9	0.11	—	0.02	0.00	0.02	0.63	0.06	5.7	43.9	0	0.3
0	7	1.05	11.1	231.3	113.8	0.14	—	0.01	0.00	0.21	0.61	0.34	6.6	0.3	0	0.3
0	5	0.16	3.8	19.0	258.4	0.05	0	0.00	0.04	0.03	0.18	0.01	3.7	0.1	0	0.1
2	5	0.00	0.5	6.7	14.6	0.01	8.0	0.00	0.02	0.01	0.00	0.00	0.5	0.1	0	0.1
1	38	1.81	58.3	280.9	304.8	1.15	13.3	0.06	1.72	0.08	1.84	0.09	15.9	3.4	0.1	1.1
0	5	0.02	0.6	8.6	437.3	0.01	0	0.00	0.00	0.02	0.23	0.00	2.4	0	0.1	0.7
0	1	0.05	0.6	6.4	31.7	0.01	4.1	0.00	0.00	0.00	0.01	0.01	0.1	0.2	0	0
0	9	0.14	4.8	95.0	192.0	0.11	4.8	0.01	0.37	0.01	0.02	0.05	1.3	0.6	0	0.3
0	4	0.43	7.3	38.7	1018.9	0.08	0	0.01	0.00	0.03	0.72	0.04	3.3	0	0	0.1
0	5	0.20	1.2	8.2	97.5	0.01	0	0.00	—	0.01	0.11	0.03	0.2	0	0	—
0	5	0.30	11.0	40.5	689.9	0.01	0	0.01	0.00	0.01	0.22	0.01	1.4	0	0	0.2
0	23	1.24	28.9	536.8	268.6	0.36	—	0.08	0.52	0.08	1.64	0.20	23.2	32.0	0	1.0
4	74	0.20	8.8	97.5	221.3	0.25	—	0.04	—	0.11	0.25	0.02	3.1	0.5	0.2	—
0	6	0.30	0.7	45.4	55.6	0.01	0.3	0.00	0.00	0.01	0.03	0.00	0.5	0.7	0	0
0	0	0.00	—	—	0	—	0	—	—	—	—	—	—	0	—	—
0	1	0.03	0.7	10.9	0.7	0.01	0	0.00	0.00	0.00	0.00	0.00	0	0	0	0
0	1	0.09	0	2.3	0.1	0.00	0	0.00	0.00	0.00	0.00	0.00	0	0	0	5.0
0	0	0.07	—	2.3	0.7	—	0	0.07	—	0.07	0.07	—	—	0.3	0	—
41	68	1.86	58.1	539.7	510.6	1.50	31.5	0.07	4.11	0.22	9.57	0.43	26.6	5.1	0.3	13.6
120	26	1.70	32.4	419.7	500.9	2.67	—	0.09	0.01	0.24	6.87	0.40	15.0	7.9	0.3	19.5
38	333	3.01	52.5	447.6	510.6	1.98	—	0.28	0.01	0.30	1.92	0.19	134.4	8.2	0.3	15.9
45	85	3.65	37.9	475.0	756.0	3.52	17.8	0.38	0.80	0.29	5.33	0.39	102.6	23.4	2.1	28.3
74	31	1.68	20.5	248.3	547.8	0.89	25.6	0.32	1.28	0.24	2.55	0.18	38.4	4.0	0.3	17.5
71	29	2.90	—	613.0	292.0	—	—	0.15	0.51	0.17	4.70	—	—	17.0	0	15.0
74	69	3.25	35.8	391.7	816.6	3.63	69.1	0.21	1.25	0.30	3.80	0.21	69.1	1.3	1.8	27.9
41	68	1.86	58.1	539.7	510.6	1.50	31.5	0.07	4.11	0.22	9.57	0.43	26.6	5.1	0.3	13.6
17	249	2.78	28.0	294.0	739.2	1.42	47.6	0.29	1.05	0.33	2.84	0.14	89.6	15.3	0.4	18.6
23	190	1.04	13.5	75.6	469.3	0.86	58.3	0.11	0.43	0.15	0.89	0.02	32.4	2.4	0.1	9.2
103	26	2.20	—	149.0	600.0	—	—	0.05	—	0.17	4.30	—	75.5	0	—	29.0
42	28	1.19	22.7	299.7	620.5	1.32	81.0	0.07	1.11	0.14	5.28	0.36	16.2	22.5	0.2	12.0
109	47	1.97	40.0	489.3	492.1	2.13	—	0.11	0.00	0.20	9.81	0.57	25.3	14.0	0.3	22.6
156	423	8.79	110.3	1182.9	880.4	6.18	—	0.72	0.00	1.05	20.16	1.20	180.1	2.7	1.3	97.6
68	66	3.32	37.8	390.6	652.7	1.94	259.6	0.39	1.05	0.39	7.25	0.23	113.4	10.3	0.2	27.0
156	51	3.26	68.3	588.0	3208.6	3.75	31.7	0.15	0.58	0.36	16.68	0.88	24.4	2.0	0.5	36.1
42	20	0.82	23.9	202.5	246.5	1.13	—	0.05	0.62	0.09	4.06	0.25	15.8	2.5	0.2	10.7
27	42	2.83	50.6	636.8	864.8	2.36	—	0.15	0.01	0.22	3.18	0.19	58.1	10.3	0.6	7.3
7	41	0.53	9.0	162.9	20.7	0.18	47.7	0.06	—	0.05	0.24	0.11	24.3	29.4	0	0.6

TABLE **A–1** **Table of Food Composition** (continued)

(Computer code is for Cengage Diet & Wellness Plus program)

D&W+ Code	Food Description	QTY	Measure	Wt (g)	H₂O (g)	Ener (cal)	Prot (g)	Carb (g)	Fiber (g)	Fat (g)	Fat Breakdown (g) Sat	Mono	Poly
MIXED FOODS, SOUPS, SANDWICHES—CONTINUED
1574	Crab cakes, from blue crab	1	item(s)	60	42.6	93	12.1	0.3	0	4.5	0.9	1.7	1.4
32144	Enchiladas with green chili sauce (enchiladas verdes)	1	item(s)	144	103.8	207	9.3	17.6	2.6	11.7	6.4	3.6	1.0
2793	Falafel patty	3	item(s)	51	17.7	170	6.8	16.2	—	9.1	1.2	5.2	2.1
28546	Fettuccine alfredo	1	cup(s)	244	88.7	279	13.1	46.1	1.4	4.2	2.2	1.0	0.4
32146	Flautas	3	item(s)	162	78.0	438	24.9	36.3	4.1	21.6	8.2	8.8	2.3
29629	Fried rice with meat or poultry	1	cup(s)	198	128.5	333	12.3	41.8	1.4	12.3	2.2	3.5	5.7
16649	General Tso chicken	1	cup(s)	146	91.0	296	18.7	16.4	0.9	17.0	4.0	6.3	5.3
1826	Green salad	¾	cup(s)	104	98.9	17	1.3	3.3	2.2	0.1	0	0	0
1814	Hummus	½	cup(s)	123	79.8	218	6.0	24.7	4.9	10.6	1.4	6.0	2.6
16650	Kung pao chicken	1	cup(s)	162	87.2	434	28.8	11.7	2.3	30.6	5.2	13.9	9.7
16622	Lamb curry	1	cup(s)	236	187.9	257	28.2	3.7	0.9	13.8	3.9	4.9	3.3
25253	Lasagna with ground beef	1	cup(s)	237	158.4	284	16.9	22.3	2.4	14.5	7.5	4.9	0.8
442	Macaroni and cheese, prepared	1	cup(s)	200	122.3	390	14.9	40.6	1.6	18.6	7.9	6.4	2.9
29637	Meat filled ravioli with tomato or meat sauce, canned	1	cup(s)	251	198.7	208	7.8	36.5	1.3	3.7	1.5	1.4	0.3
25105	Meat loaf	1	slice(s)	115	84.5	245	17.0	6.6	0.4	16.0	6.1	6.9	0.9
16646	Moo shi pork	1	cup(s)	151	76.8	512	18.9	5.3	0.6	46.4	6.9	15.8	21.2
16788	Nachos with beef, beans, cheese, tomatoes and onions	1	serving(s)	551	253.5	1576	59.1	137.5	20.4	90.8	32.6	41.9	9.4
6116	Pepperoni pizza	2	slice(s)	142	66.1	362	20.2	39.7	2.9	13.9	4.5	6.3	2.3
29601	Pizza with meat and vegetables, thin crust	2	slice(s)	158	81.4	386	16.5	36.8	2.7	19.1	7.7	8.1	2.2
655	Potato salad	½	cup(s)	125	95.0	179	3.4	14.0	1.6	10.3	1.8	3.1	4.7
25109	Salisbury steaks with mushroom sauce	1	serving(s)	135	101.8	251	17.1	9.3	0.5	15.5	6.0	6.7	0.8
16637	Shrimp creole with rice	1	cup(s)	243	176.6	309	27.0	27.7	1.2	9.2	1.7	3.6	2.9
497	Spaghetti and meatballs with tomato sauce, prepared	1	cup(s)	248	174.0	330	19.0	39.0	2.7	12.0	3.9	4.4	2.2
28585	Spicy thai noodles (pad thai)	8	ounce(s)	227	73.3	221	8.9	35.7	3.0	6.4	0.8	3.3	1.8
33073	Stir fried pork and vegetables with rice	1	cup(s)	235	173.6	348	15.4	33.5	1.9	16.3	5.6	6.9	2.6
28588	Stuffed shells	2½	item(s)	249	157.5	243	15.0	28.0	2.5	8.1	3.1	3.0	1.3
16821	Sushi with egg in seaweed	6	piece(s)	156	116.5	190	8.9	20.5	0.3	7.9	2.2	3.2	1.5
16819	Sushi with vegetables and fish	6	piece(s)	156	101.6	218	8.4	43.7	1.7	0.6	0.2	0.1	0.2
16820	Sushi with vegetables in seaweed	6	piece(s)	156	110.3	183	3.4	40.6	0.8	0.4	0.1	0.1	0.1
25266	Sweet and sour pork	¾	cup(s)	249	205.9	265	29.2	17.1	1.0	8.1	2.6	3.5	1.5
16824	Tabouli, tabbouleh or tabuli	1	cup(s)	160	123.7	198	2.6	15.9	3.7	14.9	2.0	10.9	1.6
25276	Three bean salad	½	cup(s)	99	82.2	95	1.9	9.7	2.6	5.9	0.8	1.4	3.5
160	Tuna salad	½	cup(s)	103	64.7	192	16.4	9.6	0	9.5	1.6	3.0	4.2
25241	Turkey and noodles	1	cup(s)	319	228.5	270	24.0	21.2	1.0	9.2	2.4	3.5	2.3
16794	Vegetable egg roll	2	item(s)	128	89.8	201	5.1	19.5	1.7	11.6	2.5	5.7	2.6
16818	Vegetable sushi, no fish	6	piece(s)	156	99.0	226	4.8	49.9	2.0	0.4	0.1	0.1	0.1
	SANDWICHES
1744	Bacon, lettuce and tomato with mayonnaise	1	item(s)	164	97.2	341	11.6	34.2	2.3	17.6	3.8	5.5	6.7
30287	Bologna and cheese with margarine	1	item(s)	111	45.6	345	13.4	29.3	1.2	19.3	8.1	7.0	2.4
30286	Bologna with margarine	1	item(s)	83	33.6	251	8.1	27.3	1.2	12.1	3.7	5.0	2.1
16546	Cheese	1	item(s)	83	31.0	261	9.1	27.6	1.2	12.7	5.4	4.2	2.1
8789	Cheeseburger, large, plain	1	item(s)	185	78.9	564	32.0	38.5	2.6	31.5	12.5	10.2	1.0
8624	Cheeseburger, large, with bacon, vegetables, and condiments	1	item(s)	195	91.4	550	30.8	36.8	2.5	30.9	11.9	10.6	1.3
1745	Club with bacon, chicken, tomato, lettuce, and mayonnaise	1	item(s)	246	137.5	546	31.0	48.9	3.0	24.5	5.3	7.5	9.4
1908	Cold cut submarine with cheese and vegetables	1	item(s)	228	131.8	456	21.8	51.0	2.0	18.6	6.8	8.2	2.3
30247	Corned beef	1	item(s)	130	74.9	265	18.2	25.3	1.6	9.6	3.6	3.5	1.0
25283	Egg salad	1	item(s)	126	72.1	278	10.7	28.0	1.4	13.5	2.9	4.2	5.0
16686	Fried egg	1	item(s)	96	49.7	226	10.0	26.2	1.2	8.6	2.3	3.2	1.9
16547	Grilled cheese	1	item(s)	83	27.5	291	9.2	27.9	1.2	15.8	6.0	5.7	3.0
16659	Gyro with onion and tomato	1	item(s)	105	68.3	163	12.0	20.0	1.1	3.5	1.3	1.3	0.5

PAGE KEY: A-4 = Breads/Baked Goods A-10 = Cereal/Rice/Pasta A-14 = Fruit A-20 = Vegetables/Legumes A-30 = Nuts/Seeds A-32 = Vegetarian A-34 = Dairy A-42 = Eggs A-42 = Seafood A-46 = Meats A-50 = Poultry A-50 = Processed Meats A-52 = Beverages A-56 = Fats/Oils A-58 = Sweets A-60 = Spices/Condiments/Sauces A-64 = Mixed Foods/Soups/Sandwiches A-70 = Fast Food A-90 = Convenience A-92 = Baby Foods

A

CHOL (mg)	CALC (mg)	IRON (mg)	MAGN (mg)	POTA (mg)	SODI (mg)	ZINC (mg)	VIT A (µg)	THIA (mg)	VIT E (mg α)	RIBO (mg)	NIAC (mg)	VIT B6 (mg)	FOLA (µg DFE)	VIT C (mg)	VIT B12 (µg)	SELE (µg)
90	63	0.64	19.8	194.4	198.0	2.45	34.2	0.05	—	0.04	1.74	0.10	36.6	1.7	3.6	24.4
27	266	1.07	38.5	251.4	276.3	1.26		0.07	0.02	0.16	1.27	0.17	44.6	59.3	0.2	6.0
0	28	1.74	41.8	298.4	149.9	0.76	0.5	0.07	—	0.08	0.53	0.06	47.4	0.8	0	0.5
9	218	1.83	38.4	163.9	472.9	1.24	—	0.41	0.00	0.35	2.85	0.09	225.0	1.6	0.4	38.4
73	146	2.66	61.3	222.9	885.7	3.43	0	0.10	0.10	0.16	3.00	0.26	95.7	0	1.2	36.7
103	38	2.77	33.7	196.0	833.6	1.34	41.6	0.33	1.60	0.18	4.17	0.27	146.5	3.4	0.3	22.0
66	26	1.46	23.4	248.2	849.7	1.40	29.2	0.10	1.62	0.18	6.28	0.28	23.4	12.0	0.2	19.9
0	13	0.65	11.4	178.0	26.9	0.21	59.0	0.03	—	0.05	0.56	0.08	38.3	24.0	0	0.4
0	60	1.91	35.7	212.8	297.7	1.34	0	0.10	0.92	0.06	0.49	0.49	72.6	9.7	0	3.0
65	50	1.96	63.2	427.7	907.2	1.50	38.9	0.15	4.32	0.14	13.22	0.58	42.1	7.5	0.3	23.0
90	38	2.95	40.1	493.2	495.6	6.60	—	0.08	1.29	0.28	8.03	0.21	28.3	1.4	2.9	30.4
68	233	2.22	40.1	420.1	433.6	2.70	—	0.21	0.21	0.29	3.06	0.22	91.1	15.0	0.8	21.4
34	310	2.06	40.0	258.0	784.0	2.06	180.0	0.27	0.72	0.43	2.18	0.08	100.0	0	0.5	30.6
15	35	2.10	20.1	283.6	1352.9	1.28	27.6	0.19	0.70	0.16	2.77	0.14	60.2	21.6	0.4	13.3
85	59	1.87	21.8	300.8	411.7	3.40	—	0.08	0.00	0.27	3.72	0.13	18.7	0.9	1.6	17.9
172	32	1.57	25.7	333.7	1052.5	1.82	49.8	0.49	5.39	0.36	2.88	0.31	21.1	8.0	0.8	30.0
154	948	7.32	242.4	1201.2	1862.4	10.68	259.0	0.29	7.71	0.81	6.39	1.09	148.8	16.0	2.6	44.1
28	129	1.87	17.0	305.3	533.9	1.03	105.1	0.26	—	0.46	6.09	0.11	76.7	3.3	0.4	26.1
36	258	3.14	31.6	352.3	971.7	2.02	49.0	0.37	1.13	0.37	3.77	0.19	91.6	15.6	0.6	22.8
85	24	0.81	18.8	317.5	661.3	0.38	40.0	0.09	—	0.07	1.11	0.17	8.8	12.5	0	5.1
60	74	1.94	23.8	314.5	360.5	3.45	—	0.10	0.00	0.27	3.95	0.13	20.8	0.7	1.6	17.4
180	102	4.68	63.2	413.1	330.5	1.72	94.8	0.29	2.06	0.11	4.75	0.21	121.5	12.9	1.2	49.3
89	124	3.70	—	665.0	1009.0	—	81.5	0.25	—	0.30	4.00	—	—	22.0	—	22.0
37	31	1.56	49.4	181.3	591.6	1.05	—	0.18	0.35	0.13	1.82	0.17	55.8	22.6	0.1	3.2
46	38	2.71	33.0	396.9	569.5	2.08	—	0.51	0.38	0.20	5.07	0.30	162.4	18.8	0.4	22.8
30	188	2.26	49.4	403.0	471.5	1.41	—	0.26	0.00	0.26	3.83	0.24	161.2	17.9	0.2	28.9
214	45	1.84	18.7	135.7	463.3	0.98	106.1	0.13	0.67	0.28	1.35	0.13	82.7	1.9	0.7	20.3
11	23	2.15	25.0	202.8	340.1	0.78	45.2	0.26	0.24	0.07	2.76	0.14	121.7	3.6	0.3	13.9
0	20	1.54	18.7	96.7	152.9	0.68	25.0	0.19	0.12	0.03	1.86	0.13	118.6	2.3	0	9.8
74	40	1.76	35.6	619.9	621.8	2.53	—	0.81	0.20	0.37	6.69	0.66	14.7	11.9	0.7	49.6
0	30	1.21	35.2	249.6	796.8	0.48	54.4	0.07	2.43	0.04	1.11	0.11	30.4	26.1	0	0.5
0	26	0.96	15.5	144.8	224.2	0.30	—	0.02	0.88	0.04	0.26	0.04	32.2	10.0	0	2.7
13	17	1.02	19.5	182.5	412.1	0.57	24.6	0.03	—	0.07	6.86	0.08	8.2	2.3	1.2	42.2
77	69	2.56	33.2	400.8	577.1	2.51	—	0.23	0.28	0.30	6.41	0.29	109.5	1.4	1.1	33.4
60	29	1.65	17.9	193.3	549.1	0.48	25.6	0.15	1.28	0.20	1.59	0.09	46.1	5.5	0.2	11.3
0	23	2.38	21.8	157.6	369.7	0.82	48.4	0.28	0.15	0.05	2.44	0.12	135.7	3.7	0	8.1
21	79	2.36	27.9	351.0	944.6	1.08	44.3	0.32	1.16	0.24	4.36	0.21	105.0	9.7	0.2	27.1
40	258	2.38	24.4	215.3	941.3	1.88	102.1	0.31	0.55	0.35	2.97	0.14	91.0	0.2	0.8	20.4
17	100	2.24	16.6	138.6	579.3	1.02	44.8	0.29	0.49	0.21	2.92	0.12	88.8	0.2	0.5	16.0
22	233	2.04	19.9	127.0	733.7	1.24	97.1	0.25	0.47	0.30	2.25	0.05	88.8	0	0.3	13.1
104	309	4.47	44.4	401.5	986.1	5.75	0	0.35	—	0.77	8.26	0.49	129.48	0	2.8	38.9
98	267	4.03	44.9	464.1	1314.3	5.20	0	0.33	—	0.67	8.25	0.47	122.9	1.4	2.4	6.6
71	157	4.57	46.7	464.9	1087.3	1.82	41.8	0.54	1.52	0.40	12.82	0.61	172.2	6.4	0.4	42.3
36	189	2.50	68.4	394.4	1650.7	2.57	70.7	1.00	—	0.79	5.49	0.13	109.4	12.3	1.1	30.8
46	81	3.04	19.5	127.4	1206.4	2.26	2.6	0.23	0.20	0.24	3.42	0.11	88.4	0.3	0.9	31.2
219	85	2.25	18.8	159.0	423.1	0.87	—	0.27	0.12	0.43	2.06	0.15	112.1	0.9	0.6	29.9
206	104	2.79	17.3	117.1	438.7	0.92	89.3	0.26	0.66	0.40	2.26	0.10	110.4	0	0.6	24.2
22	235	2.05	19.9	128.7	763.6	1.26	129.5	0.19	0.72	0.28	2.05	0.05	58.1	0	0.2	13.2
28	47	1.77	22.1	218.4	235.2	2.33	9.5	0.23	0.26	0.20	3.12	0.13	63.0	3.2	0.9	18.3

D&W+ Code	Food Description	QTY	Measure	Wt (g)	H₂O (g)	Ener (cal)	Prot (g)	Carb (g)	Fiber (g)	Fat (g)	Sat	Mono	Poly
											Fat Breakdown (g)		

Mixed Foods, Soups, Sandwiches—continued

D&W+ Code	Food Description	QTY	Measure	Wt (g)	H₂O (g)	Ener (cal)	Prot (g)	Carb (g)	Fiber (g)	Fat (g)	Sat	Mono	Poly
1906	Ham and cheese	1	item(s)	146	74.2	352	20.7	33.3	2.0	15.5	6.4	6.7	1.4
31890	Ham with mayonnaise	1	item(s)	112	56.3	271	13.0	27.9	1.9	11.6	2.8	4.0	4.0
756	Hamburger, double patty, large, with condiments and vegetables	1	item(s)	226	121.5	540	34.3	40.3	—	26.6	10.5	10.3	2.8
8793	Hamburger, large, plain	1	item(s)	137	57.7	426	22.6	31.7	1.5	22.9	8.4	9.9	2.1
8795	Hamburger, large, with vegetables and condiments	1	item(s)	218	121.4	512	25.8	40.0	3.1	27.4	10.4	11.4	2.2
25134	Hot chicken salad	1	item(s)	98	48.4	242	15.2	23.8	1.3	9.2	2.9	2.5	3.0
25133	Hot turkey salad	1	item(s)	98	50.1	224	15.6	23.8	1.3	6.9	2.3	1.6	2.5
1411	Hotdog with bun, plain	1	item(s)	98	52.9	242	10.4	18.0	1.6	14.5	5.1	6.9	1.7
30249	Pastrami	1	item(s)	134	71.2	328	13.4	27.8	1.6	17.7	6.1	8.3	1.2
16701	Peanut butter	1	item(s)	93	23.6	345	12.2	37.6	3.3	17.4	3.4	7.7	5.2
30306	Peanut butter and jelly	1	item(s)	93	24.2	330	10.3	41.9	2.9	14.7	2.9	6.5	4.4
1909	Roast beef submarine with mayonnaise and vegetables	1	item(s)	216	127.4	410	28.6	44.3	—	13.0	7.1	1.8	2.6
1910	Roast beef, plain	1	item(s)	139	67.6	346	21.5	33.4	1.2	13.8	3.6	6.8	1.7
1907	Steak with mayonnaise and vegetables	1	item(s)	204	104.2	459	30.3	52.0	2.3	14.1	3.8	5.3	3.3
25288	Tuna salad	1	item(s)	179	102.2	415	24.5	28.4	1.6	22.4	3.5	6.2	11.4
30283	Turkey submarine with cheese, lettuce, tomato, and mayonnaise	1	item(s)	277	168.0	529	30.4	49.4	3.0	22.8	6.8	6.0	8.6
31891	Turkey with mayonnaise	1	item(s)	143	74.5	329	28.7	26.4	1.3	11.2	2.6	2.6	4.8
	Soups												
25296	Bean	1	cup(s)	301	253.1	191	13.8	29.0	6.5	2.3	0.7	0.8	0.5
711	Bean with pork, condensed, prepared with water	1	cup(s)	253	215.9	159	7.3	21.0	7.3	5.5	1.4	2.0	1.7
713	Beef noodle, condensed, prepared with water	1	cup(s)	244	224.9	83	4.7	8.7	0.7	3.0	1.1	1.2	0.5
825	Cheese, condensed, prepared with milk	1	cup(s)	251	206.9	231	9.5	16.2	1.0	14.6	9.1	4.1	0.5
826	Chicken broth, condensed, prepared with water	1	cup(s)	244	234.1	39	4.9	0.9	0	1.4	0.4	0.6	0.3
25297	Chicken noodle soup	1	cup(s)	286	258.4	117	10.8	10.9	0.9	2.9	0.8	1.1	0.7
827	Chicken noodle, condensed, prepared with water	1	cup(s)	241	226.1	60	3.1	7.1	0.5	2.3	0.6	1.0	0.6
724	Chicken noodle, dehydrated, prepared with water	1	cup(s)	252	237.3	58	2.1	9.2	0.3	1.4	0.3	0.5	0.4
823	Cream of asparagus, condensed, prepared with milk	1	cup(s)	248	213.3	161	6.3	16.4	0.7	8.2	3.3	2.1	2.2
824	Cream of celery, condensed, prepared with milk	1	cup(s)	248	214.4	164	5.7	14.5	0.7	9.7	3.9	2.5	2.7
708	Cream of chicken, condensed, prepared with milk	1	cup(s)	248	210.4	191	7.5	15.0	0.2	11.5	4.6	4.5	1.6
715	Cream of chicken, condensed, prepared with water	1	cup(s)	244	221.1	117	3.4	9.3	0.2	7.4	2.1	3.3	1.5
709	Cream of mushroom, condensed, prepared with milk	1	cup(s)	248	215.0	166	6.2	14.0	0	9.6	3.3	2.0	1.8
716	Cream of mushroom, condensed, prepared with water	1	cup(s)	244	224.6	102	1.9	8.0	0	7.0	1.6	1.3	1.7
25298	Cream of vegetable	1	cup(s)	285	250.7	165	7.2	15.2	1.9	8.6	1.6	4.6	1.9
16689	Egg drop	1	cup(s)	244	228.9	73	7.5	1.1	0	3.8	1.1	1.5	0.6
25138	Golden squash	1	cup(s)	258	223.9	145	7.6	20.4	0.4	4.1	0.8	2.2	0.9
16663	Hot and sour	1	cup(s)	244	209.7	161	15.0	5.4	0.5	7.9	2.7	3.4	1.1
28054	Lentil chowder	1	cup(s)	244	202.8	153	11.4	27.7	12.6	0.5	0.1	0.1	0.2
28560	Macaroni and bean	1	cup(s)	246	138.8	146	5.8	22.9	5.1	3.7	0.5	2.2	0.6
714	Manhattan clam chowder, condensed, prepared with water	1	cup(s)	244	225.1	73	2.1	11.6	1.5	2.1	0.4	0.4	1.2
28561	Minestrone	1	cup(s)	241	185.4	103	4.5	16.8	4.8	2.3	0.3	1.4	0.4
717	Minestrone, condensed, prepared with water	1	cup(s)	241	220.1	82	4.3	11.2	1.0	2.5	0.6	0.7	1.1

PAGE KEY: A-4 = Breads/Baked Goods A-10 = Cereal/Rice/Pasta A-14 = Fruit A-20 = Vegetables/Legumes A-30 = Nuts/Seeds A-32 = Vegetarian A-34 = Dairy A-42 = Eggs A-42 = Seafood A-46 = Meats A-50 = Poultry A-50 = Processed Meats A-52 = Beverages A-56 = Fats/Oils A-58 = Sweets A-60 = Spices/Condiments/Sauces A-64 = Mixed Foods/Soups/Sandwiches A-70 = Fast Food A-90 = Convenience A-92 = Baby Foods

A

CHOL (mg)	CALC (mg)	IRON (mg)	MAGN (mg)	POTA (mg)	SODI (mg)	ZINC (mg)	VIT A (µg)	THIA (mg)	VIT E (mg α)	RIBO (mg)	NIAC (mg)	VIT B6 (mg)	FOLA (µg DFE)	VIT C (mg)	VIT B12 (µg)	SELE (µg)
58	130	3.24	16.1	290.5	770.9	1.37	96.4	0.30	0.29	0.48	2.68	0.20	78.8	2.8	0.5	23.1
34	91	2.47	23.5	210.6	1097.6	1.13	5.6	0.57	0.50	0.26	3.80	0.25	90.7	2.2	0.2	20.2
122	102	5.85	49.7	569.5	791.0	5.67	0	0.36	—	0.38	7.57	0.54	110.7	1.1	4.1	25.5
71	74	3.57	27.4	267.2	474.0	4.11	0	0.28	—	0.28	6.24	0.23	80.8	0	2.1	27.1
87	96	4.92	43.6	479.6	824.0	4.88	0	0.41	—	0.37	7.28	0.32	115.5	2.6	2.4	33.6
39	115	1.88	20.0	172.4	505.1	1.19	—	0.23	0.28	0.22	4.84	0.19	79.5	0.5	0.2	19.9
37	114	1.99	21.3	189.0	494.5	1.07	—	0.22	0.28	0.20	4.26	0.22	79.6	0.5	0.2	23.4
44	24	2.31	12.7	143.1	670.3	1.98	0	0.23	—	0.27	3.64	0.04	60.7	0.1	0.5	26.0
51	80	3.02	22.8	182.2	1364.1	2.70	2.7	0.28	0.26	0.26	4.97	0.14	89.8	0.3	1.0	14.3
0	110	2.92	66.0	226.0	580.3	1.32	0	0.31	2.39	0.23	6.72	0.18	130.2	0	0	13.2
0	94	2.50	56.7	198.1	492.9	1.12	0	0.26	2.01	0.20	5.66	0.15	110.7	0.1	0	11.2
73	41	2.80	67.0	330.5	844.6	4.38	30.2	0.41	—	0.41	5.96	0.32	88.6	5.6	1.8	25.7
51	54	4.22	30.6	315.5	792.3	3.39	11.1	0.37	—	0.30	5.86	0.26	68.1	2.1	1.2	29.2
73	92	5.16	49.0	524.3	797.6	4.52	0	0.40	—	0.36	7.30	0.36	128.5	5.5	1.6	42.0
59	78	2.97	35.9	316.3	724.7	1.02	—	0.27	0.34	0.26	12.07	0.46	99.6	1.8	2.4	76.9
64	307	4.59	49.9	534.6	1759.0	2.74	74.8	0.49	1.19	0.65	3.91	0.31	171.7	10.5	0.6	42.1
67	100	3.46	34.3	304.6	564.9	3.00	5.7	0.28	0.74	0.32	6.84	0.46	94.4	0	0.3	40
5	79	3.05	61.8	588.8	689.0	1.41	—	0.27	0.02	0.15	3.63	0.23	140.1	3.6	0.2	7.9
3	78	1.89	43.0	371.9	883.0	0.96	43.0	0.08	1.08	0.03	0.52	0.03	30.4	1.5	0	7.8
5	20	1.07	7.3	97.6	929.6	1.51	12.2	0.06	1.22	0.05	1.03	0.03	29.3	0.5	0.2	7.3
48	289	0.80	20.1	341.4	1019.1	0.67	358.9	0.06	—	0.33	0.50	0.07	10.0	1.3	0.4	7.0
0	10	0.51	2.4	209.8	775.9	0.24	0	0.01	0.04	0.07	3.34	0.02	4.9	0	0.2	0
24	25	1.38	16.4	340.1	774.5	0.77	—	0.15	0.02	0.16	5.57	0.13	37.2	1.8	0.3	10.2
12	14	1.59	9.6	53.0	638.7	0.38	26.5	0.13	0.07	0.10	1.30	0.04	28.9	0	0	11.6
10	5	0.50	7.6	32.8	577.1	0.20	2.5	0.20	0.12	0.07	1.08	0.02	27.7	0	0.1	9.6
22	174	0.86	19.8	359.6	1041.6	0.91	62.0	0.10	—	0.27	0.88	0.06	29.8	4.0	0.5	8.0
32	186	0.69	22.3	310.0	1009.4	0.19	114.1	0.07	—	0.24	0.43	0.06	7.4	1.5	0.5	4.7
27	181	0.67	17.4	272.8	1046.6	0.67	178.6	0.07	—	0.25	0.92	0.06	7.4	1.2	0.5	8.0
10	34	0.61	2.4	87.8	985.8	0.63	163.5	0.02	—	0.06	0.82	0.01	2.4	0.2	0.1	7.0
10	164	1.36	19.8	267.8	823.4	0.79	81.8	0.10	1.01	0.29	0.62	0.05	7.4	0.2	0.6	6.0
0	17	1.31	4.9	73.2	775.9	0.24	9.8	0.05	0.97	0.05	0.50	0.00	2.4	0	0	2.9
1	80	1.20	17.5	340.7	787.9	0.56	—	0.12	1.05	0.18	3.32	0.12	39.5	10.7	0.3	4.3
102	22	0.75	4.9	219.6	729.6	0.48	41.5	0.02	0.29	0.19	3.02	0.05	14.6	0	0.5	7.6
4	262	0.78	42.4	542.2	515.6	0.88	—	0.16	0.52	0.30	1.14	0.16	32.7	12.5	0.7	6.0
34	29	1.24	19.5	373.3	1561.6	1.43	—	0.26	0.12	0.24	4.96	0.20	14.6	0.5	0.4	19.3
0	48	4.38	59.3	626.2	26.7	1.57	—	0.24	0.06	0.12	1.87	0.32	192.7	16.1	0	3.5
0	59	1.90	32.4	275.9	531.0	0.51	—	0.16	0.37	0.12	1.44	0.10	92.3	9.1	0	8.8
2	27	1.56	9.8	180.6	551.4	0.87	48.8	0.02	1.22	0.03	0.77	0.09	9.8	3.9	3.9	9.0
0	62	1.70	29.0	287.5	442.7	0.42	—	0.09	0.23	0.09	0.70	0.07	62.0	13.3	0	3.5
2	34	0.91	7.2	313.3	911.0	0.74	118.1	0.05	—	0.04	0.94	0.09	50.6	1.2	0	8.0

A

D&W+ Code	Food Description	QTY	Measure	Wt (g)	H₂O (g)	Ener (cal)	Prot (g)	Carb (g)	Fiber (g)	Fat (g)	Fat Breakdown (g) Sat	Mono	Poly
Mixed Foods, Soups, Sandwiches—continued														
28038	Mushroom and wild rice	1	cup(s)	244	199.7	86	4.7	13.2	1.7	0.3	0	0	0.2
828	New England clam chowder, condensed, prepared with milk	1	cup(s)	248	212.2	151	8.0	18.4	0.7	5.0	2.1	0.7	0.6
28036	New England style clam chowder	1	cup(s)	244	227.5	61	3.8	8.8	1.8	0.2	0.1	0	0
28566	Old country pasta	1	cup(s)	252	183.3	146	6.5	18.3	3.6	4.5	2.0	2.4	0.9
725	Onion, dehydrated, prepared with water	1	cup(s)	246	235.7	30	0.8	6.8	0.7	0	0	0	0
16667	Shrimp gumbo	1	cup(s)	244	207.2	166	9.5	18.2	2.4	6.7	1.3	2.9	2.0
28037	Southwestern corn chowder	1	cup(s)	244	217.8	98	4.9	17.0	2.4	0.5	0.1	0.1	0.2
30282	Soybean (miso)	1	cup(s)	240	218.6	84	6.0	8.0	1.9	3.4	0.6	1.1	1.4
25140	Split pea	1	cup(s)	165	119.7	72	4.5	16.0	1.6	0.3	0.1	0	0.2
718	Split pea with ham, condensed, prepared with water	1	cup(s)	253	206.9	190	10.3	28.0	2.3	4.4	1.8	1.8	0.6
726	Tomato vegetable, dehydrated, prepared with water	1	cup(s)	253	238.4	56	2.0	10.2	0.8	0.9	0.4	0.3	0.1
710	Tomato, condensed, prepared with milk	1	cup(s)	248	213.4	136	6.2	22.0	1.5	3.2	1.8	0.9	0.3
719	Tomato, condensed, prepared with water	1	cup(s)	244	223.0	73	1.9	16.0	1.5	0.7	0.2	0.2	0.2
28595	Turkey noodle	1	cup(s)	244	216.9	114	8.1	15.1	1.9	2.4	0.3	1.1	0.7
28051	Turkey vegetable	1	cup(s)	244	220.8	96	12.2	6.6	2.0	1.1	0.3	0.2	0.3
25141	Vegetable	1	cup(s)	252	228.1	82	5.2	16.5	4.5	0.3	0	0	0.1
720	Vegetable beef, condensed, prepared with water	1	cup(s)	244	224.0	76	5.4	9.9	2.0	1.9	0.8	0.8	0.1
28598	Vegetable gumbo	1	cup(s)	252	184.5	170	4.4	28.9	3.6	4.7	0.7	3.2	0.5
721	Vegetarian vegetable, condensed, prepared with water	1	cup(s)	241	222.7	67	2.1	11.8	0.7	1.9	0.3	0.8	0.7
Fast Food														
Arby's														
36094	Au jus sauce	1	serving(s)	85	—	43	1.0	7.0	0	1.3	0.4	—	—
751	Beef 'n cheddar sandwich	1	item(s)	195	—	445	22.0	44.0	2.0	21.0	6.0	—	—
9279	Cheddar curly fries	1	serving(s)	198	—	631	8.0	73.0	7.0	37.4	6.8	—	—
34770	Chicken breast fillet sandwich, grilled	1	item(s)	233	—	414	32.0	36.0	3.0	17.0	3.0	—	—
36131	Chocolate shake, regular	1	serving(s)	397	—	507	13.0	83.0	0	13.0	8.0	—	—
36045	Curly fries, large size	1	serving(s)	198	—	631	8.0	73.0	7.0	37.0	7.0	—	—
36044	Curly fries, medium size	1	serving(s)	128	—	406	5.0	47.0	5.0	24.0	4.0	—	—
752	Ham 'n cheese sandwich	1	item(s)	167	—	304	23.0	35.0	1.0	7.0	2.0	—	—
36048	Homestyle fries, large size	1	serving(s)	213	—	566	6.0	82.0	6.0	37.0	7.0	—	—
36047	Homestyle fries, medium size	1	serving(s)	142	—	377	4.0	55.0	4.0	25.0	4.0	—	—
33465	Homestyle fries, small size	1	serving(s)	113	—	302	3.0	44.0	3.0	20.0	4.0	—	—
9249	Junior roast beef sandwich	1	item(s)	125	—	272	16.0	34.0	2.0	10.0	4.0	—	—
9251	Large roast beef sandwich	1	item(s)	281	—	547	42.0	41.0	3.0	28.0	12.0	—	—
39640	Market Fresh chicken salad with pecans sandwich	1	item(s)	322	—	769	30.0	79.0	9.0	39.0	10.0	—	—
39641	Market Fresh Martha's Vineyard salad, without dressing	1	serving(s)	330	—	277	26.0	24.0	5.0	8.0	4.0	—	—
34769	Market Fresh roast turkey and Swiss sandwich	1	serving(s)	359	—	725	45.0	75.0	5.0	30.0	8.0	—	—
9267	Market Fresh roast turkey ranch and bacon sandwich	1	serving(s)	382	—	834	49.0	75.0	5.0	38.0	11.0	—	—
39642	Market Fresh Santa Fe salad, without dressing	1	serving(s)	372	—	499	30.0	42.0	7.0	23.0	8.0	—	—
39650	Market Fresh Southwest chicken wrap	1	serving(s)	251	—	567	36.0	42.0	4.0	29.0	9.0	—	—
37021	Market Fresh Ultimate BLT sandwich	1	item(s)	294	—	779	23.0	75.0	6.0	45.0	11.0	—	—
750	Roast beef sandwich, regular	1	item(s)	154	—	320	21.0	34.0	2.0	14.0	5.0	—	—
36132	Strawberry shake, regular	1	serving(s)	397	—	498	13.0	81.0	0	13.0	8.0	—	—
2009	Super roast beef sandwich	1	item(s)	198	—	398	21.0	40.0	2.0	19.0	6.0	—	—
36130	Vanilla shake, regular	1	serving(s)	369	—	437	13.0	66.0	0	13.0	8.0	—	—
Auntie Anne's														
35371	Cheese dipping sauce	1	serving(s)	35	—	100	3.0	4.0	0	8.0	4.0	—	—
35353	Cinnamon sugar soft pretzel	1	item(s)	120	—	350	9.0	74.0	2.0	2.0	0	—	—

PAGE KEY: A-4 = Breads/Baked Goods A-10 = Cereal/Rice/Pasta A-14 = Fruit A-20 = Vegetables/Legumes A-30 = Nuts/Seeds A-32 = Vegetarian A-34 = Dairy A-42 = Eggs A-42 = Seafood A-46 = Meats A-50 = Poultry A-50 = Processed Meats A-52 = Beverages A-56 = Fats/Oils A-58 = Sweets A-60 = Spices/Condiments/Sauces A-64 = Mixed Foods/Soups/Sandwiches A-70 = Fast Food A-90 = Convenience A-92 = Baby Foods

CHOL (mg)	CALC (mg)	IRON (mg)	MAGN (mg)	POTA (mg)	SODI (mg)	ZINC (mg)	VIT A (µg)	THIA (mg)	VIT E (mg α)	RIBO (mg)	NIAC (mg)	VIT B6 (mg)	FOLA (µg DFE)	VIT C (mg)	VIT B12 (µg)	SELE (µg)
0	30	1.38	27.3	376.9	283.8	1.00	—	0.06	0.07	0.23	3.21	0.14	27.3	3.7	0.1	4.7
17	169	3.00	29.8	456.3	887.8	0.99	91.8	0.20	0.54	0.43	1.96	0.17	22.3	5.2	11.9	10.9
3	89	1.30	29.2	503.7	256.8	0.52	—	0.06	0.02	0.10	1.30	0.15	24.2	11.8	3.0	3.8
5	57	2.43	51.9	500.4	355.7	0.78	—	0.21	0.01	0.14	2.64	0.20	105.2	22.0	0.1	10.3
0	22	0.12	9.8	76.3	851.2	0.12	0	0.03	0.02	0.03	0.15	0.06	0	0.2	0	0.5
51	105	2.85	48.8	461.2	441.6	0.90	80.5	0.18	1.90	0.12	2.52	0.19	102.5	17.6	0.3	14.9
1	83	1.03	26.3	434.4	217.4	0.57	—	0.08	0.09	0.13	1.81	0.21	32.1	39.6	0.2	1.7
0	65	1.87	36.0	362.4	988.8	0.86	232.8	0.06	0.96	0.16	2.61	0.15	57.6	4.6	0.2	1.0
0	28	1.26	29.8	328.1	602.4	0.52	—	0.10	0.00	0.07	1.50	0.16	49.5	8.1	0	0.7
8	23	2.27	48.1	399.7	1006.9	1.31	22.8	0.14	—	0.07	1.47	0.06	2.5	1.5	0.3	8.0
0	20	0.60	10.1	169.5	334.0	0.20	10.1	0.06	0.43	0.09	1.26	0.06	12.7	3.0	0.1	2.0
10	166	1.36	29.8	466.2	711.8	0.84	94.2	0.09	0.44	0.31	1.35	0.15	5.0	15.6	0.6	9.2
0	20	1.31	17.1	273.3	663.7	0.29	24.4	0.04	0.41	0.07	1.23	0.10	0	15.4	0	6.1
26	28	1.40	24.1	223.8	395.9	0.75	—	0.21	0.01	0.12	2.85	0.15	65.1	7.1	0.1	13.7
21	38	1.48	25.0	423.4	348.7	0.99	—	0.09	0.01	0.09	3.64	0.27	23.9	10.6	0.2	10.3
0	40	2.08	39.1	681.5	670.3	0.67	—	0.16	0.00	0.09	2.70	0.26	36.3	22.4	0	2.2
5	20	1.09	7.3	168.4	773.5	1.51	190.3	0.03	0.58	0.04	1.00	0.07	9.8	2.4	0.3	2.7
0	56	1.85	38.9	360.2	518.4	0.64	—	0.18	0.64	0.08	1.77	0.17	107.5	21.9	0	4.1
0	24	1.06	7.2	207.3	814.6	0.45	171.1	0.05	1.39	0.04	0.90	0.05	9.6	1.4	0	4.3
0	0	—	—	—	1510.0	—	—	—	—	—	—	—	—	—	—	—
51	80	3.96	—	—	1274.0	—	—	—	—	—	—	—	—	1.8	—	—
0	80	3.24	—	—	1476.0	—	—	—	—	—	—	—	—	9.6	—	—
9	90	3.06	—	—	913.0	—	—	—	—	—	—	—	—	10.8	—	—
34	510	0.54	—	—	357.0	—	—	—	—	—	—	—	—	5.4	—	—
0	80	3.24	—	—	1476.0	—	—	—	—	—	—	—	—	9.6	—	—
0	50	1.98	—	—	949.0	—	—	—	—	—	—	—	—	6.0	—	—
35	160	2.70	—	—	1420.0	—	—	—	—	—	—	—	—	1.2	—	—
0	50	1.62	—	—	1029.0	—	—	—	—	—	—	—	—	12.6	—	—
0	30	1.08	—	—	686.0	—	—	—	—	—	—	—	—	8.4	—	—
0	30	0.90	—	—	549.0	—	—	—	—	—	—	—	—	6.6	—	—
29	60	3.06	—	—	740.0	—	0	—	—	—	—	—	—	0	—	—
102	70	6.30	—	—	1869.0	—	0	—	—	—	—	—	—	0.6	—	—
74	180	4.32	—	—	1240.0	—	—	—	—	—	—	—	—	30.0	—	—
72	200	1.62	—	—	454.0	—	—	—	—	—	—	—	—	33.6	—	—
91	360	5.22	—	—	1788.0	—	—	—	—	—	—	—	—	10.2	—	—
109	330	5.40	—	—	2258.0	—	—	—	—	—	—	—	—	11.4	—	—
59	420	3.60	—	—	1231.0	—	—	—	—	—	—	—	—	36.6	—	—
88	240	4.50	—	—	1451.0	—	—	—	—	—	—	—	—	7.8	—	—
51	170	4.68	—	—	1571.0	—	—	—	—	—	—	—	—	16.8	—	—
44	60	3.60	—	—	953.0	—	0	—	—	—	—	—	—	0	—	—
34	510	0.72	—	—	363.0	—	—	—	—	—	—	—	—	6.6	—	—
44	70	3.78	—	—	1060.0	—	—	—	—	—	—	—	—	6.0	—	—
34	510	0.36	—	—	350.0	—	—	—	—	—	—	—	—	5.4	—	—
10	100	0.00	—	—	510.0	—	—	—	—	—	—	—	—	0	—	—
0	20	1.98	—	—	410.0	—	0	—	—	—	—	—	—	0	—	—

TABLE **A-1** **Table of Food Composition** (continued)

(Computer code is for Cengage Diet & Wellness Plus program)

D&W+ Code	Food Description	QTY	Measure	Wt (g)	H₂O (g)	Ener (cal)	Prot (g)	Carb (g)	Fiber (g)	Fat (g)	Fat Breakdown (g) Sat	Mono	Poly
Fast Food—continued
35354	Cinnamon sugar soft pretzel with butter	1	item(s)	120	—	450	8.0	83.0	3.0	9.0	5.0	—	—
35372	Marinara dipping sauce	1	serving(s)	35	—	10	0	4.0	0	0	0	0	0
35357	Original soft pretzel	1	serving(s)	120	—	340	10.0	72.0	3.0	1.0	0	—	—
35358	Original soft pretzel with butter	1	item(s)	120	—	370	10.0	72.0	3.0	4.0	2.0	—	—
35359	Parmesan herb soft pretzel	1	item(s)	120	—	390	11.0	74.0	4.0	5.0	2.5	—	—
35360	Parmesan herb soft pretzel with butter	1	item(s)	120	—	440	10.0	72.0	9.0	13.0	7.0	—	—
35361	Sesame soft pretzel	1	item(s)	120	—	350	11.0	63.0	3.0	6.0	1.0	—	—
35362	Sesame soft pretzel with butter	1	item(s)	120	—	410	12.0	64.0	7.0	12.0	4.0	—	—
35364	Sour cream and onion soft pretzel	1	item(s)	120	—	310	9.0	66.0	2.0	1.0	0	—	—
35366	Sour cream and onion soft pretzel with butter	1	item(s)	120	—	340	9.0	66.0	2.0	5.0	3.0	—	—
35373	Sweet mustard dipping sauce	1	serving(s)	35	—	60	0.5	8.0	0	1.5	1.0	—	—
35367	Whole wheat soft pretzel	1	item(s)	120	—	350	11.0	72.0	7.0	1.5	0	—	—
35368	Whole wheat soft pretzel with butter	1	item(s)	120	—	370	11.0	72.0	7.0	4.5	1.5	—	—
	Boston Market
34978	Butternut squash	¾	cup(s)	143	—	140	2.0	25.0	2.0	4.5	3.0	—	—
35006	Caesar side salad	1	serving(s)	71	—	40	3.0	3.0	1.0	20.0	2.0	—	—
35013	Chicken Carver sandwich with cheese and sauce	1	item(s)	321	—	700	44.0	68.0	3.0	29.0	7.0	—	—
34979	Chicken gravy	4	ounce(s)	113	—	15	1.0	4.0	0	0.5	0	—	—
35053	Chicken noodle soup	¾	cup(s)	283	—	180	13.0	16.0	1.0	7.0	2.0	—	—
34973	Chicken pot pie	1	item(s)	425	—	800	29.0	59.0	4.0	49.0	18.0	—	—
35054	Chicken tortilla soup with toppings	¾	cup(s)	227	—	340	12.0	24.0	1.0	22.0	7.0	—	—
35007	Cole slaw	¾	cup(s)	125	—	170	2.0	21.0	2.0	9.0	2.0	—	—
35057	Cornbread	1	item(s)	45	—	130	1.0	21.0	0	3.5	1.0	—	—
34980	Creamed spinach	¾	cup(s)	191	—	280	9.0	12.0	4.0	23.0	15.0	—	—
34998	Fresh vegetable stuffing	1	cup(s)	136	—	190	3.0	25.0	2.0	8.0	1.0	—	—
34991	Garlic dill new potatoes	¾	cup(s)	156	—	140	3.0	24.0	3.0	3.0	1.0	—	—
34983	Green bean casserole	¾	cup(s)	170	—	60	2.0	9.0	2.0	2.0	1.0	—	—
34982	Green beans	¾	cup(s)	91	—	60	2.0	7.0	3.0	3.5	1.5	—	—
34984	Homestyle mashed potatoes	¾	cup(s)	221	—	210	4.0	29.0	3.0	9.0	6.0	—	—
34985	Homestyle mashed potatoes and gravy	1	cup(s)	334	—	225	5.0	33.0	3.0	9.5	6.0	—	—
34988	Hot cinnamon apples	¾	cup(s)	145	—	210	0	47.0	3.0	3.0	0	—	—
34989	Macaroni and cheese	¾	cup(s)	221	—	330	14.0	39.0	1.0	12.0	7.0	—	—
51193	Market chopped salad with dressing	1	item(s)	563	—	580	11.0	31.0	9.0	48.0	9.0	—	—
34970	Meatloaf	1	serving(s)	218	—	480	29.0	23.0	2.0	33.0	13.0	—	—
39383	Nestle Toll House chocolate chip cookie	1	item(s)	78	—	370	4.0	49.0	2.0	19.0	9.0	—	—
34965	Quarter chicken, dark meat, no skin	1	item(s)	134	—	260	30.0	2.0	0	13.0	4.0	—	—
34966	Quarter chicken, dark meat, with skin	1	item(s)	149	—	280	31.0	3.0	0	15.0	4.5	—	—
34963	Quarter chicken, white meat, no skin or wing	1	item(s)	173	—	250	41.0	4.0	0	8.0	2.5	—	—
34964	Quarter chicken, white meat, with skin and wing	1	item(s)	110	—	330	50.0	3.0	0	12.0	4.0	—	—
34968	Roasted turkey breast	5	ounce(s)	142	—	180	38.0	0	0	3.0	1.0	—	—
35011	Seasonal fresh fruit salad	1	serving(s)	142	—	60	1.0	15.0	1.0	0	0	0	0
51192	Spinach with garlic butter sauce	1	item(s)	170	—	130	5.0	9.0	5.0	9.0	6.0	—	—
34969	Spiral sliced holiday ham	8	ounce(s)	227	—	450	40.0	13.0	0	26.0	10.0	—	—
35003	Steamed vegetables	1	cup(s)	136	—	50	2.0	8.0	3.0	2.0	0	—	—
35005	Sweet corn	¾	cup(s)	176	—	170	6.0	37.0	2.0	4.0	1.0	—	—
35004	Sweet potato casserole	¾	cup(s)	198	—	460	4.0	77.0	3.0	17.0	6.0	—	—
	Burger King
29731	Biscuit with sausage, egg, and cheese	1	item(s)	191	—	610	20.0	33.0	1.0	45.0	15.0	—	—
14249	Cheeseburger	1	item(s)	133	—	330	17.0	31.0	1.0	16.0	7.0	—	—
14251	Chicken sandwich	1	item(s)	219	—	660	24.0	52.0	4.0	40.0	8.0	—	—
3808	Chicken Tenders, 8 pieces	1	serving(s)	123	—	340	19.0	21.0	0.5	20.0	5.0	—	—
14259	Chocolate shake, small	1	item(s)	315	—	470	8.0	75.0	1.0	14.0	9.0	—	—
29732	Croissanwich with sausage and cheese	1	item(s)	106	37.2	370	14.0	23.0	0.5	25.0	9.0	12.7	3.3

PAGE KEY: A-4 = Breads/Baked Goods A-10 = Cereal/Rice/Pasta A-14 = Fruit A-20 = Vegetables/Legumes A-30 = Nuts/Seeds A-32 = Vegetarian A-34 = Dairy A-42 = Eggs A-42 = Seafood A-46 = Meats A-50 = Poultry A-50 = Processed Meats A-52 = Beverages A-56 = Fats/Oils A-58 = Sweets A-60 = Spices/Condiments/Sauces A-64 = Mixed Foods/Soups/Sandwiches A-70 = Fast Food A-90 = Convenience A-92 = Baby Foods

A

CHOL (mg)	CALC (mg)	IRON (mg)	MAGN (mg)	POTA (mg)	SODI (mg)	ZINC (mg)	VIT A (µg)	THIA (mg)	VIT E (mg α)	RIBO (mg)	NIAC (mg)	VIT B6 (mg)	FOLA (µg DFE)	VIT C (mg)	VIT B12 (µg)	SELE (µg)
25	30	2.34	—	—	430.0	—	—	—	—	—	—	—	—	0	—	—
0	0	0.00	—	—	180.0	—	0	—	—	—	—	—	—	0	—	—
0	30	2.34	—	—	900.0	—	0	—	—	—	—	—	—	0	—	—
10	30	2.16	—	—	930.0	—	—	—	—	—	—	—	—	0	—	—
10	80	1.80	—	—	780.0	—	—	—	—	—	—	—	—	1.2	—	—
30	60	1.80	—	—	660.0	—	—	—	—	—	—	—	—	1.2	—	—
0	20	2.88	—	—	840.0	—	0	—	—	—	—	—	—	0	—	—
15	20	2.70	—	—	860.0	—	—	—	—	—	—	—	—	0	—	—
0	30	1.98	—	—	920.0	—	—	—	—	—	—	—	—	0	—	—
10	40	2.16	—	—	930.0	—	—	—	—	—	—	—	—	0	—	—
40	0	0.00	—	—	120.0	—	0	—	—	—	—	—	—	0	—	—
0	30	1.98	—	—	1100.0	—	0	—	—	—	—	—	—	0	—	—
10	30	2.34	—	—	1120.0	—	—	—	—	—	—	—	—	0	—	—
10	59	0.80	—	—	35.0	—	—	—	—	—	—	—	—	22.2	—	—
0	60	0.43	—	—	75.0	—	—	—	—	—	—	—	—	5.4	—	—
90	211	2.85	—	—	1560.0	—	—	—	—	—	—	—	—	15.8	—	—
0	0	0.00	—	—	570.0	—	0	—	—	—	—	—	—	0	—	—
55	0	1.07	—	—	220.0	—	—	—	—	—	—	—	—	1.8	—	—
115	40	4.50	—	—	800.0	—	—	—	—	—	—	—	—	1.2	—	—
45	123	1.32	—	—	1310.0	—	—	—	—	—	—	—	—	18.4	—	—
10	41	0.48	—	—	270.0	—	—	—	—	—	—	—	—	24.5	—	—
5	0	0.71	—	—	220.0	—	0	—	—	—	—	—	—	0	—	—
70	264	2.84	—	—	580.0	—	—	—	—	—	—	—	—	9.5	—	—
0	41	1.48	—	—	580.0	—	—	—	—	—	—	—	—	2.5	—	—
0	0	0.85	—	—	120.0	—	0	—	—	—	—	—	—	14.3	—	—
5	20	0.72	—	—	620.0	—	—	—	—	—	—	—	—	2.4	—	—
0	43	0.38	—	—	180.0	—	—	—	—	—	—	—	—	5.1	—	—
25	51	0.46	—	—	660.0	—	—	—	—	—	—	—	—	19.2	—	—
25	100	0.59	—	—	1230.0	—	—	—	—	—	—	—	—	24.9	—	—
0	16	0.28	—	—	15.0	—	—	—	—	—	—	—	—	0	—	—
30	345	1.65	—	—	1290.0	—	—	—	—	—	—	—	—	0	—	—
10	—	—	—	—	2010.0	—	—	—	—	—	—	—	—	—	—	—
125	140	3.77	—	—	970.0	—	—	—	—	—	—	—	—	1.8	—	—
20	0	1.32	—	—	340.0	—	—	—	—	—	—	—	—	0	—	—
155	0	1.52	—	—	260.0	—	0	—	—	—	—	—	—	0	—	—
155	0	2.14	—	—	660.0	—	0	—	—	—	—	—	—	0	—	—
125	0	0.89	—	—	480.0	—	0	—	—	—	—	—	—	0	—	—
165	0	0.78	—	—	960.0	—	0	—	—	—	—	—	—	0	—	—
70	20	1.80	—	—	620.0	—	0	—	—	—	—	—	—	0	—	—
0	16	0.29	—	—	20.0	—	—	—	—	—	—	—	—	29.5	—	—
20	—	—	—	—	200.0	—	—	—	—	—	—	—	—	—	—	—
140	0	1.73	—	—	2230.0	—	0	—	—	—	—	—	—	0	—	—
0	53	0.46	—	—	45.0	—	—	—	—	—	—	—	—	24.0	—	—
0	0	0.43	—	—	95.0	—	—	—	—	—	—	—	—	5.8	—	—
20	44	1.18	—	—	210.0	—	—	—	—	—	—	—	—	9.8	—	—
210	250	2.70	—	—	1620.0	—	89.9	—	—	—	—	—	—	0	—	—
55	150	2.70	—	—	780.0	—	—	0.24	—	0.31	4.17	—	—	1.2	—	—
70	64	2.89	—	—	1440.0	—	—	0.50	—	0.32	10.29	—	—	0	—	—
55	20	0.72	—	—	960.0	—	—	0.14	—	0.11	10.93	—	—	0	—	—
55	333	0.79	—	—	350.0	—	—	0.11	—	0.61	0.26	—	—	2.7	0	—
50	99	1.78	20.1	217.3	810.0	1.51	—	0.34	1.03	0.33	4.33	—	—	0	0.6	22.2

A

D&W+ Code	Food Description	QTY	Measure	Wt (g)	H₂O (g)	Ener (cal)	Prot (g)	Carb (g)	Fiber (g)	Fat (g)	Fat Breakdown (g)		
											Sat	Mono	Poly
Fast Food—continued													
14261	Croissanwich with sausage, egg, and cheese	1	item(s)	159	71.4	470	19.0	26.0	0.5	32.0	11.0	15.8	6.1
3809	Double cheeseburger	1	item(s)	189	—	500	30.0	31.0	1.0	29.0	14.0	—	—
14244	Double Whopper sandwich	1	item(s)	373	—	900	47.0	51.0	3.0	57.0	19.0	—	—
14245	Double Whopper with cheese sandwich	1	item(s)	398	—	990	52.0	52.0	3.0	64.0	24.0	—	—
14250	Fish Filet sandwich	1	item(s)	250	—	630	24.0	67.0	4.0	30.0	6.0	—	—
14255	French fries, medium, salted	1	serving(s)	116	—	360	4.0	41.0	4.0	20.0	4.5	—	—
14262	French toast sticks, 5 pieces	1	serving(s)	112	37.6	390	6.0	46.0	2.0	20.0	4.5	10.6	2.9
14248	Hamburger	1	item(s)	121	—	290	15.0	30.0	1.0	12.0	4.5	—	—
14263	Hash brown rounds, small	1	serving(s)	75	27.1	230	2.0	23.0	2.0	15.0	4.0	—	—
14256	Onion rings, medium	1	serving(s)	91	—	320	4.0	40.0	3.0	16.0	4.0	—	—
39000	Tendercrisp chicken sandwich	1	item(s)	286	—	780	25.0	73.0	4.0	43.0	8.0	—	—
37514	TenderGrill chicken sandwich	1	item(s)	258	—	450	37.0	53.0	4.0	10.0	2.0	—	—
14258	Vanilla shake, small	1	item(s)	296	—	400	8.0	57.0	0	15.0	9.0	—	—
1736	Whopper sandwich	1	item(s)	290	—	670	28.0	51.0	3.0	39.0	11.0	—	—
14243	Whopper with cheese sandwich	1	item(s)	315	—	760	33.0	52.0	3.0	47.0	16.0	—	—
	Carl's Jr												
33962	Carl's bacon Swiss crispy chicken sandwich	1	item(s)	268	—	750	31.0	91.0	—	28.0	28.0	—	—
10801	Carl's Catch fish sandwich	1	item(s)	215	—	560	19.0	58.0	2.0	27.0	7.0	—	1.9
10862	Carl's Famous Star hamburger	1	item(s)	254	—	590	24.0	50.0	3.0	32.0	9.0	—	—
10785	Charbroiled chicken club sandwich	1	item(s)	270	—	550	42.0	43.0	4.0	23.0	7.0	—	2.9
10866	Charbroiled chicken salad	1	item(s)	437	—	330	34.0	17.0	5.0	7.0	4.0	—	1.0
10855	Charbroiled Santa Fe chicken sandwich	1	item(s)	266	—	610	38.0	43.0	4.0	32.0	8.0	—	—
10790	Chicken stars, 6 pieces	1	serving(s)	85	—	260	13.0	14.0	1.0	16.0	4.0	—	1.6
34864	Chocolate shake, small	1	serving(s)	595	—	540	15.0	98.0	0	11.0	7.0	—	—
10797	Crisscut fries	1	serving(s)	139	—	410	5.0	43.0	4.0	24.0	5.0	—	—
10799	Double Western Bacon cheeseburger	1	item(s)	308	—	920	51.0	65.0	2.0	50	21.0	—	6.6
14238	French fries, small	1	serving(s)	92	—	290	5.0	37.0	3.0	14.0	3.0	—	—
10798	French toast dips without syrup, 5 pieces	1	serving(s)	155	—	370	8.0	49.0	0	17.0	5.0	—	1.4
10802	Onion rings	1	serving(s)	128	—	440	7.0	53.0	3.0	22.0	5.0	—	0.8
34858	Spicy chicken sandwich	1	item(s)	198	—	480	14.0	48.0	2.0	26.0	5.0	—	—
34867	Strawberry shake, small	1	serving(s)	595	—	520	14.0	93.0	0	11.0	7.0	—	—
10865	Super Star hamburger	1	item(s)	348	—	790	41.0	52.0	3.0	47.0	14.0	—	—
38925	The Six Dollar burger	1	item(s)	429	—	1010	40.0	60.0	3.0	66.0	26.0	—	—
10818	Vanilla shake, small	1	item(s)	398	—	314	10.0	51.5	0	7.4	4.7	—	—
10770	Western Bacon cheeseburger	1	item(s)	225	—	660	32.0	64.0	2.0	30.0	12.0	—	4.8
	Chick-Fil-A												
38746	Biscuit with bacon, egg, and cheese	1	item(s)	163	—	470	18.0	39.0	1.0	26.0	9.0	—	—
38747	Biscuit with egg	1	item(s)	135	—	350	11.0	38.0	1.0	16.0	4.5	—	—
38748	Biscuit with egg and cheese	1	item(s)	149	—	400	14.0	38.0	1.0	21.0	7.0	—	—
38753	Biscuit with gravy	1	item(s)	192	—	330	5.0	43.0	1.0	15.0	4.0	—	—
38752	Biscuit with sausage, egg, and cheese	1	item(s)	212	—	620	22.0	39.0	2.0	42.0	14.0	—	—
38771	Carrot and raisin salad	1	item(s)	113	—	170	1.0	28.0	2.0	6.0	1.0	—	—
38761	Chargrilled chicken Cool Wrap	1	item(s)	245	—	390	29.0	54.0	3.0	7.0	3.0	—	—
38766	Chargrilled chicken garden salad	1	item(s)	275	—	180	22.0	9.0	3.0	6.0	3.0	—	—
38758	Chargrilled chicken sandwich	1	item(s)	193	—	270	28.0	33.0	3.0	3.5	1.0	—	—
38742	Chicken biscuit	1	item(s)	145	—	420	18.0	44.0	2.0	19.0	4.5	—	—
38743	Chicken biscuit with cheese	1	item(s)	159	—	470	21.0	45.0	2.0	23.0	8.0	—	—
38762	Chicken Caesar Cool Wrap	1	item(s)	227	—	460	36.0	52.0	3.0	10.0	6.0	—	—
38757	Chicken deluxe sandwich	1	item(s)	208	—	420	28.0	39.0	2.0	16.0	3.5	—	—
38764	Chicken salad sandwich on wheat bun	1	item(s)	153	—	350	20.0	32.0	5.0	15.0	3.0	—	—
38756	Chicken sandwich	1	item(s)	170	—	410	28.0	38.0	1.0	16.0	3.5	—	—
38768	Chick-n-Strip salad	1	item(s)	327	—	400	34.0	21.0	4.0	20.0	6.0	—	—
38763	Chick-n-Strips	4	item(s)	127	—	300	28.0	14.0	1.0	15.0	2.5	—	—
38770	Cole slaw	1	item(s)	128	—	260	2.0	17.0	2.0	21.0	3.5	—	—
38776	Diet lemonade, small	1	cup(s)	255	—	25	0	5.0	0	0	0	0	0

PAGE KEY: A-4 = Breads/Baked Goods A-10 = Cereal/Rice/Pasta A-14 = Fruit A-20 = Vegetables/Legumes A-30 = Nuts/Seeds A-32 = Vegetarian A-34 = Dairy A-42 = Eggs A-42 = Seafood A-46 = Meats A-50 = Poultry A-50 = Processed Meats A-52 = Beverages A-56 = Fats/Oils A-58 = Sweets A-60 = Spices/Condiments/Sauces A-64 = Mixed Foods/Soups/Sandwiches A-70 = Fast Food A-90 = Convenience A-92 = Baby Foods

A

CHOL (mg)	CALC (mg)	IRON (mg)	MAGN (mg)	POTA (mg)	SODI (mg)	ZINC (mg)	VIT A (µg)	THIA (mg)	VIT E (mg α)	RIBO (mg)	NIAC (mg)	VIT B6 (mg)	FOLA (µg DFE)	VIT C (mg)	VIT B12 (µg)	SELE (µg)
180	146	2.63	28.6	313.2	1060.0	2.08	—	0.38	1.66	0.51	4.72	0.28	—	0	1.1	38.0
105	250	4.50	—	—	1030.0	—	—	0.26	—	0.44	6.37	—	—	1.2	—	—
175	150	8.07	—	—	1090.0	—	—	0.39	—	0.59	11.05	—	—	9.0	—	—
195	299	8.08	—	—	1520.0	—	—	0.39	—	0.66	11.03	—	—	9.0	—	—
60	101	3.62	—	—	1380.0	—	—	—	—	—	—	—	—	3.6	—	—
0	20	0.71	—	—	590.0	—	0	0.15	—	0.48	2.30	—	—	8.9	—	—
0	60	1.80	21.3	124.3	440.0	0.57	—	0.31	0.98	0.19	2.88	0.05	—	0	0	13.7
40	80	2.70	—	—	560.0	—	—	0.25	—	0.28	4.25	—	—	1.2	—	—
0	0	0.36	—	—	450.0	—	0	0.11	0.83	0.06	1.35	0.17	—	1.2	—	—
0	100	0.00	—	—	460.0	—	0	0.14	—	0.09	2.32	—	—	0	—	—
75	79	4.43	—	—	1730.0	—	—	—	—	—	—	—	—	8.9	—	—
75	57	6.82	—	—	1210.0	—	—	—	—	—	—	—	—	5.7	—	—
60	348	0.00	—	—	240.0	—	—	0.11	—	0.63	0.21	—	—	2.4	0	—
51	100	5.38	—	—	1020.0	—	—	0.38	—	0.43	7.30	—	—	9.0	—	—
115	249	5.38	—	—	1450.0	—	—	0.38	—	0.51	7.28	—	—	9.0	—	—
80	200	5.40	—	—	1900.0	—	—	—	—	—	—	—	—	2.4	—	—
80	150	2.70	—	—	990.0	—	60.0	—	—	—	—	—	—	2.4	—	—
70	100	4.50	—	—	910.0	—	—	—	—	—	—	—	—	6.0	—	—
95	200	3.60	—	—	1330.0	—	—	—	—	—	—	—	—	9.0	—	—
75	200	1.80	—	—	880.0	—	—	—	—	—	—	—	—	30.0	—	—
100	200	3.60	—	—	1440.0	—	—	—	—	—	—	—	—	9.0	—	—
35	19	1.02	—	—	470.0	—	0	—	—	—	—	—	—	0	—	—
45	600	1.08	—	—	360.0	—	0	—	—	—	—	—	—	0	—	—
0	20	1.80	—	—	950.0	—	0	—	—	—	—	—	—	12.0	—	—
155	300	7.20	—	—	1730.0	—	—	—	—	—	—	—	—	1.2	—	—
0	0	1.08	—	—	170.0	—	0	—	—	—	—	—	—	21.0	—	—
3	0	0.00	—	—	470.0	—	0	0.25	—	0.23	2.00	—	—	0	—	—
0	20	0.72	—	—	700.0	—	0	—	—	—	—	—	—	3.6	—	—
40	100	3.60	—	—	1220.0	—	—	—	—	—	—	—	—	6.0	—	—
45	600	0.00	—	—	340.0	—	0	—	—	—	—	—	—	0	—	—
130	100	7.20	—	—	980.0	—	—	—	—	—	—	—	—	9.0	—	—
145	279	4.29	—	—	1960.0	—	—	—	—	—	—	—	—	16.7	—	—
30	401	0.00	—	—	234.0	—	0	—	—	—	—	—	—	0	—	—
85	200	5.40	—	—	1410.0	—	60.0	—	—	—	—	—	—	1.2	—	—
270	150	2.70	—	—	1190.0	—	—	—	—	—	—	—	—	0	—	—
240	80	2.70	—	—	740.0	—	—	—	—	—	—	—	—	0	—	—
255	150	2.70	—	—	970.0	—	—	—	—	—	—	—	—	0	—	—
5	60	1.80	—	—	930.0	—	0	—	—	—	—	—	—	0	—	—
300	200	3.60	—	—	1360.0	—	—	—	—	—	—	—	—	0	—	—
10	40	0.36	—	—	110.0	—	—	—	—	—	—	—	—	4.8	—	—
65	200	3.60	—	—	1020.0	—	—	—	—	—	—	—	—	6.0	—	—
65	150	0.72	—	—	620.0	—	—	—	—	—	—	—	—	30	—	—
65	80	2.70	—	—	940.0	—	—	—	—	—	—	—	—	6.0	—	—
35	60	2.70	—	—	1270.0	—	0	—	—	—	—	—	—	0	—	—
50	150	2.70	—	—	1500.0	—	—	—	—	—	—	—	—	0	—	—
80	500	3.60	—	—	1350.0	—	—	—	—	—	—	—	—	1.2	—	—
60	100	2.70	—	—	1300.0	—	—	—	—	—	—	—	—	2.4	—	—
65	150	1.80	—	—	880.0	—	—	—	—	—	—	—	—	0	—	—
60	100	2.70	—	—	1300.0	—	—	—	—	—	—	—	—	0	—	—
80	150	1.44	—	—	1070.0	—	—	—	—	—	—	—	—	6.0	—	—
65	40	1.44	—	—	940.0	—	—	—	—	—	—	—	—	0	—	—
25	60	0.36	—	—	220.0	—	—	—	—	—	—	—	—	36.0	—	—
0	0	0.36	—	—	5.0	—	0	—	—	—	—	—	—	15.0	—	—

(Computer code is for Cengage Diet & Wellness Plus program)

D&W+ Code	FOOD DESCRIPTION	QTY	MEASURE	WT (g)	H₂O (g)	ENER (cal)	PROT (g)	CARB (g)	FIBER (g)	FAT (g)	FAT BREAKDOWN (g)		
											SAT	MONO	POLY
	FAST FOOD—CONTINUED												
38755	Hashbrowns	1	serving(s)	84	—	260	2.0	25.0	3.0	17.0	3.5	—	—
38765	Hearty breast of chicken soup	1	cup(s)	241	—	140	8.0	18.0	1.0	3.5	1.0	—	—
38741	Hot buttered biscuit	1	item(s)	79	—	270	4.0	38.0	1.0	12.0	3.0	—	—
38778	IceDream, small cone	1	item(s)	135	—	160	4.0	28.0	0	4.0	2.0	—	—
38774	IceDream, small cup	1	serving(s)	227	—	240	6.0	41.0	0	6.0	3.5	—	—
38775	Lemonade, small	1	cup(s)	255	—	170	0	41.0	0	0.5	0	—	—
38777	Nuggets	8	item(s)	113	—	260	26.0	12.0	0.5	12.0	2.5	—	—
38769	Side salad	1	item(s)	108	—	60	3.0	4.0	2.0	3.0	1.5	—	—
38767	Southwest chargrilled salad	1	item(s)	303	—	240	25.0	17.0	5.0	8.0	3.5	—	—
40481	Spicy chicken cool wrap	1	serving(s)	230	—	380	30.0	52.0	3.0	6.0	3.0	—	—
38772	Waffle potato fries, small, salted	1	serving(s)	85	—	270	3.0	34.0	4.0	13.0	3.0	—	—
	CINNABON												
39572	Caramellata Chill w/whipped cream	16	fluid ounce(s)	480	—	406	10.0	61.0	0	14.0	8.0	—	—
39571	Cinnabon Bites	1	serving(s)	149	—	510	8.0	77.0	2.0	19.0	5.0	—	—
39570	Cinnabon Stix	5	item(s)	85	—	379	6.0	41.0	1.0	21.0	6.0	—	—
39567	Classic roll	1	item(s)	221	—	813	15.0	117.0	4.0	32.0	8.0	—	—
39568	Minibon	1	item(s)	92	—	339	6.0	49.0	2.0	13.0	3.0	—	—
39573	Mochalatta Chill w/whipped cream	16	fluid ounce(s)	480	—	362	9.0	55.0	0	13.0	8.0	—	—
39569	Pecanbon	1	item(s)	272	—	1100	16.0	141.0	8.0	56.0	10.0	—	—
	DAIRY QUEEN												
1466	Banana split	1	item(s)	369	—	510	8.0	96.0	3.0	12.0	8.0	—	—
38552	Brownie Earthquake®	1	serving(s)	304	—	740	10.0	112.0	0	27.0	16.0	—	—
38561	Chocolate chip cookie dough blizzard,® small	1	item(s)	319	—	720	12.0	105.0	0	28.0	14.0	—	—
1464	Chocolate malt, small	1	item(s)	418	—	640	15.0	111.0	1.0	16.0	11.0	—	—
38541	Chocolate shake, small	1	item(s)	397	—	560	13.0	93.0	1.0	15.0	10.0	—	—
17257	Chocolate soft serve	½	cup(s)	94	—	150	4.0	22.0	0	5.0	3.5	—	—
1463	Chocolate sundae, small	1	item(s)	163	—	280	5.0	49.0	0	7.0	4.5	—	—
1462	Dipped cone, small	1	item(s)	156	—	340	6.0	42.0	1.0	17.0	9.0	4.0	3.0
38555	Oreo cookies blizzard, small	1	item(s)	283	—	570	11.0	83.0	0.5	21.0	10.0	—	—
38547	Royal Treats Peanut Buster® Parfait	1	item(s)	305	—	730	16.0	99.0	2.0	31.0	17.0	—	—
17256	Vanilla soft serve	½	cup(s)	94	—	140	3.0	22.0	0	4.5	3.0	—	—
	DOMINO'S												
31606	Barbeque buffalo wings	1	item(s)	25	—	50	6.0	2.0	0	2.5	0.5	—	—
31604	Breadsticks	1	item(s)	30	—	115	2.0	12.0	0	6.3	1.1	—	—
37551	Buffalo Chicken Kickers	1	item(s)	24	—	47	4.0	3.0	0	2.0	0.5	—	—
37548	CinnaStix	1	item(s)	30	—	123	2.0	15.0	1.0	6.1	1.1	—	—
37549	Dot, cinnamon	1	item(s)	28	7.6	99	1.9	14.9	0.7	3.7	0.7	—	—
31605	Double cheesy bread	1	item(s)	35	—	123	4.0	13.0	0	6.5	1.9	—	—
31607	Hot buffalo wings	1	item(s)	25	—	45	5.0	1.0	0	2.5	0.5	—	—
	DOMINO'S CLASSIC HAND TOSSED PIZZA												
31573	America's favorite feast, 12″	1	slice(s)	102	—	257	10.0	29.0	2.0	11.5	4.5	—	—
31574	America's favorite feast, 14″	1	slice(s)	141	—	353	14.0	39.0	2.0	16.0	6.0	—	—
37543	Bacon cheeseburger feast, 12″	1	slice(s)	99	—	273	12.0	28.0	2.0	13.0	5.5	—	—
37545	Bacon cheeseburger feast, 14″	1	slice(s)	137	—	379	17.0	38.0	2.0	18.0	8.0	—	—
37546	Barbeque feast, 12″	1	slice(s)	96	—	252	11.0	31.0	1.0	10.0	4.5	—	—
37547	Barbeque feast, 14″	1	slice(s)	131	—	344	14.0	43.0	2.0	13.5	6.0	—	—
31569	Cheese, 12″	1	slice(s)	55	—	160	6.0	28.0	1.0	3.0	1.0	—	—
31570	Cheese, 14″	1	slice(s)	75	—	220	8.0	38.0	2.0	4.0	1.0	—	—
37538	Deluxe feast, 12″	1	slice(s)	201	101.8	465	19.5	57.4	3.5	18.2	7.7	—	—
37540	Deluxe feast, 14″	1	slice(s)	273	138.4	627	26.4	78.3	4.7	24.1	10.2	—	—
31685	Deluxe, 12″	1	slice(s)	100	—	234	9.0	29.0	2.0	9.5	3.5	—	—
31694	Deluxe, 14″	1	slice(s)	136	—	316	13.0	39.0	2.0	12.5	5.0	—	—
31686	Extravaganzza, 12″	1	slice(s)	122	—	289	13.0	30.0	2.0	14.0	5.5	—	—
31695	Extravaganzza, 14″	1	slice(s)	165	—	388	17.0	40.0	3.0	18.5	7.5	—	—
31575	Hawaiian feast, 12″	1	slice(s)	102	—	223	10.0	30.0	2.0	8.0	3.5	—	—
31576	Hawaiian feast, 14″	1	slice(s)	141	—	309	14.0	41.0	2.0	11.0	4.5	—	—
31687	Meatzza, 12″	1	slice(s)	108	—	281	13.0	29.0	2.0	13.5	5.5	—	—

PAGE KEY: A-4 = Breads/Baked Goods A-10 = Cereal/Rice/Pasta A-14 = Fruit A-20 = Vegetables/Legumes A-30 = Nuts/Seeds A-32 = Vegetarian
A-34 = Dairy A-42 = Eggs A-42 = Seafood A-46 = Meats A-50 = Poultry A-50 = Processed Meats A-52 = Beverages A-56 = Fats/Oils A-58 = Sweets
A-60 = Spices/Condiments/Sauces A-64 = Mixed Foods/Soups/Sandwiches A-70 = Fast Food A-90 = Convenience A-92 = Baby Foods

A

CHOL (mg)	CALC (mg)	IRON (mg)	MAGN (mg)	POTA (mg)	SODI (mg)	ZINC (mg)	VIT A (µg)	THIA (mg)	VIT E (mg α)	RIBO (mg)	NIAC (mg)	VIT B6 (mg)	FOLA (µg DFE)	VIT C (mg)	VIT B12 (µg)	SELE (µg)
5	20	0.72	—	—	380.0	—	—	—	—	—	—	—	—	0	—	—
25	40	1.08	—	—	900.0	—	—	—	—	—	—	—	—	0	—	—
0	60	1.80	—	—	660.0	—	0	—	—	—	—	—	—	0	—	—
15	100	0.36	—	—	80.0	—	—	—	—	—	—	—	—	0	—	—
25	200	0.36	—	—	105.0	—	—	—	—	—	—	—	—	0	—	—
0	0	0.36	—	—	10.0	—	0	—	—	—	—	—	—	15.0	—	—
70	40	1.08	—	—	1090.0	—	0	—	—	—	—	—	—	0	—	—
10	100	0.00	—	—	75.0	—	—	—	—	—	—	—	—	15.0	—	—
60	200	1.08	—	—	770.0	—	—	—	—	—	—	—	—	24.0	—	—
60	200	3.60	—	—	1090.0	—	—	—	—	—	—	—	—	3.6	—	—
0	20	1.08	—	—	115.0	—	0	—	—	—	—	—	—	1.2	—	—
46	—	—	—	—	187.0	—	—	—	—	—	—	—	—	—	—	—
35	—	—	—	—	530.0	—	—	—	—	—	—	—	—	—	—	—
16	—	—	—	—	413.0	—	—	—	—	—	—	—	—	—	—	—
67	—	—	—	—	801.0	—	—	—	—	—	—	—	—	—	—	—
27	—	—	—	—	337.0	—	—	—	—	—	—	—	—	—	—	—
46	—	—	—	—	252.0	—	—	—	—	—	—	—	—	—	—	—
63	—	—	—	—	600.0	—	—	—	—	—	—	—	—	—	—	—
30	250	1.80	—	—	180.0	—	—	—	—	—	—	—	—	15.0	—	—
50	250	1.80	—	—	350.0	—	—	—	—	—	—	—	—	0	—	—
50	350	2.70	—	—	370.0	—	—	—	—	—	—	—	—	1.2	—	—
55	450	1.80	—	—	340.0	—	—	—	—	—	—	—	—	2.4	—	—
50	450	1.44	—	—	280.0	—	—	—	—	—	—	—	—	2.4	—	—
15	100	0.72	—	—	75.0	—	—	—	—	—	—	—	—	0	—	—
20	200	1.08	—	—	140.0	—	—	—	—	—	—	—	—	0	—	—
20	200	1.08	—	—	130.0	—	—	—	—	—	—	—	—	1.2	—	—
40	350	2.70	—	—	430.0	—	—	—	—	—	—	—	—	1.2	—	—
35	300	1.80	—	—	400.0	—	—	—	—	—	—	—	—	1.2	—	—
15	150	0.72	—	—	70.0	—	—	—	—	—	—	—	—	0	—	—
26	10	0.36	—	—	175.5	—	—	—	—	—	—	—	—	0	—	—
0	0	0.72	—	—	122.1	—	—	—	—	—	—	—	—	0	—	—
9	0	0.00	—	—	162.5	—	—	—	—	—	—	—	—	0	—	—
0	0	0.72	—	—	111.4	—	—	—	—	—	—	—	—	0	—	—
0	6	0.59	—	—	85.7	—	—	—	—	—	—	—	—	0	—	—
6	40	0.72	—	—	162.3	—	—	—	—	—	—	—	—	0	—	—
26	10	0.36	—	—	254.5	—	—	—	—	—	—	—	—	1.2	—	—
22	100	1.80	—	—	625.5	—	—	—	—	—	—	—	—	0.6	—	—
31	140	2.52	—	—	865.5	—	—	—	—	—	—	—	—	0.6	—	—
27	140	1.80	—	—	634.0	—	—	—	—	—	—	—	—	0	—	—
38	190	2.52	—	—	900.0	—	—	—	—	—	—	—	—	0	—	—
20	140	1.62	—	—	600.0	—	—	—	—	—	—	—	—	0.6	—	—
27	190	2.16	—	—	831.5	—	—	—	—	—	—	—	—	0.6	—	—
0	0	1.80	—	—	110.0	—	0	—	—	—	—	—	—	0	—	—
0	0	2.70	—	—	150.0	—	0	—	—	—	—	—	—	0	—	—
40	199	3.56	—	—	1063.1	—	—	—	—	—	—	—	—	1.4	—	—
53	276	4.84	—	—	1432.2	—	—	—	—	—	—	—	—	1.8	—	—
17	100	1.80	—	—	541.5	—	—	—	—	—	—	—	—	0.6	—	—
23	130	2.34	—	—	728.5	—	—	—	—	—	—	—	—	1.2	—	—
28	140	1.98	—	—	764.0	—	—	—	—	—	—	—	—	0.6	—	—
37	190	2.70	—	—	1014.0	—	—	—	—	—	—	—	—	1.2	—	—
16	130	1.62	—	—	546.5	—	—	—	—	—	—	—	—	1.2	—	—
23	180	2.34	—	—	765.0	—	—	—	—	—	—	—	—	1.2	—	—
28	130	1.80	—	—	739.5	—	—	—	—	—	—	—	—	0	—	—

D&W+ Code	Food Description	QTY	Measure	Wt (g)	H₂0 (g)	Ener (cal)	Prot (g)	Carb (g)	Fiber (g)	Fat (g)	Fat Breakdown (g)		
											Sat	Mono	Poly
Fast Food—continued													
31696	Meatzza, 14"	1	slice(s)	146	—	378	17.0	39.0	2.0	18.0	7.5	—	—
31571	Pepperoni feast, extra pepperoni and cheese, 12"	1	slice(s)	98	—	265	11.0	28.0	2.0	12.5	5.0	—	—
31572	Pepperoni feast, extra pepperoni and cheese, 14"	1	slice(s)	135	—	363	16.0	39.0	2.0	17.0	7.0	—	—
31577	Vegi feast, 12"	1	slice(s)	102	—	218	9.0	29.0	2.0	8.0	3.5	—	—
31578	Vegi feast, 14"	1	slice(s)	139	—	300	13.0	40.0	3.0	11.0	4.5	—	—
	Domino's thin crust pizza												
31583	America's favorite, 12"	1	slice(s)	72	—	208	8.0	15.0	1.0	13.5	5.0	—	—
31584	America's favorite, 14"	1	slice(s)	100	—	285	11.0	20.0	2.0	18.5	7.0	—	—
31579	Cheese, 12"	1	slice(s)	49	—	137	5.0	14.0	1.0	7.0	2.5	—	—
31580	Cheese, 14"	1	slice(s)	68	27.0	214	8.8	19.0	1.4	11.4	4.6	2.9	2.5
31688	Deluxe, 12"	1	slice(s)	70	—	185	7.0	15.0	1.0	11.5	4.0	—	—
31697	Deluxe, 14"	1	slice(s)	94	—	248	10.0	20.0	2.0	15.0	5.5	—	—
31689	Extravaganzza, 12"	1	slice(s)	92	—	240	11.0	16.0	1.0	15.5	6.0	—	—
31698	Extravaganzza, 14"	1	slice(s)	123	—	320	14.0	21.0	2.0	20.5	8.0	—	—
31585	Hawaiian, 12"	1	slice(s)	71	—	174	8.0	16.0	1.0	9.5	3.5	—	—
31586	Hawaiian, 14"	1	slice(s)	100	—	240	11.0	21.0	2.0	13.0	5.0	—	—
31690	Meatzza, 12"	1	slice(s)	78	—	232	11.0	15.0	1.0	15.0	6.0	—	—
31699	Meatzza, 14"	1	slice(s)	104	—	310	14.0	20.0	2.0	20	8.0	—	—
31581	Pepperoni, extra pepperoni and cheese, 12"	1	slice(s)	68	—	216	9.0	14.0	1.0	14.0	5.5	—	—
31582	Pepperoni, extra pepperoni and cheese, 14"	1	slice(s)	93	—	295	13.0	20.0	1.0	19.0	7.5	—	—
31587	Vegi, 12"	1	slice(s)	71	—	168	7.0	15.0	1.0	9.5	3.5	—	—
31588	Vegi, 14"	1	slice(s)	97	—	231	10.0	21.0	2.0	13.5	5.0	—	—
	Domino's Ultimate deep dish pizza												
31596	America's favorite, 12"	1	slice(s)	115	—	309	12.0	29.0	2.0	17.0	6.0	—	—
31702	America's favorite, 14"	1	slice(s)	162	—	433	17.0	42.0	3.0	23.5	8.0	—	—
31590	Cheese, 12"	1	slice(s)	90	—	238	9.0	28.0	2.0	11.0	3.5	—	—
31591	Cheese, 14"	1	slice(s)	128	53.9	351	14.5	41.0	2.9	13.2	5.2	3.8	2.5
31589	Cheese, 6"	1	item(s)	215	—	598	22.9	68.4	3.9	27.6	9.9	—	—
31691	Deluxe, 12"	1	slice(s)	122	—	287	11.0	29.0	2.0	15.0	5.0	—	—
31700	Deluxe, 14"	1	slice(s)	156	—	396	15.0	42.0	3.0	20.0	7.0	—	—
31692	Extravaganzza, 12"	1	slice(s)	136	—	341	14.0	30.0	2.0	19.0	7.0	—	—
31701	Extravaganzza, 14"	1	slice(s)	186	—	468	20.0	43.0	3.0	25.5	9.5	—	—
31599	Hawaiian, 12"	1	slice(s)	114	—	275	12.0	30.0	2.0	13.0	5.0	—	—
31600	Hawaiian, 14"	1	slice(s)	162	—	389	17.0	43.0	3.0	18.0	6.5	—	—
31693	Meatzza, 12"	1	slice(s)	121	—	333	14.0	29.0	2.0	19.0	7.0	—	—
31703	Meatzza, 14"	1	slice(s)	167	—	458	19.0	42.0	3.0	25.0	9.5	—	—
31593	Pepperoni, extra pepperoni and cheese, 12"	1	slice(s)	110	—	317	13.0	29.0	2.0	17.5	6.5	—	—
31594	Pepperoni, extra pepperoni and cheese, 14"	1	slice(s)	155	—	443	18.0	42.0	3.0	24.0	9.0	—	—
31602	Vegi, 12"	1	slice(s)	114	—	270	11.0	30.0	2.0	13.5	5.0	—	—
31603	Vegi, 14"	1	slice(s)	159	—	380	15.0	43.0	3.0	18.0	6.5	—	—
31598	With ham and pineapple tidbits, 6"	1	item(s)	430	—	619	25.2	69.9	4.0	28.3	10.2	—	—
31595	With Italian sausage, 6"	1	item(s)	430	—	642	24.8	69.6	4.2	31.1	11.3	—	—
31592	With pepperoni, 6"	1	item(s)	430	—	647	25.1	68.5	3.9	32.0	11.7	—	—
31601	With vegetables, 6"	1	item(s)	430	—	619	23.4	70.8	4.6	28.7	10.1	—	—
	In-N-Out Burger												
34391	Cheeseburger with mustard and ketchup	1	serving(s)	268	—	400	22.0	41.0	3.0	18.0	9.0	—	—
34374	Cheeseburger	1	serving(s)	268	—	480	22.0	39.0	3.0	27.0	10.0	—	—

PAGE KEY: A-4 = Breads/Baked Goods A-10 = Cereal/Rice/Pasta A-14 = Fruit A-20 = Vegetables/Legumes A-30 = Nuts/Seeds A-32 = Vegetarian A-34 = Dairy A-42 = Eggs A-42 = Seafood A-46 = Meats A-50 = Poultry A-50 = Processed Meats A-52 = Beverages A-56 = Fats/Oils A-58 = Sweets A-60 = Spices/Condiments/Sauces A-64 = Mixed Foods/Soups/Sandwiches A-70 = Fast Food A-90 = Convenience A-92 = Baby Foods

A

CHOL (mg)	CALC (mg)	IRON (mg)	MAGN (mg)	POTA (mg)	SODI (mg)	ZINC (mg)	VIT A (µg)	THIA (mg)	VIT E (mg α)	RIBO (mg)	NIAC (mg)	VIT B6 (mg)	FOLA (µg DFE)	VIT C (mg)	VIT B12 (µg)	SELE (µg)
37	190	2.52	—	—	983.5	—	—	—	—	—	—	—	—	0	—	—
24	130	1.62	—	—	670.0	—	70.9	—	—	—	—	—	—	0	—	—
33	180	2.34	—	—	920.0	—	104.7	—	—	—	—	—	—	0	—	—
13	130	1.62	—	—	489.0	—	—	—	—	—	—	—	—	0.6	—	—
18	180	2.34	—	—	678.0	—	—	—	—	—	—	—	—	0.6	—	—
23	100	0.90	—	—	533.0	—	—	—	—	—	—	—	—	2.4	—	—
32	140	1.26	—	—	736.5	—	—	—	—	—	—	—	—	3.0	—	—
10	90	0.54	—	—	292.5	—	60.0	—	—	—	—	—	—	1.8	—	—
14	151	0.48	17.7	125.1	338.0	0.02	64.6	0.05	1.01	0.07	0.69	—	—	2.4	0.5	24.1
19	100	0.90	—	—	449.0	—	—	—	—	—	—	—	—	2.4	—	—
24	130	1.08	—	—	601.0	—	—	—	—	—	—	—	—	3.6	—	—
29	140	1.08	—	—	671.5	—	—	—	—	—	—	—	—	2.4	—	—
38	190	1.44	—	—	886.5	—	—	—	—	—	—	—	—	3.6	—	—
17	130	0.72	—	—	454.0	—	—	—	—	—	—	—	—	3.0	—	—
24	180	0.90	—	—	637.5	—	—	—	—	—	—	—	—	3.6	—	—
29	140	0.90	—	—	647.0	—	—	—	—	—	—	—	—	1.8	—	—
38	190	1.26	—	—	865.5	—	—	—	—	—	—	—	—	2.4	—	—
26	130	0.72	—	—	577.0	—	80.0	—	—	—	—	—	—	1.8	—	—
35	80	1.08	—	—	792.5	—	105.8	—	—	—	—	—	—	2.4	—	—
14	130	0.72	—	—	396.5	—	—	—	—	—	—	—	—	2.4	—	—
19	180	1.08	—	—	550.5	—	—	—	—	—	—	—	—	3.0	—	—
25	120	2.34	—	—	796.5	—	—	—	—	—	—	—	—	0.6	—	—
34	170	3.24	—	—	1110.0	—	—	—	—	—	—	—	—	0.6	—	—
11	110	1.98	—	—	555.5	—	70.0	—	—	—	—	—	—	0	—	—
18	189	3.78	32.0	209.9	718.1	1.75	99.8	0.29	1.13	0.31	5.44	—	—	0	0.6	45.6
36	295	4.67	—	—	1341.4	—	174.0	—	—	—	—	—	—	0.5	—	—
20	120	2.16	—	—	712.0	—	—	—	—	—	—	—	—	1.2	—	—
26	170	3.06	—	—	974.5	—	—	—	—	—	—	—	—	1.2	—	—
31	160	2.52	—	—	934.5	—	—	—	—	—	—	—	—	1.2	—	—
40	220	3.42	—	—	1260.0	—	—	—	—	—	—	—	—	1.2	—	—
19	150	1.98	—	—	717.0	—	—	—	—	—	—	—	—	1.2	—	—
26	210	2.88	—	—	1011.0	—	—	—	—	—	—	—	—	1.8	—	—
31	160	2.34	—	—	910.5	—	—	—	—	—	—	—	—	0	—	—
40	220	3.24	—	—	1230.0	—	—	—	—	—	—	—	—	0.6	—	—
27	150	2.16	—	—	840.5	—	86.5	—	—	—	—	—	—	0	—	—
37	220	3.06	—	—	1166.0	—	115.4	—	—	—	—	—	—	0.6	—	—
15	150	2.16	—	—	659.5	—	—	—	—	—	—	—	—	0.6	—	—
21	220	3.06	—	—	924.0	—	—	—	—	—	—	—	—	1.2	—	—
43	298	4.84	—	—	1497.8	—	—	—	—	—	—	—	—	1.5	—	—
45	302	4.89	—	—	1478.1	—	—	—	—	—	—	—	—	0.6	—	—
47	299	4.81	—	—	1523.7	—	167.9	—	—	—	—	—	—	0.6	—	—
36	307	5.10	—	—	1472.5	—	—	—	—	—	—	—	—	4.7	—	—
60	200	3.60	—	—	1080.0	—	—	—	—	—	—	—	—	12.0	—	—
60	200	3.60	—	—	1000.0	—	—	—	—	—	—	—	—	9.0	—	—

(Computer code is for Cengage Diet & Wellness Plus program)

D&W+ Code	Food Description	QTY	Measure	Wt (g)	H₂0 (g)	Ener (cal)	Prot (g)	Carb (g)	Fiber (g)	Fat (g)	Sat	Mono	Poly
											Fat Breakdown (g)		

Fast Food—continued

D&W+ Code	Food Description	QTY	Measure	Wt (g)	H₂0 (g)	Ener (cal)	Prot (g)	Carb (g)	Fiber (g)	Fat (g)	Sat	Mono	Poly
34390	Cheeseburger, lettuce leaves instead of buns	1	serving(s)	300	—	330	18.0	11.0	3.0	25.0	9.0	—	—
34377	Chocolate shake	1	serving(s)	425	—	690	9.0	83.0	0	36.0	24.0	—	—
34375	Double-Double cheeseburger	1	serving(s)	330	—	670	37.0	39.0	3.0	41.0	18.0	—	—
34393	Double-Double cheeseburger with mustard and ketchup	1	serving(s)	330	—	590	37.0	41.0	3.0	32.0	17.0	—	—
34392	Double-Double cheeseburger, lettuce leaves instead of buns	1	serving(s)	362	—	520	33.0	11.0	3.0	39.0	17.0	—	—
34376	French fries	1	serving(s)	125	—	400	7.0	54.0	2.0	18.0	5.0	—	—
34373	Hamburger	1	item(s)	243	—	390	16.0	39.0	3.0	19.0	5.0	—	—
34389	Hamburger with mustard and ketchup	1	serving(s)	243	—	310	16.0	41.0	3.0	10.0	4.0	—	—
34388	Hamburger, lettuce leaves instead of buns	1	serving(s)	275	—	240	13.0	11.0	3.0	17.0	4.0	—	—
34379	Strawberry shake	1	serving(s)	425	—	690	9.0	91.0	0	33.0	22.0	—	—
34378	Vanilla shake	1	serving(s)	425	—	680	9.0	78.0	0	37.0	25.0	—	—

Jack in the Box

D&W+ Code	Food Description	QTY	Measure	Wt (g)	H₂0 (g)	Ener (cal)	Prot (g)	Carb (g)	Fiber (g)	Fat (g)	Sat	Mono	Poly
30392	Bacon ultimate cheeseburger	1	item(s)	338	—	1090	46.0	53.0	2.0	77.0	30.0	—	—
1740	Breakfast Jack	1	item(s)	125	—	290	17.0	29.0	1.0	12.0	4.5	—	—
14074	Cheeseburger	1	item(s)	131	—	350	18.0	31.0	1.0	17.0	8.0	—	—
14106	Chicken breast strips, 4 pieces	1	serving(s)	201	—	500	35.0	36.0	3.0	25.0	6.0	—	—
37241	Chicken club salad, plain, without salad dressing	1	serving(s)	431	—	300	27.0	13.0	4.0	15.0	6.0	—	—
14064	Chicken sandwich	1	item(s)	145	—	400	15.0	38.0	2.0	21.0	4.5	—	—
14111	Chocolate ice cream shake, small	1	serving(s)	414	—	880	14.0	107.0	1.0	45.0	31.0	—	—
14073	Hamburger	1	item(s)	118	—	310	16.0	30.0	1.0	14.0	6.0	—	—
14090	Hash browns	1	serving(s)	57	—	150	1.0	13.0	2.0	10.0	2.5	—	—
14072	Jack's Spicy Chicken sandwich	1	item(s)	270	—	620	25.0	61.0	4.0	31.0	6.0	—	—
1468	Jumbo Jack hamburger	1	item(s)	261	—	600	21.0	51.0	3.0	35.0	12.0	—	—
1469	Jumbo Jack hamburger with cheese	1	item(s)	286	—	690	25.0	54.0	3.0	42.0	16.0	—	—
14099	Natural cut french fries, large	1	serving(s)	196	—	530	8.0	69.0	5.0	25.0	6.0	—	—
14098	Natural cut french fries, medium	1	serving(s)	133	—	360	5.0	47.0	4.0	17.0	4.0	—	—
1470	Onion rings	1	serving(s)	119	—	500	6.0	51.0	3.0	30.0	6.0	—	—
33141	Sausage, egg, and cheese biscuit	1	item(s)	234	—	740	27.0	35.0	2.0	55.0	17.0	—	—
14095	Seasoned curly fries, medium	1	serving(s)	125	—	400	6.0	45.0	5.0	23.0	5.0	—	—
14077	Sourdough Jack	1	item(s)	245	—	710	27.0	36.0	3.0	51.0	18.0	—	—
37249	Southwest chicken salad, plain, without salad dressing	1	serving(s)	488	—	300	24.0	29.0	7.0	11.0	5.0	—	—
14112	Strawberry ice cream shake, small	1	serving(s)	417	—	880	13.0	105.0	0	44.0	31.0	—	—
14078	Ultimate cheeseburger	1	item(s)	323	—	1010	40.0	53.0	2.0	71.0	28.0	—	—
14110	Vanilla ice cream shake, small	1	serving(s)	379	—	790	13.0	83.0	0	44.0	31.0	—	—

Jamba Juice

D&W+ Code	Food Description	QTY	Measure	Wt (g)	H₂0 (g)	Ener (cal)	Prot (g)	Carb (g)	Fiber (g)	Fat (g)	Sat	Mono	Poly
31645	Aloha Pineapple smoothie	24	fluid ounce(s)	730	—	500	8.0	117.0	4.0	1.5	1.0	—	—
31646	Banana Berry smoothie	24	fluid ounce(s)	719	—	480	5.0	112.0	4.0	1.0	0	—	—
31656	Berry Lime Sublime smoothie	24	fluid ounce(s)	728	—	460	3.0	106.0	5.0	2.0	1.0	—	—
31647	Caribbean Passion smoothie	24	fluid ounce(s)	730	—	440	4.0	102.0	4.0	2.0	1.0	—	—
38422	Carrot juice	16	fluid ounce(s)	472	—	100	3.0	23.0	0	0.5	0	—	—
31648	Chocolate Moo'd smoothie	24	fluid ounce(s)	634	—	720	17.0	148.0	3.0	8.0	5.0	—	—
31649	Citrus Squeeze smoothie	24	fluid ounce(s)	727	—	470	5.0	110.0	4.0	2.0	1.0	—	—
31651	Coldbuster smoothie	24	fluid ounce(s)	724	—	430	5.0	100.0	5.0	2.5	1.0	—	—
31652	Cranberry Craze smoothie	24	fluid ounce(s)	793	—	460	6.0	104.0	4.0	0.5	0	—	—
31654	Jamba Powerboost smoothie	24	fluid ounce(s)	738	—	440	6.0	105.0	6.0	1.0	0	—	—
38423	Lemonade	16	fluid ounce(s)	483	—	300	1.0	75.0	0	0	0	0	0
31657	Mango-a-go-go smoothie	24	fluid ounce(s)	690	—	440	3.0	104.0	4.0	1.5	0.5	—	—
38424	Orange juice, freshly squeezed	16	fluid ounce(s)	496	—	220	3.0	52.0	0.5	1.0	0	—	—
38426	Orange/carrot juice	16	fluid ounce(s)	484	—	160	3.0	37.0	0	1.0	0	—	—
31660	Orange-a-peel smoothie	24	fluid ounce(s)	726	—	440	8.0	102.0	5.0	1.5	0	—	—
31662	Peach Pleasure smoothie	24	fluid ounce(s)	720	—	460	4.0	108.0	4.0	2.0	1.0	—	—
31665	Protein Berry Pizzaz smoothie	24	fluid ounce(s)	710	—	440	20.0	92.0	5.0	1.5	0	—	—
31668	Razzmatazz smoothie	24	fluid ounce(s)	730	—	480	3.0	112.0	4.0	2.0	1.0	—	—
31669	Strawberries Wild smoothie	24	fluid ounce(s)	725	—	450	6.0	105.0	4.0	0.5	0	—	—
38421	Strawberry Tsunami smoothie	24	fluid ounce(s)	740	—	530	4.0	128.0	4.0	2.0	1.0	—	—

PAGE KEY: A-4 = Breads/Baked Goods A-10 = Cereal/Rice/Pasta A-14 = Fruit A-20 = Vegetables/Legumes A-30 = Nuts/Seeds A-32 = Vegetarian A-34 = Dairy A-42 = Eggs A-42 = Seafood A-46 = Meats A-50 = Poultry A-50 = Processed Meats A-52 = Beverages A-56 = Fats/Oils A-58 = Sweets A-60 = Spices/Condiments/Sauces A-64 = Mixed Foods/Soups/Sandwiches A-70 = Fast Food A-90 = Convenience A-92 = Baby Foods

A

CHOL (mg)	CALC (mg)	IRON (mg)	MAGN (mg)	POTA (mg)	SODI (mg)	ZINC (mg)	VIT A (µg)	THIA (mg)	VIT E (mg α)	RIBO (mg)	NIAC (mg)	VIT B6 (mg)	FOLA (µg DFE)	VIT C (mg)	VIT B12 (µg)	SELE (µg)
60	200	2.70	—	—	720.0	—	—	—	—	—	—	—	—	12.0	—	—
95	300	0.72	—	—	350.0	—	—	—	—	—	—	—	—	0	—	—
120	350	5.40	—	—	1440.0	—	—	—	—	—	—	—	—	9.0	—	—
115	350	5.40	—	—	1520.0	—	—	—	—	—	—	—	—	12.0	—	—
120	350	4.50	—	—	1160.0	—	—	—	—	—	—	—	—	12.0	—	—
0	20	1.80	—	—	245.0	—	0	—	—	—	—	—	—	0	—	—
40	40	3.60	—	—	650.0	—	—	—	—	—	—	—	—	9.0	—	—
35	40	3.60	—	—	730.0	—	—	—	—	—	—	—	—	12.0	—	—
40	40	2.70	—	—	370.0	—	—	—	—	—	—	—	—	12.0	—	—
85	300	0.00	—	—	280.0	—	—	—	—	—	—	—	—	0	—	—
90	300	0.00	—	—	390.0	—	—	—	—	—	—	—	—	0	—	—
140	308	7.38	—	540.0	2040.0	—	—	—	—	—	—	—	—	0.6	—	—
220	145	3.48	—	210.0	760.0	—	—	—	—	—	—	—	—	3.5	—	—
50	151	3.61	—	270.0	790.0	—	40.2	—	—	—	—	—	—	0	—	—
80	18	1.60	—	530.0	1260.0	—	—	—	—	—	—	—	—	1.1	—	—
65	280	3.35	—	560.0	880.0	—	—	—	—	—	—	—	—	50.4	—	—
35	100	2.70	—	240.0	730.0	—	—	—	—	—	—	—	—	4.8	—	—
135	460	0.47	—	840.0	330.0	—	—	—	—	—	—	—	—	0	—	—
40	100	3.60	—	250.0	600.0	—	0	—	—	—	—	—	—	0	—	—
0	10	0.18	—	190.0	230.0	—	0	—	—	—	—	—	—	0	—	—
50	150	1.80	—	450.0	1100.0	—	—	—	—	—	—	—	—	9.0	—	—
45	164	4.92	—	380.0	940.0	—	—	—	—	—	—	—	—	9.8	—	—
70	234	4.20	—	410.0	1310.0	—	—	—	—	—	—	—	—	8.4	—	—
0	20	1.42	—	1240.0	870.0	—	0	—	—	—	—	—	—	8.9	—	—
0	19	1.01	—	840.0	590.0	—	0	—	—	—	—	—	—	5.6	—	—
0	40	2.70	—	140.0	420.0	—	40.0	—	—	—	—	—	—	18.0	—	—
280	88	2.36	—	310.0	1430.0	—	—	—	—	—	—	—	—	0	—	—
0	40	1.80	—	580.0	890.0	—	—	—	—	—	—	—	—	0	—	—
75	200	4.50	—	430.0	1230.0	—	—	—	—	—	—	—	—	9.0	—	—
55	274	4.10	—	670.0	860.0	—	—	—	—	—	—	—	—	43.8	—	—
135	466	0.00	—	750.0	290.0	—	—	—	—	—	—	—	—	0	—	—
125	308	7.39	—	480.0	1580.0	—	—	—	—	—	—	—	—	0.6	—	—
135	532	0.00	—	750.0	280.0	—	—	—	—	—	—	—	—	0	—	—
5	200	1.80	60.0	1000.0	30.0	0.30	—	0.37	—	0.34	2.00	0.60	60.0	102.0	0	1.4
0	200	1.44	40.0	1010.0	115.0	0.60	—	0.09	—	0.25	0.80	0.70	24.0	15.0	0.2	1.4
5	200	1.80	16.0	510.0	35.0	0.30	—	0.06	—	0.25	6.00	0.70	140.0	54.0	0	1.4
5	100	1.80	24.0	810.0	60.0	0.30	—	0.09	—	0.25	5.00	0.50	100.0	78.0	0	1.4
0	150	2.70	80.0	1030.0	250.0	0.90	—	0.52	—	0.25	5.00	0.70	80.0	18.0	0	5.6
30	500	1.08	60.0	810.0	380.0	1.50	—	0.22	—	0.76	0.40	0.16	16.0	6.0	1.5	4.2
5	100	1.80	80.0	1170.0	35.0	0.30	—	0.37	—	0.34	1.90	0.60	100.0	180.0	0	1.4
5	100	1.08	60.0	1260.0	35.0	16.50	—	0.37	—	0.34	3.00	0.40	121.5	1302.0	0	1.4
0	250	1.44	16.0	500.0	50.0	0.30	—	0.03	—	0.25	5.00	0.60	120.0	54.0	0	1.4
0	1200	1.80	480.0	1070.0	45.0	16.50	—	5.55	—	6.12	68.00	7.40	640.0	288.0	10.8	77.0
0	20	0.00	8.0	200.0	10.0	0.00	—	0.03	—	0.17	14.00	1.80	320.0	36.0	0	0
5	100	1.08	24.0	780.0	50.0	0.30	—	0.15	—	0.25	5.00	0.70	120.0	72.0	0	1.4
0	60	1.08	60.0	990.0	0	0.30	—	0.45	—	0.13	2.00	0.20	160.0	246.0	0	0
0	100	1.80	60.0	1010.0	125.0	0.60	—	0.45	—	0.25	3.00	0.50	120.0	132.0	0	2.8
0	250	1.80	80.0	1300.0	160.0	0.90	—	0.45	—	0.42	2.00	0.50	140.0	240.0	0.6	1.4
5	100	0.72	32.0	740.0	60.0	0.30	—	0.06	—	0.25	4.00	0.60	80.0	18.0	0	1.4
0	1100	2.62	60.0	650.0	240.0	0.58	—	0.08	—	0.17	1.20	0.70	58.3	60.0	0	5.6
5	150	1.80	32.0	810.0	70.0	0.30	—	0.09	—	0.34	6.00	1.00	160.0	60.0	0	1.4
5	250	1.80	40.0	1050.0	180.0	0.90	—	0.12	—	0.34	0.80	0.40	40.0	60.0	0.6	1.4
5	100	1.08	24.0	480.0	10.0	0.30	—	0.06	—	0.34	14.00	1.80	320.0	90.0	0	1.4

(Computer code is for Cengage Diet & Wellness Plus program)

D&W+ Code	Food Description	QTY	Measure	Wt (g)	H₂0 (g)	Ener (cal)	Prot (g)	Carb (g)	Fiber (g)	Fat (g)	Fat Breakdown (g) Sat	Mono	Poly
	Fast Food—continued												
38427	Vibrant C juice	16	fluid ounce(s)	448	—	210	2.0	50.0	1.0	0	0	0	0
38428	Wheatgrass juice, freshly squeezed	1	ounce(s)	28	—	5	0.5	1.0	0	0	0	0	0
	Kentucky Fried Chicken (KFC)												
31850	BBQ baked beans	1	serving(s)	136	—	220	8.0	45.0	7.0	1.0	0	—	—
31853	Biscuit	1	item(s)	57	—	220	4.0	24.0	1.0	11.0	2.5	—	—
51223	Boneless Fiery Buffalo Wings	6	item(s)	211	—	530	30.0	44.0	3.0	26.0	5.0	—	—
39386	Boneless Honey BBQ Wings	6	item(s)	213	—	570	30.0	54.0	5.0	26.0	5.0	—	—
51224	Boneless Sweet & Spicy Wings	6	item(s)	203	—	550	30.0	50.0	3.0	26.0	5.0	—	—
31851	Cole slaw	1	serving(s)	130	—	180	1.0	22.0	3.0	10.0	1.5	—	—
31842	Colonel's Crispy Strips	3	item(s)	151	—	370	28.0	17.0	1.0	20.0	4.0	—	—
31849	Corn on the cob	1	item(s)	162	—	150	5.0	26.0	7.0	3.0	1.0	—	—
51221	Double Crunch sandwich	1	item(s)	213	—	520	27.0	39.0	3.0	29.0	5.0	—	—
3761	Extra Crispy chicken, breast	1	item(s)	162	—	370	33.0	10.0	2.0	22.0	5.0	—	—
3762	Extra Crispy chicken, drumstick	1	item(s)	60	—	150	12.0	4.0	0	10.0	2.5	—	—
3763	Extra Crispy chicken, thigh	1	item(s)	114	—	290	17.0	16.0	1.0	18.0	4.0	—	—
3764	Extra Crispy chicken, whole wing	1	item(s)	52	—	150	11.0	11.0	1.0	7.0	1.5	—	—
51218	Famous Bowls mashed potatoes with gravy	1	serving(s)	531	—	720	26.0	79.0	6.0	34.0	9.0	—	—
51219	Famous Bowls rice with gravy	1	serving(s)	384	—	610	25.0	67.0	5.0	27.0	8.0	—	—
31841	Honey BBQ chicken sandwich	1	item(s)	147	—	290	23.0	40.0	2.0	4.0	1.0	—	—
31833	Honey BBQ wing pieces	6	item(s)	157	—	460	27.0	26.0	3.0	27.0	6.0	—	—
10859	Hot wings pieces	6	piece(s)	134	—	450	26.0	19.0	2.0	30.0	7.0	—	—
42382	KFC Snacker sandwich	1	serving(s)	119	—	320	14.0	29.0	2.0	17.0	3.0	—	—
31848	Macaroni and cheese	1	serving(s)	136	—	180	8.0	18.0	0	8.0	3.5	—	—
31847	Mashed potatoes with gravy	1	serving(s)	151	—	140	2.0	20.0	1.0	5.0	1.0	—	—
10825	Original Recipe chicken, breast	1	item(s)	161	—	340	38.0	9.0	0	17.0	4.0	—	—
10826	Original Recipe chicken, drumstick	1	item(s)	59	—	140	13.0	3.0	0	8.0	2.0	—	—
10827	Original Recipe chicken, thigh	1	item(s)	126	—	350	19.0	7.0	1.0	27.0	7.0	—	—
10828	Original Recipe chicken, whole wing	1	item(s)	47	—	140	10.0	4.0	0	9.0	2.0	—	—
51222	Oven roasted Twister chicken wrap	1	item(s)	269	—	520	30.0	46.0	4.0	23.0	3.5	—	—
31844	Popcorn chicken, small or individual	1	item(s)	114	—	370	19.0	21.0	2.0	24.0	4.5	—	—
31852	Potato salad	1	serving(s)	128	—	180	2.0	22.0	2.0	9.0	1.5	—	—
10845	Potato wedges, small	1	serving(s)	102	—	250	4.0	32.0	3.0	12.0	2.0	—	—
31839	Tender Roast chicken sandwich with sauce	1	item(s)	236	—	430	37.0	29.0	2.0	18.0	3.5	—	—
	Long John Silver												
39392	Baked cod	1	serving(s)	101	—	120	22.0	1.0	0	4.5	1.0	—	—
3777	Batter dipped fish sandwich	1	item(s)	177	—	470	18.0	48.0	3.0	23.0	5.0	—	—
37568	Battered fish	1	item(s)	92	—	260	12.0	17.0	0.5	16.0	4.0	—	—
37569	Breaded clams	1	serving(s)	85	—	240	8.0	22.0	1.0	13.0	2.0	—	—
37566	Chicken plank	1	item(s)	52	—	140	8.0	9.0	0.5	8.0	2.0	—	—
39404	Clam chowder	1	item(s)	227	—	220	9.0	23.0	0	10.0	4.0	—	—
39398	Cocktail sauce	1	ounce(s)	28	—	25	0	6.0	0	0	0	0	0
3770	Coleslaw	1	serving(s)	113	—	200	1.0	15.0	3.0	15.0	2.5	1.8	4.1
39400	French fries, large	1	item(s)	142	—	390	4.0	56.0	5.0	17.0	4.0	—	—
3774	Fries, regular	1	serving(s)	85	—	230	3.0	34.0	3.0	10.0	2.5	—	—
3779	Hushpuppy	1	piece(s)	23	—	60	1.0	9.0	1.0	2.5	0.5	—	—
3781	Shrimp, batter-dipped, 1 piece	1	piece(s)	14	—	45	2.0	3.0	0	3.0	1.0	—	—
39399	Tartar sauce	1	ounce(s)	28	—	100	0	4.0	0	9.0	1.5	—	—
39395	Ultimate Fish sandwich	1	item(s)	199	—	530	21.0	49.0	3.0	28.0	8.0	—	—
	McDonald's												
50828	Asian salad with grilled chicken	1	item(s)	362	—	290	31.0	23.0	6.0	10.0	1.0	—	—
2247	Barbecue sauce	1	item(s)	28	—	45	0	11.0	0	0	0	0	0
737	Big Mac hamburger	1	item(s)	219	—	560	25.0	47.0	3.0	30.0	10.0	—	—
29777	Caesar salad dressing	1	package(s)	44	—	150	1.0	5.0	0	13.0	2.5	—	—
38391	Caesar salad with grilled chicken, no dressing	1	serving(s)	278	230.6	181	26.4	10.5	3.1	6.0	2.9	1.7	0.8
38393	Caesar salad without chicken, no dressing	1	serving(s)	190	170.4	84	6.0	8.1	3.0	3.9	2.2	0.9	0.3
738	Cheeseburger	1	item(s)	119	—	310	15.0	35.0	1.0	12.0	6.0	—	—
29775	Chicken McGrill sandwich	1	item(s)	213	—	400	27.0	38.0	3.0	16.0	3.0	—	—

PAGE KEY: A-4 = Breads/Baked Goods A-10 = Cereal/Rice/Pasta A-14 = Fruit A-20 = Vegetables/Legumes A-30 = Nuts/Seeds A-32 = Vegetarian A-34 = Dairy A-42 = Eggs A-42 = Seafood A-46 = Meats A-50 = Poultry A-50 = Processed Meats A-52 = Beverages A-56 = Fats/Oils A-58 = Sweets A-60 = Spices/Condiments/Sauces A-64 = Mixed Foods/Soups/Sandwiches A-70 = Fast Food A-90 = Convenience A-92 = Baby Foods

A

CHOL (mg)	CALC (mg)	IRON (mg)	MAGN (mg)	POTA (mg)	SODI (mg)	ZINC (mg)	VIT A (µg)	THIA (mg)	VIT E (mg α)	RIBO (mg)	NIAC (mg)	VIT B6 (mg)	FOLA (µg DFE)	VIT C (mg)	VIT B12 (µg)	SELE (µg)
0	20	1.08	40.0	720.0	0	0.30	—	0.30	—	0.10	1.60	0.40	80.0	678.0	0	0
0	0	1.80	8.0	80.0	0	0.00	0	0.03	—	0.03	0.40	0.04	16.0	3.6	0	2.8
0	100	2.70	—	—	730.0	—	—	—	—	—	—	—	—	1.2	—	—
0	40	1.80	—	—	640.0	—	—	—	—	—	—	—	—	0	—	—
65	40	1.80	—	—	2670.0	—	—	—	—	—	—	—	—	1.2	—	—
65	40	1.80	—	—	2210.0	—	—	—	—	—	—	—	—	1.2	—	—
65	60	1.80	—	—	2000.0	—	—	—	—	—	—	—	—	1.2	—	—
5	40	0.72	—	—	270.0	—	—	—	—	—	—	—	—	12.0	—	—
65	40	1.44	—	—	1220.0	—	0	—	—	—	—	—	—	1.2	—	—
0	60	1.08	—	—	10.0	—	—	—	—	—	—	—	—	6.0	—	—
55	100	2.70	—	—	1220.0	—	—	—	—	—	—	—	—	6.0	—	—
85	20	2.70	—	—	1020.0	—	—	—	—	—	—	—	—	1.2	—	—
55	0	1.44	—	—	300.0	—	0	—	—	—	—	—	—	0	—	—
95	20	2.70	—	—	700.0	—	—	—	—	—	—	—	—	—	—	—
45	20	1.08	—	—	340.0	—	—	—	—	—	—	—	—	0	—	—
35	200	5.40	—	—	2330.0	—	—	—	—	—	—	—	—	6.0	—	—
35	200	4.50	—	—	2130.0	—	—	—	—	—	—	—	—	6.0	—	—
60	80	2.70	—	—	710.0	—	—	—	—	—	—	—	—	2.4	—	—
140	40	1.80	—	—	970.0	—	—	—	—	—	—	—	—	21.0	—	—
115	40	1.44	—	—	990.0	—	—	—	—	—	—	—	—	1.2	—	—
25	60	2.70	—	—	690.0	—	—	—	—	—	—	—	—	2.4	—	—
15	150	0.72	—	—	800.0	—	—	—	—	—	—	—	—	1.2	—	—
0	40	1.44	—	—	560.0	—	—	—	—	—	—	—	—	1.2	—	—
135	20	2.70	—	—	960.0	—	—	—	—	—	—	—	—	6.0	—	—
70	20	1.08	—	—	340.0	—	—	—	—	—	—	—	—	0	—	—
110	20	2.70	—	—	870.0	—	—	—	—	—	—	—	—	1.2	—	—
50	20	1.44	—	—	350.0	—	0	—	—	—	—	—	—	1.2	—	—
60	40	6.30	—	—	1380.0	—	—	—	—	—	—	—	—	15.0	—	—
25	40	1.80	—	—	1110.0	—	0	—	—	—	—	—	—	0	—	—
5	0	0.36	—	—	470.0	—	—	—	—	—	—	—	—	6.0	—	—
0	20	1.08	—	—	700.0	—	0	—	—	—	—	—	—	0	—	—
80	80	2.70	—	—	1180.0	—	—	—	—	—	—	—	—	9.0	—	—
90	20	0.72	—	—	240.0	—	—	—	—	—	—	—	—	0	—	—
45	60	2.70	—	—	1210.0	—	—	—	—	—	—	—	—	2.4	—	—
35	20	0.72	—	—	790.0	—	—	—	—	—	—	—	—	4.8	—	—
10	20	1.08	—	—	1110.0	—	0	—	—	—	—	—	—	0	—	—
20	0	0.72	—	—	480.0	—	0	—	—	—	—	—	—	2.4	—	—
25	150	0.72	—	—	810.0	—	—	—	—	—	—	—	—	0	—	—
0	0	0.00	—	—	250.0	—	—	—	—	—	—	—	—	0	—	—
20	40	0.36	—	222.7	340.0	0.70	—	0.07	—	0.08	2.34	—	—	18.0	—	—
0	0	0.00	—	—	580.0	—	0	—	—	—	—	—	—	24.0	—	—
0	0	0.00	—	370.0	350.0	0.30	0	0.09	—	0.01	1.60	—	—	15.0	—	—
0	20	0.36	—	—	200.0	—	0	—	—	—	—	—	—	0	—	—
15	0	0.00	—	—	160.0	—	0	—	—	—	—	—	—	1.2	—	—
15	0	0.00	—	—	250.0	—	0	—	—	—	—	—	—	0	—	—
60	150	2.70	—	—	1400.0	—	—	—	—	—	—	—	—	4.8	—	—
65	150	3.60	—	—	890.0	—	—	—	—	—	—	—	—	54.0	—	—
0	0	0.00	—	55.0	260.0	—	—	—	—	—	—	—	—	0	—	—
80	250	4.50	—	400.0	1010.0	—	—	—	—	—	—	—	—	1.2	—	—
10	40	0.18	—	30.0	400.0	—	—	—	—	—	—	—	—	0.6	—	—
67	178	1.77	—	708.9	767.3	—	—	0.15	—	0.19	10.62	—	127.9	29.2	0.2	—
10	163	1.15	17.1	410.4	157.7	—	—	0.08	—	0.07	0.40	—	102.6	26.8	0	0.4
40	200	2.70	—	240.0	740.0	—	60.0	—	—	—	—	—	—	1.2	—	—
70	150	2.70	—	510.0	1010.0	—	—	—	—	—	—	—	—	6.0	—	—

D&W+ Code	Food Description	QTY	Measure	Wt (g)	H₂O (g)	Ener (cal)	Prot (g)	Carb (g)	Fiber (g)	Fat (g)	Fat Breakdown (g)		
											Sat	Mono	Poly
Fast Food—continued													
1873	Chicken McNuggets, 6 piece	1	serving(s)	96	—	250	15.0	15.0	0	15.0	3.0	—	—
3792	Chicken McNuggets, 4 piece	1	serving(s)	64	—	170	10.0	10.0	0	10.0	2.0	—	—
29774	Crispy chicken sandwich	1	item(s)	232	121.8	500	27.0	63.0	3.0	16.0	3.0	5.7	7.4
743	Egg McMuffin	1	item(s)	139	76.8	300	17.0	30.0	2.0	12.0	4.5	3.8	2.5
742	Filet-O-Fish sandwich	1	item(s)	141	—	400	14.0	42.0	1.0	18.0	4.0	—	—
2257	French fries, large	1	serving(s)	170	—	570	6.0	70.0	7.0	30.0	6.0	—	—
1872	French fries, small	1	serving(s)	74	—	250	2.0	30.0	3.0	13.0	2.5	—	—
33822	Fruit 'n Yogurt Parfait	1	item(s)	149	111.2	160	4.0	31.0	1.0	2.0	1.0	0.2	0.1
739	Hamburger	1	item(s)	105	—	260	13.0	33.0	1.0	9.0	3.5	—	—
2003	Hash browns	1	item(s)	53	—	140	1.0	15.0	2.0	8.0	1.5	—	—
2249	Honey sauce	1	item(s)	14	—	50	0	12.0	0	0	0	0	0
38397	Newman's Own creamy Caesar salad dressing	1	item(s)	59	32.5	190	2.0	4.0	0	18.0	3.5	4.6	9.6
38398	Newman's Own low fat balsamic vinaigrette salad dressing	1	item(s)	44	29.1	40	0	4.0	0	3.0	0	1.0	1.2
38399	Newman's Own ranch salad dressing	1	item(s)	59	30.1	170	1.0	9.0	0	15.0	2.5	9.0	3.7
1874	Plain Hotcakes with syrup and margarine	3	item(s)	221	—	600	9.0	102.0	2.0	17.0	4.0	—	—
740	Quarter Pounder hamburger	1	item(s)	171	—	420	24.0	40.0	3.0	18.0	7.0	—	—
741	Quarter Pounder hamburger with cheese	1	item(s)	199	—	510	29.0	43.0	3.0	25.0	12.0	—	—
2005	Sausage McMuffin with egg	1	item(s)	165	82.4	450	20.0	31.0	2.0	27.0	10.0	10.9	4.6
50831	Side salad	1	item(s)	87	—	20	1.0	4.0	1.0	0	0	0	0
Pizza Hut													
39009	Hot chicken wings	2	item(s)	57	—	110	11.0	1.0	0	6.0	2.0	—	—
14025	Meat Lovers hand tossed pizza	1	slice(s)	118	—	300	15.0	29.0	2.0	13.0	6.0	—	—
14026	Meat Lovers pan pizza	1	slice(s)	123	—	340	15.0	29.0	2.0	19.0	7.0	—	—
31009	Meat Lovers stuffed crust pizza	1	slice(s)	169	—	450	21.0	43.0	3.0	21.0	10.0	—	—
14024	Meat Lovers thin 'n crispy pizza	1	slice(s)	98	—	270	13.0	21.0	2.0	14.0	6.0	—	—
14031	Pepperoni Lovers hand tossed pizza	1	slice(s)	113	—	300	15.0	30.0	2.0	13.0	7.0	—	—
14032	Pepperoni Lovers pan pizza	1	slice(s)	118	—	340	15.0	29.0	2.0	19.0	7.0	—	—
31011	Pepperoni Lovers stuffed crust pizza	1	slice(s)	163	—	420	21.0	43.0	3.0	19.0	10.0	—	—
14030	Pepperoni Lovers thin 'n crispy pizza	1	slice(s)	92	—	260	13.0	21.0	2.0	14.0	7.0	—	—
10834	Personal Pan pepperoni pizza	1	slice(s)	61	—	170	7.0	18.0	0.5	8.0	3.0	—	—
10842	Personal Pan supreme pizza	1	slice(s)	77	—	190	8.0	19.0	1.0	9.0	3.5	—	—
39013	Personal Pan Veggie Lovers pizza	1	slice(s)	69	—	150	6.0	19.0	1.0	6.0	2.0	—	—
14028	Veggie Lovers hand tossed pizza	1	slice(s)	118	—	220	10.0	31.0	2.0	6.0	3.0	—	—
14029	Veggie Lovers pan pizza	1	slice(s)	119	—	260	10.0	30.0	2.0	12.0	4.0	—	—
31010	Veggie Lovers stuffed crust pizza	1	slice(s)	172	—	360	16.0	45.0	3.0	14.0	7.0	—	—
14027	Veggie Lovers thin 'n crispy pizza	1	slice(s)	101	—	180	8.0	23.0	2.0	7.0	3.0	—	—
39012	Wing blue cheese dipping sauce	1	item(s)	43	—	230	2.0	2.0	0	24.0	5.0	—	—
39011	Wing ranch dipping sauce	1	item(s)	43	—	210	0.5	4.0	0	22.0	3.5	—	—
Starbucks													
38052	Cappuccino, tall	12	fluid ounce(s)	360	—	120	7.0	10.0	0	6.0	4.0	—	—
38053	Cappuccino, tall nonfat	12	fluid ounce(s)	360	—	80	7.0	11.0	0	0	0	0	0
38054	Cappuccino, tall soymilk	12	fluid ounce(s)	360	—	100	5.0	13.0	0.5	2.5	0	—	—
38059	Cinnamon spice mocha, tall nonfat w/o whipped cream	12	fluid ounce(s)	360	—	170	11.0	32.0	0	0.5	—	—	—
38057	Cinnamon spice mocha, tall w/ whipped cream	12	fluid ounce(s)	360	—	320	10.0	31.0	0	17.0	11.0	—	—
38051	Espresso, single shot	1	fluid ounce(s)	30	—	5	0	1.0	0	0	0	0	0
38088	Flavored syrup, 1 pump	1	serving(s)	10	—	20	0	5.0	0	0	0	0	0
32562	Frappuccino bottled coffee drink, mocha	9½	fluid ounce(s)	298	—	190	6.0	39.0	3.0	3.0	2.0	—	—
32561	Frappuccino coffee drink, all bottled flavors	9½	fluid ounce(s)	281	—	190	7.0	35.0	0	3.5	2.5	—	—
38073	Frappuccino, mocha	12	fluid ounce(s)	360	—	220	5.0	44.0	0	3.0	1.5	—	—
38067	Frappuccino, tall caramel w/o whipped cream	12	fluid ounce(s)	360	—	210	4.0	43.0	0	2.5	1.5	—	—
38070	Frappuccino, tall coffee	12	fluid ounce(s)	360	—	190	4.0	38.0	0	2.5	1.5	—	—
39894	Frappuccino, tall coffee, light blend	12	fluid ounce(s)	360	—	110	5.0	22.0	2.0	1.0	0	—	—

PAGE KEY: A-4 = Breads/Baked Goods A-10 = Cereal/Rice/Pasta A-14 = Fruit A-20 = Vegetables/Legumes A-30 = Nuts/Seeds A-32 = Vegetarian A-34 = Dairy A-42 = Eggs A-42 = Seafood A-46 = Meats A-50 = Poultry A-50 = Processed Meats A-52 = Beverages A-56 = Fats/Oils A-58 = Sweets A-60 = Spices/Condiments/Sauces A-64 = Mixed Foods/Soups/Sandwiches A-70 = Fast Food A-90 = Convenience A-92 = Baby Foods

A

CHOL (mg)	CALC (mg)	IRON (mg)	MAGN (mg)	POTA (mg)	SODI (mg)	ZINC (mg)	VIT A (µg)	THIA (mg)	VIT E (mg α)	RIBO (mg)	NIAC (mg)	VIT B6 (mg)	FOLA (µg DFE)	VIT C (mg)	VIT B12 (µg)	SELE (µg)
35	20	0.72	—	240.0	670.0	—	—	—	—	—	—	—	—	1.2	—	—
25	0	0.36	—	160.0	450.0	—	—	—	—	—	—	—	—	1.2	—	—
60	80	3.60	62.6	526.6	1380.0	1.53	41.8	0.46	2.27	0.39	12.85	—	94.2	6.0	0.4	—
230	300	2.70	26.4	218.2	860.0	1.59	—	0.36	0.82	0.51	4.31	0.20	109.8	1.2	0.9	—
40	150	1.80	—	250.0	640.0	—	36.2	—	—	—	—	—	—	0	—	—
0	20	1.80	—	—	330.0	—	0	—	—	—	—	—	—	9.0	—	—
0	20	0.72	—	—	140.0	—	0	—	—	—	—	—	—	3.6	—	—
5	150	0.67	20.9	248.8	85.0	0.53	0	0.06	—	0.17	0.35	—	19.4	9.0	0.3	—
30	150	2.70	—	210.0	530.0	—	5.0	—	—	—	—	—	—	1.2	—	—
0	0	0.36	—	210.0	290.0	—	0	—	—	—	—	—	—	1.2	—	—
0	0	0.00	—	0	0	—	0	—	—	—	—	—	—	0	—	—
20	61	0.00	3.0	16.0	500.0	0.20	—	0.01	15.43	0.02	0.01	0.64	2.4	0	0.1	0.1
0	4	0.00	1.3	8.8	730.0	0.01	—	0.00	0.00	0.00	0.00	0.00	0	2.4	0	0
0	40	0.00	1.8	70.4	530.0	0.03	0	0.01	—	0.08	0.01	0.02	0.6	0	0	0.2
20	150	2.70	—	280.0	620.0	—	—	—	—	—	—	—	—	0	—	—
70	150	4.50	—	390.0	730.0	—	10.0	—	—	—	—	—	—	1.2	—	—
95	300	4.50	—	440.0	1150.0	—	100.0	—	—	—	—	—	—	1.2	—	—
255	300	3.60	29.7	282.2	950.0	2.01	—	0.43	0.82	0.56	4.83	0.24	—	0	1.2	—
0	20	0.72	—	—	10.0	—	—	—	—	—	—	—	—	15.0	—	—
70	0	0.36	—	—	450.0	—	—	—	—	—	—	—	—	—	—	—
35	150	1.80	—	—	760.0	—	—	—	—	—	—	—	—	6.0	—	—
35	150	2.70	—	—	750.0	—	—	—	—	—	—	—	—	6.0	—	—
55	250	2.70	—	—	1250.0	—	—	—	—	—	—	—	—	9.0	—	—
35	150	1.44	—	—	740.0	—	—	—	—	—	—	—	—	6.0	—	—
40	200	1.80	—	—	710.0	—	57.7	—	—	—	—	—	—	2.4	—	—
40	200	2.70	—	—	700.0	—	57.7	—	—	—	—	—	—	2.4	—	—
55	300	2.70	—	—	1120.0	—	—	—	—	—	—	—	—	3.6	—	—
40	200	1.44	—	—	690.0	—	58.0	—	—	—	—	—	—	2.4	—	—
15	80	1.44	—	—	340.0	—	38.5	—	—	—	—	—	—	1.4	—	—
20	80	1.86	—	—	420.0	—	—	—	—	—	—	—	—	3.6	—	—
10	80	1.80	—	—	280.0	—	—	—	—	—	—	—	—	3.6	—	—
15	150	1.80	—	—	490.0	—	—	—	—	—	—	—	—	9.0	—	—
15	150	2.70	—	—	470.0	—	—	—	—	—	—	—	—	9.0	—	—
35	250	2.70	—	—	980.0	—	—	—	—	—	—	—	—	9.0	—	—
15	150	1.44	—	—	480.0	—	—	—	—	—	—	—	—	9.0	—	—
25	20	0.00	—	—	550.0	—	0	—	—	—	—	—	—	0	—	—
10	0	0.00	—	—	340.0	—	0	—	—	—	—	—	—	0	—	—
25	250	0.00	—	—	95.0	—	—	—	—	—	—	—	—	1.2	0	—
3	200	0.00	—	—	100.0	—	—	—	—	—	—	—	—	0	0	—
0	250	0.72	—	—	75.0	—	—	—	—	—	—	—	—	0	0	—
5	300	0.72	—	—	150.0	—	—	—	—	—	—	—	—	0	0	—
70	350	1.08	—	—	140.0	—	—	—	—	—	—	—	—	2.4	0	—
0	0	0.00	—	—	0	—	0	—	—	—	—	—	—	0	0	—
0	0	0.00	—	—	0	—	0	—	—	—	—	—	—	0	0	—
12	219	1.08	—	530.0	110.0	—	—	—	—	—	—	—	—	0	—	—
15	250	0.36	—	510.0	105.0	—	—	—	—	—	—	—	—	0	0	—
10	150	0.72	—	—	180.0	—	—	—	—	—	—	—	—	0	0	—
10	150	0.00	—	—	180.0	—	—	—	—	—	—	—	—	0	0	—
10	150	0.00	—	—	180.0	—	—	—	—	—	—	—	—	0	0	—
0	150	0.00	—	—	220.0	—	—	—	—	—	—	—	—	0	—	—

(Computer code is for Cengage Diet & Wellness Plus program)

A

D&W+ Code	Food Description	QTY	Measure	Wt (g)	H₂O (g)	Ener (cal)	Prot (g)	Carb (g)	Fiber (g)	Fat (g)	Fat Breakdown (g)		
											Sat	Mono	Poly
Fast Food—continued													
38071	Frappuccino, tall espresso	12	fluid ounce(s)	360	—	160	4.0	33.0	0	2.0	1.5	—	—
39897	Frappuccino, tall mocha, light blend	12	fluid ounce(s)	360	—	140	5.0	28.0	3.0	1.5	0	—	—
39887	Frappuccino, tall Strawberries and Creme, w/o whipped cream	12	fluid ounce(s)	360	—	330	10.0	65.0	0	3.5	1.0	—	—
38063	Frappuccino, tall Tazo chai creme w/o whipped cream	12	fluid ounce(s)	360	—	280	10.0	52.0	0	3.5	1.0	—	—
38066	Frappuccino, tall Tazoberry	12	fluid ounce(s)	360	—	140	0.5	36.0	0.5	0	0	0	0
38065	Frappuccino, tall Tazoberry Crème	12	fluid ounce(s)	360	—	240	4.0	54.0	0.5	1.0	0	—	—
38080	Frappuccino, tall vanilla w/o whipped cream	12	fluid ounce(s)	360	—	270	10.0	51.0	0	3.5	1.0	—	—
39898	Frappuccino, tall white chocolate mocha, light blend	12	fluid ounce(s)	360	—	160	6.0	32.0	2.0	2.0	1.0	—	—
38074	Frappuccino, tall white chocolate w/o whipped cream	12	fluid ounce(s)	360	—	240	5.0	48.0	0	3.5	2.5	—	—
39883	Java Chip Frappuccino, tall w/o whipped cream	12	fluid ounce(s)	360	—	270	5.0	51.0	1.0	7.0	4.5	—	—
33111	Latte, tall w/nonfat milk	12	fluid ounce(s)	360	335.3	120	12.0	18.0	0	0	0	0	0
33112	Latte, tall w/whole milk	12	fluid ounce(s)	360	—	200	11.0	16.0	0	11.0	7.0	—	—
33109	Macchiato, tall caramel w/nonfat milk	12	fluid ounce(s)	360	—	170	11.0	30.0	0	1.0	0	—	—
33110	Macchiato, tall caramel w/whole milk	12	fluid ounce(s)	360	—	240	10.0	28.0	0	10.0	6.0	—	—
33107	Mocha coffee drink, tall nonfat, w/o whipped cream	12	fluid ounce(s)	360	—	170	11.0	33.0	1.0	1.5	0	—	—
38089	Mocha syrup	1	serving(s)	17	—	25	1.0	6.0	0	0.5	0	—	—
33108	Mocha, tall mocha w/whole milk	12	fluid ounce(s)	360	—	310	10.0	32.0	1.0	17.0	10.0	—	—
38042	Steamed apple cider, tall	12	fluid ounce(s)	360	—	180	0	45.0	0	0	0	0	0
38087	Tazo chai black tea, soymilk, tall	12	fluid ounce(s)	360	—	190	4.0	39.0	0.5	2.0	0	—	—
38084	Tazo chai black tea, tall	12	fluid ounce(s)	360	—	210	6.0	36.0	0	5.0	3.5	—	—
38083	Tazo chai black tea, tall nonfat	12	fluid ounce(s)	360	—	170	6.0	37.0	0	0	0	0	0
38076	Tazo iced tea, tall	12	fluid ounce(s)	360	—	60	0	16.0	0	0	0	0	0
38077	Tazo tea, grande lemonade	16	fluid ounce(s)	480	—	120	0	31.0	0	0	0	0	0
38045	Vanilla crème steamed nonfat milk, tall w/whipped cream	12	fluid ounce(s)	360	—	260	11.0	33.0	0	8.0	5.0	—	—
38046	Vanilla crème steamed soymilk, tall w/whipped cream	12	fluid ounce(s)	360	—	300	8.0	37.0	1.0	12.0	6.0	—	—
38044	Vanilla crème steamed whole milk, tall w/whipped cream	12	fluid ounce(s)	360	—	330	10.0	31.0	0	18.0	11.0	—	—
38090	Whipped cream	1	serving(s)	27	—	100	0	2.0	0	9.0	6.0	—	—
38062	White chocolate mocha, tall nonfat w/o whipped cream	12	fluid ounce(s)	360	—	260	12.0	45.0	0	4.0	3.0	—	—
38061	White chocolate mocha, tall w/ whipped cream	12	fluid ounce(s)	360	—	410	11.0	44.0	0	20.0	13.0	—	—
38048	White hot chocolate, tall nonfat w/o whipped cream	12	fluid ounce(s)	360	—	300	15.0	51.0	0	4.5	3.5	—	—
38050	White hot chocolate, tall soymilk w/ whipped cream	12	fluid ounce(s)	360	—	420	11.0	56.0	1.0	16.0	9.0	—	—
38047	White hot chocolate, tall w/whipped cream	12	fluid ounce(s)	360	—	460	13.0	50.0	0	22.0	15.0	—	—
	Subway												
15842	Cheese steak sandwich, 6", wheat bread	1	item(s)	250	—	360	24.0	47.0	5.0	10.0	4.5	—	—
40478	Chicken and bacon ranch sandwich, 6", white or wheat bread	1	serving(s)	297	—	540	36.0	47.0	5.0	25.0	10.0	—	—
38622	Chicken and bacon ranch wrap with cheese	1	item(s)	257	—	440	41.0	18.0	9.0	27.0	10.0	—	—
32045	Chocolate chip cookie	1	item(s)	45	—	210	2.0	30.0	1.0	10.0	6.0	—	—
32048	Chocolate chip M&M cookie	1	item(s)	45	—	210	2.0	32.0	0.5	10.0	5.0	—	—
32049	Chocolate chunk cookie	1	item(s)	45	—	220	2.0	30.0	0.5	10.0	5.0	—	—
4024	Classic Italian B.M.T. sandwich, 6", white bread	1	item(s)	236	—	440	22.0	45.0	2.0	21.0	8.5	—	—

CHOL (mg)	CALC (mg)	IRON (mg)	MAGN (mg)	POTA (mg)	SODI (mg)	ZINC (mg)	VIT A (µg)	THIA (mg)	VIT E (mg α)	RIBO (mg)	NIAC (mg)	VIT B6 (mg)	FOLA (µg DFE)	VIT C (mg)	VIT B12 (µg)	SELE (µg)
10	100	0.00	—	—	160.0	—	—	—	—	—	—	—	—	0	0	—
0	150	0.72	—	—	220.0	—	—	—	—	—	—	—	—	0	—	—
3	350	0.00	—	—	270.0	—	—	—	—	—	—	—	—	21.0	—	—
3	350	0.00	—	—	270.0	—	—	—	—	—	—	—	—	3.6	0	—
0	0	0.00	—	—	30.0	—	0	—	—	—	—	—	—	0	0	—
0	150	0.00	—	—	125.0	—	0	—	—	—	—	—	—	1.2	0	—
3	350	0.00	—	—	370.0	—	—	—	—	—	—	—	—	3.6	0	—
3	150	0.00	—	—	250.0	—	—	—	—	—	—	—	—	0	—	—
10	150	0.00	—	—	210.0	—	—	—	—	—	—	—	—	0	0	—
10	150	1.44	—	—	220.0	—	—	—	—	—	—	—	—	0	—	—
5	350	0.00	39.8	—	170.0	1.35	—	0.12	—	0.47	0.36	0.13	17.5	0	1.3	—
45	400	0.00	46.6	—	160.0	1.28	—	0.12	—	0.54	0.34	0.14	16.8	2.4	1.2	—
5	300	0.00	—	—	160.0	—	—	—	—	—	—	—	—	1.2	—	—
30	300	0.00	—	—	135.0	—	—	—	—	—	—	—	—	2.4	—	—
5	300	2.70	—	—	135.0	—	—	—	—	—	—	—	—	0	—	—
0	0	0.72	—	—	0	—	0	—	—	—	—	—	—	0	0	—
55	300	2.70	—	—	115.0	—	—	—	—	—	—	—	—	0	—	—
0	0	1.08	—	—	15.0	—	0	—	—	—	—	—	—	0	0	—
0	200	0.72	—	—	70.0	—	—	—	—	—	—	—	—	0	0	—
20	200	0.36	—	—	85.0	—	—	—	—	—	—	—	—	1.2	0	—
5	200	0.36	—	—	95.0	—	—	—	—	—	—	—	—	0	0	—
0	0	0.00	—	—	0	—	0	—	—	—	—	—	—	0	0	—
0	0	0.00	—	—	15.0	—	0	—	—	—	—	—	—	4.8	0	—
35	350	0.00	—	—	170.0	—	—	—	—	—	—	—	—	0	0	—
30	400	1.44	—	—	130.0	—	—	—	—	—	—	—	—	0	—	—
65	350	0.00	—	—	140.0	—	—	—	—	—	—	—	—	0	0	—
40	0	0.00	—	—	10.0	—	—	—	—	—	—	—	—	0	0	—
5	400	0.00	—	—	210.0	—	—	—	—	—	—	—	—	0	0	—
70	400	0.00	—	—	210.0	—	—	—	—	—	—	—	—	2.4	0	—
10	450	0.00	—	—	250.0	—	—	—	—	—	—	—	—	0	0	—
35	500	1.44	—	—	210.0	—	—	—	—	—	—	—	—	0	0	—
75	500	0.00	—	—	250.0	—	—	—	—	—	—	—	—	3.6	0	—
35	150	8.10	—	—	1090.0	—	—	—	—	—	—	—	—	18.0	—	—
90	250	4.50	—	—	1400.0	—	—	—	—	—	—	—	—	21.0	—	—
90	300	2.70	—	—	1680.0	—	—	—	—	—	—	—	—	9.0	—	—
15	0	1.08	—	—	150.0	—	—	—	—	—	—	—	—	0	—	—
10	20	1.00	—	—	100.0	—	—	—	—	—	—	—	—	0	—	—
10	0	1.00	—	—	100.0	—	—	—	—	—	—	—	—	0	—	—
55	150	2.70	—	—	1770.0	—	—	—	—	—	—	—	—	16.8	—	—

(Computer code is for Cengage Diet & Wellness Plus program)

D&W+ Code	Food Description	QTY	Measure	Wt (g)	H₂O (g)	Ener (cal)	Prot (g)	Carb (g)	Fiber (g)	Fat (g)	Fat Breakdown (g) Sat	Mono	Poly
	Fast Food—continued												
15838	Classic tuna sandwich, 6″, wheat bread	1	item(s)	250	—	530	22.0	45.0	4.0	31.0	7.0	—	—
15837	Classic tuna sandwich, 6″, white bread	1	item(s)	243	—	520	21.0	43.0	2.0	31.0	7.5	—	—
16397	Club salad, no dressing and croutons	1	item(s)	412	—	160	18.0	15.0	4.0	4.0	1.5	—	—
3422	Club sandwich, 6″, white bread	1	item(s)	250	—	310	23.0	45.0	2.0	6.0	2.5	—	—
4030	Cold cut combo sandwich, 6″, white bread	1	item(s)	242	—	400	20.0	45.0	2.0	17.0	7.5	—	—
34030	Ham and egg breakfast sandwich	1	item(s)	142	—	310	16.0	35.0	3.0	13.0	3.5	—	—
3885	Ham sandwich, 6″, white bread	1	item(s)	238	—	310	17.0	52.0	2.0	5.0	2.0	—	—
3888	Meatball marinara sandwich, 6″, wheat bread	1	item(s)	377	—	560	24.0	63.0	7.0	24.0	11.0	—	—
4651	Meatball sandwich, 6″, white bread	1	item(s)	370	—	550	23.0	61.0	5.0	24.0	11.5	—	—
15839	Melt sandwich, 6″, white bread	1	item(s)	260	—	410	25.0	47.0	4.0	15.0	5.0	—	—
32046	Oatmeal raisin cookie	1	item(s)	45	—	200	3.0	30.0	1.0	8.0	4.0	—	—
16379	Oven-roasted chicken breast sandwich, 6″, wheat bread	1	item(s)	238	—	330	24.0	48.0	5.0	5.0	1.5	—	—
32047	Peanut butter cookie	1	item(s)	45	—	220	4.0	26.0	1.0	12.0	5.0	—	—
4655	Roast beef sandwich, 6″, wheat bread	1	item(s)	224	—	290	19.0	45.0	4.0	5.0	2.0	—	—
3957	Roast beef sandwich, 6″, white bread	1	item(s)	217	—	280	18.0	43.0	2.0	5.0	2.5	—	—
16378	Roasted chicken breast, 6″, white bread	1	item(s)	231	—	320	23.0	46.0	3.0	5.0	2.0	—	—
34028	Southwest steak and cheese sandwich, 6″, Italian bread	1	item(s)	271	—	450	24.0	48.0	6.0	20.0	6.0	—	—
4032	Spicy Italian sandwich, 6″, white bread	1	item(s)	220	—	470	20.0	43.0	2.0	25.0	9.5	—	—
4031	Steak and cheese sandwich, 6″, white bread	1	item(s)	243	—	350	23.0	45.0	3.0	10.0	5.0	—	—
32050	Sugar cookie	1	item(s)	45	—	220	2.0	28.0	0.5	12.0	6.0	—	—
40477	Sweet onion chicken teriyaki sandwich, 6″, white or wheat bread	1	serving(s)	281	—	370	26.0	59.0	4.0	5.0	1.5	—	—
38623	Turkey breast and bacon melt wrap with chipotle sauce	1	item(s)	228	—	380	31.0	20.0	9.0	24.0	7.0	—	—
15834	Turkey breast and ham sandwich, 6″, white bread	1	item(s)	227	—	280	19.0	45.0	2.0	5.0	2.0	—	—
16376	Turkey breast sandwich, 6″, white bread	1	item(s)	217	—	270	17.0	44.0	2.0	4.5	2.0	—	—
15841	Veggie Delite sandwich, 6″, wheat bread	1	item(s)	167	—	230	9.0	44.0	4.0	3.0	1.0	—	—
16375	Veggie Delite, 6″, white bread	1	item(s)	160	—	220	8.0	42.0	2.0	3.0	1.5	—	—
32051	White chip macadamia nut cookie	1	item(s)	45	—	220	2.0	29.0	0.5	11.0	5.0	—	—
	Taco Bell												
29906	7-Layer burrito	1	item(s)	283	—	490	17.0	65.0	9.0	18.0	7.0	—	—
744	Bean burrito	1	item(s)	198	—	340	13.0	54.0	8.0	9.0	3.5	—	—
749	Beef burrito supreme	1	item(s)	248	—	410	17.0	51.0	7.0	17.0	8.0	—	—
33417	Beef Chalupa Supreme	1	item(s)	153	—	380	14.0	30.0	3.0	23.0	7.0	—	—
34474	Beef Gordita Baja	1	item(s)	153	—	340	13.0	29.0	4.0	19.0	5.0	—	—
29910	Beef Gordita Supreme	1	item(s)	153	—	310	14.0	29.0	3.0	16.0	6.0	—	—
2014	Beef soft taco	1	item(s)	99	—	200	10.0	21.0	3.0	9.0	4.0	—	—
10860	Beef soft taco supreme	1	item(s)	135	—	250	11.0	23.0	3.0	13.0	6.0	—	—
34472	Chicken burrito supreme	1	item(s)	248	—	390	20.0	49.0	6.0	13.0	6.0	—	—
33418	Chicken Chalupa Supreme	1	item(s)	153	—	360	17.0	29.0	2.0	20.0	5.0	—	—
34475	Chicken Gordita Baja	1	item(s)	153	—	320	17.0	28.0	3.0	16.0	3.5	—	—
29909	Chicken quesadilla	1	item(s)	184	—	520	28.0	40.0	3.0	28.0	12.0	—	—
29907	Chili cheese burrito	1	item(s)	156	—	390	16.0	40.0	3.0	18.0	9.0	—	—
10794	Cinnamon twists	1	serving(s)	35	—	170	1.0	26.0	1.0	7.0	0	—	—
29911	Grilled chicken Gordita Supreme	1	item(s)	153	—	290	17.0	28.0	2.0	12.0	5.0	—	—
14463	Grilled chicken soft taco	1	item(s)	99	—	190	14.0	19.0	1.0	6.0	2.5	—	—

PAGE KEY: A-4 = Breads/Baked Goods A-10 = Cereal/Rice/Pasta A-14 = Fruit A-20 = Vegetables/Legumes A-30 = Nuts/Seeds A-32 = Vegetarian
A-34 = Dairy A-42 = Eggs A-42 = Seafood A-46 = Meats A-50 = Poultry A-50 = Processed Meats A-52 = Beverages A-56 = Fats/Oils A-58 = Sweets
A-60 = Spices/Condiments/Sauces A-64 = Mixed Foods/Soups/Sandwiches A-70 = Fast Food A-90 = Convenience A-92 = Baby Foods

A

CHOL (mg)	CALC (mg)	IRON (mg)	MAGN (mg)	POTA (mg)	SODI (mg)	ZINC (mg)	VIT A (µg)	THIA (mg)	VIT E (mg α)	RIBO (mg)	NIAC (mg)	VIT B6 (mg)	FOLA (µg DFE)	VIT C (mg)	VIT B12 (µg)	SELE (µg)
45	100	5.40	—	—	1030.0	—	—	—	—	—	—	—	—	21.0	—	—
45	100	3.60	—	—	1010.0	—	—	—	—	—	—	—	—	16.8	—	—
35	60	3.60	—	—	880.0	—	—	—	—	—	—	—	—	30.0	—	—
35	60	3.60	—	—	1290.0	—	—	—	—	—	—	—	—	13.8	—	—
60	150	3.60	—	—	1530.0	—	—	—	—	—	—	—	—	16.8	—	—
190	80	4.50	—	—	720.0	—	66.7	—	—	—	—	—	—	3.6	—	—
25	60	2.70	—	—	1375.0	—	—	—	—	—	—	—	—	13.8	—	—
45	200	7.20	—	—	1610.0	—	—	—	—	—	—	—	—	36.0	—	—
45	200	5.40	—	—	1590.0	—	—	—	—	—	—	—	—	31.8	—	—
45	150	5.40	—	—	1720.0	—	—	—	—	—	—	—	—	24.0	—	—
15	20	1.08	—	—	170.0	—	—	—	—	—	—	—	—	0	—	—
45	60	4.50	—	—	1020.0	—	—	—	—	—	—	—	—	18.0	—	—
15	20	0.72	—	—	200.0	—	—	—	—	—	—	—	—	0	—	—
20	60	6.30	—	—	920.0	—	—	—	—	—	—	—	—	18.0	—	—
20	60	4.50	—	—	900.0	—	—	—	—	—	—	—	—	13.8	—	—
45	60	2.70	—	—	1000.0	—	—	—	—	—	—	—	—	13.8	—	—
45	150	8.10	—	—	1310.0	—	—	—	—	—	—	—	—	21.0	—	—
55	60	2.70	—	—	1650.0	—	—	—	—	—	—	—	—	16.8	—	—
35	150	6.30	—	—	1070.0	—	—	—	—	—	—	—	—	13.8	—	—
15	0	0.72	—	—	140.0	—	—	—	—	—	—	—	—	0	—	—
50	80	4.50	—	—	1220.0	—	—	—	—	—	—	—	—	24.0	—	—
50	200	2.70	—	—	1780.0	—	—	—	—	—	—	—	—	6.0	—	—
25	60	2.70	—	—	1210.0	—	—	—	—	—	—	—	—	13.8	—	—
20	60	2.70	—	—	1000.0	—	—	—	—	—	—	—	—	13.8	—	—
0	60	4.50	—	—	520.0	—	—	—	—	—	—	—	—	18.0	—	—
0	60	2.70	—	—	500.0	—	—	—	—	—	—	—	—	13.8	—	—
15	20	0.72	—	—	160.0	—	—	—	—	—	—	—	—	0	—	—
25	250	5.40	—	—	1350.0	—	—	—	—	—	—	—	—	15.0	—	—
5	200	4.50	—	—	1190.0	—	5.9	—	—	—	—	—	—	4.8	—	—
40	200	4.50	—	—	1340.0	—	9.9	—	—	—	—	—	—	6.0	—	—
40	150	2.70	—	—	620.0	—	—	—	—	—	—	—	—	3.6	—	—
35	100	2.70	—	—	780.0	—	—	—	—	—	—	—	—	2.4	—	—
40	150	2.70	—	—	620.0	—	—	—	—	—	—	—	—	3.6	—	—
25	100	1.80	—	—	630.0	—	—	—	—	—	—	—	—	1.2	—	—
40	150	2.70	—	—	650.0	—	—	—	—	—	—	—	—	3.6	—	—
45	200	4.50	—	—	1360.0	—	—	—	—	—	—	—	—	9.0	—	—
45	100	2.70	—	—	650.0	—	—	—	—	—	—	—	—	4.8	—	—
40	100	1.80	—	—	800.0	—	—	—	—	—	—	—	—	3.6	—	—
75	450	3.60	—	—	1420.0	—	—	—	—	—	—	—	—	1.2	—	—
40	300	1.80	—	—	1080.0	—	—	—	—	—	—	—	—	0	—	—
0	0	0.37	—	—	200.0	—	0	—	—	—	—	—	—	0	—	—
45	150	1.80	—	—	650.0	—	—	—	—	—	—	—	—	4.8	—	—
30	100	1.08	—	—	550.0	—	14.6	—	—	—	—	—	—	1.2	—	—

D&W+ Code	Food Description	QTY	Measure	WT (g)	H₂O (g)	Ener (cal)	Prot (g)	Carb (g)	Fiber (g)	Fat (g)	Sat	Mono	Poly
Fast Food—continued													
29912	Grilled steak Gordita Supreme	1	item(s)	153	—	290	15.0	28.0	2.0	13.0	5.0	—	—
29904	Grilled steak soft taco	1	item(s)	128	—	270	12.0	20.0	2.0	16.0	4.5	—	—
29905	Grilled steak soft taco supreme	1	item(s)	135	—	235	13.0	21.0	1.0	11.0	6.0	—	—
2021	Mexican pizza	1	serving(s)	216	—	530	20.0	42.0	7.0	30.0	8.0	—	—
29894	Mexican rice	1	serving(s)	131	—	170	6.0	23.0	1.0	11.0	3.0	—	—
10772	Meximelt	1	serving(s)	128	—	280	15.0	22.0	3.0	14.0	7.0	—	—
2011	Nachos	1	serving(s)	99	—	330	4.0	32.0	2.0	21.0	3.5	—	—
2012	Nachos Bellgrande	1	serving(s)	308	—	770	19.0	77.0	12.0	44.0	9.0	—	—
2023	Pintos 'n cheese	1	serving(s)	128	—	150	9.0	19.0	7.0	6.0	3.0	—	—
34473	Steak burrito supreme	1	item(s)	248	—	380	18.0	49.0	6.0	14.0	7.0	—	—
33419	Steak Chalupa Supreme	1	item(s)	153	—	360	15.0	28.0	2.0	21.0	6.0	—	—
747	Taco	1	item(s)	78	—	170	8.0	13.0	3.0	10.0	3.5	—	—
2015	Taco salad with salsa, with shell	1	serving(s)	548	—	840	30.0	80.0	15.0	45.0	11.0	—	—
14459	Taco supreme	1	item(s)	113	—	210	9.0	15.0	3.0	13.0	6.0	—	—
748	Tostada	1	item(s)	170	—	230	11.0	27.0	7.0	10.0	3.5	—	—
Convenience Meals													
Banquet													
29961	Barbeque chicken meal	1	item(s)	281	—	330	16.0	37.0	2.0	13.0	3.0	—	—
14788	Boneless white fried chicken meal	1	item(s)	286	—	310	10.0	21.0	4.0	20.0	5.0	—	—
29960	Fish sticks meal	1	item(s)	207	—	470	13.0	58.0	1.0	20.0	3.5	—	—
29957	Lasagna with meat sauce meal	1	item(s)	312	—	320	15.0	46.0	7.0	9.0	4.0	—	—
14777	Macaroni and cheese meal	1	item(s)	340	—	420	15.0	57.0	5.0	14.0	8.0	—	—
1741	Meatloaf meal	1	item(s)	269	—	240	14.0	20.0	4.0	11.0	4.0	—	—
39418	Pepperoni pizza meal	1	item(s)	191	—	480	11.0	56.0	5.0	23.0	8.0	—	—
33759	Roasted white turkey meal	1	item(s)	255	—	230	14.0	30.0	5.0	6.0	2.0	—	—
1743	Salisbury steak meal	1	item(s)	269	196.9	380	12.0	28.0	3.0	24.0	12.0	—	—
Budget Gourmet													
1914	Cheese manicotti with meat sauce entrée	1	item(s)	284	194.0	420	18.0	38.0	4.0	22.0	11.0	6.0	1.3
1915	Chicken with fettucini entrée	1	item(s)	284	—	380	20.0	33.0	3.0	19.0	10.0	—	—
3986	Light beef stroganoff entrée	1	item(s)	248	177.0	290	20.0	32.0	3.0	7.0	4.0	—	—
3996	Light sirloin of beef in herb sauce entrée	1	item(s)	269	214.0	260	19.0	30.0	5.0	7.0	4.0	2.3	0.3
3987	Light vegetable lasagna entrée	1	item(s)	298	227.0	290	15.0	36.0	4.8	9.0	1.8	0.9	0.6
Healthy Choice													
9425	Cheese French bread pizza	1	item(s)	170	—	340	22.0	51.0	5.0	5.0	1.5	—	—
9306	Chicken enchilada suprema meal	1	item(s)	320	251.5	360	13.0	59.0	8.0	7.0	3.0	2.0	2.0
3821	Familiar Favorites lasagna bake with meat sauce entrée	1	item(s)	255	—	270	13.0	38.0	4.0	7.0	2.5	—	—
13744	Familiar Favorites sesame chicken with vegetables and rice entrée	1	item(s)	255	—	260	17.0	34.0	4.0	6.0	2.0	2.0	2.0
9316	Lemon pepper fish meal	1	item(s)	303	—	280	11.0	49.0	5.0	5.0	2.0	1.0	2.0
9322	Traditional salisbury steak meal	1	item(s)	354	250.3	360	23.0	45.0	5.0	9.0	3.5	4.0	1.0
9359	Traditional turkey breasts meal	1	item(s)	298	—	330	21.0	50.0	4.0	5.0	2.0	1.5	1.5
Stouffers													
2313	Cheese French bread pizza	1	serving(s)	294	—	380	15.0	43.0	3.0	16.0	6.0	—	—
11138	Cheese manicotti with tomato sauce entrée	1	item(s)	255	—	360	18.0	41.0	2.0	14.0	6.0	—	—
2366	Chicken pot pie entrée	1	item(s)	284	—	740	23.0	56.0	4.0	47.0	18.0	12.4	10.5
11116	Homestyle baked chicken breast with mashed potatoes and gravy entrée	1	item(s)	252	—	270	21.0	21.0	2.0	11.0	3.5	—	—
11146	Homestyle beef pot roast and potatoes entrée	1	item(s)	252	—	260	16.0	24.0	3.0	11.0	4.0	—	—
11152	Homestyle roast turkey breast with stuffing and mashed potatoes entrée	1	item(s)	273	—	290	16.0	30.0	2.0	12.0	3.5	—	—
11043	Lean Cuisine Comfort Classics baked chicken and whipped potatoes and stuffing entrée	1	item(s)	245	—	240	15.0	34.0	3.0	4.5	1.0	2.0	1.0
11046	Lean Cuisine Comfort Classics honey mustard chicken with rice pilaf entrée	1	item(s)	227	—	250	17.0	37.0	1.0	4.0	1.0	1.0	1.0

PAGE KEY: A-4 = Breads/Baked Goods   A-10 = Cereal/Rice/Pasta   A-14 = Fruit   A-20 = Vegetables/Legumes   A-30 = Nuts/Seeds   A-32 = Vegetarian   A-34 = Dairy   A-42 = Eggs   A-42 = Seafood   A-46 = Meats   A-50 = Poultry   A-50 = Processed Meats   A-52 = Beverages   A-56 = Fats/Oils   A-58 = Sweets   A-60 = Spices/Condiments/Sauces   A-64 = Mixed Foods/Soups/Sandwiches   A-70 = Fast Food   A-90 = Convenience   A-92 = Baby Foods

A

CHOL (mg)	CALC (mg)	IRON (mg)	MAGN (mg)	POTA (mg)	SODI (mg)	ZINC (mg)	VIT A (µg)	THIA (mg)	VIT E (mg α)	RIBO (mg)	NIAC (mg)	VIT B_6 (mg)	FOLA (µg DFE)	VIT C (mg)	VIT B_{12} (µg)	SELE (µg)
40	100	2.70	—	—	530.0	—	—	—	—	—	—	—	—	3.6	—	—
35	100	2.70	—	—	660.0	—	—	—	—	—	—	—	—	3.6	—	—
35	120	1.44	—	—	565.0	—	29.2	—	—	—	—	—	—	3.6	—	—
40	350	3.60	—	—	1000.0	—	—	—	—	—	—	—	—	4.8	—	—
15	100	1.44	—	—	790.0	—	—	—	—	—	—	—	—	3.6	—	—
40	250	2.70	—	—	880.0	—	—	—	—	—	—	—	—	2.4	—	—
3	80	0.71	—	—	530.0	—	0	—	—	—	—	—	—	0	—	—
35	200	3.60	—	—	1280.0	—	—	—	—	—	—	—	—	4.8	—	—
15	150	1.44	—	—	670.0	—	—	—	—	—	—	—	—	3.6	—	—
35	200	4.50	—	—	1250.0	—	9.9	—	—	—	—	—	—	9.0	—	—
40	100	2.70	—	—	530.0	—	—	—	—	—	—	—	—	3.6	—	—
25	80	1.08	—	—	350.0	—	—	—	—	—	—	—	—	1.2	—	—
65	450	7.20	—	—	1780.0	—	—	—	—	—	—	—	—	12.0	—	—
40	100	1.08	—	—	370.0	—	—	—	—	—	—	—	—	3.6	—	—
15	200	1.80	—	—	730.0	—	—	—	—	—	—	—	—	4.8	—	—
																—
50	40	1.08	—	—	1210.0	—	0	—	—	—	—	—	—	4.8	—	—
45	80	1.44	—	—	1200.0	—	—	—	—	—	—	—	—	18.0	—	—
55	20	1.44	—	—	710.0	—	—	—	—	—	—	—	—	0	—	—
20	100	2.70	—	—	1170.0	—	—	—	—	—	—	—	—	0	—	—
20	150	1.44	—	—	1330.0	—	0	—	—	—	—	—	—	0	—	—
30	0	1.80	—	—	1040.0	—	0	—	—	—	—	—	—	0	—	—
35	150	1.80	—	—	870.0	—	0	—	—	—	—	—	—	0	—	—
25	60	1.80	—	—	1070.0	—	—	—	—	—	—	—	—	3.6	—	—
60	40	1.44	—	—	1140.0	—	0	—	—	—	—	—	—	0	—	—
85	300	2.70	45.4	484.0	810.0	2.29	—	0.45	—	0.51	4.00	0.22	30.7	0	0.7	—
85	100	2.70	—	—	810.0	—	—	0.15	—	0.42	6.00	—	—	0	—	—
35	40	1.80	38.9	280.0	580.0	4.71	—	0.17	—	0.36	4.28	0.27	18.9	2.4	2.5	—
30	40	1.80	57.7	540.0	850.0	4.81	—	0.15	—	0.29	5.53	0.37	38.4	6.0	1.6	—
15	283	3.03	78.5	420.0	780.0	1.39	—	0.22	—	0.45	3.13	0.32	74.8	59.1	0.2	—
10	350	3.60	—	—	600.0	—	—	—	—	—	—	—	—	0	—	—
30	40	1.44	—	—	580.0	—	—	—	—	—	—	—	—	3.6	—	—
20	100	1.80	—	—	600.0	—	—	—	—	—	—	—	—	0	—	—
35	18	0.72	—	—	580.0	—	—	—	—	—	—	—	—	12.0	—	—
35	20	0.36	—	—	580.0	—	—	—	—	—	—	—	—	30.0	—	—
45	80	2.70	—	—	580.0	—	—	—	—	—	—	—	—	21.0	—	—
35	40	1.80	—	—	600.0	—	—	—	—	—	—	—	—	0	—	—
30	200	1.80	—	230.0	660.0	—	—	—	—	—	—	—	—	2.4	—	—
70	250	1.44	—	550.0	920.0	—	—	—	—	—	—	—	—	6.0	—	—
65	150	2.70	—	—	1170.0	—	—	—	—	—	—	—	—	2.4	—	—
55	20	0.72	—	490.0	770.0	—	0	—	—	—	—	—	—	0	—	—
35	20	1.80	—	800.0	960.0	—	—	—	—	—	—	—	—	6.0	—	—
45	40	1.08	—	490.0	970.0	—	—	—	—	—	—	—	—	3.6	—	—
25	40	1.16	—	500.0	650.0	—	—	—	—	—	—	—	—	3.6	—	—
30	64	0.38	—	370.0	650.0	—	—	—	—	—	—	—	—	0	—	—

TABLE **A–1** **Table of Food Composition** *(continued)*

(Computer code is for Cengage Diet & Wellness Plus program)

D&W+ Code	Food Description	QTY	Measure	Wt (g)	H₂0 (g)	Ener (cal)	Prot (g)	Carb (g)	Fiber (g)	Fat (g)	Fat Breakdown (g) Sat	Mono	Poly
Convenience Meals—continued													
9479	Lean Cuisine Deluxe French bread pizza	1	item(s)	174	—	310	16.0	44.0	3.0	9.0	3.5	0.5	0.5
360	Lean Cuisine One Dish Favorites chicken chow mein with rice	1	item(s)	255	—	190	13.0	29.0	2.0	2.5	0.5	1.0	0.5
11054	Lean Cuisine One Dish Favorites chicken enchilada Suiza with Mexican-style rice	1	serving(s)	255	—	270	10.0	47.0	3.0	4.5	2.0	1.5	1.0
9467	Lean Cuisine One Dish Favorites fettucini alfredo entrée	1	item(s)	262	—	270	13.0	39.0	2.0	7.0	3.5	2.0	1.0
11055	Lean Cuisine One Dish Favorites lasagna with meat sauce entrée	1	item(s)	298	—	320	19.0	44.0	4.0	7.0	3.0	2.0	0.5
Weight Watchers													
11164	Smart Ones chicken enchiladas Suiza entrée	1	item(s)	255	—	340	12.0	38.0	3.0	10.0	4.5	—	—
39763	Smart Ones chicken oriental entrée	1	item(s)	255	—	230	15.0	34.0	3.0	4.5	1.0	—	—
11187	Smart Ones pepperoni pizza	1	item(s)	198	—	400	22.0	58.0	4.0	9.0	3.0	—	—
39765	Smart Ones spaghetti bolognese entrée	1	item(s)	326	—	280	17.0	43.0	5.0	5.0	2.0	—	—
31512	Smart Ones spicy Szechuan style vegetables and chicken	1	item(s)	255	—	220	11.0	34.0	4.0	5.0	1.0	—	—
Baby Foods													
787	Apple juice	4	fluid ounce(s)	127	111.6	60	0	14.8	0.1	0.1	0	0	0
778	Applesauce, strained	4	tablespoon(s)	64	56.7	26	0.1	6.9	1.1	0.1	0	0	0
779	Bananas with tapioca, strained	4	tablespoon(s)	60	50.4	34	0.2	9.2	1.0	0	0	0	0
604	Carrots, strained	4	tablespoon(s)	56	51.7	15	0.4	3.4	1.0	0.1	0	0	0
770	Chicken noodle dinner, strained	4	tablespoon(s)	64	54.8	42	1.7	5.8	1.3	1.3	0.4	0.5	0.3
801	Green beans, strained	4	tablespoon(s)	60	55.1	16	0.7	3.8	1.3	0.1	0	0	0
910	Human milk, mature	2	fluid ounce(s)	62	53.9	43	0.6	4.2	0	2.7	1.2	1.0	0.3
760	Mixed cereal, prepared with whole milk	4	ounce(s)	113	84.6	128	5.4	18.0	1.5	4.0	2.2	1.2	0.4
772	Mixed vegetable dinner, strained	2	ounce(s)	57	50.3	23	0.7	5.4	0.8	0	—	—	0
762	Rice cereal, prepared with whole milk	4	ounce(s)	113	84.6	130	4.4	18.9	0.1	4.1	2.6	1.0	0.2
758	Teething biscuits	1	item(s)	11	0.7	44	1.0	8.6	0.2	0.6	0.2	0.2	0.1

PAGE KEY: A-4 = Breads/Baked Goods A-10 = Cereal/Rice/Pasta A-14 = Fruit A-20 = Vegetables/Legumes A-30 = Nuts/Seeds A-32 = Vegetarian A-34 = Dairy A-42 = Eggs A-42 = Seafood A-46 = Meats A-50 = Poultry A-50 = Processed Meats A-52 = Beverages A-56 = Fats/Oils A-58 = Sweets A-60 = Spices/Condiments/Sauces A-64 = Mixed Foods/Soups/Sandwiches A-70 = Fast Food A-90 = Convenience A-92 = Baby Foods

A

CHOL (mg)	CALC (mg)	IRON (mg)	MAGN (mg)	POTA (mg)	SODI (mg)	ZINC (mg)	VIT A (µg)	THIA (mg)	VIT E (mg α)	RIBO (mg)	NIAC (mg)	VIT B_6 (mg)	FOLA (µg DFE)	VIT C (mg)	VIT B_{12} (µg)	SELE (µg)
20	150	2.70	—	300.0	700.0	—	—	—	—	—	—	—	—	15.0	—	—
25	40	0.72	—	380.0	650.0	—	—	—	—	—	—	—	—	2.4	—	
20	150	0.72	—	350.0	510.0	—	—	—	—	—	—	—	—	2.4		
15	200	0.72	—	290.0	690.0	—	0	—	—	—	—	—	—	0	—	—
30	250	1.47	—	610.0	690.0	—	—	—	—	—	—	—	—	2.4	—	—
40	200	0.72	—	—	800.0	—	—	—	—	—	—	—	—	2.4	—	—
35	40	0.72	—	—	790.0	—	—	—	—	—	—	—	—	6.0	—	—
15	200	1.08	—	401.0	700.0	—	69.1	—	—	—	—	—	—	4.8	—	—
15	150	3.60	—	—	670.0	—	—	—	—	—	—	—	—	9.0	—	—
10	40	1.44	—	—	890.0	—	—	—	—	—	—	—	—	0	—	—
0	5	0.72	3.8	115.4	3.8	0.03	1.3	0.01	0.76	0.02	0.10	0.03	0	73.4	0	0.1
0	3	0.12	1.9	45.4	1.3	0.01	0.6	0.01	0.36	0.02	0.04	0.02	1.3	24.5	0	0.2
0	3	0.12	6.0	52.8	5.4	0.04	1.2	0.01	0.36	0.02	0.08	0.04	3.6	10.0	0	0.4
0	12	0.20	5.0	109.8	20.7	0.08	320.9	0.01	0.29	0.02	0.25	0.04	8.4	3.2	0	0.1
10	17	0.40	9.0	89.0	14.7	0.32	70.4	0.03	0.12	0.04	0.44	0.04	8.3	0	0	2.4
0	23	0.40	12.0	87.6	3.0	0.12	10.8	0.02	0.04	0.04	0.20	0.02	14.4	0.2	0	0
9	20	0.02	1.8	31.4	10.5	0.10	37.6	0.01	0.04	0.02	0.10	0.01	3.1	3.1	0	1.1
12	249	11.82	30.6	225.7	53.3	0.80	28.4	0.49	—	0.65	6.54	0.07	10.2	1.4	0.3	
—	12	0.18	6.2	68.6	4.5	0.08	77.1	0.01	—	0.02	0.28	0.04	4.5	1.6	0	0.4
12	271	13.82	51.0	215.5	52.2	0.72	24.9	0.52	—	0.56	5.90	0.12	6.8	1.4	0.3	4.0
0	11	0.39	3.9	35.5	28.4	0.10	3.1	0.02	0.02	0.05	0.47	0.01	7.6	1.0	0	2.6

Dietary Guidelines

The Dietary Guidelines for Americans is the centerpiece of the USDA's nutrition advice system, described in Chapter 2. Table B–1 presents the overarching themes that informed the 2015–2020 Dietary Guidelines. The World Health Organization is the source of nutrition guidance for many of the world's populations. These nutrient intake recommendations set the basis for country-specific dietary guidance, and they are listed in Table B–2.

TABLE B–1 Six Themes of the Dietary Guidelines for Americans Committee Report, 2015

These overarching themes provided the scientific basis of evidence for the Dietary Guidelines 2015.

The nation has serious health problems.	117 million people suffer from one or more preventable diseases related to poor diet and physical inactivity, a profile evident over two decades and disproportionately among low-income people.
A large gap exists between actual and optimal food intake patterns.	Suboptimal dietary patterns are *causally* related to poor health, and few, if any, improvements are evident over recent decades (see Figure 2–4, p. 39). Access to affordable, healthy foods is unequal. The prevailing food environment is characterized by abundant highly processed, convenient, low-cost, energy-dense, nutrient-poor foods, making change difficult.
Optimal food intake patterns are known.	Strong links exist between a healthy dietary pattern and good health; this pattern is higher in vegetables, fruits, whole grains, low-fat or nonfat dairy, seafood, legumes, and nuts; moderate in alcohol (among adults who drink); lower in red and processed meats; and low in refined grains and sugar-sweetened foods and drinks.
Individuals can make the needed changes.	Eating behaviors are modifiable, particularly with tools like the Dietary Guidelines for Americans and the Physical Activity Guidelines for Americans. Sound behavioral interventions can help people make needed changes.
Public policy affects population-wide behaviors.	Environmental and policy changes affecting child care, schools, and work sites effectively change population-wide diets, particularly when combined with other programs, such as nutrition education, parent engagement, food labeling, nutrition standards, and behavioral interventions.
Diet choices can affect the environment.	Sustainability of healthy dietary patterns, as well as the safety of key dietary constituents, was examined. Healthy dietary patterns that are higher in plant-based foods, such as vegetables, fruits, whole grains, legumes, nuts, and seeds, while lower in calories and animal-based foods are associated with more favorable environmental outcomes (see Chapter 15 for details).

Source: U.S. Department of Agriculture and U.S. Department of Health and Human Services, Scientific Report of the 2015 Dietary Guidelines Advisory Committee *(2015), B-2:1–3, available at www.health.gov.*

TABLE B–2 World Health Organization (WHO) Nutrient Intake Guidelines, 2015

WHO has assessed the relationships between diet and the development of chronic diseases. Its recommendations include these:

- Energy: sufficient to support growth, physical activity, and a healthy body weight (BMI between 18.5 and 24.9) and to avoid weight gain greater than 11 lb (5 kg) during adult life
- Total fat: 15% to 35% of total energy
- Saturated fatty acids: <10% of total energy
- Polyunsaturated fatty acids: 6% to 11% of total energy
- Omega-6 polyunsaturated fatty acids: 2.5% to 9% of total energy
- Omega-3 polyunsaturated fatty acids: 0.5% to 2% of total energy
- *Trans*-fatty acids: <1% of total energy
- Total carbohydrate: 55% to 75% of total energy
- Sugars: <10% of total energy (< 5% of total energy would provide additional health benefits)
- Protein: 10% to 15% of total energy
- Cholesterol: <300 mg/day
- Salt (sodium): <5 g salt/day (<2 g sodium/day), appropriately iodized
- Fruits and vegetables: ≥400 g/day (about 1 lb)
- Total dietary fiber: >25 g/day from foods
- Physical activity: 1 hr of moderate-intensity activity, such as walking, on most days of the week

Source: Compiled from tables available at www.who.int/publications/guidelines/nutrition/en/index.html and www.who.int/nutrition/publications/guidelines/sugars_intake/en/.

Aids to Calculations

Mathematical problems have been worked out for you as examples at appropriate places in the text. This Appendix aims to help with the use of the metric system and with those problems not fully explained elsewhere.

Conversion Factors

Conversion factors are useful mathematical tools in everyday calculations, like the ones encountered in the study of nutrition. A conversion factor is a fraction in which the numerator (top) and the denominator (bottom) express the same quantity in different units. For example, 2.2 pounds (lb) and 1 kilogram (kg) are equivalent; they express the same weight. The conversion factor used to change pounds to kilograms or vice versa is:

$$\frac{2.2 \text{ lb}}{1 \text{ kg}} \quad \text{or} \quad \frac{1 \text{ kg}}{2.2 \text{ lb}}$$

Because both factors equal 1, measurements can be multiplied by the factor without changing the value of the measurement. Thus, the units can be changed.

The correct factor to use in a problem is the one with the unit you are seeking in the numerator (top) of the fraction. Following are some examples of problems commonly encountered in nutrition study; they illustrate the usefulness of conversion factors.

Example 1

Convert the weight of 130 pounds to kilograms.

1. Choose the conversion factor in which the unit you are seeking is on top:

$$\frac{1 \text{ kg}}{2.2 \text{ lb}}$$

2. Multiply 130 pounds by the factor:

$$130 \text{ lb} \times \frac{1 \text{ kg}}{2.2 \text{ lb}} = \frac{130 \text{ kg}}{2.2}$$

$$= 59 \text{ kg (rounded off to the nearest whole number)}$$

Example 2

How many grams (g) of saturated fat are contained in a 3-ounce (oz) hamburger?

1. Appendix A shows that a 4-ounce hamburger contains 7 grams of saturated fat. You are seeking grams of saturated fat; therefore, the conversion factor is:

$$\frac{7 \text{ g saturated fat}}{4 \text{ oz hamburger}}$$

2. Multiply 3 ounces of hamburger by the conversion factor:

$$3 \text{ oz hamburger} \times \frac{7 \text{ g saturated fat}}{4 \text{ oz hamburger}} = \frac{3 \times 7}{4} = \frac{21}{4}$$

$$= 5 \text{ g saturated fat (rounded off to the nearest whole number)}$$

Energy Units

1 calorie* (cal) = 4.2 kilojoules

1 millijoule (MJ) = 240 cal

1 kilojoule (kJ) = 0.24 cal

1 gram (g) carbohydrate = 4 cal = 17 kJ

1 g fat = 9 cal = 37 kJ

1 g protein = 4 cal = 17 kJ

1 g alcohol = 7 cal = 29 kJ

Nutrient Unit Conversions

Sodium

To convert milligrams of sodium to grams of salt:

mg sodium ÷ 400 = g of salt

The reverse is also true:

g salt × 400 = mg sodium

Folate

To convert micrograms (μg) of synthetic folate in supplements and enriched foods to Dietary Folate Equivalents (μg DFE):

μg synthetic folate × 1.7 = μg DFE

For naturally occurring folate, assign each microgram of folate a value of 1 μg DFE:

μg folate = μg DFE

Example 3

Consider a pregnant woman who takes a supplement and eats a bowl of fortified cornflakes, 2 slices of fortified bread, and a cup of fortified pasta.

1. From the supplement and fortified foods, she obtains synthetic folate:

Supplement	100 μg folate
Fortified cornflakes	100 μg folate
Fortified bread	40 μg folate
Fortified pasta	60 μg folate
	300 μg folate

2. To calculate the DFE, multiply the amount of synthetic folate by 1.7:

    300 μg × 1.7 = 510 μg DFE

3. Now add the naturally occurring folate from the other foods in her diet—in this example, another 90 μg of folate.

    510 μg DFE + 90 μg = 600 μg DFE

Notice that if we had not converted synthetic folate from supplements and fortified foods to DFE, then this woman's

intake would appear to fall short of the 600 μg recommendation for pregnancy (300 μg + 90 μg = 390 μg). But as this example shows, her intake does meet the recommendation.

Vitamin A

Equivalencies for vitamin A:

1 μg RAE = 1 μg retinol
= 12 μg beta-carotene
= 24 μg other vitamin A carotenoids

1 international unit (IU) = 0.3 μg retinol
= 3.6 μg beta-carotene
= 7.2 μg other vitamin A carotenoids

To convert older RE values to micrograms RAE:

1 μg RE retinol = 1 μg RAE retinol

6 μg RE beta-carotene = 12 μg RAE beta-carotene

12 μg RE other vitamin A carotenoids = 24 μg RAE other vitamin A carotenoids

International Units (IU)

To convert IU to:

- μg vitamin D: divide by 40 or multiply by 0.025.
- 1 IU natural vitamin E = 0.67 mg alpha-tocopherol.
- 1 IU synthetic vitamin E = 0.45 mg alpha-tocopherol.
- vitamin A, see above.

Percentages

A percentage is a comparison between a number of items (perhaps your intake of energy) and a standard number (perhaps the number of calories recommended for your age and gender—your energy DRI). The standard number is the number you divide by. The answer you get after the division must be multiplied by 100 to be stated as a percentage (percent means "per 100").

Example 4

What percentage of the DRI recommendation for energy is your energy intake?

1. Find your energy DRI value on the inside front cover. We'll use 2,368 calories to demonstrate.

2. Total your energy intake for a day—for example, 1,200 calories.

3. Divide your calorie intake by the DRI value:

    1,200 cal (your intake) ÷ 2,368 cal (DRI) = 0.507

4. Multiply your answer by 100 to state it as a percentage:

    0.507 × 100 = 50.7 = 51% (rounded off to the nearest whole number)

In some problems in nutrition, the percentage may be more than 100. For example, suppose your daily intake of

---

Throughout this book and in the appendixes, the term calorie is used to mean kilocalorie. Thus, when converting calories to kilojoules, do not enlarge the calorie values—they are kilocalorie values.

vitamin A is 3,200 and your DRI is 900 μg. Your intake as a percentage of the DRI is more than 100 percent (that is, you consume more than 100 percent of your recommendation for vitamin A). The following calculations show your vitamin A intake as a percentage of the DRI value:

$$3,200 \div 900 = 3.6 \text{ (rounded)}$$
$$3.6 \times 100 = 360\% \text{ of DRI}$$

Example 5

Food labels express nutrients and energy contents of foods as percentages of the Daily Values. If a serving of a food contains 200 milligrams of calcium, for example, what percentage of the calcium Daily Value does the food provide?

1. Find the calcium Daily Value on the inside back cover, page Y.
2. Divide the milligrams of calcium in the food by the Daily Value standard:

$$\frac{200}{1,300} = 0.15 \text{ (rounded)}$$

3. Multiply by 100:

$$0.15 \times 100 = 15\% \text{ of the Daily Value}$$

Example 6

This example demonstrates how to calculate the percentage of fat in a day's meals.

1. Recall the general formula for finding percentages of calories from a nutrient:

(one nutrient's calories ÷ total calories) × 100 =
the percentage of calories from that nutrient

2. Say a day's meals provide 1,754 calories and 54 grams of fat. First, convert fat grams to fat calories:

$$54 \text{ g} \times 9 \text{ cal per g} = 486 \text{ cal from fat}$$

3. Then apply the general formula for finding percentage of calories from fat:

(fat calories ÷ total calories) × 100 =
percentage of calories from fat
$$(486 \div 1,754) \times 100 = 27.7 \text{ (28\%, rounded)}$$

Weights and Measures

Length

1 inch (in.) = 2.54 centimeters (cm)
1 foot (ft) = 30.48 cm
1 meter (m) = 39.37 in

Temperature

	Celsius†	Fahrenheit	
Steam	100°C	212°F	Steam
Body temperature	37°C	98.6°F	Body temperature
Ice	0°C	32°F	Ice

- To find degrees Fahrenheit (°F) when you know degrees Celsius (°C), multiply by 9/5 and then add 32.

- To find degrees Celsius (°C) when you know degrees Fahrenheit (°F), subtract 32 and then multiply by 5/9.

Volume

Used to measure fluids or pourable dry substances such as cereal.

1 milliliter (ml) = ⅕ teaspoon or 0.034 fluid ounce or ¹⁄₁,₀₀₀ liter
1 deciliter (dL) = ¹⁄₁₀ liter
1 teaspoon (tsp or t) = 5 ml or about 5 grams (weight) salt
1 tablespoon (tbs or T) = 3 tsp or 15 ml
1 ounce, fluid (fl oz) = 2 tbs or 30 ml
1 cup (c) = 8 fl oz or 16 tbs or 250 ml
1 quart (qt) = 32 fl oz or 4 c or 0.95 liter
1 liter (L) = 1.06 qt or 1,000 ml
1 gallon (gal) = 16 c or 4 qt or 128 fl oz or 3.79 L

Weight

1 microgram (μg or mcg) = ¹⁄₁,₀₀₀ milligram
1 milligram (mg) = 1,000 mcg or ¹⁄₁,₀₀₀ gram
1 gram (g) = 1,000 mg or ¹⁄₁,₀₀₀ kilogram
1 ounce, weight (oz) = about 28 g or ¹⁄₁₆ pound
1 pound (lb) = 16 oz (wt) or about 454 g
1 kilogram (kg) = 1,000 g or 2.2 lb

---

†Also known as centigrade.

Food Lists for Diabetes and Weight Management

Chapter 2 introduces meal planning principles, and this Appendix provides details from the 2014 *Choose Your Foods: Food Lists for Diabetes* and the 2014 *Choose Your Foods: Food Lists for Weight Management.* These lists can help people with diabetes to manage their blood glucose levels by controlling the amount and kinds of carbohydrates they consume. The lists can also help in planning diets for weight management by controlling calorie intake.

The Food Lists

The Food Lists sort foods by their proportions of carbohydrate, fat, and protein. These lists also fall into groups that reflect the dominant energy nutrient (Table D–1, p. D-2). For example, the Carbohydrates include these Food Lists:

- Starch
- Fruits
- Milk
- Nonstarchy Vegetables
- Sweets, Desserts, and Other Carbohydrates

Any food on a list can be traded for any other food on the same list without significantly affecting the intake of energy nutrients or total calories. The term *choice* is used throughout the lists to describe a certain quantity of food within a group of similar foods.

Serving Sizes

The serving sizes have been carefully adjusted and defined so that a serving of any food on a given list provides roughly the same amount of carbohydrate, fat, and protein—and therefore total energy. For example, a person may select 17 small grapes or ½ large grapefruit as one fruit serving, and either would provide roughly 15 grams of carbohydrate and 60 calories. A whole grapefruit, however, would count as 2 fruit servings.

  To apply the system successfully, users must become familiar with the specified serving sizes. A convenient way to remember the serving sizes and energy values is to keep in mind a typical item from each list (review Table D–1).

The Foods on the Lists

Foods do not always appear on the Food Lists where you might first expect to find them. They are grouped according to their energy-nutrient contents rather than by their source, their outward appearance, or their vitamin and mineral contents. For example, cheeses are found among the meats on the Protein lists (not Milk and Milk Substitutes) because, like meats, cheeses contribute energy from protein and fat but provide negligible carbohydrate. For similar reasons, starchy vegetables such as corn, green peas, and potatoes are found on the Starch list with breads and cereals, not with the vegetables. Diet planners learn to view mixtures of foods, such as casseroles and soups, as combinations of foods from different lists.

Controlling Energy, Fat, and Sodium

The Food Lists help people control their energy intakes by paying close attention to serving sizes. Also, people wanting to lose weight can limit foods from the Sweets, Desserts, and Other Carbohydrates and Fats lists, and they might choose to avoid the Alcohol list altogether. The Free Foods list provide low-calorie choices.

The lists alert consumers to foods that are unexpectedly high in fat. For example, the Starch list specifies which grain products contain added fat (such as biscuits) by marking them with a symbol to indicate extra fat (the symbols are explained in the table keys). In addition, foods on the Milk and Milk Substitutes and Protein lists are separated into categories based on their fat contents (review Table D–1). The Protein list also includes plant-based proteins, which tend to be rich in fiber. Notice that many of these foods (p. D-9) bear the symbol for "good source of fiber."

People wanting to control the sodium in their diets can begin by eliminating any foods bearing the "high in sodium" symbol. In most cases, the symbol identifies foods that, in one serving, provide 480 milligrams or more of sodium. Foods on the Combination Foods and Fast Foods lists that bear the symbol provide more than 600 milligrams of sodium. Take time to explore the Food Lists (Tables D–2 through D–12). Doing so can provide a new focus on the energy-yielding nutrients that everyday foods provide.

TABLE D–1 The Food Lists

This table shows the amounts of nutrients and energy in one choice from each list.

Food Lists	Typical Item/Serving Size	Carbohydrate (g)	Protein (g)	Fat (g)	Energy[a] (cal)
Carbohydrates					
Starch[b]	1 slice bread	15	3	1	80
Fruits	1 small apple	15	—	—	60
Milk and milk substitutes					
Fat-free, low-fat (1%)	1 c fat-free milk	12	8	0–3	100
Reduced-fat (2%)	1 c reduced-fat milk	12	8	5	120
Whole	1 c whole milk	12	8	8	160
Nonstarchy vegetables	½ c cooked carrots	5	2	—	25
Sweets, desserts, and other carbohydrates	5 vanilla wafers	15	varies	varies	varies
Protein					
Lean	1 oz chicken (no skin)	—	7	2	45
Medium-fat	1 oz ground beef	—	7	5	75
High-fat	1 oz pork sausage	—	7	8	100
Plant-based	½ c tofu	varies	7	varies	varies
Fats	1 tsp olive oil	—	—	5	45
Alcohol	12 fl oz beer	varies	—	—	100

[a]The energy value for each food list represents an approximate average for the group and does not reflect the precise number of grams of carbohydrate, protein, and fat. For example, a slice of bread contains 15 grams of carbohydrate (60 calories), 3 grams of protein (12 calories), and 1 gram of fat (9 calories)—rounded to 80 calories for ease in calculating. A ½ cup of nonstarchy vegetables contains 5 grams of carbohydrate (20 calories) and 2 grams of protein (8 calories), which has been rounded down to 25 calories.

[b]The Starch list includes cereals, grains and pasta, breads, crackers and snacks, starchy vegetables (such as corn, green peas, and potatoes), and legumes (dried beans, peas, and lentils).

The Starch list includes breads, cereals, grains (including pasta and rice), starchy vegetables, crackers and snacks, and legumes (beans, peas, and lentils).

1 starch choice = 15 grams carbohydrate, 3 grams protein, 1 gram fat, and 80 calories.

Note: In general, one starch choice is ½ cup of cooked cereal, grain, or starchy vegetable; ⅓ cup of cooked rice or pasta; 1 ounce of bread product, such as 1 slice of bread; ¾ to 1 ounce of most snack foods.

Food	Serving Size	Food	Serving Size
Bread		**Starchy Vegetables** (continued)	
Bagel	¼ large bagel (1 oz)	Cassava or dasheen	⅓ cup
! Biscuit	1 (2½ in. across)	Corn	½ cup
Breads, loaf-type		on cob	4- to 4½-in. piece (½ large)
white, whole-grain, French, Italian, pumpernickel,	1 slice (1 oz)	✓ Hominy	¾ cup
rye, sourdough, unfrosted raisin or cinnamon		✓ Mixed vegetables with corn or peas	1 cup
✓ reduced-calorie, light	2 slices (1½ oz)	Marinara, pasta, or spaghetti sauce	½ cup
Breads, flat-type (flatbreads)		✓ Parsnips	½ cup
chapati	1 oz	✓ Peas, green	½ cup
ciabatta	1 oz	Plantain	⅓ cup
naan	3¼-in. square (1 oz)	Potato	
pita (6 in. across)	½ pita	baked with skin	¼ large (3 oz)
roti	1 oz	boiled, all kinds	½ cup or ½ medium (3 oz)
✓ sandwich flat buns, whole-wheat	1 bun (1½ oz)	! mashed, with milk and fat	½ cup
! taco shell	2 (each 5 in. across)	French-fried (oven-baked)c	1 cup (2 oz)
tortilla, corn	1 small (6 in. across)	✓ Pumpkin puree, canned, no sugar added	¾ cup
tortilla, flour (white or whole-wheat)	1 small (6 in. across) or ⅓ large	✓ Squash, winter (acorn, butternut)	1 cup
	(10 in. across)	✓ Succotash	½ cup
Cornbread	1¾-in. cube (1½ oz)	Yam or sweet potato, plain	½ cup (3½ oz)
English muffin	½ muffin	**Crackers and Snacks**	
Hot dog bun or hamburger bun	½ bun (¾ oz)	Crackers	
Pancake	1 (4 in. across, ¼ in. thick)	animal	8
Roll, plain	1 small (1 oz)	✓ crispbread	2–5 pieces (¾ oz)
! Stuffing, bread	⅓ cup	graham, 2½-in. square	3
Waffle	1 (4-in. square or 4 in. across)	nut and rice	10
Cereals		oyster	20
✓ Bran cereal (twigs, buds, or flakes)	½ cup	! round, butter-type	6
Cooked cereals (oats, oatmeal)	½ cup	saltine-type	6
Granola cereal	¼ cup	! sandwich-style, cheese or peanut	3
Grits, cooked	½ cup	butter filling	
Muesli	¼ cup	whole-wheat, baked	5 regular 1½-in. squares or
Puffed cereal	1½ cups		10 thins (¾ oz)
Shredded wheat, plain	½ cup	Granola or snack bar	1 (¾ oz)
Sugar-coated cereal	½ cup	Matzoh, all shapes and sizes	¾ oz
Unsweetened, ready-to-eat cereal	¾ cup	Melba toast	4 (2 in. by 4 in.)
Grainsa		Popcorn	
Barley	⅓ cup	✓ no fat added	3 cups
Bran, dry		!! with butter added	3 cups
✓ oat	¼ cup	Pretzels	¾ oz
✓ wheat	½ cup	Rice cakes	2 (4 in. across)
✓ Bulgur	½ cup	Snack chips	
Couscous	⅓ cup	baked (potato, pita)	~8 (¾ oz)
Kasha	½ cup	!! regular (tortilla, potato)	~13 (1 oz)
Millet	⅓ cup	**Beans, Peas, and Lentilsd**	
Pasta, white or whole-wheat	⅓ cup	The choices on this list count as 1 starch + 1 lean protein.	
Polenta	⅓ cup	✓ Baked beans, canned	⅓ cup
Quinoa, all colors	⅓ cup	✓ Beans (black, garbanzo, kidney, lima,	½ cup
Rice, all colors and types	⅓ cup	navy, pinto, white), cooked or canned,	
Tabbouleh (tabouli), prepared	½ cup	drained and rinsed	
Wheat germ, dry	3 tbs	✓ Lentils (any color), cooked	½ cup
Wild rice	½ cup	✓ Peas (black-eyed and split), cooked or canned,	½ cup
Starchy Vegetablesb		drained and rinsed	
Breadfruit	¼ cup	🅂 ✓ Refried beans, canned	½ cup

aServing sizes are for cooked grains unless otherwise noted. bServing sizes are for cooked vegetables. cRestaurant-style French fries are on the Fast Foods list. dAlso found on the Protein list.

Key:	
✓ = Good source of fiber. 3 g/serving	!! — Extra fat: +10 g/serving
! = Extra fat: +5 g/serving	🅂 = High in sodium: ≥480 mg/serving

TABLE D–3 Fruits

Fruit[a]

The Fruits list includes fresh, frozen, canned, and dried fruits and fruit juices.

1 fruit choice = 15 grams carbohydrate, 0 grams protein, 0 grams fat, and 60 calories.

Note: In general, one fruit choice is ½ cup of canned or frozen fruit or unsweetened fruit juice; 1 small fresh fruit (¾ to 1 cup); 2 tablespoons of dried fruit.

Food	Serving Size
Apple, unpeeled	1 small (4 oz)
Apples, dried	4 rings
Applesauce, unsweetened	½ cup
Apricots	
canned	½ cup
dried	8 halves
fresh	4 (5½ oz total)
Banana	1 extra-small, ~4 in. long (4 oz)
✓ Blackberries	1 cup
Blueberries	¾ cup
Cantaloupe	1 cup diced
Cherries	
sweet, canned	½ cup
sweet, fresh	12 (3½ oz)
Dates	3 small (deglet noor) or 1 large (medjool)
Dried fruits (blueberries, cherries, cranberries, mixed fruit, raisins)	2 tbs
Figs	
dried	3 small
✓ fresh	1½ large or 2 medium (3½ oz)
Fruit cocktail	½ cup
Grapefruit	
fresh	½ large (5½ oz)
sections, canned	¾ cup
Grapes	17 small (3 oz)
✓ Guava	2 small (2½ oz total)
Honeydew melon	1 cup diced
Kiwi	½ cup sliced
Loquat	¾ cup cubed
Mandarin oranges, canned	¾ cup
Mango	½ small (5½ oz) or ½ cup
Nectarine	1 medium (5½ oz)
✓ Orange	1 medium (6½ oz)
Papaya	½ (8 oz) or 1 cup cubed
Peaches	
canned	½ cup
fresh	1 medium (6 oz)
Pears	
canned	½ cup
✓ fresh	½ large (4 oz)
Pineapple	
canned	½ cup
fresh	¾ cup
Plantain, extra-ripe (black), raw	¼ (2¼ oz)
Plums	
canned	½ cup
dried (prunes)	3
fresh	2 small (5 oz total)
Pomegranate seeds (arils)	½ cup
✓ Raspberries	1 cup
✓ Strawberries	1¼ cup whole
Tangerine	1 large (6 oz)
Watermelon	1¼ cups diced
Fruit Juice	
Apple juice/cider	½ cup
Fruit juice blends, 100% juice	⅓ cup
Grape juice	⅓ cup
Grapefruit juice	½ cup
Orange juice	½ cup
Pineapple juice	½ cup
Pomegranate juice	½ cup
Prune juice	⅓ cup

[a]The weights listed include skin, core, seeds, and rind.

Key:
✓ = Good source of fiber: >3 g/serving

Food Lists for Diabetes and Weight Management

TABLE D–4 Milk and Milk Substitutes

The Milk and Milk Substitutes list groups milks and yogurts based on the amount of fat they contain.

1 fat-free (skim) or low-fat (1%) milk = 12 grams carbohydrate, 8 grams protein, 0–3 grams fat, and 100 calories.

1 reduced-fat milk choice = 12 grams carbohydrate, 8 grams protein, 5 grams fat, and 120 calories.

1 whole milk choice = 12 grams carbohydrate, 8 grams protein, 8 grams fat, and 160 calories.

1 carbohydrate choice adds 15 grams carbohydrate and about 70 calories.

1 fat choice adds 5 grams fat and 45 calories.

Note: Cheeses are on the Protein list because they are rich in protein and have very little carbohydrate. Butter, cream, coffee creamers, almond milk, and unsweetened coconut milk lack protein and so are listed with the Fats. Ice cream and frozen yogurt are on the Sweets, Desserts, and Other Carbohydrates list.

Food	Serving Size	Choices per Serving
Milk and Yogurts		
Fat-free (skim) or low-fat (1%)		
milk, buttermilk, acidophilus milk, lactose-free milk	1 cup	1 fat-free milk
evaporated milk	½ cup	1 fat-free milk
yogurt, plain or Greek; may be sweetened with artificial sweetener	⅔ cup (6 oz)	1 fat-free milk
chocolate milk	1 cup	1 fat-free milk + 1 carbohydrate
Reduced-fat (2%)		
milk, acidophilus milk, kefir, lactose-free milk	1 cup	1 reduced-fat milk
yogurt, plain	⅔ cup (6 oz)	1 reduced-fat milk
Whole		
milk, buttermilk, goat's milk	1 cup	1 whole milk
evaporated milk	½ cup	1 whole milk
yogurt, plain	1 cup (8 oz)	1 whole milk
chocolate milk	1 cup	1 whole milk + 1 carbohydrate
Other Milk Foods and Milk Substitutes		
Eggnog		
fat-free	⅓ cup	1 carbohydrate
low-fat	⅓ cup	1 carbohydrate + ½ fat
whole milk	⅓ cup	1 carbohydrate + 1 fat
Rice drink		
plain, fat-free	1 cup	1 carbohydrate
flavored, low-fat	1 cup	2 carbohydrates
Soy milk		
light or low-fat, plain	1 cup	½ carbohydrate + ½ fat
regular, plain	1 cup	½ carbohydrate + 1 fat
Yogurt with fruit, low-fat	⅔ cup (6 oz)	1 fat-free milk + 1 carbohydrate

TABLE D–5 Nonstarchy Vegetables

The Nonstarchy Vegetables list includes vegetables that contain small amounts of carbohydrates and few calories; starchy vegetables that contain higher amounts of carbohydrate and calories are found on the Starch list. Salad greens (like arugula, chicory, endive, escarole, lettuce, radicchio, romaine, and watercress) are on the Free Foods list.

1 nonstarchy vegetable choice = 5 grams carbohydrate, 2 grams protein, 0 grams fat, and 25 calories.

Note: In general, one nonstarchy vegetable choice is ½ cup of cooked vegetables or vegetable juice or 1 cup of raw vegetables. Count 3 cups of raw vegetables or 1½ cups of cooked nonstarchy vegetables as one carbohydrate choice.

Amaranth leaves (Chinese spinach)	Hearts of palm
Artichoke	✓ Jicama
Artichoke hearts (no oil)	Kale
Asparagus	Kohlrabi
Baby corn	Leeks
Bamboo shoots	Mixed vegetables (without starchy vegetables, legumes,
Bean sprouts (alfalfa, mung, soybean)	or pasta)
Beans (green, wax, Italian, yard-long)	Mushrooms, all kinds, fresh
Beets	Okra
Broccoli	Onions
Broccoli slaw, packaged, no dressing	Pea pods
✓ Brussels sprouts	Peppers (all varieties)
Cabbage (green, red, bok choy, Chinese)	Radishes
✓ Carrots	Rutabaga
Cauliflower	s Sauerkraut, drained and rinsed
Celery	Spinach
Chayote	Squash, summer varieties (yellow, pattypan, crookneck, zucchini)
Coleslaw, packaged, no dressing	Sugar snap peas
Cucumber	Swiss chard
Daikon	Tomato
Eggplant	Tomatoes, canned
Fennel	s Tomato sauce (unsweetened)
Gourds (bitter, bottle, luffa, bitter melon)	Tomato/vegetable juice
Green onions or scallions	Turnips
Greens (collard, dandelion, mustard, purslane, turnip)	Water chestnuts

Key:
✓ = Good source of fiber: >3 g/serving
s = High in sodium: ≥480 mg/serving

TABLE D–6 Sweets, Desserts, and Other Carbohydrates

The Sweets, Desserts, and Other Carbohydrates list contains foods with added sugars, added fats, or both, and their total calories vary accordingly.

1 carbohydrate choice = 15 grams carbohydrate and about 70 calories.

1 fat choice = 5 grams fat and 45 calories.

Food	Serving Size	Choices per Serving
Beverages, Soda, and Sports Drinks		
Cranberry juice cocktail	½ cup	1 carbohydrate
Fruit drink or lemonade	1 cup (8 oz)	2 carbohydrates
Hot chocolate, regular	1 envelope (2 tbs or ¾ oz) added to 8 oz water	1 carbohydrate
Soft drink (soda), regular	1 can (12 oz)	2½ carbohydrates
Sports drink (fluid replacement type)	1 cup (8 oz)	1 carbohydrate
Brownies, Cake, Cookies, Gelatin, Pie, and Pudding		
Biscotti	1 oz	1 carbohydrate + 1 fat
Brownie, small, unfrosted	1½-in. square, ⅞-in. high (~1 oz)	1 carbohydrate + 1 fat
Cake		
angel food, unfrosted	1⁄12 of cake (~2 oz)	2 carbohydrates
frosted	2-in. square (~2 oz)	2 carbohydrates + 1 fat
unfrosted	2-in. square (~1 oz)	1 carbohydrate + 1 fat
Cookies		
100-calorie pack	1 oz	1 carbohydrate + ½ fat
chocolate chip cookies	2, 2¼ in. across	1 carbohydrate + 2 fats
gingersnaps	3 small, 1½ in. across	1 carbohydrate
large cookie	1, 6 in. across (~3 oz)	4 carbohydrates + 3 fats
sandwich cookies with crème filling	2 small (~⅔ oz)	1 carbohydrate + 1 fat
sugar-free cookies	1 large or 3 small (¾ to 1 oz)	1 carbohydrate + 1–2 fats
vanilla wafer	5	1 carbohydrate + 1 fat
Cupcake, frosted	1 small (~1¾ oz)	2 carbohydrates + 1–1½ fats
Flan	½ cup	2½ carbohydrates + 1 fat

TABLE D–6 Sweets, Desserts, and Other Carbohydrates (*continued*)

Food	Serving Size	Choices per Serving
Brownies, Cake, Cookies, Gelatin, Pie, and Pudding (continued)		
Fruit cobbler	½ cup (3½ oz)	3 carbohydrates + 1 fat
Gelatin, regular	½ cup	1 carbohydrate
Pie		
commercially prepared fruit, 2 crusts	⅙ of 8-in. pie	3 carbohydrates + 2 fats
pumpkin or custard	⅛ of 8-in. pie	1½ carbohydrates + 1½ fats
Pudding		
regular (made with reduced-fat milk)	½ cup	2 carbohydrates
sugar-free or sugar- and fat-free (made with fat-free milk)	½ cup	1 carbohydrate
Candy, Spreads, Sweets, Sweeteners, Syrups, and Toppings		
Blended sweeteners (mixtures of artificial sweeteners and sugar)	1½ tbs	1 carbohydrate
Candy		
chocolate, dark or milk type	1 oz	1 carbohydrate + 2 fats
chocolate "kisses"	5 pieces	1 carbohydrate + 1 fat
hard	3 pieces	1 carbohydrate
Coffee creamer, nondairy type		
powdered, flavored	4 tsp	½ carbohydrate + ½ fat
liquid, flavored	2 tbs	1 carbohydrate
Fruit snacks, chewy (pureed fruit concentrate)	1 roll (¾ oz)	1 carbohydrate
Fruit spreads, 100% fruit	1½ tbs	1 carbohydrate
Honey	1 tbs	1 carbohydrate
Jam or jelly, regular	1 tbs	1 carbohydrate
Sugar	1 tbs	1 carbohydrate
Syrup		
chocolate	2 tbs	2 carbohydrates
light (pancake-type)	2 tbs	1 carbohydrate
regular (pancake-type)	1 tbs	1 carbohydrate
Condiments and Sauces		
Barbecue sauce	3 tbs	1 carbohydrate
Cranberry sauce, jellied	¼ cup	1½ carbohydrates
ⓢ Curry sauce	1 oz	1 carbohydrate + 1 fat
ⓢ Gravy, canned or bottled	½ cup	½ carbohydrate + ½ fat
Hoisin sauce	1 tbs	½ carbohydrate
Marinade	1 tbs	½ carbohydrate
Plum sauce	1 tbs	½ carbohydrate
Salad dressing, fat-free, cream-based	3 tbs	1 carbohydrate
Sweet-and-sour sauce	3 tbs	1 carbohydrate
Doughnuts, Muffins, Pastries, and Sweet Breads		
Banana nut bread	1-in. slice (2 oz)	2 carbohydrates + 1 fat
Doughnut		
cake, plain	1 medium (1½ oz)	1½ carbohydrates + 2 fats
hole	2 (1 oz)	1 carbohydrate + 1 fat
yeast-type, glazed	1, 3¾ in. across (2 oz)	2 carbohydrates + 2 fats
Muffin		
regular	1 (4 oz)	4 carbohydrates + 2½ fats
lower-fat	1 (4 oz)	4 carbohydrates + ½ fat
Scone	1 (4 oz)	4 carbohydrates + 3 fats
Sweet roll or Danish	1 (2½ oz)	2½ carbohydrates + 2 fats
Frozen Bars, Frozen Desserts, Frozen Yogurt, and Ice Cream		
Frozen pops	1	½ carbohydrate
Fruit juice bars, frozen, 100% juice	1 (3 oz)	1 carbohydrate
Ice cream		
fat-free	½ cup	1½ carbohydrates
light	½ cup	1 carbohydrate + 1 fat
no-sugar-added	½ cup	1 carbohydrate + 1 fat
regular	½ cup	1 carbohydrate + 2 fats
Sherbet, sorbet	½ cup	2 carbohydrates
Yogurt, frozen		
fat-free	⅓ cup	1 carbohydrate
regular	½ cup	1 carbohydrate + 0–1 fat
Greek, lower-fat or fat-free	½ cup	1½ carbohydrates

Key:
ⓢ = High in sodium: ≥480 mg/serving

TABLE D–7 Protein

The Protein list groups foods based on the amount of fat they contain.
1 lean protein choice = 0 grams carbohydrate, 7 grams protein, 2 grams fat, and 45 calories.
1 medium-fat protein choice = 0 grams carbohydrate, 7 grams protein, 5 grams fat, and 75 calories.
1 high-fat protein choice = 0 grams carbohydrate, 7 grams protein, 8 grams fat, and 100 calories.

Food	Serving Size	Food	Serving Size
Lean Protein		**Medium-Fat Protein**	
Beef: ground (90% or higher lean/10% or lower fat); select or choice grades trimmed of fat, such as roast (chuck, round, rump, sirloin), steak (cubed, flank, porterhouse, T-bone), tenderloin	1 oz	Beef trimmed of visible fat: ground beef (85% or lower lean/15% or higher fat), corned beef, meatloaf, prime cuts of beef (rib roast), short ribs, tongue	1 oz
s Beef jerky	½ oz	Cheeses with 4–7 g fat/oz: feta, mozzarella, pasteurized processed cheese spread, reduced-fat cheeses	1 oz
Cheeses with ≥3 g fat/oz	1 oz	Cheese, ricotta (regular or part-skim)	¼ cup (2 oz)
Curd-style cheeses: cottage-type (all kinds); ricotta (fat-free or light)	¼ cup (2 oz)	Egg	1
Egg substitutes, plain	¼ cup	Fish: any fried	1 oz
Egg whites	2	Lamb: ground, rib roast	1 oz
Fish		Pork: cutlet, ground, shoulder roast	1 oz
fresh or frozen, such as catfish, cod, flounder, haddock, halibut, orange roughy, tilapia, trout	1 oz	Poultry with skin: chicken, dove, pheasant, turkey, wild duck, or goose; fried chicken	1 oz
salmon, fresh or canned	1 oz	s Sausage with 4–7 g fat/oz	1 oz
sardines, canned	2 small	**High-Fat Protein**	
tuna, fresh or canned in water or oil and drained	1 oz	These foods are high in saturated fat, cholesterol, and calories and may raise blood cholesterol levels if eaten on a regular basis. Try to eat 3 or fewer choices from this group per week.	
s smoked: herring or salmon (lox)	1 oz	Bacon, pork	2 slices (1 oz each before cooking)
Game: buffalo, ostrich, rabbit, venison	1 oz		
s Hot dog[a] with ≤3 g fat/oz	1 (1¾ oz)	s Bacon, turkey	3 slices (½ oz each before cooking)
Lamb: chop, leg, or roast	1 oz		
Organ meats: heart, kidney, liver[b]	1 oz	Cheese, regular: American, blue-veined, brie, cheddar, hard goat, Monterey jack, Parmesan, queso, and Swiss	1 oz
Oysters, fresh or frozen	6 medium		
Pork, lean		! Hot dog: beef, pork, or combination	1 (10 per 1 lb-sized package)
s Canadian bacon	1 oz		
s ham	1 oz	Hot dog: turkey or chicken	1 (10 per 1 lb-sized package)
rib or loin chop/roast, tenderloin	1 oz		
Poultry, without skin: chicken; Cornish hen; domestic duck or goose (well-drained of fat); turkey; lean ground turkey or chicken	1 oz	Pork: sausage, spareribs	1 oz
s Processed sandwich meats with ≤3 g fat/oz: chipped beef, thin-sliced deli meats, turkey ham, turkey pastrami	1 oz	s Processed sandwich meats with ≥8 g fat/oz: bologna, hard salami, pastrami	1 oz
s Sausage with ≤3 g fat/oz	1 oz	s Sausage with ≥8 g fat/oz: bratwurst, chorizo, Italian, knockwurst, Polish, smoked, summer	1 oz
Shellfish: clams, crab, imitation shellfish, lobster, scallops, shrimp	1 oz		
Veal: cutlet (no breading), loin chop, roast	1 oz		

[a]May contain carbohydrate.

[b]May be high in cholesterol.

Key:
! = Extra fat
s = High in sodium: ≥480 mg/serving (based on the sodium content of a typical 3-oz serving of meat, unless 1 oz or 2 oz is the normal serving size)

TABLE D-7 Protein (continued)

Plant-Based Protein

Beans, peas, and lentils are also on the Starch list; nut butters in small amounts are on the Fats list. Because carbohydrate content varies among plant-based proteins, read food labels.
1 plant-based protein choice = variable grams carbohydrate, 7 grams protein, variable grams fat, and variable calories.

Food	Serving Size	Choices per Serving
"Bacon" strips, soy-based	2 (½ oz)	1 lean protein
✓ Baked beans, canned	⅓ cup	1 starch + 1 lean protein
✓ Beans (black, garbanzo, kidney, lima, navy, pinto, white), cooked or canned, drained and rinsed	⅓ cup	1 starch + 1 lean protein
"Beef" or "sausage" crumbles, meatless	1 oz	1 lean protein
"Chicken" nuggets, soy-based	2 (1½ oz)	½ carbohydrate + 1 medium-fat protein
✓ Edamame, shelled	½ cup	½ carbohydrate + 1 lean protein
Falafel (spiced chickpea and wheat patties)	3 patties (~2 in. across)	1 carbohydrate + 1 high-fat protein
Hot dog, meatless, soy-based	1 hot dog (1½ oz)	1 lean protein
✓ Hummus	⅓ cup	1 carbohydrate + 1 medium-fat protein
✓ Lentils, any color, cooked or canned, drained and rinsed	½ cup	1 starch + 1 lean protein
Meatless burger, soy-based	3 oz	½ carbohydrate + 2 lean proteins
✓ Meatless burger, vegetable- and starch-based	1 patty (~2½ oz)	½ carbohydrate + 1 lean protein
Meatless deli slices	1 oz	1 lean protein
Mycoprotein ("chicken" tenders or crumbles), meatless	2 oz	½ carbohydrate + 1 lean protein
Nut spreads: almond butter, cashew butter, peanut butter, soy nut butter	1 tbs	1 high fat protein
✓ Peas (black-eyed and split peas), cooked or canned, drained and rinsed	½ cup	1 starch + 1 lean protein
✓ ⓢ Refried beans, canned	½ cup	1 starch + 1 lean protein
"Sausage" breakfast-type patties, meatless	1 (1½ oz)	1 medium-fat protein
Soy nuts, unsalted	¾ oz	½ carbohydrate + 1 medium-fat protein
Tempeh, plain, unflavored	¼ cup (1½ oz)	1 medium-fat protein
Tofu	½ cup (4 oz)	1 medium-fat protein
Tofu, light	½ cup (4 oz)	1 lean protein

Key:
✓ = Good source of fiber: >3 g/serving   ⓢ = High in sodium: ≥480 mg/serving

TABLE D-8 Fats

Fats and oils have mixtures of unsaturated (polyunsaturated and monounsaturated) and saturated fats. Foods on the Fats list are grouped together based on the major type of fat they contain.
1 fat choice = 0 grams carbohydrate, 0 grams protein, 5 grams fat, and 45 calories.
NOTE: In general, one fat choice is 1 teaspoon of oil or solid fat or 1 tablespoon of salad dressing.
When used in large amounts, bacon and nut butters are counted as high-fat protein choices (see Protein list). Fat-free salad dressings are on the Sweets, Desserts, and Other Carbohydrates list.
Fat-free products such as margarines, salad dressings, mayonnaise, sour cream, and cream cheese are on the Free Foods list.

Food	Serving Size	Food	Serving Size
Unsaturated Fats—Monounsaturated Fats		**Unsaturated Fats—Polyunsaturated Fats**	
Almond milk (unsweetened)	1 cup	Margarine	
Avocado, medium	2 tbs (1 oz)	lower-fat spread (30–50% vegetable oil, *trans* fat–free)	1 tbs
Nut butters (*trans* fat-free): almond butter, cashew butter, peanut butter (smooth or crunchy)	1½ tsp	stick, tub, or squeeze (*trans* fat–free)	1 tsp
		Mayonnaise	
Nuts		reduced-fat	1 tbs
almonds	6 nuts	regular	1 tsp
Brazil	2 nuts	Mayonnaise-style salad dressing	
cashews	6 nuts	reduced-fat	1 tbs
filberts (hazelnuts)	5 nuts	regular	2 tsp
macadamia	3 nuts	Nuts	
mixed (50% peanuts)	6 nuts	pignolia (pine nuts)	1 tbs
peanuts	10 nuts	walnuts, English	4 halves
pecans	4 halves	Oil: corn, cottonseed, flaxseed, grapeseed, safflower, soybean, sunflower	1 tsp
pistachios	16 nuts		
Oil: canola, olive, peanut	1 tsp	Salad dressing	
Olives		reduced-fat[a]	2 tbs
black (ripe)	8	regular	1 tbs
green, stuffed	10 large	Seeds	
Spread, plant stanol ester-type		flaxseed, ground	1½ tbs
light	1 tbs	pumpkin, sesame, sunflower	1 tbs
regular	2 tsp	Tahini or sesame paste	2 tsp

[a]May contain carbohydrate.

(continued)

TABLE D–8 Fats (continued)

Food	Serving Size	Food	Serving Size
Saturated Fats		**Saturated Fats** (continued)	
Bacon, cooked, regular or turkey	1 slice	Cream	
Butter		half-and-half	2 tbs
reduced-fat	1 tbs	heavy	1 tbs
stick	1 tsp	light	1½ tbs
whipped	2 tsp	whipped	2 tbs
Butter blends made with oil		Cream cheese	
reduced-fat or light	1 tbs	reduced-fat	1½ tbs (¾ oz)
regular	1½ tsp	regular	1 tbs (½ oz)
Chitterlings, boiled	2 tbs (½ oz)	Lard	1 tsp
Coconut, sweetened, shredded	2 tbs	Oil: coconut, palm, palm kernel	1 tsp
Coconut milk, canned, thick		Salt pork	¼ oz
light	⅓ cup	Shortening, solid	1 tsp
regular	1½ tbs	Sour cream	
Coconut milk beverage (thin), unsweetened	1 cup	reduced-fat or light	3 tbs
		regular	2 tbs

TABLE D–9 Free Foods

Most foods on the Free Foods list should be limited to 3 servings per day and eaten throughout the day. Eating all 3 servings at one time could raise blood glucose levels. Food and drink choices listed without a serving size can be eaten whenever you like.

1 free food choice = ≤5 grams carbohydrate and ≤20 calories.

Food	Serving Size	Food	Serving Size
Low-Carbohydrate Foods		**Condiments** (continued)	
Candy, hard (regular or sugar-free)	1 piece	Hot pepper sauce	
Fruits: cranberries or rhubarb, sweetened with sugar substitute	½ cup	Lemon juice	
Gelatin dessert, sugar-free, any flavor		Miso	1½ tsp
Gum, sugar-free		Mustard	
Jam or jelly, light or no-sugar-added	2 tsp	honey	1 tbs
Salad greens (such as arugula, chicory, endive, escarole, leaf or iceberg lettuce, purslane,		brown, Dijon, horseradish-flavored, wasabi-flavored, or yellow	
romaine, radicchio, spinach, watercress)		Parmesan cheese, grated	1 tbs
Sugar substitutes (artificial sweeteners)		Pickle relish (dill or sweet)	1 tbs
Syrup, sugar-free	2 tbs	Pickles	
Vegetables: any **raw** nonstarchy vegetables (such as broccoli,	½ cup	🧂 dill	1½ medium
cabbage, carrots, cucumber, tomato)		sweet, bread and butter	2 slices
Vegetables: any **cooked** nonstarchy vegetables (such as carrots,	¼ cup	sweet, gherkin	¾ oz
cauliflower, green beans)		Pimento	
Reduced-Fat or Fat-Free Foods		Salsa	¼ cup
Cream cheese, fat-free	1 tbs (½ oz)	🧂 Soy sauce, light or regular	1 tbs
Coffee creamers, nondairy		Sweet-and-sour sauce	2 tsp
liquid, flavored	1½ tsp	Taco sauce	1 tbs
liquid, sugar-free, flavored	4 tsp	Vinegar	
powdered, flavored	1 tsp	Worcestershire sauce	
powdered, sugar-free, flavored	2 tsp	Yogurt, any type	2 tbs
Margarine spread		**Drinks/Mixes**	
fat-free	1 tbs	🧂 Bouillon, broth, consommé	
reduced-fat	1 tsp	Bouillon or broth, low-sodium	
Mayonnaise		Carbonated or mineral water	
fat-free	1 tbs	Club soda	
reduced-fat	1 tsp	Cocoa powder, unsweetened	1 tbs
Mayonnaise-style salad dressing		Coffee, unsweetened or with sugar substitute	
fat-free	1 tbs	Diet soft drinks, sugar-free	
reduced-fat	2 tsp	Drink mixes (powder or liquid drops), sugar-free	
Salad dressing		Tea, unsweetened or with sugar substitute	
fat-free	1 tbs	Tonic water, sugar-free	
fat-free, Italian	2 tbs	Water	
Sour cream, fat-free or reduced-fat	1 tbs	Water, flavored, sugar-free	
Whipped topping		**Seasonings**	
light or fat-free	2 tbs	Flavoring extracts (for example, vanilla, almond, or peppermint)	
regular	1 tbs	Garlic, fresh or powder	
Condiments		Herbs, fresh or dried	
Barbecue sauce	2 tsp	Kelp	
Catsup (ketchup)	1 tbs	Nonstick cooking spray	
Chili sauce, sweet, tomato-type	2 tsp	Spices	
Horseradish		Wine, used in cooking	

Key:
🧂 = High in sodium: ≥480 mg/serving

TABLE D-10 Combination Foods

Many foods are eaten in various combinations, such as casseroles. Because "combination" foods do not fit into any one choice list, this list of choices provides some typical combination foods.
1 carbohydrate choice = 15 grams carbohydrate and about 70 calories.

Food	Serving Size	Choices per Serving
Entrees		
⑤ Casserole-type entrees (tuna noodle, lasagna, spaghetti with meatballs, chili with beans, macaroni and cheese)	1 cup (8 oz)	2 carbohydrates + 2 medium-fat proteins
⑤ Stews (beef/other meats and vegetables)	1 cup (8 oz)	1 carbohydrate + 1 medium-fat protein + 0–3 fats
Frozen Meals/Entrees		
⑤ ✓ Burrito (beef and bean)	1 (5 oz)	3 carbohydrates + 1 lean protein + 2 fats
Dinner-type healthy meal (includes dessert and is usually <400 cal)	~9–12 oz	2–3 carbohydrates + 1–2 lean proteins + 1 fat
"Healthy"-type entree (usually <300 cal)	~7–10 oz	2 carbohydrates + 2 lean proteins
Pizza		
⑤ cheese/vegetarian, thin crust	¼ of a 12-in. pizza (4½–5 oz)	2 carbohydrates + 2 medium-fat proteins
⑤ meat topping, thin crust	¼ of a 12-in. pizza (5 oz)	2 carbohydrates + 2 medium-fat proteins + 1½ fats
⑤ cheese/vegetarian or meat topping, rising crust	⅙ of a 12-in. pizza (4 oz)	2½ carbohydrates + 2 medium-fat proteins
⑤ Pocket sandwich	1 sandwich (4½ oz)	3 carbohydrates + 1 lean protein + 1–2 fats
⑤ Pot pie	1 (7 oz)	3 carbohydrates + 1 medium-fat protein + 3 fats
Salads (Deli-Style)		
Coleslaw	½ cup	1 carbohydrate + 1½ fats
Macaroni/pasta salad	½ cup	2 carbohydrates + 3 fats
⑤ Potato salad	½ cup	1½–2 carbohydrates + 1–2 fats
Tuna salad or chicken salad	½ cup (3½ oz)	½ carbohydrate + 2 lean proteins + 1 fat
Soups		
⑤ ✓ Bean, lentil, or split pea soup	1 cup (8 oz)	1½ carbohydrates + 1 lean protein
⑤ Chowder (made with milk)	1 cup (8 oz)	1 carbohydrate + 1 lean protein + 1½ fats
⑤ Cream soup (made with water)	1 cup (8 oz)	1 carbohydrate + 1 fat
⑤ Miso soup	1 cup (8 oz)	½ carbohydrate + 1 lean protein
⑤ Ramen noodle soup	1 cup (8 oz)	2 carbohydrates + 2 fats
Rice soup/porridge (congee)	1 cup (8 oz)	1 carbohydrate
⑤ Tomato soup (made with water), borscht	1 cup (8 oz)	1 carbohydrate
⑤ Vegetable beef, chicken, noodle, or other broth-type soup (including "healthy"-type soups, such as those lower in sodium and/or fat)	1 cup (8 oz)	1 carbohydrate + 1 lean protein

Key:
✓ = Good source of fiber: >3 g/serving
⑤ = High in sodium: ≥600 mg/serving for main dishes/meals and ≥480 mg/serving for side dishes

TABLE D-11 Fast Foods

The choices in the Fast Foods list are not specific fast-food meals or items but are estimates based on popular foods. Ask the restaurant or check its website for nutrition information about your favorite fast foods.
1 carbohydrate choice = 15 grams carbohydrate and about 70 calories.

Food	Serving Size	Choices per Serving
Main Dishes/Entrees		
Chicken		
⑤ breast, breaded and fried[a]	1 (~7 oz)	1 carbohydrate + 6 medium-fat proteins
breast, meat only[b]	1	4 lean proteins
drumstick, breaded and fried[a]	1 (~2½ oz)	½ carbohydrate + 2 medium-fat proteins
drumstick, meat only[b]	1	1 lean protein + ½ fat
⑤ nuggets or tenders	6 (~3½ oz)	1 carbohydrate + 2 medium-fat proteins + 1 fat
⑤ thigh, breaded and fried[a]	1 (~5 oz)	1 carbohydrate + 3 medium-fat proteins + 2 fats
thigh, meat only[b]	1	2 lean proteins + ½ fat
wing, breaded and fried[a]	1 wing (~2 oz)	½ carbohydrate + 2 medium-fat proteins
wing, meat only[b]	1 wing	1 lean protein
⑤ ✓ Main dish salad (grilled chicken-type, no dressing or croutons)	1 salad (~11½ oz)	1 carbohydrate + 4 lean proteins

[a]Definition and weight refer to food **with** bone, skin, and breading.
[b]Definition refers to food **without** bone, skin, and breading.

(continued)

TABLE D–11 **Fast Foods** (*continued*)

Food	Serving Size	Choices per Serving
Pizza		
s cheese, pepperoni, or sausage, regular or thick crust	⅛ of a 14-in. pizza (~4 oz)	2½ carbohydrates + 1 high-fat protein + 1 fat
s cheese, pepperoni, or sausage, thin crust	⅛ of a 14-in. pizza (~2¾ oz)	1½ carbohydrates + 1 high-fat protein + 1 fat
s cheese, meat, and vegetable, regular crust	⅛ of a 14-in. pizza (~5 oz)	2½ carbohydrates + 2 high-fat proteins
Asian		
s Beef/chicken/shrimp with vegetables in sauce	1 cup (~6 oz)	1 carbohydrate + 2 lean proteins + 1 fat
Egg roll, meat	1 egg roll (~3 oz)	1½ carbohydrates + 1 lean protein + 1½ fats
Fried rice, meatless	1 cup	2½ carbohydrates + 2 fats
Fortune cookie	1	½ carbohydrate
s Hot-and-sour soup	1 cup	½ carbohydrate + ½ fat
s Meat with sweet sauce	1 cup (~6 oz)	3½ carbohydrates + 3 medium-fat proteins + 3 fats
s Noodles and vegetables in sauce (chow mein, lo mein)	1 cup	2 carbohydrates + 2 fats
Mexican		
s ✓ Burrito with beans and cheese	1 small (~6 oz)	3½ carbohydrates + 1 medium-fat protein + 1 fat
s Nachos with cheese	1 small order (~8)	2½ carbohydrates + 1 high-fat protein + 2 fats
s Quesadilla, cheese only	1 small order (~5 oz)	2½ carbohydrates + 3 high-fat proteins
Taco, crisp, with meat and cheese	1 small (~3 oz)	1 carbohydrate + 1 medium-fat protein + ½ fat
s ✓ Taco salad with chicken and tortilla bowl	1 salad (1 lb including bowl)	3½ carbohydrates + 4 medium-fat proteins + 3 fats
s Tostada with beans and cheese	1 small (~5 oz)	2 carbohydrates + 1 high-fat protein
Sandwiches		
Breakfast sandwiches		
s breakfast burrito with sausage, egg, cheese	1 (~4 oz)	1½ carbohydrates + 2 high-fat proteins
s egg, cheese, meat on an English muffin	1	2 carbohydrates + 3 medium-fat proteins + ½ fat
s egg, cheese, meat on a biscuit	1	2 carbohydrates + 3 medium-fat proteins + 2 fats
s sausage biscuit sandwich	1	2 carbohydrates + 1 high-fat protein + 4 fats
Chicken sandwiches		
s grilled with bun, lettuce, tomatoes, spread	1 (~7½ oz)	3 carbohydrates + 4 lean proteins
s crispy, with bun, lettuce, tomatoes, spread	1 (~6 oz)	3 carbohydrates + 2 lean proteins + 3½ fats
Fish sandwich with tartar sauce and cheese	1 (5 oz)	2½ carbohydrates + 2 medium-fat proteins + 1½ fats
Hamburger		
regular with bun and condiments (catsup, mustard, onion, pickle)	1 (~3½ oz)	2 carbohydrates + 1 medium-fat protein + 1 fat
s 4 oz meat with cheese, bun, and condiments (catsup, mustard, onion, pickle)	1 (~8½ oz)	3 carbohydrates + 4 medium-fat proteins + 2½ fats
Hot dog with bun, plain	1 (~3½ oz)	1½ carbohydrates + 1 high-fat protein + 2 fats
Submarine sandwich (no cheese or sauce)		
s <6 g fat	1 6-in. sub	3 carbohydrates + 2 lean proteins
s regular	1 6-in. sub	3 carbohydrates + 2 lean proteins + 1 fat
s Wrap, grilled chicken, vegetables, cheese, and spread	1 small (~4–5 oz)	2 carbohydrates + 2 lean proteins + 1½ fats
Sides/Appetizers		
s ! French fries	1 small order (~3½ oz)	2½ carbohydrates + 2 fats
	1 medium order (~5 oz)	3½ carbohydrates + 3 fats
	1 large order (~6 oz)	4½ carbohydrates + 4 fats
s Hash browns	1 cup/medium order (~5 oz)	3 carbohydrates + 6 fats
s Onion rings	1 serving (8–9 rings, ~4 oz)	3½ carbohydrates + 4 fats
Salad, side (no dressing, croutons, or cheese)	1 small	1 nonstarchy vegetable
Beverages and Desserts		
Coffee, latte (fat-free milk)	1 small (~12 oz)	1 fat-free milk
Coffee, mocha (fat-free milk, no whipped cream)	1 small (~12 oz)	1 fat-free milk + 1 carbohydrate
Milkshake, any flavor	1 small (~12 oz)	5½ carbohydrates + 3 fats
	1 medium (~16 oz)	7 carbohydrates + 4 fats
	1 large (~22 oz)	10 carbohydrates + 5 fats
Soft-serve ice cream cone	1 small	2 carbohydrates + ½ fat

Key:
✓ = Good source of fiber: >3 g/serving

! = Extra fat

s = High in sodium: ≥600 mg/serving for main dishes/meals and ≥480 mg/serving for side dishes

TABLE D-12 Alcohol

NOTE: For those who choose to drink alcohol, guidelines suggest limiting alcohol intake to 1 drink or less per day for women and 2 drinks or less per day for men. To reduce the risk of low blood glucose (hypoglycemia), especially when taking insulin or a diabetes pill that increases insulin, alcohol should always be consumed with food, not alone. While alcohol, by itself, does not directly affect blood glucose, be aware of the carbohydrate (for example, in mixed drinks, beer, and wine) that may raise blood glucose.

1 alcohol equivalent (½ oz ethanol) = 100 calories.

1 carbohydrate choice = 15 g carb and about 70 calories.

Alcoholic Beverage[a]	Serving Size	Choices per Serving
Beer		
light (<4.5% abv)	12 fl oz	1 alcohol equivalent + ½ carbohydrate
regular (~5% abv)	12 fl oz	1 alcohol equivalent + 1 carbohydrate
dark (>5.7% abv)	12 fl oz	1 alcohol equivalent + 1–1½ carbohydrates
Distilled spirits (80 or 86 proof): vodka, rum, gin, whiskey, tequila	1½ fl oz	1 alcohol equivalent
Liqueur, coffee (53 proof)	1 fl oz	½ alcohol equivalent + 1 carbohydrate
Sake	1 fl oz	½ alcohol equivalent
Wine		
champagne/sparkling	5 fl oz	1 alcohol equivalent
dessert (sherry)	3½ fl oz	1 alcohol equivalent + 1 carbohydrate
dry, red or white (10% abv)	5 fl oz	1 alcohol equivalent

[a] "% abv" refers to the percentage of alcohol by volume.

The Food Lists are the basis of a meal planning system designed by a committee of the American Diabetes Association and the Academy of Nutrition and Dietetics. While originally designed for people with diabetes and others who must follow special diets, the Food Lists are based on principles of good nutrition that apply to everyone. © 2014 by the American Diabetes Association and the Academy of Nutrition and Dietetics.

TABLE E–1 USDA Healthy U.S.-Style Eating Patterns

(recommended daily intake amounts, weekly amounts for vegetable and protein foods subgroups)

Energy Level of Pattern[a,b]	1,000	1,200	1,400	1,600	1,800	2,000	2,200	2,400	2,600	2,800	3,000	3,200
Food Group[c]												
Fruits	1 c	1 c	1½ c	1½ c	1½ c	2 c	2 c	2 c	2 c	2½ c	2½ c	2½ c
Vegetables[d]	1 c	1½ c	1½ c	2 c	2½ c	2½ c	3 c	3 c	3½ c	3½ c	4 c	4 c
Dark green vegetables (c/wk)	½	1	1	1½	1½	1½	2	2	2½	2½	2½	2½
Red/orange vegetables (c/wk)	2½	3	3	4	5½	5½	6	6	7	7	7½	7½
Dry beans and peas (c/wk)	½	½	½	1	1½	1½	2	2	2½	2½	3	3
Starchy vegetables (c/wk)	2	3½	3½	4	5	5	6	6	7	7	8	8
Other vegetables (c/wk)	1½	2½	2½	3½	4	4	5	5	5½	5½	7	7
Grains[e]	3 oz-eq	4 oz-eq	5 oz-eq	5 oz-eq	6 oz-eq	6 oz-eq	7 oz-eq	8 oz-eq	9 oz-eq	10 oz-eq	10 oz-eq	10 oz-eq
Whole grains	1½ oz-eq	2 oz-eq	2½ oz-eq	3 oz-eq	3 oz-eq	3 oz-eq	3½ oz-eq	4 oz-eq	4½ oz-eq	5 oz-eq	5 oz-eq	5 oz-eq
Other grains	1½ oz-eq	2 oz-eq	2½ oz-eq	2 oz-eq	3 oz-eq	3 oz-eq	3½ oz-eq	4 oz-eq	4½ oz-eq	5 oz-eq	5 oz-eq	5 oz-eq
Protein Foods[d]	2 oz-eq	3 oz-eq	4 oz-eq	5 oz-eq	5 oz-eq	5½ oz-eq	6 oz-eq	6½ oz-eq	6½ oz-eq	7 oz-eq	7 oz-eq	7 oz-eq
Meat, poultry, eggs (oz/wk)	10	14	19	23	23	26	28	31	31	33	33	33
Seafood (oz/wk)	3	4	6	8	8	8	9	10	10	10	10	10
Nuts seeds, soy (oz/wk)	2	2	3	4	4	5	5	5	5	6	6	6
Dairy	2 c	2.5 c	2.5 c	3 c	3 c	3 c	3 c	3 c	3 c	3 c	3 c	3 c
Oils	15 g	17 g	17 g	22 g	24 g	27 g	29 g	31 g	34 g	36 g	44 g	51 g
Limit on Calories for Other Uses, calories (% of calories)[e]	150 (15%)	100 (8%)	110 (8%)	130 (8%)	170 (9%)	270 (14%)	280 (13%)	350 (15%)	380 (15%)	400 (14%)	470 (16%)	610 (19%)

[a]Food group amounts shown in cup (c) or ounce equivalents (oz-eq). Oils, solid fats, and added sugars are shown in grams (g).

[b]Eating patterns at 1,000, 1,200, and 1,400 calories meet the nutritional needs of children ages 2 to 8 years. Patterns from 1,600 to 3,200 calories meet the nutritional needs of children ages 9 years and older and adults. If a child ages 4 to 8 years needs more calories and, therefore, is following a pattern at 1,600 calories or more, the recommended amount from the dairy group can be 2½ cups per day. Children ages 9 years and older and adults should not use the 1,000, 1,200, or 1,400 calorie patterns.

[c]Quantity equivalents for each food group are:
- Grains, 1 ounce equivalent is: ½ cup cooked rice, pasta, or cooked cereal; 1 ounce dry pasta or rice; 1 slice bread; 1 small muffin (1 oz); 1 cup ready-to-eat cereal flakes.
- Fruits and Vegetables, 1 cup equivalent is: 1 cup raw or cooked fruit or vegetable, 1 cup fruit or vegetable juice, 2 cups leafy salad greens.
- Protein Foods, 1 ounce equivalent is: 1 ounce lean meat, poultry, or fish; 1 egg; ¼ cup cooked dry beans or tofu; 1 tbs peanut butter; ½ ounce nuts or seeds.
- Dairy, 1 cup equivalent is: 1 cup milk or yogurt, 1½ ounces natural cheese such as Cheddar cheese or 2 ounces of processed cheese.

[d]Vegetable and protein foods subgroup amounts are shown in this table as weekly amounts, because it would be difficult for consumers to select foods from all subgroups daily.

[e]Whole-grain subgroup amounts shown in this table are minimums. More whole grains up to all of the grains recommended may be selected, with offsetting decreases in the amounts of enriched refined grains.

The DASH Eating Plan at 1,600-, 2,000-, 2,600-, and 3,100-Calorie Levels[a]

The number of daily servings to choose from each food group depends on a person's energy requirement (see Chapter 9).

Food Group	1,600 Calories	2,000 Calories	2,600 Calories	3,100 Calories	Serving Sizes	Examples and Notes	Significance of Each Food Group to the DASH Eating Plan
Grains[b]	6 servings	7–8 servings	10–11 servings	12–13 servings	1 slice bread, 1 oz dry cereal,[c] ½ cup cooked rice, pasta, or cereal	Whole-wheat bread, English muffin, pita bread, bagel, cereals, grits, oatmeal, crackers, unsalted pretzels, popcorn	Major sources of energy and fiber
Vegetables	3–4 servings	4–5 servings	5–6 servings	6 servings	1 cup raw leafy vegetable, ½ cup cooked vegetable, 6 oz vegetable juice	Tomatoes, potatoes, carrots, green peas, squash, broccoli, turnip greens, collards, kale, spinach, artichokes, green beans, lima beans, sweet potatoes	Rich sources of potassium, magnesium, and fiber
Fruits	4 servings	4–5 servings	5–6 servings	6 servings	6 oz fruit juice, 1 medium fruit, ¼ cup dried fruit, ½ cup fresh, frozen, or canned fruit	Apricots, bananas, dates, grapes, oranges, orange juice, grapefruit, grapefruit juice, mangoes, melons, peaches, pineapples, prunes, raisins, strawberries, tangerines	Important sources of potassium, magnesium, and fiber
Low-fat or fat-free dairy foods	2–3 servings	2–3 servings	3 servings	3–4 servings	8 oz milk, 1 cup yogurt, 1½ oz cheese	Fat-free or low-fat milk, fat-free or low-fat buttermilk, fat-free or low-fat regular or frozen yogurt, low-fat and fat-free cheese	Major sources of calcium and protein
Meat, poultry, fish	1–2 servings	2 or fewer servings	2 servings	2–3 servings	3 oz cooked meats, poultry, or fish	Select only lean; trim away visible fats; broil, roast, or boil instead of frying; remove skin from poultry	Rich sources of protein and magnesium
Nuts, seeds, legumes	3–4 servings/week	4–5 servings/week	1 serving	1 serving	⅓ cup or 1½ oz nuts, 2 Tbsp or ½ oz seeds, ½ cup cooked dry beans or peas	Almonds, filberts, mixed nuts, peanuts, walnuts, sunflower seeds, kidney beans, lentils	Rich sources of energy, magnesium, potassium, protein, and fiber
Fat and oils[d]	2 servings	2–3 servings	3 servings	4 servings	1 tsp soft margarine, 1 Tbsp low-fat mayonnaise, 2 Tbsp light salad dressing, 1 tsp vegetable oil	Soft margarine, low-fat mayonnaise, light salad dressing, vegetable oil (such as olive, corn, canola, or safflower)	DASH has 27 percent of calories as fat (low in saturated fat), including fat in or added to foods
Sweets	0 servings	5 servings/week	2 servings	2 servings	1 Tbsp sugar, 1 Tbsp jelly or jam, ½ oz jelly beans, 8 oz lemonade	Maple syrup, sugar, jelly, jam, fruit-flavored gelatin, jelly beans, hard candy, fruit punch, sorbet, ices	Sweets should be low in fat

[a]NIH publication No. 03–4082; Karanja NM et al. JADA 8:S19–27, 1999.

[b]Equals ½–1¼ cups, depending on cereal type. Check the product's Nutrition Facts label.

[c]Whole grains are recommended for most servings to meet fiber recommendations.

[d]Fat content changes serving counts for fats and oils: For example, 1 Tbsp of regular salad dressing equals 1 serving; 1 Tbsp of a low-fat dressing equals ½ serving; 1 Tbsp of a fat-free dressing equals 0 servings.

TABLE E-3 Healthy Vegetarian Eating Patterns

Vegans can use this pattern by replacing all dairy choices with fortified soy beverages (soymilk) or other fortified plant-based dairy substitutes.

Calorie Level of Pattern[a]	1,000	1,200	1,400	1,600	1,800	2,000	2,200	2,400	2,600	2,800	3,000	3,200
Food Group[b]	**Daily Amount**[c] of Food From Each Group (vegetable and protein foods subgroup amounts are per week)											
Vegetables	1 c-eq	1½ c-eq	1½ c-eq	2 c-eq	2½ c-eq	2½ c-eq	3 c-eq	3 c-eq	3½ c-eq	3½ c-eq	4 c-eq	4 c-eq
Dark-green vegetables (c-eq/wk)	½	1	1	1½	1½	1½	2	2	2½	2½	2½	2½
Red and orange vegetables (c-eq/wk)	2½	3	3	4	5½	5½	6	6	7	7	7½	7½
Legumes (beans and peas) (c-eq/wk)[d]	½	½	½	1	1½	1½	2	2	2½	2½	3	3
Starchy vegetables (c-eq/wk)	2	3½	3½	4	5	5	6	6	7	7	8	8
Other vegetables (c-eq/wk)	1½	2½	2½	3½	4	4	5	5	5½	5½	7	7
Fruits	1 c-eq	1 c-eq	1½ c-eq	1½ c-eq	1½ c-eq	2 c-eq	2 c-eq	2 c-eq	2 c-eq	2½ c-eq	2½ c-eq	2½ c-eq
Grains	3 oz-eq	4 oz-eq	5 oz-eq	5½ oz-eq	6½ oz-eq	6½ oz-eq	7½ oz-eq	8½ oz-eq	9½ oz-eq	10½ oz-eq	10½ oz-eq	10½ oz-eq
Whole grains[e] (oz-eq/day)	1½	2	2½	3	3½	3½	4	4½	5	5½	5½	5½
Refined grains (oz-eq/day)	1½	2	2½	2½	3	3	3½	4	4½	5	5	5
Dairy	2 c-eq	2.5 c-eq	2.5 c-eq	3 c-eq	3 c-eq	3 c-eq	3 c-eq	3 c-eq	3 c-eq	3 c-eq	3 c-eq	3 c-eq
Protein Foods	1 oz-eq	1½ oz-eq	2 oz-eq	2½ oz-eq	3 oz-eq	3½ oz-eq	3½ oz-eq	4 oz-eq	4½ oz-eq	5 oz-eq	5½ oz-eq	6 oz-eq
Eggs (oz-eq/wk)	2	3	3	3	3	3	3	3	3	4	4	4
Legumes (beans and peas) (oz-eq/wk)[d]	1	2	4	4	6	6	6	8	9	10	11	12
Soy products (oz-eq/wk)	2	3	4	6	6	8	8	9	10	11	12	13
Nuts and seeds (oz-eq/wk)	2	2	3	5	6	7	7	8	9	10	12	13
Oils	15 g	17 g	17 g	22 g	24 g	27 g	29 g	31 g	34 g	36 g	44 g	51 g
Limit on Calories for Other Uses, calories (% of calories)	190 (19%)	170 (14%)	190 (14%)	180 (11%)	190 (11%)	290 (15%)	330 (15%)	390 (16%)	390 (15%)	400 (14%)	440 (15%)	550 (17%)

[a,b,c]See Table E–1 notes.

[d]About half of total legumes are shown as vegetables, in cup-eq, and half as protein foods, in oz-eq. Total legumes in the Patterns, in cup-eq, is the amount in the vegetable group plus the amount in protein foods group (in oz-eq) divided by 4.

[e]See Table E–1 notes.

TABLE E–4 Healthy Mediterranean-Style Eating Patterns

Calorie Level of Pattern[a]	1,000	1,200	1,400	1,600	1,800	2,000	2,200	2,400	2,600	2,800	3,000	3,200
Food Group[b]	Daily Amount[c] of Food From Each Group (vegetable and protein foods subgroup amounts are per week)											
Vegetables	1 c-eq	1½ c-eq	1½ c-eq	2 c-eq	2½ c-eq	2½ c-eq	3 c-eq	3 c-eq	3½ c-eq	3½ c-eq	4 c-eq	4 c-eq
Dark-green vegetables (c-eq/wk)	½	1	1	1½	1½	1½	2	2	2½	2½	2½	2½
Red and orange vegetables (c-eq/wk)	2½	3	3	4	5½	5½	6	6	7	7	7½	7½
Legumes (beans and peas) (c-eq/wk)	½	½	½	1	1½	1½	2	2	2½	2½	3	3
Starchy vegetables (c-eq/wk)	2	3½	3½	4	5	5	6	6	7	7	8	8
Other vegetables (c-eq/wk)	1½	2½	2½	3½	4	4	5	5	5½	5½	7	7
Fruits	1 c-eq	1 c-eq	1½ c-eq	2 c-eq	2 c-eq	2½ c-eq	2½ c-eq	2½ c-eq	2½ c-eq	3 c-eq	3 c-eq	3 c-eq
Grains	3 oz-eq	4 oz-eq	5 oz-eq	5 oz-eq	6 oz-eq	6 oz-eq	7 oz-eq	8 oz-eq	9 oz-eq	10 oz-eq	10 oz-eq	10 oz-eq
Whole grains[d] (oz-eq/day)	1½	2	2½	3	3	3	3½	4	4½	5	5	5
Refined grains (oz-eq/day)	1½	2	2½	2	3	3	3½	4	4½	5	5	5
Dairy	2 c-eq	2½ c-eq	2½ c-eq	2 c-eq	2 c-eq	2 c-eq	2 c-eq	2½ c-eq	2½ c-eq	2½ c-eq	2½ c-eq	2½ c-eq
Protein Foods	2 oz-eq	3 oz-eq	4 oz-eq	5½ oz-eq	6 oz-eq	6½ oz-eq	7 oz-eq	7½ oz-eq	7½ oz-eq	8 oz-eq	8 oz-eq	8 oz-eq
Seafood (oz-eq/wk)[e]	3	4	6	11	15	15	16	16	17	17	17	17
Meats, poultry, eggs (oz-eq/wk)	10	14	19	23	23	26	28	31	31	33	33	33
Nuts, seeds, soy products (oz-eq/wk)	2	2	3	4	4	5	5	5	5	6	6	6
Oils	15 g	17 g	17 g	22 g	24 g	27 g	29 g	31 g	34 g	36 g	44 g	51 g
Limit on Calories for Other Uses, calories (% of calories)	150 (15%)	100 (8%)	110 (8%)	140 (9%)	160 (9%)	260 (13%)	270 (12%)	300 (13%)	330 (13%)	350 (13%)	430 (14%)	570 (18%)

[a,b,c,d]See Table E–1, notes a through d.

[e]The U.S. Food and Drug Administration (FDA) and the U.S. Environmental Protection Agency (EPA) provide joint guidance regarding seafood consumption for women who are pregnant or breastfeeding and young children. For more information, see the FDA or EPA websites www.FDA.gov/fishadvice; www.EPA.gov/fishadvice.

TABLE E–5 Three USDA Eating Patterns Compared

Three USDA Eating Patterns (Healthy U.S.-Style, Healthy Vegetarian, and Healthy Mediterranean-Style) are recognized as useful for meeting the ideals of the Dietary Guidelines for Americans. The columns below compare them at the 2,000-calorie level.

Food Group	Healthy U.S.-Style Pattern	Healthy Vegetarian Pattern	Healthy Mediterranean Pattern
Fruit	2 c per day	2 c per day	2½ c per day
Vegetables	2½ c per day	2½ c per day	2½ c per day
Legumes	1½ c per wk	3 c per wk	1½ c per wk
Whole Grains	3 oz-eq per day	3 oz-eq per day	3 oz-eq per day
Dairy	3 c per day	3 c per day	2 c per day
Protein Foods	5½ oz-eq per day	3½ oz-eq per day	6½ oz-eq per day
Meat	12½ oz-eq/wk	—	12½ oz-eq/wk
Poultry	10½ oz-eq/wk	—	10½ oz-eq/wk
Seafood	8 oz-eq/wk	—	15 oz-eq/wk
Eggs	3 oz-eq/wk	3 oz-eq/wk	3 oz-eq/wk
Nuts/seeds	4 oz-eq/wk	7 oz-eq/wk	4 oz-eq/wk
Processed soy	½ oz-eq/wk	8 oz-eq/wk	½ oz-eq/wk
Oils	27 g per day	27 g per day	27 g per day

Source: U.S. Department of Agriculture and U.S. Department of Health and Human Services, Scientific Report of the 2015 Dietary Guidelines Advisory Committee, *2015, D-1: 125, available at www.health.gov.*

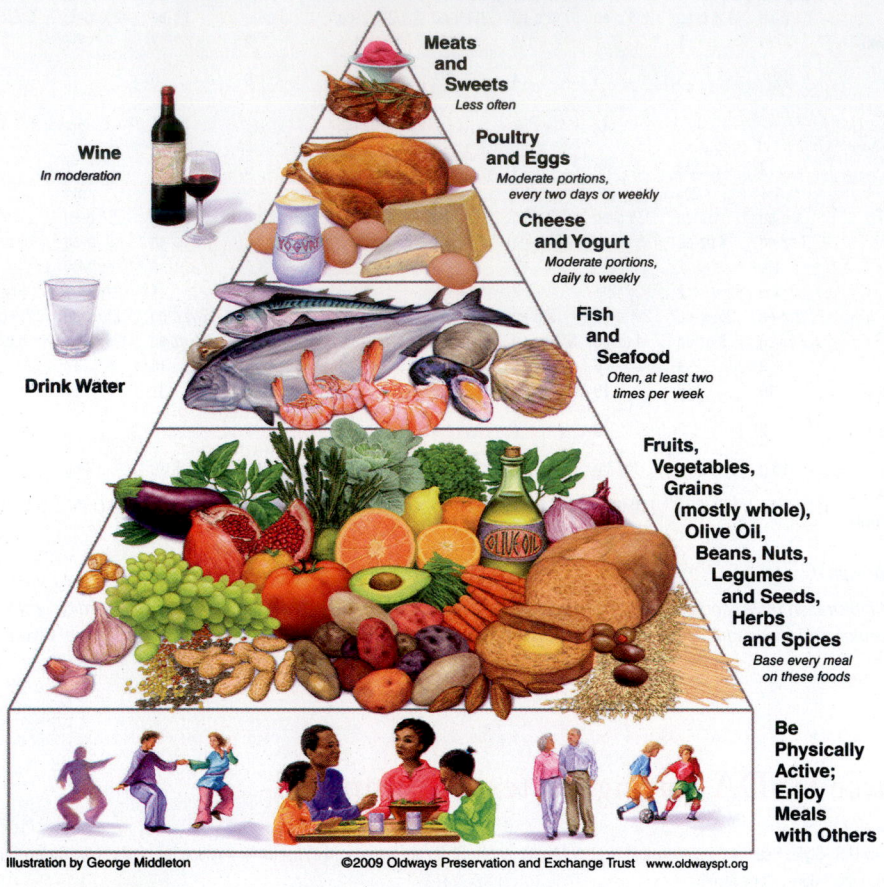

Mediterranean Diet Pyramid
A contemporary approach to delicious, healthy eating

Meats and Sweets
Less often

Wine
In moderation

Poultry and Eggs
Moderate portions, every two days or weekly

Cheese and Yogurt
Moderate portions, daily to weekly

Drink Water

Fish and Seafood
Often, at least two times per week

Fruits, Vegetables, Grains (mostly whole), Olive Oil, Beans, Nuts, Legumes and Seeds, Herbs and Spices
Base every meal on these foods

Be Physically Active; Enjoy Meals with Others

Illustration by George Middleton   ©2009 Oldways Preservation and Exchange Trust www.oldwayspt.org

FIGURE E–1 **A Mediterranean Diet Pyramid**

TABLE E–6 Ideas for Healthy Mediterranean-Style Meals

As a general rule, fill half your plate with vegetables, a fourth with whole grains, and a quarter with protein foods. Eat fish or seafood 1–2 times a week, and choose baked, steamed, grilled, or poached preparations over fried. One day a week, substitute vegetable proteins for all meats.

Choose this	Instead of this
Breakfast	
Whole fruit pieces; cut fruit or fruit salad without added sugar	Fruit juice; fruit salad with sugars or marshmallows
Low-sugar whole-grain granola (no hydrogenated oils) with nuts and dried fruit; oatmeal (including instant oatmeal) with apples, cinnamon, or a teaspoon of berry or other fruit jam	Commercial high-sugar granola with hydrogenated oils; refined, sugar-sweetened, ready-to-eat cereal
Mediterranean protein foods (peanut butter, hummus, egg, yogurt); turkey, chicken, or soy breakfast sausages	Sausage, bacon, breakfast steak
100% whole-grain toasted bread slice, bagel, or English muffin with hummus, mashed avocado, or nut butter	Refined white toast with butter and jelly
Omelet with sautéed onions, mushrooms, broccoli, or leftover vegetables, or cooked or smoked salmon with a sprinkle of hard cheese, salsa, or olive tapenade	Omelet with sausage or ham and cheese
Smoothies with milk or fortified soy milk, frozen overripe bananas, and berries (a handful of spinach or other greens blends well and adds a fresh flavor and nutrients)	High-sugar commercial smoothies; milkshakes with ice cream, chocolate syrup
Plain yogurt or Greek yogurt with fresh fruit, homemade granola, or a teaspoon of fruit jam or syrup	Commercial sugar-sweetened yogurt
Lunch	
Creative salads with a variety of ingredients: nuts, beans, fish, hard cheese sprinkles, olives, or berries and other fruit	Repetitive, boring lettuce and tomato salads
Canned tuna, sardines, or mackerel (olive oil or water packed) mixed with hummus, lemon juice, and seasonings; add chopped apple or dried cranberries for sweetness	Canned fish salads made with regular mayonnaise and sugar-sweetened pickle relish
Whole-grain crackers, wraps, or breads	Refined flour crackers, wraps, or breads
Whole-grain wheat flour or corn tortillas for burritos, wraps, and quesadillas	Refined flour tortillas
Tapenades, avocado, or hummus spread on sandwiches	Mayonnaise for sandwiches (or choose a mayonnaise made with olive oil)
Broth-based vegetable soups (preferably low-sodium) with whole-grain pasta	Cream-based soups with refined starches
Vegetarian pizza with tomatoes, olives, spinach, artichokes, or other vegetables on whole-grain crust	Sausage, pepperoni, or hamburger pizza on refined flour crust
Supper	
Whole-grain pasta or fortified "extra protein" pasta (½ to 1 c for most adults), with beans or seafood and tomato sauce, garlic, onions, artichokes, frozen peas, or other vegetables to fill in the plate	Refined flour pasta with cream, butter, and cheese sauces
Turkey burgers (made with ground turkey breast and oatmeal); chicken or turkey Italian sausage; serve burgers or sausages with wilted spinach and sliced tomatoes on a whole-grain bun	Ground beef burgers; pork Italian sausage; refined white buns
Prepared salsa for topping potatoes, beans, veggie burgers, rice, or eggs	Creamy, cheesy sauces
Poultry or seafood; limited lean red meat	Frequent use of fatty beef, lamb, or pork

Source: Many of these ideas and more can be found at http://oldwayspt.org/.

Chapter 1

1. Position of the Academy of Nutrition and Dietetics: Total diet approach to healthy eating, *Journal of the Academy of Nutrition and Dietetics* 113 (2013): 307–317.

2. U.S. Department of Health and Human Services, *Healthy People 2020* (Washington, D.C.: U.S. Government Printing Office, 2010), available at www.healthypeople.gov.

3. Healthy People 2020 Leading Health Indicators: Nutrition, Physical Activity, and Obesity, May 2014, available at http://www.healthypeople.gov/sites/default/files/HP2020_LHI_Nut_PhysActiv.pdf.

4. Centers for Disease Control and Prevention, Adults meeting fruit and vegetable intake recommendations—United States, 2013, *Morbidity and Mortality Weekly Report* 64 (2015): 709–713.

5. Position of the American Dietetic Association: Functional foods, *Journal of the American Dietetic Association* 113 (2013): 1096–1103.

6. Position of the Academy of Nutrition and Dietetics: Total diet approach to healthy eating, 2013.

7. S. L. Connor, Think globally, practice locally: Culturally competent dietetics, *Journal of the Academy of Nutrition and Dietetics* 115 (2015): S55; Academy Quality Management Committee and Scope of Practice Subcommittee, Academy of Nutrition and Dietetics: Scope of practice in nutrition and dietetics, *Journal of the Academy of Nutrition and Dietetics* 113 (2013): S11–S16.

8. L. Hebden and coauthors, You are what you choose to eat: Factors influencing young adults' food selection behaviour, *Journal of Human Nutrition and Dietetics* (2015), epub, doi:10.1111/jhn.12312; International Food Information Council Foundation, *2013 Food and Health Survey: Consumer Attitudes toward Food Safety, Nutrition, and Health* (Washington, D.C.: International Food Information Council Foundation, May 2013), available at www.foodinsight.org.

9. H. W. Wu and R. Sturm, Changes in the energy and sodium content of main entrées in US chain restaurants from 2010 to 2011, *Journal of the Academy of Nutrition and Dietetics* 114 (2014): 209–219; H. W. Wu and R. Sturm, What's on the menu? A review of the energy and nutritional content of US chain restaurant menus, *Public Health Nutrition* 16 (2013): 87–96.

10. C. Jacquier and coauthors, Improving the effectiveness of nutritional information policies: Assessment of unconscious pleasure mechanisms involved in food-choice decisions, *Nutrition Reviews* 70 (2012): 118–131.

11. E. Robinson and coauthors, What everyone else is eating: A systematic review and meta-analysis of the effect of informational eating norms on eating behavior, *Journal of the Academy of Nutrition and Dietetics* 114 (2014): 414–429.

12. B. Liebman, What's the catch? Why the latest study is rarely the final answer, *Nutrition Action Health Letter*, April 2014, pp. 1, 3.

13. D. Quagliani and M. Hermann, Communicating accurate food and nutrition information: Practice paper of the Academy of Nutrition and Dietetics (abstract), *Journal of the Academy of Nutrition and Dietetics* 112 (2012): 759, epub ahead of print, doi:10.1016/j.jand.2012.03.006.

14. U.S. Department of Agriculture, Monitoring America's nutritional health, *Agricultural Research*, March 2012, pp. 4–23.

15. J. Di Noia, Defining powerhouse fruits and vegetables: A nutrient density approach, *Preventing Chronic Disease* 11 (2014), epub, doi:http://dx.doi.org/10.5888/pcd11.130390.

16. Position of the Academy of Nutrition and Dietetics: Total diet approach to healthy eating, 2013.

Consumer's Guide 1

1. D. Quagliani and M. Hermann, Communicating accurate food and nutrition information: Practice paper of the Academy of Nutrition and Dietetics (abstract), *Journal of the Academy of Nutrition and Dietetics* 112 (2012): 759, epub ahead of print, doi:10.1016/j.jand.2012.03.006.

2. M. Chang, Should meta-analyses trump observational studies? *American Journal of Clinical Nutrition* 97 (2013): 237–238.

Controversy 1

1. D. Quagliani and M. Hermann, Communicating accurate food and nutrition information: Practice paper of the Academy of Nutrition and Dietetics (abstract), *Journal of the Academy of Nutrition and Dietetics* 112 (2012): 759, epub ahead of print, doi:10.1016/j.jand.2012.03.006.

2. L. McKeever and coauthors, Demystifying the search button: A comprehensive PubMed search strategy for performing an exhaustive literature review, *Journal of Parenteral and Enteral Nutrition* (2015), epub ahead of print, doi:10.1177/0148607115593791.

3. S. Barrett, Where to get professional nutrition advice, *Quackwatch*, October 14, 2012, available at www.quackwatch.com.

4. S. H. Laramee and M. Tate, Dietetics Workforce Demand Study Task Force supplement: An introduction, *Journal of the Academy of Nutrition and Dietetics* 112 (2012): S7–S9.

5. Academy Quality Management Committee and Scope of Practice Subcommittee, Academy of Nutrition and Dietetics: Scope of practice for the Registered Dietitian, *Journal of the Academy of Nutrition and Dietetics* 113 (2013): S17–S28.

Chapter 2

1. Standing Committee on the Scientific Evaluation of Dietary Reference Intakes, Food and Nutrition Board, Institute of Medicine, *Dietary Reference Intakes: Applications in Dietary Assessment* (Washington, D.C.: National Academies Press, 2000), pp. 5–7.

2. P. R. Trumbo and coauthors, Dietary reference intakes: Cases of appropriate and inappropriate uses, *Nutrition Reviews* 71 (2013): 657–664.

3. U.S. Department of Agriculture and U.S. Department of Health and Human Services, *Scientific Report of the 2015 Dietary Guidelines Advisory Committee* (2015), C:15, available at www.health.gov.

4. Food and Drug Administration, Food labeling: Revision of the nutrition and supplement facts labels (Docket No. FDA–2012–N–1210), *Federal Register* 79 (2014): 11880–11987.

5. U.S. Department of Health and Human Services and U.S. Department of Agriculture, *2015–2020 Dietary Guidelines for Americans,* 8th edition (2015), available at http://health.gov/dietaryguidelines/2015/guidelines/.

6. R. D. Whitehead and coauthors, You are what you eat: Within-subject increases in fruit and vegetable consumption confer beneficial skin-color changes, *PLoS ONE* 7 (2012), epub, doi:10.1371/journal.pone.0032988.

7. U.S. Department of Health and Human Services, *2008 Physical Activity Guidelines for Americans* (Washington, D.C.: U.S. Department of Health and Human Services, 2008), available at www.health.gov/paguidelines/default.aspx.

8. U.S. Department of Agriculture and U.S. Department of Health and Human Services, *Scientific Report of the 2015 Dietary Guidelines Advisory Committee* (2015), E-5:4; S. J. Nielsen and coauthors, *Calories Consumed from Alcoholic Beverages by U.S. Adults, 2007–2010* (NCHS Data Brief 110) (Hyattsville, Md.: National Center for Health Statistics, November 2012), available at www.cdc.gov/nchs/data/databriefs/db110.htm.

9. R. C. Post and coauthors, What's new on MyPlate? A new message, redesigned web site,

and SuperTracker debut, *Journal of the Academy of Nutrition and Dietetics* 112 (2012): 18–22.

10. R. M. Bliss, Nutrient data in time for the new year, *Agricultural Research*, January 2012, pp. 20–21.

11. Food and Drug Administration, Food labeling, 2014.

12. M. S. Edge and coauthors, The impact of variation in a fact-based front-of-package nutrition labeling system on consumer comprehension, *Journal of the Academy of Nutrition and Dietetics* 114 (2014): 843–854.

13. E. A. Wartella and coauthors, *Front-of-Package Nutrition Rating Systems and Symbols: Promoting Healthier Choices* (Washington, D.C.: National Academies Press, 2011), available at www.iom.edu/Reports/2011/Front-of-Package-Nutrition-Rating-Systems-and-Symbols-Promoting-Healthier-Choices.aspx.

Consumer's Guide 2

1. Economic Research Service, U.S. Department of Agriculture, Food expenditures, 2013, available at http://www.ers.usda.gov/topics/food-choices-health/food-consumption-demand/food-away-from-home.aspx.

2. R. M. Morrison, L. Mancino, and J. N. Variyam, Will calorie labeling in restaurants make a difference? Amber Waves, March 2011, available at www.ers.usda.gov/AmberWaves.

Controversy 2

1. E. E. Devore and coauthors, Dietary intakes of berries and flavonoids in relation to cognitive decline, *Annals of Neurology* 72 (2012): 135–143; R. J. Williams and J. P. E. Spencer, Flavonoids, cognition, and dementia: Actions, mechanisms, and potential therapeutic utility for Alzheimer disease, *Free Radical Biology and Medicine* 52 (2012): 35–45.

2. Devore and coauthors, Dietary intakes of berries and flavonoids, 2012.

3. A. L. Macready and coauthors, Flavonoid-rich fruit and vegetables improve microvascular reactivity and inflammatory status in men at risk of cardiovascular disease—FLAVURS: A randomized controlled trial, *American Journal of Clinical Nutrition* 99 (2014): 479–489.

4. G. Annuzzi and coauthors, Diets naturally rich in polyphenols improve fasting and postprandial dyslipidemia and reduce oxidative stress: A randomized controlled trial, *American Journal of Clinical Nutrition* 99 (2014): 463–471.

5. N. M. Wedick and coauthors, Dietary flavonoid intakes and risk of type 2 diabetes in US men and women, *American Journal of Clinical Nutrition* 95 (2012): 925–933.

6. C. S. Kwok and coauthors, Habitual chocolate consumption and risk of cardiovascular disease among health men and women, *Heart* (2015), epub ahead of print, doi:10.1136/heartjnl-2014-307050; C. Matsumoto and coauthors, Chocolate consumption and risk of diabetes mellitus in the Physicians' Health Study, *American Journal of Clinical Nutrition* 101 (2015): 362–367; D. Esser and coauthors, Dark chocolate consumption improves leukocyte

adhesion factors and vascular function in overweight men, *FASEB Journal* 28 (2014): 1466–1473; L. M. Ostertag and coauthors, Flavan-3-ol-enriched dark chocolate and white chocolate improve acute measures of platelet function in a gender-specific way—a randomized-controlled human intervention trial, *Molecular Nutrition and Food Research* 57 (2013): 191–202.

7. A. Scholey and L. Owen, Effects of chocolate on cognitive function and mood: A systematic review, Nutrition Reviews 71 (2013): 665–681; A. N. Sokolov and coauthors, Chocolate and the brain: Neurobiological impact of cocoa flavanols on cognition and behavior, Neuroscience and Biobehavioral Reviews 37 (2013): 2445–2453.

8. D. Rodriguez-Lewa and coauthors, Potent antihypertensive action of dietary flaxseed in hypertensive patients, *Hypertension* 62 (2013): 1081–1089.

9. H. B. Mabrok and coauthors, Lignan transformation by gut bacteria lowers tumor burden in a gnotobiotic rat model of breast cancer, *Carcinogenesis* 33 (2012): 203–208.

10. S. E. McCann and coauthors, Dietary intakes of total and specific lignans are associated with clinical breast tumor characteristics, *Journal of Nutrition* 142 (2012): 91–98.

11. M. Azrad and coauthors, Flaxseed-derived enterolactone is inversely associated with tumor cell proliferation in men with localized prostate cancer, *Journal of Medicinal Food* 16 (2013): 357–360.

12. B. Zhu and coauthors, Allium vegetables and garlic supplements do not reduce risk of colorectal cancer, based on meta-analysis of prospective studies, *Clinical Gastroenterology and Hepatology* (2014), epub ahead of print, doi:10.1016/j.cgh.2014.03.019.; S. Meng and coauthors, No association between garlic intake and risk of colorectal cancer, *Cancer Epidemiology* 37 (2013): 152–155.

13. N. Mehrotra, S. Gaur, and A. Petrova, Health care practices of the foreign born Asian Indians in the United States: A community based survey, *Journal of Community Health* 37 (2012): 328–334.

14. A. Bakhtiary and coauthors, Effects of soy on metabolic biomarkers of cardiovascular disease in elderly women with metabolic syndrome, *Archives of Iranian Medicine* 15 (2012): 462–468; M. S. Miraghajani and coauthors, Soy milk consumption and blood pressure among type 2 diabetic patients with nephropathy, *Journal of Renal Nutrition: The Official Journal of the Council on Renal Nutrition of the National Kidney Foundation* 23 (2013): 277–282.

15. H. Gylling and coauthors, Plant sterols and plant stanols in the management of dyslipidaemia and prevention of cardiovascular disease, *Atherosclerosis* 232 (2014): 346–360.

16. G. L. Arellano-Martinez and coauthors, Soya protein stimulates bile acid excretion by the liver and intestine through direct and indirect pathways influenced by the presence of dietary cholesterol, *British Journal of Nutrition* 111 (2014): 2059–2066.

17. P. Dey and coauthors, Insight into the mechanisms of action of estrogen receptor β in the breast, prostate, colon, and CNS, *Journal of Molecular Endocrinology* 51 (2013): T61–T74.

18. S. Mahabir, Association between diet during preadolescence and adolescence and risk for breast cancer during adulthood, *Journal of Adolescent Health* 52 (2013): S30–S35.

19. Y. F. Zhang and coauthors, Positive effects of soy isoflavone food on survival of breast cancer patients in China, *Asian Pacific Journal of Cancer Prevention* 13 (2012): 479–482.

20. S. J. Nechuta and coauthors, Soy food intake after diagnosis of breast cancer and survival: An in-depth analysis of combined evidence from cohort studies of U.S. and Chinese women, *American Journal of Clinical Nutrition* 96 (2012): 123–132; S. A. Khan and coauthors, Soy isoflavones supplementation for breast cancer risk reduction: A randomized phase II trial, *Cancer Prevention Research* 5 (2012): 309–319.

21. K. Taku and coauthors, Extracted or synthesized soybean isoflavones reduce menopausal hot flash frequency and severity: Systematic review and meta-analysis of randomized controlled trials, *Menopause* 19 (2012): 776–790; S. Bedell, M. Nachtigall, and F. Naftolin, The pros and cons of plant estrogens for menopause, *Journal of Steroid Biochemistry and Molecular Biology* 139 (2014): 225–236.

22. X. X. Chi and T. Zhang, The effects of soy isoflavones in bone density in north region of climacteric Chinese women, *Journal of Clinical Biochemistry and Nutrition* 53 (2013): 102–107; V. S. Lagari and S. Levis, Phytoestrogens in the prevention of postmenopausal bone loss, *Journal of Clinical Densitometry: The Official Journal of the International Society for Clinical Densitometry* 16 (2013): 445–449.

23. R. Bosviel and coauthors, Can soy phytoestrogens decrease DNA methylation in BRCA1 and BRCA2 oncosuppressor genes in breast cancer? *Omics* 16 (2012): 235–244; T. T. Rajah and coauthors, Physiological concentrations of genistein and 17β-estradiol inhibit MDA-MB231 breast cancer cell growth by increasing BAX/BCL-2 and reducing pERK1/2, *Anticancer Research* 32 (2012): 1181–1191.

24. H. Fritz and coauthors, Soy, red clover, and isoflavones and breast cancer: A systematic review, *PLOS ONE* 8 (2013), doi:10.1371/journal.pone.0081968.

25. L. H. Kushi and coauthors, American Cancer Society guidelines on nutrition and physical activity for cancer prevention: Reducing the risk of cancer with healthy food choices and physical activity, *CA: A Cancer Journal for Clinicians* 62 (2012): 30–67; M. McCullough, The bottom line on soy and breast cancer risk, Expert Voices: Timely Insight on Cancer Topics from the Experts of the American Cancer Society, August 2, 2012, available at http://www.cancer.org/cancer/news/expertvoices/post/2012/08/02/the-bottom-line-on-soy-and-breast-cancer-risk.aspx.

26. K. Sahin and coauthors, Orally administered lycopene attenuates diethylnitrosamine-induced hepatocarcinogenesis in rats by modulating

Nrf-2/HO-1 and Akt-mTOR pathways, *Nutrition and Cancer* 66 (2014): 590–598.

27. X. Li and J. Xu, Meta-analysis of the association between dietary lycopene intake and ovarian cancer risk in postmenopausal women, *Scientific Reports* 4 (2014): 4885.

28. W. Stahl and H. Sies, Photoprotection by dietary carotenoids: Concept, mechanisms, evidence and future development, *Molecular Nutrition & Food Research* 56 (2012): 287–295.

29. J. Virtamo and coauthors, Effects of α-tocopherol and β-carotene supplementation on cancer incidence and mortality: 18-year postintervention follow-up of the Alpha-tocopherol, Beta-carotene Cancer Prevention Study, *International Journal of Cancer* 135 (2014): 178–185.

30. S. Nechuta and coauthors, Prospective cohort study of tea consumption and risk of digestive system cancers: Results from the Shanghai Women's Health Study, *American Journal of Clinical Nutrition* 96 (2012): 1056–1063.

31. S. C. Larsson, J. Virtamo, and A. Wolk, Black tea consumption and risk of stroke in women and men, *Annals of Epidemiology* 23 (2013): 157–160.

32. S. Khalesi and coauthors, Green tea catechins and blood pressure: A systematic review and meta-analysis of randomised controlled trials, *European Journal of Nutrition* (2014), epub ahead of print.

33. I. C. Hou and coauthors, Green tea and the risk of gastric cancer: Epidemiological evidence, *World Journal of Gastroenterology* 19 (2013): 3713–3722.

34. A. Murakami, Dose-dependent functionality and toxicity of green tea polyphenols in experimental rodents, *Archives of Biochemistry and Biophysics* 557 (2014): 3–10; A. Jain and coauthors, Tea and human health: The dark shadows, *Toxicology Letters* 220 (2013): 82–87.

35. C. S. Yang and E. Pan, The effects of green tea polyphenols on drug metabolism, *Expert Opinion on Drug Metabolism and Toxicology* 8 (2012): 677–689.

36. L. M. Vislocky and M. L. Fernandez, Grapes and grape products: Their role in health, *Nutrition Today* 48 (2013): 47–51.

37. K. Liu and coauthors, Effect of resveratrol on glucose control and insulin sensitivity: A meta-analysis of 11 randomized controlled trials, *American Journal of Clinical Nutrition* 99 (2014): 1510–1519; S. Sheth and coauthors, Resveratrol reduces prostate cancer growth and metastasis by inhibiting the Akt/MicroRNA-21 pathway, *PLoS ONE* 7 (2012), doi:10.1371/journal.pone.0051655.

38. Y. Liu and coauthors, Effect of resveratrol on blood pressure: A meta-analysis of randomized controlled trials, *Clinical Nutrition* 34 (2015): 27–34; J. Tomé-Carneiro and coauthors, One-year consumption of a grape nutraceutical containing resveratrol improves the inflammatory and fibrinolytic status of patients in primary prevention of cardiovascular disease, *American Journal of Cardiology* 110 (2012): 356–363; B. Wang and coauthors, Resveratrol prevents suppression of regulatory T-cell production, oxidative stress,

and inflammation of mice prone or resistant to high-fat diet–induced obesity, *Nutrition Research* 33 (2013): 971–981.

39. Y. Liu and coauthors, Effect of resveratrol on blood pressure: A meta-analysis of randomized controlled trials, *Clinical Nutrition* (2014), epub ahead of print, doi:10.1016/j.clnu.2014.03.009.

40. K. L. Hector, M. Lagisz, and S. Nakagawa, The effect of resveratrol on longevity across species: A meta-analysis, *Biology Letters* 8 (2012): 790–793.

41. R. Estruch and coauthors, Primary prevention of cardiovascular disease with a Mediterranean diet, *New England Journal of Medicine* 368 (2013): 1279–1290.

42. R. D. Semba and coauthors, Resveratrol levels and all-cause mortality in older community-dwelling adults, *JAMA: Internal Medicine* 174 (2014): 1077–1084; S. D. Anton and coauthors, Safety and metabolic outcomes of resveratrol supplementation in older adults: Results of a twelve-week, placebo-controlled pilot study, *Experimental Gerontology* 57 (2014): 181–187.

43. W. M. de Vos and E. A. J. de Vos, Role of the intestinal microbiome in health and disease: From correlation to causation, *Nutrition Reviews* 70 (2012): S45–S56.

44. S. Chatterjee and coauthors, Randomised placebo-controlled double blind multicentric trial on efficacy and safety of Lactobacillus acidophilus LA-5 and Bifidobacterium BB-12 for prevention of antibiotic-associated diarrhoea, *Journal of the Association of Physicians of India* 61 (2013): 708–712.

45. N. Upadhyay and V. Moudgal, Probiotics: A review, *Journal of Clinical Outcomes Management* 19 (2012): 76–84.

46. H. J. Flint, The impact of nutrition on the human microbiome, *Nutrition Reviews* 70 (2012): S10–S13.

47. A. M. Brownawell and coauthors, Prebiotics and the health benefits of fiber: Current regulatory status, future research, and goals, *Journal of Nutrition* 142 (2012): 962–974; M. A. Conlon and coauthors, Resistant starches protect against colonic DNA damage and alter microbiota and gene expression in rats fed a Western diet, *Journal of Nutrition* 142 (2012): 832–840.

48. T. Bohn, Dietary factors affecting polyphenol bioavailability, *Nutrition Reviews* 72 (2014): 429–452.

49. C. Gerhauser, Epigenetic impact of dietary isothiocyanates in cancer chemoprevention, *Current Opinion in Clinical Nutrition and Metabolic Care* 16 (2013): 405–410; C. Zhang and coauthors, Sulforaphane enhances Nrf2 expression in prostate cancer TRAMP C1 cells through epigenetic regulation, *Biochemical Pharmacology* 85 (2013): 1398–1404.

50. A. Soare and coauthors, Multiple dietary supplements do not affect metabolic and cardiovascular health, *Aging* 6 (2014): 149–157.

51. J. I. Boullata and L. M. Hudson, Drug-nutrient interactions: A broad view with implications for practice, *Journal of the Academy of Nutrition and Dietetics* 112 (2012): 506–517.

52. S. K. Nordeen and coauthors, Endocrine disrupting activities of the flavonoid nutraceuticals luteolin and quercetin, *Hormones & Cancer* 4 (2013): 293–300.

53. S. Takahashi and coauthors, A randomized clinical trial to evaluate the preventive effect of cranberry juice (UR65) for patients with recurrent urinary tract infection, *Journal of Infection and Chemotherapy* 19 (2013): 112–117; C. H. Wang and coauthors, Cranberry-containing products for prevention of urinary tract infections in susceptible populations: A systematic review and meta-analysis of randomized controlled trials, *JAMA: Internal Medicine* 172 (2012): 988–996.

54. K. M. Crowe, C. Francis, and Academy of Nutrition and Dietetics, Position of the Academy of Nutrition and Dietetics: Functional foods, *Journal of the Academy of Nutrition and Dietetics* 113 (2013): 1096–1103.

Chapter 3

1. I. R. Stienstra and coauthors, The inflammasome puts obesity in the danger zone, *Cell Metabolism* 15 (2012): 10–18.

2. A. K. Ventura and J. Worobey, Early influences on the development of food preferences, *Current Biology* 23 (2013): R401–R408.

3. A. Drewnowski and coauthors, Sweetness and food preference, *Journal of Nutrition* 142 (2012): 1142S–1148S.

4. R. Shamir and S. M. Donovan, Introduction to the Second Global Summit on the Health Effects of Yogurt, *Nutrition Reviews* 73 (2015): 1–3; A. Kuwahara, Contributions of colonic short-chain fatty acid receptors in energy homeostasis, *Frontiers in Endocrinology* 5 (2014), epub, doi:10.3389/fendo.2014.00144.

5. K. Tuohy and D. Del Rio, eds., *Diet-Microbe Interactions in the Gut* (San Diego, Calif.: Academic Press, 2014).

6. J. Bienenstock, W. Kunze, and P. Forsythe, Microbiota and the gut-brain axis, *Nutrition Reviews* 73 (2015): 28–31; D. S. Spasova and C. D. Surh, Blowing on embers: Commensal microbiota and our immune system, *Frontiers in Immunology* 5 (2014), epub, doi:10.3389/fimmu.2014.00318.

7. C. M. Ferreira and coauthors, The central role of the gut microbiota in chronic inflammatory diseases, *Journal of Immunology Research* (2014), epub, doi:10.1155/2014/689492; Y. J. Lee and K. S. Park, Irritable bowel syndrome: Emerging paradigm in pathophysiology, *World Journal of Gastroenterology* 20 (2014): 2456–2469; H. Zeng, D. L. Lazarova, and M. Bordonaro, Mechanisms linking dietary fiber, gut microbiota and colon cancer prevention, *World Journal of Gastrointestinal Oncology* 6 (2014): 41–51; I. Moreno-Indias and coauthors, Impact of the gut microbiota on the development of obesity and type 2 diabetes mellitus, *Frontiers in Microbiology* 5 (2014), epub, doi:10.3389/fmicb.2014.00190.

8. S. J. Spechler, Barrett's esophagus and risk of esophageal cancer: A clinical review, *Journal of the American Medical Association* 310 (2013): 627–636.

9. G. Basilisco and M. Coletta, Chronic constipation: A critical review, *Digestive and Liver Disease* 45 (2013): 886–893.

10. Y. J. Lee and K. S. Park, Irritable bowel syndrome: Emerging paradigm in pathophysiology, *World Journal of Gastroenterology* 20 (2014): 2456–2469.

11. T. Wilkins and coauthors, Diagnosis and management of IBS in adults, *American Family Physician* 86 (2012): 419–426.

Controversy 3

1. M. Stahre and coauthors, Contribution of excessive alcohol consumption to deaths and years of potential life lost in the United States, *Preventing Chronic Disease* 11 (2014), doi:http://dx.doi.org/10.5888/pcd11.130293; K. Gonzales and coauthors, Alcohol-attributable deaths and years of potential life lost—11 states, 2006–2010, *Morbidity and Mortality Weekly Report* 63 (2014): 213–216.

2. S. J. Nielsen and coauthors, *Calories Consumed from Alcoholic Beverages by U.S. Adults, 2007–2010* (NCHS Data Brief 110) (Hyattsville, Md.: National Center for Health Statistics, November 2012), available at www.cdc.gov/nchs/data/databriefs/db110.htm.

3. Centers for Disease Control and Prevention, Binge drinking, Facts Sheets, updated January 2014, available at www.cdc.gov/alcohol/fact-sheets/binge-drinking.htm.

4. Centers for Disease Control and Prevention, Vital signs: Binge drinking prevalence, frequency, and intensity among adults—United States, 2010, *Morbidity and Mortality Weekly Report* 61 (2012): 14–19.

5. J. H. O'Keefe and coauthors, Alcohol and cardiovascular health: The dose makes the poison … or the remedy, *Mayo Clinic Proceedings* 89 (2014): 382–393; E. Nova and coauthors, Potential health benefits of moderate alcohol consumption: Current perspectives in research, *Proceedings of the Nutrition Society* 71 (2012): 307–315; M. Krenz and R. J. Korthuis, Moderate ethanol ingestion and cardiovascular protection: From epidemiologic associations to cellular mechanisms, *Journal of Molecular and Cellular Cardiology* 52 (2012): 93–104.

6. M. V. Holmes and coauthors, Association between alcohol and cardiovascular disease: Mendelian randomisation analysis based on individual participant data, *British Medical Journal* 349 (2014), epub, doi:10.1136/bmj.g4164; G. Chiva-Blanch and coauthors, Effects of wine, alcohol and polyphenols on cardiovascular disease risk factors: Evidences from human studies, *Alcohol and Alcoholism* 48 (2013): 270–277; Krenz and Korthuis, Moderate ethanol ingestion and cardiovascular protection, 2012.

7. C. S. Knott and coauthors, All cause mortality for age specific alcohol consumption guidelines: Pooled analyses of up to 10 population based cohorts, *British Medical Journal* 350 (2015), epub, doi: 10.1136/bmj.h384.

8. A. K. Piazza-Gardner, T. J. Gaffud, and A. E. Barry, The impact of alcohol on Alzheimer's disease: A systematic review, *Aging and Mental Health* 17 (2013): 133–146; F. Panza and coauthors, Alcohol consumption in mild cognitive impairment and dementia: Harmful or neuroprotective? *International Journal of Geriatric Psychiatry* 27 (2012): 1218–1238.

9. A. D. Plunk and coauthors, Alcohol consumption, heavy drinking, and mortality: Rethinking the j-shaped curve, *Alcohol Clinical and Experimental Research* 38 (2014): 471–478.

10. J. Martin and coauthors, Alcohol-attributable mortality in Ireland, *Alcohol and Alcoholism* 45 (2010): 379–386.

11. O'Keefe and coauthors, Alcohol and cardiovascular health, 2014.

12. Supporting evidence: L. C. Del Gobbo and coauthors, Contribution of major lifestyle risk factors for incident heart failure in older adults: The Cardiovascular Health Study, *JACC: Heart Failure* 3 (2015): 520–528; S. Arranz and coauthors, Wine, beer, alcohol and polyphenols on cardiovascular disease and cancer, *Nutrients* 4 (2012): 759–781; Krenz and Korthuis, Moderate ethanol ingestion and cardiovascular protection, 2012; Refuting evidence: A. Gonçalves and coauthors, Relationship between alcohol consumption and cardiac structure and function in the elderly, *Epidemiology* (2015), epub ahead of print, doi:10.1161/circimaging.114.002846.

13. G. Siasos and coauthors, Favorable effects of concord grape juice on endothelial function and arterial stiffness in healthy smokers, *American Journal of Hypertension* 27 (2014): 38–45; L. M. Vislocky and M. L. Fernandez, Grapes and grape products: Their role in health, *Nutrition Today* 48 (2013): 47–51.

14. M. Varela-Rey and coauthors, Alcohol, DNA methylation, and cancer, *Alcohol Research* 35 (2013): 25–35; D. E. Nelson and coauthors, Alcohol-attributable cancer deaths and years of potential life lost in the United States, *American Journal of Public Health* 103 (2013): 641–648.

15. USDA, *Scientific Report of the 2015 Dietary Guidelines for Americans Committee* (2015), A-4, available at www.health.gov/dietaryguidelines/2015-scientific-report/.

16. D. Tonelo, R. Providência, and L. Gonçalves, Holiday heart syndrome revisited after 34 years, *Arquivos Brasileiros de Cardiologia* 10 (2013): 183–189.

17. Centers for Disease Control and Prevention, Alcohol Poisoning Deaths—United States, 2010–2012, *Morbidity and Mortality Weekly Report* 63 (2015):1238–1242.

18. Centers for Disease Control and Prevention, Binge drinking, 2012.

19. World Health Organization, *Global Status Report on Alcohol and Health* (Geneva, Switzerland: World Health Organization, 2014).

20. R. McKetin and A. Coen, The effect of energy drinks on the urge to drink alcohol in young adults, *Alcoholism: Clinical and Experimental Research* 38 (2014): 2279–2285.

21. Y. Liang and coauthors, Alcohol consumption and the risk of incident atrial fibrillation among people with cardiovascular disease, *Canadian Medical Association Journal* 16 (2012): E857–E866.

22. Centers for Disease Control and Prevention, National Center for Injury Prevention and Control (NCIPC), www.cdc.gov.

23. Nelson and coauthors, Alcohol-attributable cancer deaths and years of potential life lost in the United States, 2013.

24. Y. Liu and coauthors, Alcohol intake between menarche and first pregnancy: A prospective study of breast cancer risk, *Journal of the National Cancer Institute* 105 (2013): 1571–1578; H. K. Seitz and coauthors, Epidemiology and pathophysiology of alcohol and breast cancer: Update 2012, *Alcohol and Alcoholism* 47 (2012): 204–212.

25. J. F. Gonzales and coauthors, Applying the precautionary principle to nutrition and cancer, *Journal of the American College of Nutrition* 33 (2014): 239–246.

26. C. A. Downs and coauthors, Chronic alcohol ingestion changes the landscape of the alveolar epithelium, *Biomed Research International* (2013), epub, doi:10.1155/2013/470217.

27. S. Lourenco, A. Oliveira, and C. Lopes, The effect of current and lifetime alcohol consumption on overall and central obesity, *European Journal of Clinical Nutrition* 66 (2012): 813–818.

Chapter 4

1. Position of the Academy of Nutrition and Dietetics: Use of nutritive and nonnutritive sweeteners, *Journal of the Academy of Nutrition and Dietetics* 112 (2012): 739–758.

2. G. Tang and coauthors, Meta-analysis of the association between whole grain intake and coronary heart disease risk, *American Journal of Cardiology* 115 (2015): 625–629; P. Vitaglione and coauthors, Whole-grain wheat consumption reduces inflammation in a randomized controlled trial on overweight and obese subjects with unhealthy dietary and lifestyle behaviors: Role of polyphenols bound to cereal dietary fiber, *American Journal of Clinical Nutrition* 101 (2015): 251–261; J. Slavin, Fiber and prebiotics: Mechanism and health benefits, *Nutrients* 5 (2013): 1417–1435.

3. J. W. McRorie, Evidence-based approach to fiber supplements and clinically meaningful health benefits, Part I, *Nutrition Today* 50 (2015): 82–89; J. W. McRorie, Evidence-based approach to fiber supplements and clinically meaningful health benefits, Part II, *Nutrition Today* 50 (2015): 90–97.

4. H. Zeng, D. L. Lazarova, and M. Bordonaro, Mechanisms linking dietary fiber, gut microbiota and colon cancer prevention, *World Journal of Gastrointestinal Oncology* 6 (2014): 41–51; F. De Vadder and coauthors, Microbiota-generated metabolites promote metabolic benefits via gut-brain neural circuits, *Cell* 156 (2014): 84–96.

5. 2013 AHA/ACC Guideline on Lifestyle Management to Reduce Cardiovascular Risk: A report of the American College of Cardiology/American Heart Association Task Force on Practice Guidelines, *Circulation* 129 (2014): S76–S99; D. E. Threapleton and coauthors,

Dietary fibre intake and risk of cardiovascular disease: Systematic review and meta-analysis, *British Medical Journal* 347 (2013), doi:10.1136/bmj.f6879.

6. A. Whitehead and coauthors, Cholesterol-lowering effects of oat β-glucan: A meta-analysis of randomized controlled trials, *American Journal of Clinical Nutrition* (2014), epub ahead of print, doi:10.3945/ajcn.114.086108.

7. F. M. Silva and coauthors, Fiber intake and glycemic control in patients with type 2 diabetes mellitus: A systematic review with meta-analysis of randomized controlled trials, *Nutrition Reviews* 71 (2013): 790–801.

8. J. Tan and coauthors, The role of short-chain fatty acids in health and disease, *Advances in Immunology* 121 (2014): 91–119; A. M. Brownawell and coauthors, Prebiotics and the health benefits of fiber: Current regulatory status, future research, and goals, *Journal of Nutrition* 142 (2012): 962–974.

9. A. W. Templeton and L. L. Strate, Updates in diverticular disease, *Current Gastroenterology Reports* 15 (2013), epub, doi:10.1007/s11894-013-0339-z; A. F. Peery and coauthors, A high-fiber diet does not protect against asymptomatic diverticulosis, *Gastroenterology* 142 (2012): 266–272.

10. Department of Health and Human Services, Centers for Disease Control and Prevention, and National Cancer Institute, United States cancer statistics: 1999–2007 incidence and mortality web-based report, 2010, available at www.cdc.gov/uscs.

11. N. Murphy and coauthors, Dietary fibre intake and risks of cancers of the colon and rectum in the European Prospective Investigation into Cancer and Nutrition (EPIC), *PLoS ONE* 7 (2012): e39361, doi:10.1371/journal.pone.0039361.

12. Zeng, Lazarova, and Bordonaro, Mechanisms linking dietary fiber, gut microbiota and colon cancer prevention, 2014.

13. Tan and coauthors, The role of short-chain fatty acids in health and disease, 2014; J. Slavin, Fiber and prebiotics: Mechanisms and health benefits, *Nutrients* 5 (2013): 1417–1435.

14. M. K. Hoy and J. D. Goldman, Fiber intake of the U.S. population: What we eat in America, NHANES 2009–2010 (Food Surveys Research Group Dietary Data Brief 12), September 2014, available at www.ars.usda.gov/SP2UserFiles/Place/80400530/pdf/DBrief/12_fiber_intake_0910.pdf.

15. M. Kristensen and coauthors, Whole grain compared with refined wheat decreases the percentage of body fat following a 12-week, energy-restricted dietary intervention in post-menopausal women, *Journal of Nutrition* 142 (2012): 710–716.

16. P. G. Williams, Evaluation of the evidence between consumption of refined grains and health outcomes, *Nutrition Reviews* 70 (2012): 80–99.

17. D. F. Birt and coauthors, Resistant starch: Promise for improving human health, *Advances in Nutrition* 4 (2013): 587–601.

18. R. K. Bailey and coauthors, Lactose intolerance and health disparities among African Americans and Hispanic Americans: An updated consensus statement, *Journal of the National Medical Association* 105 (2013): 112–117.

19. C. M. Weaver, How sound is the science behind the dietary recommendations for dairy? *American Journal of Clinical Nutrition* 99 (2014): 1217S–1222S; Bailey and coauthors, Lactose intolerance and health disparities among African Americans and Hispanic Americans, 2013; R. P. Heaney, Dairy intake, dietary adequacy, and lactose intolerance, *Advances in Nutrition* 4 (2013): 151–156.

20. D. A. Saviano, Lactose digestion from yogurt: Mechanism and relevance, *American Journal of Clinical Nutrition* 99 (2014): 1251S–1255S.

21. K. Sevastianova and coauthors, Effect of short-term carbohydrate overfeeding and long-term weight loss on liver fat in overweight humans, *American Journal of Clinical Nutrition* 96 (2012): 727–734.

22. P. Klein, I. Tyrlikova, and G. C. Mathews, Dietary treatment in adults with refractory epilepsy: A review, *Neurology* 83 (2014): 1978–1985.

23. Standing Committee on the Scientific Evaluation of Dietary Reference Intakes, *Dietary Reference Intakes for Energy, Carbohydrate, Fiber, Fat, Fatty Acids, Cholesterol, Protein, and Amino Acids* (National Academies Press: Washington, D.C., 2002/2005), pp. 265–338.

24. S. N. Bhupathiraju and coauthors, Glycemic index, glycemic load, and risk of type 2 diabetes: Results from 3 large US cohorts and an updated meta-analysis, *American Journal of Clinical Nutrition* 100 (2014): 218–232; E. S. Eshak and coauthors, Rice consumption is not associated with risk of cardiovascular disease morbidity or mortality in Japanese men and women: A large population-based, prospective cohort study, *American Journal of Clinical Nutrition* 100 (2014): 199–207; J. M. Jones, Glycemic index, *Nutrition Today* 47 (2012): 207–213; M. L. Wheeler and coauthors, Macronutrients, food groups, and eating patterns in the management of diabetes: A systematic review of the literature, 2010, *Diabetes Care* 35 (2012): 434–445.

25. A. S. Kristo, N. R. Matthan, and A. H. Lichtenstein, Effects of diets differing in glycemic index and glycemic load on cardiovascular risk factors: Review of randomized controlled-feeding trials, *Nutrients* 5 (2013): 1071–1080.

26. A. E. Buyken and coauthors, Association between carbohydrate quality and inflammatory markers: Systematic review of observational and interventional studies, *American Journal of Clinical Nutrition* 99 (2014): 813–833; L. M. Goff and coauthors, Low glycaemic index diet and blood lipids: A systematic review and meta-analysis of randomised controlled trials, *Nutrition, Metabolism, and Cardiovascular Diseases* 23 (2013): 1–10.

27. Bhupathiraju and coauthors, Glycemic index, glycemic load, and risk of type 2 diabetes, 2014.

28. A. B. Evert and coauthors, Nutrition therapy recommendations for management of adults with diabetes, *Diabetes Care* 37 (2014): S120–S143.

29. F. M. Sacks and coauthors, Effects of high vs low glycemic index of dietary carbohydrate on cardiovascular disease risk, *Journal of the American Medical Association* 312 (2014): 2531–2541.

30. F. M. Silva and coauthors, Fiber intake and glycemic control in patients with type 2 diabetes mellitus: A systematic review with meta-analysis of randomized controlled trials, *Nutrition Reviews* 71 (2013): 790–801.

31. Centers for Disease Control and Prevention, *National Diabetes Statistics Report: Estimates of Diabetes and Its Burden in the United States* (Atlanta: U.S. Department of Health and Human Services, 2014), available at www.cdc.gov/diabetes/pubs/statsreport14/national-diabetes-report-web.pdf.

32. L. Perreault and coauthors, Effect of regression from prediabetes to normal glucose regulation on long-term reduction in diabetes risk: Results from the Diabetes Prevention Program Outcomes Study, *Lancet* 379 (2012): 2243–2251; A. G. Tabák and coauthors, Prediabetes: A high-risk state for diabetes development, *Lancet* 379 (2012): 2279–2290.

33. X. Zhuo and coauthors, Alternative HbA1c cutoffs to identify high-risk adults for diabetes prevention, *American Journal of Preventive Medicine* 42 (2012): 374–381.

34. J. M. Lawrence and coauthors, Trends in incidence of type 1 diabetes among non-Hispanic white youth in the U.S., 2002–2009, *Diabetes* 63 (2014): 3938–3945.

35. R. Aathira and V. Jain, Advances in management of type 1 diabetes mellitus, *World Journal of Diabetes* 5 (2014): 689–696, S. J. Russell and coauthors, Outpatient glycemic control with a bionic pancreas in type 1 diabetes, *New England Journal of Medicine* 371 (2014): 313–325.

36. K. J. Basile and coauthors, Genetic susceptibility to type 2 diabetes and obesity: Follow-up findings from genome-wide association studies, *International Journal of Endocrinology* 2014 (2014), epub, doi:10.1155/2014/769671.

37. J. A. Wali, H. E. Thomas, and A. P. Sutherland, Linking obesity with type 2 diabetes: The role of T-bet, *Diabetes, Metabolic Syndrome, and Obesity: Targets and Therapy* 7 (2014): 331–340.

38. E. S. Koeck and coauthors, Adipocyte exosomes induce transforming growth factor beta pathway dysregulation in hepatocytes: A novel paradigm for obesity-related liver disease, *Journal of Surgical Research* (2014), epub ahead of print, doi:10.1016/j.jss.2014.06.050; N. Sattar and J. M. Gill, Type 2 diabetes as a disease of ectopic fat? *BMC Medicine* 12 (2014), epub, doi:10.1186/s12916-014-0123-4.

39. E. M. Balk and coauthors, Combined diet and physical activity promotion programs to prevent type 2 diabetes among persons at increased risk: A systematic review for the Community Preventive Services Task Force, *Annals of Internal Medicine* (2015), epub ahead of print, doi:10.7326/M15-0452; K. C. Portero and coauthors, Therapeutic interventions to reduce the risk of progression from prediabetes to type 2 diabetes mellitus, *Therapeutics and Clinical*

Risk Management 10 (2014): 173–188; E. Q. Ye and coauthors, Greater whole-grain intake is associated with lower risk of type 2 diabetes, cardiovascular disease, and weight gain, *Journal of Nutrition* 142 (2012): 1304–1313.

40. S. Ding and coauthors, Adjustable gastric band surgery or medical management in patients with type 2 diabetes: A randomized clinical trial, *Journal of Clinical Endocrinology and Metabolism* (2015), epub ahead of print, doi:10.1210/jc.2015-1443; L. Sjöström and coauthors, Association of bariatric surgery with long-term remission of type 2 diabetes and with microvascular and macrovascular complications, *Journal of the American Medical Association* 311 (2014): 2297–2304; D. E. Arterburn and coauthors, A multisite study of long-term remission and relapse of type 2 diabetes mellitus following gastric bypass, *Obesity Surgery* 23 (2013): 93–102.

41. M. J. Franz, J. L. Boucher, and A. B. Evert, Evidence-based diabetes nutrition therapy recommendations are effective: The key is individualization, *Diabetes, Metabolic Syndrome, and Obesity: Targets and Therapy* 7 (2014): 65–72.

42. Evert and coauthors, Nutrition therapy recommendations for management of adults with diabetes, 2014.

43. C. K. Roberts, J. P. Little, and J. P. Thyfault, Modification of insulin sensitivity and glycemic control by activity and exercise, *Medicine & Science in Sports & Exercise* 45 (2013): 1868–1877; H. Naci and J. P. A. Ioannidis, Comparative effectiveness of exercise and drug interventions on mortality outcomes: Metaepidemiological study, *British Medical Journal* 347 (2013), f5577, doi:http://dx.doi.org/10.1136/bmj.f5577.

Consumer's Guide 4

1. U.S. Department of Health and Human Services and U.S. Department of Agriculture, *2015–2020 Dietary Guidelines for Americans*, 8th edition (2015), available at http://health.gov/dietaryguidelines/2015/guidelines/.

2. P. G. Williams, Evaluation of the evidence between consumption of refined grains and health outcomes, *Nutrition Reviews* 70 (2012): 80–99.

Controversy 4

1. World Health Organization, *Guideline: Sugars Intake for Adults and Children* (Geneva: World Health Organization, 2015), available at http://who.int/nutrition/publications/guidelines/sugars_intake/en/; U.S. Department of Health and Human Services and U.S. Department of Agriculture, *2015–2020 Dietary Guidelines for Americans*, 8th edition (2015), available at http://health.gov/dietaryguidelines/2015/guidelines/.

2. U.S. Department of Agriculture, Agricultural Research Service, Nutrient intakes from food, 2008, available at www.ars.usda.gov/ba/bhnrc/fsrg.

3. Q. Yang and coauthors, Added sugar intake and cardiovascular diseases mortality among U.S. adults, *JAMA Internal Medicine* 174 (2014): 516–524.

4. U. Ladabaum and coauthors, Obesity, abdominal obesity, physical activity, and caloric intake in U.S. adults: 1988–2010, *American Journal of Medicine* (February 2014), epub ahead of print, doi:http://dx.doi.org/10.1016/j.amjmed.2014.02.026.

5. B. Lin and R. Morrison, ERS's food consumption and nutrient intake data—Tools for assessing Americans' diets, *Amber Waves*, August 2014, available at www.ers.usda.gov/publications.aspx.

6. S. C. Bundrick and coauthors, Soda consumption during ad libitum food intake predicts weight change, *Journal of the Academy of Nutrition and Dietetics* 114 (2014): 444–449; L. T. Morenga, S. Mallard, and J. Mann, Dietary sugars and body weight: Systematic review and meta-analyses of randomised controlled trials and cohort studies, *British Medical Journal* 100 (2014): 65–79; J. Massougbodji and coauthors, Reviews examining sugar-sweetened beverages and body weight: Correlates of the quality and conclusions, *American Journal of Clinical Nutrition* 99 (2014): 1096–1104; F. B. Hu, Resolved: There is sufficient scientific evidence that decreasing sugar-sweetened beverage consumption will reduce the prevalence of obesity and obesity-related diseases, *Obesity Reviews* 14 (2013): 606–619; V. S. Malik and coauthors, Sugar-sweetened beverages and weight gain in children and adults: A systematic review and meta-analysis, *American Journal of Clinical Nutrition* 98 (2013): 1084–1102.

7. M. S. Estimé, B. Lutz, and F. Strobe, Trade as a structural driver of dietary risk factors for noncommunicable diseases in the Pacific: An analysis of household income and expenditure survey data, *Globalization and Health* 10 (2014), doi:10.1186/1744-8603-10-48; B. M. Popkin, L. S. Adair, and S. W. Ng, Global nutrition transition and the pandemic of obesity in developing countries, *Nutrition Reviews* 70 (2012): 3–21; A. Pan, V. Malik, and F. B. Hu, Exporting diabetes to Asia: The impact of Western-style fast food (Editorial), *Circulation* 126 (2012): 163–165.

8. N. I. Toufel-Shone and coauthors, Demographic characteristics and food choices of participants in the Special Diabetes Program for American Indians Diabetes Prevention Demonstration Project, *Ethnicity and Health* (June 2014), epub ahead of print, doi:10.1080/13557858.2014.921890.

9. A. M. Fretts and coauthors, Associations of processed meat and unprocessed red meat intake with incident diabetes: The Strong Heart Family Study, *American Journal of Clinical Nutrition* 95 (2012): 752–758.

10. J. L. Sievenpiper and R. J. de Souza, Are sugar-sweetened beverages the whole story? *American Journal of Clinical Nutrition* 98 (2013): 261–263.

11. A. S. Go and coauthors, Heart disease and stroke statistics—2013 update: A report from the American Heart Association, *Circulation* 127 (2013): e6–e245.

12. M. Siervo and coauthors, Sugar consumption and global prevalence of obesity and hypertension: An ecological analysis, *Public Health Nutrition* 17 (2014): 587–596; L. A. Te Morenga and coauthors, Dietary sugars and cardiometabolic risk: Systematic review and meta-analyses of randomized controlled trials of the effects on blood pressure and lipids, *American Journal of Clinical Nutrition* 100 (2014): 65–79.

13. A. H. Malik and coauthors, Impact of sugar-sweetened beverages on blood pressure, *American Journal of Cardiology* 113 (2014): 1574–1580.

14. K. P. Kell and coauthors, Added sugars in the diet are positively associated with diastolic blood pressure and triglycerides in children, *American Journal of Clinical Nutrition* 100 (2014): 46–52.

15. V. Ha and coauthors, Fructose-containing sugars, blood pressure, and cardiometabolic risk: A critical review, *Current Hypertension Reports* 15 (2013): 281–297.

16. G. A. Bray and B. M. Popkin, Dietary sugar and body weight: Have we reached a crisis in the epidemic of obesity and diabetes? *Diabetes Care* 37 (2014): 950–956.

17. B. A. Cassady, R. V. Considine, and R. D. Mattes, Beverage consumption, appetite, and energy intake: What did you expect? *American Journal of Clinical Nutrition* 95 (2012): 587–593.

18. L. B. Sørensen and coauthors, Sucrose compared with artificial sweeteners: A clinical intervention study of effects on energy intake, appetite, and energy expenditure after 10 wk of supplementation in overweight subjects, *American Journal of Clinical Nutrition* 100 (2014): 36–45; F. Tate and coauthors, Replacing caloric beverages with water or diet beverages for weight loss in adults: Main results of the Choose Healthy Options Consciously Everyday (CHOICE) randomized clinical trial, *American Journal of Clinical Nutrition* 95 (2012): 555–563.

19. Bray and Popkin, Dietary sugar and body weight, 2014; A. Bebollo and coauthors, Way back for fructose and liver metabolism: Bench side to molecular insights, *World Journal of Gastroenterology* 18 (2012), epub, doi:10.3748/wjg.v18.i45.6552; K. L. Stanhope, Role of fructose-containing sugars in the epidemics of obesity and metabolic syndrome, *Annual Review of Medicine* 63 (2012): 19.1–19.15.

20. D. S. Ludwig, Examining the health effects of fructose, *Journal of the American Medical Association* 310 (2013): 33–34.

21. A. Kolderup and B. Svihus, Fructose metabolism and relation to atherosclerosis, type 2 diabetes, and obesity, *Journal of Nutrition and Metabolism* (2015), epub, doi.org/10.2255/2015/823081.

22. J. Lowndes and coauthors, The effect of normally consumed amounts of sucrose or high fructose corn syrup on lipid profiles, body composition, and related parameters in overweight/obese subjects, *Nutrients* 6 (2014): 1128–1144.

23. Kolderup and Svihus, Fructose metabolism and relation to atherosclerosis, type 2 diabetes, and obesity, 2015.

24. L. de Koning and coauthors, Sweetened beverages consumption, incident coronary heart

disease and biomarkers of risk in men, *Circulation* 125 (2012): 1735–1741.

25. R. Kelishadi, M. Mansourian, and M. Heidari-Beni, Association of fructose consumption and components of metabolic syndrome in human studies: A systematic review and meta-analysis, *Nutrition* 30 (2014): 503–510.

26. K. Stanhope and coauthors, A dose-response study of consuming high fructose corn syrup-sweetened beverages on lipid/lipoprotein risk factors for cardiovascular disease in young adults, *American Journal of Clinical Nutrition* 101 (2015): 1144–1154; A. K. Lee and coauthors, Consumption of less than 10% of total energy from added sugars is associated with increasing HDL in females during adolescence: A longitudinal analysis, *Journal of the American Heart Association* 3 (2014), doi:10.1161/JAHA.113.000615.

27. K. L. Stanhope and coauthors, A dose-response study of consuming high-fructose corn syrup-sweetened beverages on lipid/lipoprotein risk factors for cardiovascular disease in young adults, 2015.

28. M. Del Ben and coauthors, Modern approach to the clinical management of non-alcoholic fatty liver disease, *World Journal of Gastroenterology* 20 (2014): 8341–8350.

29. R. J. Johnson and coauthors, Sugar, uric acid, and the etiology of diabetes and obesity, *Diabetes* 62 (2013): 3307–3315.

30. J. Ma and coauthors, Sugar-sweetened beverage, diet soda, and fatty liver disease in the Framingham Heart Study cohorts, *Journal of Hepatology* (2015), epub ahead of print, doi:http://dx.doi.org/10.1016/j.jhep2015.03.032; M. Chung and coauthors, Fructose, high-fructose corn syrup, sucrose, and nonalcoholic fatty liver disease or indexes of liver health: A systematic review and meta-analysis, *American Journal of Clinical Nutrition* 100 (2014): 833–849.

31. J. M. Rippe, The metabolic and endocrine response and health implication of consuming sugar-sweetened beverages: Findings from recent randomized controlled trials, *Advances in Nutrition* 4 (2013): 677–686.

32. U.S. Department of Health and Human Services and U.S. Department of Agriculture, 2015-2020 Dietary Guidelines for Americans, 8th edition (2015), available at http://health.gov/dietaryguidelines/2015/guidelines/.

Chapter 5

1. A. T. Ryan and coauthors, Effects of intraduodenal lipid and protein on gut motility and hormone release, glycemia, appetite, and energy intake in lean men, *American Journal of Clinical Nutrition* 98 (2013): 300–311.

2. D. Piomelli, A fatty gut feeling, *Trends in Endocrinology and Metabolism* 24 (2013): 332–341.

3. A. Romano and coauthors, High dietary fat intake influences the activation of specific hindbrain and hypothalamic nuclei by the satiety factor oleoylethanolamide, *Physiology and Behavior* (2014), epub ahead of print, doi:10.1016/j.physbeh.2014.04.03; F. A. Duca, Y. Sakar, and M. Covasasa, The modulatory role of high fat feeding on gastrointestinal signals in obesity, *Journal of Nutritional Biochemistry* 24 (2013): 1663–1677.

4. Position of the Academy of Nutrition and Dietetics: Dietary fatty acids for healthy adults, *Journal of the Academy of Nutrition and Dietetics* 114 (2014): 136–153.

5. A. Shaghaghi, S. S. Aburnweis, and P. J. Jones, Cholesterol-lowering efficacy of plant sterols/stanols provided in capsule and tablet formats: Results of a systematic review and meta-analysis, *Journal of the Academy of Nutrition and Dietetics* 113 (2013): 494–503.

6. G. A. Bray and coauthors, Effect of protein overfeeding on energy expenditure measured in a metabolic chamber, *American Journal of Clinical Nutrition* 101 (2015): 496–505; D. E. Berryman and coauthors, Control of energy balance, in M. H. Stipanuk and M. A. Caudill, *Biochemical, Physiological, and Molecular Aspects of Human Nutrition* (St. Louis, Mo: Saunders, 2013), pp. 501–518.

7. G. Michas, R. Micha, and A. Zampelas, Dietary fats and cardiovascular disease: Putting together the pieces of a complicated puzzle, *Atherosclerosis* 234 (2014): 320–328.

8. R. H. Eckel and coauthors, 2013 AHA/ACC Guideline on Lifestyle Management to Reduce Cardiovascular Risk: A report of the American College of Cardiology/American Heart Association Task Force on Practice Guidelines, *Circulation* 129 (2014): S76–S99 A. S. Go and coauthors, Heart disease and stroke statistics—2014 Update: A report from the American Heart Association, *Circulation* 129 (2014): e28–e292.

9. National Center for Health Statistics, Age-adjusted kilocalorie and macronutrient intake among adults aged ≥20 years, by sex—National Health and Nutrition Examination Survey, United States, 2007–2008, *Morbidity and Mortality Weekly Report* 60 (2011): 252.

10. I. Castro-Quezada, B. Roman-Vinas, and L. Serra-Majem, The Mediterranean diet and nutritional adequacy: A review, *Nutrients* 6 (2014): 231–248; M. A. Martinez and M. Bes-Rastrollo, Dietary patterns, Mediterranean diet, and cardiovascular disease, *Current Opinion in Lipidology* 25 (2014): 20–26; I. R. Estruch and coauthors, Primary prevention of cardiovascular disease with a Mediterranean diet, *New England Journal of Medicine* 368 (2013): 1279–1290.

11. M. L. Bertoia and coauthors, Mediterranean and Dietary Approaches to Stop Hypertension dietary patterns and risk of sudden cardiac death in postmenopausal women, *American Journal of Clinical Nutrition* 99 (2014): 344–351; E. Ros and coauthors, Mediterranean diet and cardiovascular health: Teachings of the PREDIMED study, *Advances in Nutrition* 5 (2014): 330S–336S; H. Gardener and coauthors, Mediterranean diet and carotid atherosclerosis in the Northern Manhattan Study, *Atherosclerosis* 234 (2014): 303–310.

12. R. C. Albuquerque, V. T. Baltar, and D. M. Marchioni, Breast cancer and dietary patterns: A systematic review, *Nutrition Reviews* 72 (2014): 1–17; K. Esposito and coauthors, The effects of a Mediterranean diet on need for diabetes drugs and remission of newly diagnosed type 2 diabetes: Follow-up of a randomized trial, *Diabetes Care* 37 (2014): 1824–1830; L. Ilianna and coauthors, Mediterranean diet, cognitive function, and dementia: A systematic review, *Epidemiology* 24 (2013): 479–489.

13. W. Annema and A. von Eckardstein, High-density lipoproteins: Multifunctional but vulnerable protections from atherosclerosis, *Circulation Journal* 77 (2013): 2432–2448; G. Kellner-Weibel and M. de la Llera-Moya, Update on HDL receptors and cellular cholesterol transport, *Current Atherosclerosis Reports* 13 (2011): 233–241.

14. Go and coauthors, Heart disease and stroke statistics—2014 update, 2014.

15. R. H. Eckel and coauthors, 2013 AHA/ACC Guideline on Lifestyle Management to Reduce Cardiovascular Risk: A report of the American College of Cardiology/American Heart Association Task Force on Practice Guidelines, 2014; D. J. McNamara, Dietary cholesterol, heart disease risk and cognitive dissonance, *Proceedings of the Nutrition Society* 73 (2014): 161–166.

16. J. Y. Shin and coauthors, Egg consumption in relation to risk of cardiovascular disease and diabetes: A systematic review and meta-analysis, *American Journal of Clinical Nutrition* 98 (2013): 146–159; J. D. Spence, D. J. Jenkins, and J. Davignon, Egg yolk consumption and carotid plaque, *Atherosclerosis* 224 (2012): 469–473.

17. E. V. Kulina and coauthors, *Trends in High LDL Cholesterol, Cholesterol-Lowering Medication Use, and Dietary Saturated-Fat Intake: United States,* 1976–2010 (NCHS Data Brief 117) (Hyattsville, MD: National Center for Health Statistics, March 2013), available at http://www.cdc.gov/nchs/data/databriefs/db117.pdf.

18. M. D. Carroll and coauthors, *Total and High-Density Lipoprotein Cholesterol in Adults: National Health and Nutrition Examination Survey, 2011–2012* (NCHS Data Brief 132) (Hyattsville, Md: National Center for Health Statistics, 2013), available from www.cdc.gov/nchs/data/databriefs/db132.pdf.

19. K. M. Ali and coauthors, Cardiovascular disease risk reduction by raising HDL cholesterol—Current therapies and future opportunities, *British Journal of Pharmacology*, 167 (2012): 1177–1194.

20. H. Ohnishi and Y. Saito, Eicosapentaenoic acid (EPA) reduces cardiovascular events: Relationship with the EPA/arachidonic acid ratio, *Journal of Atherosclerosis and Thrombosis* 20 (2013): 861–877.

21. T. A. Mori, Conference on "Dietary Strategies for the Management of Cardiovascular Risk," Dietary n-3 PUFA and CVD: A review of the evidence, *Proceedings of the Nutrition Society* 73 (2014): 57–64; K. Takada and coauthors, Effects of eicosapentaenoic acid on platelet function in patients taking long-term aspirin following coronary stent implantation, *International*

Heart Journal 55 (2014): 228–233; M. van Bilsen and A. Planavila, Fatty acids and cardiac disease: Fuel carrying a message, *Acta Physiologica* 211 (2014): 476–490; W. S. Harris, T. D. Dayspring, and T. J. Moran, Omega-3 fatty acids and cardiovascular disease: New developments and applications, *Postgraduate Medicine* 125 (2013): 100–113.

22. H. R. Superko and coauthors, Omega-3 fatty acid blood levels: Clinical significance and Controversy, *Circulation* 128 (2013): 2154–2161.

23. D. Kromhout and J. de Goede, Update on cardiometabolic health effects of ω-3 fatty acids, *Current Opinion in Lipidology* 25 (2014): 85–90; D. Mozaffarian and coauthors, Plasma phospholipid long-chain omega-3 fatty acids and total cause-specific mortality in older adults: The Cardiovascular Health Study, *Annals of Internal Medicine* 158 (2013): 515–525; E. C. Rizos and coauthors, Association between omega-3 fatty acid supplementation and risk of major cardiovascular disease events, *Journal of the American Medical Association* 308 (2012): 1024–1033.

24. M. Azrad, C. Turgeon, and W. Denmark-Wahnefried, Current evidence linking polyunsaturated fatty acids with cancer risk and progression, *Frontiers in Oncology* (September 2013), epub, doi:10.3389/fonc.2013.0024; J. Zhen and coauthors, Intake of fish and marine n-3 polyunsaturated fatty acids and risk of breast cancer: Meta-analysis of data from 21 independent prospective cohort studies, *British Medical Journal* 346 (2013), epub, doi:10.1136/bmj.f3706; K. He and coauthors, Types of fish consumed and fish preparation methods in relation to pancreatic cancer incidence: The VITAL cohort study, *American Journal of Epidemiology* 177 (2013): 152–160.

25. T. M. Brasky and coauthors, Associations of long-chain ω-3 fatty acids and fish intake with endometrial cancer risk in the VITamins And Lifestyle cohort, *American Journal of Clinical Nutrition* 99 (2014): 599–608.

26. D. W. Luchtman and C. Song, Cognitive enhancement by omega-3 fatty acids from childhood to old age: Findings from animal and clinical studies, *Neuropharmacology*, 64 (2013): 550–565; A. P. Simopoulos, Evolutionary aspects of diet: The omega-6/omega-3 ratio and the brain, *Molecular Neurobiology* 44 (2011): 203–215.

27. M. Hennebelle and coauthors, Omega-3 polyunsaturated fatty acids and chronic stress-induced modulations of glutamatergic neurotransmission in the hippocampus, *Nutrition Reviews* 72 (2014): 99–112; J. V. Pottala and coauthors, Higher RBC EPA + DHA corresponds with larger total brain and hippocampal volumes: WHIMS–MRI study, *Neurology* 82 (2014): 435–442.

28. R. S. Kuipers and coauthors, Fetal intrauterine whole body linoleic, arachidonic, and docosahexaenoic acid contents and accretion rates, *Prostaglandins, Leukotrienes, and Essential Fatty Acids* 86 (2012): 13–20; M. Guxens and coauthors, Breastfeeding, long-chain polyunsaturated fatty acids in colostrums, and infant mental development, *Pediatrics* 128 (2011): e880–e889; M. B. Imhoff-Kunsch and coauthors, Prenatal docosahexaenoic acid supplementation and infant morbidity: Randomized controlled trial, *Pediatrics* 128 (2011): e505–e515.

29. S. K. Orr and coauthors, Lipid metabolism: Polyunsaturated fatty acids, in M. H. Stipanuk and M. A. Caudill, *Biochemical, Physiological, and Molecular Aspects of Human Nutrition* (St. Louis, Mo.: Saunders, 2013), pp. 416–433.

30. U.S. Department of Agriculture and U.S. Department of Health and Human Services, *Dietary Guidelines for Americans 2010* (Washington, D.C.: U.S. Government Printing Office, December 2010), available at www.dietaryguidelines.gov.

31. Y. Papanikolaou and coauthors, U.S. adults are not meeting recommended levels for fish and mega-3 fatty acid intake: Results of an analysis using observational data from NHANES 2003–2008, *Nutrition* 13 (2014), open access, doi:10.1186/1475-2891-13-31.

32. B. B. Albert and coauthors, Supplementation with a blend of krill and salmon oil is associated with increased metabolic risk in overweight men, *American Journal of Clinical Nutrition* 102 (2015): 49–57; C. von Schacky, Omega-3 index and cardiovascular health, *Nutrients* 6 (2014): 799–814.

33. K. Lane and coauthors, Bioavailability and potential uses of vegetarian sources of omega-3 fatty acids: A review of the literature, *Critical Reviews in Food Science and Nutrition* 54 (2014): 572–579; R. J. Deckelbaum and C. Torrejon, The omega-3 fatty acid nutritional landscape: Health benefits and sources, *Journal of Nutrition* 142 (2012): 587S–591S.

34. R. Ganguly and G. N. Pierce, The toxicity of dietary *trans* fats, *Food and Chemical Toxicology* 78 (2015): 170–176; J. N. Kiage and coauthors, Intake of *trans* fat and all-cause mortality in the Reasons for Geographical and Racial Differences in Stroke (REGARDS) cohort, *American Journal of Clinical Nutrition* 97 (2013): 1121–1128; F. Imamura and coauthors, Novel circulating fatty acid patterns and risk of cardiovascular disease: The Cardiovascular Health Study, *American Journal of Clinical Nutrition* 96 (2012): 1252–1261.

35. R. Ganguly and G. N. Pierce, The toxicity of dietary *trans* fats, 2015; I. A. Brouwer, A. J. Wanders, and M. B Katan, *Trans* fatty acids and cardiovascular health: Research completed? *European Journal of Clinical Nutrition* 67 (2013): 541–547.

36. F. O. Otite and coauthors, Trends in *trans* fatty acids reformulations of US supermarket and brand-name foods from 2007 through 2011, *Preventing Chronic Disease* 10 (2013): 120198.

37. A. Baylin, Secular trends in *trans* fatty acids: Decreased *trans* fatty acids in the food supply are reflected in decreased *trans* fatty acids in plasma, *American Journal of Clinical Nutrition* 97 (2013): 665–666.

38. F. Mohamedshah and J. Ruff, IFT addresses sodium, sugars, and fats for DGAC, *Food Technology*, May 2014, available at http://www.ift.org /Food-Technology/Past-Issues/2014/May/Columns /SCIENCE-AND-POLICY-INITIATIVES.aspx.

39. W. H. Dietz and K. S. Scanlon, Eliminating the use of partially hydrogenated oil in food production and preparation, *Journal of the American Medical Association* 308 (2012): 143–144.

40. USDA Nutrient Data Laboratory, Release 27, available at http://ndb.nal.usda.gov/ndb /search/list.

41. S. Bulotta and coauthors, Beneficial effects of the olive oil phenolic components oleuropein and hydroxytyrosol: Focus on protection against cardiovascular and metabolic diseases, *Journal of Translational Medicine* 12 (2014), doi:10.1186/ s12967-014-0219-9.

42. H. N. Luu and coauthors, Prospective evaluation of the association of nut/peanut consumption with total and cause-specific mortality, *JAMA Internal Medicine* (2015), epub ahead of print, doi: 10.1001/jamainternmed.2014.8347; A. Afshin and coauthors, Consumption of nuts and legumes and risk of incident ischemic heart disease, stroke, and diabetes: A systematic review and meta-analysis, *American Journal of Clinical Nutrition* 100 (2014): 278–288; C. Luo and coauthors, Nut consumption and risk of type 2 diabetes, cardiovascular disease, and all-cause mortality: A systematic review and meta-analysis, *American Journal of Clinical Nutrition* 100 (2014): 256–269; J. Salas-Salvadó and coauthors, Nuts in the prevention and treatment of metabolic syndrome, *American Journal of Clinical Nutrition* 100 (2014): 399S–407S.

43. J. A. Novotny, S. K. Gebauer, and D. J. Baer, Discrepancy between the Atwater factor predicted and empirically measured energy values of almonds in human diets, *American Journal of Clinical Nutrition* 96 (2012): 296–301.

Consumer's Guide 5

1. I. E. Amara and coauthors, Acute mercury toxicity modulates cytochrome P450, soluble epoxide hydrolase, and their associated arachidonic acid metabolites in C57BI/6 mouse heart, *Toxicology Letter* 226 (2014): 53–63.

2. D. Mozaffarian and coauthors, Mercury exposure and risk of hypertension in US men and women in two prospective cohorts, *Hypertension* 60 (2012): 645–652.

3. E. C. Somers and coauthors, Mercury exposure and antinuclear antibodies among females of reproductive age in the United States: NHANES, *Environmental Health Perspectives* (2015), epub ahead of print, doi:10.1289/ ehp.1408751; D. Mozaffarian and coauthors, Methylmercury exposure and incident diabetes in U.S. men and women in two prospective cohorts, *Diabetes Care* 36 (2013): 3578–3584.

4. Fish: What pregnant women and parents should know (Draft updated advice by FDA and EPA), June 2014, available at www.fda .gov/food/foodborneillnesscontaminants/metals /ucm393070.htm.

5. Fish: What pregnant women and parents should know, June 2014.

6. D. B. Jump, C. M. Depner, and S. Tripathy, Omega-3 fatty acid supplementation and cardiovascular disease, *Journal of Lipid Research* 53 (2012): 2525–2545.

Controversy 5

1. A. Yngve, A historical perspective of the understanding of the link between diet and coronary heart disease, *American Journal of Lifestyle Medicine* 3 (2009): 35S–38S.

2. National Center for Health Statistics, Anthropometric reference data for children and adults: United States, 2007–2010, published 2013, available at www.cdc.gov/nchs/data/series /sr_11/sr11_252.pdf; E. S. Ford and W. H. Dietz, Trends in energy intake among adults in the United States: Findings from NHANES, *American Journal of Clinical Nutrition* 97 (2013): 848–853.

3. A. Keys, *Seven Countries: A Multivariate Analysis of Death and Coronary Heart Disease* (Cambridge, Mass.: Harvard University Press, 1980).

4. U.S. Department of Agriculture and U.S. Department of Health and Human Services, Scientific report of the 2015 Dietary Guidelines Advisory Committee, 2015, D-6:11, available at www.health.gov.

5. M. R. Flock, J. A. Fleming, and P. M. Kris-Etherton, Macronutrient replacement options for saturated fat: Effects on cardiovascular health, *Current Opinion in Lipidology* 25 (2014): 67–74.

6. U.S. Department of Agriculture and U.S. Department of Health and Human Services, Scientific report of the 2015 Dietary Guidelines Advisory Committee, 2015, D-6:15, available at www.health.gov.

7. U.S. Department of Agriculture and U.S. Department of Health and Human Services, Scientific report of the 2015 Dietary Guidelines Advisory Committee, 2015, A:3–5, available at www.health.gov.

8. A. M. Fretts and coauthors, Plasma phospholipid saturated fatty acids and incident atrial fibrillation: The Cardiovascular Health Study, *Journal of the American Heart Association* (2014), epub, doi:10l1161/JAHA.114.000889; Flock, Fleming, and Kris-Etherton, Macronutrient replacement options for saturated fat, 2014.

9. R. H. Eckel and coauthors, 2013 AHA/ACC guideline on lifestyle management to reduce cardiovascular risk: A report of the American College of Cardiology/American Heart Association Task Force on Practice Guidelines, *Circulation* 129 (2014): S76–S99.

10. L. Hooper and coauthors, Reduced or modified dietary fat for preventing cardiovascular disease, *Cochrane Database Systematic Reviews* (2012), epub, doi:10.1002/14651858.CD002137.pub2.

11. J. A. Nettleton, P. Legrand, and R. P. Mensink, ISSFAL 2014 debate: Is it time to update saturated fat recommendations? *Annals of Nutrition and Metabolism* (2015), epub, doi:10.1159/000371585; G. Michas, R. Micha, and A. Zampelas, Dietary fats and cardiovascular disease: Putting together the pieces of a complicated puzzle, *Atherosclerosis* 234 (2014): 320–328; G. D. Lawrence, Dietary fats and health: Dietary recommendations in the context of scientific evidence, *Advances in Nutrition* 4 (2013): 294–302.

12. U. Ravnskov and coauthors, The questionable benefits of exchanging saturated fat with polyunsaturated fat, *Mayo Clinic Proceedings* 89 (2014): 451–453; National Cancer Institute, Sources of saturated fat, stearic acid, and cholesterol raising fat among the US population, 2005–2006, updated April 11, 2014, available at http://appliedresearch.cancer.gov/diet /foodsources/sat-fat/.

13. B. H. Rice, Dairy and cardiovascular disease: A review of recent observational research, *Current Nutrition Reports* 3 (2014): 130–138.

14. B. Walsh, Eat butter: Scientists labeled fat the enemy: Why they were wrong, *Time*, June 23, 2014; M. Bittman, Butter is back, *New York Times*, March 26, 2014, p. A-23.

15. R. Chowdhury and coauthors, Association of dietary, circulating, and supplement fatty acids with coronary risk, *Annals of Internal Medicine* 160 (2014): 398–407.

16. Comments and response, *Annals of Internal Medicine* 161 (2014): 453–459; M. Katan, as interviewed in B. Liebman, Fat under fire: New findings or shaky science? *Nutrition Action Healthletter*, May 2014, pp. 3–7; D. Kromhout and coauthors, The confusion about dietary fatty acids recommendations for CHD prevention, *British Journal of Nutrition* 106 (2011): 627–632.

17. U.S. Department of Agriculture and U.S. Department of Health and Human Services, Scientific report of the 2015 Dietary Guidelines Advisory Committee, 2015, D-6:16, available at www.health.gov.

18. N. G. Puaschitz and coauthors, Dietary intake of saturated fat is not associated with risk of coronary events or mortality in patients with established coronary artery disease, *Journal of Nutrition* 145 (2015): 299–305.

19. B. Haring and coauthors, Healthy dietary interventions and lipoprotein (a) plasma levels: Results from the Omni Heart Trial, *PLOS ONE* (2014), epub, doi:10.1371/journal.pone.0114859.

20. J. A. Dias and coauthors, A high quality diet is associated with reduced systemic inflammation in middle-aged individuals, *Atherosclerosis* 238 (2015): 38–44.

21. U.S. Department of Health and Human Services and U.S. Department of Agriculture, *2015–2020 Dietary Guidelines for Americans*, 8th edition (2015), available at http://health .gov/dietaryguidelines/2015/guidelines/.

Chapter 6

1. Standing Committee on the Scientific Evaluation of Dietary Reference Intakes, Food and Nutrition Board, Institute of Medicine, *Dietary Reference Intakes for Energy, Carbohydrate, Fiber, Fat, Fatty Acids, Cholesterol, Protein, and Amino Acids* (Washington, D.C.: National Academies Press, 2002/2005), pp. 589–768.

2. S. Chakravorty and T. N. Williams, Sickle cell disease: A neglected chronic disease of increasing global health importance, *Archives of Disease in Childhood* (2014): epub ahead of print, doi:10.1136/archdischild-2013-303773.

3. N. M. Sales, P. B. Pelegrini, and M. C. Goersch, Nutrigenomics: Definitions and advances of this new science, *Journal of Nutrition and Metabolism* (2014): epub ahead of print, doi:10.1155/2014/202759.

4. Position of the Academy of Nutrition and Dietetics, Dietitians of Canada, and the American College of Sports Medicine, Nutrition and athletic performance, *Journal of the Academy of Nutrition and Dietetics* 109 (2009): 509–527 (under revision); S. M. Phillips, Dietary protein requirements and adaptive advantages in athletes, *British Journal of Nutrition* 108 (2012): epub, doi:10.1017/S0007114512002516.

5. E. Arentson-Lantz and coauthors, Protein: A nutrient in focus, *Applied Physiology, Nutrition, and Metabolism* 40 (2015): 755–761; N. R. Rodriguez and S. L. Miller, Effective translation of current dietary guidance: Understanding and communication the concepts of minimal and optimal levels of dietary protein, *American Journal of Clinical Nutrition* 101 (2015): 1353S–1358S; M. Rafii and coauthors, Dietary protein requirement of female adults >65 years determined by the indicator amino acid oxidation technique is higher than current recommendations, *Journal of Nutrition* 145 (2015): 18–24; A. N. Pedersen and T. Cederholm, Health effects of protein intake in healthy elderly populations: A systematic literature review, *Food and Nutrition Research* 58 (2014): epub, doi:10.3402/fnr.v58.23364.

6. G. Kreymann and coauthors, The ratio of energy expenditure to nitrogen loss in diverse patient groups—A systematic review, *Clinical Nutrition* 31 (2012): 168–175.

7. Centers for Disease Control and Prevention, Diet/Nutrition, Fast Facts, June 2014, available at www.cdc.gov/nchs/fastats/diet.htm.

8. A. Belza and coauthors, Contribution of gastroenteropancreatic appetite hormones to protein-induced satiety, *American Journal of Clinical Nutrition* 97 (2013): 980–989; M. Journel and coauthors, Brain responses to high-protein diets, *Advances in Nutrition* 3 (2012): 322–329.

9. A. Pan and coauthors, Red meat consumption and mortality, *Archives of Internal Medicine* 172 (2012): 555–563.

10. S. C. Larsson and A. Wolk, Red and processed meat consumption and risk of pancreatic cancer: Meta-analysis of prospective studies, *British Journal of Cancer* 106 (2012): 603–607; A. M. Bernstein and coauthors, Dietary protein sources and the risk of stroke in men and women, *Stroke* 43 (2012): 637–644.

11. P. Hernández-Alonso and coauthors, High dietary protein intake is associated with an increased body weight and total death risk, *Clinical Nutrition* (2015), epub ahead of print, doi: 10.1016/j.clnu.2015.03.016; A. M. Fretts and coauthors, Associations of processed meat and unprocessed red meat intake with incident diabetes: The Strong Heart Family Study,

American Journal of Clinical Nutrition 95 (2012): 752–758.

12. Hernández-Alonso and coauthors, High dietary protein intake is associated with an increased body weight and total death risk, 2015; T. Huang and coauthors, Cardiovascular disease mortality and cancer incidence in vegetarians: A meta-analysis and systematic review, *Annals of Nutrition and Metabolism* 60 (2012): 233–240.

13. J. A. Beto, W. E. Ramirez, and V. K. Bansal, Medial nutrition therapy in adults with chronic kidney disease: Integrating evidence and consensus into practice for the generalist Registered Dietitian Nutritionist, *Journal of the Academy of Nutrition and Dietetics* 114 (2014): 1077–1087; M. Giordano and coauthors, Long-term effects of moderate protein diet on renal function and low-grade inflammation in older adults with type 2 diabetes and chronic kidney disease, *Nutrition* 30 (2014): 1045–1049; S. Ohkawa and coauthors, Attenuation of the activated mammalian target of rapamycin pathway might be associated with renal function reserve by a low-protein diet in the rat remnant kidney model, *Nutrition Research* 33 (2013): 761–771.

14. D. H. Pesta and V. T. Samuel, A high-protein diet for reducing body fat: Mechanisms and possible caveats, *Nutrition and Metabolism* 11 (2014), epub, doi: 10.1186/1743-7075-11-53.

15. J. M. Beasley and coauthors, Biomarker-calibrated protein intake and bone health in the Women's Health Initiative clinical trials and observational study, *American Journal of Clinical Nutrition* 99 (2014): 934–940; T. Remer, D. Krupp, and L. Shi, Dietary protein's and dietary acid load's influence on bone health, *Critical Reviews in Food Science and Nutrition* 54 (2014): 1140–1150.

16. World Health Organization, International Agency for Research on Cancer, IARC Monographs evaluate consumption of red meat and processed meat, Press release no. 240, October 2015, available at http://www.iarc.fr/en/media-centre/pr/2015/pdfs/pr240_E.pdf; P. J. Tárraga López, J. S. Albero, and J. A. Rodríguez-Montes, Primary and secondary prevention of colorectal cancer, *Clinical Medicine Insights: Gastroenterology* 14 (2014): 33–46; E. Kim, D. Coelho, and F. P. Blachier, Review of the association between meat consumption and risk of colorectal cancer, *Nutrition Research* 33 (2013): 983–994; S. C. Larsson and A. Wolk, Red and processed meat consumption and risk of pancreatic cancer: Meta-analysis of prospective studies, *British Journal of Cancer* 106 (2012): 603–607.

17. N. J. Wierdsma and coauthors, Vitamin and mineral deficiencies are highly prevalent in newly diagnosed celiac disease patients, *Nutrients* 5 (2013): 39753992.

18. A Fasano and coauthors, Nonceliac gluten sensitivity, Gastroenterology 148 (2015): 1195–1204; L. Eli, L. Roncoroni, and M. T. Bardella, Non-celiac gluten sensitivity: Time for sifting the grain, *World Journal of Gastroenterology* 21 (2015): 8221–8226; M. M. Leonard and B. Vasagar, US perspective on gluten-related diseases, *Clinical and Experimental Gastroenterology*

7 (2014), epub, doi:10.2147/CEG.S54567; A. D. Sabatino and G. R. Corazza, Non-celiac gluten sensitivity: Sense or sensibility? *Annals of Internal Medicine* 156 (2012): 309–311; M. Pietzak, Celiac disease, wheat allergy, and gluten sensitivity: When gluten free is not a fad, *Journal of Parenteral and Enteral Nutrition* 36 (2012): 68S–75S.

19. K. E. Lundin, Non-celiac gluten sensitivity—Why worry? *BMC Medicine* 12 (2014), epub, doi:10.1186/1741-7015-12-86.

20. T. A. Kabbani and coauthors, Body mass index and the risk of obesity in coeliac disease treated with the gluten-free diet, *Alimentary Pharmacology and Therapeutics* 35 (2012): 723–729.

21. E. Lionetti and coauthors, Celiac disease from a global perspective, *Best Practice and Research: Clinical Gastroenterology* 29 (2015): 365–379; A. Rubio-Tapia and coauthors, The prevalence of celiac disease in the United States, *American Journal of Gastroenterology* 107 (2012): 1538–1544.

Consumer's Guide 6

1. H. J. Leidy and coauthors, The role of protein in weight loss and maintenance, *American Journal of Clinical Nutrition* (2015), epub ahead of print, doi: 10.3945/ajcn.114.084038; D. H. Pesta and V. T. Samuel, A high-protein diet for reducing body fat: Mechanisms and possible caveats, *Nutrition and Metabolism* 11 (2014), epub, doi: 10.1186/1743-7075-11-53; A. Belza and coauthors, Contribution of gastroenteropancreatic appetite hormones to protein-induced satiety, *American Journal of Clinical Nutrition* 97 (2013): 980–989.

2. P. B. Pencharz, R. Elango, and R. O. Ball, Determination of the Tolerable Upper Intake Level of leucine in adult men, *Journal of Nutrition* 142 (2012): 2220S–2224S.

3. D. Seshadri and D. De, Nails in nutritional deficiencies, *Indian Journal of Dermatology, Venereology, and Leprology* 78 (2012): 237–241.

4. J. D. Fernstrom, Effects and side effects associated with the non-nutritional use of tryptophan by humans, *Journal of Nutrition* 142 (2012): 2236S–2244S.

5. H. Y. Guo and coauthors, Hyperhomocysteinemia independently causes and promotes atherosclerosis in LDL receptor-deficient mice, *Journal of Geriatric Cardiology* 11 (2014): 74–78; R. H. Mendes and coauthors, Moderate hyperhomocysteinemia provokes dysfunction of cardiovascular autonomic system and liver oxidative stress in rats, *Autonomic Neuroscience: Basic and Clinical* 180 (2014): 43–47.

6. A. Timcheh-Hariri and coauthors, Toxic hepatitis in a group of 20 male body-builders taking dietary supplements, *Food and Chemical Toxicology* 50 (2012): 3826–3832.

7. L. Wandrag and coauthors, Impact of supplementation with amino acids or their metabolites on muscle wasting in patients with critical illness or other muscle wasting illness: A systematic review, *Journal of Human Nutrition and Dietetics* 28 (2015): 313–330; E. Ridley, D. Gantner, and V. Pellegrino, Nutrition therapy in critically ill patients: A review of current evidence for clinicians, *Clinical Nutrition* (2014), epub, doi:10.1016/j.clnu.2014.12.008.

8. J. I. Boullata and L. M. Hudson, Drug-nutrient interactions: A broad view with implications for practice, *Journal of the Academy of Nutrition and Dietetics* 112 (2012): 506–507.

9. Standing Committee on the Scientific Evaluation of Dietary Reference Intakes, Food and Nutrition Board, Institute of Medicine, *Dietary Reference Intakes for Energy, Carbohydrate, Fiber, Fat, Fatty Acids, Cholesterol, Protein, and Amino Acids* (Washington, D.C.: National Academies Press, 2002/2005), pp. 589–768.

Controversy 6

1. M. J. Orlich and G. E. Frasier, Vegetarian diets in the Adventist Health Study 2: A review of initial published findings, *American Journal of Clinical Nutrition* 100 (2014): 353S–358S; A. Pan and coauthors, Red meat consumption and mortality: Results from 2 prospective cohort studies, *Archives of Internal Medicine* 172 (2012): 555–563.

2. Position of the Academy of Nutrition and Dietetics: Vegetarian diets, *Journal of the Academy of Nutrition and Dietetics* 115 (2015): 801–810; N. S. Rizzo and coauthors, Nutrient profiles of vegetarian and nonvegetarian dietary patterns, *Journal of the Academy of Nutrition and Dietetics* 114 (2014): 1610–1619.

3. X. Wang and coauthors, Fruit and vegetable consumption and mortality from all causes, cardiovascular disease, and cancer: Systematic review and dose-response meta-analysis of prospective cohort studies, *British Medical Journal* 349 (2014), epub, doi:10.1136/bmj.g4490.

4. O. Oyebode and coauthors, Fruit and vegetable consumption and all-cause, cancer and CVD mortality: Analysis of Health Survey for England data, *Journal of Epidemiology and Community Health* 68 (2014): 856–862.

5. P. N. Singh and coauthors, Global epidemiology of obesity, vegetarian dietary patterns, and noncommunicable disease in Asian Indians, *American Journal of Clinical Nutrition* 100 (2014): 359S–364S.

6. F. L. Crow and coauthors, Risk of hospitalization or death from ischemic heart disease among British vegetarians and nonvegetarians: Results from the EPIC-Oxford cohort study, *American Journal of Clinical Nutrition* 97 (2013): 597–603; Pan and coauthors, Red meat consumption and mortality, 2012.

7. Y. Yokoyama and coauthors, Vegetarian diets and blood pressure: A meta-analysis, *JAMA Internal Medicine* 174 (2014): 577–587.

8. World Health Organization, International Agency for Research on Cancer, IARC Monographs evaluate consumption of red meat and processed meat, Press release no. 240, October 2015, available at http://www.iarc.fr/en/media-centre/pr/2015/pdfs/pr240_E.pdf; M. J. Orlich and coauthors, Vegetarian dietary paterns and the risk of colorectal cancers, *JAMA Internal Medicine* 175 (2015): 767–776; D. Demeyer and coauthors, Mechanisms linking colorectal cancer to the consumption of (processed) red meat: A review, *Food Science and Nutrition,* (2015), epub ahead of print,

doi: www.tandfonline.com/action/showCit-Formats?doi=10.1080/10408398.2013.873886; J. C. Figueiredo and coauthors, Genome-wide diet-gene interaction analyses for risk of colorectal cancer, *PLoS Genetics* 10 (2014), epub, doi:10.1371/journal.pgen.1004228.

9. T. J. Key and coauthors, Cancer in British vegetarians: Updated analyses of 4998 incident cancers in a cohort of 32,491 meat eaters, 8612 fish eaters, 18,298 vegetarians, and 2246 vegans, *American Journal of Clinical Nutrition* 100 (2014): 378S–385S.

10. Orlich and Frasier, Vegetarian diets in the Adventist Health Study 2, 2014; T. Huang and coauthors, Cardiovascular disease mortality and cancer incidence in vegetarians: A meta-analysis and systematic review, *Annals of Nutrition and Metabolism* 60 (2012): 233–240; C. T. McEvoy, N. Temple, and J. V. Woodside, Vegetarian diets, low-meat diets and health: A review, *Public Health Nutrition* 15 (2012): 2287–2294; Pan and coauthors, Red meat consumption and mortality, 2012; B. Magalhães and coauthors, Dietary patterns and colorectal cancer: Systematic review and meta-analysis, *European Journal of Cancer Prevention* 21 (2012): 15–23; L. M. Ferrucci and coauthors, Meat consumption and the risk of incident distal colon and rectal adenoma, *British Journal of Cancer* 106 (2012): 608–616.

11. R. Pawlak, S. E. Lester, and T. Babatunde, The prevalence of cobalamin deficiency among vegetarians assessed by serum vitamin B_{12}: A review of literature, *European Journal of Clinical Nutrition* 68 (2014): 541–548; R. Pawlak and coauthors, How prevalent is vitamin B12 deficiency among vegetarians? *Nutrition Reviews* 71 (2013): 110–117.

12. C. Kocaoglu and coauthors, Cerebral atrophy in a vitamin B_{12}-deficient infant of a vegetarian mother, *Journal of Health, Population, and Nutrition* 32 (2014): 367–371.

13. G. J. Lee and coauthors, Consumption of non-cow's milk beverages and serum vitamin D levels in early childhood, *Canadian Medical Association Journal* 186 (2014): 1287–1293; N. F. Krebs and coauthors, Meat consumption is associated with less stunting among toddlers in four diverse low-income settings, *Food and Nutrition Bulletin* 32 (2011): 185–191; M. Van Winckel and coauthors, Clinical practice: Vegetarian infant and child nutrition, *European Journal of Pediatrics* 170 (2011): 1489–1494.

14. R. S. Gibson, A. M. Heath, and E. A. Szymlek-Gay, Is iron and zinc nutrition a concern for vegetarian infants and young children in industrialized nations? *American Journal of Clinical Nutrition* 100 (2014): 459S–468S.

15. P. D. Genaro and coauthors, Dietary protein intake in elderly women: Association with muscle and bone mass, *Nutrition in Clinical Practice* (2014), epub ahead of print, doi:10.1177/0884533614545404.

16. K. L. Tucker, Vegetarian diets and bone status, *American Journal of Clinical Nutrition* 100 (2014): 329S–335S.

17. M. Foster and coauthors, Effect of vegetarian diets on zinc status: A systematic review

and meta-analysis of studies in humans, *Journal of Science in Food and Agriculture* 93 (2013): 2362–2371.

Chapter 7

1. Sy and coauthors, Effects of physiolochemical properties of carotenoids on their bioaccessibility, intestinal cell uptake, and blood and tissue concentrations, *Molecular Nutrition and Food Research* 56 (2012): 1385–1397.

2. J. von Lintig, Metabolism of carotenoids and retinoids related to vision, *Journal of Biological Chemistry* 287 (2012): 1627–1634.

3. C. Rochette-Egly, Retinoic acid signaling and mouse embryonic stem cell differentiation: Cross talk between genomic and non-genomic effects of RA, *Biochemica et Biophysica Acta* (2014), epub ahead of print; C. Skazik and coauthors, Downregulation of STRA6 expression in epidermal keratinocytes leads to hyperproliferation-associated differentiation in both in vitro and in vivo skin models, *Journal of Investigative Dermatology* 134 (2014): 1579–1588; G. Bakdash and coauthors, Retinoic acid primes human dendritic cells to induce gut-homing, IL-10-producing regulatory T cells, *Mucosal Immunology* (2014), epub ahead of print; J. C. Saari, Vitamin A metabolism in rod and cone visual cycles, *Annual Review of Nutrition* 32 (2012): 125–145.

4. S. A. van de Pavert and coauthors, Maternal retinoids control type 3 innate lymphoid cells and set the offspring immunity, *Nature* 508 (2014): 123–127; M. Rhinn and P. Dolle, Retinoic acid signaling during development, *Development* 139 (2012): 843–858.

5. L. B. da Rocha, F. Pichi, and C. Y. Lowder, Night blindness and Crohn's disease, *International Ophthalmology* (2014), epub ahead of print; S. Akhtar and coauthors, Prevalence of vitamin A deficiency in South Asia: Causes, outcomes, and possible remedies, *Journal of Health, Population, and Nutrition* 31 (2013): 413–423.

6. J. C. Sherwin and coauthors, Epidemiology of vitamin A deficiency and xerophthalmia in at-risk populations, *Transactions of the Royal Society of Tropical Medicine and Hygiene* 106 (2012): 205–214.

7. A. Sommer, Preventing blindness and saving lives: The century of vitamin A, *Journal of the American Medical Association Ophthalmology* 132 (2014): 115–117; Sherwin and coauthors, Epidemiology of vitamin A deficiency and xerophthalmia in at-risk populations, 2012.

8. D. C. Berry and coauthors, Retinoic acid upregulates preadipocyte genes to block adipogenesis and suppress diet-induced obesity, *Diabetes* 61 (2012): 1112–1121; Rhinn and Dolle, Retinoic acid signaling during development, 2012.

9. C. A. Klebanoff and coauthors, Retinoic acid controls the homeostasis of pre-cDC-derived splenic and intestinal dendritic cells, *Journal of Experimental Medicine* 210 (2013): 1961–1976; A. C. Ross, Vitamin A and retinoic acid in T cell-related immunity, *American Journal of Clinical Nutrition* 96 (2012): 1166S–1172S.

10. World Health Organization, Measles factsheet, updated February 2014, available at www.who.int/mediacentre/factsheets, f286.

11. E. Samarut and C. Rochette-Egly, Nuclear retinoic acid receptors: Conductors of the retinoic acid symphony during development, *Journal of Molecular and Cellular Endocrinology* 348 (2012): 348–360; R. K. Kam and coauthors, Retinoic acid synthesis and functions in early embryonic development, *Cell and Bioscience* 2 (2012): 11.

12. S. Pinkaew and coauthors, Triple-fortified rice containing vitamin A reduced marginal vitamin A deficiency and increased vitamin A liver stored in school-aged Thai children, *Journal of Nutrition* 144 (2014): 519–524.

13. Centers for Disease Control and Prevention, Measles (Rubeola), in *CDC Health Information for International Travel (The Yellow Book)* (New York: Oxford University Press, 2014), available at www.cdc.gov.

14. R. L. Bailey and coauthors, Examination of vitamin intakes among US adults by dietary supplement use, *Journal of the Academy of Nutrition and Dietetics* 112 (2012): 657–663; Y. A. Shakur and coauthors, A comparison of micronutrient inadequacy and risk of high micronutrient intakes among vitamin and mineral supplement users and nonusers in Canada, *Journal of Nutrition* 142 (2012): 534–540.

15. N. B. Duerbeck and D. D. Dowling, Vitamin A: Too much of a good thing? *Obstetrical & Gynecological Survey* 67 (2012): 122–128; N. Hovdenak and K. Haram, Influence of mineral and vitamin supplements on pregnancy outcome, *European Journal of Obstetrics & Gynecology and Reproductive Biology* 164 (2012): 127–132.

16. N. Prevost and J. C. English, Isotretinoin: Update on controversial issues, *Journal of Pediatric and Adolescent Gynecology* 26 (2013): 290–293.

17. Y. Wang and coauthors, Dietary carotenoids are associated with cardiovascular disease risk biomarkers mediated by serum carotenoid concentrations, *Journal of Nutrition* 144 (2014): 1067–1074; E. M. Abdel-Aal and coauthors, Dietary sources of lutein and zeaxanthin carotenoids and their role in eye health, *Nutrients* 5 (2013): 1169–1185; W. Stahl and H. Sies, β-Carotene and other carotenoids in protection from sunlight, *American Journal of Clinical Nutrition* 96 (2012): 1179S–1184S; D. Aune and coauthors, Dietary compared with blood concentration of carotenoids and breast cancer risk: A systematic review and meta-analysis of prospective studies, *American Journal of Clinical Nutrition* 356 (2012): 356–373.

18. C. J. Chiu and coauthors, The relationship of major American dietary patterns to age-related macular degeneration, *American Journal of Ophthalmology* 158 (2014): 118–127.

19. W. Andreatta and S. El-Sherbiny, Evidence-based nutritional advice for patients affected by age-related macular degeneration, *Ophthalmologica* 231 (2014): 185–190; M. D. Pinazo-Duran and coauthors, Do nutrition supplements have a role in age macular degeneration prevention? *Journal of Ophthalmology* (2014), epub,

doi:10.1155/2014/901686; J. R. Evans and J. G. Lawrenson, Antioxidant vitamin and mineral supplements for preventing age-related macular degeneration, *Cochrane Database Systematic Reviews* (2012), epub, doi:10.1002/14651858. CD000253.pub3.

20. R. D. Whitehead and coauthors, You are what you eat: Within-subject increases in fruit and vegetable consumption confer beneficial skin-color changes, *PLoS ONE* 7 (2012), epub, doi:10.1371/journal.pone.0032988.

21. V. Ganji, X. Zhang, and V. Tangpricha, Serum 25-hydroxyvitamin D concentrations and prevalence estimates of hypovitaminosis D in the U.S. population based on assay-adjusted data, *Journal of Nutrition* 142 (2012): 498–507.

22. L. Lieben and coauthors, Normocalcemia is maintained in mice under conditions of calcium malabsorption by vitamin D-induced inhibition of bone mineralization, *Journal of Clinical Investigation* 122 (2012): 1803–1815.

23. P. R. Ebeling, Vitamin D and bone health: Epidemiologic studies, *BoneKEy Reports* 3 (2014): 511.

24. G. J. Fung and coauthors, Vitamin D intake is inversely related to risk of developing metabolic syndrome in African American and white men and women over 20 y: The Coronary Artery Risk Development in Young Adults Study, *American Journal of Clinical Nutrition* 96 (2012): 24–29; I. Laaski, Vitamin D and respiratory infections in adults, *Proceedings of the Nutrition Society* 71 (2012): 90–97; Y. Liss and W. H. Frishman, Vitamin D: A cardioprotective agent? *Cardiology in Review* 20 (2012): 38–44; A. Zittermann and coauthors, Vitamin D deficiency and mortality risk in the general population: A meta-analysis of prospective cohort studies, *American Journal of Clinical Nutrition* 95 (2012): 91–100.

25. N. H. Golden, S. A. Abrams, and Committee on Nutrition, Optimizing bone health in children and adolescents, *Pediatrics* 134 (2014): e1229–e1243; J. Czech-Kowalska and coauthors, Impact of vitamin D supplementation during lactation on vitamin D status and body composition of mother-infant pairs: A MAVID randomized controlled trial, *PLOS ONE* 9 (2014): e107708; U.S. Preventive Services Task Force, Vitamin D and calcium supplementation to prevent cancer and osteoporotic fractures (Draft recommendations), August 2012, available at www.uspreventiveservicestaskforce.org/uspstf12/vitamind/vitdart.htm.

26. S. J. Wimalawansa, Vitamin D in the new millennium, *Current Osteoporosis Reports* 10 (2012): 4–15; C. B. Turer, H. Lin, and G. Flores, Prevalence of vitamin D deficiency among overweight and obese US children, *Pediatrics* 131 (2013): e152–e161.

27. T. D. Thacher and coauthors, Increasing incidence of nutritional rickets: A population-based study in Olmsted County, Minnesota, *Mayo Clinic Proceedings* 88 (2013): 176–183.

28. K. Shikino, M. Ikusaka, and T. Yamashita, Vitamin D-deficient osteomalacia due to excessive self-restrictions for atopic dermatitis, *The BMJ* (2014), doi:10.1136/bcr-2014-204558.

29. L. D. Gillespie and coauthors, Interventions for preventing falls in older people living in the community, *Cochrane Database of Systematic Reviews* 9 (2012): CD007146, doi:10.1002/14651858.CD007146.pub3; U.S. Preventive Services Task Force, Vitamin D and calcium supplementation to prevent cancer and osteoporotic fractures, 2012; V. A. Moyer and the U.S. Preventive Services Task Force, Prevention of falls in community-dwelling older adults: U.S. Preventive Services Task Force recommendation statement, *Annals of Internal Medicine* 157 (2012): 197–204.

30. L. Samuel and L. N. Borrell, The effect of body mass index on adequacy of serum 25-hydroxyvitamin D levels in US adults: The National Health and Nutrition Examination Survey 2001 to 2006, *Annals of Epidemiology* 24 (2014): 781–784.

31. Turer and coauthors, Prevalence of vitamin D deficiency among overweight and obese US children, 2013.

32. K. S. Vimaleswaran and coauthors, Causal relationship between obesity and vitamin D status: Bi-directional Mendelian randomization analysis of multiple cohorts, *PLoS Medicine* 10 (2013): e1001383.

33. A. T. Drincic and coauthors, Volumetric dilution, rather than sequestration best explains the low vitamin D status of obesity, *Obesity* 20 (2012): 1444–1448; J. E. Heller and coauthors, Relation between vitamin D status and body composition in collegiate athletes, *International Journal of Sports Nutrition, Exercise, and Metabolism* (2014), epub ahead of print; S. J. Mutt and coauthors, Vitamin D and adipose tissue—More than storage, *Frontiers in Physiology* 24 (2014): 228.

34. F. Alshahrani and N. Aljohani, Vitamin D: Deficiency, sufficiency and toxicity, *Nutrients* 5 (2013): 3605–3616.

35. H. Ketha and coauthors, Iatrogenic vitamin D toxicity in an infant: A case report and review of literature, *Journal of Steroid Biochemistry and Molecular Biology* 148 (2015): 14–18; J. R. Genzen, Hypercalcemic crisis due to vitamin D toxicity, *Lab Medicine* 45 (2014): 147–150; S. M. Alsanad, E. M. Williamson, and R. L. Howard, Cancer patients at risk of herb/food supplement-drug interactions: A systematic review, *Phytotherapy Research* 28 (2014): 1749–1755; Committee on Dietary Reference Intakes, *Dietary Reference Intakes for Calcium and Vitamin D* (Washington, D.C.: National Academies Press, 2011), pp. 125–344.

36. A. K. Kasahara, R. J. Singh, and A. Noymer, Vitamin D (25OHD) serum seasonality in the United States, PLOS ONE 8 (2013): e65785; D. A. Wahl and coauthors, A global representation of vitamin D status in healthy populations, *Archives of Osteoporosis* 7 (2012): 155–172.

37. Committee on Dietary Reference Intakes, *Dietary Reference Intakes for Calcium and Vitamin D*, 2011, p. 6.

38. E. M. Brouwer-Brolsma and coauthors, Vitamin D: Do we get enough? *Osteoporosis International* 24 (2013): 1567–1577; P. Pramyothin and M. F. Holick, Vitamin D supplementation: Guidelines and evidence for subclinical deficiency, *Current Opinion in Gastroenterology* 28 (2012): 139–150.

39. H. L. Kristensen, E. Rosenqvist, and J. Jacobsen, Increase in vitamin D(2) by UV-B exposure during the growth phase of white button mushroom (agaricua bisporus), *Food and Nutrition Research* 56 (2012), doi:10.3402/fnr.v56i0.7114.

40. F. Mangialasche and coauthors, Tocopherols and tocotrienols plasma levels are associated with cognitive impairment, *Neurobiology of Aging* 33 (2012): 2282–2290; V. K. Singh, L. A. Beattie, and T. M. Seed, Vitamin E: Tocopherols and tocotrienols as potential radiation countermeasures, *Journal of Radiation Research* 54 (2013): 973–988; V. Patel and coauthors, Oral tocotrienols are transported to human tissues and delay the progression of the model for end-stage liver disease score in patients, *Journal of Nutrition* 142 (2012): 513–519.

41. P. R. Di and S. Cuzzocrea, Reactive oxygen species, inflammation, and lung diseases, *Current Pharmaceutical Design* 18 (2012): 3889–3900; Y. W. Kim, X. Z. West, and T. V. Byzova, Inflammation and oxidative stress in angiogenesis and vascular disease, *Journal of Molecular Medicine* 91 (2013): 323–328.

42. E. Giraldo and coauthors, Aβ and tau toxicities in Alzheimer's are linked via oxidative stress-induced p38 activation: Protective role of vitamin E, *Redox Biology* 2 (2014): 873–877; J. Virtamo and coauthors, Effects of α-tocopherol and β-carotene supplementation on cancer incidence and mortality: 18-year postintervention follow-up of the Alpha-tocopherol, Beta-carotene Cancer Prevention Study, *International Journal of Cancer* 135 (2014): 178–185; M. F. Rossato and coauthors, Anti-inflammatory effects of vitamin E on adjuvant-induced arthritis in rats, *Inflammation* (2014), epub ahead of print, PMID: 25120238.

43. Y. Gopalan and coauthors, Clinical investigation of the effects of palm vitamin E tocotrienols on brain white matter, *Stroke* 45 (2014): 1422–1428; T. H. Kang and coauthors, Treatment of tumors with vitamin E suppresses myeloid derived suppressor cells and enhances CD8+ T cell-mediated antitumor effects, *PLOS ONE* 9 (2014): e103562.

44. M. J. Stanger and coauthors, Anticoagulant activity of select dietary supplements, *Nutrition Reviews* 70 (2012): 107–117.

45. G. Bjelakovic and coauthors, Antioxidant supplements for prevention of mortality in healthy participants and patients with various diseases, *Cochrane Database of Sytematic Reviews* 3 (2012): CD007176.

46. S. Jiang and coauthors, Meta-analysis: Low-dose intake of vitamin E combined with other vitamins or minerals may decrease all-cause mortality, *Journal of Nutritional Science and Vitaminology* 60 (2014): 194–205; Virtamo and

coauthors, Effects of α-tocopherol and β-carotene supplementation on cancer incidence and mortality, 2014.

47. U.S. Department of Agriculture and U.S. Department of Health and Human Services, Scientific report of the 2015 Dietary Guidelines Advisory Committee, 2015, D-1:8, available at www.health.gov; P. Borel, D. Preveraud, and C. Desmarchelier, Bioavailability of vitamin E in humans: An update, *Nutrition Reviews* 71 (2013): 319–331; U.S. Department of Agriculture, Agricultural Research Service, What we eat in America: NHANES 2009–2010, Table 1, Nutrient intakes from food: Mean amounts consumed per individual, by gender and age, in the United States, 2009–2010, available at www.ars.usda.gov.

48. E. M. Hawes and A. J. Viera, Anticoagulation: Managing adverse events in patients receiving anticoagulation and perioperative care, *FP Essentials* 422 (2014): 31–39.

49. A. Urano and coauthors, Vitamin K deficiency evaluated by serum levels of undercarboxylated osteocalcin in patients with anorexia nervosa with bone loss, *Journal of Clinical Nutrition* (2014), doi:10.1016/j.clnu.2014.04.016; T. Matsumoto, T. Miyakawa, and D. Yamamoto, Effects of vitamin K on the morphometric and material properties of bone in the tibiae of growing rats, *Metabolism Clinical and Experimental* 61 (2012): 407–414.

50. A. C. Torbergsen and coauthors, Vitamin K1 and 25(OH)D are independently and synergistically associated with a risk for hip fracture in an elderly population: A case control study, *Journal of Clinical Nutrition* (2014), doi:10.1016/j.clnu.2014.01.016.

51. M. S. Hamidi and A. M. Cheung, Vitamin K and musculoskeletal health in postmenopausal women, *Molecular Nutrition and Food Research* 58 (2014): 1647–1657; C. M. Gundberg, J. B. Lian, and S. L. Booth, Vitamin K-dependent carboxylation of osteocalcin: Friend or foe? *Advances in Nutrition* 3 (2012): 149–157.

52. V. Sahni, F. Y. Lai, and S. E. MacDonald, Neonatal vitamin K refusal and nonimmunization, *Journal of Pediatrics* (2014), epub ahead of print; M. J. Shearer, X. Fu, and S. L. Booth, Vitamin K nutrition, metabolism, and requirements: Current concepts and future research, *Advances in Nutrition* 3 (2012): 182–195.

53. R. Schulte and coauthors, Rise in late onset vitamin K deficiency bleeding in young infants because of omission or refusal of prophylaxis at birth, *Pediatric Neurology* 50 (2014): 564–568; Centers for Disease Control and Prevention, Notes from the field: Late vitamin K deficiency bleeding in infants whose parents declined vitamin K prophylaxis—Tennessee, 2013, *Morbidity and Mortality Weekly Report* 62 (2013): 901–902.

54. P. G. Cocate and coauthors, Fruit and vegetable intake and related nutrients are associated with oxidative stress markers in middle-aged men, *Journal of Nutrition* 30 (2014): 660–665; M. F. Garcia-Saura and coauthors, Nitroso-redox status and vascular function in marginal and severe ascorbate deficiency, *Antioxidants and Redox Signaling* 17 (2012): 937–950.

55. J. J. Yin and coauthors, Dual role of selected antioxidants found in dietary supplements: Crossover between anti- and pro-oxidant activities in the presence of copper, *Journal of Agricultural and Food Chemistry* 60 (2012): 2554–2561.

56. P. H. Lin, W. Aronson, and S. J. Freedland, Nutrition, dietary interventions and prostate cancer: The latest evidence, *BMC Medicine* 13 (2015), epub, doi:10.1186/s12916-014-0234-y.

57. G. M. Allan and B. Arroll, Prevention and treatment of the common cold: Making sense of the evidence, *Canadian Medical Association Journal* 186 (2014): 190–199; H. Hemila and E. Chalker, Vitamin C for preventing and treating the common cold, *Cochrane Database of Systematic Reviews* 31 (2013): CD000980, doi:10.1002/14651858.

58. S. M. Bozonet and coauthors, Enhanced human neutrophil vitamin C status, chemotaxis and oxidant generation following dietary supplementation with vitamin C-rich SunGold kiwifruit, *Nutrients* 7 (2015): 2574–2588.

59. J. Ong and R. Randhawa, Scurvy in an alcoholic patient treated with intravenous vitamins, *British Medical Journal Case Reports* (2014), doi:10.1136/bcr-2013-009479; P. Zammit, Vitamin C deficiency in an elderly adult, *Journal of the American Geriatrics Society* 61 (2013): 657–658.

60. S. Yaich and coauthors, Secondary oxalosis due to excess vitamin C intake: A cause of graft loss in a renal transplant recipient, *Saudi Journal of Kidney Diseases and Transplantation* 25 (2014): 113–116; L. D. Thomas and coauthors, Ascorbic acid supplements and kidney stone incidence among men: A prospective study, *Journal of the American Medical Association* 173 (2013): 386–388.

61. E. Isenberg-Grzeda, H. E. Kutner, and S. E. Nicolson, Wernicke-Korsakoff-syndrome: Under-recognized and under-treated, *Journal of Psychosomatics* 53 (2012): 507–516.

62. Y. P. Wang and coauthors, Riboflavin supplementation improves energy metabolism in mice exposed to acute hypoxia, *Physiological Research* 63 (2014): 341–350.

63. A. A. Badawy, Pellagra and alcoholism: A biochemical perspective, *Alcohol and Alcoholism* 49 (2014): 238–250.

64. G. P. Frank and coauthors, Pellagra: A non-communicable disease of poverty, *Tropical Doctor* 42 (2012): 182–184; B. Kavitha, R. Balasubramanian, and T. Kumar, Electrocardiographic enigma of a classical disease: Pellagra, *Tropical Doctor* 42 (2012): 211–213.

65. D. MacKay, J. Hathcock, and E. Guarneri, Niacin: Chemical forms, bioavailability, and health effects, *Nutrition Reviews* 70 (2012): 357–366.

66. A. L. Catapano and coauthors, Combination therapy in dyslipidemia: Where are we now? *Atherosclerosis* 237 (2014): 319–335; J. E. Digby, N. Ruparelia, and R. P. Choudhury, Niacin in cardiovascular disease: Recent preclinical and clinical developments, *Arteriosclerosis, Thrombosis, and Vascular Biology* 32 (2012): 582–588.

67. S. Tuteja and D. J. Rader, Dyslipidemia: Cardiovascular prevention—End of the road for niacin? *Nature Reviews Endocrinology* (2014), epub ahead of print, doi:10.1038/nrendo.2014.159.

68. Tuteja and Rader, Dyslipidemia, 2014.

69. T. J. Anderson and coauthors, Safety profile of extended-release niacin in the AIM–HIGH trial, *New England Journal of Medicine* 371 (2014): 288–290.

70. R. P. da Silva and coauthors, Novel insights on interactions between folate and lipid metabolism, *BioFactors* 40 (2014): 277–283; S. C. Kalhan and S. E. Marczewski, Methionine, homocysteine, one carbon metabolism and fetal growth, *Reviews in Endocrine and Metabolic Disorders* 13 (2012): 109–119.

71. B. A. Jennings and G. Willis, How folate metabolism affects colorectal cancer development and treatment: A story of heterogeneity and pleiotropy, *Cancer Letters* 356 (2015), epub, doi:10.1016/j.canlet.2014.02.024; M. Tio and coauthors, Folate intake and the risk of prostate cancer: A systematic review and meta-analysis, *Prostate Cancer and Prostatic Diseases* 17 (2014): 213–219; K. C. Strickland, N. I. Krupenko, and S. A. Krupenko, Molecular mechanisms underlying the potentially adverse effects of folate, *Clinical Chemistry and Laboratory Medicine* 51 (2013): 607–616.

72. A. E. Czeizel and coauthors, Folate deficiency and folic acid supplementation: The prevention of neural-tube defects and congenital heart defects, *Nutrients* 5 (2013): 4760–4775.

73. C. M. Marchetta and coauthors, Assessing the association between natural food folate intake and blood folate concentrations: A systematic review and Bayesian meta-analysis of trials and observational studies, *Nutrients* 7 (2015): 2663–2686.

74. C. M. Pfeiffer and coauthors, Estimation of trends in serum and RBC folate in the U.S. population from pre- to postfortification using assay-adjusted data from the NHANES 1988–2010, *Journal of Nutrition* 142 (2012): 886–893; Centers for Disease Control and Prevention, Executive Summary, Second National Report on Biochemical Indicators of Diet and Nutrition in the U.S. Population, 2012, available at www.cdc.gov/nutritionreport/.

75. S. P. Stabler, Clinical practice: Vitamin B12 deficiency, *New England Journal of Medicine* 368 (2013): 149–160; P. Gudgeon and R. Cavalcanti, Folate testing in hospital patients, *American Journal of Medicine* (2014), doi:10.1016/j.amjmed.2014.08.020.

76. J. Choi and coauthors, Contemporary issues surrounding folic acid fortification initiatives, *Preventive Nutrition and Food Science* 19 (2014): 247–260.

77. C. M. Pfeiffer and coauthors, Assessing vitamin status in large population surveys by measuring biomarkers and dietary intake—Two case

studies: Folate and vitamin D, *Food and Nutrition Research* 56 (2012), doi:10.3402/fnr.v56i0.5944.

78. N. Farahi and A. Zolotor, Recommendations for preconception counseling and care, *American Family Physician* 88 (2013): 499–506.

79. R. Carmel, Subclinical cobalamin deficiency, *Current Opinion in Gastroenterology* 28 (2012): 151–158.

80. U. Grober, K. Kisters, and J. Schmidt, Neuroenhancement with vitamin B12—Underestimated neurological significance, *Nutrients* 5 (2013): 5031–5045; J. G. Walker and coauthors, Oral folic acid and vitamin B-12 supplementation to prevent cognitive decline in community-dwelling older adults with depressive symptoms—The Beyond Ageing Project: A randomized controlled trial, *American Journal of Clinical Nutrition* 95 (2012): 194–203.

81. A. Hunt, D. Harrington, and S. Robinson, Vitamin B12 deficiency, *British Medical Journal* 349 (2014): g5226; A. Permoda-Osip and coauthors, Hyperhomocysteinemia in bipolar depression: Clinical and biochemical correlates, *Neuropsychobiology* 68 (2013):193–196.

82. M. L. Schubert, Gastric secretion, *Current Opinions in Gastroenterology* 30 (2014): 578–582; R. Kozyraki and O. Cases, Vitamin B12 absorption: Mammalian physiology and acquired and inherited disorders, *Biochimie* 95 (2013): 1002–1007; Moore and coauthors, Cognitive impairment and vitamin B12, 2012.

83. M. L. Tung and L. K. Tan, Long term use of metformin leading to vitamin B 12 deficiency, *Diabetes Research and Clinical Practice* 104 (2014): e75–e76.

84. B. Debreceni and L. Debreceni, The role of homocysteine-lowering B-vitamins in the primary prevention of cardiovascular disease, *Cardiovascular Therapeutics* 32 (2014): 130–138; G. Lurie and coauthors, Prediagnostic plasma pyridoxal 5'-phosphate (vitamin b6) levels and invasive breast carcinoma risk: The multiethnic cohort, *Cancer Epidemiology, Biomarkers, and Prevention* 21 (2012): 1942–1948.

85. J. Zempleni and coauthors, Novel roles of holocarboxylase synthetase in gene regulation and intermediary metabolism, *Nutrition Reviews* 72 (2014): 369–376.

86. J. A. Ash and coauthors, Maternal choline supplementation improves spatial mapping and increases basal forebrain cholinergic neuron number and size in aged Ts65Dn mice, *Neurobiology of Disease* 70 (2014): 32–42; J. Yan and coauthors, Pregnancy alters cholione dynamics: Results of a randomized trial using stable isotope methodology in pregnant and nonpregnant women, *American Journal of Clinical Nutrition* 98 (2013): 1459–1467; S. H. Zeisel, Nutrition in pregnancy: The argument for including a source of choline, *International Journal of Women's Health* 5 (2013): 193–199.

87. Zeisel, Nutrition in pregnancy, 2013.

88. S. B. Procter and C. G. Campbell, Position of the Academy of Nutrition and Dietetics: Nutrition and lifestyle for a healthy pregnancy outcome, *Journal of the Academy of Nutrition and Dietetics* 114 (2014): 1099–1103.

89. D. R. Jacobs and L. C. Tapsell, Food synergy: The key to a healthy diet, *Proceedings of the Nutrition Society* 72 (2013): 200–206; H. Boeing and coauthors, Critical review: Vegetables and fruit in the prevention of chronic diseases, *European Journal of Nutrition* 51 (2012): 637–663.

Consumer's Guide 7

1. U.S. Department of Agriculture and U.S. Department of Health and Human Services, Scientific report of the 2015 Dietary Guidelines Advisory Committee, 2015, D-1:27, available at www.health.gov; L. J. Black and coauthors, An updated systematic review and meta-analysis of the efficacy of vitamin D food fortification, *Journal of Nutrition* 142 (2012): 1102–1108.

2. J. I. Boullata, Vitamin D supplementation: A pharmacologic perspective, *Current Opinion in Clinical Nutrition & Metabolic Care* 15 (2012): 677–684.

3. D. V. Dudenkov and coauthors, Changing incidence of serum 25-hydroxyvitamin D values above 50 ng/mL: A 10-year population-based study, *Mayo Clinic Proceedings* 90 (2015): 577–587; U.S. Preventive Services Task Force, Vitamin D and calcium supplementation to prevent fractures in adults: Recommendation statement, *American Family Physician* 89 (2014), epub.

4. D. E. Godar and coauthors, Solar UV doses of young Americans and vitamin D3 production, *Environmental Health Perspectives* 120 (2012): 139–143.

5. S. Kannan and H. W. Lim, Photoprotection and vitamin D: A review, *Photodermatology, Photoimmunology and Photomedicine* 30 (2014): 137–145; E. Linos and coauthors, Sun protective behaviors and vitamin D levels in the US population: NHANES 2003–2006, *Cancer Causes and Control* 23 (2012): 133–140.

6. U.S. Department of Agriculture and U.S. Department of Health and Human Services, Scientific report of the 2015 Dietary Guidelines Advisory Committee, 2015, D-1:27, 31, available at www.health.gov.

Controversy 7

1. M. L. Garcia-Cazarin and coauthors, Dietary supplement research portfolio at the NIH, 2009–2011, *Journal of Nutrition* 144 (2014): 414–418; R. L. Bailey and coauthors, Examination of vitamin intakes among US adults by dietary supplement use, *Journal of the Academy of Nutrition and Dietetics* 112 (2012): 657–663.

2. Centers for Disease Control and Prevention, Notes from the field: Late vitamin K deficiency in infants whose parents declined vitamin K prophylaxis—Tennessee, 2013, *Morbidity and Mortality Weekly Report* 62 (2013): 901–902; M. J. Shearer, X. Fu, and S. L. Booth, Vitamin K nutrition, metabolism, and requirements: Current concepts and future research, *Advances in Nutrition* 3 (2012): 182–195.

3. J. R. Cherry-Bukowiec, Optimizing nutrition therapy to enhance mobility in critically ill patients, *Critical Care Nursing Quarterly* 36 (2013): 28–36; W. Manzanares, P. L. Langlois, and G. Hardy, Update on antioxidant

micronutrients in the critically ill, *Current Opinion in Clinical Nutrition and Metabolic Care* 16 (2013): 719–725; J. I. Mechanick and coauthors, Clinical practice guidelines for the perioperative nutritional, metabolic, and nonsurgical support of the bariatric surgery patient—2013 update: Cosponsored by American Association of Clinical Endocrinologists, The Obesity Society, and American Society for Metabolic and Bariatric Surgery, *Obesity* 21 (2013): S1–S27.

4. R. L. Bailey and coauthors, Examination of vitamin intakes among US adults by dietary supplement use, *Journal of the Academy of Nutrition and Dietetics* 112 (2012): 657–663; Y. A. Shakur and coauthors, A comparison of micronutrient inadequacy and risk of high micronutrient intakes among vitamin and mineral supplement users and nonusers in Canada, *Journal of Nutrition* 142 (2012): 534–540.

5. A. Timcheh-Hariri and coauthors, Toxic hepatitis in a group of 20 male body-builders taking dietary supplements, *Food and Chemical Toxicology* 50 (2012): 3826–3832.

6. J. M. Mowry and coauthors, 2012 annual report of the American Association of Poison Control Centers' National Poison Data System (NPDS): 30th annual report, *Clinical Toxicology* 51 (2013): 949–1229.

7. FDA, Letter to manufacturers of dietary supplements, December 15, 2010, available at www.fda.gov.

8. S. J. Genuis and coauthors, Toxic element contamination of natural health products and pharmaceutical preparations, *PLoS One* 7 (2012): e49676; L. Foster and coauthors, Multiple dosing of ephedra-free dietary supplements: Hemodynamic, electrocardiographic, and bacterial contamination effects, *Clinical Pharmacology and Therapeutics* 93 (2013): 267–274.

9. ConsumerLab.com, Product review: Multivitamin and mulitmineral supplements review, 2014, available at www.consumerlab.com.

10. P. Gusev and coauthors, Over-the-counter prenatal multivitamin/mineral products: Chemical analysis for the dietary supplement ingredient database, *Journal of the Federation of American Societies for Experimental Biology* 28 (2014): 809.3.

11. P. A. Cohen and coauthors, Presence of banned drugs in dietary supplements following FDA recalls, *Journal of the American Medical Association* 312 (2014): 1691–1693.

12. D. R. Jacobs, L. C. Tapsell, and N. J. Temple, Food synergy: The key to balancing the nutrition research effort, *Public Health Reviews* 33 (2012): 507–529.

13. K. M. Wesa and coauthors, Serum 25-hydroxy vitamin D and survival in advanced colorectal cancer: A retrospective analysis, *Nutrition and Cancer* (2015): 1–7, epub ahead of print.

14. G. Bjelakovic and coauthors, Vitamin D supplementation for prevention of cancer in adults, *Cochrane Database of Systematic Reviews* 6 (2014): CD007469, doi:10.1002/14651858. CD007469.pub2; Committee on Dietary Reference Intakes, *Dietary Reference Intakes for Calcium*

and *Vitamin D* (Washington, D.C.: National Academies Press, 2011), pp. 125–344.

15. U.S. Preventive Services Task Force, Vitamin D and calcium supplementation to prevent cancer and osteoporotic fractures (Draft recommendations), August 2012, available at www.uspreventiveservicestaskforce.org/uspstf12/vitamind/vitdart.htm.

16. M. J. Bolland, A. Grey, and I. R. Reid, Calcium supplements and cardiovascular risk: 5 years on, *Therapeutic Advances in Drug Safety* 4 (2013): 199–210; H. D. Sesso and coauthors, Multivitamins in the prevention of cardiovascular disease in men: The Physician's Health Study II randomized controlled trial, *Journal of the American Medical Association* 308 (2012): 1802–1803; H. Macpherson, A. Pipingas, and M. P. Pase, Multivitamin-multimineral supplementation and mortality: A meta-analysis of randomized controlled trials, *American Journal of Clinical Nutrition* 97 (2013): 437–444; S. P. Fortmann and coauthors, Vitamin and mineral supplements in the primary prevention of cardiovascular disease and cancer: An updated systematic evidence review for the U.S. Preventive Services Task Force, *Annals of Internal Medicine* 159 (2013): 824–834; M. E. Martinez and coauthors, Dietary supplements and cancer prevention: Balancing potential benefits against proven harms, *Journal of the National Cancer Institute* 104 (2012): 732–739.

17. X. Wang and coauthors, Dietary calcium intake and mortality risk from cardiovascular disease and all causes: A meta-analysis of prospective cohort studies, *BioMed Central Medicine* 12 (2014): 158; M. P. Rayman, Selenium and human health, *Lancet* 379 (2012): 1256–1268.

18. J. Z. Selin and coauthors, High-dose supplements of vitamins C and E, low-dose multivitamins, and the risk of age-related cataract: A population-based prospective cohort study of men, *American Journal of Epidemiology* 177 (2013): 548–555; S. P. Juraschek and coauthors, Effects of vitamin C supplementation on blood pressure: A meta-analysis of randomized controlled trials, *American Journal of Clinical Nutrition* 95 (2012): 1079–1088.

19. Y. H. Cui, C. X. Jing, and H. W. Pan, Association of blood antioxidants and vitamins with risk of age-related cataract: A meta-analysis of observational studies, *American Journal of Clinical Nutrition* 98 (2013): 778–786; M. C. Mathew, A. M. Ervin, and R. M. Davis, Antioxidant vitamin supplementation for preventing and slowing the progression of age-related cataract, *Cochrane Database of Systematic Reviews* 6 (2012): CD004567, doi:10.1002/14651858.CD004567.pub2.

20. J. Tinkel, H. Hassanain, and S. Khouri, Cardiovascular antioxidant therapy: A review of supplements, pharmacotherapies, and mechanisms, *Cardiology in Review* 20 (2012): 77–83.

21. A. W. Ashor and coauthors, Effect of vitamin C and vitamin E supplementation on endothelial function: A systematic review and meta-analysis of randomised controlled trials, *British Journal of Nutrition* 113 (2015): 1182–1194; C. U. Chae and coauthors, Vitamin E supplementation and the risk of heart failure in women, *Circulation: Heart Failure* 5 (2012): 176–182.

22. A. J. Curtis and coauthors, Vitamin E supplementation and mortality in healthy people: A meta-analysis of randomised controlled trials, *Cardiovascular Drugs and Therapy* 28 (2014): 563–573; Y. Wang, O. K. Chun, and W. O. Song, Plasma and dietary antioxidant status as cardiovascular disease risk factors: A review of human studies, *Nutrients* 5 (2013): 2969–3004.

23. B. Debreceni and L. Debreceni, Why do homocysteine-lowering B vitamin and antioxidant E vitamin supplements appear to be ineffective in the prevention of cardiovascular diseases? *Cardiovascular Therapeutics* 30 (2012): 227–233.

24. S. M. Jeurnink and coauthors, Plasma carotenoids, vitamin C, retinol and tocopherols levels and pancreatic cancer risk within the European Prospective Investigation into Cancer and Nutrition: A nested case-control study: Plasma micronutrients and pancreatic cancer risk, *International Journal of Cancer* (2014), epub ahead of print, doi:10.1002/ijc.29175; C. S. Yang, N. Suh, and A. T. Kong, Does vitamin E prevent or promote cancer? *Cancer Prevention Research* 5 (2012): 701–705.

25. V. A. Moyer and the U.S. Preventive Services Task Force, Vitamin, mineral, and multivitamin supplements for the primary prevention of cardiovascular disease and cancer: U.S. Preventive Services Task Force recommendation statement, *Annals of Internal Medicine* 160 (2014): 558–564.

Chapter 8

1. U.S. Department of Health and Human Services and U.S. Department of Agriculture, *2015–2020 Dietary Guidelines for Americans*, 8th edition (2015), available at http://health.gov/dietaryguidelines/2015/guidelines/.

2. W. C. Bae and coauthors, Quantitative ultra-short echo time (UTE) MRI of human cortical bone: Correlation with porosity and biomechanical properties, *Journal of Bone and Mineral Research* 27 (2012): 848–857.

3. J. D. Louden, Regulation of fluid and electrolyte balance, *Anaesthesia and Intensive Care Medicine* 13 (2012): 302–308.

4. S. N. Cheuvront and R. W. Kenefick, Dehydration: Physiology, assessment, and performance effects, *Comprehensive Physiology* 4 (2014): 257–285.

5. A. Drewnowski, C. D. Rehm, and F. Constant, Water and beverage consumption among adults in the United States: Cross-sectional study using data from NHANES 2005–2010, *Biomed Central Public Health* 13 (2013): 1068, doi:10.1186/1471-2458-13-1068; S. M. Shirreffs, Global patterns of water intake: How intake data affect recommendations, *Nutrition Reviews* 70 (2012): S98–S100.

6. Drewnowski, Rehm, and Constant, Water and beverage consumption among adults in the United States, 2013; Shirreffs, Global patterns of water intake, 2012.

7. United Nations, Water cooperation facts and figures, 2013, available at www.unwater.org/water-cooperation-2013/water-cooperation/facts-and-figures/en/.

8. U.S. Environmental Protection Agency, Actions you can take to reduce lead in drinking water, 2013, available at water.epa.gov/drink/info/lead/lead1.cfm.

9. Y. Zhao and coauthors, Occurrence and formation of chloro- and bromo-benzoquinones during drinking water disinfection, *Water Research* 46 (2012): 4351–4360; P. A. Neale and coauthors, Bioanalytical assessment of the formation of disinfection byproducts in a drinking water treatment plant, *Environmental Science and Technology* 46 (2012): 10317–10325.

10. U.S. Food and Drug Administration, Bottled water everywhere: Keeping it safe, 2013, available at www.fda.gov/ForConsumers/Consumer Updates.

11. U.S. Food and Drug Administration, FDA regulates the safety of bottled water beverages including flavored water and nutrient-added water beverages, Food Facts, 2014, available at www.fda.gov/food/foodborneillnesscontaminants/buystoreservesafefood/ucm046894.htm; Natural Resources Defense Council, Bottled water: Pure drink or pure hype?, 2013, available at www.nrdc.org/water/drinking/bw/bwinx.asp.

12. U.S. Food and Drug Administration, Code of federal regulations, Title 21—Food and drugs, Part 129 Processing and bottling of bottled drinking water, 2014, available at www.accessdata.fda.gov/scripts/cdrh/cfdocs/cfcfr/cfrsearch.cfm?cfrpart=129&showfr=1.

13. U.S. Department of Agriculture and U.S. Department of Health and Human Services, Scientific report of the 2015 Dietary Guidelines Advisory Committee, 2015, D-6:8–15, available at www.health.gov; S. Agarwal and coauthors, Comparison of prevalence of inadequate nutrient intake based on body weight status of adults in the United States: An analysis of NHANES 2001–2008, *Journal of the American College of Nutrition* 7 (2015): 1–9; C. E. O'Neil and coauthors, Ethnic disparities among food sources of energy and nutrients of public health concern and nutrients to limit in adults in the United State: NHANES 2003–2006, *Food and Nutrition Research* 58 (2014): 15784.

14. T. C. Wallace, M. McBurney, and V. L. Fulgoni, Multivitamin/mineral supplement contribution to micronutrient intakes in the United States, 2007–2010, *Journal of the American College of Nutrition* 33 (2014): 94–102.

15. P. A. James and coauthors, 2014 evidence-based guideline for the management of high blood pressure in adults: Report from the panel members appointed to the eighth Joint National Committee (JNC 8), *Journal of the American Medical Association* 311 (2014): 507–520.

16. L. Moore-Schiltz and coauthors, Dietary intake of calcium and magnesium and the metabolic syndrome in the National Health and Nutrition Examination (NHANES) 2001–2010 data, *British Journal of Nutrition* 114 (2015):

924–935; Y. Park and J. Kim, Association of dietary vitamin D and calcium with genetic polymorphisms in colorectal neoplasia, *Journal of Cancer Prevention* 20 (2015): 97–105.

17. J. A. Beto, The role of calcium in aging, *Clinical Nutrition Research* 4 (2015): 1–8.

18. P. Burckhardt, Calcium revisited: Part 1, *BoneKEy Reports* 2 (2013): 433; Committee on Dietary Reference Intakes, Dietary Reference Intakes for Calcium and Vitamin D (Washington, D.C.: National Academies Press, 2011), pp. 2–4.

19. L. R. Brun, M. L. Brance, and A. Rigalli, Luminal calcium concentration controls intestinal calcium absorption by modification of intestinal alkaline phosphatase activity, *British Journal of Nutrition* 108 (2012): 229–233.

20. Brun, Brance, and Rigalli, Luminal calcium concentration controls intestinal calcium absorption, 2012.

21. J. Gao and coauthors, Age-related regional deterioration patterns and changes in nanoscale characterizations of trabeculae in the femoral head, *Experimental Gerontology* 62C (2015): 63–72; R. D. Jackson and W. J. Mysiw, Insights into the epidemiology of postmenopausal osteoporosis: The Women's Health Initiative, *Seminars in Reproductive Medicine* 32 (2014): 454–462.

22. R. Zhao, Z. Xu, and M. Zhao, Antiresorptive agents increase the effects of exercise on preventing postmenopausal bone loss in women: A meta-analysis, *PLOS ONE* 10 (2015): e0116729.

23. U.S. Department of Agriculture and U.S. Department of Health and Human Services, Scientific report of the 2015 Dietary Guidelines Advisory Committee, 2015, D-1:15, available at www.health.gov; Burckhardt, Calcium revisited: Part 1, 2013.

24. Q. Xiao and coauthors, Dietary and supplemental calcium intake and cardiovascular disease mortality: The National Institutes of Health–AARP diet and health study, *JAMA Internal Medicine* 173 (2013): 639–646; V. A. Moyer and the U.S. Preventive Services Task Force, Vitamin D and calcium supplementation to prevent fractures in adults: U.S. Preventive Services Task Force recommendation statement, *Annals of Internal Medicine* 158 (2013): 691–696.

25. U.S. Department of Health and Human Services and U.S. Department of Agriculture, *2015–2020 Dietary Guidelines for Americans*, 8th edition (2015), available at http://health.gov/dietaryguidelines/2015/guidelines/.

26. E. Takeda and coauthors, Dietary phosphorus in bone health and quality of life, *Nutrition Reviews* 70 (2012): 311–321.

27. J. Uribarri and M. S. Calvo, Dietary phosphorus intake and health, *American Journal of Clinical Nutrition* 99 (2014): 247–248.

28. Takeda and coauthors, Dietary phosphorus in bone health and quality of life, 2012.

29. J. Sahni and A. M. Scharenberg, The SLC41 family of MgtE-like magnesium transporters, *Molecular Aspects of Medicine* 34 (2013): 620–628.

30. P. L. Lutsey and coauthors, Serum magnesium, phosphorus, and calcium are associated with risk of incident heart failure: The Atherosclerosis Risk in Communities (ARIC) study, *American Journal of Clinical Nutrition* 100 (2014): 756–764; D. Kolte and coauthors, Role of magnesium in cardiovascular diseases, *Cardiology in Review* 22 (2014): 182–192.

31. S. N. Adebamowo and coauthors, Association between intakes of magnesium, potassium, and calcium and risk of stroke: 2 cohorts of US women and updated meta-analysis, *American Journal of Clinical Nutrition* 101 (2015): 1269–1277; Lutsey and coauthors, Serum magnesium, phosphorus, and calcium are associated with risk of incident heart failure, 2014; S. Karadas and coauthors, Serum levels of trace elements and heavy metals in patients with acute hemorrhagic stroke, *Journal of Membrane Biology* 247 (2014): 175–180; S. C. Larsson, N. Orsini, and A. Wolk, Dietary magnesium intake and risk of stroke: A meta-analysis of prospective studies, *American Journal of Clinical Nutrition* 95 (2012): 362–366.

32. U.S. Department of Agriculture and U.S. Department of Health and Human Services, Scientific report of the 2015 Dietary Guidelines Advisory Committee, 2015, D-1:9–11, available at www.health.gov; S. Castiglioni and coauthors, Magnesium and osteoporosis: Current state of knowledge and future research directions, *Nutrients* 5 (2013): 3022–3033.

33. U.S. Department of Agriculture and U.S. Department of Health and Human Services, Scientific report of the 2015 Dietary Guidelines Advisory Committee, 2015, A-2, available at www.health.gov; A. Rosanoff, C. M. Weaver, and R. K. Rude, Suboptimal magnesium status in the United States: Are the health consequences underestimated? *Nutrition Reviews* 70 (2012): 153–164.

34. J. Otten, J. P. Hellwig, and L. D. Meyers, eds., *Dietary Reference Intakes: The Essential Guide to Nutrient Requirements* (Washington, D.C.: National Academies Press, 2006), p. 340.

35. U.S. Department of Agriculture and U.S. Department of Health and Human Services, Scientific report of the 2015 Dietary Guidelines Advisory Committee, 2015, D-1:27, available at www.health.gov.

36. M. J. Hannon and J. G. Verbalis, Sodium homeostasis and bone, *Current Opinion in Nephrology and Hypertension* 23 (2014): 370–376; C. Kruse, P. Eiken, and P. Vestergaard, Hyponatremia and osteoporosis: Insights from the Danish National Patient Registry, *Osteoporosis International* (2014), epub ahead of print.

37. Standing Committee on the Scientific Evaluation of Dietary Reference Intakes, Food and Nutrition Board, Institute of Medicine, *Dietary Reference Intakes*, 2006.

38. Centers for Disease Control and Prevention, Trends in the prevalence of excess dietary sodium intake—United States, 2003–2010, *Morbidity and Mortality Weekly Report* 62 (2013): 1021–1025; M. E. Cogswell and coauthors, Sodium and potassium intakes among US adults:

NHANES 2003–2008, *American Journal of Clinical Nutrition* 96 (2012): 647–657.

39. U.S. Department of Agriculture and U.S. Department of Health and Human Services, Scientific report of the 2015 Dietary Guidelines Advisory Committee, 2015, D-6:4, available at www.health.gov; M. D. Ritchey and coauthors, Million hearts: Prevalence of leading cardiovascular disease risk factors—United States, 2005–2012, *Morbidity and Mortality Weekly Report* 63 (2014): 462–467.

40. U.S. Department of Agriculture and U.S. Department of Health and Human Services, Scientific report of the 2015 Dietary Guidelines Advisory Committee, 2015, D-6:5, available at www.health.gov; R. H. Eckel and coauthors, 2013 AHA/ACC Guideline on Lifestyle Management to Reduce Cardiovascular Risk, *Circulation* 129 (2014): S76–S99.

41. U.S. Department of Agriculture and U.S. Department of Health and Human Services, Scientific report of the 2015 Dietary Guidelines Advisory Committee, 2015, D-6:5, available at www.health.gov.

42. B. M. Davy, T. M. Halliday, and K. P. Davy, Sodium intake and blood pressure: New controversies, new labels … new guidelines? *Journal of the Academy of Nutrition and Dietetics* 115 (2015): 200–203; R. H. Eckel and coauthors, 2013 AHA/ACC Guideline on Lifestyle Management to Reduce Cardiovascular Risk, 2013.

43. V. Reddy and coauthors, High sodium causes hypertension: Evidence from clinical trials and animal experiments, *Journal of Integrative Medicine* 13 (2015): 1–8; D. Mozaffarian and coauthors, Global sodium consumption and death from cardiovascular causes, *New England Journal of Medicine* 371 (2014): 624–634; H. Gardener and coauthors, Dietary sodium and risk of stroke in the Northern Manhattan Study, *Stroke* 43 (2012): 1200–1205.

44. W. B. Farquhar and coauthors, Dietary sodium and health: More than just blood pressure, *Journal of the American College of Cardiology* 65 (2015): 1042–1050; M. P. Blaustein and coauthors, How NaCl raises blood pressure: A new paradigm for the pathogenesis of salt-dependent hypertension, *American Journal of Physiology: Heart and Circulatory Physiology* 302 (2012): H1031–H1049; J. P. Forman and coauthors, Association between sodium intake and change in uric acid, urine albumin excretion, and the risk of developing hypertension, *Circulation* 125 (2012): 3108–3116.

45. Q. Chan, J. Stamler, and P. Elliott, Dietary factors and higher blood pressure in African-Americans, *Current Hypertension Reports* 17 (2015), epub, doi:10.1007/s11906-014-0517-x.

46. V. Ponzo and coauthors, Blood pressure and sodium intake from snacks in adolescents, *European Journal of Clinical Nutrition* 16 (2015): 681–686; C. A. Anderson and coauthors, Commentary on making sense of the science of sodium, *Nutrition Today* 50 (2015): 66–71;

Forman and coauthors, Association between sodium intake and change in uric acid, urine albumin excretion, and the risk of developing hypertension, 2012; Standing Committee on the Scientific Evaluation of Dietary Reference Intakes, Food and Nutrition Board, Institute of Medicine, Dietary Reference Intakes, 2006.

47. L. Brian and coauthors, Institute of Medicine of the National Academies, *Sodium Intake in Populations: Assessment of the Evidence* (National Academies Press: Washington D.C., 2013), p. 7; S. Doaei and M. Gholamalizadeh, The association of genetic variations with sensitivity of blood pressure to dietary salt: A narrative literature review, *ARYA Atherosclerosis* 10 (2014): 169–174; R. M. Carey and coauthors, Salt sensitivity of blood pressure is associated with polymorphisms in the sodium-bicarbonate cotransporter, *Hypertension* 60 (2012): 1359–1366.

48. Y. Wang and coauthors, Genetic variants in renalase and blood pressure responses to dietary salt and potassium interventions: A family-based association study, *Kidney and Blood Pressure Research* 39 (2014): 497–506.

49. U.S. Department of Agriculture and U.S. Department of Health and Human Services, Scientific report of the 2015 Dietary Guidelines Advisory Committee, 2015, D-2:9–11, available at www.health.gov; M. Siervo and coauthors, Effects of the Dietary Approach to Stop Hypertension (DASH) diet on cardiovascular risk factors: A systematic review and meta-analysis, *British Journal of Nutrition* 113 (2015): 1–15; P. Saneei and coauthors, Influence of Dietary Approaches to Stop Hypertension (DASH) diet on blood pressure: A systematic review and meta-analysis on randomized controlled trials, *Nutrition, Metabolism, and Cardiovascular Diseases* 24 (2014): 1253–1261.

50. S. M. Park and coauthors, High dietary sodium intake assessed by 24-hour urine specimen increase urinary calcium excretion and bone resorption marker, *Journal of Bone Metabolism* 21 (2014): 189–194.

51. Farquhar and coauthors, Dietary sodium and health: More than just blood pressure, 2015; J. A. Gaddy and coauthors, High dietary salt intake exacerbates Helicobacter pylori-induced gastric carcinogenesis, *Infection and Immunity* 81 (2013): 2258–2267; L. D'Elia and coauthors, Habitual salt intake and risk of gastric cancer: A meta-analysis of prospective studies, *Clinical Nutrition* 31 (2012): 489–498.

52. M. D. Ritchey and coauthors, *Million hearts*, 2014; A. Drewnowski, M. Maillot, and C. Rehm, Reducing the sodium-potassium ratio in the US diet: A challenge for public health, *American Journal of Clinical Nutrition* 96 (2012): 439–444.

53. C. Gillespie and coauthors, Sodium content in major brands of US packaged foods, *American Journal of Clinical Nutrition* 101 (2015): 344–353; M. Maillot, P. Monsivais, and A. Drewnowski, Food pattern modeling shows that the 2010 Dietary Guidelines for sodium and potassium cannot be met simultaneously, *Nutrition Research* 33 (2013): 188–194.

54. U.S. Department of Agriculture and U.S. Department of Health and Human Services, Scientific report of the 2015 Dietary Guidelines Advisory Committee, 2015, D-6:4–5, available at www.health.gov.

55. C. Gillespie and coauthors, Sodium content in major brands of US packaged foods, 2009, *American Journal of Clinical Nutrition* 101 (2015): 344–353; M. F. Jacobson, S. Havas, and R. McCarter, Changes in sodium levels in processed and restaurant foods, 2005 to 2011, *Journal of the American Medical Association Internal Medicine* 173 (2013): 1285–1291.

56. L. J. Appel and coauthors, Population-wide sodium reduction: The bumpy road from evidence to policy, *Annals of Epidemiology* 22 (2012): 417–425.

57. R. S. Sebastian and coauthors, Sandwiches are major contributors of sodium in the diets of American adults: Results from What We Eat in America, National Health and Nutrition Examination Survey 2009–2010, *Journal of the Academy of Nutrition and Dietetics* 115 (2015): 272–277; U.S. Department of Agriculture and U.S. Department of Health and Human Services, Scientific report of the 2015 Dietary Guidelines Advisory Committee, 2015, D-1:39, 43–44, available at www.health.gov; Centers for Disease Control and Prevention, Vital signs: Food categories contributing the most to sodium consumption—United States, 2007–2008, *Morbidity and Mortality Weekly Report* 61 (2012): 92–98.

58. Adebamowo and coauthors, Association between intakes of magnesium, potassium, and calcium and risk of stroke: 2 cohorts of US women and updated meta-analysis, 2015; H. J. Adrogue and N. E. Madias, The impact of sodium and potassium on hypertension risk, *Seminars in Nephrology* 34 (2014): 257–272; L. D'Elia and coauthors, Potassium-rich diet and risk of stroke: Updated meta-analysis, *Nutrition, Metabolism, and Cardiovascular Diseases* 24 (2014): 585–587; N. J. Aburto and coauthors, Effect of increased potassium intake on cardiovascular risk factors and disease: Systematic review and meta-analyses, *British Medical Journal* 346 (2013): f1378.

59. U.S. Department of Health and Human Services and U.S. Department of Agriculture, *2015–2020 Dietary Guidelines for Americans*, 8th edition (2015), available at http://health.gov/dietaryguidelines/2015/guidelines/.

60. U.S. Department of Agriculture and U.S. Department of Health and Human Services, Scientific report of the 2015 Dietary Guidelines Advisory Committee, 2015, D-1:9–16, available at www.health.gov; N. Tian and coauthors, Sodium and potassium intakes among US infants and preschool children, 2003–2010, *American Journal of Clinical Nutrition* 98 (2013): 1113–1122; Cogswell and coauthors, Sodium and potassium intakes among US adults, 2012.

61. K. Stolarz-Skrzypek and coauthors, Sodium and potassium and the pathogenesis of hypertension, *Current Hypertension Reports* 15 (2013): 122–130.

62. M. B. Zimmermann and M. Andersson, Update on iodine status worldwide, *Current Opinion in Endocrinology, Diabetes and Obesity* 19 (2012): 382–387; M. Andersson, V. Karumbunathan, and M. B. Zimmermann, Global iodine status in 2011 and trends over the past decade, *Journal of Nutrition* 142 (2012): 744–750.

63. J. H. Lazarus, The importance of iodine in public health, Environmental Geochemistry and Health 37 (2015): 605–618; M. B. Zimmermann, The effects of iodine deficiency in pregnancy and infancy, *Paediatric and Perinatal Epidemiology* 26 (2012): 108–117.

64. K. Redman and coauthors, Iodine deficiency and the brain: Effects and mechanisms, *Critical Reviews in Food Science and Nutrition* (2015), epub ahead of print, doi.10.1080.10408398.2014.922042; P. N. Taylor and coauthors, Therapy of endocrine disease: Impact of iodine supplementation in mild-to-moderate iodine deficiency: Systematic review and meta-analysis, *European Journal of Endocrinology* 170 (2013): R1–R15.

65. M. B. Zimmermann, Iodine deficiency and excess in children: Worldwide status in 2013, *Endocrine Practice* 19 (2013): 839–846.

66. Standing Committee on the Scientific Evaluation of Dietary Reference Intakes, Food and Nutrition Board, Institute of Medicine, *Dietary Reference Intakes for Vitamin A, Vitamin K, Arsenic, Boron, Chromium, Copper, Iodine, Iron, Manganese, Molybdenum, Nickel, Silicon, Vanadium, and Zinc* (Washington, D.C.: National Academies Press, 2001), p. 258.

67. Z. Sang and coauthors, Exploration of the safe upper level of iodine intake in euthyroid Chinese adults: A randomized double-blind trial, *American Journal of Clinical Nutrition* 95 (2012): 367–373.

68. S. I. Borucki Castro and coauthors, Effects of iodine intake and teat-dipping practices on milk iodine concentrations in dairy cows, *Journal of Dairy Science* 95 (2012): 213–220.

69. C. G. Perrine and coauthors, Intakes of dairy products and dietary supplements are positively associated with iodine status among U.S. children, *Journal of Nutrition* 143 (2013): 1155–1160; E. N. Pearce, M. Andersson, and M. B. Zimmermann, Global iodine nutrition: Where do we stand in 2013? *Thyroid* 23 (2013): 523–528.

70. H. Padmanabhan, M. J. Brookes, and T. Iqbal, Iron and colorectal cancer: Evidence from in vitro and animal studies, *Nutrition Reviews* 73 (2015): 308–317; H. Aljwaid and coauthors, Non-transferrin-bound iron is associated with biomarkers of oxidative stress, inflammation, and endothelial dysfunction in type 2 diabetes, *Journal of Diabetes Complications* (2015), epub ahead of print, doi:http://dx.doi.org/10.1016/j.jdiacomp.2015.05.017; J. Milonski and coauthors, DNA damage and oxidant-antioxidant status in blood of patients with head and neck cancer, *DNA and Cell Biology* (2014), epub ahead of print.

71. S. Gulec, G. J. Anderson, and J. F. Collins, Mechanistic and regulatory aspects of intestinal iron absorption, *American Journal of Physiology—Gastrointestinal and Liver Physiology* 307 (2014): G397–G409; G. J. Anderson and F. Wang, Essential but toxic: Controlling the flux of iron in the body, *Clinical and Experimental Pharmacology and Physiology* 39 (2012): 719–724.

72. U.S. Department of Health and Human Services, National Institutes of Health, Office of Dietary Supplements, Iron: Dietary supplement fact sheet, 2014, available at http://ods.od.nih.gov/factsheets/Iron-HealthProfessional/.

73. C. Cao and K. O. O'Brien, Pregnancy and iron homeostasis: An update, *Nutrition Reviews* 71 (2013): 35–51; A. A. Khalafallah and A. E. Dennis, Iron deficiency anaemia in pregnancy and postpartum: Pathophysiology and effect of oral versus intravenous iron therapy, *Journal of Pregnancy* (2012): 630519, doi:10.1155/2012/630519.

74. L. Tussing-Humphreys and coauthors, Rethinking iron regulation and assessment in iron deficiency, anemia of chronic disease, and obesity: Introducing hepcidin, *Journal of the Academy of Nutrition and Dietetics* 112 (2012): 391–400.

75. T. Konz, M. Montes-Bayon, and S. Vaulont, Hepcidin quantification: Methods and utility in diagnosis, *Metallomics* 6 (2014): 1583–1590; N. Zhao, A. Zhang, and C. A. Enns, Iron regulation by hepcidin, *Journal of Clinical Investigation* 123 (2013): 2337–2343.

76. U.S. Department of Agriculture and U.S. Department of Health and Human Services, Scientific report of the 2015 Dietary Guidelines Advisory Committee, 2015, D-1:33, available at www.health.gov; C. Cao and coauthors, Duodenal absorption and tissue utilization of dietary heme and nonheme iron differ in rats, *Journal of Nutrition* 144 (2014): 1710–1717; M. F. Young and coauthors, Maternal hepcidin is associated with placental transfer of iron derived from dietary heme and nonheme sources, *Journal of Nutrition* 142 (2012): 33–39.

77. I. Jauregui-Lobera, Iron deficiency and cognitive functions, *Neuropsychiatric Disease and Treatment* 10 (2014): 2087–2095; S. K. Berglund and coauthors, Effects of iron supplementation of LBW infants on cognition and behavior at 3 years, *Pediatrics* 131 (2013): 47–55.

78. J. L. Miller, Iron deficiency anemia: A common and curable disease, *Perspectives in Medicine* 3 (2013): doi:10.1101/cshperspect.a011866; P. Vaucher and coauthors, Effect of iron supplementation on fatigue in nonanemic menstruating women with low ferritin: A randomized controlled trial, *Canadian Medical Association Journal* 184 (2012): 1247–1254.

79. M. Low and coauthors, Effects of daily iron supplementation in primary-school-aged children: Systematic review and meta-analysis of randomized controlled trials, *Canadian Medical Association Journal* 185 (2013): E791–E802; Berglund and coauthors, Effects of iron supplementation of LBW infants on cognition and behavior at 3 years, 2013.

80. A. J. Greig and coauthors, Iron deficiency, cognition, mental health and fatigue in women of childbearing age: A systematic review, *Journal of Nutritional Science* 2 (2013): e14.

81. D. Howarth, Pica—A case report, *Australian Family Physician* 42 (2013): 299–300.

82. Miller, Iron deficiency anemia, 2013.

83. T. Sonnweber and coauthors, High-fat diet causes iron deficiency via hepcidin-independent reduction of duodenal iron absorption, *Journal of Nutritional Biochemistry* 23 (2012): 1600–1608.

84. M. Khanbhai and coauthors, The prevalence of iron deficiency anaemia in patients undergoing bariatric surgery, *Obesity Research & Clinical Practice* 9 (2015): 45–49; R. T. Hamza, A. I. Hamed, and R. R. Kharshoum, Iron homeostasis and serum hepcidin-25 levels in obese children and adolescents: Relation to body mass index, *Hormone Research in Paediatrics* 80 (2013): 11–17.

85. U.S. Department of Agriculture and U.S. Department of Health and Human Services, Scientific report of the 2015 Dietary Guidelines Advisory Committee, 2015, D-1:16–17, available at www.health.gov; M. Mesias, I. Seiquer, and M. P. Navarro, Iron nutrition in adolescence, *Critical Reviews in Food Science and Nutrition* 53 (2013): 1226–1237.

86. J. Bertinato and coauthors, Diet-induced obese rats have higher iron requirements and are more vulnerable to iron deficiency, *European Journal of Nutrition* 53 (2014): 885–895; A. A. Nikovorov and coauthors, Mutual interaction between iron homeostasis and obesity pathogenesis, *Journal of Trace Elements in Medicine and Biology* (2014), doi:10.1016/j.jtemb.2014.05.005.

87. World Health Organization, Micronutrient deficiencies: Iron deficiency anaemia, 2015, available at www.who.int/nutrition/topics/ida/en/; Miller, Iron deficiency anemia, 2013.

88. T. Asano and coauthors, Possible involvement of iron-induced oxidative insults in neurodegeneration, *Neuroscience Letters* 588 (2015): 29–35; R. J. Castellani and coauthors, The role of iron as a mediator of oxidative stress in Alzheimer disease, *Biofactors* 38 (2012): 133–138.

89. H. Padmanabhan, M. J. Brookes, and T. Iqbal, Iron and colorectal cancer: evidence from in vitro and animal studies, *Nutrition Reviews* 73 (2015): 308–317.

90. R. J. Salgia and K. Brown, Diagnosis and management of hereditary hemochromatosis, *Clinics in Liver Disease* 19 (2015): 187–198; C. E. McLaren and coauthors, Exome sequencing in HFE C282Y homozygous men with extreme phenotypes identifies a GNPAT variant associated with severe iron overload, *Hepatology* (2015), doi:10.1002/hep.27711; B. K. Crownover and C. J. Covey, Hereditary hemochromatosis, *American Family Physician* 87 (2013): 183–190.

91. M. L. Maia and coauthors, Invariant natural killer T cells are reduced in hereditary hemochromatosis patients, *Journal of Clinical Immunology* (2014), epub ahead of print, doi:10.1007/s10875-014-0118-0.

92. J. Snakar and coauthors, Near fatal iron intoxication managed conservatively, *British Medical Journal Case Reports* (2013), doi: 10.1136/bcr-2012-007670.

93. A. S. Prasad, Discovery of human zinc deficiency: Its impact on human health and disease, *Advances in Nutrition* 4 (2013): 176–190; W. Maret, Zinc biochemistry: From a single zinc enzyme to a key element of life, *Advances in Nutrition* 4 (2013): 82–91.

94. F. Wang and coauthors, Zinc might prevent heat-induced hepatic injury by activating the Nrf2-antioxidant in mice, *Biological Trace Element Research* (2015), epub ahead of print, doi:10.1007/s12011-015-0228-4; P. I. Oteiza, Zinc and the modulation of redox homeostasis, *Free Radical Biology and Medicine* 53 (2012): 1748–1759.

95. D. C. Hamm, E. R. Bondra, and M. M. Harrison, Transcriptional activation is a conserved feature of the early embryonic factor Zelda that requires a cluster of four zinc fingers for DNA binding and a low-complexity activation domain, *Journal of Biological Chemistry* (2014), epub ahead of print, pii:jbc.M114.602292; S. D. Gower-Winter and C. W. Levenson, Zinc in the central nervous system: From molecules to behavior, *Biofactors* 38 (2012): 186–193.

96. N. F. Krebs, L. V. Miller, and K. M. Hambidge, Zinc deficiency in infants and children: A review of its complex and synergistic interactions, *Paediatrics and International Child Health* 34 (2014): 279–288; J. J. Heller and coauthors, Restriction of IL-22-producing T cell responses and differential regulation of regulatory T cell compartments by zinc finger transcription factor Ikaros, *Journal of Immunology* 193 (2014): 3934–3946.

97. S. C. Liberato, G. Singh, and K. Mulholland, Zinc supplementation in young children: A review of the literature focusing on diarrhoea prevention and treatment, *Clinical Nutrition* (2014), epub ahead of print, doi:10.1016/j.clnu.2014.08.002.

98. Liberato and coauthors, Zinc supplementation in young children, 2014; E. Mayo-Wilson and coauthors, Zinc supplementation for preventing mortality, morbidity, and growth failure in children aged 6 months to 12 years of age, *Cochrane Database of Systematic Reviews* (2014), doi:10.1002/14651858.CD009384.pub2.

99. L. M. Lamberti and coauthors, Oral zinc supplementation for the treatment of acute diarrhea in children: A systematic review and meta-analysis, *Nutrients* 5 (2013): 4715–4740; M. E. Penny, Zinc supplementation in public health, *Annals of Nutrition and Metabolism* 62 (2013): 31–42.

100. R. R. Das and M. Singh, Oral zinc for the common cold, *Journal of the American Medical Association* 311 (2014): 1440–1441; U.S. Food and Drug Administration, FDA advises consumers not to use certain Zicam cold remedies: Intranasal zinc product linked to loss of sense of smell, Press Announcements, April 2013, available at www.fda.gov/NewsEvents/Newsroom/PressAnnouncements/2009/ucm167065.htm; M. Science and coauthors, Zinc for the treatment

of the common cold: A systematic review and meta-analysis of randomized controlled trials, *Canadian Medical Association* 184 (2012): E551–E561.

101. B. Farmer, Nutritional adequacy of plant-based diets for weight management: Observations from the NHANES, *American Journal of Clinical Nutrition* 100 (2014): 365S–368S; M. Foster and coauthors, Effect of vegetarian diets on zinc status: A systematic review and meta-analysis of studies in humans, *Journal of the Science of Food and Agriculture* 93 (2013): 2362–2371.

102. L. H. Duntas and S. Benvenga, Selenium: An element for life, *Endocrine* (2014), epub ahead of print, doi:10.1007/s12020-014-0477-6; P. Sabino, S. Stranges, and P. Strazzullo, Does selenium matter in cardiometabolic disorders? A short review of the evidence, *Journal of Endocrinological Investigation* 36 (2013): 21–27.

103. A. H. Rose and P. R. Hoffmann, Selenoproteins and cardiovascular stress, *Thrombosis and Haemostasis* 113 (2014), epub ahead of print; Z. Zhang, J. Zhang, and J. Xiao, Selenoproteins and selenium status in bone physiology and pathology, *Biochemica et Biophysica Acta* 1840 (2014): 3246–3256.

104. K. E. Geillinger and coauthors, Hepatic metabolite profiles in mice with a suboptimal selenium status, *Journal of Nutritional Biochemistry* 25 (2014): 914–922; J. Kohrle, Selenium and the thyroid, *Current Opinion in Endocrinology, Diabetes, and Obesity* 20 (2013): 441–448.

105. F. Brigo and coauthors, Selenium supplementation for primary prevention of cardiovascular disease: Proof of no effectiveness, *Nutrition, Metabolism, and Cardiovascular Diseases* 24 (2014): e2–e3; K. Rees and coauthors, Selenium supplementation for the primary prevention of cardiovascular disease, *Cochrane Database of Systematic Reviews* 1 (2013): CD009671.

106. N. Babaknejad and coauthors, The relationship between selenium levels and breast cancer: A systematic review and meta-analysis, *Biological Trace Element Research* 159 (2014): 1–7; R. Hurst and coauthors, Selenium and prostate cancer: Systematic review and meta-analysis, *American Journal of Clinical Nutrition* 96 (2012): 111–122; M. P. Rayman, Selenium and human health, *Lancet* 379 (2012): 1256–1268.

107. M. Vinceti and coauthors, Selenium for preventing cancer, *Cochrane Database of Systematic Reviews* 3 (2014): CD005195; S. A. Kenfield and coauthors, Selenium supplementation and prostate cancer mortality, *Journal of the National Cancer Institute* 107 (2014): 360.

108. C. Junshi, An original discovery: Selenium deficiency and keshan disease (an endemic heart disease), *Asia Pacific Journal of Clinical Nutrition* 21 (2012): 320–326.

109. J. S. Morris and S. B. Crane, Selenium toxicity from a misformulated dietary supplement, adverse health effects, and the temporal response in the nail biologic monitor, *Nutrients* 5 (2013): 1024–1057.

110. E. J. Joy and coauthors, Soil type influences crop mineral composition in Malawi, *Science of*
the Total Environment 505 (2015): 587–595; Rayman, Selenium and human health, 2012.

111. X. H. Yin and coauthors, Exposure to fluoride in drinking water and hip fracture risk: A meta-analysis of observational studies, *PLoS One* (2015), epub, doi: 10.1371/journal.pone.0126488; L. Huo and coauthors, Fluoride promotes viability and differentiation of osteoblast-like Saos-2 cells via BMP/Smads signaling pathway, *Biological Trace Element Research* 155 (2013): 142–149; Position of the Academy of Nutrition and Dietetics, The impact of fluoride on health, *Journal of the Academy of Nutrition and Dietetics* 112 (2012): 1443–1453.

112. V. C. Marinho and coauthors, Fluoride varnishes for preventing dental caries in children and adolescents, *Cochrane Database of Systematic Reviews* 7 (2013): CD002279; Position of the Academy of Nutrition and Dietetics, The impact of fluoride on health, 2012.

113. J. P. Brown and coauthors, The dynamic behavior of the early dental caries lesion in caries-active adults and implications, *Community Dentistry and Oral Epidemiology* (2015), doi:10.1111/cdoe.

114. S. A. Moimaz and coauthors, Dental fluorosis and its influence on children's life, *Brazilian Oral Research* 29 (2015): 1–7.

115. S. B. Gopalakrishnan and G. Viswanathan, Assessment of fluoride-induced changes on physicochemical and structural properties of bone and the impact of calcium on its control in rabbits, *Journal of Bone Mineral Metabolism* 30 (2012): 154–163.

116. N. Kakumanu and S. D. Rao, Skeletal fluorosis due to excessive tea drinking, *New England Journal of Medicine* 368 (2013): 1140; J. Aaseth, G. Boivin, and O. Andersen, Osteoporosis and trace elements—An overview, *Journal of Trace Elements in Medicine and Biology* 26 (2012): 149–152.

117. National Cancer Institute, Fact sheet: Fluoridated water, February 21, 2012, available at www.cancer.gov.

118. D. M. Proctor and coauthors, Assessment of the mode of action for hexavalent chromium-induced lung cancer following inhalation exposures, *Toxicology* 325 (2014): 160–179.

119. N. J. Hoffman and coauthors, Chromium enhances insulin responsiveness via AMPK, *Journal of Nutritional Biochemistry* 25 (2014): 565–572; Y. Hua and coauthors, Molecular mechanisms of chromium in alleviating insulin resistance, *Journal of Nutritional Biochemistry* 23 (2012): 313–319.

120. S. Zlatic and coauthors, Molecular basis of neurodegeneration and neurodevelopmental defects in Menkes disease, *Neurobiology of Disease* (2015), doi:10.1016/j.nbd.2014.12.024; O. Bandmann, K. H. Weiss, and S. G. Kaler, Wilson's disease and other neurological copper disorders, *Lancet Neurology* 14 (2015): 103–113.

121. C. L. Frankenfeld and coauthors, Dietary intake measured from a self-administered, online 24-hour recall system compared with 4-day diet records in an adult US population, *Journal of the Academy of Nutrition and Dietetics*
112 (2012): 1642–1647; Standing Committee on the Scientific Evaluation of Dietary Reference Intakes, Food and Nutrition Board, Institute of Medicine, *Dietary Reference Intakes for Vitamin A, Vitamin K, Arsenic, Boron, Chromium, Copper, Iodine, Iron, Manganese, Molybdenum, Nickel, Silicon, Vanadium, and Zinc*, 2001, p. 245.

122. Wallace, McBurney, and Fulgoni, Multivitamin/mineral supplement contribution to micronutrient intakes in the United States, 2014.

123. A. R. Mangels, Bone nutrients for vegetarians, *American Journal of Clinical Nutrition* 100 (2014): 469S–475S.

Consumer's Guide 8

1. A. Qaseem and coauthors, Dietary and pharmacologic management to prevent recurrent nephrolothiasis in adults: A clinical practice guideline from the American College of Physicians, *Annals of Internal Medicine* 161 (2014): 659–667.

2. D. F. Tate and coauthors, Replacing caloric beverages with water or diet beverages for weight loss in adults: Main results of the Choose Healthy Options Consciously Everyday (CHOICE) randomized clinical trial, *American Journal of Clinical Nutrition* 95 (2012): 555–563; A. Pan and coauthors, Changes in water and beverage intake and long-term weight changes: Results from three prospective cohort studies, *International Journal of Obesity* 37 (2013): 1378–1385.

3. Q. Yang and coauthors, Added sugar intake and cardiovascular diseases mortality among US adults, *Journal of the American Medical Association Internal Medicine* 174 (2014): 516–524; P. J. Huth and coauthors, Major food sources of calories, added sugars, and saturated fat and their contribution to essential nutrient intakes in the U.S. diet: Data from the National Health and Nutrition Examination Survey (2003–2006), *Nutrition Journal* 12 (2013): 116.

Controversy 8

1. N. C. Wright and coauthors, The recent prevalence of osteoporosis and low bone mass in the United States based on bone mineral density at the femoral neck or lumbar spine, *Journal of Bone Mineral Research* 29 (2014): 2520–2526; A. C. Looker and coauthors, Osteoporosis or low bone mass at the femur neck or lumbar spine in older adults: United States, 2005–2008, National Center for Health Statistics data brief number 93 (2012), available at http://www.cdc.gov/nchs/data/databriefs/db93.htm#findings.

2. J. A. Cauley, Public health impact of osteoporosis, *Journals of Gerontology* 68 (2013): 1243–1251.

3. G. R. Clark and E. L. Duncan, The genetics of osteoporosis, *British Medical Bulletin* (2015), epub ahead of print; J. B. Richards, H. Zheng, and T. D. Spector, Genetics of osteoporosis from genome-wide association studies: Advances and challenges, *Nature Reviews Genetics* 13 (2012): 576–588.

4. M. Pekkinen and coauthors, Vitamin D binding protein genotype is associated with serum

25-hydroxyvitamin D and PTH concentrations, as well as bone health in children and adolescents in Finland, *PLOS ONE* 9 (2014): e87292; C. Holroyd and coauthors, Epigenetic influences in the developmental origins of osteoporosis, *Osteoporosis International* 23 (2012): 401–410.

5. D. Feskanich, A. J. Flint, and W. C. Willett, Physical activity and inactivity and risk of hip fractures in men, *American Journal of Public Health* 104 (2014): e75–e81; Holroyd and coauthors, Epigenetic influences in the developmental origins of osteoporosis, 2012; S. Levis and V. S. Lagari, The role of diet in osteoporosis prevention and management, *Current Osteoporosis Reports* 10 (2012): 296–302.

6. P. Andreopoulou and R. S. Bockman, Management of postmenopausal osteoporosis, *Annual Review of Medicine* 66 (2015): 329–342; A. Giusti and G. Bianchi, Treatment of primary osteoporosis in men, *Clinical Interventions in Aging* 10 (2014): 105–115.

7. N. Kurtoglu-Aksoy and coauthors, Implications of premature ovarian failure on bone turnover markers and bone mineral density, *Clinical and Experimental Obstetrics and Gynecology* 41 (2014): 149–153; O. Svenjme and coauthors, Early menopause and risk of osteoporosis, fracture and mortality: A 34-year prospective observational study in 390 women, *BJOG: An International Journal of Obstetrics and Gynaecology* 119 (2012): 810–816.

8. T. Willson and coauthors, The clinical epidemiology of male osteoporosis: A review of the recent literature, *Clinical Epidemiology* 7 (2015): 65–76; A. D. Manthripragada and coauthors, Fracture incidence in a large cohort of men age 30 years and older with osteoporosis, *Osteoporosis International* (2015), epub ahead of print.

9. N. Iucif and coauthors, Association between plasma testosterone level and bone mineral density in healthy elderly men, *Journal of the American Geriatrics Society* 62 (2014): 981–982; L. Modekilde, P. Vestergaard, and L. Rejnmark, The pathogenesis, treatment and prevention of osteoporosis in men, *Drugs* 73 (2013): 15–29.

10. E. Nieschlag, Current topics in testosterone replacement of hypogonadal men, *Best Practice and Research: Clinical Endocrinology and Metabolism* 29 (2015): 77–90; F. Oury, A crosstalk between bone and gonads, *Annals of the New York Academy of Sciences* 1260 (2012): 1–7.

11. P. Zhang and coauthors, Visceral adiposity is negatively associated with bone density and muscle attenuation, *American Journal of Clinical Nutrition* 101 (2015): 337–343; P. Y. Liu and coauthors, New insight into fat, muscle and bone relationship in women: Determining the threshold at which body fat assumes negative relationship with bone mineral density, *International Journal of Preventive Medicine* 5 (2014): 1452–1463.

12. J. M. Lappe and coauthors, The longitudinal effects of physical activity and dietary calcium on bone mass accrual across stages of pubertal development, *Journal of Bone and Mineral Research* 30 (2015): 156–164.

13. K. G. Avin and coauthors, Biomechanical aspects of the muscle-bone interaction, *Current Osteoporosis Reports* 13 (2015): 1–8; A. Seabra and coauthors, Muscle strength and soccer practice as major determinants of bone mineral density on adolescents, *Joint Bone Spine* 79 (2012): 403–408; N. K. LeBrasseur and coauthors, Skeletal muscle mass is associated with bone geometry and microstructure and serum IGFBP-2 levels in adult women and men, *Journal of Bone and Mineral Research* (2012), epub ahead of print, doi:10.1002/jbmr.1666.

14. A. A. Shanb and E. F. Youssef, The impact of adding weight-bearing exercise versus nonweight bearing programs to the medical treatment of elderly patients with osteoporosis, *Journal of Family and Community Medicine* 21 (2014): 176–181; M. Behringer and coauthors, Effects of weight-bearing activities on bone mineral content and density in children and adolescents: A meta-analysis, *Journal of Bone and Mineral Research* 29 (2014): 467–478.

15. R. I. Ray and coauthors, Predictors of poor clinical outcome following hip fracture in middle aged-patients, *Injury* (2014), doi:10.1016/j.injury.2014.11.005; V. Yoon, N. M. Maalouf, and K. Sakhaee, The effects of smoking on bone metabolism, *Osteoporosis International* 23 (2012): 2081–2092.

16. J. A. Marrone and coauthors, Moderate alcohol intake lowers biochemical markers of bone turnover in postmenopausal women, *Menopause* 19 (2012): 974–979.

17. G. W. Gaddini and coauthors, Twelve months of voluntary heavy alcohol consumption in male rhesus macaques suppresses intracortical bone remodeling, *Bone* 71 (2015): 227–236; D. B. Maurel and coauthors, Alcohol and bone: Review of dose effects and mechanisms, *Osteoporosis International* 23 (2012): 1–16.

18. M. Halfon, O. Phan, and D. Teta, Vitamin D: A review on its effects on muscle strength, the risk of fall, and frailty, *BioMed Research International* (2015), epub, doi.org/10.1155/2015/953241; V. A. Moyer and the U.S. Preventive Services Task Force, Vitamin D and calcium supplementation to prevent fractures in adults: U.S. Preventive Services Task Force recommendation statement, *Annals of Internal Medicine* 158 (2013): 691–696.

19. P. D. Genaro and coauthors, Dietary protein intake in elderly women: Association with muscle and bone mass, *Nutrition in Clinical Practice* (2014), epub ahead of print.

20. T. Hu and coauthors, Protein intake and lumbar bone density: The multi-ethnic study of atherosclerosis (MESA), *British Journal of Nutrition* 112 (2014): 1384–1392.

21. T. Remer, D. Krupp, and L. Shi, Dietary protein's and dietary acid load's influence on bone health, *Critical Reviews in Food Science and Nutrition* 54 (2014): 1140–1150; J. Calvez and coauthors, Protein intake, calcium balance and health consequences, *European Journal of Clinical Nutrition* 66 (2012): 281–295.

22. K. L. Tucker, Vegetarian diets and bone status, *American Journal of Clinical Nutrition* 100 (2014): 329S–335S; A. R. Mangels, Bone nutrients for vegetarians, *American Journal of Clinical Nutrition* 100 (2014): 469S–475S.

23. J. Lappe and coauthors, Effect of a combination of genistein, polyunsaturated fatty acids and vitamins D3 and K1 on bone mineral density in postmenopausal women: A randomized, placebo-controlled, double-blind pilot study, *European Journal of Nutrition* 52 (2013): 203–215; M. Bevilacqua and coauthors, Effect of a mixture of calcium, vitamin D, inulin and soy isoflavones on bone metabolism in post-menopausal women: A retrospective analysis, *Aging Clinical and Experimental Research* 25 (2013): 611–617.

24. S. M. Park and coauthors, Effect of high dietary sodium on bone turnover markers and urinary calcium excretion in Korean postmenopausal women with low bone mass, *European Journal of Clinical Nutrition* (2015), doi:10.1038/ejcn.2014.284.

25. M. S. Yatabe and coauthors, Effects of a high-sodium diet on renal tubule Ca2+ transporter and claudin expression in Wistar-Kyoto rats, *BioMed Central Nephrology* 13 (2012): 160; W. Pan and coauthors, The epithelial sodium/proton exchanger, NHE3, is necessary for renal and intestinal calcium (re)absorption, *American Journal of Physiology* 302 (2012): F943–F956.

26. M. S. Calvo and J. Uribarri, Public health impact of dietary phosphorus excess on bone and cardiovascular health in the general population, *American Journal of Clinical Nutrition* 98 (2013): 6–15; E. Takeda and coauthors, Dietary phosphorus in bone health and quality of life, *Nutrition Reviews* 70 (2012): 311–321.

27. M. H. Knapen and coauthors, Three-year low-dose menaquinone-7 supplementation helps decrease bone loss in healthy postmenopausal women, *Osteoporosis International* 24 (2013): 2499–2507; Y. Fang and coauthors, Effect of vitamin K on bone mineral density: A meta-analysis of randomized controlled trials, *Journal of Bone and Mineral Metabolism* 30 (2012): 60–68.

28. T. S. Orchard and coauthors, Magnesium intake, bone mineral density, and fractures: Results from the Women's Health Initiative Observational Study, *American Journal of Clinical Nutrition* 99 (2014): 926–933.

29. M. S. LeBoff and coauthors, VITAL-Bone Health: Rationale and design of two ancillary studies evaluating the effects of vitamin D and/or omega-3 fatty acid supplements on incident fractures and bone health outcomes in the VITamin D and OmegA-3 Trial, *Contemporary Clinical Trials* (2015), doi:10.1016/j.cct.2015.01.007; T. S. Orchard and coauthors, A systematic review of omega-3 fatty acids and osteoporosis, *British Journal of Nutrition* 107 (2012): S253–S260.

30. S. Nayak and coauthors, Systematic review and meta-analysis of the performance of clinical risk assessment instruments for screening for osteoporosis or low bone density, *Osteoporosis International* (2015), epub ahead of print; K. H. Rubin and coauthors, Risk assessment tools to identify women with increased risk of

osteoporotic fracture: Complexity or simplicity? A systematic review, *Journal of Bone and Mineral Research* 28 (2013): 1701–1717.

31. M. R. McClung and coauthors, Romosozumab in postmenopausal women with low bone mineral density, *New England Journal of Medicine* 370 (2014): 412–420.

32. M. McClung and coauthors, Bisphosphonate therapy for osteoporosis: Benefits, risks, and drug holiday, *American Journal of Medicine* 126 (2013): 13–20; J. J. Body and coauthors, Extraskeletal benefits and risks of calcium, vitamin D and anti-osteoporosis medications, *Osteoporosis International* 23 (2012): S1–S23.

33. J. Aaseth, G. Boivin, and O. Andersen, Osteoporosis and trace elements—An overview, *Journal of Trace Elements in Medicine and Biology* 26 (2012): 149–152.

34. J. Hess and J. Slavin, Snacking for a cause: Nutritional insufficiencies and excesses of U.S. children: A critical review of food consumption patterns and macronutrient and micronutrient intake of U.S. children, *Nutrients* 6 (2014): 4750–4759.

35. L. P. Piodi, A. Poloni, and F. M. Ulivieri, Managing osteoporosis in ulcerative colitis: Something new? *World Journal of Gastroenterology* 20 (2014): 14087–14098.

36. J. R. Lewis and coauthors, The effects of calcium supplementation on verified coronary heart disease hospitalization and death in postmenopausal women: A collaborative meta-analysis of randomized controlled trials, *Journal of Bone and Mineral Research* 30 (2015): 165–175; R. L. Prentice and coauthors, Health risks and benefits from calcium and vitamin D supplementation: Women's Health Initiative clinical trial and cohort study, *Osteoporosis International* 24 (2013): 567–580; E. J. Samelson and coauthors, Calcium intake is not associated with increased coronary artery calcification: The Framingham Study, *American Journal of Clinical Nutrition* 96 (2012): 1274–1280; L. Kuanrong and coauthors, Associations of dietary calcium intake and calcium supplementation with myocardial infarction and stroke risk and overall cardiovascular mortality in the Heidelberg cohort of the European Prospective Investigation into Cancer and nutrition study (EPIC-Heidelberg), *Heart* 98 (2012): 920–925.

37. V. A. Moyer and the U.S. Preventive Services Task Force, Vitamin D and calcium supplementation to prevent fractures in adults, 2013.

38. U.S. Department of Agriculture and U.S. Department of Health and Human Services, Scientific report of the 2015 Dietary Guidelines Advisory Committee, 2015, D-1:18, available at www.health.gov; C. L. Taylor and L. D. Meyers, Perspectives and progress on upper levels of intake in the United States, *Journal of Nutrition* 142 (2012): 2207S–2211S.

39. K. Michaelsson and coauthors, Long term calcium intake and rates of all cause and cardiovascular mortality: Community based prospective longitudinal cohort study, *British Medical Journal* 346 (2013): f228, doi: 10.1136/bmj.f228.

40. U.S. Department of Agriculture and U.S. Department of Health and Human Services, Scientific report of the 2015 Dietary Guidelines Advisory Committee, 2015, D-1:18, available at www.health.gov.

41. U.S. Department of Agriculture and U.S. Department of Health and Human Services, Scientific report of the 2015 Dietary Guidelines Advisory Committee, 2015, D-1:31–33, available at www.health.gov; C. M. Weaver, How sound is the science behind the dietary recommendations for dairy? *American Journal of Clinical Nutrition* 99 (2014): 1217S–1222S.

Chapter 9

1. Centers for Disease Control and Prevention, Obesity and overweight, FastStats, 2015, available at www.cdc.gov/nchs/fastats/obesity-overweight.htm; C. D. Fryar, M. D. Carroll, and C. L. Ogden, Prevalence of overweight, obesity, and extreme obesity among adults: United States, 1960–1962 through 2011–2012, NCHS Health E-Stats, 2014, available at www.cdc.gov.

2. B. M. Popkin, L. S. Adair, and S. W. Ng, Global nutrition transition and the pandemic of obesity in developing countries, *Nutrition Reviews* 70 (2012): 3–21.

3. W. Dietz, Current epidemiology of obesity in the United States, in *The Current State of Obesity Solutions in the United States* (Washington, D.C.: National Academies Press, 2014), pp. 5–14.

4. C. D. Fryar and C. L. Ogden, Prevalence of underweight among adults aged 20 and over: United States, 1960–1962 through 2011–2012, NCHS Health E-Stats, updated September 2014, available at www.cdc.gov/nchs/data/hestat/underweight_adult_11_12/underweight_adult_11_12.htm.

5. T. M. Valentijn and coauthors, The obesity paradox in the surgical population, *Surgeon* 11 (2013): 169–176.

6. Centers for Disease Control and Prevention, Obesity is common, serious and costly, Obesity and Overweight Facts, updated September 2014, available at www.cdc.gov/obesity/data/adult.html; S. A. Grover and coauthors, Years of life lost and healthy life-years lost from diabetes and cardiovascular disease in overweight and obese people: A modeling study, *Lancet* (2014), epub ahead of print, doi:10.1016/S2213-8587(14)70229-3.

7. A. V. Patel, J. S. Hildebrand, and S. M. Gapstur, Body mass index and all-cause mortality in a large prospective cohort of white and black U.S. adults, *PLOS ONE* 9 (2014), epub, doi:10.1371/journal.pone.0109153.

8. K. Bhaskaran and coauthors, 22 specific cancers: A population-based cohort study of 5.24 million UK adults, *Lancet* 384 (2014): 255–265; M. Bastien and coauthors, Overview of epidemiology and contribution of obesity to cardiovascular disease, *Progress in Cardiovascular Diseases* 56 (2014): 369–381; V. G. Gilby and T. A. Ajith, Role of adipokines and peroxisome proliferator-activated receptors in nonalcoholic fatty liver disease, *World Journal of Hepatology* 6

(2014): 570–579; Centers for Disease Control and Prevention, The health effects of overweight and obesity, Healthy Weight, updated December 2013, available at www.cdc.gov/healthyweight/effects/.

9. N. Sattar and J. M. R. Gill, Type 2 diabetes as a disease of ectopic fat? *BMC Medicine* 12 (2014), epub, doi:10.1186/s12916-014-0123-4.

10. H. J. Yoo and K. M. Choi, Adipokines as a novel link between obesity and atherosclerosis, *World Journal of Diabetes* 5 (2014): 357–363.

11. M. Lee, Y. Wu, and S. K. Fried, Adipose tissue heterogeneity: Implication of depot differences in adipose tissue for obesity complications, *Molecular Aspects of Medicine* 34 (2013): 1–11.

12. I. Imayama and coauthors, Effects of a caloric restriction weight loss diet and exercise on inflammatory biomarkers in overweight/obese postmenopausal women: A randomized controlled trial, *Cancer Research* 72 (2012): 2314–2326.

13. Bastien and coauthors, Overview of epidemiology and contribution of obesity to cardiovascular disease, 2014; J. R. Cerhan and coauthors, A pooled analysis of waist circumference and mortality in 650,000 adults, *Mayo Clinic Proceedings* 89 (2014): 335–345.

14. D. Mozaffarian and coauthors, Heart disease and stroke statistics—2015 update: A report from the American Heart Association, *Circulation* 131 (2015), epub ahead of print, doi: 10.1161/CIR.0000000000000152.

15. P. Singh and coauthors, Effects of weight gain and weight loss on regional fat distribution, *American Journal of Clinical Nutrition* 96 (2012): 229–233.

16. T. Kondoh and coauthors, Association of dietary factors with abdominal subcutaneous and visceral adiposity in Japanese men, *Obesity Research and Clinical Practice* 8 (2014): e16–e25; N. T. Bendsen and coauthors, Is beer consumption related to measures of abdominal and general obesity? A systematic review and meta-analysis, *Nutrition Reviews* 71(2013): 67–87; U. Ladabaum and coauthors, Obesity, abdominal obesity, physical activity, and caloric intake in U.S. adults: 1988–2010, *American Journal of Medicine* 127 (2014): 717–727; K. H. Kim and coauthors, Alcohol consumption and its relation to visceral and subcutaneous adipose tissues in healthy male Koreans, *Annals of Nutrition and Metabolism* 60 (2012): 52–61.

17. American College of Cardiology/American Heart Association Task Force on Practice Guidelines and the Obesity Society, Executive summary: Guidelines (2013) for the management of overweight and obesity in adults, *Obesity* 22 (2014): S5–S39.

18. E. Fabbrini and coauthors, Metabolically normal obese people are protected from adverse effects following weight gain, *Journal of Clinical Investigation* (2015), epub, doi:10.1172/JCI78425.

19. C. K. Kramer, B. Zinman, and R. Retnakaran, Are metabolically healthy overweight and obesity benign conditions? A systematic review and meta-analysis, *Annals of Internal*

Medicine 159 (2014): 758–769; J. H. Goedecke and L. K. Micklesfield, The effect of exercise on obesity, body fat distribution and risk for type 2 diabetes, *Medicine and Sport Science* 60 (2014): 82–93; A. Philipsen and coauthors, Associations of objectively measured physical activity and abdominal fat distribution, *Medicine and Science in Sports and Exercise* (2014), epub ahead of print, PMID:25207926.

20. S. R. Karasu, Of mind and matter: Psychological dimensions of obesity, *American Journal of Psychotherapy* 66 (2012): 111–128.

21. E. Manzato and coauthors, Risk factors for weight gain: A longitudinal study in non-weight loss treatment-seeking overweight adults, *Eating and Weight Disorders* (2015), epub ahead of print, doi:10.1007/s40519-014-0174-8; A. R. Sutin and A. Terracciano, Perceived weight discrimination and obesity, *PLOS ONE* (2014), epub, doi:10.1371/journal.pone.0070048; G. M. Coelho, Prevention of eating disorders in female athletes, *Journal of Sports Medicine* (2014), epub, doi:10.2147/OAJSM.S36528.

22. K. D. Hall and coauthors, Energy balance and its components: Implications for body weight regulation, *American Journal of Clinical Nutrition* 95 (2012): 989–994.

23. D. M. Thomas and coauthors, Time to correctly predict the amount of weight loss with dieting, *Journal of the Academy of Nutrition and Dietetics* 114 (2014): 857–861.

24. Standing Committee on the Scientific Evaluation of Dietary Reference Intakes, Food and Nutrition Board, Institute of Medicine, *Dietary Reference Intakes for Energy, Carbohydrate, Fiber, Fat, Fatty Acids, Cholesterol, Protein, and Amino Acids* (Washington, D.C.: National Academies Press, 2002/2005), p. 107.

25. N. R. Shah and E. R. Braverman, Measuring adiposity in patients: The utility of body mass index (BMI), percent body fat, and leptin, *PLoS ONE* 7 (2012), epub, doi:10.1371/journal.pone.0033308.

26. M. Heo and coauthors, Percentage of body fat cutoffs by sex, age, and race-ethnicity in the US adult population from NHANES 1999–2004, *American Journal of Clinical Nutrition* 95 (2012): 594–602.

27. Mozaffarian and coauthors, Heart disease and stroke statistics—2015 update, 2015.

28. C. Delporte, Structure and physiological actions of ghrelin, *Scientifica* (2013), epub, doi:10.1155/2013/518909.

29. J. A. Parker and J. R. Bloom, Hypothalamic neuropeptides and the regulation of appetite, *Neuropharmacology* (2012), epub, doi:org/10.1016/j.neuropharm.2012.02.004.

30. L. Sominsky and S. J. Spencer, Eating behavior and stress: A pathway to obesity, *Frontiers in Psychology* 5 (2014), epub, doi:10.3389/fpsyg.2014.00434.

31. M. A. Deluca, Habituation of the responsiveness of mesolimbic and mesocortical dopamine transmission to taste stimuli, *Frontiers in Integrative Neuroscience* 8 (2014), epub, doi:10.3389/fnint.2014.00021.

32. M. B. Allison and M. G. Myers Jr., Connecting leptin signaling to biological function, *Journal of Endocrinology* 223 (2014), epub, doi:10.1530/JOE-14-0404; C. Sobrino Crespo and coauthors, Peptides and food intake, *Frontiers in Endocrinology* 5 (2014), epub, doi:10.3389/fendo.2014.00058R.

33. H. K. Park and R. S. Ahima, Physiology of leptin: Energy homeostasis, neuroendocrine function and metabolism, *Metabolism* (2014), epub ahead of print, doi:10.1016/j.metabol.2014.08.004.

34. M. Journel and coauthors, Brain responses to high-protein diets, *Advances in Nutrition* 3 (2012): 322–329; A. M. Johnstone, Safety and efficacy of high-protein diets for weight loss, *Proceedings of the Nutrition Society* 71 (2012): 339–349.

35. C. J. Rebello and coauthors, Acute effect of oatmeal on subjective measures of appetite and satiety compared to a ready-to-eat breakfast cereal: A randomized crossover trial, *Journal of the American College of Nutrition* 32 (2013): 272–279.

36. T. S. Bruna and coauthors, A systematic review and meta-analysis of the prebiotics and synbiotics effects on glycaemia, insulin concentrations and lipid parameters in adult patients with overweight or obesity, *Clinical Nutrition* (2014), epub ahead of print, doi:http://dx.doi.org/10.1016/j.clnu.2014.10.004.

37. R. J. de Souza and coauthors, Effects of 4 weight-loss diets differing in fat, protein, and carbohydrate on fat mass, lean mass, visceral adipose tissue, and hepatic fat: Results from the POUNDS LOST trial, *American Journal of Clinical Nutrition* 95 (2012): 614–625.

38. Hall and coauthors, Energy balance and its components, 2012.

39. E. Ferrannini, M. Rosenbaum, and R. O. Leibel, The threshold shift paradigm of obesity: Evidence from surgically induced weight loss, *American Journal of Clinical Nutrition* 100 (2014): 996–1002.

40. S. Kajimura and M. Saito, A new era in brown adipose tissue biology: Molecular control of brown fat development and energy homeostasis, *Annual Review of Physiology* 76 (2014): 225–249.

41. I. Shimizu and coauthors, Vascular rarefaction mediates whitening of brown fat in obesity, *Journal of Clinical Investigation* 124 (2014): 2099–2112.

42. P. Lee and coauthors, Irisin and FGF21 are cold-induced endocrine activators of brown fat function in humans, *Cell Metabolism* 19 (2014): 302–309; Y. Oiq and coauthors, Eosinophils and type 2 cytokine signaling in macrophages orchestrate development of functional beige fat, *Cell* 157 (2014): 1292–1308; J. Wu and coauthors, Beige adipocytes are a distinct type of thermogenic fat cell in mouse and human, *Cell* 150 (2012): 366–376.

43. C. Graham, A. Mullen, and K. Whelan, Obesity and the gastrointestinal microbiota: A review of associations and mechanisms, *Nutrition Reviews* 73 (2015): 376–385; P. Carthage, M. B. Moran, and F. Shanahan, Gut microbiota and obesity: Role in aetiology and potential therapeutic target, *Best Practice and Research: Clinical Gastroenterology* 28 (2014): 585–597; V. Tremoroli and F. Bäckhed, Functional interactions between the gut microbiota and host metabolism, *Nature* 489 (2012): 242–249.

44. J. Aron-Wisnewsky and K. Clément, Gut microbiota in obesity and type-2 diabetes: Links with diet and weight loss intervention, in E. J. Schiffrin, P. Marteau, and D. Brassart (eds.), *Intestinal Microbiota in Health and Disease: Modern Concepts* (Boca Raton, Fla.: CRC Press, 2014), pp. 307–324.

45. S. A. Joyce and coauthors, Regulation of host weight gain and lipid metabolism by bacterial bile acid modification in the gut, *Proceedings of the National Academy of Sciences* 111 (2014): 7421–7426; M. Remely and coauthors, Effects of short chain fatty acid producing bacteria on epigenetic regulation of FFAR3 in type 2 diabetes and obesity, *Gene* 537 (2014): 85–92.

46. L. C. Kong and coauthors, Dietary patterns differently associate with inflammation and gut microbiota in overweight and obese subjects, *PLOS ONE* 9 (2014), epub, doi:10.1371/journal.pone.0109434; Y. Sanz and A. Moya-Pérez, Microbiota, inflammation, and obesity, *Advances in Experimental Medicine and Biology* 817 (2014): 291–317.

47. E. Ishikawa and coauthors, Ethnic diversity of gut microbiota: Species characterization of Bacteroides fragilis group and genus Bifidobacterium in healthy Belgian adults, and comparison with data from Japanese subjects, *Journal of Bioscience and Bioengineering* 116 (2013): 265–270; Ł. Grzśkowiak and coauthors, Distinct gut microbiota in southeastern African and northern European infants, *Journal of Pediatric Gastroenterology and Nutrition* 54 (2012): 812–816.

48. M. J. Khan and coauthors, Unraveling the role of the gut microbiota in obesity; Cause or effect? *Proceedings of the Nutrition Society* 73 (2014), epub, doi.org/10.1017/S0029665114000329; A. Cotillard and coauthors, Dietary intervention impact on gut microbial gene richness, *Nature* 500 (2013): 585–588.

49. A. E. Locke and coauthors, Genetic studies of body mass index yield new insights for obesity biology, *Nature* 518 (2015), epub ahead of print, doi:10.1038/nature14177; S. E. Ozanne, Epigenetic signatures of obesity, *New England Journal of Medicine* 372 (2015): 973–974.

50. P. Dominguez-Salas and coauthors, Maternal nutrition at conception modulates DNA methylation of human metastable epialleles, *Nature Communications* (2014), epub, doi:10.1038/ncomms4746; C. Lavebratt, M. Almgren, and T. J. Ekström, Epigenetic regulation in obesity, *International Journal of Obesity* 36 (2012): 757–765.

51. T. South and coauthors, Rats eat a cafeteria-style diet to excess but eat smaller amounts and less frequently when tested with chow, *PLOS ONE* 9 (2014), epub, doi:10.1371/journal.pone.0093506.

52. A. C. Reichelt, M. J. Morris, and R. R. Westbrook, Cafeteria diet impairs expression of sensory-specific satiety and stimulus-outcome learning, *Frontiers in Psychology* 5 (2014), epub, doi:10.3389/fpsyg.2014.00852.

53. Sominsky and Spencer, Eating behavior and stress, 2014; M. Singh, Mood, food, and obesity, *Frontiers in Psychology* 5 (2014), epub, doi:10.3389/fpsyg.2014.00925; S. Carnell and coauthors, Appetitive traits from infancy to adolescence: Using behavioral and neural measures to investigate obesity risk, *Physiology and Behavior* 121 (2013), epub, doi:10.1016/j.physbeh.2013.02.015; C. J. Moore and S. A. Cunningham, Social position, psychological stress, and obesity: A systematic review, *Journal of the Academy of Nutrition and Dietetics* 112 (2012): 518–526.

54. B. Wansink and J. Kim, Bad popcorn in big buckets: Portion size can influence intakes as much as taste, *Journal of Nutrition Education and Behavior* 37 (2005): 242–245.

55. B. Wansink, K. van Ittersum, and C. R. Payne, Larger bowl size increases the amount of cereal children request, consume, and waste, *Journal of Pediatrics* 164 (2014): 323–326.

56. K. Blum, P. K. Thanos, and M. S. Gold, Dopamine and glucose, obesity, and reward deficiency syndrome, *Frontiers in Psychology* 5 (2014), epub, doi:103389/fpsyc.2014.00919.

57. G. Wang and coauthors, Brain dopamine and obesity, *Lancet* 357 (2001): 354–357.

58. Reichelt, Morris, and Westbrook, Cafeteria diet impairs expression of sensory-specific satiety and stimulus-outcome learning, 2014.

59. L. Epstein and coauthors, Food reinforcement and obesity: Psychological moderators, *Appetite* 58 (2012): 157–162.

60. J. S. Schiller and coauthors, Summary health statistics for U.S. adults: National Health Interview Survey, *Vital and Health Statistics* 10 (2012): 1–217.

61. L. Yang and coauthors, Occupational sitting and weight status in a diverse sample of employees in midwest metropolitan cities, 2012–2013, *Preventing Chronic Disease* 11 (2014), epub, doi:10.5888/pcd11.140286; H. P. van der Ploeg and coauthors, Sitting time and all-cause mortality risk in 222,497 Australian adults, *Archives of Internal Medicine* 172 (2012): 494–500.

62. J. F. Salis, Role of built environments in physical activity, obesity, and cardiovascular disease, *Circulation* 125 (2012): 729–737.

63. C. Larson and coauthors, Development of a community-sensitive strategy to increase availability of fresh fruits and vegetables in Nashville's urban food deserts, *Preventing Chronic Disease* 10 (2014), epub, doi:10.5888/pcd10.130008; N. M. Wedick and coauthors, Access to healthy food stores modifies effect of a dietary intervention, *American Journal of Preventive Medicine* (2014), epub, doi:10.1016/j.amepre.2014.08.020.

64. T. Dubowitz and coauthors, Are our actions aligned with our evidence? The skinny on changing the landscape of obesity, *Obesity (Silver Spring)* 21 (2013): 419–420.

65. Institute of Medicine, Committee on Accelerating Progress in Obesity Prevention, *Accelerating Progress in Obesity Prevention: Solving the Weight of the Nation* (Washington, D.C.: National Academies Press, 2012), available at www.nap.edu.

66. J. Cawley, D. Dragone, and S. Von Hinke Kessler Scholder, The demand for cigarettes as derived from the demand for weight loss: A theoretical and empirical investigation, *Health Economics* (2014), epub ahead of print, doi:10.1002/hec.3118.

67. J. W. Carbone, J. P. McClung, and S. M. Pasiakos, Skeletal muscle responses to negative energy balance: Effects of dietary protein, *Advances in Nutrition* 3 (2012): 119–126.

68. de Souza and coauthors, Effects of 4 weight-loss diets differing in fat, protein, and carbohydrate on fat mass, lean mass, visceral adipose tissue, and hepatic fat, 2012.

69. L. Li, Z. Wang, and Z. Zuo, Chronic intermittent fasting improves cognitive functions and brain structures in mice. *PLOS ONE* 8 (2013), epub, doi:10.1371/journal.pone.0066069.

70. R. E. Patterson and coauthors, Intermittent fasting and human metabolic health, *Journal of the Academy of Nutrition and Dietetics* 115 (2015): 1203–1212; R. M. Elliott and coauthors, Transcriptome analysis of peripheral blood mononuclear cells in human subjects following a 36 h fast provides evidence of effects on genes regulating inflammation, apoptosis and energy metabolism, *Genes and Nutrition* 9 (2014), epub, doi:10.1007/s12263-014-0432-4.

71. S. Kumar and G. Kaur, Intermittent fasting dietary restriction regimen negatively influences reproduction in young rats: A study of hypothalamo-hypophysial-gonadal axis, *PLOS ONE* 8 (2013), epub, doi:10.1371/journal.pone.0052416; J. Karbowska and Z. Kochan, Intermittent fasting up-regulates Fsp27/Cidec gene expression in white adipose tissue, *Nutrition* 28 (2012): 294–299.

72. B. Wansink, A. Tal, and M. Shimizu, First foods most: After 18-hour fast, people drawn to starches first and vegetables last, *Archives of Internal Medicine* 172 (2012): 961–963.

73. Bendsen and coauthors, Is beer consumption related to measures of abdominal and general obesity?, 2013; S. Lourenco, A. Oliveira, and C. Lopes, The effect of current and lifetime alcohol consumption on overall and central obesity, *European Journal of Clinical Nutrition* 66 (2012): 813–818.

74. A. Fildes and coauthors, Probability of an obese person attaining normal body weight: Cohort study using electronic health records, *American Journal of Public Health* (2015), epub ahead of print, doi:10.2105/AJPH.2015.302773; American College of Cardiology/American Heart Association Task Force on Practice Guidelines and the Obesity Society, Executive summary: Guidelines (2013) for the management of overweight and obesity in adults, 2014.

75. U.S. Department of Agriculture and U.S. Department of Health and Human Services, Scientific report of the 2015 Dietary Guidelines Advisory Committee, 2015, D-2:66, available at www.health.gov; D. J. Johns and coauthors, Diet or exercise interventions vs combined behavioral weight management programs: A systematic review and meta-analysis of direct comparisons, *Journal of the Academy of Nutrition and Dietetics* 114 (2014): 1557–1568.

76. S. B. Heymsfield and coauthors, Energy content of weight loss: Kinetic features during voluntary caloric restriction, *Metabolism* 61 (2012): 937–943.

77. J. M. Nicklas and coauthors, Successful weight loss among obese U.S. adults, *American Journal of Preventive Medicine* 42 (2012): 481–485.

78. American College of Cardiology/American Heart Association Task Force on Practice Guidelines and the Obesity Society, Executive summary: Guidelines (2013) for the management of overweight and obesity in adults, 2014.

79. Position of the Academy of Nutrition and Dietetics: Interventions for the treatment of overweight and obesity in adults, *Journal of the Academy of Nutrition and Dietetics* 116 (2016): 129–147; American College of Cardiology/American Heart Association Task Force on Practice Guidelines and the Obesity Society, Executive summary: Guidelines (2013) for the management of overweight and obesity in adults, 2014.

80. U.S. Department of Agriculture and U.S. Department of Health and Human Services, Scientific report of the 2015 Dietary Guidelines Advisory Committee, 2015, D-2:43, available at www.health.gov; U.S. Department of Agriculture, Evidence Analysis Library Division, A series of systematic reviews on the relationship between dietary patterns and health outcomes (2014), available at www.nel.gov/vault/2440/web/files/DietaryPatterns/DPRptFullFinal.pdf; N. D. Barnard, S. M. Levin, and Y. Yokoyama, A systematic review and meta-analysis of changes in body weight in clinical trials of vegetarian diets, *Journal of the Academy of Nutrition and Dietetics* 115 (2015): 954–969; J. D. Smith and coauthors, Changes in intake of protein foods, carbohdrate amount and quality, and long-term weight change: Results from 3 prospective cohorts, *American Journal of Clinical Nutrition* (2015), epub ahead of print, doi: 10.3945/ajcn.114.100867.

81. C. L. Jackson and F. B. Hu, Long-term associations of nut consumption with body weight and obesity, *American Journal of Clinical Nutrition* 100 (2014): 408S–411S; G. Flores-Mateo and coauthors, Nut intake and adiposity: Meta-analysis of clinical trials, *American Journal of Clinical Nutrition* 97 (2013): 1346–1355.

82. J. W. Carbone, J. P. McClung, and S. M. Pasiakos, Skeletal muscle responses to negative energy balance: Effects of dietary protein, *Advances in Nutrition* 3 (2012): 119–126.

83. H. Stewart and R. M. Morrison, New regulations will inform consumers about calories in restaurant foods, Amber Waves, 2015, available at www.ers.usda.gov/amber-waves.aspx; U.S. Food and Drug Administration, How many calories? Look at the menu, Consumer Health

Information, November 2014, available at www.fda.gov/consumer.

84. S. Kucukgoncu, M. Midura, and C. Tek, Optimal management of night eating syndrome: challenges and solutions, *Neuropsychiatric Disease and Treatment* 11 (2015): 751–760.

85. R. Pérez-Escamilla and coauthors, Dietary energy density and body weight in adults and children: A systematic review, *Journal of the Academy of Nutrition and Dietetics* 112 (2012): 671–684.

86. L. B. Sørensen and coauthors, Sucrose compared with artificial sweeteners: A clinical intervention study of effects on energy intake, appetite, and energy expenditure after 10 wk of supplementation in overweight subjects, *American Journal of Clinical Nutrition* 100 (2014): 36–45; R. Muckelbauer and coauthors, Association between water consumption and body weight outcomes: A systematic review, *American Journal of Clinical Nutrition* 98 (2013): 282–299; D. F. Tate and coauthors, Replacing caloric beverages with water or diet beverages for weight loss in adults: Main results of the Choose Healthy Options Consciously Everyday (CHOICE) randomized clinical trial, *American Journal of Clinical Nutrition* 95 (2012): 555–563.

87. J. Suez and coauthors, Artificial sweeteners induce glucose intolerance by altering the gut microbiota, *Nature* 514 (2014): 181–186.

88. E. Green and C. Murphy, Altered processing of sweet taste in the brain of diet soda drinkers, *Physiology and Behavior* 107 (2012): 560–567.

89. M. Chen and coauthors, Effects of dairy intake on body weight and fat: A meta-analysis of randomized controlled trials, *American Journal of Clinical Nutrition* 96 (2012): 735–747.

90. K. Deighton and D. J. Stensel, Creating an acute energy deficit without stimulating compensatory increases in appetite: Is there an optimal exercise protocol? *Proceedings of the Nutrition Society* 73 (2014): 352–358; K. J. Guelfi and coauthors, Beneficial effects of 12 weeks of aerobic compared with resistance exercise training on perceived appetite in previously sedentary overweight and obese men, *Metabolism* 62 (2012): 235–243.

91. J. Zibellini and coauthors, Does diet-induced weight loss lead to bone loss in overweight or obese adults? A systematic review and meta-analysis of clinical trials, *Journal of Bone and Mineral Research* (2015), epub ahead of print, doi:10.1002/jbmr.2564; A. R. Josse and coauthors, Diets higher in dairy foods and dietary protein support bone health during diet- and exercise-induced weight loss in overweight and obese premenopausal women, *Journal of Clinical Endocrinology and Metabolism* 97 (2012): 251–260.

92. T. Baranowski, Are active video games useful to combat obesity? (editorial) *American Journal of Clinical Nutrition* 101 (2015): 1107–1108; A. Gribbon and coauthors, Active video games and energy balance in male adolescents: a randomized crossover trial, *American Journal of Clinical Nutrition* 101 (2015): 1126–1134; P. C. Douris and coauthors, Comparison between

Nintendo Wii fit aerobics and traditional aerobic exercise in sedentary young adults, *Journal of Strength and Conditioning Research* 26 (2012): 1052–1057.

93. Nicklas and coauthors, Successful weight loss among obese U.S. adults, 2012.

94. U.S. Food and Drug Administration, Beware of products promising miracle weight loss, Consumer Health Information, 2015, available at ww.fda.gov/consumer.

95. M. C. Cheung and coauthors, Surgical options for weight loss, in S. Thaller and M. Cohen (eds.), *Cosmetic Surgery after Massive Weight Loss* (London: J. P. Medical, 2013), pp. 1–10.

96. P. E. O'Brien and coauthors, Long-term outcomes after bariatric surgery: Fifteen-year follow-up of adjustable gastric banding and a systematic review of the bariatric surgical literature, *Annals of Surgery* 257 (2013): 87–94.

97. L. Sjöström and coauthors, Association of bariatric surgery with long-term remission of type 2 diabetes and with microvascular and macrovascular complications, *Journal of the American Medical Association* 311 (2014): 2297–2304; S. Brethauer and coauthors, Can diabetes be surgically cured? Long-term metabolic effects of bariatric surgery in obese patients with type 2 diabetes mellitus, *Annals of Surgery* 258 (2013): 628–637.

98. V. Tremaroli and coauthors, Roux-en-Y gastric bypass and vertical banded gastroplasty induce long-term changes on the human gut microbiome contributing to fat mass regulation, *Cancer Bioenergetics* 22 (2015): 228–238; A. P. Liou and coauthors, Conserved shifts in the gut microbiota due to gastric bypass reduce host weight and adiposity, *Science Translational Medicine* (2014), epub, doi:10.1126/scitranslmed.3005687; L. C. Kong and coauthors, Gut microbiota after gastric bypass in human obesity: Increased richness and associations of bacterial genera with adipose tissue genes, *American Journal of Clinical Nutrition* 98 (2013): 16–24.

99. B. Finan and coauthors, A rationally designed monomeric peptide triagonist corrects obesity and diabetes in rodents, *Nature Medicine* (2014), epub ahead of print, doi:10.1038/nm.3761.

100. U.S. Food and Drug Administration, FDA targets gastric band weight-loss claims, Consumer Health Information, December 2011, updated July 2014, available at www.fda.gov/ForConsumers/ConsumerUpdates.

101. J. Tack and E. Deloose, Complications of bariatric surgery: Dumping syndrome, reflux and vitamin deficiencies, *Best Practice and Research Clinical Gastroenterology* 28 (2014): 741–749; P. G. de Moura-Grec and coauthors, Impact of bariatric surgery on oral health conditions: 6-months cohort study, *International Dental Journal* 64 (2014): 144–149; T. Weiderman and R. Heuberger, The nutritional status of the bariatric patient and its effect on periodonal disease, *Bariatric Surgical Practice and Patient Care* 8 (2013): 161–165.

102. A. A. AlHassany, Night blindness due to vitamin A deficiency associated with copper deficiency myelopathy secondary to bowel bypass surgery, *BMJ Case Reports* (2014) epub, doi:10.1136/bcr-2013-202478; C. Karefylakis and coauthors, Vitamin D status 10 years after primary gastric bypass: Gravely high prevalence of hypovitaminosis D and raised PTH levels, *Obesity Surgery* 24 (2014): 343–348; R. A. Guerreiro and R. Ribeiro, Ophthalmic complications of bariatric surgery, *Obesity Surgery* (2014), epub ahead of print, doi:10.1007/s11685-014-1472-y.

103. E. Saltzman and J. P. Karl, Nutrient deficiencies after gastric bypass surgery, *Annual Review of Nutrition* 33 (2013): 183–203; V. L. Gloy and coauthors, Bariatric surgery versus non-surgical treatment for obesity: A systematic review and meta-analysis of randomised controlled trials, *British Medical Journal* 347 (2013), epub, doi:10.1136/bmj.f5934.

104. United States Department of Agriculture, FDA approves non-surgical temporary balloon device to treat obesity, FDA News Release, July 2015, available at www.fda.gov/NewsEvents/Newsroom/PressAnnouncements/ucm456296.htm.

105. Y. R. Krishna and coauthors, Acute liver failure caused by "fat burners" and dietary supplements: A case report and literature review, *Canadian Journal of Gastroenterology* 25 (2011): 157–160.

106. P. S. MacLean and coauthors, NIH working group report: Innovative research to improve maintenance of weight loss, *Obesity* (2014), epub ahead of print, doi:10.1002/oby.20967; J. P. Moreno and C. A. Johnston, Successful habits of weight losers, *American Journal of Lifestyle Medicine* 6 (2012): 113–115.

107. C. Mason, History of weight cycling does not impede future weight loss or metabolic improvements in postmenopausal women, 62 (2013): 127–136; K. H. Pietiläinen and coauthors, Does dieting make you fat? A twin study, *International Journal of Obesity* 36 (2012): 456–464.

108. J. P. Montani, Y. Schutz, and A. G. Dulloo, Dieting and weight cycling as risk factors for cardometabolic diseases: Who is really at risk? *Obesity Reviews* 16 (2015): 7–18.

109. L. E. Burke and coauthors, Current science on consumer use of mobile health for cardiovascular disease prevention: A scientific statement fro the American Heart Association, *Circulation* (2015), epub ahead of print, doi:10.1161/CIR.0000000000000232; K. O. Hwang and coauthors, Website usage and weight loss in a free commercial online weight loss program: Retrospective cohort study, *Journal of Medical Internet Research* 15 (2013), epub, doi:10.2196/jmir.2195.

110. E. Robinson and coauthors, A systematic review and meta-analysis examining the effect of eating rate on energy intake and hunger, *American Journal of Clinical Nutrition* 100 (2014): 123–151.

111. N. R. Reyes and coauthors, Similarities and differences between weight loss maintainers and

regainers: A qualitative analysis, *Journal of the Academy of Nutrition and Dietetics* 112 (2012): 499–505.

Consumer's Guide 9

1. J. M. Nicklas and coauthors, Successful weight loss among obese U.S. adults, *American Journal of Preventive Medicine* 42 (2012): 481–485.

2. R. D. Grave and coauthors, A randomized trial of energy-restricted high-protein versus high-carbohydrate, low-fat diet in morbid obesity, *Obesity* 21 (2013): 1774–1778; J. de Souza and coauthors, Effects of 4 weight-loss diets differing in fat, protein, and carbohydrate on fat mass, lean mass, visceral adipose tissue, and hepatic fat: Results from the POUNDS LOST trial, *American Journal of Clinical Nutrition* 95 (2012): 614–625.

3. U.S. Department of Agriculture and U.S. Department of Health and Human Services, Scientific report of the 2015 Dietary Guidelines Advisory Committee, 2015, D-2:7, available at www.health.gov.

4. A. M. Johnstone, Safety and efficacy of high-protein diets for weight loss, *Proceedings of the Nutrition Society* 71 (2012): 339–349.

5. H. J. Leidy and coauthors, The role of protein in weight loss and maintenance, *American Journal of Clinical Nutrition* 101 (2015): 1320S–1329S; A. Astrup, A. Raben, and N. Gieker, The role of higher protein diets in weight control and obesity-related comorbidities, *International Journal of Obesity* 39 (2015): 721–726; E. A. Martens and M. S. Westerterp-Plantenga, Protein diets, body weight loss and weight maintenance, *Current Opinion in Clinical Nutrition and Metabolic Care* 17 (2014): 75–79; D. H. Pesta and V. T. Samuel, A high-protein diet for reducing body fat: Mechanisms and possible caveats, *Nutrition and Metabolism* 11 (2014), epub, doi:10.1186/1743-7075-11-53.

6. D. L. Layman and coauthors, Defining meal requirements for protein to optimize metabolic roles of amino acids, *American Journal of Clinical Nutrition* 101 (2015): 1330S–1338S; A. J. Hector and coauthors, Whey protein supplementation preserves postprandial myofibrillar protein synthesis during short-term energy restriction in overweight and obese adults, *Journal of Nutrition* (2015), epub, doi:10.3945/jn.114.200832.

7. Leidy and coauthors, The role of protein in weight loss and maintenance, 2015.

8. J. D. Smith and coauthors, Changes in intake of protein foods, carbohdrate amount and quality, and long-term weight change: Results from 3 prospective cohorts, *American Journal of Clinical Nutrition* (2015), epub ahead of print, doi:10.3945/ajcn.114.100867.

9. L. Schwingshackl and G. Hoffmann, Comparison of effects of long-term low-fat vs high-fat diets on blood lipid levels in overweight or obese patients: A systematic review and meta-analysis, *Journal of the Academy of Nutrition and Dietetics* 113 (2013): 1640–1661; C. B. Ebbeling and coauthors, Effects of dietary composition on energy expenditure during weight-loss maintenance, *Journal of the American Medical Association* 307 (2012): 2627–2634; P. Lagiou and coauthors, Low carbohydrate–high protein diet and incidence of cardiovascular diseases in Swedish women: Prospective cohort study, *British Medical Journal* 344 (2012), epub, doi:10.1136/bmj.e4026.

10. J. Merino and coauthors, Negative effect of a low-carbohydrate, high-protein, high-fat diet on small peripheral artery reactivity in patients with increased cardiovascular risk, *British Journal of Nutrition* 109 (2013): 1241–1247.

11. P. Hernández-Alonso and coauthors, High dietary protein intake is associated with an increased body weight and total death risk, *Clinical Nutrition* (2015), epub ahead of print, doi.org/10.1016/j.clnu.2015.03.016; H. Noto and coauthors, Low-carbohydrate diets and all-cause mortality: A systematic review and meta-analysis of observational studies, *PLOS ONE* 8 (2013), epub, doi:10.1371/journal.pone.0055030.

Controversy 9

1. Academy of Nutrition and Dietetics, Understanding eating disorders, December 2012, available at www.eatright.org.

2. K. Campbell and R. Peebles, Eating disorders in children and adolescents: State of the art review, *Pediatrics* 134 (2014): 582–592.

3. B. Herpertz-Dahlmann and coauthors, Eating disorder symptoms do not just disappear: The implications of adolescent eating-disordered behaviour for body weight and mental health in young adulthood, *European Child and Adolescent Psychiatry* (2014), epub ahead of print, doi:10.1007/s00787-014-0610-3.

4. A. A. Rikani and coauthors, A critique of the literature on etiology of eating disorders, *Annals of Neurosciences* 20 (2013): 157–161.

5. K. M. Pike, H. W. Hoek, and P. E. Dunne, Cultural trends and eating disorders, *Current Opinion in Psychiatry* 27 (2014): 436–442; G. L. Whitcomb, J. Arcelus, and J. Chen, Can cognitive dissonance methods developed in the West for combating the "thin idea" help slow the rapidly increasing prevalence of eating disorders in non-Western cultures? *Shanghai Archives of Psychiatry* 25 (2013): 332–340.

6. A. G. Mabe, K. J. Forney, and P. K. Keel, Do you "like" my photo? Facebook use maintains eating disorder risk, *International Journal of Eating Disorders* 47 (2014): 516–523; A. Dakanalis and coauthors, The developmental effects of media-ideal internalization and self-objectification processes on adolescents' negative body-feelings, dietary restraint, and binge eating, *European Child and Adolescent Psychiatry* (2014), epub ahead of print, doi:10.1007/s00787-014-0649-1.

7. M. Martinsen and coauthors, Preventing eating disorders among young elite athletes: A randomized controlled trial, *Medicine and Science in Sports and Exercise* 46 (2014): 435–447.

8. G. M. Coelho and coauthors, Prevention of eating disorders in female athletes, *Open Access Journal of Sports Medicine* 5 (2014): 105–113; A. E. Field and coauthors, Body image and eating disorders in males, *Journal of the American Medical Association* 312 (2014): 2156–2157.

9. D. Neumark-Sztainer and M. E. Eisenberg, Body image concerns, muscle-enhancing behaviors, and eating disorders in males, *Journal of the American Medical Association* 312 (2014): 2156–2157.

10. M. J. de Souza and coauthors, 2014 Female Athlete Triad Coalition consensus statement on treatment and return to play of the Female Athlete Triad, *British Journal of Sports Medicine* 48 (2014), epub, doi:10.1136/bjsports-2013-093218; M. Payne and J. T. Kirchner, Should you suspect the female athlete triad? *Journal of Family Practice* 63 (2014): 187–192.

11. M. T. Barrack and coauthors, Higher incidence of bone stress injuries with increasing female athlete triad–related risk factors: A prospective multisite study of exercising girls and women, *American Journal of Sports Medicine* 42 (2014): 949–958.

12. Position of the American Dietetic Association, Nutrition intervention in the treatment of eating disorders, *Journal of the American Dietetic Association* (2011): 1236–1241 (reaffirmed).

13. *Diagnostic and Statistical Manual of Mental Disorders*, 5th edition (Washington, D.C.: American Psychiatric Association, 2013), prepublication, available at www.dsm5.org/ProposedRevision/Pages/FeedingandEatingDisorders.aspx.

14. M. Misra and A. Klibanski, Anorexia nervosa and bone, *Journal of Endocrinology* 221 (2014): R163–R176; A. P. Winston, The clinical biochemistry of anorexia nervosa, *Annals of Clinical Biochemistry* 49 (2012): 132–143.

15. C. Stheneur, S. Bergeron, and A. L. Lapeyraque, Renal complications in anorexia nervosa, *Eating and Weight Disorders* 19 (2014): 455–460.

16. D. Modan-Moses and coauthors, High prevalence of vitamin D deficiency and insufficiency in adolescent inpatients diagnosed with eating disorders, *International Journal of Eating Disorders* (2014), epub, doi:10.1002/eat.22347; W. Renthal, I. Marin-Valencia, and P. A. Evans, Thiamine deficiency secondary to anorexia nervosa: An uncommon cause of peripheral neuropathy and Wernicke encephalopathy in adolescence, *Pediatric Neurology* 51 (2014): 100–103.

17. L. M. de Barse and coauthors, Does maternal history of eating disorders predict mothers' feeding practices and preschoolers' emotional eating? *Appetite* 85 (2015): 1–7.

18. A. Keshaviah and coauthors, Re-examining premature mortality in anorexia nervosa: A meta-analysis redux, *Comprehensive Psychiatry* 55 (2014): 1773–1784; G. Di Cola and coauthors, Cardiovascular disorders in anorexia nervosa and potential therapeutic targets, *Internal and Emergency Medicine* 9 (2014): 717–721.

19. Position of the American Dietetic Association, Nutrition intervention in the treatment of eating disorders, 2011.

20. A. E. Kass, R. P. Kolko, and D. E. Wilfley, Psychological treatments for eating disorders, *Current Opinion in Psychology* 26 (2013): 549–555;

F

Position of the American Dietetic Association, Nutrition intervention in the treatment of eating disorders, 2011.

21. E. Marzola and coauthors, Nutritional rehabilitation in anorexia nervosa: Review of the literature and implications for treatment, *BMC Psychiatry* 290 (2013), epub, doi:10.1186/1471-244X-13-290.

22. B. T. Walsh, The enigmatic persistence of anorexia nervosa, *American Journal of Psychiatry* 170 (2013): 477–484.

23. *Diagnostic and Statistical Manual of Mental Disorders*, 2013.

24. S. E. Racine and coauthors, Examining associations between negative urgency and key components of objective binge episodes, *International Journal of Eating Disorders* (2015), epub ahead of print, doi:10.1002/eat.22412; Position of the American Dietetic Association, Nutrition intervention in the treatment of eating disorders, 2011.

25. D. Mitchison and P. J. Hay, The epidemiology of eating disorders: Genetic, environmental, and societal factors, *Clinical Epidemiology* 6 (2014): 89–97; E. M. Stephen and coauthors, Adolescent risk factors for purging in young women: Findings from national longitudinal study of adolescent health, *Journal of Eating Disorders* (2014), epub, doi:10.1186/2050-2974-2-1.

26. K. Campbell and R. Peebles, Eating disorders in children and adolescents: State of the art review, 2014.

27. M. J. Krantz and coauthors, Factors influencing QT prolongation in patients hospitalized with severe anorexia nervosa, *General Hospital Psychiatry* 34 (2012): 173–177.

28. A. Raevuori and coauthors, Highly increased risk of type 2 diabetes in patients with binge eating disorder and bulimia nervosa, *International Journal of Eating Disorders* (2014), epub ahead of print, doi:10.1002/eat.22334.

29. D. G. Smith and T. W. Robbins, The neurobiological underpinnings of obesity and binge eating: A rationale for adopting the food addiction model, *Biological Psychiatry* 73 (2013): 804–810; N. D. Volkow and coauthors, Obesity and addiction: Neurobiological overlaps, *Obesity Reviews* 14 (2013): 2–18.

30. A. Meule and A. N. Gearhardt, Food addiction in the light of DSM-5, *Nutrients* 6 (2014): 3653–3671; A. J. Flint and coauthors, Food-addiction scale measurement in 2 cohorts of middle-aged and older women, *American Journal of Clinical Nutrition* 99 (2014): 578–586.

31. N. M. Avena, M. E. Bocarsly, and B. G. Hoebel, Animal models of sugar and fat bingeing: Relationship to food addiction and increased body weight, *Methods in Molecular Biology* 829 (2012): 351–365.

32. M. E. Bocarsly and coauthors, GS 455534 selectively suppresses binge eating of palatable food and attenuates dopamine release in the accumbens of sugar-bingeing rats, *Behavioral Pharmacology* 25 (2014): 147–157; N. A. Hadad and L. A. Knackstedt, Addicted to palatable foods: Comparing the neurobiology of bulimia nervosa to that of drug addiction, *Psychopharmacology* 231 (2014): 1897–1912.

Chapter 10

1. K. Gebel and coauthors, Effect of moderate to vigorous physical activity on all-cause mortality in middle-aged and older Australians, *JAMA Internal Medicine* (2015), epub ahead of print, doi:10.1001/jamainternmed.2015.0541; M. Renier and coauthors, Long-term health benefits of physical activity—A systematic review of longitudinal studies, *BMC Public Health* 13 (2013), epub, doi:10.1186/1471-2458-13-813.

2. C. D. Harris and coauthors, Adult participation in aerobic and muscle strengthening physical activities—United States, 2011, *Morbidity and Mortality Weekly Report* 62 (2013): 326–330.

3. U. Ladabaum and coauthors, Obesity, abdominal obesity, physical activity, and caloric intake in U.S. adults: 1988–2010, *American Journal of Medicine* 127 (2014): 717–727.

4. B. Bond and coauthors, Exercise intensity and the protection from postprandial vascular dysfunction in adolescents, *Heart and Circulatory Physiology* (2015), epub, doi:10.1152/ajpheart.00074.2015; M. Catoire and S. Kersten, The search for exercise factors in humans, *FASEB Journal* 29 (2015):1615–1628; R. Y. Aysano and coauthors, Acute effects of physical exercise in type 2 diabetes: A review, *World Journal of Diabetes* 15 (2014): 659–665; K. Iizuka, T. Machida, and M. Hirafuji, Skeletal muscle is an endocrine organ, *Journal of Pharmacological Sciences* 125 (2014): 125–131.

5. J. O. Chen and coauthors, Irisin: A new molecular marker and target in metabolic disorder, *Lipids in Health and Disease* 14 (2015), epub ahead of print, doi:10.1186/1476-511X-14-2; S. Raschke and J. Eckel, Adipo-myokines: Two sides of the same coin—Mediators of inflammation and mediators of exercise, *Mediators of Inflammation* (2013), epub, doi:10.1155/2013/320724.

6. D. Bishop-Bailey, Mechanisms governing the health and performance benefits of exercise, *British Journal of Pharmacology* 170 (2013): 1153–1166; P. Boström and coauthors, A PGC1-α-dependent myokine that drives brown-fat-like development of white fat and thermogenesis, *Nature* 481 (2012): 463–468; B. K. Pedersen, A muscular twist on the fate of fat, *New England Journal of Medicine* 366 (2012): 1544–1545.

7. U.S. Department of Health and Human Services, 2008 Physical Activity Guidelines for Americans (Washington, D.C.: U.S. Department of Health and Human Services, 2008), available at www.health.gov/paguidelines/default.aspx.

8. M. E. Armstrong and coauthors, Frequent physical activity may not reduce vascular disease risk as much as moderate activity: Large prospective study of UK women, *Circulation* (2015), epub ahead of print, 114.010296; U. Ekelund and coauthors, Physical activity and all-cause mortality across levels of overall and abdominal adiposity in European men and women: The European Prospective Investigation into Cancer and Nutrition Study (EPIC), *American Journal of Clinical Nutrition* (2015), epub ahead of print, doi:10.3945/ajcn.114.100065; C. Y. Wu and coauthors, The association of physical activity with all-cause, cardiovascular, and cancer mortality among older adults, *Preventive Medicine* (2015), epub ahead of print, doi:10.1016/j.ypmed.2014.12.023.

9. D. L. Swift and coauthors, The role of exercise and physical activity in weight loss and maintenance, *Progress in Cardiovascular Diseases* 56 (2014): 441–447; Nicklas and coauthors, Successful weight loss among obese U.S. adults, *American Journal of Preventive Medicine* 48 (2012): 1–5.

10. American College of Sports Medicine, Position stand: Quantity and quality of exercise for developing and maintaining cardiorespiratory, musculoskeletal, and neuromotor fitness in apparently healthy adults: Guidance for prescribing exercise, *Medicine and Science in Sports and Exercise* 43 (2011): 1334–1359.

11. S. Phillips, Building an "optimal diet": Putting protein into practice, presented at the Academy of Nutrition and Dietetics' Food and Nutrition Conference and Expo, Atlanta, October 2014; B. E. Phillips, D. S. Hill, and P. J. Atherton, Regulation of muscle protein synthesis in humans, *Current Opinion in Clinical Nutrition and Metabolic Care* 15 (2012): 58–63.

12. P. J. Atherton and K. Smith, Muscle protein synthesis in response to nutrition and exercise, *Journal of Physiology* 590 (2012): 1049–1057.

13. American College of Sports Medicine, Position stand: Progression models in resistance training for healthy adults, *Medicine and Science in Sports and Exercise* 41 (2009): 687–708.

14. American College of Sports Medicine, Position stand: Quantity and quality of exercise for developing and maintaining cardiorespiratory, musculoskeletal, and neuromotor fitness in apparently healthy adults, 2011.

15. C. H. Murphy, A. J. Hector, and S. M. Phillips, Considerations for protein intake in managing weight loss in athletes, *European Journal of Sport Science* 15 (2015): 21–28; T. A. Churchward-Venne and coauthors, Role of protein and amino acids in promoting lean mass accretion with resistance exercise and attenuating lean mass loss during energy deficit in humans, *Amino Acids* 45 (2013): 231–240.

16. C. Y. Wu and coauthors, The association of physical activity with all-cause, cardiovascular, and cancer mortality among older adults, *Preventive Medicine* (2015), epub ahead of print, doi:10.1016/j.ypmed.2014.12.023; P. Kokkinos, Physical activity, health benefits, and mortality risk, *ISRN Cardiology* (2012), epub, doi:10.5402/2012/718789.

17. M. Amann, Pulmonary system limitations to endurance exercise performance in humans, *Experimental Physiology* 97 (2012): 311–318.

18. A. C. McKee and coauthors, The neuropathology of sport, *Acta Neuropathologica* 127 (2014): 29–51; J. Calatayud and coauthors, Exercise and ankle sprain injuries: A comprehensive review, *Physician and Sportsmedicine* 42

(2014): 88–93; M. Leppänen and coauthors, Interventions to prevent sports related injuries: A systematic review and meta-analysis of randomised controlled trials, *Sports Medicine* 44 (2014): 473–486; K. G. Harmon and coauthors, American Medical Society for Sports Medicine position statement: Concussion in sport, *British Journal of Sports Medicine* 47 (2013): 15–26.

19. American College of Sports Medicine, *ACSM's Guidelines for Exercise Testing and Prescription*, 9th ed. (Philadelphia: Lippincott, Williams, and Wilkins, 2014).

20. J. S. Baker, M. C. McCormick, and R. A. Robergs, Interaction among skeletal muscle metabolic energy systems during intense exercise, *Journal of Nutrition and Metabolism* (2010), epub, doi:10.1155/2010/905612.

21. S. Kuzmiak-Glancy and W. T. Willis, Skeletal muscle fuel selection occurs at the mitochondrial level, *Journal of Experimental Biology* 217 (2014): 1993–2003.

22. D. G. Burt and coauthors, Effects of exercise-induced muscle damage on resting metabolic rate, submaximal running and post-exercise oxygen consumption, *European Journal of Sport Science* 14 (2014): 337–344; G. C. Henderson, Sexual dimorphism in the effects of exercise on metabolism of lipids to support resting metabolism, *Frontiers in Endocrinology* 5 (2014), epub, doi:10.3389/fendo.2014.00162.

23. I. Larsen and coauthors, High- and moderate-intensity aerobic exercise and excess post-exercise oxygen consumption in men with metabolic syndrome, *Scandinavian Journal of Medicine & Science in Sports* 24 (2014): e174–e179.

24. C. J. Ramnanan and coauthors, Physiologic action of glucagon on liver glucose metabolism, *Diabetes, Obesity, and Metabolism* 13 (2011): 118–125.

25. J. Bergstrom and coauthors, Diet, muscle glycogen and physical performance, *Acta Physiologica Scandanavica* 71 (1967): 140–150.

26. K. J. Stuempfle and coauthors, Race diet of finishers and non-finishers in a 100 mile (161 km) mountain footrace, *Journal of the American College of Nutrition* 30 (2011): 529–535.

27. Position of the American Dietetic Association, Dietitians of Canada, and the American College of Sports Medicine: Nutrition and Athletic Performance, *Journal of the Academy of Nutrition and Dietetics* 109 (2009): 509–527, reaffirmed 2015.

28. K. A. Pollak and coauthors, Exogenously applied muscle metabolites synergistically evoke sensations of muscle fatigue and pain in human subjects, *Experimental Physiology* 99 (2014): 368–380.

29. G. van Hall, Lactate kinetics in human tissues at rest and during exercise, *Acta Physiologica* 199 (2012): 499–508.

30. J. F. Moxnes and Ø. Sandbakk, The kinetics of lactate production and removal during whole-body exercise, *Theoretical Biology and Medical Modeling* 9 (2012), epub, doi:10.1186/1742-4682-9-7.

31. K. D. Gejl and coauthors, Muscle glycogen content modifies SR Ca2+ release rate in elite endurance athletes, *Medicine and Science in Sports and Exercise* 46 (2014): 496–505; N. Ørtenblad, H. Westerblad, and J. Nielsen, Muscle glycogen stores and fatigue, *Journal of Physiology* 18 (2013): 4405–4413.

32. J. Finsterer, Biomarkers of peripheral muscle fatigue during exercise, *BMC Musculoskeletal Disorders* 13 (2013), epub, doi:10.1186/1471-2474-13-218.

33. T. D. Noakes, Fatigue is a brain-derived emotion that regulates the exercise behavior to ensure the protection of whole body homeostasis, *Frontiers in Physiology*, April 2012, epub, doi:10.3389/phys.2012.00082.

34. Position of the American Dietetic Association, Dietitians of Canada, and the American College of Sports Medicine, Nutrition and athletic performance, *Journal of the American Dietetic Association* 109 (2009): 509–527.

35. J. D. Bartlett, J. A. Hawley, and J. P. Morton, Carbohydrate availability and exercise training adaptation: Too much of a good thing? *European Journal of Sport Science* 15 (2015): 3–12; L. M. Margolis and S. M. Pasiakos, Optimizing intramuscular adaptations to aerobic exercise: Effects of carbohydrate restriction and protein supplementation on mitochondrial biogenesis, *Advances in Nutrition* 4 (2013): 657–664.

36. N. M. Cermak and L. J. van Loon, The use of carbohydrates during exercise as an ergogenic aid, *Sports Medicine* 43 (2013): 1139–1155.

37. A. Jeukendrup, The new carbohydrate recommendations, *Nestlé Nutrition Institute Workshop Series* 75 (2013): 63–71.

38. E. Prado de Oliveira, R. C. Burnini, and A. Jeukendrup, Gastrointestinal complaints during exercise: Prevalence, etiology, and nutritional recommendations, *Sports Medicine* 44 (2014): S79–S85.

39. N. M. Cermak and L. J. van Loon, The use of carbohydrates during exercise as an ergogenic aid, *Sports Medicine* 43 (2013): 1139–1155; Position of the American Dietetic Association, Dietitians of Canada, and the American College of Sports Medicine, Nutrition and athletic performance, 2009, reaffirmed 2015.

40. L. L. Spriet, New insights into the interaction of carbohydrate and fat metabolism during exercise, *Sports Medicine* 44 (2014): S87–S96.

41. T. A. Astorino and coauthors, Effect of two doses of interval training on maximal fat oxidation in sedentary women, *Medicine and Science in Sports and Exercise* 45 (2013): 1878–1886; L. H. Willis and coauthors, Effects of aerobic and/or resistance training on body mass and fat mass in overweight or obese adults, *Journal of Applied Physiology* 113 (2012): 1831–1837.

42. R. J. Maughan and S. M. Shirreffs, Nutrition for sports performance: Issues and opportunities, *Proceedings of the Nutrition Society* 71 (2012): 112–119.

43. Position of the American Dietetic Association, Dietitians of Canada, and the American College of Sports Medicine, Nutrition and athletic performance, 2009.

44. M. Martorell and coauthors, Docosahexaenoic acid supplementation promotes erythrocyte antioxidant defense and reduces protein nitrosative damage in male athletes, *Lipids* 50 (2015): 131–148; F. M. DiLorenzo, C. J. Drager, and J. W. Rankin, Docosahexaenoic acid affects markers of inflammation and muscle damage after eccentric exercise, *Journal of Strength and Conditioning Research* 28 (2014): 2768–2774.

45. T. A. Churchward-Venne, N. A. Burd, and S. M. Phillips, Nutrition regulation of muscle protein synthesis with resistance exercise: Strategies to enhance anabolism, *Nutrition and Metabolism* 9 (2012), epub, doi:10.1186/1743-7075-9-40.

46. D. M. Camera and coauthors, Protein ingestion increases myofibrillar protein synthesis after concurrent exercise, *Medicine and Science in Sports and Exercise* 47 (2015): 82–91; D. K. Layman and coauthors, Defining meal requirements for protein to optimize metabolic roles of amino acids, *American Journal of Clinical Nutrition* 101 (2015): 1330S–1338S.

47. Churchward-Venne, Burd, and Phillips, Nutrition regulation of muscle protein synthesis with resistance exercise, 2012.

48. J. L. Areta and coauthors, Timing and distribution of protein ingestion during prolonged recovery from resistance exercise alters myofibrillar protein synthesis, *Journal of Physiology* 591 (2013): 2319–2331.

49. C. J. Mitchell and coauthors, Acute post-exercise myofibrillar protein synthesis is not correlated with resistance training-induced muscle hypertrophy in young men, *PLOS ONE* 9 (2014), epub, doi:10.1371/journal.pone.0089431.

50. T. M. McLellan, S. M. Pasiakos, and H. R. Lieberman, Effects of protein in combination with carbohydrate supplements on acute or repeat endurance exercise performance: A systematic review, *Sports Medicine* 44 (2014): 535–550.

51. Selected issues for nutrition and the athlete: A team physician consensus statement, *Medicine and Science in Sports and Exercise* 45 (2013): 2378–2386.

52. Position of the American Dietetic Association, Dietitians of Canada, and the American College of Sports Medicine, Nutrition and Athletic Performance, 2009.

53. N. R. Rodriguez and S. L. Miller, Effective translation of current dietary guidance: Understanding and communicating the concepts of minimal and optimal levels of dietary protein, *American Journal of Clinical Nutrition* 101 (2015): 1353S–1358S.

54. D. Villacis and coauthors, Prevalence of abnormal vitamin D levels among Division I NCAA athletes, *Sports Health* 6 (2014): 340–347; F. Farrokhyar and coauthors, Prevalence of vitamin D inadequacy in athletes: A systematic review and meta-analysis, *Sports Medicine* (2014), epub ahead of print, doi:10.1007/s40279-014-0267-6.

55. K. Janakiraman, S. Shenoy, and J. S. Sandhu, Firm insoles effectively reduce hemolysis in runners during long distance running—A comparative study, *Sports Medicine, Arthroscopy,*

Rehabilitation, Therapy and Technology 3 (2011), epub, doi:10.1186/1758–255–3–12.

56. G. Lippi and coauthors, Foot-strike haemolysis after a 60-km ultramarathon, *Blood Transfusion* 10 (2012): 377–383.

57. W. Kong, G. Gao, and Y. Chang, Hepcidin and sports anemia, *Cell and Bioscience* 4 (2014), epub, doi:10.1186/2045-3701-4-19.

58. D. M. DellaValle and J. D. Haas, Iron supplementation improves energetic efficiency in iron-depleted female rowers, *Medicine and Science in Sports and Exercise* 46 (2014): 1204–1215; S. Pasricha and coauthors, Iron supplementation benefits physical performance in women of reproductive age: A systematic review and meta-analysis, *Journal of Nutrition* (2014), epub ahead of print, doi:10.3945/jn.113.189589.

59. Executive summary of National Athletic Trainers' Association position statement on exertional heat illnesses, 2014, available at www.nata.org/sites/default/files/Heat-Illness-Executive-Summary.pdf.

60. Centers for Disease Control and Prevention, Hypothermia-related deaths—Wisconsin, 2014 and United States, 2003–2013, *Morbidity and Mortality Weekly Report* 64 (2015): 141–143.

61. C. A. Rosenbloom and E. J. Coleman (eds.), *Sports Nutrition: A Practice Manual for Professionals* (Chicago: Academy of Nutrition and Dietetics, 2012), pp. 106–127; Position of the American Dietetic Association, Dietitians of Canada, and the American College of Sports Medicine, Nutrition and Athletic Performance, 2009.

62. N. Yamashita and coauthors, Two percent hypohydration does not impair self- selected high-intensity intermittent exercise performance, *Journal of Strength and Conditioning Research* 29 (2015): 116–125; C. N. Bardis and coauthors, Mild hypohydration decreases cycling performance in the heat, *Medicine and Science in Sports and Exercise* 45 (2013): 1782–1789.

63. E. L. Earhart and coauthors, Effects of oral sodium supplementation on indices of thermoregulation in trained, endurance athletes, *Journal of Sports Science and Medicine* 14 (2015): 172–178.

64. E. R. Parr and coauthors, Alcohol ingestion impairs maximal post-exercise rates of myofibrillar protein synthesis following a single bout of concurrent training, *PLOS ONE* 9 (2014), epub, doi:10.1371/journal.pone.0088384.

65. Position of the American Dietetic Association, Dietitians of Canada, and the American College of Sports Medicine, Nutrition and Athletic Performance, 2009.

66. C. Rosenbloom, Food and fluid guidelines before, during, and after exercise, *Nutrition Today* 47 (2012): 63–69.

67. W. R. Lunn and coauthors, Chocolate milk and endurance exercise recovery: Protein balance, glycogen, and performance, *Medicine and Science in Sports and Exercise* 44 (2012): 682–691.

68. B. Besbrow and coauthors, Comparing the rehydration potential of different milk-based drinks to a carbohydrate-electrolyte beverage, *Applied Physiology and Nutrition Metabolism* 39 (2014): 1366–1372.

Controversy 10

1. M. Comassi and coauthors, Acute effects of different degrees of ultra-endurance exercise on systemic inflammatory responses, *Internal Medicine Journal* 45 (2015): 74–79.

2. C. L. Draeger and coauthors, Controversies of antioxidant vitamins supplementation in exercise: Ergogenic or ergolytic effects in humans? *Journal of the International Society of Sports Nutrition* 11 (2014), epub, doi:10.1186/1550-2783-11-4; T. D. Scribbans and coauthors, Resveratrol supplementation does not augment performance adaptations or fibre-type-specific responses to high-intensity interval training in humans, *Applied Physiology, Nutrition, and Metabolism* 39 (2014): 1305–1313.

3. R. C. Leonardo-Mendonça and coauthors, Redox status and antioxidant response in professional cyclists during training, *European Journal of Sport Science* 14 (2014): 830–838; S. K. Powers and coauthors, Exercise-induced improvements in myocardial antioxidant capacity: The antioxidant players and cardioprotection, *Free Radical Research* 48 (2014): 43–51; G. Sharifi, A. B. Najafabadi, and F. E. Ghashghaei, Oxidative stress and total antioxidant capacity in handball players, *Advances in Biomedical Research* 3 (2014), epub, doi:10.4103/2277-9175.139538.

4. G. Paulsen and coauthors, Vitamin C and E supplementation alters protein signaling after a strength training session, but not muscle growth during 10 weeks of training, *Journal of Physiology* 592 (2014): 5391–5408.

5. R. Meeusen, B. Roelands, and L. L. Spriet, Caffeine, exercise and the brain, *Nestlé Nutrition Institute Workshop Series* 76 (2013): 1–12; T. A. Astorino and coauthors, Increases in cycling performance in response to caffeine ingestion are repeatable, *Nutrition Research* 32 (2012): 78–84.

6. R. S. Cruz and coauthors, Caffeine affects time to exhaustion and substrate oxidation during cycling at maiximal lactate steady state, *Nutrients* 7 (2015): 5254–5264; S. M. An, J. S. Park and S. H. Kim, Effect of energy drink dose on exercise capacity, heart rate recovery and heart rate variability after high-intensity exercise, *Journal of Exercise Nutrition and Biochemistry* 18 (2014): 31–39; C. F. Hurley, D. L. Hatfield, and D. A. Riebe, The effect of caffeine ingestion on delayed onset muscle soreness, *Journal of Strength and Conditioning Research* 27 (2013): 3101–3109.

7. Astorino and coauthors, Increases in cycling performance in response to caffeine ingestion are repeatable, 2012.

8. P. Jain and coauthors, A comparison of sports and energy drinks—Physiochemical properties and enamel dissolution, *General Dentistry* 60 (2012): 190–197; W. Doyle and coauthors, The effects of energy beverages on cultured cells, *Food and Chemical Toxicology* 50 (2012): 3759–3768.

9. S. Bull and coauthors, Extensive literature search as preparatory work for the safety assessment for caffeine (EFSA supporting publication 2015:EN-561), 2015, available at www.efsa.europa.eu/en/supporting/doc/561e.pdf; A. B. Hodgson, R. K. Randell, and A. E. Jeukendrup, The metabolic and performance effects of caffeine compared to coffee during endurance exercise, *PLOS ONE* 8 (2013), epub, doi:10.1371/journal.pone.0059561.

10. K. Novakova and coauthors, Effect of L-carnitine supplementation on the body carnitine pool, skeletal muscle energy metabolism and physical performance in male vegetarians, *European Journal of Nutrition* (2015), epub ahead of print, doi:10.1007/s00394-015-0838-9.

11. L. W. Judge and coauthors, Creatine usage and education of track and field throwers at NCAA Division I universities, *Journal of Strength and Conditioning Research* (2014), epub ahead of print, doi:10.1519/JSC.0000000000000818.

12. C. L. Camic and coauthors, The effects of polyethylene glycosylated creatine supplementation on anaerobic performance measure and body composition, *Journal of Strength and Conditioning Research* 28 (2014): 825–833; M. C. Devries and S. M. Phillips, Creatine supplementation during resistance training in older adults—A meta-analysis, *Medicine and Science in Sports and Exercise* 46 (2014): 1194–1203.

13. Devries and Phillips, Creatine supplementation during resistance training in older adults, 2014; Judge and coauthors, Creatine usage and education of track and field throwers at NCAA Division I universities, 2014.

14. A. Nasseri and A. Jafari, Effects of creatine supplementation along with resistance training on urinary formaldehyde and serum enzymes in wrestlers, *Journal of Sports Medicine and Physical Fitness* (2014), epub ahead of print, PMID:25286897.

15. L. M. Burke, Practical considerations for bicarbonate loading and sports performance, *Nestlé Nutrition Institute Workshop Series* 75 (2013): 15–26.

16. P. M. Bellinger, β-alanine supplementation for athletic performance: An update, *Journal of Strength and Conditioning Research* 28 (2014): 1751–1770; R. M. Hobson and coauthors, Effects of β-alanine supplementation on exercise performance: A meta-analysis, *Amino Acids* 43 (2012): 25–37; A. E. Smith and coauthors, Exercise-induced oxidative stress: The effects of β-alanine supplementation in women, *Amino Acids* 43 (2012): 77–90; A. E. Smith-Ryan and coauthors, High-velocity intermittent running: Effects of beta-alanine supplementation, *Journal of Strength and Conditioning Research* 26 (2012): 2798–2805.

17. P. M. Bellinger and C. L. Minahan, Performance effects of acute β-alanine induced paresthesia in competitive cyclists, *European Journal of Sport Science* 30 (2015): 1–8.

18. T. A. Churchward-Venne and coauthors, Leucine supplementation of a low-protein mixed macronutrient beverage enhances myofibrillar protein synthesis in young men: A double-blind, randomized trial, *American Journal of Clinical Nutrition* 99 (2014): 276–286.

19. T. A. Churchward-Venne, N. A. Burd, and S. M. Phillips, Nutrition regulation of muscle protein synthesis with resistance exercise: Strategies to enhance anabolism, *Nutrition and Metabolism* 9 (2012), epub, doi:10.1186/1743-7075-9-40; N. Gwacham and D. R. Wagner, Acute effects of a caffeine-taurine energy drink on repeated sprint performance of American college football players, *International Journal of Sport Nutrition and Exercise Metabolism* 22 (2012): 109–116.

20. L. E. Norton and coauthors, Leucine content of dietary proteins is a determinant of postprandial skeletal muscle protein synthesis in adult rats, *Nutrition and Metabolism* 9 (2012), epub, doi:10.1186/1743-7075-9-67.

21. N. Babault and coauthors, Pea proteins oral supplementation promotes muscle thickness gains during resistance training: A double-blind, randomized, placebo-controlled clinical trial vs. whey protein, *Journal of the International Society of Sports Nutrition* 12 (2015), epub, doi:10.1186/s12970-014-0064-5.

22. S. M. Pasiakos, T. M. McLellan, and H. R. Lieberman, The effects of protein supplements on muscle mass, strength, and aerobic and anaerobic power in healthy adults: A systematic review, *Sports Medicine* 45 (2015): 111–131.

23. P. A. Cohen, J. C. Travis, and B. J. Venhuis, A synthetic stimulant never tested in humans, 1,3-dimethylbutylamine (DMBA) is identified in multiple dietary supplements, *Drug Testing and Analysis* 7 (2015): 83–87.

24. M. E. Arensberg and coauthors, Summit on Human Performance and Dietary Supplements summary report, *Nutrition Today* 49 (2014): 7–15.

Chapter 11

1. D. F. Warner and V. Mizrahi, Complex genetics of drug resistance in Mycobacterium tuberculosis, *Nature Genetics* 45 (2013): 1107–1108; W. G. van Panhuis and coauthors, Contagious diseases in the United States from 1888 to the present, *New England Journal of Medicine* 369 (2013): 2152–2158.

2. N. J. Afacan, C. D. Fjell, and R. E. Hancock, A systems biology approach to nutritional immunology—Focus on innate immunity, *Molecular Aspects of Medicine* 33 (2012): 14–25; I. Laaksi, Vitamin D and respiratory infection in adults, *Proceedings of the Nutrition Society* 71 (2012): 90–97.

3. D. L. Hoyert and J. Xu, Deaths: Preliminary data for 2011, *National Vital Statistics Reports* 61, no. 6 (2012): 1–50.

4. P. C. Calder, Feeding the immune system, *Proceedings of the Nutrition Society* 72 (2013): 299–309; Afacan, Fjell, and Hancock, A systems biology approach to nutritional immunology, 2012; Laaksi, Vitamin D and respiratory infection in adults, 2012.

5. Calder, Feeding the immune system, 2013; O. P. Garcia, Effect of vitamin A deficiency on the immune response in obesity, *Proceedings of the Nutrition Society* 71 (2012): 290–297.

6. H. Haase and L. Rink, Multiple impacts of zinc on immune function, *Metallomics* 6 (2014): 1175–1180; S. Hojyo and coauthors, Zinc transporter SLC39A10/ZIP10 controls humoral immunity by modulating B-cell receptor signal strength, *Proceedings of the National Academy of Sciences of the United States of America* 111 (2014): 11786–11791; N. W. Solomons, Update on zinc biology, *Annals of Nutrition and Metabolism* 62 (2013): 8–17; Calder, Feeding the immune system, 2013.

7. P. K. Mankal and D. P. Kotler, From wasting to obesity, changes in nutritional concerns in HIV/AIDS, *Endocrinology and Metabolism Clinics of North America* 43 (2014): 647–663; Position of the American Dietetic Association: Nutrition intervention and human immunodeficiency virus infection, *Journal of the American Dietetic Association* 110 (2010): 1105–1119.

8. N. Esser and coauthors, Inflammation as a link between obesity, metabolic syndrome and type 2 diabetes, *Diabetes Research and Clinical Practice* 105 (2014): 141–150; M. El Assar, J. Angulo, and L. Rodriquez-Manas, Oxidative stress and vascular inflammation in aging, *Free Radical Biology and Medicine* 65 (2013): 380–401.

9. R. H. Eckel and coauthors, 2013 AHA/ACC guideline on lifestyle management to reduce cardiovascular risk, *Circulation* 129 (2014): S76–S99; B. Spring and coauthors, Healthy lifestyle change and subclinical atherosclerosis in young adults: Coronary Artery Risk Development in Young Adults (CARDIA) study, *Circulation* 130 (2014): 10–17; Position of the Academy of Nutrition and Dietetics: The role of nutrition in health promotion and chronic disease prevention, *Journal of the Academy of Nutrition and Dietetics* 113 (2013): 972–979; J. D. Berry and coauthors, Lifetime risks of cardiovascular disease, *New England Journal of Medicine* 366 (2012): 321–329; L. H. Kushi and coauthors, American Cancer Society guidelines on nutrition and physical activity for cancer prevention, *CA: Cancer Journal for Clinicians* 62 (2012): 30–67.

10. A. Fardet and Y. Boirie, Associations between diet-related diseases and impaired physiological mechanisms: A holistic approach based on meta-analyses to identify targets for preventive nutrition, *Nutrition Reviews* 71 (2013): 643–656.

11. A. S. Go and coauthors, Heart disease and stroke statistics—2014 update: A report from the American Heart Association, *Circulation* 129 (2014): e28–e292.

12. Go and coauthors, Heart disease and stroke statistics—2014 update, 2014.

13. Go and coauthors, Heart disease and stroke statistics—2014 update, 2014.

14. American Heart Association, Menopause and Heart Disease, updated May 28, 2015, available at www.heart.org/HEARTORG/Conditions/More/MyHeartandStrokeNews/Menopause-and-Heart-Disease_UCM_448432_Article.jsp.

15. U.S. Department of Agriculture and U. S. Department of Health and Human Services, *Scientific Report of the 2015 Dietary Guidelines Advisory Committee* (2015): Table D2.3, 43, available at www.health.gov; Eckel and coauthors, 2013 AHA/ACC guideline on lifestyle management to reduce cardiovascular risk, 2014; E. Lopez-Garcia and coauthors, The Mediterranean-style dietary pattern and mortality among men and women with cardiovascular disease, *American Journal of Clinical Nutrition* 99 (2014): 172–180; P. M. Kris-Etherton, Walnuts decrease risk of cardiovascular disease: A summary of efficacy and biologic mechanisms, *Journal of Nutrition* 144 (2014): 547S–554S; S. N. Bhupathiraju and coauthors, Quantity and variety in fruit and vegetable intake and risk of coronary heart disease, *American Journal of Clinical Nutrition* 98 (2013): 1514–1523.

16. M. da Silva Afonso and coauthors, The impact of dietary fatty acids on macrophage cholesterol homeostasis, *Journal of Nutritional Biochemistry* 25 (2014): 95–103.

17. A. A. Kalanuria, P. Nyquist, and G. Ling, The prevention and regression of atherosclerotic plaques: Emerging treatments, *Vascular Health and Risk Management* 8 (2012): 549–561.

18. B. Messner and D. Bernhard, Smoking and cardiovascular disease: Mechanisms of endothelial dysfunction and early atherogenesis, *Arteriosclerosis, Thrombosis, and Vascular Biology* 34 (2014): 509–515; Kalanuria, Nyquist, and Ling, The prevention and regression of atherosclerotic plaques, 2012.

19. Kalanuria, Nyquist, and Ling, The prevention and regression of atherosclerotic plaques, 2012.

20. D. Kromhout and J. De Goede, Update on cardiometabolic effects of ω-3 fatty acids, *Current Opinion in Lipidology* 25 (2014): 85–90; L. G. Gao and coauthors, Influence of omega-3 polyunsaturated fatty acid-supplementation on platelet aggregation in humans: A meta-analysis of randomized controlled trials, *Atherosclerosis* 226 (2013): 328–334; B. J. McEwen and coauthors, Effects of omega-3 polyunsaturated fatty acids on platelet function in healthy subjects and subjects with cardiovascular disease, *Seminars in Thrombosis and Hemostasis* 39 (2013): 25–32.

21. Kromhout and De Goede, Update on cardiometabolic effects of ω-3 fatty acids, 2014; O. A. Khawaja, J. M. Gaziano, and L. Djoussè, N-3 fatty acids for prevention of cardiovascular disease, *Current Atherosclerosis Reports* 16 (2014): 450–457; M. Dessi and coauthors, Atherosclerosis, dyslipidemia, and inflammation: The significant role of polyunsaturated fatty acids, *ISRN Inflammation* (2013), doi:10.1155/2013/191823; M. C. de Oliveira Otto and coauthors, Circulating and dietary omega-3 and omega-6 polyunsaturated fatty acids and incidence of CVD in the Multi-Ethnic Study of Atherosclerosis, *Journal of the American Heart Association* 2 (2013): e000506.

22. Go and coauthors, Heart disease and stroke statistics—2014 update, 2014.

23. Go and coauthors, Heart disease and stroke statistics—2014 update, 2014; Q. Yang and coauthors, Trends in cardiovascular health metrics and association with all-cause and CVD mortality,

Journal of the American Medical Association 307 (2012): 1273–1283.

24. J. D. Berry and coauthors, Lifetime risks of cardiovascular disease, *New England Journal of Medicine* 366 (2012): 321–329.

25. Go and coauthors, Heart disease and stroke statistics—2014 update, 2014.

26. Go and coauthors, Heart disease and stroke statistics—2014 update, 2014.

27. E. Incalcaterra and coauthors, Pro-inflammatory genetic markers of atherosclerosis, *Current Atherosclerosis Reports* 15 (2013): 329–335; F. C. McGillicuddy and H. M. Roche, Nutritional status, genetic susceptibility, and insulin resistance—Important precedents to atherosclerosis, *Molecular Nutrition and Food Research* 56 (2012): 1173–1184.

28. R. C. Hoogeveen and coauthors, Small dense low-density lipoprotein cholesterol concentrations predict risk for coronary heart disease: The Atherosclerosis Risk in Communities (ARIC) study, *Arteriosclerosis, Thrombosis, and Vascular Biology* 34 (2014): 1069–1077; N. B. Allen and coauthors, Blood pressure trajectories in early adulthood and subclinical atherosclerosis in middle age, *Journal of the American Medical Association* 311 (2014): 490–497.

29. C. G. Santos-Gallego and R. S. Rosenson, Role of HDL in those with diabetes, *Current Cardiology Reports* 16 (2014): 512; M. H. Davidson, HDL and CETP inhibition: Will this DEFINE the future? *Current Treatment Options in Cardiovascular Medicine* 14 (2012): 384–390; K. Mahdy Ali and coauthors, Cardiovascular disease risk reduction by raising HDL cholesterol—Current therapies and future opportunities, *British Journal of Pharmacology* 167 (2012): 1177–1194; D. Kothapalli and coauthors, Cardiovascular protection by apoE and apoE-HDL linked to suppression of ECM gene expression and arterial stiffening, *Cell Reports* 2 (2012): 1–13.

30. B. F. Voight and coauthors, Plasma HDL cholesterol and risk of myocardial infarction: A Mendelian randomisation study, *Lancet* 380 (2012): 572–580.

31. P. Burchardt and coauthors, Low-density lipoprotein, its susceptibility to oxidation and the role of lipoprotein-associated phospholipase A2 and carboxyl ester lipase lipases in atherosclerotic plaque formation, *Archives of Medical Science* 9 (2013): 151–158; Kalanuria, Nyquist, and LIng, The prevention and regression of atherosclerotic plaques, 2012.

32. Kalanuria, Nyquist, and Ling, The prevention and regression of atherosclerotic plaques, 2012.

33. M. Miller and coauthors, Triglycerides and cardiovascular disease: A scientific statement from the American Heart Association, *Circulation* 123 (2011): 2292–2333.

34. Go and coauthors, Heart disease and stroke statistics—2014 update, 2014; P. A. James and coauthors, 2014 evidence-based guidelines for the management of high blood pressure in adults: Report from the panel members appointed to the Eighth Joint National Committee (JNCS),

Journal of the American Medical Association 311 (2014): 507–520.

35. American Diabetes Association, Position statement: Diagnosis and classification of diabetes mellitus, *Diabetes Care* 37 (2014): S81–S90.

36. B. A. Larsen and coauthors, Associations of physical activity and sedentary behavior with regional fat deposition, *Medicine and Science in Sports and Exercise* 46 (2014): 520–528; C. P. Earnest and coauthors, Aerobic and strength training in concomitant metabolic syndrome and type 2 diabetes, *Medicine and Science in Sports and Exercise* 46 (2014): 1293–1301; C. K. Roberts, J. P. Little, and J. P. Thyfault, Modification of insulin sensitivity and glycemic control by activity and exercise, *Medicine and Science in Sports and Exercise* 45 (2013): 1868–1877; S. W. Farrell, C. E. Finley, and S. M. Grundy, Cardiorespiratory fitness, LDL cholesterol, and CHD mortality in men, *Medicine and Science in Sports and Exercise* 44 (2012): 2132–2137; M. Hamer and coauthors, Physical activity and cardiovascular mortality risk: Possible protective mechanisms? *Medicine and Science in Sports and Exercise* 44 (2012): 84–88.

37. P. Nestel, Trans fatty acids: Are its cardiovascular risks fully appreciated? *Clinical Therapeutics* 36 (2014): 315–321; J. N. Kiage and coauthors, Intake of trans fat and all-cause mortality in the Reasons for Geographical and Racial Differences in Stroke (REGARDS) cohort, *American Journal of Clinical Nutrition* 97 (2013): 1121–1128.

38. D. P. Redlinger and coauthors, How effective are current dietary guidelines for cardiovascular disease prevention in healthy middle-aged and older men and women? A randomized controlled trial, *Ameircan Journal of Clinical Nutrition* 101 (2015): 922–930; D. Mozaffarian and coauthors, Heart disease and stroke statistics—2015 update: A report from the American Heart Association, *Circulation* 131 (2015): e76–e86; Eckel and coauthors, 2013 AHA/ACC guideline on lifestyle management to reduce cardiovascular risk, 2014.

39. Lopez-Garcia and coauthors, The Mediterranean-style dietary pattern and mortality among men and women with cardiovascular disease, 2014; Kris-Etherton, Walnuts decrease risk of cardiovascular disease, 2014; Bhupathiraju and coauthors, Quantity and variety in fruit and vegetable intake and risk of coronary heart disease, 2013; Dessi and coauthors, Atherosclerosis, dyslipidemia, and inflammation, 2013.

40. Go and coauthors, Heart disease and stroke statistics–2014 update, 2014; A. R. Aroor and coauthors, Maladaptive immune and inflammatory pathways lead to cardiovascular insulin resistance, *Metabolism* 62 (2013): 1543–1552.

41. M. Santaniemi and coauthors, Metabolic syndrome in the prediction of cardiovascular events: The potential additive role of hsCRP and adiponectin, *European Journal of Preventive Cardiology* 21 (2014): 1242–1248; S. M. Grundy, Pre-diabetes, metabolic syndrome, and cardiovascular risk, *Journal of the American College of Cardiology* 59 (2012): 635–643.

42. M. Exley and coauthors, The interplay between the immune system and adipose in obesity, *Journal of Endocrinology* (September 16, 2014), epub ahead of print; P. Bhargava and C. H. Lee, Role and function of macrophages in metabolic syndrome, *Biochemical Journal* 442 (2012): 253–262; R. Lorenzet and coauthors, Thrombosis and obesity: Cellular bases, *Thrombosis Research* 129 (2012): 285–289.

43. Go and coauthors, Heart disease and stroke statistics—2014 update, 2014.

44. J. R. Cerhan and coauthors, A pooled analysis of waist circumference and mortality in 650,000 adults, *Mayo Clinic Proceedings* 89 (2014): 335–345; N. M. Al-Daghri and coauthors, Visceral adiposity index is highly associated with adiponectin values and glycaemic disturbances, *European Journal of Clinical Investigation* 43 (2013): 183–189; H. E. Bays and coauthors, Obesity, adiposity, and dyslipidemia: A consensus statement from the National Lipid Association, *Journal of Clinical Lipidology* 7 (2013): 304–383; C. K. Kramer, B. Zinman, and R. Retnakaran, Are metabolically healthy overweight and obesity benign conditions? A systematic review and meta-analysis, *Annals of Internal Medicine* 159 (2013): 758–769; L. Landsberg and coauthors, Obesity-related hypertension: Pathogenesis, cardiovascular risk, and treatment: A position paper of The Obesity Society and the American Society of Hypertension, *Journal of Clinical Hypertension* 15 (2013): 14–33.

45. J. Clarke and I. Janssen, Sporadic and bouted physical activity and the metabolic syndrome in adults, *Medicine and Science in Sports and Exercise* 46 (2014): 76–83; C. H. Lin and coauthors, Moderate physical activity level as a protective factor against metabolic syndrome in middle-aged and older women, *Journal of Clinical Nursing* (September 25, 2014), doi:10.1111/jcn.12683; S. W. Farrell, C. E. Finley, and S. M. Grundy, Cardiorespiratory fitness, LDL cholesterol, and CHD mortality in men, *Medicine and Science in Sports and Exercise* 44 (2012): 2132–2137; M. Hamer and coauthors, Physical activity and cardiovascular mortality risk: Possible protective mechanisms? *Medicine and Science in Sports and Exercise* 44 (2012): 84–88; S. Liu and coauthors, Blood pressure responses to acute and chronic exercise are related in prehypertension, *Medicine and Science in Sports and Exercise* 44 (2012): 1644–1652.

46. D. C. Goff and coauthors, 2013 ACC/AHA guidelines on the assessment of cardiovascular risk: A report of the American College of Cardiology/American Heart Association Task Force on Practice Guidelines, *Circulation* 129 (2014): S49–S73; Eckel and coauthors, 2013 AHA/ACC guideline on lifestyle management to reduce cardiovascular risk, 2014; N. J. Stone and coauthors, ACC/AHA guideline on the treatment of blood cholesterol to reduce atherosclerotic cardiovascular risk in adults: A report of the American College of Cardiology/American Heart Association Task Force on Practice Guidelines, *Circulation* 129 (2014): S1–S45.

47. Go and coauthors, Heart disease and stroke statistics—2014 update, 2014; Eckel and coauthors, 2013 AHA/ACC guideline on lifestyle management to reduce cardiovascular risk, 2014; A. Akesson and coauthors, Low-risk diet and lifestyle habits in the primary prevention of myocardial infarction in men, *Journal of the American College of Cardiology* 64 (2014): 1299–1306.

48. O. Oyebode and coauthors, Fruit and vegetable consumption and all-cause, cancer, and CVD mortality: Analysis of Health Survey for England data, *Journal of Epidemiology and Community Health* 68 (2014): 856–862; X. Wang and coauthors, Fruit and vegetable consumption and mortality from all causes, cardiovascular disease, and cancer: Systematic review and dose-response meta-analysis of prospective cohort studies, *BMJ* (2014), doi:10.1136/bmj.g4490; E. Garcia-Fernandez and coauthors, Mediterranean diet and cardiodiabesity: A review, *Nutrients* 6 (2014): 3474–3500; Bhupathiraju and coauthors, Quantity and variety in fruit and vegetable intake and risk of coronary heart disease, 2013; P. Guallar-Castillón and coauthors, Major dietary patterns and risk of coronary heart disease in middle-aged persons from a Mediterranean country: The EPIC–Spain cohort study, *Nutrition, Metabolism, and Cardiovascular Diseases* 22 (2012): 192–199.

49. Go and coauthors, Heart disease and stroke statistics—2014; L. de Koning and coauthors, Sweetened beverage consumption, incident coronary heart disease and biomarkers of risk in men, *Circulation* 125 (2012): 1735–1741.

50. Miller and coauthors, Triglycerides and cardiovascular disease: A scientific statement from the American Heart Association, 2011.

51. Khawaja, Gaziano, and Djoussè, N-3 fatty acids for prevention of cardiovascular disease, 2014; C. von Schacky, Omega-3 index and cardiovascular health, *Nutrients* 6 (2014): 799–814; Dessi and coauthors, Atherosclerosis, dyslipidemia, and inflammation, 2013.

52. S. M. Kwak and coauthors, Efficacy of omega-3 fatty acid supplements (eicosapentaenoic acid and docosahexaenoic acid) in the secondary prevention of cardiovascular disease, *Archives of Internal Medicine* 172 (2012): 686–694.

53. Go and coauthors, Heart disease and stroke statistics—2014 update, 2014.

54. Go and coauthors, Heart disease and stroke statistics—2014 update, 2014.

55. Y. Huang and coauthors, Prehypertension and the risk of stroke: A meta-analysis, *Neurology* 82 (2014): 1153–1161.

56. Go and coauthors, Heart disease and stroke statistics—2014 update, 2014.

57. Landsberg and coauthors, Obesity-related hypertension: Pathogenesis, cardiovascular risk, and treatment, 2013; C. W. Mende, Obesity and hypertension: A common coexistence, *Journal of Clinical Hypertension* 14 (2012): 137–138.

58. T. A. Kotchen, A. W. Cowley, and E. D. Frohlich, Salt in health and disease—A delicate balance, *New England Journal of Medicine* 368 (2013): 1229–1237; P. K. Whelton and coauthors, AHA presidential advisory: Sodium,

blood pressure, and cardiovascular disease, *Circulation* 126 (2012): 2880–2889.

59. C. Koliaki and N. Datsilambros, Dietary sodium, potassium, and alcohol: Key players in the pathophysiology, prevention, and treatment of human hypertension, *Nutrition Reviews* 71 (2013): 402–411.

60. Eckel and coauthors, 2013 AHA/ACC guideline on lifestyle management to reduce cardiovascular risk, 2014; D. E. Epstein and coauthors, Determinants and consequences of adherence to the Dietary Approaches to Stop Hypertension diet in African-American and white adults with high blood pressure: Results from the ENCORE trial, *Journal of the Academy of Nutrition and Dietetics* 112 (2012): 1763–1773.

61. Landsberg and coauthors, Obesity-related hypertension: Pathogenesis, cardiovascular risk, and treatment, 2013.

62. J. E. Sharman, A. La Gerche, and J. S. Coombes, Exercise and cardiovascular risk in patients with hypertension, *American Journal of Hypertension* (October 10, 2014), epub ahead of print; D. T. Lackland and J. H. Voeks, Metabolic syndrome and hypertension: Regular exercise as part of lifestyle management, *Current Hypertension Reports* 16 (2014): 492.

63. Kotchen, Cowley, and Frohlich, Salt in health and disease, 2013; Whelton and coauthors, AHA presidential advisory: Sodium, blood pressure, and cardiovascular disease, 2012.

64. Eckel and coauthors, 2013 AHA/ACC guideline on lifestyle management to reduce cardiovascular risk, 2014

65. Whelton and coauthors, AHA presidential advisory: Sodium, blood pressure, and cardiovascular disease, 2012.

66. Whelton and coauthors, AHA presidential advisory: Sodium, blood pressure, and cardiovascular disease, 2012.

67. Koliaki and Katsilambros, Dietary sodium, potassium, and alcohol, 2013.

68. N. J. Aburto and coauthors, Effect of increased potassium intake on cardiovascular risk factors and disease: Systematic review and meta-analysis, *BMJ* (April 3, 2013), doi:10.1136/bmj.f1378; Koliaki and Katsilambros, Dietary sodium, potassium, and alcohol, 2013.

69. American Cancer Society, *Cancer Facts and Figures 2014* (Atlanta, Ga.: American Cancer Society, 2014), available at www.cancer.org/research/cancerfactsstatistics/cancerfactsfigures2014/index.

70. R. Siegel, D. Naishadham, and A. Jemal, Cancer statistics, 2012, *CA: Cancer Journal for Clinicians* 62 (2012): 10–29.

71. J. F. Gonzales and coauthors, Applying the precautionary principle to nutrition and cancer, *Journal of the American College of Nutrition* 33 (2014): 239–246; Oyebode and coauthors, Fruit and vegetable consumption and all-cause, cancer, and CVD mortality, 2014; D. Romaguera and coauthors, Is concordance with World Cancer Research Fund/American Institute for Cancer research guidelines for cancer prevention related to subsequent risk of cancer? Results from the EPIC study, *American Journal of Clinical Nutrition*

96 (2012): 150–163; Kushi and coauthors, American Cancer Society guidelines on nutrition and physical activity for cancer prevention, 2012; C. Eheman and coauthors, Annual report to the nation on the status of cancer, 1975–2008, featuring cancers associated with excess weight and lack of sufficient physical activity, *Cancer* 118 (2012): 2338–2366.

72. T. A. Hastert and coauthors, Adherence to the WCRF/AICR cancer prevention recommendations and cancer-specific mortality: Results from the Vitamins and Lifestyle (VITAL) study, *Cancer Causes and Control* 25 (2014): 541–552; G. Supic, M. Jagodic, and Z. Magic, Epigenetics: A new link between nutrition and cancer, *Nutrition and Cancer* 65 (2013): 781–792; L. J. Rasmussen-Torvik and coauthors, Ideal cardiovascular health is inversely associated with incident cancer: The Atherosclerosis Risk in Communities study, *Circulation* 127 (2013): 1270–1275; American Institute for Cancer Research, One in three cancer cases can be prevented, November 9, 2012, available at www.aicr.org/learn-more-about-cancer/infographics-prevention.html; Kushi and coauthors, American Cancer Society guidelines on nutrition and physical activity for cancer prevention, 2012; L. D'Elia and coauthors, Habitual salt intake and risk of gastric cancer: A meta-analysis of prospective studies, *Clinical Nutrition* 31 (2012): 489–498.

73. S. Ghosh and coauthors, Association of obesity and circulating adipose stromal cells among breast cancer survivors, *Molecular Biology Reports* 41 (2014): 2907–2916; R. Z. Stolzenberg-Solomon and coauthors, Lifetime adiposity and risk of pancreatic cancer in the NIH–AARP Diet and Health Study cohort, *American Journal of Clinical Nutrition* 98 (2013): 1057–1065; Eheman and coauthors, Annual report to the nation on the status of cancer, 1975–2008, 2012.

74. K. B. Michels, The rise and fall of breast cancer rates, *BMJ* 344 (2012), epub, doi:10.1136/bmj.d8003.

75. Kushi and coauthors, American Cancer Society guidelines on nutrition and physical activity for cancer prevention, 2012.

76. D. T. Fisher, M. M. Appenheimer, and S. S. Evans, The two faces of IL-6 in the tumor environment, *Seminars in Immunology* 26 (2014): 38–47.

77. W. C. Willett, T. Key, and I. Romieu, Diet, obesity, and physical activity, in B. W. Stewart and C. P. Wild (eds.), *World Cancer Report* (Lyon, France: International Agency for Research on Cancer, 2014), pp. 124–133; Kushi and coauthors, American Cancer Society guidelines on nutrition and physical activity for cancer prevention, 2012.

78. A. E. Harvey and coauthors, Calorie restriction decreases murine and human pancreatic tumor cell growth, nuclear factor-kB activation, and inflammation-related gene expression in an insulin-like growth factor-1-dependent manner, *PLOS ONE* 9 (2014): e94151; S. D. Hursting and coauthors, Calorie restriction and cancer prevention: A mechanistic perspective, *Cancer and Metabolism* 1 (2013): 10.

79. Willett, Key, and Romieu, Diet, obesity, and physical activity, 2014; Stolzenberg-Solomon and coauthors, Lifetime adiposity and risk of pancreatic cancer in the NIH–AARP Diet and Health Study, 2013; Kushi and coauthors, American Cancer Society guidelines on nutrition and physical activity for cancer prevention, 2012.

80. Ghosh and coauthors, Association of obesity and circulating adipose stromal cells among breast cancer survivors, 2014; Kushi and coauthors, American Cancer Society guidelines on nutrition and physical activity for cancer prevention, 2012.

81. T. Boyle and coauthors, Physical activity and risks of proximal and distal colon cancers: A systematic review and meta-analysis, *Journal of the National Cancer Institute* 104 (2012): 1548–1561; Kushi and coauthors, American Cancer Society guidelines on nutrition and physical activity for cancer prevention, 2012.

82. Willett, Key, and Romieu, Diet, obesity, and physical activity, 2014; Kushi and coauthors, American Cancer Society guidelines on nutrition and physical activity for cancer prevention, 2012.

83. C. D. Castro and J. A. Castro, Alcohol drinking and mammary cancer: Pathogenesis and potential dietary preventive alternatives, *World Journal of Clinical Oncology* 5 (2014): 713–729; Kushi and coauthors, American Cancer Society guidelines on nutrition and physical activity for cancer prevention, 2012.

84. Kushi and coauthors, American Cancer Society guidelines on nutrition and physical activity for cancer prevention, 2012.

85. T. M. Brasky and coauthors, Associations of long-chain ω-3 fatty acids and fish intake endometrial cancer risk in the VITamins And Lifestyle cohort, *American Journal of Clinical Nutrition* 99 (2014): 599–608; E. D. Kantor and coauthors, Long-chain omega-3 polyunsaturated fatty acid intake and risk of colorectal cancer, *Nutrition and Cancer* 66 (2014): 716–727; N. M. Iyegar, C. A. Hudis, and A. Gucalp, Omega-3 fatty acids for the prevention of breast cancer: An update and state of the science, *Current Breast Cancer Reports* 5 (2013): 247–254; K. Jing, T. Wu, and K. Lim, Omega-3 polyunsaturated fatty acids and cancer, *Anticancer Agents in Medicinal Chemistry* 13 (2013): 1162–1177.

86. World Health Organization, International Agency for Research on Cancer, IARC Monographs evaluate consumption of red meat and processed meat, Press release no. 240, October 2015, available at http://www.iarc.fr/en/media-centre/pr/2015/pdfs/pr240_E.pdf; D. Demeyer and coauthors, Mechanisms linking colorectal cancer to the consumption of (processed) red meat: A review, *Critical Reviews in Food Science and Nutrition* 2015, doi: 10.1080/10408398.2013.873886; Z. Abid, A. J. Cross, and R. Sinha, Meat, dairy, and cancer, *American Journal of Clinical Nutrition* 100 (2014): 386S–393S; D. Aune and coauthors, Red and processed meat intake and risk of colorectal adenomas: A systematic review and meta-analysis of epidemiological studies, *Cancer Causes and Control: CCC* 24 (2013): 611–627.

87. Abid, Cross, and Sinha, Meat, dairy, and cancer, 2014; Di Maso and coauthors, Red meat and cancer risk in a network of case-control studies focusing on cooking practices, 2013; Kushi and coauthors, American Cancer Society guidelines on nutrition and physical activity for cancer prevention, 2012.

88. Abid, Cross, and Rashmi, Meat, dairy, and cancer, 2014; Willett, Key, and Romieu, Diet, obesity, and physical activity, 2014; Kim, Coelho, and Blachier, Review of the association between meat consumption and risk of colorectal cancer, 2013.

89. Abid, Cross, and Rashmi, Meat, dairy, and cancer, 2014; Kim, Coelho, and Blachier, Review of the association between meat consumption and risk of colorectal cancer, 2013.

90. Centers for Disease Control and Prevention, National Center for Environmental Health, Executive summary, Second national report on biochemical indicators of diet and nutrition in the U.S. population, 2012, available at www.cdc.gov/nutritionreport.

91. T. Norat and coauthors, Fruits and vegetables: Updating the epidemiologic evidence for WCRF/AICR lifestyle recommendations for cancer prevention, *Cancer Treatment and Research* 159 (2014): 35–50; Oyebode and coauthors, Fruit and vegetable consumption and all-cause, cancer, and CVD mortality, 2014; H. M. Chen and coauthors, Decreased dietary fiber intake and structural alteration of gut microbiota in patients with advanced colorectal adenoma, *American Journal of Clinical Nutrition* 97 (2013): 1044–1052; N. Murphy and coauthors, Dietary fibre intake and risks of cancers of the colon and rectum in the European Prospective Investigation into Cancer and Nutrition (EPIC), *PLoS ONE* 7 (2012): e39361; Kushi and coauthors, American Cancer Society guidelines on nutrition and physical activity for cancer prevention, 2012.

92. Q. Xiao and coauthors, Intakes of folate, methionine, vitamin B6, and vitamin B12 with risk of esophageal and gastric cancer in a large cohort study, *British Journal of Cancer* 110 (2014): 1328–1333; P. J. Tarraga López, J. S. Albero, and J. A. Rodriguez-Montes, Primary and secondary prevention of colorectal cancer, *Clinical Medicine Insights: Gastroenterology* 7 (2014): 33–46; Supic, Jagodic, and Magic, Epigenetics, 2013.

93. A. Galas, M. Augustyniak, and E. Sochacka-Tatara, Does dietary calcium interact with dietary fiber against colorectal cancer? A case-control study in Central Europe, *Nutrition Journal* 12 (2013): 134.

94. J. Hooda, A. Shah, and L. Zhang, Heme, an essential nutrient from dietary proteins, critically impacts diverse physiological and pathological processes, *Nutrients* 6 (2014): 1080–1102.

95. Norat and coauthors, Fruits and vegetables, 2014; Oyebode and coauthors, Fruit and vegetable consumption and all-cause, cancer, and CVD mortality, 2014.

96. Supic, Jagodic, and Magic, Epigenetics, 2013; M. González-Vallinas and coauthors, Dietary phytochemicals in cancer prevention and therapy: A complementary approach with promising perspectives, *Nutrition Reviews* 71 (2013): 585–599.

Consumer's Guide 11

1. C. M. Luberto and coauthors, Integrative medicine for treating depression: An update on the latest evidence, *Current Psychiatric Reports* 15 (2013): 391.

2. P. A. Offit, Studying complementary and alternative therapies, *Journal of the American Medical Association* 307 (2012): 1803–1804.

3. D. Singh, R. Gupta, and S. A. Saraf, Herbs—Are they safe enough? An overview, *Critical Reviews in Food Science and Nutrition* 52 (2012): 876–898.

4. A. J. Vickers and K. Linde, Acupuncture for chronic pain, *Journal of the American Medical Association* 311 (2014): 955–956.

5. Offit, Studying complementary and alternative therapies, 2012.

6. S. G. Newmaster and coauthors, DNA barcoding detects contamination and substitution in North American herbal products, *BMC Medicine* 11 (2013): 222.

7. P. Hore and coauthors, Lead poisoning in pregnant women who used Ayurvedic medications from India—New York City, 2011–2012, *Morbidity and Mortality Weekly Report* 61 (2012): 641–646.

8. Singh, Gupta, and Saraf, Herbs—Are they safe enough? An overview, 2012.

9. National Institutes of Health, National Center for Complementary and Alternative Medicine, Herbs at a glance, Ginkgo, available at http://nccam.nih.gov/health/ginkgo/ataglance.htm; site updated June 2013.

10. T. A. Arcury and coauthors, Attitudes of older adults regarding disclosure of complementary therapy use to conventional physicians, *Journal of Applied Gerontology* 32 (2013): 627–645; J. Ge and coauthors, Patient-physician communication about complementary and alternative medicine in a radiation oncology setting, *International Journal of Radiation, Oncology, Biology, Physics* 85 (2013): e1–e6.

Controversy 11

1. Position of the Academy of Nutrition and Dietetics: Nutritional genomics, *Journal of the Academy of Nutrition and Dietetics* 114 (2014): 299–319.

2. T. Ge and coauthors, Massively expedited genome-wide heritability analysis (MEGHA), *Proceedings of the National Academy of Sciences of the United States* 112 (2015): 2479–2484; B. Rabbani, M. Tekin, and N. Mahdieh, The promise of whole-exome sequencing in medical genetics, *Journal of Human Genetics* 59 (2014): 5–59; J. S. Berg and coauthors, Processes and preliminary outputs for identification of actionable genes as incidental findings in genomic sequence data in the Clinical Sequencing Exploratory Research Consortium, *Genetics in Medicine* 15 (2013): 860–867.

3. F. E. Dewey and coauthors, Clinical interpretation and implications of whole-genome

sequencing, *Journal of the American Medical Association* 311 (2014): 1035–1044.

4. Position of the Academy of Nutrition and Dietetics: Nutritional genomics, 2014.

5. E. Callaway, Epigenomics starts to make its mark, *Nature* 509 (2014): 33; C. Lavebratt, M. Almgren, and T. J. Estróm, Epigenetic regulation in obesity, *International Journal of Obesity* 36 (2012): 757–765.

6. G. Supic, M. Jagodic, and Z. Magic, Epigenetics: A new link between nutrition and cancer, *Nutrition and Cancer* 65 (2013): 781–792; C. Gerhauser, Epigenetic impact of dietary isothiocyanates in cancer chemoprevention, *Current Opinion in Clinical Nutrition and Metabolic Care* 16 (2013): 405–410.

7. S. I. Khan and coauthors, Epigenetic events associated with breast cancer and their prevention by dietary components targeting the epigenome, *Chemical Research in Toxicology* 25 (2012): 61–73.

8. L. K. Park, S. Fiso, and S. Choi, Nutritional influences on epigenetics and age-related disease, *Proceedings of the Nutrition Society* 71 (2012): 75–83.

9. R. Dominguez-Salas and coauthors, Maternal nutrition at conception modulates DNA methylation of human metastable epialleles, *Nature Communications* (2014), epub, doi:10.1038/ncomms4746; J. Zhang and coauthors, DNA methylation: The pivotal interaction between early-life nutrition and glucose metabolism in later life, *British Journal of Nutrition* 112 (2014): 1850–1857.

10. Y. Zhang and coauthors, Global hypomethylation in hepatocellular carcinoma and its relationship to aflatoxin B exposure, *World Journal of Hepatology* 4 (2012): 169–175.

11. Federal Trade Commission, Direct-to-consumer genetic tests, 2014, available at www.consumer.ftc.gov/articles/0166-direct-consumer-genetic-tests.

12. R. Poinhos and coauthors, Psychological determinants of consumer acceptance of personalised nutrition in 9 European countries, *PLOS ONE* (2014), epub, doi:10.1371/journal.pone.0110614.

13. Position of the Academy of Nutrition and Dietetics: Nutritional genomics, 2014.

14. U.S. Food and Drug Administration, 23andme, Inc., Inspections, Compliance, Enforcement, and Criminal Investigations, November 22, 2013, available at www.fda.gov/ICECI/EnforcementActions/WarningLetters/2013/ucm376296.htm.

15. R. C. Green and N. Farahany, Regulation: The FDA is overcautious on consumer genomics, *Nature* 505 (2014): 286–287.

16. J. Sharfstein, FDA regulation of laboratory-developed diagnostic tests: Protect the public, advance the science, *Journal of the American Medical Association* 313 (2015): 667–668.

17. L. Kuanrong and coauthors, Associations of dietary calcium intake and calcium supplementation with myocardial infarction and stroke risk and overall cardiovascular mortality in the Heidelberg cohort of the European Prospective Investigation into Cancer and Nutrition study (EPIC–Heidelberg), *Heart* 98 (2012): 920–925.

Chapter 12

1. Position of the Academy of Nutrition and Dietetics: Food and water safety, *Journal of the Academy of Nutrition and Dietetics* 114 (2014): 1819–1829.

2. Centers for Disease Control and Prevention, Foodborne illness, foodborne disease (sometimes called "Food Poisoning"), 2014, available at www.cdc.gov/foodsafety/facts.html.

3. U.S. Food and Drug Administration, Food Safety Modernization Act (FSMA), 2015, available at www.fda.gov/Food/GuidanceRegulation/FSMA/.

4. Centers for Disease Control and Prevention, Incidence and trends of infection with pathogens transmitted commonly through food—Foodborne Diseases Active Surveillance Network, 10 U.S. sites, 2006–2013, *Morbidity and Mortality Weekly Report* 63 (2014): 328–332.

5. Centers for Disease Control and Prevention, List of multistate foodborne outbreak investigations, 2015, available at www.cdc.gov/foodsafety/outbreaks/multistate-outbreaks/outbreaks-list.html.

6. FDA guards against food spoilage, contamination, Consumer Updates, 2014, available at www.fda.gov/consumer; USDA announces additional food safety requirements, new inspection system for poultry products, 2014, available at www.usda.gov/wps/portal/usda/usdamediafb?contentid=2014/07/0163.xml&printable=true&contentidonly=true.

7. C. P. Gerba and coauthors, Bacterial occurrence in kitchen hand towels, *Food Protection Trends* 34 (2014): 312–317.

8. E. L. Larson, B. Chen, and K. A. Baxter, Analysis of alcohol-based hand sanitizer delivery systems: Efficacy of foam, gel, and wipes against influenza A (H1N1) virus on hands, *American Journal of Infection Control* 40 (2012): 806–809.

9. S. H. Kim and coauthors, Growth and migration of LNCzP prostate cancer cells are promoted by triclosan and benzophenone-1 via an androgen receptor signaling pathway, *Environmental Toxicology and Pharmacology* 39 (2015): 568–576; M. T. Dinwiddie, P. D. Terry, and J. Chen, Recent evidence regarding triclosan and cancer risk, *International Journal of Environmental Research and Public Health* 11 (2014): 2209–2217.

10. Centers for Disease Control and Prevention, Foodborne illness, foodborne disease, 2014, available at www.cdc.gov/foodsafety/facts.html.

11. B. Sikorska and coauthors, B. Creutzfeldt-Jakob disease, *Advances in Experimental Medicine and Biology* 724 (2012): 76–90.

12. S. J. Chai and coauthors, *Salmonella enterica* serotype Enteritidis: Increasing incidence of domestically acquired infections, *Clinical Infectious Diseases* 54 (2012): S488–S497.

13. W. Wang, M. Li, and Y. Li, Intervention strategies for reducing *Vibrio Parahaemolyticus* in seafood: A review, *Journal of Food Science* 80 (2015): R10–R19.

14. L. H. Gould, E. Munai, and C. B. Behravesh, Outbreaks attributed to cheese: Differences between outbreaks caused by unpasteurized and pasteurized dairy products, United States, 1998–2011, *Foodborne Pathogens and Disease* 11 (2014): 545–551; Centers for Disease Control and Prevention, Majority of dairy-related disease outbreaks linked to raw milk, 2012, available at www.cdc.gov/media/releases/2012/p0221_raw_milk_outbreak.html.

15. U.S. Department of Agriculture and U.S. Department of Health and Human Services, Scientific report of the 2015 Dietary Guidelines Advisory Committee, 2015, A-4, available at www.health.gov.

16. Centers for Disease Control and Prevention, Multistate outbreak of Listeriosis linked to whole cantaloupes from Jensen farms, Colorado, August 2012, available at www.cdc.gov/listeria/outbreaks/cantaloupes-jensen-farms/082712/.

17. Centers for Disease Control and Prevention, Foodborne illness, foodborne disease, 2014, available at www.cdc.gov/foodsafety/facts.html.

18. Position of the Academy of Nutrition and Dietetics: Food and water safety, 2014; G. Botticella and coauthors, *Listeria monocyogenes*, biofilm formation and fresh cut produce, in A. Mendez-Vilas (ed.), *Microbial Pathogens and Strategies for Combating Them: Science, Technology, and Education* (Badajoz, Spain: Formatex Research Center, 2013), pp. 114–123.

19. U.S. Food and Drug Administration, Sprouts Safety Alliance, February 28, 2012, available at www.fda.gov/Food/FoodSafety/FSMA/ucm293429.htm.

20. Centers for Disease Control and Prevention, Multistate outbreak of Shiga toxin–producing *Escherichia coli* O121 infections linked to raw clover sprouts, 2014, available at www.cdc.gov/ecoli/2014/0121-05-14/index.html.

21. U.S. Food and Drug Administration, Foreign Food Facility Inspection Program questions & answers, 2014, available at www.fda.gov/Food/ComplianceEnforcement/Inspections/ucm211823.htm.

22. U.S. Department of Agriculture, Agricultural Marketing Service, Country of origin labeling, 2014, available at www.ams.usda.gov/AMSv1.0/cool.

23. U.S. Department of Agriculture, Keeping "bag" lunches safe, 2013, available at www.fsis.usda.gov.

24. U.S. Food and Drug Administration, Food irradiation: What you need to know, 2014, available at www.fda.gov/Food/ResourcesForYou/Consumers/ucm261680.htm.

25. U.S. Food and Drug Administration, Kinetics of microbial inactivation for alternative food processing technologies— High pressure processing, 2014, available at www.fda.gov/Food/FoodScienceResearch/SafePracticesforFoodProcesses/ucm101456.htm.

26. L. Zhu and coauthors, Apple, carrot, and hibiscus edible films containing the plant antimicrobials carvacrol and cinnamaldehyde inactivate *Salmonella* Newport on organic leafy greens in sealed plastic bags, *Journal of Food Science* 79

(2014): M61–M66; M. K. Morsy and coauthors, Incorporation of essential oils and nanoparticles in pullulan films to control foodborne pathogens on meat and poultry products, *Journal of Food Science* 79 (2014): M675–M684.

27. M. J. Tijhuis and coauthors, State of the art in benefit-risk analysis: Food and nutrition, *Food and Chemical Toxicology* 50 (2012): 5–25.

28. C. K. Winter and J. M. Katz, Dietary exposure to pesticide residues from commodities alleged to contain the highest contamination levels, *Journal of Toxicology* 2011 (2011): 589–674.

29. World Health Organization, *Antimicrobial Resistance: Global Report on Surveillance* (Geneva: WHO, 2014), pp. 3–6; C. Nathan and O. Cars, Antibiotic resistance— Problems, progress, and prospects, *New England Journal of Medicine* 371 (2014): 1761–1763; Institute of Medicine, *Antimicrobial Resistance: A Problem without Borders* (Washington, DC: National Academies Press, 2014).

30. L. B. Price and coauthors, *Staphylococcus aureus* CC398: Host adaptation and emergence of methicillin resistance in livestock, *mBio* 3 (2012): e00305–11.

31. C. G. Gay, Strategies that work: Alternatives to antibiotics in animal health, *Agricultural Research*, May/June 2012, pp. 4–7.

32. U.S. Food and Drug Administration, FDA annual summary report on antimicrobials sold or distributed in 2012 for use in food-producing animals, 2014, available at www.fda.gov /downloads/ForIndustry/UserFees /AnimalDrugUserFeeActADUFA/UCM416983.pdf.

33. K. E. Nachman and coauthors, Arsenic species in poultry feather meal, *Science of the Total Environment* 417–418 (2012): 183–188.

34. U.S. Food and Drug Administration, Arsenic in apple juice, 2013, available at www.fda .gov/food/foodborneillnesscontaminants/metals /ucm280209.htm; U.S. Food and Drug Administration, FDA looks for answers on arsenic in rice, Consumer Updates, September 2012, available at www.fda.gov/ForConsumers /ConsumerUpdates/ucm319827.htm.

35. U.S. Food and Drug Administration, FDA explores impact of arsenic in rice, 2013, available at www.fda.gov/forconsumers/consumerupdates /ucm352569.htm.

36. S. Munera-Picazo and coauthors, Inorganic and total arsenic contents in rice-based foods for children with celiac disease, *Journal of Food Science* 79 (2014), epub ahead of print, doi:10.1111/1750-3841.12310.

37. K. M. Rice and coauthors, Environmental mercury and its toxic effects, *Journal of Preventive Medicine and Public Health,* 47 (2014): 74–83.

38. P. W. Drevnick, C. H. Lamborg, and M. J. Horgan, Increase in mercury in Pacific yellowfin tuna, *Environmental Toxicology* (2015), epub ahead of print, doi:10.1002/etc.2883.

39. T. G. Neltner and coauthors, Navigating the U.S. food additive regulatory program, *Comprehensive Reviews in Food Science and Food Safety* 10 (2011): 342–368.

40. K. Kindy, Food additives on the rise as FDA scrutiny wanes, *Washington Post,* August 17, 2015, available at www.washingtonpost.com /national/food-additives-on-the-rise-as-fda -scrutiny-wanes/2014/08/17/828e9bf8 -1cb2-11e4-ab7b-696c295ddfd1_story.html.

41. Z. Abid, A. J. Cross, and R. Sinha, Meat, dairy, and cancer, *American Journal of Clinical Nutrition* 100 (2014): 386S–393S; E. Kim, D. Coelho, and Francois Blachier, Review of the association between meat consumption and colorectal cancer, *Nutrition Research* 33 (2013): 983–994.

42. Position of the Academy of Nutrition and Dietetics: Use of nutritive and nonnutritive sweeteners, *Journal of the Academy of Nutrition and Dietetics* 112 (2012): 739–758.

43. J. Suez and coauthors, Artificial sweeteners induce glucose intolerance by altering the gut microbiota, *Nature* 514 (2014): 181–186.

44. T. Sathyapain and coauthors, Aspartame sensitivity? A double blind randomised crossover study, *PLOS ONE* 10 (2015), epub, doi:10.1371/ journal.pone.0116212; U.S. Department of Agriculture and U.S. Department of Health and Human Services, Scientific report of the 2015 Dietary Guidelines Advisory Committee, 2015, D-5:35–41, available at www.health.gov; American Cancer Institute, Aspartame, 2014, available at www.cancer.org/cancer/cancercauses /othercarcinogens/athome/aspartame; M. L. McCullough and coauthors, Artificially and sugar-sweetened carbonated beverage consumption is not associated with risk of lymphoid neoplasms in older men and women, *Journal of Nutrition* 144 (2014): 2041–2049.

45. M. Lee, MSG: Can an amino acid really be harmful? *Clinical Correlations* (2014), epub, available at www.clinicalcorrelations.org/?p=7655.

46. U. Masic and M. R. Yeomans, Umami flavor enhances appetite but also increases satiety, *American Journal of Clinical Nutrition* 100 (2014): 532–538; N. Bhadri and coauthors, Amelioration of behavioural, biochemical, and neurophysiological deficits by combination of monosodium glutamate with resveratrol/alpha-lipoic acids/ coenzyme Q10 in rat model of cisplatin-induced peripheral neuropathy, *Scientific World Journal* (2013), epub, doi:10.1155/2013/565813.

47. B. Mole, Doubts grow over BPA replacement, *Science News*, April 4, 2015, p. 10; S. Bae and Y. Hung, Exposure to bisphenol A from drinking canned beverage increases blood pressure, *Hypertension* (2014), epub ahead of print, doi:10.1161.HYPERTENSIONAHA.114.0461; D. Melzer and coauthors, Urinary bisphenol A concentration and risk of future coronary artery disease in apparently healthy men and women, *Circulation* 125 (2012): 1482–1490.

48. U.S. Food and Drug Administration, Bisphenol A (BPA): Use in food contact application, 2015, available at www.fda.gov/NewsEvents /PublicHealthFocus/ucm064437.htm#summary.

49. J. M. Poti and coauthors, Is the degree of food processing and convenience linked with the nutritional quality of the foods purchased by US households? *American Journal of Clinical Nutrition* 101 (2015): 1251–1262; C. M. Weaver and coauthors, Processed foods: Contribution to nutrition, *American Journal of Clinical Nutrition* 99 (2014): 1525–1542.

Consumer's Guide 12

1. Institute of Food Technology, U.S. organic food sales totaled $32.3 B in 2013, 2014, available at www.ift.org/food-technology /daily-news/2014/may/15/us-organic-food-sales -totaled-$32-b-in-2013.aspx.

2. J. L. Wan-chen and coauthors, You taste what you see: Do organic labels bias taste perceptions? *Food Quality and Preference* 29 (2013): 33–39.

3. M. Baran'ski and coauthors, Higher antioxidant and lower cadmium concentrations and lower incidence of pesticide residues in organically grown crops: A systematic literature review and meta-analysis, *British Journal of Nutrition* 112 (2014): 794–811.

4. C. L. Curl and coauthors, Estimating pesticide exposure from dietary intake and organic food choices: The Multi-ethnic Study of Atherosclerosis (MESA), *Environmental Health Perspectives* (2015), epub, doi:10.1289/ ehp.1408197.

5. C. Smith-Spangler and coauthors, Are organic foods safer or healthier than conventional alternatives? A systematic review, *Annals of Internal Medicine* 157 (2012): 348–366.

6. American Academy of Pediatrics, Pesticide exposure in children, *Pediatrics* 130 (2012): e1765–e1788.

7. Environmental Working Group, Shoppers guide to pesticides in produce, 2015, available at www.ewg.org/foodnews/.

8. R. Reiss and coauthors, Estimation of cancer risks and benefits associated with a potential increased consumption of fruits and vegetables, *Food and Chemical Toxicology*, 2012, epub ahead of print, doi:10.1016/j.fct.2012.08.055.

9. Ø. Ueland and coauthors, State of the art in benefit-risk analysis: Consumer perception, *Food and Chemical Toxicology* 50 (2012): 67–76.

10. U.S. Department of Agriculture and U.S. Department of Health and Human Services, Scientific report of the 2015 Dietary Guidelines Advisory Committee, 2015, A-4, available at www.health.gov.

11. Barański and coauthors, Higher antioxidant and lower cadmium concentrations and lower incidence of pesticide residues in organically grown crops, 2014; A. Vallverdú-Queralt and coauthors, Is there any difference between the phenolic content of organic and conventional tomato juices? *Food Chemistry* 130 (2012): 222–227.

12. S. C. Marine and coauthors, The growing season, but not the farming system, is a food safety risk determinant for leafy greens in the mid-Atlantic region of the United States, *Applied Environmental Microbiology* (2015), epub ahead of print, doi:10.1128/AEM.00051- 15; J. M. Millman and coauthors, Prevalence of antibiotic-resistant *E. coli* in retail chicken: Comparing conventional, organic, kosher, and raised without antibiotics, *F1000Research* (2013), epub, doi:10.12688/ f1000research.2-155.v2.

Notes

Controversy 12

1. Ø. Ueland and coauthors, State of the art in benefit-risk analysis: Consumer perception, *Food and Chemical Toxicology* 50 (2012): 67–76.

2. U.S. Department of Agriculture, Agricultural biotechnology: Glossary of agricultural biotechnology terms, 2013, available at www.usda.gov.

3. D. R. Schilling, Genetically engineered "spider goat" spins out elastic material superior to Kevlar, *Industry Tap into News,* May 2014, available at www.industrytap.com/genetically-engineered-spider-goat-spins-elastic-material-superior-kevlar/19392.

4. Hypoallergenic peanuts: Who cares and why? Accessed March 2015, epub available at www.ncat.edu/academics/schools-colleges1/saes/agresearch/impacts/NCAT%20-%20Ibrahim%20ph.pdf.

5. E. Waltz, USDA approves next-generation GM potato, *Nature Biotechnology* 33 (2015): 12–13.

6. G. Tang and coauthors, β-Carotene in golden rice is as good as β-carotene in oil at providing vitamin A to children, *American Journal of Clinical Nutrition* 98 (2012): 658–664.

7. M. R. La Frano and coauthors, Bioavailability of iron, zinc, and provitamin A carotenoids in biofortified staple crops, *Nutrition Reviews* 72 (2014): 289–307; E. Leyva-Guerrero and coauthors, Iron and protein biofortification of cassava: Lessons learned, *Current Opinion in Biotechnology* 23 (2012): 257–264.

8. H. Jin and coauthors, Engineering biofuel tolerance in non-native producing microorganisms, *Biotechnology Advances* 32 (2014): 541–548.

9. U.S. Department of Agriculture, Natural Resources Conservation Service, USDA–Natural Resources Conservation Service (NRCS) expands project to control pigweed on cotton crops, 2012, available at www.ga.nrcs.usda.gov/news/Pigweed_Project_2012_Extended.html.

10. Union of Concerned Scientists, Protect our food: A campaign to take the harm out of pharma and industrial crops, available at www.ucsusa.org/food_and_environment/genetic_engineering/protect-our-food.html.

11. M. V. DiLeo and coauthors, An assessment of the relative influences of genetic background, functional diversity at major regulatory genes, and transgenic constructs on the tomato fruit metabolome, *Plant Genome* 7 (2014), epub, doi:10.3835/plantgenome2013.06.0021.

12. International Food Information Council Foundation, A guide to understanding modern agricultural biotechnology, 2013, available at www.foodinsight.org/sites/default/files/Undstg%20Modern%20Ag%20Biotechnology.pdf.

13. J. Fernandez-Cornejo and coauthors, *Genetically Engineered Crops in the United States* (Economic Research Report 162) (Washington, D.C.: U.S. Department of Agriculture, 2014), pp. 24–26.

14. GMO foods: What you need to know, *Consumer Reports*, March 2015, available at www.consumerreports.org/cro/magazine/2015/02/gmo-foods-what-you-need-to-know/index.htm.

15. C. N. Kanchiswamy and coauthors, Differential expression of CPKs and cytosolic Ca^2 + variation in resistant and susceptible apple cultivars *(Malus x domestica)* in response to the pathogen *Erwinia amylovora* and mechanical wounding, *BMC Genomics* 14 (2013), epub, doi:10.1186/1471-2164-14-760.

Chapter 13

1. T. K. Jensen and coauthors, Habitual alcohol consumption associated with reduced semen quality and changes in reproductive hormones: A cross-sectional study among 1221 young Danish men, *BMJ Open* 4 (2014): e005462; P. Zareba and coauthors, Semen quality in relation to antioxidant intake in a healthy male population, *Fertility and Sterility* 100 (2013): 1572–1579; R. Sharma and coauthors, Lifestyle factors and reproductive health: Taking control of your fertility, *Reproductive Biology and Endocrinology* 11 (2013): 66.

2. E. Gresham and coauthors, Effects of dietary interventions on neonatal and infant outcomes: A systematic review and meta-analysis, *American Journal of Clinical Nutrition* 100 (2014): 1298–1321; T. A. Simas and coauthors, Prepregnancy weight, gestational weight gain, and risk of growth affected neonates, *Journal of Women's Health* 21 (2012): 410–417.

3. T. L. Crume and coauthors, The long-term impact of intrauterine growth restriction in a diverse U.S. cohort of children: The EPOCH study, *Obesity* 22 (2014): 608–615; M. R. Skilton and coauthors, Fetal growth, omega-3 (n-3) fatty acids, and progression of subclinical atherosclerosis: Preventing fetal origins of disease? The Cardiovascular Risk in Young Finns Study, *American Journal of Clinical Nutrition* 97 (2013): 58–65; A. F. M. van Abeelen and coauthors, Survival effects of prenatal famine exposure, *American Journal of Clinical Nutrition* 95 (2012): 179–183; J. L. Tarry-Adkins and S. E. Ozanne, Mechanisms of early life programming: Current knowledge and future directions, *American Journal of Clinical Nutrition* 94 (2011): 1765S–1771S.

4. A. Lahat and coauthors, ADHD among young adults born at extremely low birth weight: The role of fluid intelligence in childhood, *Frontiers in Psychology* 19 (2014): 446; S. K. Berglund and coauthors, Effects of iron supplementation of LBW infants on cognition and behavior at 3 years, *Pediatrics* 131 (2013): 47–55; P. Munck and coauthors, Stability of cognitive outcome from 2 to 5 years of age in very low birth weight children, *Pediatrics* 129 (2012): 503–508.

5. M. J. K. Osterman and coauthors, Annual summary of vital statistics: 2012–2013, *Pediatrics* 135 (2015): 1115–1125.

6. Position of the Academy of Nutrition and Dietetics: Nutrition and lifestyle for a healthy pregnancy outcome, *Journal of the Academy of Nutrition and Dietetics* 114 (2014): 1099–1103; N. Kozuki, A. C. Lee, and J. Katz, Moderate to severe, but not mild, maternal anemia is associated with increased risk of small-for-gestational-age outcomes, *Journal of Nutrition* 142 (2012): 358–362.

7. R. Retnakaran and coauthors, Effect of maternal weight, adipokines, glucose intolerance and lipids on infant birth weight among women without gestational diabetes mellitus, *Canadian Medical Association Journal* 184 (2012): 1353–1360.

8. J. F. Mission, N. E. Marshall, and A. B. Caughey, Obesity in pregnancy: A big problem and getting bigger, *Obstetrical and Gynecological Survey* 68 (2013): 389–399; Retnakaran and coauthors, Effect of maternal weight, adipokines, glucose intolerance and lipids on infant birth weight among women without gestational diabetes mellitus, 2012.

9. D. M. McMahon and coauthors, Maternal obesity, folate intake, and neural tube defects in offspring, *Birth Defects Research. Part A, Clinical and Molecular Teratology* 97 (2013): 115–122; V. R. da Silva and coauthors, Obesity affects short-term folate pharmacokinetics in women of childbearing age, *International Journal of Obesity* 37 (2013): 1608–1610; A. Correa and J. Marcinkevage, Prepregnancy obesity and the risk of birth defects: An update, *Nutrition Reviews* 71 (2013): S68–S77; Position of the American Dietetic Association and American Society for Nutrition, Obesity, reproduction, and pregnancy outcomes, *Journal of the American Dietetic Association* 109 (2009): 918–927, reaffirmed 2013.

10. Mission, Marshall, and Caughey, Obesity in pregnancy, 2013; P. M. Nodine and M. Hastings-Tolsma, Maternal obesity: Improving pregnancy outcomes, *MCN: The American Journal of Maternal Child Nursing* 37 (2012): 110–115.

11. Correa and Marcinkevage, Prepregnancy obesity and the risk of birth defects, 2013.

12. E. Larqué and coauthors, Placental fatty acid transfer: A key factor in fetal growth, *Annals of Nutrition and Metabolism* 64 (2014): 247–253; A. N. Sferruzzi-Perri and coauthors, Hormonal and nutritional drivers of intrauterine growth, *Current Opinion in Clinical Nutrition and Metabolic Care* 16 (2013): 298–309.

13. van Abeelen and coauthors, Survival effects of prenatal famine exposure, 2012; M. L. de Gusmão Correia and coauthors, Developmental origins of health and disease: Experimental and human evidence of fetal programming for metabolic syndrome, *Journal of Human Hypertension* 26 (2012): 405–419.

14. Standing Committee on the Scientific Evaluation of Dietary Reference Intakes, Food and Nutrition Board, Institute of Medicine, *Dietary Reference Intakes for Energy, Carbohydrate, Fiber, Fat, Fatty Acids, Cholesterol, Protein, and Amino Acids* (Washington, D.C.: National Academies Press, 2005), pp. 185–194.

15. M. L. Blumfield and coauthors, Systematic review and meta-analysis of energy and macronutrient intakes during pregnancy in developed countries, *Nutrition Reviews* 70 (2012): 322–336.

16. V. Leventakou and coauthors, Fish intake during pregnancy, fetal growth, and gestational length in 19 European cohort studies, *American Journal of Clinical Nutrition* 99 (2014): 506–516;

K. A. Mulder, D. J. King, and S. M. Innis, Omega-3 fatty acid deficiency in infants before birth identified using a randomized trial of maternal DHA supplementation in pregnancy, *PLOS ONE* 9 (2014): e83764.

17. Centers for Disease Control and Prevention, Birth defects COUNT, updated December 24, 2014, available at www.cdc.gov/ncbddd/folicacid/global.html.

18. Centers for Disease Control and Prevention, Birth defects COUNT, updated December 24, 2014, available at www.cdc.gov/ncbddd/folicacid/global.html.

19. R. Molina-Solana and coauthors, Current concepts on the effect of environmental factors on cleft lip and palate, *International Journal of Oral and Maxillofacial Surgery* 42 (2013): 177–184; D. Kelly, T. O'Dowd, and U. Reulbach, Use of folic acid supplements and risk of cleft lip and palate in infants: A population-based cohort study, *British Journal of General Practice* 62 (2012): e466–e472.

20. P. Dominguez-Salas and coauthors, Maternal nutritional status, C (1) metabolism and offspring DNA methylations: A review of current evidence in human subjects, *Proceedings of the Nutrition Society* 71 (2012): 154–165.

21. S. H. Zeisel, Nutrition in pregnancy: The argument for including a source of choline, *International Journal of Women's Health* 22 (2013): 193–199.

22. B. E. Young and coauthors, Maternal vitamin D status and calcium intake interact to affect fetal skeletal growth in utero in pregnant adolescents, *American Journal of Clinical Nutrition* 95 (2012): 1103–1112.

23. C. R. Peterson and D. Ayoub, Congenital rickets due to vitamin D deficiency in the mothers, *Clinical Nutrition* (2014), doi:10.1016/j.clnu.2014.12.006.

24. Committee on Dietary Reference Intakes, *Dietary Reference Intakes for Calcium and Vitamin D* (Washington, D.C.: National Academies Press, 2011).

25. M. K. Ozias and coauthors, Typical prenatal vitamin D supplement intake does not prevent decrease of plasma 25-hydroxyvitamin D at birth, *Journal of the American College of Nutrition* 33 (2014): 394–399.

26. Committee on Dietary Reference Intakes, *Dietary Reference Intakes for Calcium and Vitamin D*, 2011, pp. 242–250.

27. A. N. Hacker, E. B. Fung, and J. C. King, Role of calcium during pregnancy: Maternal and fetal needs, *Nutrition Reviews* 70 (2012): 397–409.

28. Position of the Academy of Nutrition and Dietetics: Nutrition and lifestyle for a healthy pregnancy outcome, 2014; C. Cao and K. O. O'Brien, Pregnancy and iron homeostasis: An update, *Nutrition Reviews* 71 (2013): 35–51.

29. Position of the Academy of Nutrition and Dietetics: Nutrition and lifestyle for a healthy pregnancy outcome, 2014.

30. L. Englund-Ögge and coauthors, Maternal dietary patterns and preterm delivery: Results from large prospective cohort study, *BMJ* 348

(2014): g1446; J. A. Grieger, L. E. Grzeskowiak, and V. L. Clifton, Preconception dietary patterns in human pregnancies are associated with preterm delivery, *Journal of Nutrition* 144 (2014): 1075–1080.

31. C. G. Campbell and L. L. Kaiser, Practice paper of the Academy of Nutrition and Dietetics: Nutrition and lifestyle for a healthy pregnancy outcome, July 2014, available at www.eatright.org/members/practicepapers/.

32. WIC—The Special Supplemental Nutrition Program for Women, Infants, and Children, updated April 2014, available at www.fns.usda.gov/sites/default/files/WIC-fact-sheet.pdf.

33. Position of the Academy of Nutrition and Dietetics: Nutrition and lifestyle for a healthy pregnancy outcome, 2014.

34. Position of the American Dietetic Association and American Society for Nutrition: Obesity, reproduction, and pregnancy outcomes, 2009, reaffirmed 2012.

35. C. K. McClure and coauthors, Associations between gestational weight gain and BMI, abdominal adiposity, and traditional measures of cardiometabolic risk in mothers 8 y postpartum, *American Journal of Clinical Nutrition* 98 (2013): 1218–1225; A. M. Siega-Riz and G. L. Gray, Gestational weight gain recommendations in the context of the obesity epidemic, *Nutrition Reviews* 71 (2013): S26–S30; Position of the American Dietetic Association and American Society for Nutrition: Obesity, reproduction, and pregnancy outcomes, 2009, reaffirmed 2012.

36. Position of the Academy of Nutrition and Dietetics: Nutrition and lifestyle for a healthy pregnancy outcome, 2014.

37. S. T. Harris and coauthors, Exercise during pregnancy and its association with gestational weight gain, *Maternal and Child Health Journal* 19 (2015): 528–537; R. Barakat and coauthors, A program of exercise throughout pregnancy: Is it safe to mother and newborn? *American Journal of Health Promotion* 29 (2014): 2–8; S. M. Ruchat and coauthors, Nutrition and exercise reduce excessive weight gain in normal-weight pregnant women, *Medicine and Science in Sports and Exercise* 44 (2012): 1419–1426.

38. U.S. Department of Health and Human Services, Trends in teen pregnancy and childbearing, updated February 13, 2015, available at www.hhs.gov/ash/oah/adolescent-health-topics/reproductive-health/teen-pregnancy/trends.html; One in 5 teens giving birth already has a child, *Journal of the American Medical Association* 309 (2013): 1987.

39. S. V. Dean and coauthors, Preconception care: Nutritional risks and interventions, *Reproductive Health* 11 (2014): S3.

40. J. L. Bottorff and coauthors, Tobacco and alcohol use in the context of adolescent pregnancy and postpartum: A scoping review of the literature, *Health and Social Care in the Community* 22 (2014): 561–574.

41. R. W. Corbett and K. M. Kolasa, Pica and weight gain in pregnancy, *Nutrition Today* 49 (2014): 101–108.

42. A. Matthews and coauthors, Interventions for nausea and vomiting in early pregnancy, *Cochrane Database of Systemic Reviews* 3 (2014): CD007575.

43. V. T. Tong and coauthors, Trends in smoking before, during, and after pregnancy—Pregnancy Risk Assessment Monitoring System, United States, 40 sites, 2000–2010, *Morbidity and Mortality Weekly Report* 62 (2013): 1–19.

44. S. Phelan, Smoking cessation in pregnancy, *Obstetrics and Gynecology Clinics of North America* 41 (2014): 255–266; E. Stéphan-Blanchard and coauthors, Perinatal nicotine/smoking exposure and carotid chemoreceptors during development, *Respiratory Physiology & Neurobiology* 185 (2013): 110–119.

45. M. N. Kooijman and coauthors, Fetal smoke exposure and kidney outcomes in school-aged children, *American Journal of Kidney Disease* (2015), doi:10.1053/j.ajkd.2014.12.008; C. Metayer and coauthors, Tobacco smoke exposure and the risk of childhood acute lymphoblastic and myeloid leukemias by cytogenetic subtype, *Cancer Epidemiology, Biomarkers, and Prevention* 22 (2013): 1600–1611.

46. C. C. Geerts and coauthors, Parental smoking and vascular damage in their 5-year-old children, *Pediatrics* 129 (2012): 45–54.

47. E. M. Hollams and coauthors, Persistent effects of maternal smoking during pregnancy on lung function and asthma in adolescents, *American Journal of Respiratory and Critical Care Medicine* 189 (2014): 401–407; H. Burke and coauthors, Prenatal and passive smoke exposure and incidence of asthma and wheeze: Systematic review and meta-analysis, *Pediatrics* 129 (2012): 735–744.

48. J. M. Van Nguyen and H. A. Abenhaim, Sudden infant death syndrome: Review for the obstetric care provider, *American Journal of Perinatology* 30 (2013): 703–714; A. M. Lavezzi and coauthors, Vulnerability of fourth ventricle choroid plexus in sudden unexplained fetal and infant death syndromes related to smoking mothers, *International Journal of Developmental Neuroscience* 31 (2013): 319–327; F. L. Trachtenberg and coauthors, Risk factor changes for sudden infant death syndrome after initiation of back-to-sleep campaign, *Pediatrics* 129 (2012): 630–638.

49. Campbell and Kaiser, Practice paper of the Academy of Nutrition and Dietetics: Nutrition and lifestyle for a healthy pregnancy outcome, July 2014; G. Dante and coauthors, Herb remedies during pregnancy: A systematic review of controlled clinical trials, *Journal of Maternal-Fetal and Neonatal Medicine* 26 (2013): 306–312.

50. M. Neri and coauthors, Drugs of abuse in pregnancy, poor neonatal development, and future neurodegeneration: Is oxidative stress the culprit? *Current Pharmaceutical Design* 21 (2015): 1358–1368; L. L. LaGasse and coauthors, Prenatal methamphetamine exposure and childhood behavior at 3 and 5 years of age, *Pediatrics* 129 (2012): 681–688.

51. S. Buckingham-Howes and coauthors, Systematic review of prenatal cocaine exposure and

Notes

adolescent development, *Pediatrics* 131 (2013): e1917–e1936.

52. U.S. Department of Agriculture and U.S. Department of Health and Human Services, Scientific report of the 2015 Dietary Guidelines Advisory Committee, 2015, D:5–19, available at www.health.gov; U.S. Food and Drug Administration, New advice: Some women and young children should eat more fish, June 18, 2014, available at www.fda.gov/ForConsumers/ConsumerUpdates/ucm397443.htm.

53. U.S. Food and Drug Administration, New advice: Some women and young children should eat more fish, June 18, 2014.

54. Position of the Academy of Nutrition and Dietetics: Nutrition and lifestyle for a healthy pregnancy outcome, 2014; Position of the Academy of Nutrition and Dietetics: Use of nutritive and nonnutritive sweeteners, *Journal of the Academy of Nutrition and Dietetics* 112 (2012): 739–758.

55. American College of Obstetricians and Gynecologists, Nutrition during pregnancy: Frequently asked questions, April 2014, available at www.acog.org/Patients/FAQs/Nutrition-During-Pregnancy#extra; M. Jarosz, R. Wierzejska, and M. Siuba, Maternal caffeine intake and its effect on pregnancy outcome, *European Journal of Obstetrics and Gynecology and Reproductive Biology* 160 (2012): 156–160.

56. D. C. Greenwood and coauthors, Caffeine intake during pregnancy and adverse birth outcomes: A systematic review and dose-response meta-analysis, *European Journal of Epidemiology* 29 (2014): 725–734.

57. A. T. Hoyt and coauthors, Maternal caffeine consumption and small for gestational age births: Results from a population-based case-control study, *Maternal and Child Health Journal* 18 (2014): 1540–1551; L. W. Chen and coauthors, Maternal caffeine intake during pregnancy is associated with risk of low birth weight: A systematic review and dose-response meta-analysis, *BMC Medicine* 12 (2014): 174.

58. Centers for Disease Control, Fetal alcohol spectrum disorders, updated January 28, 2015, available at www.cdc.gov/ncbddd/fasd/data.html.

59. C. M. Marchetta and coauthors, Alcohol use and binge drinking among women of childbearing age—United States, 2006–2010, *Morbidity and Mortality Weekly Report* 61 (2012): 534–538.

60. K. L. Eckstrand and coauthors, Persistent dose-dependent changes in brain structure in young adults with low-to-moderate alcohol exposure in utero, *Alcoholism: Clinical and Experimental Research* 36 (2012): 1892–1902.

61. H. S. Feldman and coauthors, Prenatal alcohol exposure patterns and alcohol-related birth defects and growth deficiencies: A prospective study, *Alcoholism: Clinical and Experimental Research* 36 (2012): 670–676.

62. Position statement: Standards of medical care in diabetes—2015, *Diabetes Care* 38 (2015): S1–S93.

63. Position statement: Standards of medical care in diabetes—2015, published 2015.

64. A. Jeyabalan, Epidemiology of preeclampsia: Impact of obesity, *Nutrition Reviews* 71 (2013): S18–S25; R. Mustafa and coauthors, A comprehensive review of hypertension in pregnancy, *Journal of Pregnancy* (2012), doi:10.1155/2012/105918.

65. Mustafa and coauthors, A comprehensive review of hypertension in pregnancy, 2012.

66. Jeyabalan, Epidemiology of preeclampsia, 2013.

67. Mustafa and coauthors, A comprehensive review of hypertension in pregnancy, 2012.

68. Jeyabalan, Epidemiology of preeclampsia, 2013.

69. H. N. Moussa, S. E. Arian, and B. M Sibai, Management of hypertensive disorders in pregnancy, *Women's Health* 10 (2014): 385–404.

70. Committee on Dietary Reference Intakes, *Dietary Reference Intakes for Calcium and Vitamin D*, 2011, pp. 256–257.

71. A. K. Ventura and J. Worobey, Early influences on the development of food preferences, *Current Biology* 23 (2013): R401–R406; J. A. Mennella and J. C. Trabulsi, Complementary foods and flavor experiences: Setting the foundation, *Annals of Nutrition and Metabolism* 60 (2012): 40–50.

72. D. M. Fleischer and coauthors, Primary prevention of allergic disease through nutritional interventions, *Journal of Allergy and Clinical Immunology: In Practice* 1 (2013): 29–36.

73. R. Sámano and coauthors, Effects of breastfeeding on weight loss and recovery of pregestational weight in adolescent and adult mothers, *Food and Nutrition Bulletin* 34 (2013): 123–130.

74. A. J. Daley and coauthors, Maternal exercise and growth in breastfed infants: A meta-analysis of randomized controlled trials, *Pediatrics* 130 (2012): 108–114.

75. American Academy of Pediatrics, Policy statement: Breastfeeding and the use of human milk, *Pediatrics* 129 (2012): e827–e841, available at www.pediatrics.org/content/129/3/e827.full.

76. Centers for Disease Control and Prevention, Tobacco use and pregnancy, updated August 5, 2014, available at www.cdc.gov/reproductivehealth/tobaccousepregnancy/.

77. P. Bachour and coauthors, Effects of smoking mother's age, body mass index, and parity number on lipid, protein, and secretory immunoglobulin A concentration of human milk, *Breastfeeding Medicine* 7 (2012): 179–188.

78. Centers for Disease Control and Prevention, Health effects of secondhand smoke, updated March 5, 2014, available at www.cdc.gov/tobacco/data_statistics/fact_sheets/secondhand_smoke/health_effects; J. D. Thacher and coauthors, Pre- and postnatal exposure to parental smoking and allergic disease through adolescence, *Pediatrics* 134 (2014): 428–434.

79. Breastfeeding, in American Academy of Pediatrics, *Pediatric Nutrition*, 7th ed., ed. R. E. Kleinman (Elk Grove Village, Ill.: American Academy of Pediatrics, 2014), pp. 41–59; American Academy of Pediatrics, Policy statement: Breastfeeding and the use of human milk, 2012

80. American Academy of Pediatrics, Policy statement: Breastfeeding and the use of human milk, 2012.

81. American Academy of Pediatrics, Policy statement: Breastfeeding and the use of human milk, 2012.

82. Formula feeding of term infants, in American Academy of Pediatrics, *Pediatric Nutrition*, 7th ed., ed. R. E. Kleinman (Elk Grove Village, Ill.: American Academy of Pediatrics, 2014), pp. 61–81.

83. Position of the Academy of Nutrition and Dietetics: Promoting and supporting breastfeeding, *Journal of the Academy of Nutrition and Dietetics* 115 (2015): 444–449; Breastfeeding, in American Academy of Pediatrics, *Pediatric Nutrition*, 2014.

84. Position of the Academy of Nutrition and Dietetics: Promoting and supporting breastfeeding, 2015; Breastfeeding, in American Academy of Pediatrics, *Pediatric Nutrition*, 2014.

85. Breastfeeding, in American Academy of Pediatrics, *Pediatric Nutrition*, 2014; American Academy of Pediatrics, Policy statement: Breastfeeding and the use of human milk, 2012.

86. J. T. Smilowitz and coauthors, Breast milk oligosaccharides: Structure-function relationships in the neonate, *Annual Review of Nutrition* 34 (2014): 143–169; P. V. Jeurink and coauthors, Mechanisms underlying immune effects of dietary oligosaccharides, *American Journal of Clinical Nutrition* 98 (2013): 572S–577S.

87. Fat and fatty acids, in American Academy of Pediatrics, *Pediatric Nutrition*, 7th ed., ed. R. E. Kleinman (Elk Grove Village, Ill.: American Academy of Pediatrics, 2014), pp. 407–434; S. M. Innis, Impact of maternal diet on human milk composition and neurological development of infants, *American Journal of Clinical Nutrition* 99 (2014): 734S–741S; J. T. Brenna and S. E. Carlson, Docosahexaenoic acid and human brain development: Evidence that a dietary supply is needed for optimal development, *Journal of Human Evolution* 77 (2014): 99–106.

88. P. Willatts and coauthors, Effects of long-chain PUFA supplementation in infant formula on cognitive function in later childhood, *American Journal of Clinical Nutrition* 98 (2013): 536S–542S; A. Qawasmi, A. Landeros-Weisenberger, and M. H. Bloch, Meta-analysis of LCPUFA supplementation of infant formula and visual acuity, *Pediatrics* 131 (2013): e262–e272.

89. Willatts and coauthors, Effects of long-chain PUFA supplementation in infant formula on cognitive function in later childhood, 2013.

90. Fat-soluble vitamins, in American Academy of Pediatrics, *Pediatric Nutrition*, 7th ed., ed. R. E. Kleinman (Elk Grove Village, Ill.: American Academy of Pediatrics, 2014), pp. 495–515.

91. Fat-soluble vitamins, in American Academy of Pediatrics, *Pediatric Nutrition*, 2014.

92. S. Gallo and coauthors, Effect of different dosages of oral vitamin D supplementation on vitamin D status in healthy, breastfed infants, *Journal of the American Medical Association* 309 (2013): 1785–1792; American Academy of

Pediatrics, Policy statement: Breastfeeding and the use of human milk, 2012.

93. Position of the Academy of Nutrition and Dietetics: Promoting and supporting breastfeeding, 2015; Breastfeeding, in American Academy of Pediatrics, *Pediatric Nutrition*, 2014; Smilowitz and coauthors, Breast milk oligosaccharides, 2014; D. E. W. Chatterton and coauthors, Anti-inflammatory mechanisms of bioactive milk proteins in the intestine of newborns, *International Journal of Biochemistry and Cell Biology* 45 (2013): 1730–1747; B. Lonnerdal, Bioactive proteins in breast milk, *Journal of Paediatrics and Child Health* 49 (Supp. S1) (2013): 1–7.

94. B. M. Jakaitis and P. W. Denning, Human breast milk and the gastrointestinal innate immune system, *Clinics in Perinatology* 41 (2014): 423–435; Breastfeeding, in American Academy of Pediatrics, *Pediatric Nutrition*, 2014.

95. D. M. Fleischer and coauthors, Primary prevention of allergic disease through nutritional interventions, *Journal of Allergy and Clinical Immunology: In Practice* 1 (2013): 29–36; Breastfeeding, in American Academy of Pediatrics, *Pediatric Nutrition*, 2014.

96. R. A. Darnall and coauthors, American Academy of Pediatrics' Task Force on SIDS fully supports breastfeeding, *Breastfeeding Medicine* 9 (2014): 486–487.

97. C. M. Lefebvre and R. M. John, The effect of breastfeeding on childhood overweight and obesity: A systematic review of the literature, *Journal of the American Association of Nurse Practitioners* 26 (2014): 386–401; R. J. Hancox and coauthors, Association between breastfeeding and body mass index at age 6–7 years in an international survey, *Pediatric Obesity* (2014), doi:10.1111/jpo.266; K. Casazza, J. R. Fernandez, and D. B. Allison, Modest protective effects of breast-feeding on obesity, *Nutrition Today* 47 (2012): 33–38.

98. Lefebvre and John, The effect of breastfeeding on childhood overweight and obesity, 2014; Casazza, Fernandez, and Allison, Modest protective effects of breast-feeding on obesity, 2012.

99. S. Cao and coauthors, Infant feeding effects on early neurocognitive development in Asian children, *American Journal of Clinical Nutrition* 101 (2015): 326–336; M. B. Belfort and coauthors, Infant feeding and childhood cognition at ages 3 and 7 years: Effects of breastfeeding duration and exclusivity, *JAMA Pediatrics* 167 (2013): 836–844; M. A. Quigley and coauthors, Breastfeeding is associated with improved child cognitive development: A population-based cohort study, *Journal of Pediatrics* 160 (2012): 25–32.

100. Formula feeding of term infants, in American Academy of Pediatrics, *Pediatric Nutrition*, 2014.

101. Formula feeding of term infants, in American Academy of Pediatrics, *Pediatric Nutrition*, 2014.

102. Formula feeding of term infants, in American Academy of Pediatrics, *Pediatric Nutrition*, 2014.

103. Formula feeding of term infants, in American Academy of Pediatrics, *Pediatric Nutrition*, 2014.

104. Complementary feeding, in American Academy of Pediatrics, *Pediatric Nutrition*, 7th ed., ed. R. E. Kleinman (Elk Grove Village, Ill.: American Academy of Pediatrics, 2014), pp. 123–139.

105. Complementary feeding, in American Academy of Pediatrics, *Pediatric Nutrition*, 2014.

106. Complementary feeding, in American Academy of Pediatrics, *Pediatric Nutrition*, 2014; H. Przyrembel, Timing of introduction of complementary food: Short- and long-term health consequences, *Annals of Nutrition and Metabolism* 60 (supp.) (2012): 8–20.

107. Complementary feeding, in American Academy of Pediatrics, *Pediatric Nutrition*, 2014.

108. Complementary feeding, in American Academy of Pediatrics, *Pediatric Nutrition*, 2014.

109. Feeding the child, in American Academy of Pediatrics, *Pediatric Nutrition*, 7th ed., ed. R. E. Kleinman (Elk Grove Village, Ill.: American Academy of Pediatrics, 2014), pp. 143–173.

110. Feeding the child, in American Academy of Pediatrics, *Pediatric Nutrition*, 2014.

111. Complementary feeding, in American Academy of Pediatrics, *Pediatric Nutrition*, 2014.

Consumer's Guide 13

1. R. L. Dunn and coauthors, Engaging field-based professionals in a qualitative assessment of barriers and positive contributors to breastfeeding using the social ecological model, *Maternal and Child Health Journal* 19 (2015): 6–16; A. Brown, Maternal trait personality and breastfeeding duration: The importance of confidence and social support, *Journal of Advanced Nursing* 70 (2014): 587–598; A. S. Teich, J. Barnett, and K. Bonuck, Women's perceptions of breastfeeding barriers in early postpartum period: A qualitative analysis nested in two randomized controlled trials, *Breastfeeding Medicine* 9 (2014): 9–15.

2. Position of the Academy of Nutrition and Dietetics: Promoting and supporting breastfeeding, *Journal of the Academy of Nutrition and Dietetics* 115 (2015): 444–449; Centers for Disease Control and Prevention, Breastfeeding report card, United States/2014, available at www.cdc.gov/breastfeeding/pdf/2014breastfeedingreportcard.pdf.

3. U. S. Department of Health and Human Services, Healthy People, 2020, available at www.healthypeople.gov.

Controversy 13

1. C. L. Ogden and coauthors, Prevalence of child and adult obesity in the United States, 2011–2012, *Journal of the American Medical Association* 311 (2014): 806–814.

2. E. Estrada and coauthors, Children's Hospital Association consensus statements for comorbidities of childhood obesity, *Childhood Obesity* 10 (2014): 304–317; T. Reinehr, Type 2 diabetes mellitus in children and adolescents, *World Journal of Diabetes* 4 (2013): 270–281.

3. M. Ng and coauthors, Global, regional, and national prevalence of overweight and obesity in children and adults during 1980–2013: A systematic analysis for the Global Burden of Disease Study 2013, *Lancet* (2014): 766–781.

4. R. J. Iannotti and J. Wang, Trends in physical activity, sedentary behavior, diet, and BMI among US adolescents, 2001–2009, *Pediatrics* 132 (2013): 606–614.

5. Ogden and coauthors, Prevalence of child and adult obesity in the United States, 2011–2012, 2014.

6. R. J. Iannotti and J. Wang, Patterns of physical activity, sedentary behavior and diet in US adolescents, *Journal of Adolescent Health* 53 (2013): 280–286.

7. A. M. Linabery and coauthors, Stronger influence of maternal than paternal obesity on infant and early childhood body mass index: The Fels Longitudinal Study, *Pediatric Obesity* 8 (2013): 159–169.

8. J. C. Jones-Smith and coauthors, Socioeconomic status and trajectory of overweight from birth to mid-childhood: The Early Childhood Longitudinal Study-Birth Cohort, *PLOS ONE* (2014), epub, doi:10.1371/journal.pone.0100181.

9. Y. Yang, J. D. Goldhaber-Fiebert, and L. M. Wein, Analyzing screening policies for childhood obesity, *Management Science* 59 (2013): 782–795.

10. K. E. Rhee, R. McEachern, and E. Jelalian, Parent readiness to change differs for overweight child dietary and physical activity behaviors, *Journal of the Academy of Nutrition and Dietetics* (2014), epub, doi:10.1016/j.jand.2014.04.029.

11. Y. S. Danielsen and coauthors, Factors associated with low self-esteem in children with overweight, *Obesity Facts* (2012), epub, doi:10.1159/000338333.

12. E. M. Throop and coauthors, Pass the popcorn: "Obesogenic" behaviors and stigma in children's movies, *Obesity* 22 (2014): 1694–1700.

13. Centers for Disease Control and Prevention, Healthy weight—It's not a diet, it's a lifestyle!: About BMI for Children and Teens, 2014, available at www.cdc.gov.

14. A. I. Patel and coauthors, Under-diagnosis of pediatric obesity during outpatient preventive care visits, *Academic Pediatrics* 10 (2010): 405–409.

15. J. D. Goldhaber-Fiebert and coauthors, The utility of childhood and adolescent obesity assessment in relation to adult health, *Medical Decision Making* 33 (2013): 163–175; D. M. Harrington and coauthors, BMI percentiles for the identification of abdominal obesity and metabolic risk in children and adolescents: Evidence in support of the CDC 95% percentile, *European Journal of Clinical Nutrition* 67 (2013): 218–222.

16. Mayo Clinic, Diseases and conditions: Type 2 diabetes in children: Definition, 2015, available at www.mayoclinic.org/diseases-conditions/type-2-diabetes-in-children/basics/definition/con-20030124-40k.

17. M. Juonala, J. S. Viikari, and O. T. Raitakari, Main findings from the prospective Cardiovascular Risk in Young Finns Study, *Current Opinion in Lipidology* 24 (2013): 57–64.

18. Juonala, Viikari, and Raitakari, Main findings from the prospective Cardiovascular Risk in Young Finns Study, 2013.

19. D. Jacobson and B. M. Melnyk, A primary care healthy choices intervention program for overweight and obese school-age children and their parents, *Journal of Pediatric Health Care* 26 (2012): 126–138.

20. W. L. Chan She Ping-Delfos and coauthors, Use of the Dietary Guideline Index to assess cardiometabolic risk in adolescents, *British Journal of Nutrition* 113 (2015): 1741–1752; Kids Health, Cholesterol and your child, 2015, available at http://kidshealth.org/parent/medical/heart/cholesterol.html.

21. M. Barton, Childhood obesity: A life-long health risk, *Acta Pharmacologica Sinica* 2 (2012): 189–193.

22. S. Stabouli, S. Papakatsika, and V. Kotsis, The role of obesity, salt and exercise on blood pressure in children and adolescents, *Expert Review of Cardiovascular Therapy* 9 (2011): 753–761.

23. M. R. Lent and coauthors, Corner store purchases made by adults, adolescents and children: Items, nutritional characteristics and amount spent, *Public Health Nutrition* (2014), epub, doi:10.1017/S1368980014001670.

24. B. Y. Rollins and coauthors, Maternal controlling feeding practices and girls' inhibitory control interact to predict changes in BMI and eating in the absence of hunger from 5 to 7 y, *American Journal of Clinical Nutrition* 99 (2014): 249–257.

25. Iannotti and Wang, Patterns of physical activity, sedentary behavior and diet in US adolescents, 2013.

26. American Academy of Pediatrics, Media and children, 2015, available at www.aap.org.

27. Centers for Disease Control and Prevention, Healthy weight—It's not a diet, it's a lifestyle!: Tips for parents—Ideas to help children maintain a healthy body weight, 2014, available at www.cdc.gov; Child Trends Data Bank, Watching television, 2014, available at www.childtrends.org/?indicators=watching-television; D. S. Bickham and coauthors, Characteristics of screen media use associated with higher BMI in young adolescents, *Pediatrics* 131 (2013): 935–941; A. C. Nielsen Co., Television watching statistics, 2013, available at www.statisticbrain.com/television-watching-statistics/.

28. Bickham and coauthors, Characteristics of screen media use associated with higher BMI in young adolescents, 2013.

29. A. G. LeBlanc and coauthors, Systematic review of sedentary behaviour and health indicators in the early years (aged 0–4years), *Applied Physiology, Nutrition and Metabolism* 37 (2012): 753–772.

30. Bickham and coauthors, Characteristics of screen media use associated with higher BMI in young adolescents, 2013; S. Marsh, M. C. Ni,

and R. Maddison, The non-advertising effects of screen-based sedentary activities on acute eating behaviours in children, adolescents, and young adults: A systematic review, *Appetite* 71 (2013): 259–273.

31. M. Skatrud-Mickelson, A. M. Adachi-Mejia, and L. A. Sutherland, Tween sex differences in snacking preferences during television viewing, *Journal of the American Dietetic Association* 111 (2011): 1385–1390.

32. American Heart Association, Unhealthy and unregulated: Food advertising and marketing to children, Advocacy Fact Sheet, 2012, available at www.heart.org/idc/groups/heart-public/@wcm/@adv/documents/downloadable/ucm_301781.pdf.

33. A. C. Nielsen Co., Television watching statistics, 2013, available at www.statisticbrain.com/television-watching-statistics/.

34. Yale Rudd Center for Food Policy & Obesity, Fast food FACTS score 2013: Measuring progress in nutrition and marketing to children and teens, 2013, available at www.fastfoodmarketing.org.

35. L. Hebden, L. King, and B. Kelly, Art of persuasion: An analysis of techniques used to market foods to children, *Journal of Paediatrics and Child Health* 47 (2011): 776–782.

36. J. L. Harris and coauthors, US food company branded advergames on the Internet: Children's exposure and effects on snack consumption, *Journal of Children and Media* 6 (2012): 51–68.

37. American Psychological Association, The impact of food advertising on childhood obesity, 2015, available at www.apa.org/topics/kids-media/food.aspx; K. L. Keller and coauthors, The impact of food branding on children's eating behavior and obesity, *Physiology & Behavior* 106 (2012): 379–386; J. A. Kotler, J. M. Schiffman, and K. G. Hanson, The influence of media characters on children's food choices, *Journal of Health Communication* 17 (2012): 886–898.

38. Council of Better Business Bureaus, Children's Food and Beverage Advertising Initiative, 2015, available at www.bbb.org/council/the-national-partner-program/national-advertising-review-services/childrens-food-and-beverage-advertising-initiative/.

39. J. L. Harris and coauthors, Redefining "child-directed advertising" to reduce unhealthy television food advertising, *American Journal of Preventive Medicine* 44 (2013): 358–364.

40. J. L. Harris and S. K. Graff, Protecting young people from junk food advertising: Implications of psychological research for First Amendment law, *American Journal of Public Health* 102 (2012): 214–222.

41. American Heart Association, Policy position statement on food advertising and marketing practices to children, 2015, available at www.heart.org/advocacy; World Health Organization, A framework for implementing the set of recommendations on the marketing of foods and non-alcoholic beverages to children, 2012, available at www.who.int.

42. A. H. Kristensen and coauthors, Reducing childhood obesity through U.S. federal policy: A microsimulation analysis, *American Journal of Preventive Medicine* 47 (2014): 604–612.

43. M. Hunsberger, Early feeding practices and family structure: Associations with overweight in children, *Proceedings of the Nutrition Society* 73 (2014): 132–136; R. F. Rodgers, Maternal feeding practices predict weight gain and obesogenic eating behaviors in young children: A prospective study, *International Journal of Behavioral Nutrition and Physical Activity* (2013), epub, doi:10.1186/1479-5868-10-24.

44. Mayo Clinic, Childhood obesity: Treatment and drugs, 2015, available at www.Mayoclinic.org.

45. D. E. Bock and coauthors, The Health Initiative Program for Kids (HIP Kids): Effects of a 1-year multidisciplinary lifestyle intervention on adiposity and quality of life in obese children and adolescents—A longitudinal pilot intervention study, *BMC Pediatrics* (2014), epub, doi:10.1186/s12887-014-0296-1.

46. H. Bergmeier, H. Skouteris, and M. Heatherington, Systematic research review of observational approaches used to evaluate mother–child mealtime interactions during preschool years, *American Journal of Clinical Nutrition* 101 (2015): 7–15.

47. J. Martin-Biggers and coauthors, Translating it into real life: A qualitative study of the cognitions, barriers, and supports for key obesogenic behaviors of parents of preschoolers, *BMC Public Health* 15 (2015): 189–203.

48. Bock and coauthors, The Health Initiative Program for Kids (HIP Kids), 2014; K. K. Davison and coauthors, A childhood obesity intervention developed by families for families: Results from a pilot study, *International Journal of Behavioral Nutrition and Physical Activity* (2013), epub, doi:10.1186/1479-5868-10-3.

49. R. Sherafat-Kazemzadeh, S. Z. Yanovski, and J. A. Yanovski, Pharmacotherapy for childhood obesity: Present and future prospects, *International Journal of Obesity* 37 (2013): 1–15.

50. M. Sinha and coauthors, Metabolic effects of Roux-en-Y gastric bypass in obese adolescents and young adults, *Journal of Pediatric Gastroenterology and Nutrition* 56 (2013): 528–531.

51. B. Hofmann, Bariatric surgery for obese children and adolescents: A review of the moral challenges, *BMC Medical Ethics* (2013), epub, doi:10.1186/1472-6939-14-18.

52. National Restaurant Association, Kids live well: Healthful choices, happy kids, 2012, available at http://mommacuisine.com/2012/05/11/lifestyle-kids-live-well-healthful-choices-happy-kids/.

53. U.S. Department of Agriculture and U.S. Department of Health and Human Services, Scientific report of the 2015 Dietary Guidelines Advisory Committee, 2015, D:3–7, available at www.health.gov; R. B. Ervin and coauthors, Consumption of added sugar among U.S. children and adolescents, 2005–2008 (NCHS Data Brief 87), 2012.

54. Ervin and coauthors, Consumption of added sugar among U.S. children and adolescents, 2005–2008, 2012.

55. G. M. Singh and coauthors, Estimated global, regional, and national disease burdens related to sugar-sweetened beverage consumption in 2010, *Circulation* (2015): epub ahead of print, doi:10.1161/CIRCULATIONAHA.114.010636; K. L. Stanhope and coauthors, A dose-response study of consuming high-fructose corn syrup–sweetened beverages on lipid/lipoprotein risk factors for cardiovascular disease in young adults, *American Journal of Clinical Nutrition* (2015), epub ahead of print, doi:10.3945/ajcn.114.100461; F. B. Hu, Resolved: There is sufficient scientific evidence that decreasing sugar-sweetened beverage consumption will reduce the prevalence of obesity and obesity-related diseases, *Obesity Reviews* 14 (2013): 606–619; J. C. de Ruyter and coauthors, A trial of sugar-free or sugar-sweetened beverages and body weight in children, *New England Journal of Medicine* 367 (2012): 1397–1406.

56. U. Ekelund and coauthors, Association of moderate to vigorous physical activity and sedentary time with cardiometabolic risk factors in children and adolescents, *Journal of the American Medical Association* 307 (2012): 704–712.

57. A. Bauman and R. Macniven, Are active video games useful in increasing physical activity and addressing obesity in children? *JAMA Pediatrics* 167 (2013): 676–677; J. P. Chaput and coauthors, Are active video games useful in increasing physical activity and addressing obesity in children? *JAMA Pediatrics* 167 (2013): 677–678; S. R. Smallwood and coauthors, Physiologic responses and energy expenditure of kinect active video game play in schoolchildren, *Archives of Pediatric and Adolescent Medicine* (2012), epub, doi:10.1001/archpediatrics.2012.1271.

58. S. Gahagan, The development of eating behavior: Biology and context, *Journal of Developmental and Behavioral Pediatrics* 33 (2012): 261–271; T. R. Cromley, Parent and family associations with weight-related behaviors and cognitions among overweight adolescents, *Journal of Adolescent Health* 47 (2010): 263–269.

59. B. L. Jones, B. H. Fiese, and The STRONG Kids Team, Parent routines, child routines, and family demographics associated with obesity in parents and preschool-aged children, *Frontiers in Psychology* (2014), epub, doi:10.3389/fpsyg.2014.00374.

60. Bock and coauthors, The Health Initiative Program for Kids (HIP Kids), 2014.

61. G. Antonogeorgos and coauthors, Breakfast consumption and meal frequency interaction with childhood obesity, *Pediatric Obesity* 7 (2012): 65–72.

62. A. Remington and coauthors, Increasing food acceptance in the home setting: A randomized controlled trial of parent-administered taste exposure with incentives, *American Journal of Clinical Nutrition* 95 (2012): 72–77.

Chapter 14

1. U.S. Department of Agriculture, Center for Nutrition Policy and Promotion, Diet quality of children age 2–17 years as measured by the Healthy Eating Index—2010, *Nutrition Insight* 52 (2013), epub, available at www.cnpp.usda.gov/sites/default/files/nutrition_insights_uploads/Insight52.pdf.

2. L. L. Birch and A. E. Doub, Learning to eat: Birth to age 2 y, *American Journal of Clinical Nutrition* 99 (2014): 723S–728S.

3. L. D. Ritchie, Less frequent eating predicts greater BMI and waist circumference in female adolescents, *American Journal of Clinical Nutrition* 95 (2012): 290–296.

4. R. S. Gibson, A. M. Heath, and E. A. Szymlek-Gay, Is iron and zinc nutrition a concern for vegetarian infants and young children in industrialized countries? *American Journal of Clinical Nutrition* 100 (2014): 459S–468S.

5. U.S. Department of Agriculture, Dietary Reference Intakes: Macronutrients, 2012, available at fnic.nal.usda.gov/dietary-guidance/dietary-reference-intakes/dri-tables.

6. Committee on Dietary Reference Intakes, *Dietary Reference Intakes for Energy, Carbohydrate, Fiber, Fat, Fatty Acids, Cholesterol, Protein, and Amino Acids* (Washington, D.C.: National Academies Press, 2005), Chapter 11.

7. R. L. Bailey and coauthors, Do dietary supplements improve micronutrient sufficiency in children and adolescents? *Journal of Pediatrics* 161 (2012): 837–842.

8. Committee on Dietary Reference Intakes, *Dietary Reference Intakes for Calcium and Vitamin D* (Washington, D.C.: National Academies Press, 2011), pp. 5–35.

9. D. R. Keast and coauthors, Associations between yogurt, dairy, calcium, and vitamin D intake and obesity among U.S. children aged 8–18 years: NHANES, 2005–2008, *Nutrients* 7 (2015): 1577–1593; L. Cosenza and coauthors, Calcium and vitamin D intakes in children: A randomized controlled trial, *BMC Pediatrics* 13 (2013): 86.

10. M. A. Atkinson and coauthors, Vitamin D, race, and risk for anemia in children, *Journal of Pediatrics* 164 (2014): 153–158.

11. Birch and Doub, Learning to eat, 2014; S. Lioret and coauthors, Tracking of dietary intakes in early childhood: The Melbourne Infant Program, *European Journal of Clinical Nutrition* 67 (2013): 275–281.

12. R. R. Briefel and coauthors, The Feeding Infants and Toddlers Study 2008: Study design and methods, *Journal of the Academy of Nutrition and Dietetics* 110 (2010): S16–S26.

13. J. M. Saavedra and coauthors, Lessons from the Feeding Infants and Toddlers Study in North America: What children eat, and implications for obesity prevention, *Annals of Nutrition & Metabolism* 62 (2013): 27–36.

14. L. L. Moore and coauthors, Food group intake and micronutrient adequacy in adolescent girls, *Nutrients* 4 (2012): 1692–1708.

15. C. C. Tan and S. C. Holub, Maternal feeding practices associated with food neophobia, *Appetite* 59 (2012): 483–487.

16. N. Zucker and coauthors, Psychological and psychosocial impairment in preschoolers with selective eating, *Pediatrics* (2015), epub ahead of print, doi:10.1542/peds.2014-2386; S. Monnery-Patris and coauthors, Smell differential reactivity, but not taste differential reactivity, is related to food neophobia in toddlers, *Appetite* 95 (2015): 303–309; V. Quick and coauthors, Relationships of neophobia and pickiness with dietary variety, dietary quality and diabetes management adherence in youth with type 1 diabetes, *European Journal of Clinical Nutrition* 68 (2014): 131–136.

17. Birch and Doub, Learning to eat, 2014.

18. H. H. Laroche and coauthors, Changes in diet behavior when adults become parents, *Journal of the Academy of Nutrition and Dietetics* 112 (2012): 832–839.

19. A. M. Ashman and coauthors, Maternal diet during early childhood, but not pregnancy, predicts diet quality and fruit and vegetable acceptance in offspring, *Maternal and Child Nutrition* (2014), epub ahead of print, doi:10.1111/mcn.12151; J. A. Mennella and J. C. Trabulsi, Complementary foods and flavor experiences: Setting the foundation, *Annals of Nutrition & Metabolism* 60 (2012): 40–50.

20. E. C. Radlowski and R. W. Johnson, Perinatal iron deficiency and neurocognitive development, *Frontiers in Human Neuroscience* (2013), epub, doi:10.3389/fnhum.2013.00585.

21. S. R. Pasricha and coauthors, Effect of daily iron supplementation on health in children aged 4–23 months: A systematic review and meta-analysis of randomised controlled trials, *Lancet: Global Health* (2013), epub, doi:10.1016/S2214-109X(13)70046-9.

22. Pasricha and coauthors, Effect of daily iron supplementation on health in children aged 4–23 months, 2013; P. Sant-Rayn, Should we screen for iron deficiency anemia? A review of the evidence and recent recommendations, *Pathology* 44 (2012): 139–147.

23. Centers for Disease Control and Prevention, Lead, available at www.cdc.gov/nceh/lead.

24. World Health Organization, Childhood lead poisoning, available at www.who.int/ceh/publications/childhoodpoisoning/en/.

25. World Health Organization, Childhood lead poisoning, available at www.who.int/ceh/publications/childhoodpoisoning/en/.

26. KidsHealth, Lead poisoning, 2015, available at http://kidshealth.org/parent/medical/brain/lead_poisoning.html.

27. J. Liu and coauthors, Impact of low blood lead concentrations on IQ and school performance in Chinese children, *PLOS ONE* (2013), epub, doi:10.1371/journal.pone.0065230.

28. Y. Wang, K. Wu, and W. Zhao, Blood zinc, calcium and lead levels in Chinese children aged 1–36 months, *International Journal of Clinical and Experimental Medicine* 8 (2015): 1424–1426; X. Ji and coauthors, Evaluation of blood zinc,

calcium and blood lead levels among children aged 1–36 months, *Nutricion Hospitalaria* 30 (2014): 548–551; C. S. Sim and coauthors, Iron deficiency increases blood lead levels in boys and pre-menarche girls surveyed in KNHANES 2010–2011, *Environmental Research* (2014), epub, doi:10.1016/j.envres.2014.01.004.

29. Food Allergy Research & Education, About food allergies, 2015, available at www.foodallergy.org/about-food-allergies.

30. B. I. Nwaru and coauthors, Prevalence of common food allergies in Europe: A systematic review and meta-analysis, *Allergy* 69 (2014): 992–1007; S. H. Sicherer and coauthors, The natural history of egg allergy in an observational cohort, *Journal of Allergy and Clinical Immunology* 133 (2014): 492–499; R. A. Wood and coauthors, The natural history of milk allergy in an observational cohort, *Journal of Allergy and Clinical Immunology* 131 (2013): 805–812.

31. American College of Allergy, Asthma & Immunology, Types of food allergy: Peanut allergy, 2014, available at http://acaai.org/allergies/types/food-allergies/types-food-allergy/peanut-allergy; R. M. Johnson and C. S. Barnes, Airborne concentrations of peanut protein, *Allergy and Asthma Proceedings* 34 (2013): 59–64.

32. R. Meyer and coauthors, A practical approach to vitamin and mineral supplementation in food allergic children, *Clinical and Translational Allergy* 5 (2015): 11.

33. Meyer and coauthors, A practical approach to vitamin and mineral supplementation in food allergic children, 2015; H. Mehta, M. Groetch, and J. Wang, Growth and nutritional concerns in children with food allergy, *Current Opinion in Allergy and Clinical Immunology* 13 (2013): 275–279.

34. A. W. Burks and coauthors, Oral immunotherapy for treatment of egg allergy in children, *New England Journal of Medicine* 367 (2012): 233–243.

35. U.S. Food and Drug Administration, Food allergies: What you need to know, 2014, available at www.fda.gov/Food/ResourcesForYou/Consumers/ucm079311.htm.

36. J. Barnett and coauthors, Beyond labeling: What strategies do nut allergic individuals employ to make food choices? A qualitative study, *PLOS ONE* (2013), epub, doi:10.1371/journal.pone.0055293.

37. National Institute of Allergy and Infectious Diseases, Food allergy, 2012, available at www.niaid.nih.gov/topics/foodAllergy/understanding/Pages/diagnosis.aspx.

38. M. V. Khodoun and coauthors, Rapid desensitization of mice with anti-FcγRIIb/FcγRIII mAb safely prevents IgG-mediated anaphylaxis, *Journal of Allergy and Clinical Immunology* 132 (2013): 1375–1387; U. H. Le and A. W. Burks, Oral and sublingual immunotherapy for food allergy, *Human Vaccines and Immunotherapeutics* 8 (2012): 1534–1543.

39. Y. Zhou and coauthors, Peanut allergy, allergen composition, and methods of reducing allergenicity: A review, *International Journal of Food Science* (2013), epub, doi:10.1155/2013/909140;

Y. M. Wu and coauthors, Synthesis and degradation of the major allergens in developing and germinating soybean seed, *Journal of Integrative Plant Biology* 54 (2012): 4–14.

40. Centers for Disease Control and Prevention, Attention-deficit/hyperactivity disorder (ADHD), 2014, available at cdc.gov/ncbddd/adhd/data.html; L. Batstra and A. Frances, DSM-5 further inflates attention deficit hyperactivity disorder, *Journal of Nervous and Mental Disease* 200 (2012): 486–488.

41. J. T. Nigg and K. Holton, Restriction and elimination diets in ADHD treatment, *Child and Adolescent Psychiatric Clinics* 23 (2014): 937–953; E. Hawkey and J. T. Nigg, Omega-3 fatty acid and ADHD: Blood level analysis and meta-analytic extension of supplementation trials, *Clinical Psychology Review* 34 (2014): 496–505; J. T. Nigg and K. Holton, Restriction and elimination diets in ADHD treatment, *Child and Adolescent Psychiatric Clinics of North America* 23 (2014): 937–953.

42. G. Kohlboeck and coauthors, Food intake, diet quality and behavioral problems in children: Results from the GINI-plus/LISA-plus studies, *Annals of Nutrition & Metabolism* 60 (2014): 247–256.

43. S. B. Sisson and coauthors, Television-viewing time and dietary quality among U.S. children and adults, *American Journal of Preventive Medicine* 43 (2012): 196–200.

44. M. Melchior and coauthors, Food insecurity and children's mental health: A prospective birth cohort study, *PLoS ONE* (2012), epub, doi:10.1371/journal.pone.0052615.

45. J. G. Millichap and M. M. Yee, The diet factor in attention-deficit/hyperactivity disorder, *Pediatrics* 129 (2012): 330–337.

46. W. B. Brinkman and coauthors, Shared decision-making to improve attention-deficit hyperactivity disorder care, *Patient Education and Counseling* 93 (2013): 95–101.

47. National Institute of Dental and Craniofacial Research, Dental caries (tooth decay) in children (age 2 to 11), available at http://nidcr.nih.gov/DataStatistics/FindDataByTopic/DentalCaries/DentalCariesChildren2to11.htm.

48. Position of the Academy of Nutrition and Dietetics: The impact of fluoride on health, *Journal of the Academy of Nutrition and Dietetics* 112 (2012): 1443–1453.

49. U.S. Food and Drug Administration, About dental amalgam fillings, 2009, available at www.fda.gov/MedicalDevices/ProductsandMedicalProcedures/DentalProducts/DentalAmalgam/ucm171094.htm.

50. M. S. Tonetti, T. E. Van Dyke, and Working Group 1 of the Joint EFP/AAP Workshop, Periodontitis and atherosclerotic cardiovascular disease: Consensus report of the Joint EFP/AAP Workshop on Periodontitis and Systematic Diseases, *Journal of Periodontology* 84 (2013): S24–S29.

51. S. Park and coauthors, Association of sugar-sweetened beverage intake during infancy with dental caries in 6-year olds, *Clinical Nutrition Research* 4 (2015): 9–17; S. Park and coauthors, The association of sugar-sweetened

beverage intake during infancy with sugar-sweetened beverage intake at 6 years of age, *Pediatrics* 134 (2014): S56–S62; A. Sheiham and W. P. T. James, A reappraisal of the quantitative relationship between sugar intake and dental caries: The need for new criteria for developing goals for sugar intake, *BMC Public Health* 14 (2014): 863; B. A. Dye, X. Li, and E. D. Beltran-Aguilar, Selected oral health indicators in the United States, 2005–2008 (NCHS Data Brief 96), May 2012.

52. P. J. Moynihan and S. A. Kelly, Effect on caries of restricting sugars intake: Systematic review to inform WHO guidelines, *Journal of Dental Research* 93 (2014): 8–18.

53. T. Coppinger and coauthors, Body mass, frequency of eating and breakfast consumption in 9–13-year-olds, *Journal of Human Nutrition and Dietetics* 25 (2012): 43–49.

54. K. Adolphus, C. L. Lawton, and L. Dye, The effects of breakfast on behavior and academic performance in children and adolescents, *Frontiers in Human Neuroscience* 7 (2013): 425; J. Liu and coauthors, Regular breakfast consumption is associated with increased IQ in kindergarten children, *Early Human Development* 89 (2013): 257–262; Coppinger and coauthors, Body mass, frequency of eating and breakfast consumption in 9–13-year-olds, 2012.

55. U.S. Department of Agriculture, Food and Nutrition Service, School Breakfast Program (SBP): Fact sheet, 2012, available at www.fns.usda.gov/sbp/school-breakfast-program-sbp.

56. Food Research and Action Center, National School Lunch Program, 2012–2013 participation, available at http://frac.org/federal-foodnutrition-programs/national-school-lunch-program/.

57. K. L. Hubbard and coauthors, What's in children's backpacks? Foods brought from home, *Journal of the Academy of Nutrition and Dietetics* (2014), epub, doi:10.1016/j.jand.2014.05.010; M. R. Longacre and coauthors, School food reduces household income disparities in adolescents' frequency of fruit and vegetable intake, *Preventive Medicine* 69 (2014): 202–207.

58. U.S. Department of Agriculture, Food and Nutrition Service, School Nutrition Dietary Assessment Study-IV, 2012, available at www.fns.usda.gov/school-nutrition-dietary-assessment-study-iv.

59. U.S. Department of Agriculture, Food and Nutrition Service, Nutrition standards in the National School Lunch and School Breakfast Programs: Final rule, *Federal Register* 77 (2012): 4088–4167.

60. American Academy of Pediatrics, Policy statement: Snacks, sweetened beverages, added sugars, and schools, *Pediatrics* 135 (2015): 575–583.

61. Centers for Disease Control and Prevention, Adolescent and school health: Competitive foods in schools, 2014, available at www.cdc.gov/healthyyouth/nutrition/standards.htm.

62. E. Hennessy and coauthors, State-level school competitive food and beverage laws are associated with children's weight status, *Journal*

of School Health 84 (2014): 609–616; D. R. Taber and coauthors, Weight status among adolescents in states that govern competitive food nutrition content, *Pediatrics* 130 (2012): 437–444; L. Turner and F. J. Chaloupka, Slow progress in changing the school food environment: Nationally representative results from the public and private elementary schools, *Journal of the Academy of Nutrition and Dietetics* 112 (2012): 1380–1389.

63. U.S. Department of Agriculture, Food and Nutrition Service, Nutrition standards in the National School Lunch and School Breakfast Programs: Final rule, 2012.

64. J. Utter and coauthors, Family meals among New Zealand young people: Relationships with eating behaviors and body mass index, *Journal of Nutrition Education and Behavior* 45 (2013): 3–11.

65. M. E. Harrison and coauthors, Systematic review of the effects of family meal frequency on psychosocial outcomes in youth, *Canadian Family Physician* 61 (2015): e96–e106.

66. R. Lowry and coauthors, Obesity and other correlates of physical activity and sedentary behaviors among US high school students, *Journal of Obesity* (2013), epub, doi:10.1155/2013/276318; A. S. Alberga and coauthors, Overweight and obese teenagers: Why is adolescence a critical period? *Pediatric Obesity* 7 (2012): 261–273.

67. S. E. Hadland, Weight misperception and unhealthy weight control behaviors among sexual minorities in the general adolescent population, *Journal of Adolescent Health* 54 (2014): 296–303.

68. G. Moschonis and coauthors, Association of iron depletion with menstruation and dietary intake indices in pubertal girls: The Healthy Growth Study, *BioMed Research International* (2013), epub, doi:10.1155/2013/423263.

69. Moschonis and coauthors, Association of iron depletion with menstruation and dietary intake indices in pubertal girls, 2013.

70. C. Gundersen, Food insecurity is an ongoing national concern, *Advances in Nutrition* 4 (2013): 36–41.

71. S. Stagi and coauthors, Bone metabolism in children and adolescents: Main characteristics of the determinants of peak bone mass, *Clinical Cases in Mineral and Bone Metabolism* 10 (2013): 172–179.

72. B. Gopinath and coauthors, Pattern and predictors of dairy consumption during adolescence, *Asia Pacific Journal of Clinical Nutrition* 23 (2014): 612–618.

73. R. S. Sebastian and coauthors, Fluid milk consumption in the United States: What we eat in America, NHANES 2005–2006 (Food Surveys Research Group Dietary Data Brief 3), September 2010, available at www.ars.usda.gov /SP2UserFiles/Place/12355000/pdf/Dbrief /3_milk_consumptio_0506.pdf.

74. E. Han and L. M. Powell, Consumption patterns of sugar sweetened beverages in the United States, *Journal of the Academy of Nutrition and Dietetics* (2014), epub, doi:10.1016/j. jand.2012.09.016.

75. S. H. Kim, W. K. Kim, and M. H. Kang, Effect of milk and milk products consumption on physical growth and bone mineral density in Korean adolescents, *Nutrition Research and Practice* 7 (2013): 309–314.

76. R. Katta and S. P. Desai, Diet and dermatology, *Journal of Clinical Aesthetic Dermatology* 7 (2014): 46–51.

77. J. Burris, W. Rietkerk, and K. Woolf, Relationships of self-reported dietary factors and perceived acne severity in a cohort of New York young adults, *Journal of the Academy of Nutrition and Dietetics* 114 (2014): 384–392; N. H. Ismail, Z. A. Manaf, and N. Z. Azizan, High glycemic load diet, milk and ice cream consumption are related to acne vulgaris in Malaysian young adults: A case control study, *BMC Dermatology* 12 (2012): 13.

78. I. Y. Hur and M. Reicks, Relationship between whole-grain intake, chronic disease risk indicators, and weight status among adolescents in the National Health and Nutrition Examination Survey, 1999–2004, *Academy of Nutrition and Dietetics* 112 (2012): 46–55.

79. H. A. Hoertel, M. J. Will, and H. J. Leidy, A randomized crossover, pilot study examining the effects of a normal protein vs. high protein breakfast on food cravings and reward signals in overweight/obese "breakfast skipping," late-adolescent girls, *Nutrition Journal* (2014), epub, doi:101186/1475-2891-13-80; J. M. Poti, K. J. Duffey, and B. M. Popkin, The association of fast food consumption with poor dietary outcomes and obesity among children: Is it the fast food or the remainder of the diet? *American Journal of Clinical Nutrition* 99 (2014): 162–171.

80. J. E. Holsten and coauthors, Children's food choice process in the home environment: A qualitative descriptive study, *Appetite* 58 (2012): 64–73.

81. H. J. Leidy and coauthors, Consuming high-protein soy snacks affects appetite control, satiety, and diet quality in young people and influences select aspects of mood and cognition, *Journal of Nutrition* 145 (2015): 1614–1622; X. Guo and coauthors, Differences in lifestyle behaviors, dietary habits, and familial factors among normal-weight, overweight, and obese Chinese children and adolescents, *International Journal of Behavioral Nutrition and Physical Activity* (2012), epub, doi:10.1186/1479-5868- 9-120.

82. W. Rizza, N. Veronese, and L. Fontana, What are the roles of calorie restriction and diet quality in promoting healthy longevity? *Ageing Research Reviews* 13 (2014): 38–45.

83. S. Sabia and coauthors, Influence of individual and combined healthy behaviours on successful aging, *Canadian Medical Association Journal* (2012), epub, doi:10.1503/cmaj.121080.

84. Federal Interagency Forum on Aging-Related Statistics, Older Americans 2012: Key indicators of well being: Health status, 2012, available at www.agingstats.gov/Main_Site /Data/2012_Documents/Health_Status.aspx.

85. Centers for Disease Control and Prevention, Deaths: Final Data for 2013, National Vital Statistics Reports, Volume 64, Number 2, available at http://www.cdc.gov/nchs/products/nvsr .htm.

86. S. Harper, D. Rushani, and J. S. Kaufman, Trends in the black-white life expectancy gap, 2003–2008, *Journal of the American Medical Association* 307 (2012): 2257–2259.

87. S. Emran and coauthors, Target of rapamycin signaling mediates the lifespan-extending effects of dietary restriction by essential amino acid alteration, *Aging* 6 (2014): 390–398; J. M. Murabito, R. Yuan, and K. L. Lunetta, The search for longevity and healthy aging genes: Insights from epidemiological studies and samples of long-lived individuals, *Journals of Gerontology: Series A, Biological Sciences and Medical Sciences* 67 (2012): 470–479.

88. I. M. Bensenor, R. D. Olmos, and P. A. Lotufo, Hypothyroidism in the elderly: Diagnosis and management, *Clinical Interventions in Aging* 7 (2012): 97–111; D. L. Johannsen and coauthors, Effect of short-term thyroxine administration on energy metabolism and mitochondrial efficiency in humans, *PloS ONE* (2012), epub, doi: 10.1371/journal.pone.0040837.

89. J. A. Cooper and coauthors, Longitudinal change in energy expenditure and effects on energy requirements of the elderly, *Nutrition Journal* 12 (2013): 73.

90. K. A. Intlekofer and C. W. Cotman, Exercise counteracts declining hippocampal function in aging and Alzheimer's disease, *Neurobiology of Disease* (2012), epub ahead of print, doi:10.1016/j.nbd.2012.06.011.

91. K. Anderson, C. Baraldi, and M. Supiano, Identifying failure to thrive in the long-term care setting, *Journal of the American Medical Directors Association* 13 (2012): 665.e15–665.e19.

92. E. Britton and J. T. McLaughlin, Ageing and the gut, *Proceedings of the Nutrition Society* 72 (2013): 173–177.

93. M. Bernstein, N. Munoz, and Academy of Nutrition and Dietetics, Position of the Academy of Nutrition and Dietetics: Food and nutrition for older adults: Promoting health and wellness, *Journal of the Academy of Nutrition and Dietetics* 112 (2012): 1255–1277.

94. J. Olesen, Exercise training, but not resveratrol, improves metabolic and inflammatory status in skeletal muscle of aged men, *Journal of Physiology* 592 (2014): 1873–1886; M. R. Beltran Valls and coauthors, Explosive type of moderate-resistance training induces functional, cardiovascular, and molecular adaptations in the elderly, *Age* 36 (2014): 759–772; S. Shahar and coauthors, Effectiveness of exercise and protein supplementation intervention on body composition, functional fitness, and oxidative stress among elderly Malays with sarcopenia, *Clinical Interventions in Aging* 8 (2013): 1365–1375; Y. Yang and coauthors, Resistance exercise enhances myofibrillar protein synthesis with graded intakes of whey protein in older men, *British Journal of Nutrition* 108 (2012): 1780–1788.

95. F. Sun, I. J. Norman, and A. E. While, Physical activity in older people: A systematic

review, *BMC Public Health* 13 (2013): 449; U.S. Department of Health and Human Services, Healthy People 2020: Physical activity, 2012, available at www.healthypeople.gov/2020/topicsobjectives2020/overview.aspx?topicid=33.

96. J. A. Harvey, S. F. M. Chastin, and D. A. Skelton, How sedentary are older people? A systematic review of the amount of sedentary behavior, *Journal of Aging and Physical Activity* (2014), epub, doi:10.1123/japa.2014-0164.

97. P. J. Chang, L. Wray, and Y. Lin, Social relationships, leisure activity, and health in older adults, *Health Psychology* 33 (2014): 516–523; J. Kim and coauthors, Health benefits of serious involvement in leisure activities among older Korean adults, *International Journal of Qualitative Studies on Health and Well-Being* (2014), epub, doi:10.3402/qhw.v9.24616; M. G. Stineman and coauthors, All-cause 1-, 5-, and 10-year mortality in elderly people according to activities of daily living stage, *Journal of the American Geriatrics Society* 60 (2012): 485–492.

98. M. Tieland and coauthors, Protein supplementation increases muscle mass gain during prolonged resistance-type exercise training in frail elderly people: A randomized, double-blind, placebo-controlled trial. *Journal of the American Medical Directors Association* 13 (2012): 713–719.

99. E. Arentson-Lantz and coauthors, Protein: A nutrient in focus, *Applied Physiology, Nutrition, and Metabolism* 40 (2015): 755–761; D. Paddon-Jones and coauthors, Protein and healthy aging, *American Journal of Clinical Nutrition* 101 (2015): 1339S–1345S; R. M. Daly and coauthors, Protein-enriched diet, with the use of lean red meat, combined with progressive resistance training enhances lean tissue mass and muscle strength and reduces circulating IL-6 concentrations in elderly women: A cluster randomized controlled trial, *American Journal of Clinical Nutrition* 99 (2014): 899–910; I. Kim and coauthors, Quantity of dietary protein intake, but not pattern of intake, affects net protein balance primarily through differences in protein synthesis in older adults, *American Journal of Physiology—Endocrinology and Metabolism* 308 (2014): E21–E28.

100. M. L. Dirks and coauthors, Skeletal muscle disuse atrophy is not attenuated by dietary protein supplementation in healthy older men, *Journal of Nutrition* 144 (2014): 1196–1203.

101. American College of Sports Medicine, Position stand: Exercise and physical activity for older adults, *Medicine and Science in Sports and Exercise* 41 (2009): 1510–1530.

102. Position of the Academy of Nutrition and Dietetics: Food and nutrition for older adults: Promoting health and wellness, 2012.

103. K. Dideriksen, S. Reitelseder, and L. Holm, Influence of amino acids, dietary protein, and physical activity on muscle mass development in humans, *Nutrients* 5 (2013): 852–876; Yang and coauthors, Resistance exercise enhances myofibrillar protein synthesis with graded intakes of whey protein in older men, 2012.

104. Dideriksen, Reitelseder, and Holm, Influence of amino acids, dietary protein, and physical activity on muscle mass development in humans, 2013; B. Pennings and coauthors, Amino acid absorption and subsequent muscle protein accretion following graded intakes of whey protein in elderly men, *American Journal of Physiology—Endocrinology and Metabolism* 302 (2012): E992–E999; Yang and coauthors, Resistance exercise enhances myofibrillar protein synthesis with graded intakes of whey protein in older men, 2012.

105. Q. L. Xue and coauthors, Patterns of 12-year change in physical activity levels in community-dwelling older women: Can modest levels of physical activity help older women live longer? *American Journal of Epidemiology* 176 (2012): 534–543; K. T. Morgan, Nutrition, resistance training, and sarcopenia: Their role in successful aging, *Topics in Clinical Nutrition* 27 (2012): 114–123.

106. A. R. Mobley, Identifying practical solutions to meet America's fiber needs: Proceedings from the Food & Fiber Summit, *Nutrients* 6 (2014): 2540–2551; U.S. Department of Agriculture, What We Eat in America: Nutrient intakes from food by gender and age, NHANES 2009–2010, available at www.ars.usda.gov/SP2UserFiles/Place/12355000/pdf/0910/Table_1_NIN_GEN_09.pdf.

107. Centers for Disease Control and Prevention, Arthritis: Meeting the challenge of living well: At a glance, 2014, available at www.cdc.gov.

108. L. A. Zdziarski, J. G. Wasser, and H. K. Vincent, Chronic pain management in the obese patient: A focused review of key challenges and potential exercise solutions, *Journal of Pain Research* 8 (2015): 63–77; H. Bliddal, A. R. Leeds, and R. Christensen, Osteoarthritis, obesity and weight loss: Evidence, hypotheses and horizons—A scoping review, *Obesity Reviews* 15 (2014): 578–586.

109. M. Jalili and coauthors, Beneficial role of antioxidants on clinical outcomes and erythrocyte antioxidant parameters in rheumatoid arthritis patients, *International Journal of Preventive Medicine* 5 (2014): 835–840; G. W. Reed and coauthors, Treatment of rheumatoid arthritis with marine and botanical oils: An 18-month, randomized, and double-blind trial, *Evidence-Based Complementary and Alternative Medicine: eCAM* (2014), epub, doi:10.1155/2014/857456.

110. M. C. Hochberg and coauthors, Combined chondroitin sulfate and glucosamine for painful knee osteoarthritis: A multicentre, randomised, double-blind, non-inferiority trial versus celecoxib, *Annals of the Rheumatic Diseases* (2014), epub, doi:10.1136/annrheumdis-2014-206792.

111. Y. Zhang and coauthors, Purine-rich foods intake and recurrent gout attacks, *Annals of the Rheumatic Diseases* 71 (2012): 1448–1453; E. Krishnan, B. Lingala, and V. Bhalla, Low-level lead exposure and the prevalence of gout: An observational study, *Annals of Internal Medicine* 157 (2012): 233–241.

112. Committee on Dietary Reference Intakes, *Dietary Reference Intakes for Calcium and Vitamin D* (Washington, D.C.: National Academies Press, 2011), pp. 345–402.

113. Committee on Dietary Reference Intakes, *Dietary Reference Intakes for Calcium and Vitamin D*, 2011, pp. 345–402.

114. U.S. Preventive Services Task Force, Vitamin D and calcium to prevent fractures: Preventive medication, February 2013, available at www.uspreventiveservicestaskforce.org/Page/Topic/recommendation-summary/vitamin-d-and-calcium-to-prevent-fractures-preventive-medication.

115. V. A. Moyer and the U.S. Preventive Services Task Force, Prevention of falls in community-dwelling older adults: U.S. Preventive Services Task Force recommendation statement, *Annals of Internal Medicine* 157 (2012): 197–204.

116. A. Mézière and coauthors, B_{12} deficiency increases with age in hospitalized patients: A study on 14,904 samples, *Journals of Gerontology: Series A, Biological Sciences and Medical Sciences* 69 (2014): 1576–1585.

117. S. P. Stabler, Vitamin B_{12} deficiency, *New England Journal of Medicine* 368 (2013): 149–160.

118. J. W. Eichenbaum, Geriatric vision loss due to cataracts, macular degeneration, and glaucoma, *Mount Sinai Journal of Medicine: A Journal of Translational and Personalized Medicine* 79 (2012): 276–294; M. Y. Wang and coauthors, Activity limitation due to a fear of falling in older adults with eye disease, *Investigative Ophthalmology & Visual Science* 53 (2012): 7967–7972.

119. S. L. Christ and coauthors, Longitudinal relationships among visual acuity, daily functional status, and mortality: The Salisbury Eye Evaluation Study, *JAMA Ophthalmology* 132 (2014): 1400–1406.

120. E. Y. Chew and coauthors, Lutein + zeaxanthin and omega-3 fatty acids for age-related macular degeneration: The Age-Related Eye Disease Study 2 (AREDS2) randomized clinical trial, *Journal of the American Medical Association* 309 (2013): 2005–2015.

121. J. R. Evans and J. G. Lawrenson, Antioxidant vitamin and mineral supplements for preventing age-related macular degeneration, *Cochrane Database Systematic Reviews* 6 (2012), epub, doi:10.1002/14651858.CD000253.pub3.

122. S. Rautiainen and coauthors, Total antioxidant capacity of the diet and risk of age-related cataract: A population-based prospective cohort of women, *JAMA Ophthalmology* 132 (2014): 247–252; M. Pastor-Valero, Fruit and vegetable intake and vitamins C and E are associated with a reduced prevalence of cataract in a Spanish Mediterranean population, *BMC Ophthalmology* (2013), epub, doi:10.1186/1471-2415-13-52.

123. J. Zheng Selin and coauthors, High-dose supplements of vitamins C and E, low-dose multivitamins, and the risk of age-related cataract: A population-based prospective, *American Journal of Epidemiology* 177 (2013): 548–555.

124. A. Adan, Cognitive performance and dehydration, *Journal of the American College of Nutrition* 31 (2012): 71–78.

125. M. Pae, S. N. Meydani, and D. Wu, The role of nutrition in enhancing immunity in aging, *Aging and Disease* 3 (2012): 91–129.

126. C. Baumeier and coauthors, Caloric restriction and intermittent fasting alter hepatic lipid droplet proteome and diacylglycerol species and prevent diabetes in NZO mice, *Biochimica et Biophysica Acta* 1851 (2015): 566–576; N. Makino and coauthors, Calorie restriction increases telomerase activity, enhances autophagy, and improves diastolic dysfunction in diabetic rat hearts, *Molecular and Cellular Biochemistry* 403 (2015): 1–11; S. E. Olivo-Marston and coauthors, Effects of calorie restriction and diet-induced obesity on murine colon carcinogenesis, growth and inflammatory factors, and microRNA expression, *PLOS ONE* (2014), epub, doi:10.1371/journal.pone.0094765.

127. R. J. Colman and coauthors, Caloric restriction reduces age-related and all-cause mortality in rhesus monkeys, *Nature Communications* (2014), epub, doi:10.1038/ncomms4557.

128. J. A. Mattison and coauthors, Impact of caloric restriction on health and survival in rhesus monkeys from the NIA study, *Nature* 489 (2012): 318–321.

129. J. C. Mathers, Impact of nutrition on the ageing process, *British Journal of Nutrition* 113 (2015): S18–S22; S. Steven and R. Taylor, Restoring normoglycaemia by use of a very low calorie diet in long- and short-duration Type 2 diabetes, *Diabetic Medicine* (2015), epub, doi:10.1111/dme.12722; A. R. Barnosky and coauthors, Intermittent fasting vs. daily calorie restriction for type 2 diabetes prevention: A review of human findings, *Translational Research: The Journal of Laboratory and Clinical Medicine* 164 (2014): 302–311.

130. E. L. Goldberg and coauthors, Lifespan-extending caloric restriction or mTOR inhibition impair adaptive immunity of old mice by distinct mechanisms, *Aging Cell* 14 (2015): 130–138; D. Omodei and coauthors, Immune-metabolic profiling of anorexic patients reveals an anti-oxidant and anti-inflammatory phenotype, *Metabolism* 64 (2015): 396–405.

131. Mattison and coauthors, Impact of caloric restriction on health and survival in rhesus monkeys from the NIA study, 2012.

132. D. K. Ingram and G. S. Roth, Calorie restriction mimetics: Can you have your cake and eat it, too? *Ageing Research Reviews* 20 (2015): 46–62; J. H. Park and coauthors, Daumone fed late in life improves survival and reduces hepatic inflammation and fibrosis in mice, *Aging Cell* 13 (2014): 709–718; J. P. de Magalhães and coauthors, Genome-environment interactions that modulate aging: Powerful targets for drug discovery, *Pharmacological Reviews* 64 (2012): 88–101.

133. S. S. Chang and coauthors, Association between inflammatory-related disease burden and frailty: Results from the Women's Health and Aging Studies (WHAS) I and II, *Archives of Gerontology and Geriatrics* 54 (2012): 9–15; A. Salminen and coauthors, Mitochondrial dysfunction and oxidative stress activate inflammasomes: Impact on the aging process and age-related diseases, *Cellular and Molecular Life Sciences* 69 (2012): 2999–3013.

134. R. de Oliveira and coauthors, ADIPOQ and IL6 variants are associated with a pro-inflammatory status in obeses with cardiometabolic dysfunction, *Diabetology and Metabolic Syndrome* 7 (2015): 34; A. U. Uslu and coauthors, Two new inflammatory markers associated with Disease Activity Score-28 in patients with rheumatoid arthritis: Neutrophil-lymphocyte ratio and platelet-lymphocyte ratio, *International Journal of Rheumatic Diseases* (2015), epub, doi:10.1111/1756-185X.12582; M. A. Alaiti and coauthors, Kruppel-like factors and vascular inflammation: Implications for atherosclerosis, *Current Atherosclerosis Reports* 14 (2012): 438–440; H. Wood, Alzheimer disease: Prostaglandin E(2) signaling is implicated in inflammation early in the Alzheimer disease course, *Nature Review Neurology* 8 (2012), epub, doi:10.1038/nrneurol.2012.145.

135. P. Y. Perera and coauthors, The role of interleukin-15 in inflammation and immune responses to infection: Implications for its therapeutic use, *Microbes and Infection* 14 (2012): 247–261.

136. T. Muka and coauthors, Polyunsaturated fatty acids and serum C-reactive protein: The Rotterdam Study, *American Journal of Epidemiology* (2015), epub ahead of print, doi:10.1016/j.jacc.2009.02.084; F. H. Soares and M. B. de Sousa, Different types of physical activity on inflammatory biomarkers in women with or without metabolic disorders: A systematic review, *Women Health* 53 (2013): 298–316.

137. B. Schöttker and coauthors, Oxidative stress markers and all-cause mortality at older age: A population-based cohort study, *Journals of Gerontology: Series A, Biological Sciences and Medical Sciences* 70 (2015): 518–524.

138. S. S. Jick and K. W. Hagberg, The risk of adverse outcomes in association with use of testosterone products: A cohort study using the UK-based general practice research database, *British Journal of Clinical Pharmacology* 75 (2013): 260–270; L. Xu and coauthors, Testosterone therapy and cardiovascular events among men: A systematic review and meta-analysis of placebo-controlled randomized trials, *BMC Medicine* 11 (2013): 108; W. E. Sonntag and coauthors, Diverse roles of growth hormone and insulin-like growth factor-1 in mammalian aging: Progress and controversies, *Journals of Gerontology: Series A, Biological Sciences and Medical Sciences* 67 (2012): 587–598.

139. J. A. Chen and coauthors, A multiancestral genome-wide exome array study of Alzheimer disease, frontotemporal dementia, and progressive supranuclear palsy, *JAMA Neurology* 72 (2015): 414–422; R. Guerreiro and coauthors, TREM2 variants in Alzheimer's disease, *New England Journal of Medicine* 368 (2013): 117–127; M. F. Mendez, Early-onset Alzheimer's disease: Nonamnestic subtypes and type 2 AD, *Archives of Medical Research* 43 (2012): 677–685.

140. O. van de Rest and coauthors, Dietary patterns, cognitive decline, and dementia: A systematic review, *Advances in Nutrition* 6 (2015): 154–168; A. Smyth and coauthors, Healthy eating and reduced risk of cognitive decline: A cohort from 40 countries, *Neurology* (2015), epub ahead of print, doi:10.1212/WNL.0000000000001638; L. Mosconi and coauthors, Mediterranean diet and magnetic resonance imaging-assessed brain atrophy in cognitively normal individuals at risk for Alzheimer's disease, *Journal of Prevention of Alzheimer's Disease* 1 (2014): 23–32.

141. F. Jernerén and coauthors, Brain atrophy in cognitively impaired elderly: The importance of long-chain ω-3 fatty acids and B vitamin status in a randomized controlled trial, *American Journal of Clinical Nutrition* (2015), epub ahead of print, doi:10.3945/ajcn.114.103283.

142. A. S. Prasad, Discovery of human zinc deficiency: Its impact on human health and disease, *Advances in Nutrition* 4 (2013): 176–190.

143. D. R. Galasko and coauthors, Antioxidants for Alzheimer disease: A randomized clinical trial with cerebrospinal fluid biomarker measures, *Archives of Neurology* 69 (2012): 836–841.

144. Position of the Academy of Nutrition and Dietetics: Food and nutrition for older adults: Promoting health and wellness, 2012.

145. M. Tsubota-Utsugi and coauthors, Living situations associated with poor dietary intake among healthy Japanese elderly: The Ohasama study, *Journal of Nutrition, Health & Aging* 19 (2015): 375–382; K. Tiedje and coauthors, A focus group study of healthy eating knowledge, practices, and barriers among adult and adolescent immigrants and refugees in the United States, *International Journal of Behavioral Nutrition and Physical Activity* (2014), epub, doi:10.1186/1479-5868-11-63.

146. Position of the Academy of Nutrition and Dietetics: Food and nutrition for older adults: Promoting health and wellness, 2012.

147. M. P. Levine, Loneliness and eating disorders, *Journal of Psychology* 146 (2012): 243–257; C. M. Perissinotto, I. S. Cenzer, and K. E. Covinsky, Loneliness in older persons: A predictor of functional decline, *Archives of Internal Medicine* 172 (2012): 1078–1084.

Consumer's Guide 14

1. F. W. Tolossa and M. L. Bekele, Prevalence, impacts and medical managements of premenstrual syndrome among female students: Cross-sectional study in College of Health Sciences, Mekelle University, Mekelle, northern Ethiopia, *BMC Women's Health* 14 (2014): 52.

2. P. M. Tacani and coauthors, Characterization of symptoms and edema distribution in premenstrual syndrome, *International Journal of Women's Health* 7 (2015): 297–303; Tolossa and Bekele, Prevalence, impacts and medical managements of premenstrual syndrome among female students, 2014.

3. J. Marjoribanks and coauthors, Selective serotonin reuptake inhibitors for premenstrual syndrome, *Cochrane Database of Systematic Reviews* (2013), epub, doi:10.1002/14651858.CD001396.pub3.

4. M. A. McVay and coauthors, Food cravings and food cue responding across the menstrual cycle in a non-eating disordered sample, *Appetite* 59 (2012): 591–600.

5. J. DiMatteo, S. C. Reed, and S. M. Evans, Alcohol consumption as a function of dietary restraint and the menstrual cycle in moderate/heavy ("at risk") female drinkers, *Eating Behaviors* 13 (2012): 285–288.

6. H. Sakai and K. Ohashi, Association of menstrual phase with smoking behavior, mood and menstrual phase-associated symptoms among young Japanese women smokers, *BMC Women's Health* 13 (2013):10.

7. E. R. Bertone-Johnson and coauthors, Plasma 25-hydroxyvitamin D and risk of premenstrual syndrome in a prospective cohort study, *BMC Women's Health* 14 (2014): 56; B. Obeidat and coauthors, Premenstrual symptoms in dysmenorrheic college students: Prevalence and relation to vitamin D and parathyroid hormone, *International Journal of Environmental Research and Public Health* 9 (2012): 4210–4222.

8. Bertone-Johnson and coauthors, Plasma 25-hydroxyvitamin D and risk of premenstrual syndrome in a prospective cohort study, 2014.

9. Obeidat and coauthors, Premenstrual symptoms in dysmenorrheic college students, 2012.

10. Bertone-Johnson and coauthors, Plasma 25-hydroxyvitamin D and risk of premenstrual syndrome in a prospective cohort study, 2014.

11. Tolossa and Bekele, Prevalence, impacts and medical managements of premenstrual syndrome among female students, 2014; R. E. Anglin and coauthors, Vitamin D deficiency and depression in adults: Systematic review and meta-analysis, *British Journal of Psychiatry* 202 (2013): 100–107.

12. J. A. Shaffer and coauthors, Vitamin D supplementation for depressive symptoms: A systematic review and meta-analysis of randomized controlled trials, *Psychosomatic Medicine* 76 (2014): 190–196.

13. A. Lasco, A. Catalano, and S. Benvenga, Improvement of primary dysmenorrhea caused by a single oral dose of vitamin D: Results of a randomized, double-blind, placebo-controlled study, *Archives of Internal Medicine* 172 (2012): 366–367.

14. E. R. Bertone-Johnson and J. E. Manson, Vitamin D for menstrual and pain-related disorders in women, *Archives of Internal Medicine* 172 (2012): 367–368.

15. Lasco, Catalano, and Benvenga, Improvement of primary dysmenorrhea caused by a single oral dose of vitamin D, 2012; Bertone-Johnson and Manson, Vitamin D for menstrual and pain-related disorders in women, 2012.

16. P. O. Chocano and coauthors, Intake of selected minerals and risk of premenstrual syndrome, *American Journal of Epidemiology* 177 (2013): 1118–1127.

Controversy 14

1. J. I. Boullata and L. M. Hudson, Drug–nutrient interactions: A broad view with implications for practice, *Journal of the Academy of Nutrition and Dietetics* 112 (2012): 506–517.

2. D. Singh, R. Gupta, and S. A. Saraf, Herbs—Are they safe enough? An overview, *Critical Reviews in Food Science and Nutrition* 52 (2012): 876–898.

3. D. Gnjidic and coauthors, Polypharmacy cut-off and outcomes: Five or more medicines were used to identify community-dwelling older men at risk of different adverse outcomes, *Journal of Clinical Epidemiology* 65 (2012): 989–995.

4. K. Neville and M. Ecker, Spice interactions, *Food and Nutrition,* March/April 2015, pp. 19–20.

5. B. Ge, Z. Zhang, and Z. Zuo, Updates on the clinical evidenced herb–warfarin interactions, *Evidence-Based Complementary and Alternative Medicine* (2014), epub, doi:10.1155/2014/957362; S. L. Haber, K. A. Cauthon, and E. C. Raney, Cranberry and warfarin interaction: A case report and review of literature, *Consultant Pharmacist* 27 (2012): 58–65.

6. C. J. Derry, S. Derry, and R. A. Moore, Caffeine as an analgesic adjuvant for acute pain in adults, *Cochrane Database Systematic Review* (2012), epub, doi:10.1002/14651858.

7. U.S. Department of Agriculture and U.S. Department of Health and Human Services, Scientific report of the 2015 Dietary Guidelines Advisory Committee, 2015, D-5:32–35, available at www.health.gov; S. B. Jabbar and M. G. Hanly, Fatal caffeine overdose: A case report and review of literature, *American Journal of Forensic Medicine and Pathology* 34 (2013): 321–324.

8. M. Ding and coauthors, Caffeinated and decaffeinated coffee consumption and risk of type 2 diabetes: A systematic review and a dose-response meta-analysis, *Diabetes Care* 37 (2014): 569–586; S. N. Bhupathiraju and coauthors, Caffeinated and caffeine-free beverages and risk of type 2 diabetes, *American Journal of Clinical Nutrition* 97 (2013): 155–166; J. D. Lane and coauthors, Pilot study of caffeine abstinence for control of chronic glucose in type 2 diabetes, *Journal of Caffeine Research* 2 (2012): 45–47.

9. U.S. Food and Drug Administration, Mixing medications and dietary supplements can endanger your health, Consumer Health Information, October 2014, available at www.fda.gov/consumer.

10. R. A. Breslow, C. Dong, and A. White, Prevalence of alcohol-interactive prescription medication use among current drinkers: United States, 1999–2010, *Alcoholism: Clinical and Experimental Research* (2015), epub ahead of print, doi:10.1111/acer/12633.

11. M. E. Gerich and coauthors, Medical marijuana for digestive disorders: High time to prescribe? *American Journal of Gastroenterology* 110 (2015): 208–214; P. J. Robson, Therapeutic potential of cannabinoid medicines, *Drug Testing and Analysis* 6 (2014): 24–30.

Chapter 15

1. A. Coleman-Jensen, C. Gregory, and A. Singh, Economic Research Service report summary: Household food security in the United States in 2013, September 2014, available at www.ers.usda.gov/publications/err-economic-research-report/err173.aspx.

2. Food and Agriculture Organization of the United Nations, International Fund for Agricultural Development, and World Food Programme, *The State of Food Insecurity in the World 2014: Strengthening the enabling environment for food security and nutrition* (Rome: Food and Agriculture Organization of the United Nations, 2014), p. 4.

3. U.S. Census Bureau, 2013 highlights, available at www.census.gov/hhes/www/poverty/about/overview/.

4. D. C. Martins and coauthors, Assessment of food intake, obesity, and health risk among the homeless in Rhode Island, *Public Health Nursing* (2015), epub ahead of print, doi:10.1111/phn.12180; J. Kaur, M. M. Lamb, and C. L. Ogden, The association between food insecurity and obesity in children—The National Health and Nutrition Examination Survey, *Journal of the Academy of Nutrition and Dietetics* (2015), epub ahead of print, doi:10.1016/j.jand.2015.01.003; D. S. Ludwig, S. J. Blumenthal, and W. C. Willett, Opportunities to reduce childhood hunger and obesity, *Journal of the American Medical Association* 308 (2012): 2567–2568.

5. World Health Organization, World health statistics, 2012, available at www.who.int/gho/publications/world_health_statistics/2012/en/; H. K. Seligman and coauthors, Food insecurity and glycemic control among low-income patients with type 2 diabetes, *Diabetes Care* 35 (2012): 233–238.

6. T. Dubowitz and coauthors, Are our actions aligned with our evidence? The skinny on changing the landscape of obesity, *Obesity* 21 (2013): 419–420.

7. K. Budzynska and coauthors, A food desert in Detroit: Associations with food shopping and eating behaviors, dietary intakes, and obesity, *Public Health Nutrition* 16 (2013): 2114–2123.

8. A. Carlson and E. Frazão, Food costs, diet quality and energy balance in the United States, *Physiology and Behavior* 134 (2014): 20–31; M. Rao and coauthors, Do healthier foods and diet patterns cost more than less healthy options? A systematic review and meta-analysis, *BMJ Open* 3 (2013), epub, doi:10.1136/bmjopen-2013-004277.

9. U.S. Department of Agriculture and U.S. Department of Health and Human Services, Scientific report of the 2015 Dietary Guidelines Advisory Committee, 2015, A-2, available at www.health.gov.

10. V. Olivera, U.S. Department of Agriculture, Economic Research Service, The food assistance landscape: FY 2014 annual report (EIB-137), March 2015, available at www.ers.usda.gov

/publications/eib-economic-information-bulletin/eib137.aspx.

11. Food and Agriculture Organization of the United Nations, International Fund for Agricultural Development, and World Food Programme, *The State of Food Insecurity in the World 2014*, 2014, p. 4.

12. Food and Agriculture Organization of the United Nations, World agriculture: Towards 2015/2030, Summary report, 2015, available at www.fao.org/docrep/004/y3557e/y3557e00.htm; Centers for Disease Control and Prevention, *Salmonella typhi* infections associated with contaminated water—Zimbabwe, October 2011–May 2012, *Morbidity and Mortality Weekly Report* 61 (2012): 435.

13. Food and Agriculture Organization of the United Nations, International Fund for Agricultural Development, and World Food Programme, *The State of Food Insecurity in the World 2015*, available at www.fao.org/hunger/en/.

14. Food and Agriculture Organization of the United Nations, International Fund for Agricultural Development, and World Food Programme, *The State of Food Insecurity in the World 2014*, 2014.

15. P. L. Tigga, J. Sen, and N. Mondal, Association of some socio-economic and socio-demographic variables with wasting among pre-school children of North Bengal, India, *Ethiopian Journal of Health Sciences* 25 (2015): 63–72.

16. S. M. O'Neill and coauthors, Child mortality as predicted by nutritional status and recent weight velocity in children under two in rural Africa, *Journal of Nutrition* 142 (2012): 520–525.

17. E. Andresen and coauthors, Malnutrition and elevated mortality among refugees from South Sudan, *Morbidity and Mortality Weekly Report* 63 (2014): 700; N. Gupta, Conflict, children and malnutrition in CAR, *Borgen Magazine,* February 19, 2015, available at www.borgenmagazine.com/conflict-children-malnutrition-car/; K. Fahim, Malnutrition hits millions of children in Yemen, *New York Times,* December 18, 2014, available at www.nytimes.com/2014/12/19/world/middleeast/yemen-children-starve-as-government-weakens.html?_r=0.

18. J. V. White and coauthors, Consensus statement of the Academy of Nutrition and Dietetics/American Society for Parenteral and Enteral Nutrition: Characteristics recommended for the identification and documentation of adult malnutrition (undernutrition), *Journal of the Academy of Nutrition and Dietetics* 112 (2012): 730–738.

19. World Health Organization, Nutrition: Micronutrient deficiencies, accessed 3/30/15, available at www.who.int/nutrition/topics/ida/en/.

20. Micronutrient Initiative, About hidden hunger: What is hidden hunger?, accessed 3/30/15, available at www.micronutrient.org/English/View.asp?x=573.

21. C. Shekhar, Hidden hunger: Addressing micronutrient deficiencies using improved crop varieties, *Chemistry and Biology* 20 (2013): 1305–1306; World Health Organization, *Global prevalence of vitamin A deficiency in populations at risk: 1995–2005* (Geneva: World Health Organization, 2009); Standing Committee on the Scientific Evaluation of Dietary Reference Intakes, Food and Nutrition Board, Institute of Medicine, *Dietary Reference Intakes for Vitamin A, Vitamin K, Arsenic, Boron, Chromium, Copper, Iodine, Iron, Manganese, Molybdenum, Nickel, Silicon, Vanadium, and Zinc* (Washington, D.C.: National Academies Press, 2001), pp. 4-9–4-10.

22. P. J. Becker and coauthors, Consensus statement of the Academy of Nutrition and Dietetics/American Society for Parenteral and Enteral Nutrition: Indicators recommended for the identification and documentation of pediatric malnutrition (undernutrition), *Journal of the Academy of Nutrition and Dietetics* 114 (2014): 1988–2000.

23. I. Trehan and M. J. Manary, Management of severe acute malnutrition in low-income and middle-income countries, *Archives of Disease in Childhood* 100 (2015): 283–287.

24. T. E. Forrester and coauthors, Prenatal factors contribute to the emergence of kwashiorkor or marasmus in severe undernutrition: Evidence for the predictive adaptation model, *PLoS ONE* (2012), epub, doi:10.1371/journal.pone.0035907.

25. B. de Gier and coauthors, Helminth infections and micronutrients in school-age children: A systematic review and meta-analysis, *American Journal of Clinical Nutrition* 99 (2014): 1499–1509.

26. M. Wolde, Y. Berhan, and A. Chala, Determinants of underweight, stunting and wasting among schoolchildren, *BMC Public Health* 15 (2015), epub, doi:10.1186/s12889-014-1337-2.

27. S. van der Kam and coauthors, Ready-to-use therapeutic food for catch-up growth in children after an episode of Plasmodium falciparum malaria: An open randomised controlled trial, *PLoS ONE* 7 (2012), epub, doi:10.1371/journal.pone.0035006.

28. I. Trehan and coauthors, Extending supplementary feeding for children younger than 5 years with moderate acute malnutrition leads to lower relapse rates, *Journal of Pediatric Gastroenterology and Nutrition* 60 (2015): 544–549.

29. K. N. Ryan and coauthors, A comprehensive linear programming tool to optimize formulations of ready-to-use therapeutic foods: An application to Ethiopia, *American Journal of Clinical Nutrition* 100 (2014): 1551–1558.

30. Food and Agriculture Organization of the United Nations, World agriculture: Towards 2015/2030, 2015.

31. U.S. Census Bureau, World vital events per time unit: 2015, available at www.census.gov/population/international/data/idb/worldvitalevents.php.

32. A. J. McMichael, Globalization, climate change, and human health, *New England Journal of Medicine* 368 (2015): 1335–1343; National Academies of Science and the Royal Society, Climate change evidence and causes, 2014, available at http://nas-sites.org/americasclimatechoices/events/a-discussion-on-climate-change-evidence-and-causes/.

33. United Nations, International Decade for Action: Water for life 2005–2015, available at www.un.org/waterforlifedecade/scarcity.shtml.

34. K. Minogue, Climate change expected to expand majority of ocean dead zones, *Smithsonian Science News* 5 (2014), available at http://smithsonianscience.org/2014/11/climate-change-expected-expand-majority-ocean-dead-zones/.

35. Food and Agricultural Organization of the United Nations, State of the world fisheries and aquaculture, 2014, available at www.fao.org/3/a-i3720e.pdf.

36. E. Pikitch and coauthors, *Little Fish, Big Impact: Managing a Crucial Link in Ocean Food Webs* (Washington, D.C.: Lenfest Ocean Program, 2012), available at www.larecherche.fr/content/system/media/fish.pdf.

37. U.S. Department of Agriculture and U.S. Department of Health and Human Services, Scientific report of the 2015 Dietary Guidelines Advisory Committee, 2015, D-5:17–20, available at www.health.gov.

38. Food and Agriculture Organization of the United Nations, Global food losses and food waste: Extent, causes and prevention, 2011, available at www.fao.org/ag/ags/ags-division/publications/en.

39. Environmental Protection Agency, Basic information about food waste, April 26, 2014, available at www.epa.gov.

40. U.S. Department of Agriculture and U.S. Department of Health and Human Services, Scientific report of the 2015 Dietary Guidelines Advisory Committee, 2015, D-5:9–15, available at www.health.gov.

41. National Research Council, Panel on Advancing the Science of Climate Change, *America's Climate Choices* (Washington, D.C.: National Academies Press, 2012), p. 3, available at www.nap.edu.

42. C. Vogliano, A. Steiber, and K. Brown, Linking agriculture, nutrition, and health: The role of the registered dietitian nutritionist, *Journal of the Academy of Nutrition and Dietetics* (2015), epub ahead of print, doi:10.1016/j.jand.2015.06.009.

Consumer's Guide 15

1. Federal Trade Commission, FTC issues revised "Green Guides," October 2012, available at www.ftc.gov/opa/2012/10/greenguides.shtm.

2. EPA announces 70 top performing Energy Star certified manufacturing plants in 29 states, *News Releases from Headquarters,* March 2015, available at http://yosemite.epa.gov/opa/admpress.nsf/d0cf6618525a9efb85257359003fb69d/24ff1f-b1bcd5355785257e03005d9f29!OpenDocume.

Controversy 15

1. Food and Agriculture Organization of the United Nations, World agriculture: Towards 2015/2030, Summary report, 2015, available at www.fao.org/docrep/004/y3557e/y3557e00.htm; R. O. Morawicki, *Handbook of Sustainability for*

the Food Sciences (Oxford, England: Wiley-Black-well, 2012), epub, doi:10.1002/9780470963166.ch10.

2. J. L. Lu, Effects of agricultural work practices and pesticide use on occupational health of farmers, Occupational and Environmental Medicine 71 (2014): A56–A57.

3. D. S. Reay and coauthors, Global agriculture and nitrous oxide emissions, Nature Climate Change 2 (2012): 410–416; N. Gilbert, Palm-oil boom raises conservation concerns, Nature 487 (2012): 14–15.

4. C. Brown and coauthors, Switchgrass biofuel production on reclaimed surface mines: I. Soil quality and dry matter yield. BioEnergy Research (2015), epub, doi:10.1007/s12155-015-9658-2; B. Mole, Bacteria make plants into biofuel, Science News, July 12, 2014, p. 16; J. C. Quinn and coauthors, Current large-scale US biofuel potential from microalgae cultivated in photobioreactors, BioEnergy Research 5 (2012): 49–60; C. S. Jones and S. P. Mayfield, Algae biofuels: Versatility for the future of bioenergy, Current Opinion in Biotechnology 23 (2012): 346–351.

5. D. Pimentel, Food for thought: A review of the role of energy in current and evolving agriculture, Critical Reviews in Plant Sciences 30 (2011): 35–44.

6. World Health Organization, Global and regional food consumption patterns and trends: Availability and changes in consumption of animal products, accessed April 2015, available at www.who.int/nutrition/topics/3_foodconsumption/en/index4.html.

7. U.S. Department of Agriculture and U.S. Department of Health and Human Services, Scientific report of the 2015 Dietary Guidelines Advisory Committee, 2015, D-5:9–16, available at www.health.gov.

8. U.S. Department of Agriculture, Natural Resources Conservation Service, NRCS conservation programs, 2013, available at www.nrcs.usda.gov/wps/portal/nrcs/main/national/programs/.

9. P. L. Pingali, Green revolution: Impacts, limits, and the path ahead, Proceedings of the National Academy of Sciences of the United States of America 109 (2012): 12302–12308.

10. B. Knight, Regaining ground: A conservation reserve program right-sized for the times: A report by Strategic Conservation Solutions, June 2012, available at www.ngfa.org/files/SCSReGainingGroundResearchStudyforNGFF%286-8-2012%29.pdf.

11. Cow poop to cow power: Powering Vermont, Sustainable Business.Com News, May 2013, available at www.sustainablebusiness.com/index.cfm/go/news.display/id/24846.

12. H. Blanco-Canqui, Crop residue removal for bioenergy reduces soil carbon pools: How can we offset carbon losses? BioEnergy Research 6 (2013): 358–371.

13. J. Skene, Methane moves from landfill to fuel tank, KQED Quest, January 2012, available at http://science.kqed.org/quest/2012/01/23/methane-moves-from-landfill-to-fuel-tank/.

14. U.S. Department of Agriculture and U.S. Department of Health and Human Services, Scientific report of the 2015 Dietary Guidelines Advisory Committee, 2015, D-5:9, available at www.health.gov; J. Sabaté and S. Soret, Sustainability of plant-based diets: Back to the future, American Journal of Clinical Nutrition 100 (2014): 476S–482S.

Answers to Chapter Questions
Answers to Consumer's Guide Review and Self-Check Questions

CHAPTER 1

Consumer's Guide Review

1. d
2. b
3. b

Self-Check Questions

1. False. Heart disease and cancer are influenced by many factors with genetics and diet among them.
2. c
3. d
4. a
5. a
6. a
7. T
8. c
9. b
10. False. The choice of where, as well as what, to eat is often based more on taste and social considerations than on nutrition judgments.
11. b
12. a
13. T
14. F
15. b
16. a
17. d
18. False. In this nation, profiteers selling diplomas and certificates make it easy to obtain a bogus nutrition credential.

CHAPTER 2

Consumer's Guide Review

1. False. Restaurant portions are not held to standards and should not be used as a guide for choosing portion sizes.
2. T
3. False. Most consumers overestimate both the calories and fat in restaurant foods.

Self-Check Questions

1. b
2. d
3. T

4. False. The DRI are estimates of the needs of healthy persons only. Medical problems alter nutrient needs.
5. c
6. T
7. c
8. d
9. False. People who choose to eat no meats or products taken from animals can still use the USDA Food Patterns to make their diets adequate.
10. a
11. False. A properly planned diet should include healthy snacks as part of the total daily food intake, if so desired.
12. c
13. T
14. T
15. T
16. d
17. T
18. False. Although they are natural constituents of foods, phytochemicals have not been proven safe to consume in large amounts.

CHAPTER 3

Self-Check Questions

1. a
2. False. Each gene is a blueprint that directs the production of one or more of the body's proteins, such as an enzyme.
3. c
4. a
5. b
6. T
7. T
8. d
9. c
10. d
11. False. Absorption of the majority of nutrients takes place across the specialized cells of the small intestine.
12. d
13. a
14. c

15. False. The kidneys straddle the cardiovascular system and filter the blood.
16. b
17. T
18. a
19. False. Alcohol is a natural toxin that can cause severe damage to the liver, brain, and other organs, and can be lethal in high enough doses.

CHAPTER 4

Consumer's Guide Review

1. b
2. b
3. a

Self-Check Questions

1. b
2. a
3. T
4. T
5. c
6. T
7. b
8. a
9. False. For people with diabetes, the risk of heart disease, stroke, and dying on any particular day is doubled.
10. False. Type I diabetes is most often controlled with insulin injections or an insulin pump.
11. c
12. False. Regular physical activity can help by reducing the body's fatness and heightening tissue sensitivity to insulin.
13. d
14. False. Hypoglycemia as a true disease is rare.
15. d
16. T
17. T
18. a

CHAPTER 5

Consumer's Guide Review

1. False. Methylmercury is a highly toxic industrial pollutant found in highest concentrations in the flesh of large predatory species of fish.
2. False. Children and pregnant or lactating women should strictly follow recommendations set for them and choose fish species that are rich in omega-3 fatty acids *and* lower in mercury.
3. False. Cod provides little EPA and DHA.

Self-Check Questions

1. c
2. False. In addition to providing abundant fuel, fat cushions tissues, serves as insulation, forms cell membranes, and serves as raw material, among other functions.
3. b

4. False. Vegetable and fish oils are excellent sources of polyunsaturated fats.
5. c
6. T
7. b
8. d
9. T
10. T
11. False. Chylomicrons are produced in small intestinal cells.
12. False. Consuming large amounts of saturated fatty acids elevates serum LDL cholesterol and thus *raises* the risk of heart disease and heart attack.
13. d
14. False. Fish, not supplements, is the recommended source of fish oil.
15. T
16. b
17. b
18. d
19. T
20. T
21. d

CHAPTER 6

Consumer's Guide Review

1. False. Evidence does not support taking protein supplements such as commercial shakes and energy bars to lose weight.
2. T
3. False. In high doses, tryptophan may induce nausea and skin disorders as unwanted side effects.

Self-Check Questions

1. b
2. c
3. a
4. a
5. b
6. T
7. T
8. d
9. a
10. T
11. T
12. d
13. False. Excess protein in the diet may have adverse effects, such as worsening kidney disease.
14. a
15. a
16. T
17. d
18. T
19. c
20. False. Fried banana or vegetable chips are often high in calories and saturated fat, and are best reserved for an occasional treat.

CHAPTER 7

Consumer's Guide Review

1. T
2. T
3. False. All things considered, the best and safest source of vitamin D for people in the United States is nutrient-dense foods and beverages.

Self-Check Questions

1. b
2. c
3. T
4. a
5. d
6. False. Vitamin A supplements have no effect on acne.
7. T
8. d
9. a
10. c
11. T
12. d
13. b
14. a
15. False. No study to date has conclusively demonstrated that vitamin C can prevent colds or reduce their severity.
16. d
17. c
18. T
19. a
20. b
21. b
22. False. The FDA has little control over supplement sales.

CHAPTER 8

Consumer's Guide Review

1. a
2. d
3. d

Self-Check Questions

1. d
2. False. Water intoxication occurs when too much plain water floods the body's fluids and disturbs their normal composition.
3. c
4. b
5. T
6. a
7. d
8. b
9. d
10. False. After about age 30, the bones begin to lose density.
11. T

12. c
13. b
14. a
15. False. Calcium is the most abundant mineral in the body.
16. False. The Academy of Nutrition and Dietetics, among others, recommends the consumption of fluoridated water.
17. False. Butter, cream, and cream cheese contain negligible calcium, being almost pure fat. Some vegetables, such as broccoli, are good sources of available calcium.
18. T
19. T
20. b

CHAPTER 9

Consumer's Guide Review

1. False. A diet book that addresses eicosanoids and adipokines may or may not present accurate nutrition science or effective diet advice.
2. False. Calorie deficit is a key strategy for weight loss.
3. True.

Self-Check Questions

1. d
2. T
3. b
4. False. The BMI are unsuitable for use with athletes and adults over age 65.
5. False. The thermic effect of food is believed to have negligible effects on total energy expenditure.
6. c
7. d
8. d
9. a
10. b
11. False. Genomic researchers have identified multiple genes likely to play roles in obesity development but have not so far identified a single genetic cause of common obesity.
12. T
13. d
14. a
15. T
16. T
17. a
18. b
19. False. Over-the-counter drugs for obesity most often present risk without benefit.
20. b
21. False. Disordered eating behaviors in early life set a pattern that likely continues into young adulthood.

CHAPTER 10

Consumer's Guide Review

1. a
2. a
3. b

Self-Check Questions

1. b
2. c
3. False. Weight-bearing exercise that improves muscle strength and endurance also helps maximize and maintain bone mass.
4. False. Muscle cells and tissues respond to a physical activity overload by altering the structures and metabolic equipment needed to perform the work.
5. c
6. c
7. a
8. T
9. a
10. d
11. T
12. T
13. a
14. False. Frequent nutritious between-meal snacks can help to provide some extra calories and help to maintain body weight.
15. T
16. d
17. a
18. b
19. d

CHAPTER 11

Consumer's Guide Review

1. T
2. False. The National Center for Complementary and Alternative Medicine (NCCAM) does not promote laetrile therapy.
3. T

Self-Check Questions

1. c
2. T
3. b
4. False. Chronic diseases have risk factors that show correlations with disease development but are not distinct causes.
5. d
6. b
7. False. Atherosclerosis is an accumulation of lipids within the artery wall, but it also involves a complex response of the artery to tissue damage and inflammation.
8. a
9. False. Men do have more heart attacks than women, but CVD kills more women than any other cause of death.
10. a
11. c
12. T
13. False. The prevalence of high blood pressure in African Americans is among the highest in the world.
14. T
15. d
16. T
17. False. Sufficient intakes of calcium-rich foods may help to prevent colon cancer.
18. False. The DASH diet is designed for helping people with hypertension to control the disease.
19. d
20. False. Currently, for the best chance of consuming adequate nutrients and staying healthy, people should eat a well-planned diet of whole foods, as described in Chapter 2.

CHAPTER 12

Consumer's Guide Review

1. d
2. T
3. a

Self-Check Questions

1. T
2. a
3. c
4. d
5. c
6. False. Today, the chance of getting a foodborne illness from eating produce is similar to the chance of becoming ill from eating meat, eggs, and seafood.
7. T
8. a
9. b
10. T
11. False. Nature has provided many plants used for food with natural poisons to fend off diseases, insects, and other predators.
12. False. The EPA and FDA warn of unacceptably high methylmercury levels in ocean fish and other seafood and advise all pregnant women not to eat certain types of fish.
13. T
14. c
15. c
16. d
17. T
18. b
19. b
20. T

CHAPTER 13

Consumer's Guide Review

1. False. Despite convincing advertising, no commercial formula can fully match the benefits of human milk.
2. False. Only about 23 percent of infants are still breastfeeding at 1 year of age.
3. False. Lactation consultants are employed by hospitals to help new mothers establish healthy breastfeeding relationships with their newborns and to help ensure successful long-term breastfeeding.

Self-Check Questions

1. c
2. T
3. b
4. d
5. d
6. T
7. b
8. False. The American Academy of Pediatrics urges all women to stop drinking as soon as they plan to become pregnant, and to abstain throughout the pregnancy.
9. a
10. T
11. d
12. T
13. a
14. a
15. d
16. d
17. False. There is no proof for the theory that "stuffing the baby" at bedtime will promote sleeping through the night.
18. T
19. False. In light of the developmental needs of one-year-olds, parents should discourage unacceptable behaviors, such as standing at the table or throwing food.
20. c

CHAPTER 14

Consumer's Guide Review

1. T
2. False. Ongoing research suggests that taking multivitamins, magnesium, manganese, or diuretics is *not* useful.
3. False. During the two weeks *before* menstruation, women may experience a natural, hormone-governed increase of appetite.

Self-Check Questions

1. c
2. b
3. T
4. d

5. b
6. False. Research to date does not support the idea that food allergies or intolerances cause hyperactivity in children, but studies continue.
7. c
8. c
9. c
10. b
11. d
12. a
13. T
14. False. Vitamin A absorption appears to increase with aging.
15. False. To date, no proven benefits are available from herbs or other remedies.
16. b
17. a
18. False. Most single elderly people would love an invitation to join someone for a meal.
19. d

CHAPTER 15

Consumer's Guide Review

1. False. The term *green* is loosely regulated and is meaningless without scientific evidence to back it up.
2. T
3. d

Self-Check Questions

1. b
2. a
3. c
4. d
5. T
6. a
7. T
8. c
9. False. Most children who die of malnutrition do not starve to death—they die because their health has been compromised by dehydration from infections that cause diarrhea.
10. a
11. c
12. d
13. c
14. T
15. T
16. False. The federal government, the states, local communities, big business and small companies, educators, and all individuals, including dietitians and food service managers, have many opportunities to make an impact in the fight against poverty, hunger, and environmental degradation.
17. T
18. c

Physical Activity Levels and Energy Requirements

Chapter 9 described how to calculate ranges of the estimated energy requirement (EER) for an adult by using an equation that accounts for age and gender alone. This Appendix offers a way of establishing estimated calorie needs per day by age, gender, and physical activity level, as endorsed by the *Dietary Guidelines for Americans 2015*, and based on the equations of the Committee on Dietary Reference Intakes.

Table H–1 describes activity levels for three groups of people: sedentary, moderately active, and active. Once you have identified an activity level that approximates your own, find your daily calorie need in Table H–2.

Table H–3 specifies the American College of Sports Medicine's Guidelines for Physical Fitness. These guidelines are more demanding and also more specific than USDA's Physical Activity Guidelines (Chapter 10). Table H–4 offers a sample workout program that meets or exceeds both sets of recommendations.

TABLE H–1 Sedentary, Moderately Active, and Active People

Sedentary	A lifestyle that includes only the light physical activity associated with typical day-to-day life.
Moderately active	A lifestyle that includes physical activity equivalent to walking about 1.5 to 3 miles per day at 3 to 4 miles per hour in addition to the light physical activity associated with typical day-to-day life.
Active	A lifestyle that includes physical activity equivalent to walking more than 3 miles per day at 3 to 4 miles per hour in addition to the light physical activity associated with typical day-to-day life.

Source: U.S. Department of Agriculture and U.S. Department of Health and Human Services, Dietary Guidelines for Americans 2010, available at www.dietaryguidelines.gov.

TABLE H-2 — Estimated Calorie Needs per Day by Age, Gender, and Physical Activity Level (Detailed)

Estimated amounts of calories needed to maintain calorie balance for various gender and age groups at three different levels of physical activity.[a] The estimates are rounded to the nearest 200 calories. An individual's calorie needs may be higher or lower than these average estimates.

Gender/ Activity Level	Male/ Sedentary	Male/ Moderately Active	Male/Active	Female[b]/ Sedentary	Female[b]/ Moderately Active	Female[b]/Active
Age (years)						
2	1,000	1,000	1,000	1,000	1,000	1,000
3	1,200	1,400	1,400	1,000	1,200	1,400
4	1,200	1,400	1,600	1,200	1,400	1,400
5	1,200	1,400	1,600	1,200	1,400	1,600
6	1,400	1,600	1,800	1,200	1,400	1,600
7	1,400	1,600	1,800	1,200	1,600	1,800
8	1,400	1,600	2,000	1,400	1,600	1,800
9	1,600	1,800	2,000	1,400	1,600	1,800
10	1,600	1,800	2,200	1,400	1,800	2,000
11	1,800	2,000	2,200	1,600	1,800	2,000
12	1,800	2,200	2,400	1,600	2,000	2,200
13	2,000	2,200	2,600	1,600	2,000	2,200
14	2,000	2,400	2,800	1,800	2,000	2,400
15	2,200	2,600	3,000	1,800	2,000	2,400
16	2,400	2,800	3,200	1,800	2,000	2,400
17	2,400	2,800	3,200	1,800	2,000	2,400
18	2,400	2,800	3,200	1,800	2,000	2,400
19–20	2,600	2,800	3,000	2,000	2,200	2,400
21–25	2,400	2,800	3,000	2,000	2,200	2,400
26–30	2,400	2,600	3,000	1,800	2,000	2,400
31–35	2,400	2,600	3,000	1,800	2,000	2,200
36–40	2,400	2,600	2,800	1,800	2,000	2,200
41–45	2,200	2,600	2,800	1,800	2,000	2,200
46–50	2,200	2,400	2,800	1,800	2,000	2,200
51–55	2,200	2,400	2,800	1,600	1,800	2,200
56–60	2,200	2,400	2,600	1,600	1,800	2,200
61–65	2,000	2,400	2,600	1,600	1,800	2,000
66–70	2,000	2,200	2,600	1,600	1,800	2,000
71–75	2,000	2,200	2,600	1,600	1,800	2,000
76+	2,000	2,200	2,400	1,600	1,800	2,000

[a] Based on estimated energy requirements (EER) equations, using reference heights (average) and reference weights (healthy) for each age-gender group. For children and adolescents, reference height and weight vary. For adults, the reference man is 5 feet 10 inches tall and weighs 154 pounds. The reference woman is 5 feet 4 inches tall and weighs 126 pounds. EER equations are from the Institute of Medicine, Dietary Reference Intakes for Energy, Carbohydrate, Fiber, Fat, Fatty Acids, Cholesterol, Protein, and Amino Acids (Washington, DC National Academies Press, 2002).

[b] Estimates for females do not include women who are pregnant or breastfeeding.

Source: U.S. Department of Agriculture and U.S. Department of Health and Human Services, Dietary Guidelines for Americans 2010, available at www.dietaryguidelines.gov.

TABLE H–3 American College of Sports Medicine's Guidelines for Physical Fitness

Type of Activity	Aerobic activity that uses large-muscle groups and can be maintained continuously	Resistance activity that is performed at a controlled speed and through a full range of motion	Stretching activity that uses the major muscle groups
Frequency	5 to 7 days per week	2 to 3 nonconsecutive days per week	2 to 7 days per week
Intensity	Moderate (equivalent to walking at a pace of 3 to 4 mph)[a]	Enough to enhance muscle strength and improve body composition	Enough to feel tightness or slight discomfort
Duration	At least 30 minutes per day	2 to 4 sets of 8 to 12 repetitions involving each major muscle group	2 to 4 repetitions of 15 to 30 seconds per muscle group
Examples	Running, cycling, dancing, swimming, Inline skating, rowing, power walking, cross-country skiing, kickboxing, water aerobics, jumping rope; sports activities such as basketball, soccer, racquetball, tennis, volleyball	Pull-ups, push-ups, sit-ups, weightlifting, pilates	Yoga

[a]For those who prefer vigorous-intensity aerobic activity such as walking at a very brisk pace (>4.5 mph) or running (≥5 mph), a minimum of 20 minutes per day, 3 days per week is recommended.

Source: American College of Sports Medicine position stand, Quantity and quality of exercise for developing and maintaining cardiorespiratory, musculoskeletal, and neuromotor fitness in apparently healthy adults: Guidance for prescribing exercise, Medicine and Science in Sports and Exercise 43 (2011): 1334–1359; W. L. Haskell and coauthors, Physical activity and public health: Updated recommendation for adults from the American College of Sports Medicine and the American Heart Association, Medicine in Sports & Exercise 39 (2007): 1423–1434.

TABLE H–4 A Sample Balanced Fitness Program

Monday	Tuesday	Wednesday	Thursday	Friday	Saturday or Sunday
5-min warm-up[a]	5-min warm-up[a]	5-min warm-up[a]	5-min warm-up[a]	5-min warm-up[a]	
Resistance training: chest, back, arms, and shoulders 15–45 min[b]	Resistance training: legs, core (abdomen/lower back) 15–45 min		Resistance training: chest, back, arms, and shoulders 15–45 min	Resistance training: legs, core (abdomen/lower back) 15–45 min	Active leisure pursuits: Sports, walking, hiking, biking, swimming
Moderate aerobic activity: 15–20 min	Moderate aerobic activity: 15–20 min	Moderate aerobic activity: 15–20 min	Moderate aerobic activity: 15–20 min	Moderate aerobic activity: 15–20 min	
Stretching: 5 min	Stretching: 5 min	Stretching: 5 min	Stretching: 5 min	Stretching: 5 min	

[a] The warm-up consists of a slower or less-intense version of the activity ahead and may count toward the week's total activity requirement if it is performed at moderate intensity.

[b] Lower-intensity exercise requires more time; higher-intensity exercise requires less time.

Source: Designed for Nutrition: Concepts and Controversies by P. Spencer Webb, MS, RDN, CSCS, Exercise/Human Performance Instructor, U.S. Military Special Operations Forces.

Chemical Structures: Carbohydrates, Lipids, and Amino Acids

The chapters of this book use simplified ball-and-stick models to illustrate the structures of molecules. This Appendix provides a bit more detail about the chemical notations associated with carbohydrates, lipids, amino acids, and peptides. Note that the four main types of atoms found in molecules of energy nutrients are hydrogen (H), oxygen (O), nitrogen (N), and carbon (C). Each atom has a characteristic number of bonds that it can form with other atoms:

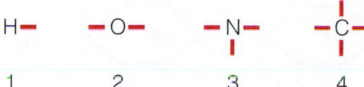

You can count the number of bonds for each atom in the molecule (ethyl alcohol) below: each H has one bond, O has two, and each C has four:

Carbohydrates

Chapter 4 described the classes of carbohydrates and demonstrated that monosaccharides can join together to form disaccharides and larger polysaccharides. Here are some of these carbohydrate structures, starting with glucose.

Glucose

The chemical notation on the left shows all of the bonds of a glucose molecule; the center and right notations show common abbreviations, with fewer illustrated bonds and hydrogen atoms.

Glucose

Glucose

Glucose

Disaccharides

When two monosaccharides are joined together, they form a disaccharide. The abbreviated chemical notations of the three disaccharides are shown below.

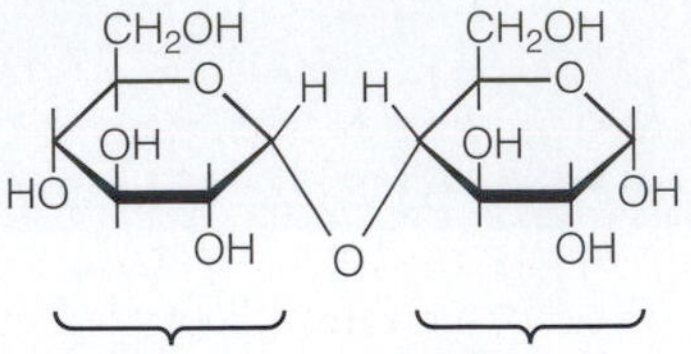

Glucose Glucose
Maltose

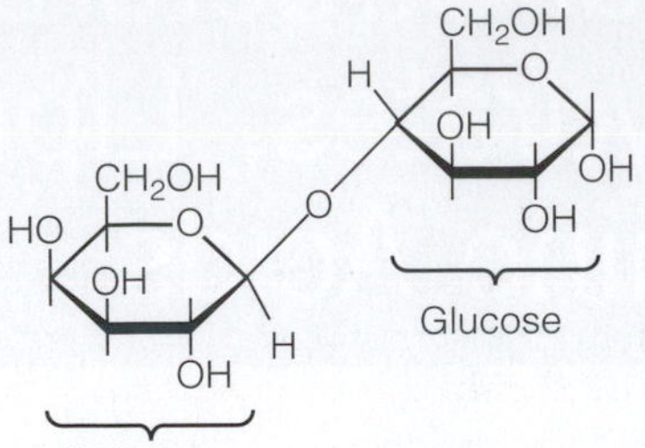

Galactose Glucose
Lactose (alpha form)

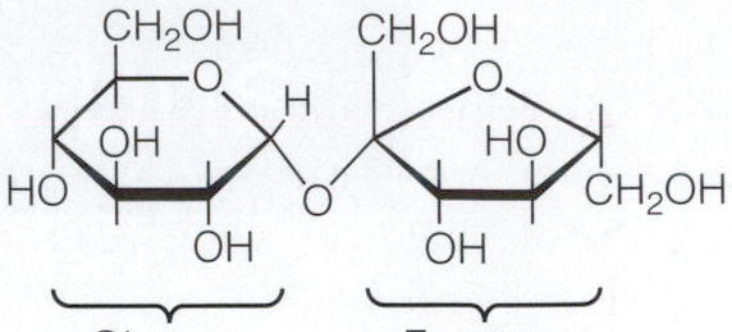

Glucose Fructose
Sucrose

Starches

Starch, glycogen, and cellulose are all long chains of glucose molecules linked together. Some starch is branched, but the structure below is an unbranched starch.

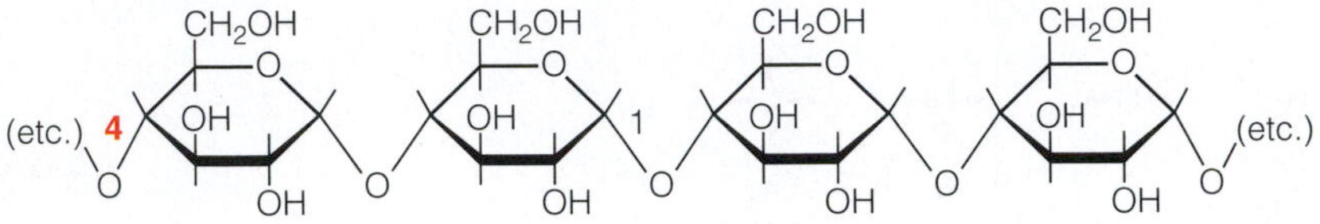

Amylose (unbranched starch)

Lipids

Chapter 5 notes that triglycerides are made up of three fatty acids attached to a glycerol molecule, forming the common fats in food and in the body. Below is a sampling of fatty acids; many others exist.

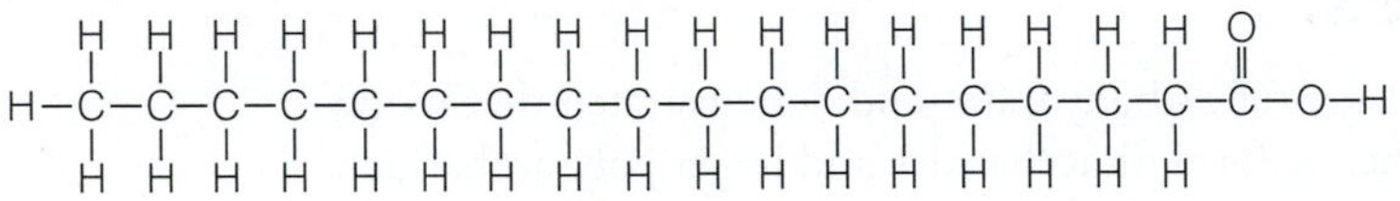

Stearic acid, an 18-carbon saturated fatty acid

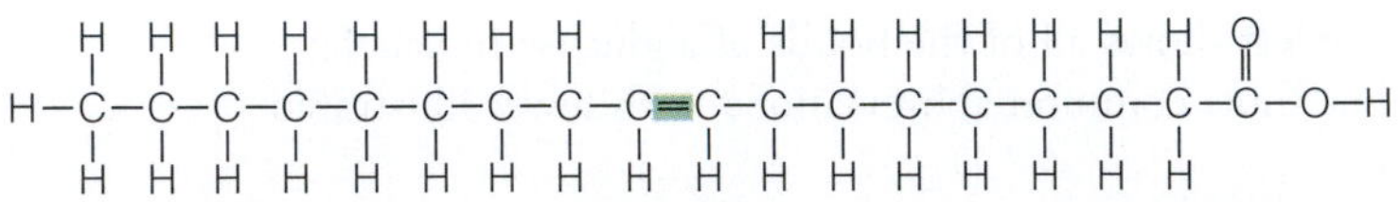

Oleic acid, an 18-carbon monounsaturated fatty acid

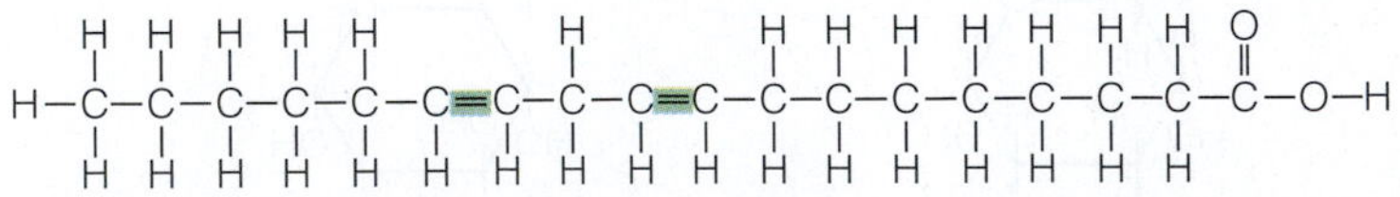

Linoleic acid, an 18-carbon polyunsaturated fatty acid

Chemical Structures: Carbohydrates, Lipids, and Amino Acids

Fatty acids join with a glycerol molecule to make a triglyceride. Glycerol is shown below.

$$
\begin{array}{c}
\text{H} \\
| \\
\text{H}-\text{C}-\text{O}-\text{H} \\
| \\
\text{H}-\text{C}-\text{O}-\text{H} \\
| \\
\text{H}-\text{C}-\text{O}-\text{H} \\
| \\
\text{H}
\end{array}
$$

Glycerol

Most triglycerides contain a mixture of more than one type of fatty acid. The simplified notation used below makes it easy to pick out points of unsaturation (double bonds) in the fatty acid structures. Note that the top fatty acid is saturated, the one below it is monounsaturated, and the third is polyunsaturated. This notation makes it appear that all fatty acids are straight-line structures, but in real fats, points of unsaturation add kinks and bends, an effect illustrated in Figure 5–4 (p. 165).

Triglyceride

A cholesterol molecule, one of the sterols, differs greatly in structure and function from the triglycerides; a molecule of cholesterol is depicted below.

Cholesterol

Amino Acids

Proteins are formed from amino acids, as Chapter 6 made clear. All amino acids have a central carbon with an amino group (NH_2), an acid group (COOH), a hydrogen (H), and a side group attached. The side group structure (shown as a blank box) varies among amino acids.

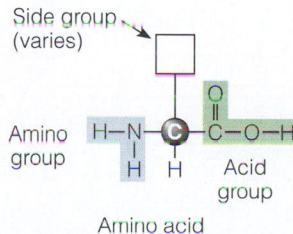

Amino acid

These are just a few of the amino acids:

Glycine   Alanine   Aspartic acid   Phenylalanine

Making dipeptides, tripeptides, and polypeptides requires joining amino acids together with peptide bonds to make a chain.

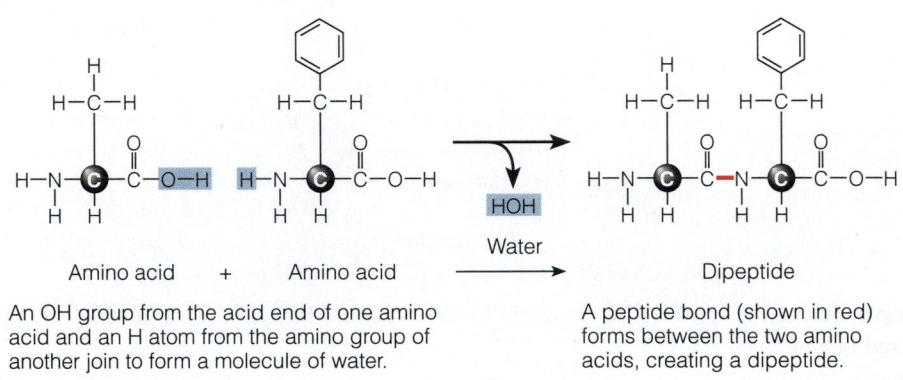

Amino acid   +   Amino acid

An OH group from the acid end of one amino acid and an H atom from the amino group of another join to form a molecule of water.

Water

Dipeptide

A peptide bond (shown in red) forms between the two amino acids, creating a dipeptide.

Glossary

A

A1C test a blood test for type 2 diabetes that measures the percentage of hemoglobin (a blood protein) with glucose attached to it. The test reflects blood glucose control over the previous few months. Also called *glycosylated hemoglobin test* or *HbA1C test* (*Hb* stands for *hemoglobin*).

absorb to take in, as nutrients are taken into the intestinal cells after digestion; the main function of the digestive tract with respect to nutrients.

Academy of Nutrition and Dietetics (AND) the professional organization of dietitians in the United States (formerly the American Dietetic Association). The Canadian equivalent is the Dietitians of Canada (DC), which operates similarly.

acceptable daily intake (ADI) the estimated amount of a sweetener that can be consumed daily over a person's lifetime without any adverse effects.

Acceptable Macronutrient Distribution Ranges (AMDR) values for carbohydrate, fat, and protein expressed as percentages of total daily caloric intake; ranges of intakes set for the energy-yielding nutrients that are sufficient to provide adequate total energy and nutrients while minimizing the risk of chronic diseases.

accredited approved; in the case of medical centers or universities, certified by an agency recognized by the U.S. Department of Education.

acetaldehyde (ass-et-AL-deh-hide) a substance to which ethanol is metabolized on its way to becoming harmless waste products that can be excreted.

acid-base balance equilibrium between acid and base concentrations in the body fluids.

acidosis (acid-DOH-sis) the condition of excess acid in the blood, indicated by a below-normal pH (*osis* means "too much").

acid reducers prescription and over-the-counter drugs that reduce the acid output of the stomach; effective for treating severe, persistent forms of heartburn but not for neutralizing acid already present. Side effects are frequent and include diarrhea, other gastrointestinal complaints, and reduction

of the stomach's capacity to destroy alcohol, thereby producing higher-than-expected blood alcohol levels from each drink. Also called *acid controllers*.

acids compounds that release hydrogens in a watery solution.

acne chronic inflammation of the skin's follicles and oil-producing glands, which leads to an accumulation of oils inside the ducts that surround hairs; usually associated with the maturation of young adults.

acupuncture (AK-you-punk-chur) a technique that involves piercing the skin with long, thin needles at specific anatomical points to relieve pain or illness. Acupuncture sometimes uses heat, pressure, friction, suction, or electromagnetic energy to stimulate the points.

added sugars sugars and syrups added to a food for any purpose, such as to add sweetness or bulk or to aid in browning (baked goods). Also called *carbohydrate sweeteners*, they include concentrated fruit juice, glucose, fructose, high-fructose corn syrup, sucrose, and other sweet carbohydrates.

additives substances that are added to foods but are not normally consumed by themselves as foods.

adequacy the dietary characteristic of providing all of the essential nutrients, fiber, and energy in amounts sufficient to maintain health and body weight.

Adequate Intakes (AI) nutrient intake goals for individuals; the recommended average daily nutrient intake level based on intakes of healthy people in a particular life stage and gender group and assumed to be adequate. Set when scientific data are insufficient to allow establishment of an RDA value.

adipokines (AD-ih-poh-kynz) protein hormones made and released by adipose tissue (fat) cells.

adipose tissue the body's fat tissue, consisting of masses of fat-storing cells and blood vessels to nourish them.

adolescence the period from the beginning of puberty until maturity.

advertorials lengthy advertisements in newspapers and magazines that read like feature articles but are written for the purpose of touting the virtues of products and may or may not be accurate.

aerobic (air-ROH-bic) requiring oxygen.

aerobic activity physical activity that involves the body's large muscles working at light to moderate intensity for a sustained period of time. Brisk walking, running, swimming, and bicycling are examples. Also called *endurance activity*.

aflatoxin (af-lah-TOX-in) a toxin from a mold that grows on corn, grains, peanuts, and tree nuts stored in warm, humid conditions; a cause of liver cancer prevalent in tropical developing nations. (To prevent it, discard shriveled, discolored, or moldy foods.)

agave syrup a carbohydrate-rich sweetener made from a Mexican plant; a higher fructose content gives some agave syrups a greater sweetening power per calorie than sucrose.

agility nimbleness; the ability to quickly change directions.

agroecology a scientific discipline that combines biological, physical, and social sciences with ecological theory to develop methods for producing food sustainably.

alcoholism a dependency on alcohol marked by compulsive, uncontrollable drinking with negative effects on physical health, family relationships, and social health.

alcohol dehydrogenase (dee-high-DRAH-gen-ace) **(ADH)** an enzyme system that breaks down alcohol. The antidiuretic hormone listed below is also abbreviated ADH.

alcohol-related birth defects (ARBD) malformations in the skeletal and organ systems (heart, kidneys, eyes, ears) associated with prenatal alcohol exposure.

alcohol-related neurodevelopmental disorder (ARND) behavioral, cognitive, or central nervous system abnormalities associated with prenatal alcohol exposure.

alkalosis (al-kah-LOH-sis) the condition of excess base in the blood, indicated by an above-normal blood pH (*alka* means "base"; *osis* means "too much").

allergy an immune reaction to a foreign substance, such as a component of food. Also called *hypersensitivity* by researchers.

alpha-lactalbumin (lact-AL-byoo-min) the chief protein in human breast milk. The chief protein in cow's milk is *casein* (CAY-seen).

amine (a-MEEN) **group** the nitrogen-containing portion of an amino acid.

amino acid chelates (KEY-lates) compounds of minerals (such as calcium) combined with amino acids in a form that favors their absorption. A chelating agent is a molecule that surrounds another molecule and can then either promote or prevent its movement from place to place (*chele* means "claw").

amino (a-MEEN-o) **acids** the building blocks of protein. Each has an amine group at one end, an acid group at the other, and a distinctive side chain.

amniotic (AM-nee-OTT-ic) **sac** the "bag of waters" in the uterus in which the fetus floats.

anabolic steroid hormones chemical messengers related to the male sex hormone testosterone that stimulate the building up of body tissues (*anabolic* means "promoting growth"; *sterol* refers to compounds chemically related to cholesterol).

anaerobic (AN-air-ROH-bic) not requiring oxygen.

anaphylactic (an-ah-feh-LACK-tick) **shock** a life-threatening whole-body allergic reaction to an offending substance.

androstenedione (AN-droh-STEEN-die-own) a precursor of testosterone that elevates both testosterone and estrogen in the blood of both males and females. Often called *andro*, it is sold with claims of producing increased muscle strength, but controlled studies disprove such claims.

anecdotal evidence information based on interesting and entertaining, but not scientific, personal accounts of events.

anemia a blood condition in which red blood cells, the body's oxygen carriers, are inadequate or impaired and so cannot meet the oxygen demands of the body.

anencephaly (an-en-SEFF-ah-lee) an uncommon and always fatal neural tube defect in which the brain fails to form.

aneurysm (AN-you-rism) the ballooning out of an artery wall at a point that is weakened by deterioration.

anorexia nervosa an eating disorder characterized by a refusal to maintain a minimally normal body weight, self-starvation to the extreme, and a disturbed perception of body weight and shape; seen (usually) in teenage girls and young women (*anorexia* means "without appetite"; *nervos* means "of nervous origin").

antacids medications that react directly and immediately with the acid of the stomach, neutralizing it. Antacids are most suitable for treating occasional heartburn.

antibiotic-resistant bacteria bacterial strains that cause increasingly common and potentially fatal infectious diseases that do not respond to standard antibiotic therapy. An example is MRSA (pronounced MER-suh), a multidrug-resistant *Staphyloccocus aureus* bacterium.

antibodies (AN-te-bod-ees) large proteins of the blood, produced by the immune system in response to an invasion of the body by foreign substances (antigens). Antibodies combine with and inactivate the antigens.

anticarcinogens compounds in foods that act in any of several ways to oppose the formation of cancer.

antidiuretic (AN-tee-dye-you-RET-ick) **hormone (ADH)** a hormone produced by the pituitary gland in response to dehydration (or a high sodium concentration in the blood). It stimulates the kidneys to reabsorb more water and so to excrete less. (This hormone should not be confused with the enzyme alcohol dehydrogenase, which is also abbreviated ADH.)

antigen a microbe or substance that is foreign to the body.

antigen a substance foreign to the body that elicits the formation of antibodies or an inflammation reaction from immune system cells. Food antigens are usually large proteins. Inflammation consists of local swelling and irritation and attracts white blood cells to the site.

antioxidant nutrients vitamins and minerals that oppose the effects of oxidants on human physical functions. The antioxidant vitamins are vitamin E, vitamin C, and beta-carotene. The mineral selenium also participates in antioxidant activities.

antioxidants (an-tee-OX-ih-dants) compounds that protect other compounds from damaging reactions involving oxygen by themselves reacting with oxygen (*anti* means "against"; *oxy* means "oxygen"). *Oxidation* is a potentially damaging effect of normal cell chemistry involving oxygen.

aorta (ay-OR-tuh) the large, primary artery that conducts blood from the heart to the body's smaller arteries.

appendicitis inflammation and/or infection of the appendix, a sac protruding from the intestine.

appetite the psychological desire to eat; a learned motivation and a positive sensation that accompanies the sight, smell, or thought of appealing foods.

appliance thermometer a thermometer that verifies the temperature of an appliance. An *oven thermometer* verifies that the oven is heating properly; a *refrigerator/freezer thermometer* tests for proper refrigerator temperature (<40°F, or <4°C) or freezer temperature (0°F, or −17°C).

aquaculture the farming of aquatic organisms for food, generally fish, mollusks, or crustaceans, that involves such activities as feeding immature organisms, providing habitat, protecting them from predators, harvesting them, and selling or consuming them.

aquifers underground rock formations containing water that can be drawn to the surface for use.

arachidonic (ah-RACK-ih-DON-ik) **acid** an omega-6 fatty acid derived from linoleic acid.

arsenic a poisonous metallic element. In trace amounts, arsenic is believed to be an essential nutrient in some animal species. Arsenic is often added to insecticides and weed killers and, in tiny amounts, to certain animal drugs.

arteries blood vessels that carry blood containing fresh oxygen supplies from the heart to the tissues.

artesian water water drawn from a well that taps a confined aquifer in which the water is under pressure.

arthritis a usually painful inflammation of joints caused by many conditions, including infections, metabolic disturbances, or injury; usually results in altered joint structure and loss of function.

artificial fats zero-energy fat replacers that are chemically synthesized to mimic the sensory and cooking qualities of naturally occurring fats but that are totally or partially resistant to digestion.

ascorbic acid one of the active forms of vitamin C (the other is *dehydroascorbic* acid); an antioxidant nutrient.

-ase (ACE) a suffix meaning *enzyme*. Categories of digestive and other enzymes and individual enzyme names often contain this suffix.

atherogenic able to initiate or promote atherosclerosis.

atherosclerosis (ath-er-oh-scler-OH-sis) the most common form of cardiovascular disease; characterized by plaque along the inner walls of the arteries (*scleros* means "hard"; *osis* means "too much"). The term *arteriosclerosis* is often used to mean the same thing.

athlete a competitor in any sport, exercise, or game requiring physical skill; for the purpose of this book, anyone who trains at a high level of physical exertion, with or without competition. From the Greek *athlein*, meaning "to contend for a prize."

atrophy (AT-tro-fee) a decrease in size (for example, of a muscle) because of disuse.

autoimmune disorder a disease in which the body develops antibodies to its own proteins and then proceeds to destroy cells containing these proteins. Examples are type 1 diabetes and lupus.

B

baby water ordinary bottled water treated with ozone to make it safe but not sterile.

balance the dietary characteristic of providing foods of a number of types in proportion to each other, such that foods rich in some nutrients do not crowd out of the diet foods that are rich in other nutrients.

balance study a laboratory study in which a person is fed a controlled diet and the intake and excretion of a nutrient are measured. Balance studies are valid only for nutrients like calcium (chemical elements) that do not change while they are in the body.

basal metabolic rate (BMR) the rate at which the body uses energy to support its basal metabolism.

basal metabolism the sum total of all the involuntary activities that are necessary to sustain life, including circulation, respiration, temperature maintenance, hormone secretion, nerve activity, and new tissue synthesis, but excluding digestion and voluntary activities. Basal metabolism is the largest component of the average person's daily energy expenditure.

bases compounds that accept hydrogens from solutions.

B-cells lymphocytes that produce antibodies. *B* stands for *bursa*, an organ in the chicken where B-cells were first identified.

beer belly central-body fatness associated with alcohol consumption.

behavior modification alteration of behavior using methods based on the theory that actions can be controlled by manipulating the environmental factors that cue, or trigger, the actions.

beriberi (berry-berry) the thiamin-deficiency disease; characterized by loss of sensation in the hands and feet, muscular weakness, advancing paralysis, and abnormal heart action.

beta-carotene an orange pigment with antioxidant activity; a vitamin A precursor made by plants and stored in human fat tissue.

bicarbonate a common alkaline chemical; a secretion of the pancreas; also the active ingredient of baking soda.

bile a cholesterol-containing digestive fluid made by the liver, stored in the gallbladder, and released into the small intestine when needed. It emulsifies fats and oils to ready them for enzymatic digestion.

binge eating disorder an eating disorder whose criteria are similar to those of bulimia nervosa, excluding purging or other compensatory behaviors.

bioaccumulation the accumulation of a contaminant in the tissues of living things at higher and higher concentrations along the food chain.

bioactive having chemical or physical properties that affect the functions of the body tissues.

bioactive food components compounds in foods, either nutrients or phytochemicals, that alter physiological processes.

biofilm a layer of microbes mixed with a sticky, protective coating of proteins and carbohydrates exuded by certain bacteria.

biotechnology the science of manipulating biological systems or organisms to modify their products or components or create new products; biotechnology includes recombinant DNA technology and traditional and accelerated selective breeding techniques.

biotin (BY-o-tin) a B vitamin; a coenzyme necessary for fat synthesis and other metabolic reactions.

bladder the sac that holds urine until time for elimination.

blind experiment an experiment in which the subjects do not know whether they are members of the experimental group or the control group. In a *double-blind experiment*, neither the subjects nor the researchers know to which group the members belong until the end of the experiment.

blood the fluid of the cardiovascular system; composed of water, red and white blood cells, other formed particles, nutrients, oxygen, and other constituents.

body composition the proportions of muscle, bone, fat, and other tissue that make up a person's total body weight.

body mass index (BMI) an indicator of health risk from obesity or underweight, calculated by dividing the weight of a person by the square of the person's height.

body system a group of related organs that work together to perform a function. Examples are the circulatory system, respiratory system, and nervous system.

bone density a measure of bone strength, the degree of mineralization of the bone matrix.

bone meal or **powdered bone** crushed or ground bone preparations intended to supply calcium to the diet. Calcium from bone is not well absorbed and is often contaminated with toxic materials such as arsenic, mercury, lead, and cadmium.

botanical pertaining to or made from plants; any drug, medicinal preparation, dietary supplement, or similar substance obtained from a plant.

bottled water drinking water sold in bottles.

botulism an often fatal foodborne illness caused by the botulinum toxin, a toxin produced by the *Clostridium botulinum* bacterium, which grows without oxygen in nonacidic canned foods.

bovine spongiform encephalopathy (BOH-vine SPUNJ-ih-form en-SEH-fal-AH-path-ee) **(BSE)** an often fatal illness of the nerves and brain observed in cattle and wild game and in people who consume affected meats. Also called *mad cow disease*.

bran the protective fibrous coating around a grain; the chief fiber donator of a grain.

broccoli sprouts the sprouted seed of *Brassica italica*, or the common broccoli plant; believed to be a functional food by virtue of its high phytochemical content.

brown adipose tissue (BAT) a type of adipose tissue abundant in hibernating animals and human infants and recently identified in human adults. Abundant pigmented enzymes of energy metabolism give BAT a dark appearance under a microscope; the enzymes release heat from fuels without accomplishing other work. Also called *brown fat*.

brown bread bread containing ingredients such as molasses that lend a brown color; may be made with any kind of flour, including white flour.

brown sugar white sugar with molasses added, 95% pure sucrose.

buffers molecules that can help to keep the pH of a solution from changing by gathering or releasing H ions.

built environment The buildings, roads, utilities, homes, fixtures, parks, and all other man-made entities that form the physical characteristics of a community.

bulimia (byoo-LEEM-ee-uh) **nervosa** recurring episodes of binge eating combined with a morbid fear of becoming fat; usually followed by self-induced vomiting or purging.

C

caffeine a stimulant that can produce alertness and reduce reaction time when used in small doses but causes headaches, trembling, an abnormally fast heart rate, and other undesirable effects in high doses.

caffeine water bottled water with caffeine added.

calcium compounds the simplest forms of purified calcium. They include calcium carbonate, citrate, gluconate, hydroxide, lactate, malate, and phosphate. These supplements vary in the amount of calcium they contain, so read the labels carefully. A 500-milligram tablet of calcium gluconate may provide only 45 milligrams of calcium, for example.

caloric effect the drop in cancer incidence seen whenever intake of food energy (calories) is restricted.

calorie control the dietary characteristic of controlling energy intake; a feature of a sound diet plan.

calories units of energy. In nutrition science, the unit used to measure the energy in foods is a kilocalorie (also called *kcalorie* or *Calorie*): it is the amount of heat energy necessary to raise the temperature of a kilogram (a liter) of water 1 degree Celsius. This book follows the common practice of using the lowercase term *calorie* (abbreviated *cal*) to mean the same thing.

cancer a group of diseases in which cells multiply out of control and disrupt normal functioning of one or more organs.

capillaries minute, weblike blood vessels that connect arteries to veins and permit transfer of materials between blood and tissues.

carbohydrase (car-boh-HIGH-drace) any of a number of enzymes that break the chemical bonds of carbohydrates.

carbohydrates compounds composed of single or multiple sugars. The name means "carbon and water," and a chemical shorthand for carbohydrate is CHO, signifying carbon (C), hydrogen (H), and oxygen (O).

carbonated water water that contains carbon dioxide gas, either naturally occurring or added, that causes bubbles to form in it; also called bubbling or sparkling water. Seltzer, soda, and tonic waters are legally soft drinks and are not regulated as water.

carcinogen (car-SIN-oh-jen) a cancer-causing substance (*carcin* means "cancer"; *gen* means "gives rise to").

carcinogenesis the origination or beginning of cancer.

cardiac output the volume of blood discharged by the heart each minute.

cardiorespiratory endurance the ability of the heart, lungs, and metabolism to sustain large-muscle exercise of moderate to high intensity for prolonged periods.

cardiovascular disease (CVD) disease of the heart and blood vessels; disease of the arteries of the heart is called *coronary heart disease* (CHD).

carnitine a nitrogen-containing compound, formed in the body from lysine and methionine, that helps transport fatty acids across the mitochondrial membrane. Carnitine is claimed to "burn" fat and spare glycogen during endurance events, but it does neither.

carotenoid (CARE-oh-ten-oyd) a member of a group of pigments in foods that range in color from light yellow to reddish orange and are chemical relatives of beta-carotene.

Many have a degree of vitamin A activity in the body.

carrying capacity the total number of living organisms that a given environment can support without deteriorating in quality.

case studies studies of individuals. In clinical settings, researchers can observe treatments and their apparent effects. To prove that a treatment has produced an effect requires simultaneous observation of an untreated similar subject (a *case control*).

catalyst a substance that speeds the rate of a chemical reaction without itself being permanently altered in the process. All enzymes are catalysts.

cataract (CAT-uh-ract) clouding of the lens of the eye that can lead to blindness. Cataracts can be caused by injury, viral infection, toxic substances, genetic disorders, and possibly some nutrient deficiencies or imbalances.

cathartic a strong laxative.

celiac (SEE-lee-ack) **disease** a disorder characterized by an abnormal immune response, weight loss, and intestinal inflammation on exposure to the dietary protein gluten; also called *gluten-sensitive enteropathy* or *celiac sprue*.

cell differentiation (dih-fer-en-she-AY-shun) the process by which immature cells are stimulated to mature and gain the ability to perform functions characteristic of their cell type.

cells the smallest units in which independent life can exist. All living things are single cells or organisms made of cells.

cellulite a term popularly used to describe dimpled fat tissue on the thighs and buttocks; not recognized in science.

central obesity excess fat in the abdomen and around the trunk.

certified diabetes educator (CDE) a health-care professional who specializes in educating people with diabetes to help them manage their disease through medical means and lifestyle changes. Work experience, extensive training, and passing an examination are required to achieve CDE status.

certified lactation consultant a health-care provider, often a registered nurse or a registered dietitian nutritionist, with specialized training and certification in breast and infant anatomy and physiology who teaches the mechanics of breastfeeding to new mothers.

cesarean (see-ZAIR-ee-un) **section** surgical childbirth, in which the infant is taken through an incision in the woman's abdomen.

chelating agents molecules that attract or bind with other molecules and are therefore useful in either preventing or promoting movement of substances from place to place.

chlorophyll the green pigment of plants that captures energy from sunlight for use in photosynthesis.

cholesterol (koh-LESS-ter-all) a member of the group of lipids known as sterols; a soft, waxy substance made in the body for a variety of purposes and also found in animal-derived foods.

choline (KOH-leen) a nutrient used to make the phospholipid lecithin and other molecules.

chronic diseases degenerative conditions or illnesses that progress slowly, are long in duration, and lack an immediate cure; chronic diseases limit functioning, productivity, and the quality and length of life. Examples include heart disease, cancer, and diabetes.

chronic hypertension in pregnant women, hypertension that is present and documented before pregnancy; in women whose prepregnancy blood pressure is unknown, the presence of sustained hypertension before 20 weeks of gestation.

chronic malnutrition malnutrition caused by long-term food deprivation; characterized in children by short height for age (stunting).

chylomicrons (KYE-low-MY-krons) lipoproteins formed when lipids from a meal cluster with carrier proteins in the cells of the intestinal lining. Chylomicrons transport food fats through the watery body fluids to the liver and other tissues.

chyme (KIME) the fluid resulting from the actions of the stomach upon a meal.

cirrhosis (seer-OH-sis) advanced liver disease, often associated with alcoholism, in which liver cells have died, hardened, turned an orange color, and permanently lost their function.

clone an individual created asexually from a single ancestor, such as a plant grown from a single stem cell; a group of genetically identical individuals descended from a single common ancestor, such as a colony of bacteria arising from a single bacterial cell; in genetics, a replica of a segment of DNA, such as a gene, produced by genetic engineering.

coconut sugar a granulated sugar composed of sucrose, glucose, and fructose; made by evaporating the sap of flower buds of coconut palm trees.

coconut water the fluid inside a young green coconut; heavily marketed for its substantial potassium content, it also provides about 45 calories per cup and little or no fat.

coenzyme (co-EN-zime) a small molecule that works with an enzyme to promote the enzyme's activity. Many coenzymes have B vitamins as part of their structure (*co* means "with").

cognitive behavioral therapy psychological therapy aimed at changing undesirable behaviors by changing underlying thought processes contributing to these behaviors; in anorexia, a goal is to replace false beliefs about body weight, eating, and self-worth with health-promoting beliefs.

cognitive skills as taught in behavior therapy, changes to conscious thoughts with the goal of improving adherence to lifestyle modifications; examples are problem-solving skills and the correction of false negative thoughts, termed *cognitive restructuring*.

collagen (COLL-a-jen) the chief protein of most connective tissues, including scars, ligaments, and tendons, and the underlying matrix on which bones and teeth are built.

colon the large intestine.

colostrum (co-LAHS-trum) a milklike secretion from the breasts during the first day or so after delivery before milk appears; rich in protective factors.

competitive foods unregulated meals, including fast foods, that compete side by side with USDA-regulated school lunches.

complementary and **alternative medicine (CAM)** a group of diverse medical and health-care systems, practices, and products that are not considered to be a part of conventional medicine. Examples include acupuncture, biofeedback, chiropractic, faith healing, and many others.

complementary foods nutrient- and energy-containing solid or semisolid foods (or liquids) fed to infants in addition to breast milk or infant formula.

complementary proteins two or more proteins whose amino acid assortments complement each other in such a way that the essential amino acids missing from one are supplied by the other.

complex carbohydrates long chains of sugar units arranged to form starch or fiber; also called *polysaccharides*.

concentrated fruit juice sweetener a concentrated sugar syrup made from dehydrated, deflavored fruit juice, commonly grape juice; used to sweeten products that can then claim to be "all fruit."

conditionally essential amino acid an amino acid that is normally nonessential but must be supplied by the diet in special circumstances when the need for it exceeds the body's ability to produce it.

confectioner's sugar finely powdered sucrose, 99.9% pure.

constipation difficult, incomplete, or infrequent bowel movements associated with discomfort in passing dry, hardened feces from the body.

control group a group of individuals who are similar in all possible respects to the group being treated in an experiment but who receive a sham treatment instead of the real one. Also called *control subjects*. See also *experimental group* and *intervention studies*.

controlled clinical trial a research study design that often reveals effects of a treatment on human beings. Health outcomes are observed in a group of people who receive the treatment and are then compared with outcomes in a control group of similar people who received a placebo (an inert or sham treatment). Ideally, neither subjects nor researchers know who receives the treatment and who gets the placebo (a double-blind study).

cornea (KOR-nee-uh) the hard, transparent membrane covering the outside of the eye.

corn sweeteners corn syrup and sugar solutions derived from corn.

corn syrup a syrup, mostly glucose, partly maltose, produced by the action of enzymes on cornstarch. Includes corn syrup solids.

correlation the simultaneous change of two factors, such as the increase of weight with increasing height (a *direct* or *positive* correlation) or the decrease of cancer incidence with increasing fiber intake (an *inverse* or *negative* correlation). A correlation between two factors suggests that one may cause the other but does not rule out the possibility that both may be caused by chance or by a third factor.

cortex the outermost layer of something. The brain's cortex is the part of the brain where conscious thought takes place.

cortical bone the ivorylike outer bone layer that forms a shell surrounding trabecular bone and that comprises the shaft of a long bone.

country of origin label (COOL) the required label stating the country of origination of certain imported fish and shellfish, certain other perishable foods, certain nuts, peanuts, and ginseng. Meats and poultry are no longer subject to COOL labeling.

creatine a nitrogen-containing compound that combines with phosphate to burn a high-energy compound stored in muscle. Some studies suggest that creatine enhances energy and stimulates muscle growth, but long-term studies are lacking; digestive side effects may occur.

cretinism (CREE-tin-ism) severe mental and physical retardation of an infant caused by the mother's iodine deficiency during pregnancy.

critical period a finite period during development in which certain events may occur that will have irreversible effects on later developmental stages. A critical period is usually a period of cell division in a body organ.

cross-contamination the contamination of a food through exposure to utensils, hands, or other surfaces that were previously in contact with a contaminated food.

cruciferous vegetables vegetables with cross-shaped blossoms—the cabbage family. Their intake is associated with low cancer rates in human populations. Examples are broccoli, brussels sprouts, cabbage, cauliflower, rutabagas, and turnips.

cuisines styles of cooking.

cultural competence having an awareness and acceptance of one's own and others' cultures and abilities, leading to effective interactions with all kinds of people.

D

Daily Values nutrient standards used on food labels and on grocery store and restaurant signs. Based on nutrient recommendations for a general 2,000-calorie diet, they allow consumers to compare foods with regard to nutrients and calorie contents.

dead zones columns of oxygen-depleted ocean water in which marine life cannot survive; often caused by algae blooms that occur when agricultural fertilizers and waste runoff enter natural waterways.

dehydration loss of water. The symptoms progress rapidly, from thirst to weakness to exhaustion and delirium, and end in death.

denaturation the irreversible change in a protein's folded shape brought about by heat, acids, bases, alcohol, salts of heavy metals, or other agents.

dental caries decay of the teeth (*caries* means "rottenness"). Also called *cavities*.

desalination (dee-SAL-ih-NAY-shun) any of a number of processes that convert salt or brackish water into fresh water for drinking, industrial use, or irrigation.

dextrose, anhydrous dextrose forms of glucose.

DHEA (dehydroepiandrosterone) a hormone made in the adrenal glands that serves as a precursor to the male hormone testosterone; recently banned by the U.S. Food and Drug Administration (FDA) because it poses the risk of life-threatening diseases, including cancer. Falsely promoted to burn fat, build muscle, and slow aging.

diabetes (dye-uh-BEET-eez) metabolic diseases characterized by elevated blood glucose and inadequate or ineffective insulin, which impair a person's ability to regulate blood glucose. The technical name is *diabetes mellitus* (*mellitus* means "honey-sweet" in Latin, referring to sugar in the urine).

dialysis (die-AL-ih-sis) in kidney disease, treatment of the blood to remove toxic substances or metabolic wastes; more properly, *hemodialysis*, meaning "dialysis of the blood."

diarrhea frequent, watery bowel movements usually caused by diet, stress, or irritation of the colon. Severe, prolonged diarrhea robs the body of fluid and certain minerals, causing dehydration and imbalances that can be dangerous if left untreated.

diastolic (dye-as-TOL-ik) **pressure** the second figure in a blood pressure reading (the "lubb" of the heartbeat is heard), which reflects the arterial pressure when the heart is between beats.

diet the foods (including beverages) a person usually eats and drinks.

dietary antioxidants compounds typically found in plant foods that significantly decrease the adverse effects of oxidation on living tissues. The major antioxidant vitamins are vitamin E, vitamin C, and beta-carotene. Many phytochemicals are also antioxidants.

dietary folate equivalent (DFE) a unit of measure expressing the amount of folate available to the body from naturally occurring sources. The measure mathematically equalizes the difference in absorption between less absorbable food folate and highly absorbable synthetic folate added to enriched foods and found in supplements.

Dietary Reference Intakes (DRI) a set of five lists of values for measuring the nutrient intakes of healthy people in the United States and Canada. The lists are Estimated Average Requirements (EAR), Recommended Dietary Allowances (RDA), Adequate Intakes (AI), Tolerable Upper Intake Levels (UL), and Acceptable Macronutrient Distribution Ranges (AMDR).

dietary supplements pills, liquids, or powders that contain purified nutrients or other ingredients.

dietetic technician a person who has completed a two-year academic degree from an accredited college or university and an approved dietetic technician program. **A dietetic technician, registered (DTR)** has also passed a national examination and maintains registration through continuing professional education.

dietitian a person trained in nutrition, food science, and diet planning. See also *registered dietitian nutritionist*.

digest to break molecules into smaller molecules; a main function of the digestive tract with respect to food.

digestive system the body system composed of organs that break down complex food particles into smaller, absorbable products. The *digestive tract* and *alimentary canal* are names for the tubular organs that extend from the mouth to the anus. The whole system, including the pancreas, liver, and gallbladder, is sometimes called the *gastrointestinal*, or *GI*, system.

dipeptides (dye-PEP-tides) protein fragments that are two amino acids long (*di* means "two").

diploma mill an organization that awards meaningless degrees without requiring students to meet educational standards. Diploma mills are not the same as diploma forgers (providing fake diplomas and certificates bearing the names of real, respected institutions). While virtually indistinguishable from authentic diplomas, forgeries can be unveiled by checking directly with the institution.

disaccharides pairs of single sugars linked together (*di* means "two").

distilled water water that has been vaporized and recondensed, leaving it free of dissolved minerals.

diuretic (dye-you-RET-ic) a compound, usually a medication, causing increased urinary water excretion; a "water pill."

diverticula (dye-ver-TIC-you-la) sacs or pouches that balloon out of the intestinal wall, caused by weakening of the muscle layers that encase the intestine. The painful inflammation of one or more of the diverticula is known as *diverticulitis*.

DNA an abbreviation for deoxyribonucleic (dee-OX-ee-RYE-bow-nu-CLAY-ick) acid, the thread-like molecule that encodes genetic information in its structure; DNA strands coil up densely to form the chromosomes.

dolomite a compound of minerals (calcium magnesium carbonate) found in limestone and marble. Dolomite is powdered and is sold as a calcium-magnesium supplement but may be contaminated with toxic minerals, is not well absorbed, and interacts adversely with absorption of other essential minerals.

dopamine (DOH-pah-meen) a neurotransmitter with many important roles in the brain, including cognition, pleasure, motivation, mood, sleep, and others.

drink a dose of any alcoholic beverage that delivers half an ounce of pure ethanol.

drug any substance that, when taken into a living organism, may modify one or more of its functions.

dual-energy X-ray absorptiometry (ab-sorp-tee-OM-eh-tree) a noninvasive method of determining total body fat, fat distribution, and bone density by passing two low-dose X-ray beams through the body. Also used in evaluation of osteoporosis. Abbreviated DEXA.

E

eating disorder a disturbance in eating behavior that jeopardizes a person's physical or psychological health.

eating pattern the combination of food and beverages that constitute an individual's complete dietary intake over time; a person's usual diet.

eclampsia (eh-CLAMP-see-ah) a severe complication during pregnancy in which seizures occur.

edamame fresh green soybeans, a source of phytoestrogens.

edema (eh-DEEM-uh) swelling of body tissue caused by leakage of fluid from the blood vessels; seen in protein deficiency (among other conditions).

eicosanoids (eye-COSS-ah-noyds) biologically active compounds that regulate body functions.

electrolytes compounds that partly dissociate in water to form ions, such as the potassium ion (K^+) and the chloride ion (Cl^-).

elemental diets diets composed of purified ingredients of known chemical composition; intended to supply all essential nutrients to people who cannot eat foods.

embolism an embolus that causes sudden closure of a blood vessel.

embolus (EM-boh-luss) a thrombus that breaks loose and travels through the blood vessels (*embol* means "to insert").

embryo (EM-bree-oh) the stage of human gestation from the third to the eighth week after conception.

emergency kitchens programs that provide prepared meals to be eaten on-site; often called *soup kitchens*.

emetic (em-ETT-ic) an agent that causes vomiting.

empty calories calories provided by added sugars and solid fats with few or no other nutrients. Other empty calorie sources include alcohol, and highly refined starches, such as corn starch or potato starch, often found in ultra-processed foods.

emulsification the process of mixing lipid with water by adding an emulsifier.

emulsifier (ee-MULL-sih-fire) a compound with both water-soluble and fat-soluble portions that can attract fats and oils into water, combining them.

endosperm the bulk of the edible part of a grain, the starchy part.

energy the capacity to do work. The energy in food is chemical energy; it can be converted to mechanical, electrical, thermal, or other forms of energy in the body. Food energy is measured in calories.

energy density a measure of the energy provided by a food relative to its weight (calories per gram).

energy drinks and **energy shots** sugar-sweetened beverages in various concentrations with supposedly ergogenic ingredients, such as vitamins, amino acids, caffeine, guarana, carnitine, ginseng, and others. The drinks are not regulated by the FDA and are often high in caffeine or other stimulants.

energy reservoir a system of high-energy compounds that hold, store, and release energy derived from the energy-yielding nutrients and transfer it to cell structures to fuel cellular activities. In exercise, the reservoir provides immediate energy sufficient for short bursts of intense physical activity.

energy-yielding nutrients the nutrients the body can use for energy—carbohydrate, fat, and protein. These also may supply building blocks for body structures. Also called *macronutrients*.

enriched foods and **fortified foods** foods to which nutrients have been added. If the starting material is a whole, basic food such as milk or whole grain, the result may be highly nutritious. If the starting material is a concentrated form of sugar or fat, the result is likely to be less nutritious.

enriched, fortified refers to the addition of nutrients to a refined food product. As defined by U.S. law, these terms mean that specified levels of thiamin, riboflavin, niacin, folate, and iron have been added to refined grains and grain products. The terms *enriched* and *fortified* can refer to the addition of more nutrients than just these five; read the label.

enterotoxins poisons that act on mucous membranes, such as those of the digestive tract.

environmental tobacco smoke the combination of exhaled smoke (mainstream smoke) and smoke from lighted cigarettes, pipes, or cigars (sidestream smoke) that enters the air and may be inhaled by other people.

enzymes (EN-zimes) proteins that facilitate chemical reactions without being changed in the process; protein catalysts.

EPA, DHA eicosapentaenoic (EYE-cossa-PENTA-ee-NO-ick) acid, docosahexaenoic (DOE-cossa-HEXA-ee-NO-ick) acid; omega-3 fatty acids made from linolenic acid in the tissues of fish.

epidemiological studies studies of populations; often used in nutrition to search for correlations between dietary habits and disease incidence; a first step in seeking nutrition-related causes of diseases.

epigenetics (ep-ih-gen-EH-tics) the science of heritable changes in gene function that occur without a change in the DNA sequence.

epigenome (ep-ih-GEE-nohm) the proteins and other molecules associated with chromosomes that affect gene expression. The epigenome is modulated by bioactive food components and other factors in ways that

can be inherited. *Epi* is a Greek prefix, meaning "above" or "on."

epinephrine (epp-ih-NEFF-rin) a hormone of the adrenal gland that counteracts anaphylactic shock by opening the airways and maintaining heartbeat and blood pressure.

epiphyseal (eh-PIFF-ih-seal) **plate** a thick, cartilage-like layer that forms new cells that are eventually calcified, lengthening the bone (*epiphysis* means "growing" in Greek).

epithelial (ep-ith-THEE-lee-ull) **tissue** the layers of the body that serve as selective barriers to environmental factors. Examples are the cornea, the skin, the respiratory tract lining, and the lining of the digestive tract.

ergogenic (ER-go-JEN-ic) **aids** products that supposedly enhance performance, although few actually do so; the term *ergogenic* implies "energy giving" (*ergo* means "work"; *genic* means "give rise to").

erythrocyte (eh-REETH-ro-sight) **hemolysis** (HEE-moh-LIE-sis, hee-MOLL-ih-sis) rupture of the red blood cells that can be caused by vitamin E deficiency (*erythro* means "red"; *cyte* means "cell"; *hemo* means "blood"; *lysis* means "breaking"). The anemia produced by the condition is *hemolytic* (HEE-moh-LIT-ick) *anemia*.

essential amino acids amino acids that either cannot be synthesized at all by the body or cannot be synthesized in amounts sufficient to meet physiological need. Also called *indispensable amino acids*.

essential fatty acids fatty acids that the body needs but cannot make and so must be obtained from the diet.

essential nutrients the nutrients the body cannot make for itself (or cannot make fast enough) from other raw materials; nutrients that must be obtained from food to prevent deficiencies.

Estimated Average Requirements (EAR) the average daily nutrient intake estimated to meet the requirement of half of the healthy individuals in a particular life stage and gender group; is used in nutrition research and policy making and is the basis upon which RDA values are set.

Estimated Energy Requirement (EER) the average dietary energy intake predicted to maintain energy balance in a healthy adult of a certain age, gender, weight, height, and level of physical activity consistent with good health.

ethanol the alcohol of alcoholic beverages, produced by the action of microorganisms on the carbohydrates of grape juice or other carbohydrate-containing fluids.

ethnic foods foods associated with particular cultural subgroups within a population.

euphoria (you-FOR-ee-uh) an inflated sense of well-being and pleasure brought on by a

moderate dose of alcohol and by some other drugs.

evaporated cane juice raw sugar from which impurities have been removed.

excess postexercise oxygen consumption (EPOC) a measure of increased metabolism (energy expenditure) that continues for minutes or hours after cessation of exercise.

exclusive breastfeeding an infant's consumption of human milk with no supplementation of any type (no water, no juice, no nonhuman milk, and no foods) except for vitamins, minerals, and medications.

exercise planned, structured, and repetitive bodily movement that promotes or maintains physical fitness.

experimental group the people or animals participating in an experiment who receive the treatment under investigation. Also called *experimental subjects*. See also *control group* and *intervention studies*.

extracellular fluid fluid residing outside the cells that transports materials to and from the cells.

extra virgin olive oil minimally processed olive oil produced by mechanical means, such as pressing (not chemical extraction), to preserve phytochemicals, green color, and flavor from the original olives. The highest grade of olive oil.

extreme obesity clinically severe overweight, presenting very high risks to health; the condition of having a BMI of 40 or above; also called *morbid obesity*.

extrusion processing techniques that transform grains, legumes, and other foods into fine particles that are cooked, shaped, colored, flavored, and often puffed, producing snacks, breakfast cereals, and other products.

F

famine widespread and extreme scarcity of food that causes starvation and death in a large portion of the population in an area.

farm share an arrangement in which a farmer offers the public a "subscription" for an allotment of the farm's products throughout the season.

fast foods restaurant foods that are available within minutes after customers order them—traditionally, hamburgers, French fries, and milkshakes; more recently, salads and other vegetable dishes as well. These foods may or may not meet people's nutrient needs, depending on the selections made and on the energy allowances and nutrient needs of the eaters.

fasting plasma glucose test a blood test that measures the current blood glucose concentration in a person who has not eaten or consumed caloric beverages for at least 8 hours;

the test can detect both diabetes and prediabetes. *Plasma* is the fluid part of whole blood.

fat cells cells that specialize in the storage of fat and form the fat tissue. Fat cells also produce fat-metabolizing enzymes; they also produce hormones involved in appetite and energy balance.

fat replacers ingredients that replace some or all of the functions of fat and may or may not provide energy.

fats lipids that are solid at room temperature (70°F or 21°C).

fatty acids organic acids composed of carbon chains of various lengths. Each fatty acid has an acid end and hydrogens attached to all of the carbon atoms of the chain.

fatty liver an early stage of liver deterioration seen in several diseases, including nonalcoholic and alcoholic liver diseases, in which fat accumulates in the liver cells.

feces waste material remaining after digestion and absorption are complete; eventually discharged from the body.

female athlete triad a potentially fatal triad of medical problems seen in female athletes: disordered eating, menstrual cessation, and osteoporosis.

fermentation the anaerobic (without oxygen) breakdown of carbohydrates by microorganisms that releases small organic compounds along with carbon dioxide and energy.

fertility the capacity of a woman to produce a normal ovum periodically and of a man to produce normal sperm; the ability to reproduce.

fetal alcohol spectrum disorders (FASD) a spectrum of physical, behavioral, and cognitive disabilities caused by prenatal alcohol exposure.

fetal alcohol syndrome (FAS) the cluster of symptoms including brain damage, growth restriction, mental retardation, and facial abnormalities seen in an infant or child whose mother consumed alcohol during her pregnancy.

fetus (FEET-us) the stage of human gestation from eight weeks after conception until the birth of an infant.

fibers the indigestible parts of plant foods, largely nonstarch polysaccharides that are not digested by human digestive enzymes, although some are digested by resident bacteria of the colon. Fibers include cellulose, hemicelluloses, pectins, gums, mucilages, and a few nonpolysaccharides such as lignin.

fibrosis (fye-BROH-sis) an intermediate stage of alcoholic liver deterioration. Liver cells lose their function and assume the characteristics of connective tissue cells (become fibrous).

fight-or-flight reaction the body's instinctive hormone- and nerve-mediated reaction to danger. Also known as the *stress response*.

filtered water water treated by filtration, usually through activated carbon filters that reduce the lead in tap water or by reverse osmosis units that force pressurized water across a membrane, removing lead, arsenic, and some microorganisms from tap water.

fitness the characteristics that enable the body to perform physical activity; more broadly, the ability to meet routine physical demands with enough reserve energy to rise to a physical challenge; or the body's ability to withstand stress of all kinds.

fitness water lightly flavored bottled water enhanced with vitamins, supposedly to enhance athletic performance.

flavonoids (FLAY-von-oyds) a common and widespread group of phytochemicals, with over 6,000 identified members; physiologic effects may include antioxidant, antiviral, anticancer, and other activities. Some flavonoids are yellow pigments in foods; *flavus* means "yellow."

flavored waters lightly flavored beverages with few or no calories, but often containing vitamins, minerals, herbs, or other unneeded substances. Not superior to plain water for athletic competition or training.

flaxseed small brown seed of the flax plant; used in baking, cereals, or other foods. Valued in nutrition as a source of fatty acids, lignans, and fiber.

flexibility the capacity of the joints to move through a full range of motion; the ability to bend and recover without injury.

fluid and electrolyte balance maintenance of the proper amounts and kinds of fluids and minerals in each compartment of the body.

fluid and electrolyte imbalance failure to maintain the proper amounts and kinds of fluids and minerals in every body compartment; a medical emergency.

fluorapatite (floor-APP-uh-tight) a crystal of bones and teeth, formed when fluoride displaces the "hydroxy" portion of hydroxyapatite. Fluorapatite resists being dissolved back into body fluid.

fluorosis (floor-OH-sis) discoloration of the teeth due to ingestion of too much fluoride during tooth development. *Skeletal fluorosis* is characterized by unusually dense but weak, fracture-prone, often malformed bones, caused by excess fluoride in bone crystals.

folate (FOH-late) a B vitamin that acts as part of a coenzyme important in the manufacture of new cells. The form added to foods and supplements is *folic acid*.

food medically, any substance that the body can take in and assimilate that will enable it to stay alive and to grow; the carrier of nourishment; socially, a more limited number of such substances defined as acceptable by each culture.

food aversion an intense dislike of a food, biological or psychological in nature, resulting from an illness or other negative experience associated with that food.

food banks facilities that collect and distribute food donations to authorized organizations feeding the hungry.

foodborne illness illness transmitted to human beings through food and water; caused by an infectious agent (*foodborne infection*) or a poisonous substance arising from microbial toxins, poisonous chemicals, or other harmful substances (*food intoxication*). Also commonly called *food poisoning*.

food contaminant any substance occurring in food by accident; any food constituent that is not normally present.

food crisis a steep decline in food availability with a proportional rise in hunger and malnutrition at the local, national, or global level.

food deserts a term used to describe urban and rural low-income neighborhoods and communities that have limited access to affordable and nutritious foods.

food group plan a diet-planning tool that sorts foods into groups based on their nutrient content and then specifies that people should eat certain minimum numbers of servings of foods from each group.

food intolerance an adverse reaction to a food or food additive not involving an immune response.

food neophobia (NEE-oh-FOE-beeah) the fear of trying new foods, common among toddlers.

food pantries community food collection programs that provide groceries to be prepared and eaten at home.

food poverty hunger occurring when enough food exists in an area but some of the people cannot obtain it because they lack money, are being deprived for political reasons, live in a country at war, or suffer from other problems such as lack of transportation.

food recovery collecting wholesome surplus food for distribution to low-income people who are hungry.

foodways the sum of a culture's habits, customs, beliefs, and preferences concerning food.

fork thermometer a utensil combining a meat fork and an instant-read food thermometer.

formaldehyde a substance to which methanol is metabolized on the way to being converted to harmless waste products that can be excreted.

fraud or **quackery** the promotion, for financial gain, of devices, treatments, services, plans, or products (including diets and supplements) claimed to improve health, wellbeing, or appearance without proof of safety or effectiveness. (The word *quackery* comes from the term *quacksalver*, meaning a person who quacks loudly about a miracle product—a lotion or a salve.)

free radicals atoms or molecules with one or more unpaired electrons that make the atom or molecule unstable and highly reactive.

fructose (FROOK-tose) a monosaccharide; sometimes known as fruit sugar (*fruct* means "fruit"; *ose* means "sugar").

fructose, galactose, glucose the monosaccharides.

fruitarian includes only raw or dried fruits, seeds, and nuts in the diet.

fufu a low-protein staple food that provides abundant starch energy to many of the world's people; fufu is made by pounding or grinding root vegetables or refined grains and cooking them to a smooth, semisolid consistency.

functional foods whole or modified foods that contain bioactive food components believed to provide health benefits, such as reduced disease risks, beyond the benefits that their nutrients confer. However, all nutritious foods can support health in some ways.

G

galactose (ga-LACK-tose) a monosaccharide; part of the disaccharide lactose (milk sugar).

gastric juice the digestive secretion of the stomach.

gastroesophageal (GAS-tro-eh-SOFF-ahjeel) **reflux disease (GERD)** a severe and chronic splashing of stomach acid and enzymes into the esophagus, throat, mouth, or airway that causes injury to those organs. Untreated GERD may increase the risk of esophageal cancer; treatment may require surgery or management with medication.

gatekeeper with respect to nutrition, a key person who controls other people's access to foods and thereby affects their nutrition profoundly. Examples are the spouse who buys and cooks the food, the parent who feeds the children, and the caregiver in a day-care center.

generally recognized as safe (GRAS) list a list, established by the FDA, of food additives long in use and believed to be safe.

genes units of a cell's inheritance; sections of the larger genetic molecule DNA (deoxyribonucleic acid). Each gene directs the making of one or more of the body's proteins.

genetically modified organism (GMO) popular term referring to an organism produced by genetic engineering; the term *genetically engineered organism (GEO)* is more scientifically accurate.

genetic engineering the direct, intentional manipulation of the genetic material of living things in order to obtain some desirable inheritable trait not present in the original organism. Also called *biotechnology*.

genetic profile the result of an analysis of genetic material that identifies unique characteristics of a person's DNA for forensic or diagnostic purposes.

genistein (GEN-ih-steen) a phytoestrogen found primarily in soybeans that both mimics and blocks the action of estrogen in the body; a type of flavonoid.

genome (GEE-nome) the full complement of genetic information in the chromosomes of a cell. In human beings, the genome consists of about 35,000 genes and supporting materials.

genomics the study of all the genes in an organism and their interactions with environmental factors.

germ the nutrient-rich inner part of a grain.

gestation the period of about 40 weeks (three trimesters) from conception to birth; the term of a pregnancy.

gestational diabetes abnormal glucose tolerance appearing during pregnancy.

gestational hypertension high blood pressure that develops in the second half of pregnancy and usually resolves after childbirth.

ghrelin (GREL-in) a hormone released by the stomach that signals the brain's hypothalamus and other regions to stimulate eating.

glucagon (GLOO-cah-gon) a hormone secreted by the pancreas that stimulates the liver to release glucose into the blood when blood glucose concentration dips.

glucose (GLOO-cose) a single sugar used in both plant and animal tissues for energy; sometimes known as blood sugar or *dextrose*.

glucose polymers compounds that supply glucose not as single molecules but linked in chains somewhat like starch. The objective is to attract less water from the body into the digestive tract.

gluten (GLOO-ten) a type of protein in certain grain foods that is toxic to the person with celiac disease.

glycemic index (GI) a ranking of foods according to their potential for raising blood glucose relative to a standard food such as glucose.

glycemic load (GL) a mathematical expression of both the glycemic index and the carbohydrate content of a food, meal, or diet.

glycerol (GLISS-er-all) an organic compound, three carbons long, of interest here because it serves as the backbone for triglycerides.

glycogen (GLY-co-gen) a highly branched polysaccharide that is made and stored by liver and muscle tissues of human beings and animals as a storage form of glucose. Glycogen is not a significant food source of carbohydrate and is not counted as one of the complex carbohydrates in foods.

goiter (GOY-ter) enlargement of the thyroid gland due to an iodine deficiency is *simple goiter*; enlargement due to an iodine excess is *toxic goiter*.

grams units of weight. A gram (g) is the weight of a cubic centimeter (cc) or milliliter (ml) of water under defined conditions of temperature and pressure. About 28 grams equal an ounce.

granulated sugar common table sugar, crystalline sucrose, 99.9% pure.

granules small grains. Starch granules are packages of starch molecules. Various plant species make starch granules of varying shapes.

greenhouse gases gases that contribute to global climate change by absorbing the sun's infrared radiation and trapping heat; examples of greenhouse gases are carbon dioxide and methane.

green revolution a series of advances in technology made in the last century that dramatically increased farm yields worldwide. The techniques rely heavily on chemical fertilizers and pesticides, along with large farm machinery.

groundwater water that comes from underground aquifers.

growth hormone a hormone (somatotropin) that promotes growth and that is produced naturally in the pituitary gland of the brain.

growth spurt the marked rapid gain in physical size usually evident around the onset of adolescence.

H

hard water water with high calcium and magnesium concentrations.

hazard a state of danger; used to refer to any circumstance in which harm is possible under normal conditions of use.

Hazard Analysis Critical Control Point (HACCP) plan a systematic plan to identify and correct potential microbial hazards in the manufacturing, distribution, and commercial use of food products. *HACCP* may be pronounced "HASS-ip."

health claims FDA-approved food label statements that link food constituents with disease or health-related conditions. Examples:

"Soluble fiber from daily oatmeal in a diet low in saturated fat and trans fat may reduce the risk of heart disease" or "A diet low in total fat may reduce the risk of some cancers."

heart attack the event in which the vessels that feed the heart muscle become closed off by an embolism, thrombus, or other cause with resulting sudden tissue death. A heart attack is also called a *myocardial infarction* (*myo* means "muscle"; *cardial* means "of the heart"; *infarct* means "tissue death").

heartburn a burning sensation in the chest (in the area of the heart) caused by backflow of stomach acid into the esophagus.

heat cramps painful cramps of the abdomen, arms, or legs, often occurring hours after exercise; associated with inadequate intake of fluid or electrolytes or heavy sweating.

heat stroke an acute and life-threatening reaction to heat buildup in the body.

heavy episodic drinking a common pattern of excessive alcohol use that elevates blood alcohol to 0.08% or above; typically, five or more drinks for men, four for women, in about two hours' time. Also called *binge drinking*.

heavy metal any of a number of mineral ions such as mercury and lead, so called because they are of relatively high atomic weight; many heavy metals are poisonous.

heme (HEEM) the iron-containing portion of the hemoglobin and myoglobin molecules.

hemoglobin (HEEM-oh-globe-in) the oxygen-carrying protein of the blood; found in the red blood cells (*hemo* means "blood"; *globin* means "spherical protein").

hemolytic-uremic (HEEM-oh-LIT-ic you-REEM-ick) **syndrome** a severe result of infection with Shiga toxin–producing *E. coli*, characterized by abnormal blood clotting with kidney failure, damage to the central nervous system and other organs, and death, especially among children.

hemorrhoids (HEM-or-oids) swollen, hardened (varicose) veins in the rectum, usually caused by the pressure resulting from constipation.

hepcidin (HEP-sid-in) a hormone secreted by the liver in response to elevated blood iron. Hepcidin reduces iron's absorption from the intestine and its release from storage.

herbal medicine a type of CAM that uses herbs and other natural substances to prevent or cure diseases or to relieve symptoms.

hernia a protrusion of an organ or part of an organ through the wall of the body chamber that normally contains the organ. An example is a *hiatal* (high-AY-tal) *hernia*, in which part of the stomach protrudes up through the diaphragm into the chest cavity, which contains the esophagus, heart, and lungs.

hiccups spasms of both the vocal cords and the diaphragm, causing periodic, audible, short, inhaled coughs. Can result from irritation of the diaphragm, indigestion, or other causes. Hiccups usually resolve in a few minutes but can have serious effects if prolonged. Breathing into a paper bag (inhaling carbon dioxide) or dissolving a teaspoon of sugar in the mouth may stop them.

high-carbohydrate energy drinks flavored commercial beverages used to restore muscle glycogen after exercise or as pregame beverages.

high-carbohydrate gels semisolid, easy-to-swallow supplements of concentrated carbohydrate, commonly with potassium and sodium added; not a fluid source.

high-density lipoproteins (HDL) lipoproteins that return cholesterol from the tissues to the liver for dismantling and disposal; contain a large proportion of protein.

high-fructose corn syrup (HFCS) a widely used commercial caloric sweetener made by adding enzymes to cornstarch to convert a portion of its glucose molecules into sweet-tasting fructose.

high-fructose corn syrup a commercial sweetener used in many foods, including soft drinks. Composed almost entirely of the monosaccharides fructose and glucose, its sweetness and caloric value are similar to sucrose.

high-quality proteins dietary proteins containing all the essential amino acids in relatively the same amounts that human beings require. They may also contain nonessential amino acids.

high-risk pregnancy a pregnancy characterized by risk factors that make it likely the birth will be complicated by premature delivery, difficult birth, retarded growth, birth defects, and early infant death. A *low-risk pregnancy* has none of these factors.

histamine a substance that participates in causing inflammation; produced by cells of the immune system as part of a local immune reaction to an antigen.

histones (HISS-tones) proteins that lend structural support to the chromosome structure and that help to activate or silence gene expression.

HIV/AIDS acquired immune deficiency syndrome; caused by infection with human immunodeficiency virus (HIV), which is transmitted primarily by sexual contact, contact with infected blood, needles shared among drug users, or fluids transferred from an infected mother to her fetus or infant.

homogenization a process by which milk fat is evenly dispersed within fluid milk; under high pressure, milk is passed through tiny nozzles to reduce the size of fat droplets and reduce their tendency to cluster and float to the top as cream.

honey a concentrated solution primarily composed of glucose and fructose, produced by enzymatic digestion of the sucrose in nectar by bees.

hormones chemical messengers secreted by a number of body organs in response to conditions that require regulation. Each hormone affects a specific organ or tissue and elicits a specific response.

hormones chemicals that are secreted by glands into the blood in response to conditions in the body that require regulation. These chemicals serve as messengers, acting on other organs to maintain constant conditions.

hourly sweat rate the amount of weight lost plus fluid consumed during exercise per hour.

hunger a consequence of food insecurity; physical discomfort, illness, weakness, or pain beyond a mild uneasy sensation arising from a prolonged involuntary lack of food.

hunger the physiological need to eat, experienced as a drive for obtaining food; an unpleasant sensation that demands relief.

husk the outer, inedible part of a grain.

hydrochloric acid a strong, corrosive acid of hydrogen and chloride atoms, produced by the stomach to assist in digestion.

hydrogenation (high-dro-gen-AY-shun) the process of adding hydrogen to unsaturated fatty acids to make fat more solid and resistant to the chemical change of oxidation.

hydroxyapatite (hi-DROX-ee-APP-uh-tight) the chief crystal of bone, formed from calcium and phosphorus.

hyperactivity (in children) a syndrome characterized by inattention, impulsiveness, and excess motor activity; usually diagnosed before age 7, lasts six months or more, and usually does not entail mental illness or mental retardation. Properly called *attention-deficit/hyperactivity disorder (ADHD)*.

hypertension high blood pressure.

hypertension higher-than-normal blood pressure.

hypertrophy (high-PURR-tro-fee) an increase in size (for example, of a muscle) in response to use.

hypoglycemia (HIGH-poh-gly-SEE-mee-ah) an abnormally low blood glucose concentration, often accompanied by symptoms such as anxiety, rapid heartbeat, and sweating.

hyponatremia (HIGH-poh-nah-TREE-mee-ah) a decreased concentration of sodium in the blood.

hypothalamus (high-poh-THAL-uh-mus) a part of the brain that senses a variety of conditions in the body, such as temperature, glucose content, salt content, and others. It signals other parts of the brain or body to adjust those conditions when necessary.

hypothermia a below-normal body temperature.

I

immune system a system of tissues and organs that defend the body against antigens, foreign materials that have penetrated the skin or body linings.

immunity protection from or resistance to a disease or infection by the development of antibodies and by the actions of cells and tissues in response to a threat.

implantation the stage of development, during the first two weeks after conception, in which the fertilized egg (fertilized ovum or zygote) embeds itself in the wall of the uterus and begins to develop.

inborn error of metabolism a genetic variation present from birth that may result in disease.

incidental additives substances that can get into food not through intentional introduction but as a result of contact with the food during growing, processing, packaging, storing, or some other stage before the food is consumed. Also called *accidental* or *indirect additives*.

infectious diseases diseases that are caused by bacteria, viruses, parasites, and other microbes and that can be transmitted from one person to another through air, water, or food; by contact; or through vector organisms such as mosquitoes and fleas.

inflammation (in-flam-MAY-shun) part of the body's immune defense against injury, infection, or allergens, marked by increased blood flow, release of chemical toxins, and attraction of white blood cells to the affected area (from the Latin *inflammare*, meaning "to flame within").

infomercials feature-length television commercials that follow the format of regular programs but are intended to convince viewers to buy products and not to educate or entertain them. The statements made may or may not be accurate.

initiation an event, probably occurring in a cell's genetic material, caused by radiation or by a chemical carcinogen that can give rise to cancer.

inositol (in-OSS-ih-tall) a nonessential nutrient found in cell membranes.

insoluble fibers the tough, fibrous structures of fruits, vegetables, and grains; indigestible food components that do not dissolve in water.

instant-read thermometer a thermometer that, when inserted into food, measures its temperature within seconds; designed to test temperature of food at intervals.

insulin a hormone secreted by the pancreas in response to a high blood glucose concentration. It assists cells in drawing glucose from the blood.

insulin resistance a condition in which a normal or high level of circulating insulin produces a less-than-normal response in muscle, liver, and adipose tissues; thought to be a metabolic consequence of obesity.

integrated pest management (IPM) management of pests using a combination of natural and biological controls and minimal or no application of pesticides.

intensity in exercise, the degree of effort required to perform a given physical activity.

Internet (the Net) a worldwide network of millions of computers linked together to share information.

intervention studies studies of populations in which observation is accompanied by experimental manipulation of some population members—for example, a study in which half of the subjects (the *experimental subjects*) follow diet advice to reduce fat intakes, while the other half (the *control subjects*) do not, and both groups' heart health is monitored.

intestine the body's long, tubular organ of digestion and the site of nutrient absorption.

intracellular fluid fluid residing inside the cells that provides the medium for cellular reactions.

intrinsic factor a factor found inside a system. The intrinsic factor necessary to prevent pernicious anemia is now known to be a compound that helps in the absorption of vitamin B_{12}.

invert sugar a mixture of glucose and fructose formed by the splitting of sucrose in an industrial process. Sold only in liquid form and sweeter than sucrose, invert sugar forms during certain cooking procedures and works to prevent crystallization of sucrose in soft candies and sweets.

ions (EYE-ons) electrically charged particles, such as sodium (positively charged) or chloride (negatively charged).

iron deficiency the condition of having depleted iron stores, which, at the extreme, causes iron-deficiency anemia.

iron-deficiency anemia a form of anemia caused by a lack of iron and characterized by red blood cell shrinkage and color loss.

Accompanying symptoms are weakness, apathy, headaches, pallor, intolerance to cold, and inability to pay attention. (For other anemias, see the index.)

iron overload the state of having more iron in the body than it needs or can handle, usually arising from a hereditary defect. Also called *hemochromatosis*.

irradiation the application of ionizing radiation to foods to reduce insect infestation or microbial contamination or to slow the ripening or sprouting process. Also called *cold pasteurization*.

irritable bowel syndrome (IBS) intermittent disturbance of bowel function, especially diarrhea or alternating diarrhea and constipation, often with abdominal cramping or bloating; managed with diet, physical activity, or relief from psychological stress. The cause is uncertain, but inflammation is often involved, and a role for an altered intestinal microbiota is suspected. IBS does not permanently harm the intestines or lead to serious diseases.

IU (international units) a measure of fat-soluble vitamin activity sometimes used in food composition tables and on supplement labels.

J

jaundice (JAWN-dis) yellowing of the skin due to spillover of the bile pigment bilirubin (bill-ee-ROO-bin) from the liver into the general circulation.

K

kefir (KEE-fur) a liquid form of yogurt, based on milk, probiotic microorganisms, and flavorings.

kefir a yogurt-based beverage.

keratin (KERR-uh-tin) the normal protein of hair and nails.

keratinization accumulation of keratin in a tissue; a sign of vitamin A deficiency.

ketone bodies acidic compounds derived from fat and certain amino acids. Normally rare in the blood, they help to feed the brain during times when too little carbohydrate is available.

ketosis (kee-TOE-sis) an undesirable high concentration of ketone bodies, such as acetone, in the blood or urine.

kidneys a pair of organs that filter wastes from the blood, make urine, and release it to the bladder for excretion from the body.

kwashiorkor (kwash-ee-OR-core, kwash-ee-or-CORE) severe malnutrition characterized by failure to grow and develop, edema, changes in the pigmentation of hair and skin, fatty liver, anemia, and apathy.

L

laboratory studies studies that are performed under tightly controlled conditions and are designed to pinpoint causes and effects. Such studies often use animals as subjects.

lactase the intestinal enzyme that splits the disaccharide lactose to monosaccharides during digestion.

lactate a compound produced during the breakdown of glucose in anaerobic metabolism.

lactation production and secretion of breast milk for the purpose of nourishing an infant.

lactoferrin (lack-toe-FERR-in) a factor in breast milk that binds iron and keeps it from supporting the growth of the infant's intestinal bacteria.

lacto-ovo vegetarian includes dairy products, eggs, vegetables, grains, legumes, fruits, and nuts; excludes flesh and seafood.

lactose a disaccharide composed of glucose and galactose; sometimes known as milk sugar (*lact* means "milk"; *ose* means "sugar").

lactose intolerance impaired ability to digest lactose due to reduced amounts of the enzyme lactase.

lactose, maltose, sucrose the disaccharides.

lacto-vegetarian includes dairy products, vegetables, grains, legumes, fruits, and nuts; excludes flesh, seafood, and eggs.

lapses periods of returning to old habits.

large intestine the portion of the intestine that completes the absorption process.

learning disability a condition resulting in an altered ability to learn basic cognitive skills such as reading, writing, and mathematics.

leavened (LEV-end) literally, "lightened" by yeast cells, which digest some carbohydrate components of the dough and leave behind bubbles of gas that make the bread rise.

lecithin (LESS-ih-thin) a phospholipid manufactured by the liver and also found in many foods; a major constituent of cell membranes.

legumes (leg-GOOMS, LEG-yooms) plants of the bean, pea, and lentil family that have roots with nodules containing special bacteria. These bacteria can trap nitrogen from the air in the soil and make it into compounds that become part of the plant's seeds. The seeds are rich in protein compared with those of most other plant foods.

leptin an appetite-suppressing hormone produced in the fat cells that conveys information about body fatness to the brain; believed to be involved in the maintenance of body composition (*leptos* means "slender").

leucine one of the essential amino acids; it is of current research interest for its role in stimulating muscle protein synthesis.

levulose an older name for fructose.

license to practice permission under state or federal law, granted on meeting specified criteria, to use a certain title (such as *dietitian*) and to offer certain services. Licensed dietitians may use the initials LD after their names.

life expectancy the average number of years lived by people in a given society.

life span the maximum number of years of life attainable by a member of a species.

lignans phytochemicals present mostly in seeds, particularly flaxseed, that are converted to phytoestrogens by intestinal bacteria and are under study as possible anticancer agents.

limiting amino acid an essential amino acid that is present in dietary protein in an insufficient amount, thereby limiting the body's ability to build protein.

linoleic (lin-oh-LAY-ic) **acid** an essential polyunsaturated fatty acid of the omega-6 family.

linolenic (lin-oh-LEN-ic) **acid** an essential polyunsaturated fatty acid of the omega-3 family. The full name of linolenic acid is *alpha-linolenic acid*.

lipase (LYE-pace) any of a number of enzymes that break the chemical bonds of fats (lipids).

lipid (LIP-id) a family of organic (carbon-containing) compounds soluble in organic solvents but not in water. Lipids include triglycerides (fats and oils), phospholipids, and sterols.

lipoic (lip-OH-ic) **acid** a nonessential nutrient.

lipoproteins (LYE-poh-PRO-teens, LIH-poh-PRO-teens) clusters of lipids associated with protein, which serve as transport vehicles for lipids in blood and lymph. The major lipoproteins include chylomicrons, VLDL, LDL, and HDL.

listeriosis a serious foodborne infection that can cause severe brain infection or death in a fetus or a newborn; caused by the bacterium *Listeria monocytogenes*, which is found in soil and water.

liver a large, lobed organ that lies just under the ribs. It filters the blood, removes and processes nutrients, manufactures materials for export to other parts of the body, and destroys toxins or stores them to keep them out of the circulatory system.

longevity long duration of life.

low birthweight a birthweight of less than 5½ pounds (2,500 grams); used as a predictor of probable health problems in the newborn and as a probable indicator of poor nutrition status of the mother before and/or during pregnancy. Low-birthweight infants may be premature (born early) or small for gestational age (suffered growth failure in the uterus).

low-density lipoproteins (LDL) lipoproteins that transport lipids from the liver to other tissues such as muscle and fat; contain a large proportion of cholesterol.

low-input agriculture agriculture practiced on a small scale using individualized approaches that vary with local conditions so as to minimize technological, fuel, and chemical inputs.

lungs the body's organs of gas exchange. Blood circulating through the lungs releases its carbon dioxide and picks up fresh oxygen to carry to the tissues.

lutein (LOO-teen) a plant pigment of yellow hue; a phytochemical believed to play roles in eye functioning and health.

lycopene (LYE-koh-peen) a pigment responsible for the red color of tomatoes and other red-hued vegetables; a phytochemical that may act as an antioxidant in the body.

lymph (lymf) the fluid that moves from the bloodstream into tissue spaces and then travels in its own vessels, which eventually drain back into the bloodstream.

lymphocytes (LIM-foh-sites) white blood cells that participate in the immune response; B-cells and T-cells.

M

macrobiotic diet a vegan diet composed mostly of whole grains, beans, and certain vegetables; taken to extremes, macrobiotic diets can compromise nutrient status.

macrophages (MACK-roh-fah-jez) large scavenger cells of the immune system that engulf debris and remove it (*macro* means "large"; *phagein* means "to eat").

macular degeneration a common, progressive loss of function of the part of the retina that is most crucial to focused vision. This degeneration often leads to blindness.

major minerals essential mineral nutrients required in the adult diet in amounts greater than 100 milligrams per day. Also called *macrominerals*.

malnutrition any condition caused by excess or deficient food energy or nutrient intake or by an imbalance of nutrients. Nutrient or energy deficiencies are forms of undernutrition; nutrient or energy excesses are forms of overnutrition.

maltose a disaccharide composed of two glucose units; sometimes known as malt sugar.

malt syrup a sweetener made from sprouted barley.

maple syrup a concentrated solution of sucrose derived from the sap of the sugar maple tree. This sugar was once common but is now usually replaced by sucrose and artificial maple flavoring.

marasmic kwashiorkor a particularly lethal form of severe acute malnutrition, in which a child's dangerously reduced lean body tissue is masked by edema, making the condition harder to detect.

marasmus (ma-RAZ-mus) severe malnutrition characterized by poor growth, dramatic weight loss, loss of body fat and muscle, and apathy. From the Greek word meaning "dying away."

margin of safety in reference to food additives, a zone between the concentration normally used and that at which a hazard exists. For common table salt, for example, the margin of safety is 1/5 (five times the amount normally used would be hazardous).

medical foods foods specially manufactured for use by people with medical disorders and administered on the advice of a physician.

medical nutrition therapy nutrition services used in the treatment of injury, illness, or other conditions; includes assessment of nutrition status and dietary intake and corrective applications of diet, counseling, and other nutrition services.

metabolic syndrome a combination of characteristic factors—high fasting blood glucose or insulin resistance, central obesity, hypertension, low blood HDL cholesterol, and elevated blood triglycerides—that greatly increase a person's risk of developing CVD. Also called *insulin resistance syndrome*.

metabolic water water generated in the tissues during the chemical breakdown of the energy-yielding nutrients in foods.

metabolism the sum of all physical and chemical changes taking place in living cells; includes all reactions by which the body obtains and spends the energy from food.

metastasis (meh-TASS-ta-sis) movement of cancer cells from one body part to another, usually by way of the body fluids.

methanol an alcohol produced in the body continually by all cells.

methyl groups (METH-il) small carbon-containing molecules that, among their activities, silence genes when applied to DNA strands by enzymes.

methylmercury any toxic compound of mercury to which a characteristic chemical structure, a methyl group, has been added, usually by bacteria in aquatic sediments. Methylmercury is readily absorbed from the intestine and causes nerve damage in people.

microbes bacteria, viruses, fungi, or other organisms invisible to the naked eye, some of which cause diseases. Also called *microorganisms*.

microbiota the mix of microbial species of a community; for example, all of the bacteria, fungi, and viruses present in the human digestive tract. The term *microbiome* refers to the collective genes of such a community.

microvilli (MY-croh-VILL-ee, MY-croh-VILL-eye) tiny, hairlike projections on each cell of every villus that greatly expand the surface area available to trap nutrient particles and absorb them into the cells (singular: microvillus).

milk anemia iron-deficiency anemia caused by drinking so much milk that iron-rich foods are displaced from the diet.

minerals naturally occurring, inorganic, homogeneous substances; chemical elements.

mineral water water from a spring or well that typically contains at least 250 parts per million (ppm) of naturally occurring minerals. Minerals give water a distinctive flavor. Many mineral waters are high in sodium.

miso fermented soybean paste used in Japanese cooking. Soy products are considered to be functional foods.

moderate drinkers people who do not drink excessively and do not behave inappropriately because of alcohol. A moderate drinker's health may or may not be harmed by alcohol over the long term.

moderation the dietary characteristic of providing constituents within set limits, not to excess.

modified atmosphere packaging (MAP) a technique used to extend the shelf life of perishable foods; the food is packaged in a gas-impermeable container from which air is removed or to which an oxygen-free gas mixture, such as carbon dioxide and nitrogen, is added to deprive microbes of oxygen.

molasses a thick brown syrup left over from the refining of sucrose from sugar cane. The major nutrient in molasses is iron, a contaminant from the machinery used in processing it.

monoglycerides (mon-oh-GLISS-er-ides) products of the digestion of lipids; a monoglyceride is a glycerol molecule with one fatty acid attached (*mono* means "one"; *glyceride* means "a compound of glycerol").

monosaccharides (mon-oh-SACK-ah-rides) single sugar units (*mono* means "one"; *saccharide* means "sugar unit").

monounsaturated fats triglycerides in which most of the fatty acids have one point of unsaturation (are monounsaturated).

monounsaturated fatty acid a fatty acid containing one point of unsaturation.

MSG symptom complex the acute, temporary, and self-limiting reactions, including burning sensations or flushing of the skin with pain and headache, experienced by sensitive people upon ingesting a large dose of MSG. Formerly called *Chinese restaurant syndrome*.

mucus (MYOO-cus) a slippery coating of the digestive tract lining (and other body linings) that protects the cells from exposure to digestive juices (and other destructive agents). The adjective form is *mucous* (same pronunciation). The digestive tract lining is a *mucous membrane*.

multi-grain a term used on food labels to indicate a food made with more than one kind of grain. Not an indicator of a whole-grain food.

muscle endurance the ability of a muscle to contract repeatedly within a given time without becoming exhausted. This muscle characteristic develops with increasing repetition rather than increasing workload and is associated with cardiorespiratory endurance.

muscle fatigue diminished force and power of muscle contractions despite consistent or increasing conscious effort to perform a physical activity.

muscle power the efficiency of a muscle contraction, measured by force and time.

muscle strength the ability of muscles to overcome physical resistance. This muscle characteristic develops with increasing work load rather than repetition and is associated with muscle size.

mutation a permanent, heritable change in an organism's DNA.

myoglobin (MYE-oh-globe-in) the oxygen-holding protein of the muscles (*myo* means "muscle").

N

National Health and Nutrition Examination Surveys (NHANES) a program of studies designed to assess the health and nutritional status of adults and children in the United States by way of interviews and physical examinations.

natural foods a term that has no legal definition but is often used to imply wholesomeness.

naturally occurring sugars sugars that are not added to a food but are present as its original constituents, such as the sugars of fruit or milk.

natural water water obtained from a spring or well that is certified to be safe and sanitary. The mineral content may not be changed, but the water may be treated in other ways, such as with ozone or by filtration.

nectars concentrated peach nectar, pear nectar, or others.

nephrons (NEFF-rons) the working units in the kidneys, consisting of intermeshed blood vessels and tubules.

neural tube the embryonic tissue that later forms the brain and spinal cord.

neural tube defect (NTD) a group of abnormalities of the brain and spinal cord apparent at birth and caused by interruption of the normal early development of the neural tube.

neurotoxins poisons that act on the cells of the nervous system.

neurotransmitters chemicals that are released at the end of a nerve cell when a nerve impulse arrives there. They diffuse across the gap to the next cell and alter the membrane of that second cell to either inhibit or excite it.

niacin a B vitamin needed in energy metabolism. Niacin can be eaten preformed or made in the body from tryptophan, one of the amino acids. Other forms of niacin are *nicotinic acid*, *niacinamide*, and *nicotinamide*.

niacin equivalents (NE) the amount of niacin present in food, including the niacin that can theoretically be made from its precursor tryptophan that is present in the food.

night blindness slow recovery of vision after exposure to flashes of bright light at night; an early symptom of vitamin A deficiency.

night eating syndrome a disturbance in the daily eating rhythm associated with obesity, characterized by more than half of the daily calories consumed after 7 p.m., frequent nighttime awakenings to eat, and a high calorie intake.

nitrogen balance the amount of nitrogen consumed compared with the amount excreted in a given time period.

nonalcoholic a term used on beverage labels, such as wine or beer, indicating that the product contains less than 0.5% alcohol. The terms *dealcoholized* and *alcohol removed* mean the same thing. *Alcohol free* means that the product contains no detectable alcohol.

non-celiac gluten sensitivity a poorly defined collection of digestive symptoms that improves with elimination of gluten from the diet.

nonheme iron dietary iron not associated with hemoglobin; the iron of plants and other sources.

nonnutritive sweeteners sweet-tasting synthetic or natural food additives that offer sweet flavor but with negligible or no calories per serving; also called *artificial sweeteners*, *intense sweeteners*, *noncaloric sweeteners*, and *very low-calorie sweeteners*.

norepinephrine (NOR-EP-ih-NEFF-rin) a compound related to epinephrine that helps to elicit the stress response.

nori a type of seaweed popular in Asian, particularly Japanese, cooking.

nucleotide (NU-klee-oh-tied) one of the subunits from which DNA and RNA are composed.

nutraceutical a term that has no legal or scientific meaning but that is sometimes used to refer to foods, nutrients, or dietary supplements believed to have medicinal effects. Often used to sell unnecessary or unproven supplements.

nutrient claims FDA-approved food label statements that describe the nutrient levels in food. Examples: "fat free" or "less sodium."

nutrient density a measure of nutrients provided per calorie of food. A *nutrient-dense food* provides vitamins, minerals, and other beneficial substances with relatively few calories.

nutrients components of food that are indispensable to the body's functioning. They provide energy, serve as building material, help maintain or repair body parts, and support growth. The nutrients include water, carbohydrate, fat, protein, vitamins, and minerals.

nutrition the study of the nutrients in foods and in the body; sometimes also the study of human behaviors related to food.

nutritional genomics the science of how food components, such as nutrients, interact with the body's genetic material.

nutritionally enhanced beverages flavored beverages that contain any of a number of nutrients, including some carbohydrate, along with protein, vitamins, minerals, herbs, or other unneeded substances. Such "enhanced waters" may not contain useful amounts of carbohydrate or electrolytes to support athletic competition or training.

Nutrition Facts on a food label, the panel of nutrition information required to appear on almost every packaged food. Grocers may also provide the information for fresh produce, meats, poultry, and seafood.

nutritionist someone who studies nutrition. Some nutritionists are RDNs, whereas others are self-described experts whose training is questionable and who are not qualified to give advice. In states with responsible legislation, the term applies only to people who have master of science (MS) or doctor of philosophy (PhD) degrees from properly accredited institutions.

O

obesity excess body weight associated with increased risk of mortality and chronic diseases; a body mass index of 30 or higher.

oils lipids that are liquid at room temperature (70°F or 21°C).

olestra a noncaloric artificial fat made from sucrose and fatty acids; formerly called *sucrose polyester*. A trade name is *Olean*.

omega-3 fatty acid a polyunsaturated fatty acid with its endmost double bond three carbons from the end of the carbon chain. Linolenic acid is an example.

omega-6 fatty acid a polyunsaturated fatty acid with its endmost double bond six carbons from the end of the carbon chain. Linoleic acid is an example.

omnivorous people who eat foods of both plant and animal origin, including animal flesh.

oral rehydration therapy (ORT) oral fluid replacement for children with severe diarrhea caused by infectious disease. A simple recipe for ORT: ½ L boiled water, 4 tsp sugar, ½ tsp salt.

organic carbon containing. Four of the six classes of nutrients are organic: carbohydrate, fat, protein, and vitamins. Organic compounds include only those made by living things and do not include compounds such as carbon dioxide, diamonds, and a few carbon salts.

organic foods foods meeting strict USDA production regulations for *organic*—that is, produced without synthetic pesticides, herbicides, fertilizers, drugs, and preservatives and without genetic engineering or irradiation.

organic gardens gardens grown with techniques of *sustainable agriculture*, such as using fertilizers made from composts and introducing predatory insects to control pests, in ways that have minimal impact on soil, water, and air quality.

organosulfur compounds a large group of phytochemicals containing the mineral sulfur. Organosulfur phytochemicals are responsible for the pungent flavors and aromas of foods belonging to the onion, leek, chive, shallot, and garlic family and are thought to stimulate cancer defenses in the body.

organs discrete structural units made of tissues that perform specific jobs. Examples are the heart, liver, and brain.

osteomalacia (OS-tee-o-mal-AY-shuh) the adult expression of vitamin D–deficiency disease, characterized by an overabundance of unmineralized bone protein (*osteo* means "bone"; *mal* means "bad"). Symptoms include bending of the spine and bowing of the legs.

osteoporosis (OSS-tee-oh-pore-OH-sis) a reduction of the bone mass of older persons in which the bones become porous and fragile (*osteo* means "bones"; *poros* means "porous"); also known as *adult bone loss*.

outbreak two or more cases of a disease arising from an identical organism acquired from a common food source within a limited time frame. Government agencies track and investigate outbreaks of foodborne illnesses, but tens of millions of individual cases go unreported each year.

outcrossing the unintended breeding of a domestic crop with a related wild species.

oven-safe thermometer a thermometer designed to remain in the food to give constant readings during cooking.

overload an extra physical demand placed on the body; an increase in the frequency, duration, or intensity of an activity. A principle of training is that for a body system to improve, it must be worked at frequencies, durations, or intensities that increase by increments.

overweight body weight above a healthy weight: BMI 25 to 29.9.

ovo-vegetarian includes eggs, vegetables, grains, legumes, fruits, and nuts; excludes flesh, seafood, and milk products.

ovum the egg, produced by the mother, that unites with a sperm from the father to produce a new individual.

oxidants compounds (such as oxygen itself) that oxidize other compounds. Compounds that prevent oxidation are called *antioxidants*, whereas those that promote it are called *prooxidants* (*anti* means "against"; *pro* means "for").

oxidation interaction of a compound with oxygen; a damaging effect by a chemically reactive form of oxygen.

oxidative stress damage inflicted on living systems by free radicals.

oyster shell a product made from the powdered shells of oysters that is sold as a calcium supplement but is not well absorbed by the digestive system.

P

palmitic acid a 16-carbon saturated fatty acid found in tropical palm oil, among other foods. Palmitic acid intake is associated with atrial fibrillation, a dangerous form of irregular heartbeat.

pancreas an organ with two main functions. One is an endocrine function—the making of hormones such as insulin, which it releases directly into the blood (*endo* means "into" the blood). The other is an exocrine function—the making of digestive enzymes, which it releases through a duct into the small intestine to assist in digestion (*exo* means "out" into a body cavity or onto the skin surface).

pancreatic juice fluid secreted by the pancreas that contains both enzymes to digest carbohydrates, fats, and proteins and sodium bicarbonate, a neutralizing agent.

pantothenic (PAN-to-THEN-ic) **acid** a B vitamin and part of a critical coenzyme needed in energy metabolism, among other roles.

partial vegetarian a term sometimes used to mean an eating style that includes seafood, poultry, eggs, dairy products, vegetables, grains, legumes, fruits, and nuts; excludes or strictly limits certain meats, such as red meats. Also called *flexitarian*.

pasteurization the treatment of milk, juices, or eggs with heat sufficient to kill certain pathogens (disease-causing microbes) commonly transmitted through these foods; not a sterilization process. Pasteurized products retain bacteria that cause spoilage.

PCBs (polychlorinated biphenyls) stable oily synthetic chemicals, once used in hundreds of U.S. industrial operations, that persist today in underwater sediments and contaminate fish and shellfish. Now banned from use in the United States, PCBs circulate globally from areas where they are still in use. PCBs cause cancer, nervous system damage, immune dysfunction, and a number of other serious health effects.

peak bone mass the highest attainable bone density for an individual; developed during the first three decades of life.

pellagra (pell-AY-gra) the niacin-deficiency disease (*pellis* means "skin"; *agra* means "rough"). Symptoms include the "4 Ds": diarrhea, dermatitis, dementia, and, ultimately, death.

peptide bond a bond that connects one amino acid with another, forming a link in a protein chain.

performance nutrition an area of nutrition science that applies its principles to maintaining health and maximizing physical performance in athletes, firefighters, military personnel, and others who must perform at high levels of physical ability. Also called *sports nutrition*.

peripheral resistance the resistance to pumped blood in the small arterial branches (arterioles) that carry blood to tissues.

peristalsis (per-ri-STALL-sis) the wavelike muscular squeezing of the esophagus, stomach, and small intestine that pushes their contents along.

pernicious (per-NISH-us) **anemia** a vitamin B_{12}–deficiency disease, caused by lack of intrinsic factor and characterized by large, immature red blood cells and damage to the nervous system (*pernicious* means "highly injurious or destructive").

persistent of a stubborn or enduring nature; with respect to food contaminants, the quality of remaining unaltered and unexcreted in plant foods or in the bodies of animals and human beings.

pesticides chemicals used to control insects, diseases, weeds, fungi, and other pests on crops and around animals. Used broadly, the term includes *herbicides* (to kill weeds), *insecticides* (to kill insects), and *fungicides* (to kill fungi).

pH a measure of acidity on a point scale. A solution with a pH of 1 is a strong acid; a solution with a pH of 7 is neutral; a solution with a pH of 14 is a strong base.

phagocytes (FAG-oh-sites) white blood cells that can ingest and destroy antigens. The process by which phagocytes engulf materials is called *phagocytosis*. The Greek word *phagein* means "to eat."

phenylketonuria an inborn error of metabolism that interferes with the body's handling of the amino acid phenylalanine, with potentially serious consequences for the brain and nervous system in infancy and childhood.

phospholipids (FOSS-foh-LIP-ids) one of the three main classes of dietary lipids. These lipids are similar to triglycerides, but each has a phosphorus-containing acid in place of one of the fatty acids. Phospholipids are present in all cell membranes.

photosynthesis the process by which green plants make carbohydrates from carbon dioxide and water using the green pigment chlorophyll to capture the sun's energy (*photo* means "light"; *synthesis* means "making").

physical activity bodily movement produced by muscle contractions that substantially increase energy expenditure.

phytates (FYE-tates) compounds present in plant foods (particularly whole grains) that bind iron and may prevent its absorption.

phytochemicals (FYE-toe-KEM-ih-cals) compounds in plants that confer color, taste, and other characteristics. Often, the bioactive food components of functional foods. *Phyto* means "plant."

phytoestrogens (FYE-toe-ESS-troh-gens) phytochemicals structurally similar to the female sex hormone estrogen. Phytoestrogens weakly mimic estrogen or modulate hormone activity in the human body.

pica (PIE-ka) a craving and intentional consumption of nonfood substances. Also known as *geophagia* (gee-oh-FAY-gee-uh) when referring to clay eating and *pagophagia* (pag-oh-FAY-gee-uh) when referring to ice craving (*geo* means "earth"; *pago* means "frost"; *phagia* means "to eat").

placebo a sham treatment often used in scientific studies; an inert, harmless medication. The *placebo effect* is the healing effect that the act of treatment, rather than the treatment itself, often has.

placenta (pla-SEN-tuh) the organ of pregnancy in which maternal blood and fetal blood circulate in close proximity and exchange nutrients and oxygen (flowing into the fetus) and wastes (picked up by the mother's blood).

plant pesticides substances produced within plant tissues that kill or repel attacking organisms.

plant sterols phytochemicals that resemble cholesterol in structure but that lower blood cholesterol, possibly by interfering with cholesterol absorption in the intestine. Plant sterols include sterol esters and stanol esters, formerly called *phytosterols*.

plaque (plack) a mass of microorganisms and their deposits on the surfaces of the teeth, a forerunner of dental caries and gum disease. The term *plaque* is also used in another connection—arterial plaque in atherosclerosis.

plaques (placks; *singular*, plaque) mounds of lipid material mixed with smooth muscle cells and calcium that develop in the artery walls in atherosclerosis (*placken* means "patch"). The same word is also used to describe the accumulation of a different kind of deposit on teeth, which promotes dental caries.

plasma the cell-free fluid part of blood and lymph.

platelets tiny cell-like fragments in the blood, important in blood clot formation (*platelet* means "little plate").

point of unsaturation a site in a molecule where the bonding is such that additional hydrogen atoms can easily be attached.

polypeptide (POL-ee-PEP-tide) protein fragments of many (more than 10) amino acids bonded together (*poly* means "many"). A peptide is a strand of amino acids.

polysaccharides another term for complex carbohydrates; compounds composed of long strands of glucose units linked together (*poly* means "many"). Also called *complex carbohydrates*.

polyunsaturated fats triglycerides in which most of the fatty acids have two or more points of unsaturation (are polyunsaturated).

polyunsaturated fatty acid a fatty acid with two or more points of unsaturation.

pop-up thermometer a disposable timing device commonly used in turkeys. The center of the device contains a spring that "pops up" when food reaches the right temperature.

prebiotic a substance that may not be digestible by the host, such as fiber, but that serves as food for probiotic bacteria and thus promotes their growth.

precursors compounds that can be converted into active vitamins. Also called *provitamins*.

prediabetes condition in which blood glucose levels are higher than normal but not high enough to be diagnosed as diabetes; a major risk factor for diabetes and cardiovascular diseases.

preeclampsia (PRE-ee-CLAMP-see-ah) a potentially dangerous condition during pregnancy characterized by hypertension and protein in the urine.

pregame meal a meal consumed in the hours before prolonged or repeated athletic training or competition to boost the glycogen stores of endurance athletes.

prehypertension borderline blood pressure between 120 over 80 and 139 over 89 millimeters of mercury, an indication that hypertension is likely to develop in the future.

premenstrual syndrome (PMS) a cluster of symptoms that some women experience prior to and during menstruation. They include, among others, abdominal cramps, back pain, swelling, headache, painful breasts, and mood changes.

prenatal (pree-NAY-tal) before birth.

prenatal supplements nutrient supplements specifically designed to provide the nutrients needed during pregnancy—particularly folate, iron, and calcium—without excesses or unneeded constituents.

pressure ulcers damage to the skin and underlying tissues as a result of unrelieved compression and poor circulation to the area; also called *bed sores*.

prion a disease agent consisting of an unusually folded protein that disrupts normal cell functioning. Prions cannot be controlled or killed by cooking or disinfecting, and the disease they cause cannot be treated; prevention is the only form of control.

probiotic a live microorganism that, when administered in adequate amounts, alters the bacterial colonies of the body in ways believed to confer a health benefit on the host.

problem drinkers or **alcohol abusers** people who suffer social, emotional, family, job-related, or other problems because of alcohol. A problem drinker is on the way to alcoholism.

processed foods foods subjected to any process, such as milling, alteration of texture, addition of additives, cooking, or others. Depending on the starting material and the process, a processed food may or may not be nutritious.

processed meats a general term for meat products preserved by smoking, curing, salting, or adding chemical chemical preservatives—for example, ham, bacon, jerky, hot dogs (including chicken and turkey), luncheon meats, salami and other sausages, SPAM, and Vienna sausages.

progressive weight training the gradual increase of a workload placed upon the body with the use of resistance.

promoters factors such as certain hormones that do not initiate cancer but speed up its development once initiation has taken place.

proof a statement of the percentage of alcohol in an alcoholic beverage. Liquor that is 100 proof is 50% alcohol, 90 proof is 45%, and so forth.

prooxidant a compound that triggers reactions involving oxygen.

protease (PRO-tee-ace) any of a number of enzymes that break the chemical bonds of proteins.

proteins compounds composed of carbon, hydrogen, oxygen, and nitrogen and arranged as strands of amino acids. Some amino acids also contain the element sulfur.

protein-sparing action the action of carbohydrate and fat in providing energy that allows protein to be used for purposes it alone can serve.

protein turnover the continuous breakdown and synthesis of body proteins involving the recycling of amino acids.

public health nutritionist a dietitian or other person with an advanced degree in nutrition who specializes in public health nutrition.

public water water from a municipal or county water system that has been treated and disinfected. Also called *tap water*.

purified water water that has been treated by distillation or other physical or chemical processes that remove dissolved solids. Because purified water contains no minerals or contaminants, it is useful for medical and research purposes.

pyloric (pye-LORE-ick) **valve** the circular muscle of the lower stomach that regulates the flow of partly digested food into the small intestine. Also called *pyloric sphincter*.

R

raw sugar the first crop of crystals harvested during sugar processing. Raw sugar cannot be sold in the United States because it contains too much filth (dirt, insect fragments, and the like). Sugar sold as "raw sugar" is actually evaporated cane juice.

reaction time the interval between stimulation and response.

ready-to-use therapeutic food (RUTF) highly caloric food products offering carbohydrate, lipid, protein, and micronutrients in a soft-textured paste used to promote rapid weight gain in malnourished people, particularly children.

recombinant bovine somatotropin (so-mat-oh-TROPE-in) **(rbST)** growth hormone of cattle, which can be produced for agricultural use by way of genetic engineering.

A *recombinant* protein arises from genetically engineered DNA. Also called *bovine growth hormone (bGH)*.

recombinant DNA (rDNA) technology a technique of genetic modification whereby scientists directly manipulate the genes of living things; includes methods of removing genes, doubling genes, introducing foreign genes, and changing gene positions to influence the growth and development of organisms.

Recommended Dietary Allowances (RDA) nutrient intake goals for individuals; the average daily nutrient intake level that meets the needs of nearly all (97 to 98 percent) healthy people in a particular life stage and gender group.

recovery drinks flavored beverages that contain protein, carbohydrate, and often other nutrients; intended to support postexercise recovery of energy fuels and muscle tissue. These can be convenient but are not superior to ordinary foods and beverages, such as chocolate milk or a sandwich, to supply carbohydrate and protein after exercise. Not intended for hydration during athletic competition or training because their high carbohydrate and protein contents may slow water absorption.

reference dose an estimate of the intake of a substance over a lifetime that is considered to be without appreciable health risk; for pesticides, the maximum amount of a residue permitted in a food. Formerly called *tolerance limit*.

refined refers to the process by which the coarse parts of food products are removed. For example, the refining of wheat into white enriched flour involves removing three of the four parts of the kernel—the chaff, the bran, and the germ—leaving only the endosperm, composed mainly of starch and a little protein.

refined grains grains and grain products from which the bran, germ, or other edible parts of whole grains have been removed; not a whole grain. Many refined grains are low in fiber and are enriched with vitamins, as required by U.S. regulations.

registered dietitian nutritionist (RDN) food and nutrition experts who have earned at least a bachelor's degree from an accredited college or university with a program approved by the Academy of Nutrition and Dietetics (or the Dietitians of Canada). The dietitian must also serve in an approved internship or coordinated program, pass the registration examination, and maintain professional competency through continuing education. Many states also require licensing of practicing dietitians. Also called *registered dietitian (RD)*.

registration listing with a professional organization that requires specific course work, experience, and passing of an examination.

requirement the amount of a nutrient that will just prevent the development of specific deficiency signs; distinguished from the DRI recommended intake value, which is a generous allowance with a margin of safety.

residues whatever remains; in the case of pesticides, those amounts that remain on or in foods when people buy and use them.

resistance training physical activity that develops muscle strength, power, endurance, and mass. Resistance can be provided by free weights, weight machines, other objects, or the person's own body weight. Also called *weight training, resistance exercise,* or *strength exercise*.

resistant starch the fraction of starch in a food that is digested slowly, or not at all, by human enzymes.

resveratrol (rez-VER-ah-trol) a phytochemical of grapes under study for potential health benefits.

retina (RET-in-uh) the layer of light-sensitive nerve cells lining the back of the inside of the eye.

retinol one of the active forms of vitamin A made from beta-carotene in animal and human bodies; an antioxidant nutrient. Other active forms are *retinal* and *retinoic acid*.

retinol activity equivalents (RAE) a new measure of the vitamin A activity of beta-carotene and other vitamin A precursors that reflects the amount of retinol that the body will derive from a food containing vitamin A precursor compounds.

rhodopsin (roh-DOP-sin) the light-sensitive pigment of the cells in the retina; it contains vitamin A (*opsin* means "visual protein").

riboflavin (RIBE-o-flay-vin) a B vitamin active in the body's energy-releasing mechanisms.

rickets the vitamin D–deficiency disease in children; characterized by abnormal growth of bone and manifested in bowed legs or knock-knees, outward-bowed chest, and knobs on the ribs.

risk factors factors known to be related to (or correlated with) diseases but not proved to be causal.

RNA (ribonucleic acid) cellular nucleic acids that play key roles in the process and control of protein synthesis.

S

safety the practical certainty that injury will not result from the use of a substance.

salts compounds composed of charged particles (ions). An example is potassium chloride (K^+Cl^-).

sarcopenia (SAR-koh-PEE-nee-ah) age-related loss of skeletal muscle mass, muscle strength, and muscle function.

satiation (SAY-she-AY-shun) the perception of fullness that builds throughout a meal, eventually reaching the degree of fullness and satisfaction that halts eating. Satiation generally determines how much food is consumed at one sitting.

satiety (sah-TIE-eh-tee) the perception of fullness that lingers in the hours after a meal and inhibits eating until the next mealtime. Satiety generally determines the length of time between meals.

saturated fats triglycerides in which most of the fatty acids are saturated.

saturated fatty acid a fatty acid carrying the maximum possible number of hydrogen atoms (having no points of unsaturation). A saturated fat is a triglyceride that contains three saturated fatty acids.

screen time sedentary time spent using an electronic device, such as a television, computer, or video game player.

scurvy the vitamin C–deficiency disease.

selective breeding a technique of genetic modification whereby organisms are chosen for reproduction based on their desirability for human purposes, such as high growth rate, high food yield, or disease resistance, with the intention of retaining or enhancing these characteristics in their offspring.

self-efficacy a person's belief in his or her ability to succeed in an undertaking.

senile dementia the loss of brain function beyond the normal loss of physical adeptness and memory that occurs with aging.

serotonin (SER-oh-TONE-in) a neurotransmitter important in sleep regulation, appetite control, and mood regulation, among other roles. Serotonin is synthesized in the body from the amino acid tryptophan with the help of vitamin B_6.

set-point theory a theory stating that the body's regulatory controls tend to maintain a particular body weight (the set point) over time, opposing efforts to lose weight by dieting.

severe acute malnutrition (SAM) malnutrition caused by recent severe food restriction; characterized in children by underweight for height (wasting).

Shiga toxin any of a group of protein toxins produced as certain bacteria strains multiply; Shiga toxins cause severe illness when absorbed by the body.

side chain the unique chemical structure attached to the backbone of each amino acid that differentiates one amino acid from another.

simple carbohydrates sugars, including both single sugar units and linked pairs of sugar units. The basic sugar unit is a molecule containing six carbon atoms, together with oxygen and hydrogen atoms.

single-use temperature indicator a disposable instant-read thermometer that changes color to indicate temperature. This type is often used in commercial food establishments to eliminate cross-contamination.

skinfold test measurement of the thickness of a fold of skin and subcutaneous fat on the back of the arm (over the triceps muscle), below the shoulder blade (subscapular), or in other places, using a caliper; also called *fatfold test*.

small intestine the 20-foot length of small-diameter intestine, below the stomach and above the large intestine, which is the major site of digestion of food and absorption of nutrients.

smoking point the temperature at which fat gives off an acrid blue gas.

SNP a type of genetic variation involving a single changed nucleotide. The letters SNP stand for *single nucleotide polymorphism*.

soft water water with a high sodium concentration.

solid fats fats that are high in saturated fat and usually not liquid at room temperature. Some common solid fats include butter, beef fat, chicken fat, pork fat, stick margarine, coconut oil, palm oil, and shortening.

solid fats fats that are high in saturated fatty acids and are usually solid at room temperature. Solid fats are found naturally in most animal foods but also can be made from vegetable oils through hydrogenation.

soluble fibers food components that readily dissolve in water, become viscous, and often impart gummy or gel-like characteristics to foods. An example is pectin from fruit, which is used to thicken jellies.

solvent a substance that dissolves another and holds it in solution.

soy milk a milklike beverage made from soybeans, claimed to be a functional food. Soy drinks should be fortified with vitamin A, vitamin D, riboflavin, and calcium to approach the nutritional equivalency of milk.

Special Supplemental Nutrition Program for Women, Infants, and Children (WIC) a USDA program offering low-income pregnant and lactating women and those with infants or preschool children coupons redeemable for specific foods that supply the nutrients deemed most necessary for growth and development.

sphincter (SFINK-ter) a circular muscle surrounding, and able to close, a body opening.

spina bifida (SPY-na BIFF-ih-duh) one of the most common types of neural tube defects, in which gaps occur in the bones of the spine. Often the spinal cord bulges and protrudes through the gaps, resulting in a number of motor and other impairments.

sports drinks flavored beverages designed to help athletes replace fluids and electrolytes and to provide carbohydrate before, during, and after physical activity, particularly endurance activities.

spring water water originating from an underground spring or well. It may be bubbly (carbonated) or "flat" or "still," meaning not carbonated. Brand names such as "Spring Pure" do not necessarily mean that the water comes from a spring.

staple foods foods used frequently or daily—for example, rice (in East and Southeast Asia) or potatoes (in Ireland). If well chosen, these foods are nutritious.

starch a plant polysaccharide composed of glucose. After cooking, starch is highly digestible by human beings; raw starch often resists digestion.

stearic acid an 18-carbon saturated fatty acid found in most animal fats. Unlike most other saturated fatty acids, it does not raise blood LDL cholesterol.

stem cell an undifferentiated cell that can mature into any of a number of specialized cell types. A stem cell of bone marrow may mature into one of many kinds of blood cells, for example.

sterols (STEER-alls) one of the three main classes of dietary lipids. Sterols have a structure similar to that of cholesterol.

stomach a muscular, elastic, pouchlike organ of the digestive tract that grinds and churns swallowed food and mixes it with acid and enzymes, forming chyme.

stone ground refers to a milling process using limestone to grind any grain, including refined grains, into flour.

stone-ground flour flour made by grinding kernels of grain between heavy wheels made of limestone, a kind of rock derived from the shells and bones of marine animals. As the stones scrape together, bits of the limestone mix with the flour, enriching it with calcium.

stroke the sudden shutting off of the blood flow to the brain by a thrombus, an embolism, or the bursting of a vessel (hemorrhage).

stroke volume the volume of oxygenated blood ejected from the heart toward body tissues at each beat.

structure-function claims legal but largely unregulated statements permitted on labels of foods and dietary supplements, describing the effect of a substance on the structure or function of the body, but that omit references to diseases. Example: "Supports immunity and digestive health" or "Builds strong bones."

stunting low height for age, indicating restriction of potential growth in children, often from chronic malnutrition.

subclinical deficiency a nutrient deficiency that has no outward clinical symptoms. Also called *marginal deficiency*.

subcutaneous fat fat stored directly under the skin (*sub* means "beneath"; *cutaneous* refers to the skin).

sucrose (SOO-crose) a disaccharide composed of glucose and fructose; sometimes known as table, beet, or cane sugar and, often, as simply *sugar*.

sugar alcohols sugarlike compounds in the chemical family *alcohol* derived from fruits or manufactured from sugar dextrose or other carbohydrates; sugar alcohols are absorbed more slowly than sugars, are metabolized differently, and do not elevate the risk of dental caries. Also called *polyols*.

sugars simple carbohydrates; that is, molecules of either single sugar units or pairs of those sugar units bonded together. By common usage, *sugar* most often refers to sucrose.

surface water water that comes from lakes, rivers, and reservoirs.

sushi a Japanese dish that consists of vinegar-flavored rice, seafood, and colorful vegetables, typically wrapped in seaweed. Some sushi contains raw fish; other sushi contains only cooked ingredients.

sustainable able to continue indefinitely; the use of resources in ways that maintain both natural resources and human life into the future; the use of natural resources at a pace that allows the earth to replace them and does not cause pollution to accumulate.

sustainable diet a diet with low environmental impact that contributes to food and nutrition security and to healthy life for present and future generations. Sustainable diets are protective and respectful of biodiversity and ecosystems; culturally acceptable; accessible; economically fair and affordable; and nutritionally adequate, safe, and healthy while optimizing natural and human resources.

systolic (sis-TOL-ik) **pressure** the first figure in a blood pressure reading (the "dupp" sound of the heartbeat's "lubb-dupp" beat is heard), which reflects arterial pressure caused by the contraction of the heart's left ventricle.

T

tannins compounds in tea (especially black tea) and coffee that bind iron. Tannins also denature proteins.

T-cells lymphocytes that attack antigens. *T* stands for the thymus gland of the neck, where the T-cells are stored and matured.

textured vegetable protein processed soybean protein used in products formulated to look and taste like meat, fish, or poultry.

thermic effect of food the body's speeded-up metabolism in response to having eaten a meal; also called *diet-induced thermogenesis*.

thermogenesis the generation and release of body heat associated with the breakdown of body fuels. *Adaptive thermogenesis* describes adjustments in energy expenditure related to changes in environment such as cold and to physiological events such as underfeeding or trauma.

thiamin (THIGH-uh-min) a B vitamin involved in the body's use of fuels.

thrombosis a thrombus that has grown enough to close off a blood vessel. A *coronary thrombosis* closes off a vessel that feeds the heart muscle. A *cerebral thrombosis* closes off a vessel that feeds the brain (*thrombo* means "clot"; the cerebrum is part of the brain).

thrombus a stationary blood clot.

thyroxine (thigh-ROX-in) a principal peptide hormone of the thyroid gland that regulates the body's rate of energy use.

tissues systems of cells working together to perform specialized tasks. Examples are muscles, nerves, blood, and bone.

tocopherol (tuh-KOFF-er-all) a kind of alcohol. The active form of vitamin E is alpha-tocopherol.

tofu (TOE-foo) a curd made from soybeans that is rich in protein, often enriched with calcium, and variable in fat content; used in many Asian and vegetarian dishes in place of meat.

Tolerable Upper Intake Levels (UL) the highest average daily nutrient intake level that is likely to pose no risk of toxicity to almost all healthy individuals of a particular life stage and gender group.

toxicity the ability of a substance to harm living organisms. All substances, even pure water or oxygen, can be toxic in high enough doses.

trabecular (tra-BECK-you-lar) **bone** the weblike structure composed of calcium-containing crystals inside a bone's solid outer shell. It provides strength and acts like a calcium storage bank.

trace minerals essential mineral nutrients required in the adult diet in amounts less than 100 milligrams per day. Also called *microminerals*.

training regular practice of an activity, which leads to physical adaptations of the body with improvement in flexibility, strength, or endurance.

trans fats fats that contain any number of unusual fatty acids—*trans*-fatty acids—formed during processing.

trans-fatty acids fatty acids with unusual shapes that can arise when hydrogens are added to the unsaturated fatty acids of polyunsaturated oils (a process known as *hydrogenation*).

transgenic organism an organism resulting from the growth of an embryonic, stem, or germ cell into which a new gene has been inserted.

triglycerides (try-GLISS-er-ides) one of the three main classes of dietary lipids and the chief form of fat in foods and in the human body. A triglyceride is made up of three units of fatty acids and one unit of glycerol (*fatty acids* and *glycerol* are defined later). In research, triglycerides are often called *triacylglycerols* (try-ay-seal-GLISS-er-ols).

trimester a period representing gestation. A trimester is about 13 to 14 weeks.

tripeptides (try-PEP-tides) protein fragments that are three amino acids long (*tri* means "three").

turbinado (ter-bih-NOD-oh) **sugar** raw sugar from which the filth has been washed; legal to sell in the United States.

type 1 diabetes the type of diabetes in which the pancreas produces no or very little insulin; often diagnosed in childhood, although some cases arise in adulthood. Formerly called *juvenile-onset* or *insulin-dependent diabetes*.

type 2 diabetes the type of diabetes in which the pancreas makes plenty of insulin but the body's cells resist insulin's action; often diagnosed in adulthood. Formerly called *adult-onset* or *non-insulin-dependent diabetes*.

U

ulcer an erosion in the topmost, and sometimes underlying, layers of cells that form a lining. Ulcers of the digestive tract commonly form in the esophagus, stomach, or upper small intestine.

ultra-high temperature a process of sterilizing food by exposing it for a short time to temperatures above those normally used in processing.

ultra-processed foods a term used to describe products of manufacturing made from industrial ingredients and additives, such as sugars, refined starches, fats, imitation flavors and colors, or industrial remnants, such as meat fats and scraps, with little or no whole food added. They are often high in fat, sugar, salt, and calories, and heavily advertised.

umbilical (um-BIL-ih-cul) **cord** the ropelike structure through which the fetus's veins and arteries reach the placenta; the route of nourishment and oxygen into the fetus and the route of waste disposal from the fetus.

unbleached flour a beige-colored refined endosperm flour with texture and nutritive qualities that approximate those of regular white flour.

underweight body weight below a healthy weight; BMI below 18.5.

unsaturated fatty acid a fatty acid that lacks some hydrogen atoms and has one or more points of unsaturation. An unsaturated fat is a triglyceride that contains one or more unsaturated fatty acids.

urban legends stories, usually false, that may travel rapidly throughout the world via the Internet, gaining strength of conviction solely on the basis of repetition.

urea (yoo-REE-uh) the principal nitrogen-excretion product of protein metabolism; generated mostly by removal of amine groups from unneeded amino acids or from amino acids being sacrificed for energy.

uterus (YOO-ter-us) the womb, the muscular organ within which the infant develops before birth.

V

variety the dietary characteristic of providing a wide selection of foods—the opposite of monotony.

vegan includes only food from plant sources: vegetables, grains, legumes, fruits, seeds, and nuts; also called strict vegetarian.

vegetarian includes plant-based foods and eliminates some or all animal-derived foods.

vegetarians people who exclude from their diets animal flesh and possibly other animal products such as milk, cheese, and eggs.

veins blood vessels that carry blood, with the carbon dioxide it has collected, from the tissues back to the heart.

very-low-density lipoproteins (VLDL) lipoproteins that transport triglycerides and other lipids from the liver to various tissues in the body.

villi (VILL-ee, VILL-eye) fingerlike projections of the sheets of cells lining the intestinal tract. The villi make the surface area much greater than it would otherwise be (*singular:* villus).

visceral fat fat stored within the abdominal cavity in association with the internal abdominal organs; also called *intra-abdominal fat* or *visceral adipose tissue*.

viscous (VISS-cuss) having a sticky, gummy, or gel-like consistency that flows relatively slowly.

vitamin B$_{12}$ a B vitamin that helps to convert folate to its active form and also helps to maintain the sheath around nerve cells. Vitamin B$_{12}$'s scientific name, not often used, is *cyanocobalamin*.

vitamin B$_6$ a B vitamin needed in protein metabolism. Its three active forms are *pyridoxine*, *pyridoxal*, and *pyridoxamine*.

vitamins organic compounds that are vital to life and indispensable to body functions but that are needed only in minute amounts; essential, noncaloric nutrients.

vitamin water bottled water with a few vitamins added; does not replace vitamins from a balanced diet and may worsen overload in people receiving vitamins from enriched food, supplements, and other enriched products such as "energy" bars.

VO$_{2max}$ the maximum rate of oxygen consumption by an individual (measured at sea level).

voluntary activities intentional activities (such as walking, sitting, or running) conducted by voluntary muscles.

W

waist circumference a measurement of abdominal girth that indicates visceral fatness.

wasting in malnutrition, thin for height, indicating recent rapid weight loss or failure to gain, often from severe acute malnutrition.

wasting the progressive, relentless loss of the body's tissues that accompanies certain diseases and shortens survival time.

water balance the balance between water intake and water excretion, which keeps the body's water content constant.

water intoxication a dangerous dilution of the body's fluids resulting from excessive ingestion of plain water. Symptoms are headache, muscular weakness, lack of concentration, poor memory, and loss of appetite.

water stress a measure of the pressure placed on water resources by human activities such as municipal water supplies, industries, power plants, and agricultural irrigation.

wean to gradually replace breast milk with infant formula or other foods appropriate to an infant's diet.

websites Internet resources composed of text and graphic files, each with a unique URL (Uniform Resource Locator) that names the site (for example, www.usda.gov).

weight cycling repeated rounds of weight loss and subsequent regain that may pose health risks; also called *yo-yo dieting*.

well water water drawn from groundwater by tapping into an aquifer.

Wernicke-Korsakoff (VER-nik-ee KOR-sah-koff) **syndrome** a cluster of symptoms involving nerve damage arising from a deficiency of the vitamin thiamin in alcoholism. Characterized by mental confusion, disorientation, memory loss, jerky eye movements, and staggering gait.

wheat bread bread made with any wheat flour, including refined enriched white flour.

wheat flour any flour made from wheat, including refined white flour.

whey (way) the watery part of milk, a by-product of cheese production. Once discarded as waste, whey is now recognized as a high-quality protein source for human consumption.

white flour an endosperm flour that has been refined and bleached for maximum softness and whiteness.

white sugar granulated sucrose, produced by dissolving, concentrating, and recrystallizing raw sugar. Also called *table sugar*.

white wheat a wheat variety developed to be paler in color than common red wheat (most familiar flours are made from red wheat). White wheat is similar to red wheat

in carbohydrate, protein, and other nutrients, but it lacks the dark and bitter, but potentially beneficial, phytochemicals of red wheat.

whole foods milk and milk products; meats and similar foods such as fish and poultry; vegetables, including dried beans and peas; fruits; and grains. These foods are generally considered to form the basis of a nutritious diet. Also called *basic foods*.

100% whole grain a label term for food in which the grain is entirely whole grain, with no added refined grains.

whole grains grains or foods made from them that contain all the essential parts and naturally occurring nutrients of the entire grain seed (except the inedible husk).

whole-wheat flour flour made from whole-wheat kernels; a whole-grain flour. Also called *graham flour*.

world food supply the quantity of food, including stores from previous harvests, available to the world's people at a given time.

World Health Organization (WHO) an agency of the United Nations charged with improving human health and preventing or controlling diseases in the world's people.

World Wide Web the Web, commonly abbreviated **www**, a graphical subset of the Internet.

X

xerophthalmia (ZEER-ahf-THALL-me-uh) progressive hardening of the cornea of the eye in advanced vitamin A deficiency that can lead to blindness (*xero* means "dry"; *ophthalm* means "eye").

xerosis (zeer-OH-sis) drying of the cornea; a symptom of vitamin A deficiency.

Z

zygote (ZYE-goat) the product of the union of ovum and sperm; a fertilized ovum.

Index

The page letters A, B, and C that stand alone refer to the tables beginning on the inside front cover. Page letters Y and Z refer to the tables on the last two pages of the book. The page numbers preceded by A through I are appendix page numbers. The boldfaced page numbers indicate definitions. Terms are also defined in the glossary. Page numbers followed by *n* indicate footnotes. Page numbers followed by *t* indicate tables. Page numbers followed by *f* indicate figures. Page numbers followed by *n* indicate footnotes.

A

A, B, C, M, V principles, 11–12

A1c test, **142**, 143*t*

AAP. *See* American Academy of Pediatrics (AAP)

Absorb, **81**

Absorption
  calcium, 307, 308, 332*f*, 524
  of carbohydrates, 129, 132
  in digestive system, 90
  of drugs and nutrients, 595–596
  of fat, 168–169, 169*f*
  of fat-soluble vitamins, 243, 243*t*
  iron, 320, 325, 409
  of protein, 209–210
  vitamin B₁₂, 273
  of water-soluble vitamins, 243*f*

Academy of Nutrition and Dietetics (AND), 26*f*, 27, **27**, **28t**, 327, 540, 613

Acceptable daily intake (ADI), **501**

Acceptable Macronutrient Distribution Ranges (AMDR), **33**, 34
  safety, 33

Accessory organs, **82f**

Accidents, 3*t*, 106, 106*f*, 430*f*

Accredited, **27**, **28**, **28t**

Accutane, 578

Acesulfame potassium, 502*t*

Acesulfame-K, 502*t*

Acetaldehyde, **101t**, **107**, 107*f*

Acid reducers, **94**

Acid-base balance, **215**, 216*t*, **305**, 308, 311, 363

Acid, 93

Acidosis, **215**

Acids, **215**

Acne, 247, **577–578**

Acquired immunodeficiency syndrome (AIDS), **431–432**, 538

Acrylamide, 456

Acupuncture, **450**, **450t**

Adapts, 394

Added sugars. *See* Sugars, added

Addiction, food supply and, 360

Additives. *See also* Sugars, added
  defensive dining and, 188, 190
  defined, **499**
  examples of, 184
  plant sterol, 190
  in processed meat, 456
  safety of, 454–455, 471, 499–505, 499*t*

Adequacy, dietary
  calories and, 21
  defined, **11**
  diet planning and, 42
  DRI and, 32, 35
  as eating pattern characteristic, 11, 12*f*
  of seafood, 182

Adequate Intakes (AI), **33**, 35, A, B

ADH. *See* Alcohol dehydrogenase (ADH)

ADHD. *See* Attention-deficit/hyperactivity disorder (ADHD)

Adipokine, **346**

Adipose tissue, **97**, 163*f*, **344**, 346, 391*t*
  See also Fat

Administration on Aging, 590

Adolescents/adolescence
  adults as gatekeepers, 578
  BMI and, Z
  calcium and, 305–306, 307
  defined, **574**
  diabetes in, 142
  eating disorders and, 383, 388
  iron and, 322–323, 576, 576*f*, 579

meat-consuming diet and, 236
  nutrition in, 574–578
  obesity in, 344
  osteoporosis in, 337, 338
  PMS in, **577**, 579–580
  pregnancy in, 528–529
  protein and, 225, 578
  supplements and, 219*t*
  vegetarian diet and, 236
  vitamin A for, 247, 578
  vitamin D for, 251, 577, 579
  weight loss and, 362

Adrenaline, 137*n*

Adults. *See also* Elderly
  adolescents and, 578
  Alzheimer's disease in, 588–589
  BMI and, 352
  BPA and, 504
  calcium and, 305, 307, 309, 331
  childhood obesity and, 553
  copper and, 328
  CVD in, 439*f*
  eating disorders in, 387
  energy restriction for, 587
  flavoring agents and, 501
  fluoride and, 326
  folate and, 271, 272
  foodborne illnesses and, 486
  food choices for, 589–590, 590–591, 592
  in good health at old age, 578, 580
  iron and, 322, 585–586, 586*t*
  life expectancy for, **580**
  life span for, **580**
  lifestyle factors for, 587
  magnesium and, 311
  niacin and, 270
  nutrient diseases in, 606
  nutrient needs for, 539*f*
  nutritional genomics and, 467–468
  nutrition in, 581–590
  obesity in, 344, 345*t*, 346
  osteoporosis in, 337*t*
  pesticides and, 492, 493
  phosphorus and, 310
  physical activity and, 392*t*, 582, 583, 588
  potassium and, 316, 586*t*
  protein and, 220*t*, 582–583, 586*t*
  sodium and, 313, 313*f*, 313*t*
  supplements for, 287*t*, 586
  underweight and, 345, 345*t*

Advantame, 502*t*

Advertorials, *24*

Aflatoxin, **488**, 513*n*

Agave syrup, **149**

Agroecological farming, 620*t*

Agroecology, **617**, 619

Agroforestry, 620*t*

AI. *See* Adequate Intakes (AI)

AIDS. *See* Acquired immunodeficiency syndrome (AIDS)

Alanine, 203*t*

Alcohol
  accidents and, 106, 106*f*
  for adults, 587
  affecting behaviors, 104*t*
  affecting liver, 108
  in body, 106
  in brain, 104, 105*f*, 109
  breakdown of, 108*f*
  caffeine and, 104
  calories from, 100, 110*t*
  cancer and, 455, 456, 458*t*
  CVD and, 443*t*
  death rate and, 3*t*, 100, 104, 430*n*
  defined, **101–102**
  diabetes and, 100, 107, D-13*t*
  "drink" and, 102
  drinking patterns with, 103
  driving ability, 105*n*
  effects of, 104, 107–108
  hangover and, 108–109
  as health benefit, 100–101
  hypertension and, 101, 446, 447*t*, 448
  lactation and, 537
  lethal dose of, 105
  long-term effects of, 109
  moderation, 448
  myths about, 108*t*
  niacin and, 269
  nutrient density and, 43
  obesity and, 346
  osteoporosis and, 337
  people who should not drink, 102*t*
  physical activity and, 414
  phytochemicals and, 66, 101
  pregnancy and, 109, 517, 525, 532–534, 532*f*, 534
  servings of, 102*f*
  stored as fat, 364*n*
  sugar, **145**, 145*t*
  thiamin and, 267
  truths about, 108*t*

Vomiting (*continued*)
   magnesium deficiency and, 311
   obesity and, 376
   potassium toxicity and, 316
   sodium deficiency and, 312
   zinc toxicity and, 325

W

Waist circumference, **347**, 348*t*, 352, 354*f*
Warfarin, 258
Wasting disease, **345**
Wasting, **607**
Water
   for adults, 585–586, 586*t*
   alcohol and, 105
   amino acids and, 204, 216*f*, 218
   artesian, **303***t*
   baby, **303***t*
   to balance loss, 296–297
   bottled, **303**
   caffeine, **303***t*
   carbonated, **303***t*
   cardiovascular system and, 74
   coconut, **303***t*
   digestive system and, 84, 86, 94–95
   distilled, **303***t*
   drinking, 298, 301–303
   EER, RDA, and AI for, A
   factors increasing need for, 298*t*
   fasting and, 362
   fat and, 162, 167, 168, 169
   features of, 294–295
   filtered, **303***t*
   fitness, **303***t*
   flavored, **413**, **413***t*
   from fluids, 298, 298*t*, 301
   fluoride and, 327*f*
   follows salt, 304
   from foods, 298, 298*t*, 301
   food safety and, 472*t*
   hard, **301**
   metabolic, **298**
   mineral, **303***t*
   natural, **303***t*
   nervous system and, 78
   as nutrient, 7*t*, 8, 294–295
   physical activity and, 410–412, 414
   public, **303***t*
   purified, **303***t*
   to quench thirst, 296–297
   soft, **301**
   spring, **303***t*
   surface, **302**, 303
   tap, 303
   vitamin, **303***t*
   ways to make appealing, 300
   weight gain and, 362
   weight loss and, 362, 369, 371
   well, **303***t*
Water balance, **296**, 296*f*, 597
Water flow, 304, 304*f*

Water intoxication, **296**, 297, 412
Water losses, 410–411
"Water pill," 362
Water purification, 303
Water sources, 302–303
Water stress, **609**
Water weight, 296, 304, 312
Water-soluble vitamins, 242, 242*t*, 243*t*, 260, 275, 277*t*–280*t*, 283
Wean, **542**
Weblogs, 26
Websites
   credible, 26*t*
   defined, **24***t*, **26**
   reliability of, 26*t*
Weight (body)
   accepting healthy, 366*t*
   achieving and maintaining healthy, 365–366, 368
   added sugars and, 156
   alcohol and, 109
   body fatness *vs.*, 352–354
   carbohydrates and, 119–120
   dehydration and, 297, 297*t*
   diabetes and, 144
   EER and, 351
   extremes of, 345–346, 346*f*
   fat and, 191
   food choices and, 13
   genetics and, 359
   nutrition and, 381
   obesity and, 359
   osteoporosis and, 337
   physical activity for healthy, 361, 381
   prepregnancy, 527*t*
   vegetarian diet and, 233
   vitamin A and, 247
   water, 296, 304, 312
Weight change, 362, 377–378
Weight control, 6*t*, 362, 379–381, 379*f*, 380*t*, 447
Weight cycling, **377**
Weight gain
   body and, 362–365
   breast milk and, 542
   carbohydrates and, 125, 143, 154–155, 365
   of children, 538–539, 538*f*, 552*f*
   chocolate for, 63
   diabetes and, 143
   during pregnancy, 526, 527*f*, 527*t*
   ghrelin and, 355
   gluten and, 226
   of infants, 538–539, 538*f*
   obesity and, 359
   preventing, 361
   strategies for, 374*t*
Weight gain, calories per lb., 154*n*
Weight loss

advertising claims, 17*f*
after pregnancy, 527
athletes and, 400
behavior modification for, 379, 380*t*
carbohydrates and, 125
CVD and, 348*t*, 441
dramatic, 368
drugs for, 374, 375*t*
fat and, 162, 172
food energy and, 400
food strategies best for, 369–372
heat stroke and, 410
indicators of urgent need for, 348*t*
lactation and, 537
moderate *vs.* rapid, 362–363, 366
obesity and, 359
physical activity in, 369, 372–373
protein and, 225, 369*t*, 370
satiety and, 357
strategies for successful, 378*t*
support for, 377–378
Weight loss dieting, 225
Weight maintenance, 139, 377
Weight management
   carbohydrates and, 125
   fat diets and, 366
   obesity and, 361
Weight reduction, 447*t*
Weight standards, 576
Weight Watchers, 368*n*, 377
Weight-loss drugs, 374, 375*t*
Weight-loss scams, 367*t*
Weights and measures, C-3
Well water, **303***t*
Wernicke-Korsakoff, **101***t*, **110**, 267
What We Eat in America survey, 17–18
Wheat bran, 311*n*
Wheat bread, **127***t*, **130**, 130*t*
Wheat flour, **127***t*
Whey, **422***t*, **424–425**
White blood cells
   folate and, 270
   immune system and, 432
White fibers, 394*n*
White flour, **127***t*, 192*t*
White sugar, **149**, 150
   See also Table sugar
White wheat, **127***t*, **130**
WHO. *See* World Health Organization (WHO)
Whole foods, **9–10**, **10***t*, 68, 176, 219, 287, 457, 507
Whole grains
   cancer and, 128, 457

carbohydrates and, 119, 121*t*, 125, 127–128, 127*f*, 130*t*, 141, 144
for children, 574
CVD and, 435, 444
DASH diet and, 459, 460*n*
defined, **119**
fat and, 191
health effects of, 128
phytochemicals and, 68
protein and, 225
sampling of, 130*t*
in USDA Eating Patterns, 42–43
in vegetarian diet, 232, 234
weight loss and, 370
Whole grains, recommendations for, 460*n*
Whole-grain cereals, 256
Whole-wheat flour, **127***t*
Wild rice, 130*t*
Willow bark, 450, 598*t*
Wilson, E. O., 613
Wine, 66, 100–101, 102, 109, 112, 501
WISEWOMAN projects, 438*n*
Women
   alcohol and, 43, 100, 102*t*, 103, 106*f*, 107, 109, 458*t*
   BMI and, 352
   BMR and, 351
   body composition of, 352*f*
   body fat and, 353
   breastfeeding, 102*t*, 179, 286
   cancer and, 455
   carbohydrates and, 121*t*, 125, 155*t*
   CVD and, 435, 438, 441
   Daily Values and, 37
   DHA and, 179
   DRI and, 35
   eating disorders in, 383, 386, 388
   EER and, 351, A
   fitness and, 409
   folate and, 272
   heart disease and, 172
   hormones and, 77
   iodine and, 319
   iron and, 322, 323
   lactating (*See* Lactating women)
   life expectancy for, 580
   magnesium and, 311
   mercury in, 182
   niacin and, 270
   obesity and, 346, 347*f*, 348, 348*f*
   osteoporosis and, 336, 337, 337*f*, 338*f*, 339
   osteoporosis in, 335, 335*f*
   phytochemicals and, 65, 66
   polyunsaturated fatty acids and, 173*t*
   poverty and, 605–606

Daily Values for Food Labels 2015

The Daily Values are standards developed by the Food and Drug Administration (FDA) for use on food labels. The values are based on 2,000 calories a day for adults and children over 4 years old. Chapter 2 provides more details.

Nutrient	Amount
Vitamins	
Biotin	30 mg
Choline	550 mg
Folate	400 µg DFE
Niacin	16 mg NE
Pantothenic acid	5 mg
Riboflavin	1.3 mg
Thiamin	1.2 mg
Vitamin A	900 µg RAE
Vitamin B_6	1.7 mg
Vitamin B_{12}	2.4 µg
Vitamin C	90 mg
Vitamin D	20 µg
Vitamin E (α-tocopherol)	15 mg
Vitamin K	120 µg

Nutrient	Amount
Minerals	
Calcium	1,300 mg
Chloride	2,300 mg
Chromium	35 µg
Copper	0.9 mg
Iodine	150 µg
Iron	18 mg
Magnesium	420 mg
Manganese	2.3 mg
Molybdenum	45 µg
Phosphorus	1,250 mg
Potassium	4,700 mg
Selenium	55 µg
Sodium	2,300 mg
Zinc	11 mg

Food Component	Amount	Calculation Factors
Fat	65 g	30% of calories
Saturated fat	20 g	10% of calories
Cholesterol	300 mg	Same regardless of calories
Carbohydrate (total)	300 g	60% of calories
Fiber	28 g	14 g per 1,000 calories
Protein	50 g	10% of calories

GLOSSARY
OF NUTRIENT MEASURES

cal calories, kcalories; a unit by which energy is measured.

g grams; a unit of weight equivalent to about 0.03 ounces.

mg milligrams; one-thousandth of a gram.

µg micrograms; one-millionth of a gram.

IU international units; an old measure of vitamin activity determined by biological methods (as opposed to new measures that are determined by direct chemical analyses). For those still using IU, the following factors can be used for conversions.

- For vitamin A, 1 IU = 0.3 µg retinol
- For vitamin D, 1 IU = 0.02 µg cholecalciferol
- For vitamin E, 1 IU = 0.67 mg α-tocopherol

mg NE milligrams niacin equivalents; a measure of niacin activity.

- 1 NE = 1 mg niacin
    = 60 mg tryptophan (an amino acid)

µg DFE micrograms dietary folate equivalents; a measure of folate activity.

- 1 µg DFE = 1 µg food folate
    = 0.6 µg folic acid from fortified food or as a supplement taken with food

µg RAE micrograms retinol activity equivalents; a measure of vitamin A activity.

- 1 µg RAE = 1 µg retinol
    = 12 µg β-carotene
    = 24 µg other vitamin A carotenoids

mmol millimoles; one-thousanth of a mole, the molecular weight of a substance. To convert mmol to mg, multiply by the atomic weight of the substance.

- For sodium, mmol × 23 = mg Na
- For chloride, mmol × 35.5 = mg Cl
- For sodium chloride, mmol × 58.5 = mg NaCl

Body Mass Index (BMI)

Find your height along the left-hand column and look across the row until you find the number that is closest to your weight. The number at the top of that column identifies your BMI. Chapter 9 describes how BMI correlates with disease risks and defines obesity. The area shaded in blue represents healthy weight ranges.

	Under-weight (<18.5)	Healthy Weight (18.5–24.9)						Overweight (25–29.9)					Obese (≥30)										
	18	19	20	21	22	23	24	25	26	27	28	29	30	31	32	33	34	35	36	37	38	39	40
Height	Body weight (pounds)																						
4'10"	86	91	96	100	105	110	115	119	124	129	134	138	143	148	153	158	162	167	172	177	181	186	191
4'11"	89	94	99	104	109	114	119	124	128	133	138	143	148	153	158	163	168	173	178	183	188	193	198
5'0"	92	97	102	107	112	118	123	128	133	138	143	148	153	158	163	168	174	179	184	189	194	199	204
5'1"	95	100	106	111	116	122	127	132	137	143	148	153	158	164	169	174	180	185	190	195	201	206	211
5'2"	98	104	109	115	120	126	131	136	142	147	153	158	164	169	175	180	186	191	196	202	207	213	218
5'3"	102	107	113	118	124	130	135	141	146	152	158	163	169	175	180	186	191	197	203	208	214	220	225
5'4"	105	110	116	122	128	134	140	145	151	157	163	169	174	180	186	192	197	204	209	215	221	227	232
5'5"	108	114	120	126	132	138	144	150	156	162	168	174	180	186	192	198	204	210	216	222	228	234	240
5'6"	112	118	124	130	136	142	148	155	161	167	173	179	186	192	198	204	210	216	223	229	235	241	247
5'7"	115	121	127	134	140	146	153	159	166	172	178	185	191	198	204	211	217	223	230	236	242	249	255
5'8"	118	125	131	138	144	151	158	164	171	177	184	190	197	203	210	216	223	230	236	243	249	256	262
5'9"	122	128	135	142	149	155	162	169	176	182	189	196	203	209	216	223	230	236	243	250	257	263	270
5'10"	126	132	139	146	153	160	167	174	181	188	195	202	209	216	222	229	236	243	250	257	264	271	278
5'11"	129	136	143	150	157	165	172	179	186	193	200	208	215	222	229	236	243	250	257	265	272	279	286
6'0"	132	140	147	154	162	169	177	184	191	199	206	213	221	228	235	242	250	258	265	272	279	287	294
6'1"	136	144	151	159	166	174	182	189	197	204	212	219	227	235	242	250	257	265	272	280	288	295	302
6'2"	141	148	155	163	171	179	186	194	202	210	218	225	233	241	249	256	264	272	280	287	295	303	311
6'3"	144	152	160	168	176	184	192	200	208	216	224	232	240	248	256	264	272	279	287	295	303	311	319
6'4"	148	156	164	172	180	189	197	205	213	221	230	238	246	254	263	271	279	287	295	304	312	320	328
6'5"	151	160	168	176	185	193	202	210	218	227	235	244	252	261	269	277	286	294	303	311	319	328	336
6'6"	155	164	172	181	190	198	207	216	224	233	241	250	259	267	276	284	293	302	310	319	328	336	345

© Cengage Learning 2014

Body Mass Index-for-Age Percentiles: Boys and Girls, Age 2 to 20

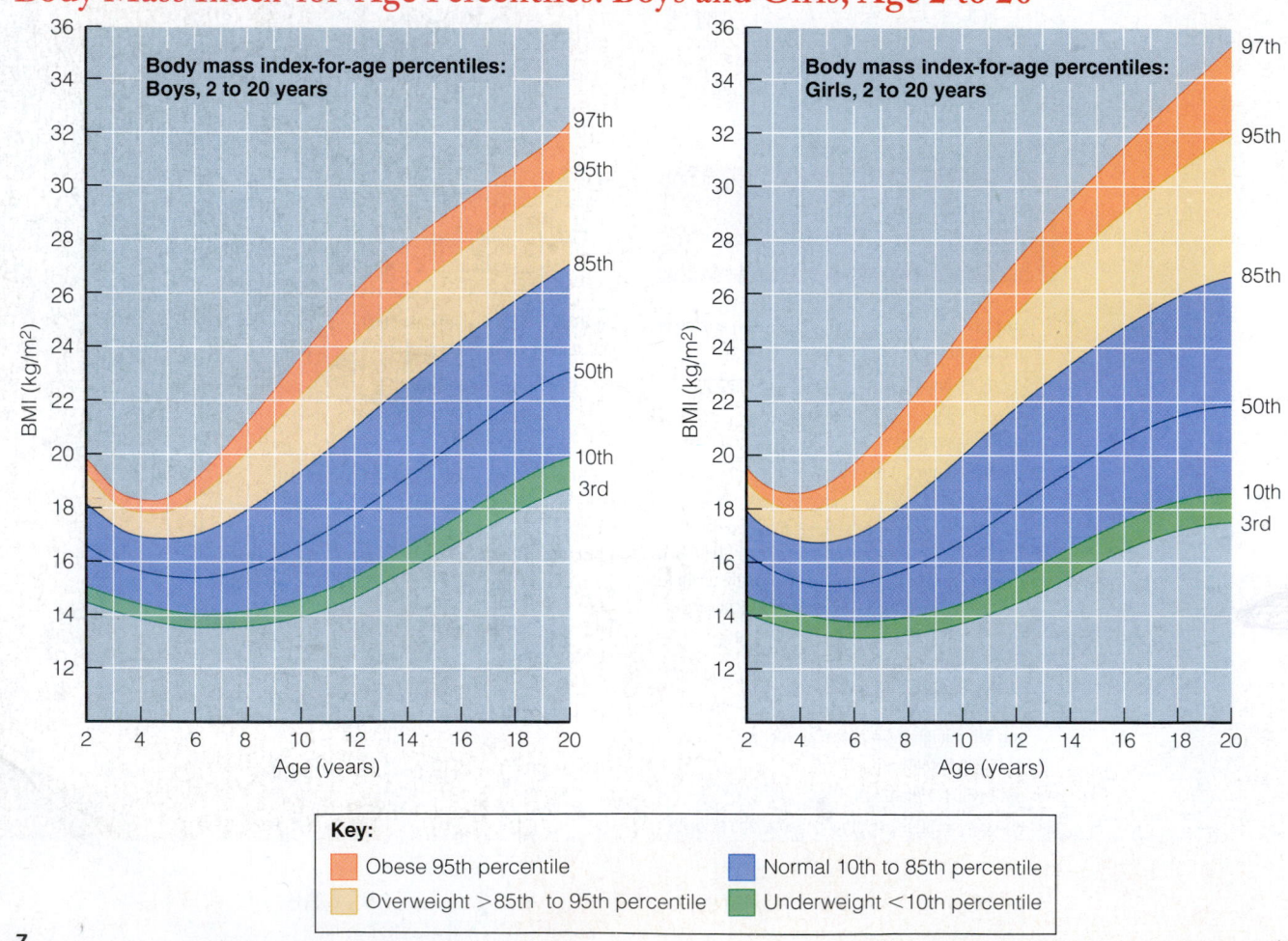

Body mass index-for-age percentiles: Boys, 2 to 20 years

Body mass index-for-age percentiles: Girls, 2 to 20 years

Key:
- Obese 95th percentile
- Overweight >85th to 95th percentile
- Normal 10th to 85th percentile
- Underweight <10th percentile